W9-AHV-022

Dietary Reference Intakes (DRIs): Tolerable Upper Intake Levels (UL),[a] Vitamins

Life-stage group	Vitamin A (μg/day)[b]	Vitamin C (mg/day)	Vitamin D (μg/day)	Vitamin E (mg/day)[c,d]	Vitamin K	Thiamin	Riboflavin	Niacin (mg/day)[d]	Vitamin B₆ (mg/day)[d]	Folate (μg/day)[d]	Vitamin B₁₂	Pantothenic acid	Biotin	Choline (g/day)	Carotenoids[e]
INFANTS															
0-6 mo	600	ND[f]	25	ND	ND	ND	ND	ND	ND	ND	ND	ND	ND	ND	ND
7-12 mo	600	ND	25	ND	ND	ND	ND	ND	ND	ND	ND	ND	ND	ND	ND
CHILDREN															
1-3 yr	600	400	50	200	ND	ND	ND	10	30	300	ND	ND	ND	1.0	ND
4-8 yr	900	650	50	300	ND	ND	ND	15	40	400	ND	ND	ND	1.0	ND
MALES, FEMALES															
9-13 yr	1700	1200	50	600	ND	ND	ND	20	60	600	ND	ND	ND	2.0	ND
14-18 yr	2800	1800	50	800	ND	ND	ND	30	80	800	ND	ND	ND	3.0	ND
19-70 yr	3000	2000	50	1000	ND	ND	ND	35	100	1000	ND	ND	ND	3.5	ND
>70 yr	3000	2000	50	1000	ND	ND	ND	35	100	1000	ND	ND	ND	3.5	ND
PREGNANT															
≤18 yr	2800	1800	50	800	ND	ND	ND	30	80	800	ND	ND	ND	3.0	ND
19-50 yr	3000	2000	50	1000	ND	ND	ND	35	100	1000	ND	ND	ND	3.5	ND
LACTATING															
≤18 yr	2800	1800	50	800	ND	ND	ND	30	80	800	ND	ND	ND	3.0	ND
19-50 yr	3000	2000	50	1000	ND	ND	ND	35	100	1000	ND	ND	ND	3.5	ND

Data from Food and Nutrition Board, Institute of Medicine: *Dietary Reference Intakes for calcium, phosphorus, magnesium, vitamin D, and fluoride* (1997); *Dietary Reference Intakes for thiamin, riboflavin, niacin, vitamin B₆, folate, vitamin B₁₂, pantothenic acid, biotin, and choline* (1998); *Dietary Reference Intakes for vitamin C, vitamin E, selenium, and carotenoids* (2000); *and Dietary Reference Intakes for vitamin A, vitamin K, arsenic, boron, chromium, copper, iodine, iron, manganese, molybdenum, nickel, silicon, vanadium, and zinc* (2001), Washington, DC, National Academies Press [www.nap.edu].

[a]UL = The maximum level of daily nutrient intake that is likely to pose no risk of adverse effects. Unless otherwise specified, the UL represents total intake from food, water, and supplements. Because of the lack of suitable data, ULs could not be established for vitamin K, thiamin, riboflavin, vitamin B₁₂, pantothenic acid, biotin, or carotenoids. In the absence of ULs, extra caution may be warranted in consuming levels above recommended intakes.

[b]As preformed vitamin A only.

[c]As alpha-tocopherol; applies to any form of supplemental alpha-tocopherol.

[d]The ULs for vitamin E, niacin, and folate apply to synthetic forms obtained from supplements, fortified foods, or a combination of the two.

[e]Beta-carotene supplements are advised only to serve as a provitamin A source for individuals at risk of vitamin A deficiency.

[f]ND = Not determinable because of lack of data of adverse effects in this age group and concern with regard to lack of ability to handle excess amounts. Source of intake should be from food only to prevent high levels of intake.

Dietary Reference Intakes (DRIs): Recommended Intakes for Individuals, Minerals

Life-stage group	Calcium (mg/day)	Chromium (µg/day)	Copper (µg/day)	Fluoride (mg/day)	Iodine (µg/day)	Iron (mg/day)	Magnesium (mg/day)	Manganese (mg/day)	Molybdenum (µg/day)	Phosphorus (mg/day)	Selenium (µg/day)	Zinc (mg/day)
INFANTS												
0-6 mo	210*	0.2*	200*	0.01*	110*	0.27*	30*	0.003*	2*	100*	15*	2*
7-12 mo	270*	5.5*	220*	0.5*	130*	**11**	75*	0.6*	3*	275*	20*	3*
CHILDREN												
1-3 yr	500*	11*	**340**	0.7*	**90**	**7**	**80**	1.2*	**17**	**460**	**20**	**3**
4-8 yr	800*	15*	**440**	1*	**90**	**10**	**130**	1.5*	**22**	**500**	**30**	**5**
MALES												
9-13 yr	1300*	25*	**700**	2*	**120**	**8**	**240**	1.9*	**34**	**1250**	**40**	**8**
14-18 yr	1300*	35*	**890**	3*	**150**	**11**	**410**	2.2*	**43**	**1250**	**55**	**11**
19-30 yr	1000*	35*	**900**	4*	**150**	**8**	**400**	2.3*	**45**	**700**	**55**	**11**
31-50 yr	1000*	35*	**900**	4*	**150**	**8**	**420**	2.3*	**45**	**700**	**55**	**11**
50-70 yr	1200*	30*	**900**	4*	**150**	**8**	**420**	2.3*	**45**	**700**	**55**	**11**
>70 yr	1200*	30*	**900**	4*	**150**	**8**	**420**	2.3*	**45**	**700**	**55**	**11**
FEMALES												
9-13 yr	1300*	21*	**700**	2*	**120**	**8**	**240**	1.6*	**34**	**1250**	**40**	**8**
14-18 yr	1300*	24*	**890**	3*	**150**	**15**	**360**	1.6*	**43**	**1250**	**55**	**9**
19-30 yr	1000*	25*	**900**	3*	**150**	**18**	**310**	1.8*	**45**	**700**	**55**	**8**
31-50 yr	1000*	25*	**900**	3*	**150**	**18**	**320**	1.8*	**45**	**700**	**55**	**8**
50-70 yr	1200*	20*	**900**	3*	**150**	**8**	**320**	1.8*	**45**	**700**	**55**	**8**
>70 yr	1200*	20*	**900**	3*	**150**	**8**	**320**	1.8*	**45**	**700**	**55**	**8**
PREGNANT												
≤18 yr	1300*	29*	**1000**	3*	**220**	**27**	**400**	2.0*	**50**	**1250**	**60**	**13**
19-30 yr	1000*	30*	**1000**	3*	**220**	**27**	**350**	2.0*	**50**	**700**	**60**	**11**
31-50 yr	1000*	30*	**1000**	3*	**220**	**27**	**360**	2.0*	**50**	**700**	**60**	**11**
LACTATING												
≤18 yr	1300*	44*	**1300**	3*	**290**	**10**	**360**	2.6*	**50**	**1250**	**70**	**14**
19-30 yr	1000*	45*	**1300**	3*	**290**	**9**	**310**	2.6*	**50**	**700**	**70**	**12**
31-50 yr	1000*	45*	**1300**	3*	**290**	**9**	**320**	2.6*	**50**	**700**	**70**	**12**

Data from Food and Nutrition Board, Institute of Medicine: *Dietary Reference Intakes for calcium, phosphorus, magnesium, vitamin D, and fluoride* (1997); *Dietary Reference Intakes for thiamin, riboflavin, niacin, vitamin B$_6$, folate, vitamin B$_{12}$, pantothenic acid, biotin, and choline* (1998); *Dietary Reference Intakes for vitamin C, vitamin E, selenium, and carotenoids* (2000); and *Dietary Reference Intakes for vitamin A, vitamin K, arsenic, boron, chromium, copper, iodine, iron, manganese, molybdenum, nickel, silicon, vanadium, and zinc* (2001), Washington, DC, National Academies Press [www.nap.edu].

Note: This table presents Recommended Dietary Allowances (RDAs) in **bold type** and Adequate Intakes (AIs) in ordinary type followed by an asterisk (*). RDAs and AIs may both be used as goals for individual intake. RDAs are set to meet the needs of almost all (97%-98%) individuals in a group. For healthy breastfed infants, the AI is the mean intake. The AI for other life-stage and gender groups is believed to cover needs of all individuals in the group, but lack of data or uncertainty in the data prevent being able to specify with confidence the percentage of individuals covered by this intake.

Dietary Reference Intakes (DRIs): Tolerable Upper Intake Levels (UL),[a] Minerals

Life-stage group	Arsenic[b]	Boron (mg/day)	Calcium (g/day)	Chromium	Copper (µg/day)	Fluoride (mg/day)	Iodine (µg/day)	Iron (mg/day)	Magnesium (mg/day)[c]	Manganese (mg/day)	Molybdenum (µg/day)	Nickel (mg/day)	Phosphorus (g/day)	Selenium (µg/day)	Silicon[d]	Vanadium (mg/day)[e]	Zinc (mg/day)
INFANTS																	
0-6 mo	ND[f]	ND	ND	ND	ND	0.7	ND	40	ND	ND	ND	ND	ND	45	ND	ND	4
7-12 mo	ND	ND	ND	ND	ND	0.9	ND	40	ND	ND	ND	ND	ND	60	ND	ND	5
CHILDREN																	
1-3 yr	ND	3	2.5	ND	1000	1.3	200	40	65	2	300	0.2	3	90	ND	ND	7
4-8 yr	ND	6	2.5	ND	3000	2.2	300	40	110	3	600	0.3	3	150	ND	ND	12
MALES, FEMALES																	
9-13 yr	ND	11	2.5	ND	5000	10	600	40	350	6	1100	0.6	4	280	ND	ND	23
14-18 yr	ND	17	2.5	ND	8000	10	900	45	350	9	1700	1.0	4	400	ND	ND	34
19-70 yr	ND	20	2.5	ND	10,000	10	1100	45	350	11	2000	1.0	4	400	ND	1.8	40
>70 yr	ND	20	2.5	ND	10,000	10	1100	45	350	11	2000	1.0	3	400	ND	1.8	40
PREGNANT																	
≤18 yr	ND	17	2.5	ND	8000	10	900	45	350	9	1700	1.0	3.5	400	ND	ND	34
19-50 yr	ND	20	2.5	ND	10,000	10	1100	45	350	11	2000	1.0	3.5	400	ND	ND	40
LACTATING																	
≤18 yr	ND	17	2.5	ND	8000	10	900	45	350	9	1700	1.0	4	400	ND	ND	34
19-50 yr	ND	20	2.5	ND	10,000	10	1100	45	350	11	2000	1.0	4	400	ND	ND	40

Data from Food and Nutrition Board, Institute of Medicine: *Dietary Reference Intakes for calcium, phosphorus, magnesium, vitamin D, and fluoride* (1997); *Dietary Reference Intakes for thiamin, riboflavin, niacin, vitamin B₆, folate, vitamin B₁₂, pantothenic acid, biotin, and choline* (1998); *Dietary Reference Intakes for vitamin C, vitamin E, selenium, and carotenoids* (2000); and *Dietary Reference Intakes for vitamin A, vitamin K, arsenic, boron, chromium, copper, iodine, iron, manganese, molybdenum, nickel, silicon, vanadium, and zinc* (2001), Washington, DC, National Academies Press [*www.nap.edu*].

[a]UL = The maximum level of daily nutrient intake that is likely to pose no risk of adverse effects. Unless otherwise specified, the UL represents total intake from food, water, and supplements. Because of lack of suitable data, ULs could not be established for arsenic, chromium, and silicon. In the absence of ULs, extra caution may be warranted in consuming levels above recommended intakes.

[b]Although the UL was not determined for arsenic, there is no justification for adding arsenic to food or supplements.

[c]The ULs for magnesium represent intake from a pharmacologic agent only and do not include intake from food or water.

[d]Although silicon has not been shown to cause adverse effects in humans, there is no justification for adding silicon to supplements.

[e]Although vanadium in food has not been shown to cause adverse effects in humans, there is no justification for adding vanadium to food, and vanadium supplements should be used with caution. The UL is based on adverse effects in laboratory animals, and these data could be used to set a UL for adults but not children and adolescents.

[f]ND = Not determinable because of lack of data of adverse effects in this age group and concern with regard to lack of ability to handle excess amounts. Source of intake should be from food only to prevent high levels of intake.

Dietary Reference Intakes (DRIs): Recommended Intakes for Individuals, Macronutrients

Life-stage group	Protein RDA/AI g/day[a]	Protein AMDR[b]	Carbohydrate RDA/AI g/day	Carbohydrate AMDR	Fiber RDA/AI g/day	Fiber AMDR	Fat RDA/AI g/day	Fat AMDR	n-6 Polyunsaturated fatty acids (linoleic acid) RDA/AI g/day	n-6 AMDR	n-3 Polyunsaturated fatty acids (α-linolenic acid) RDA/AI g/day	n-3 AMDR[d]	Saturated and trans fatty acids and cholesterol RDA/AI g/day	Sat. AMDR
INFANTS														
0-6 mo	9.1	ND[c]	60	ND	ND	—	31	—	4.4	ND	0.5	ND	—	—
7-12 mo	13.5	ND	95	ND	ND	—	30	—	4.6	ND	0.5	ND	—	—
CHILDREN														
1-3 yr	13	5-20	130	45-65	19	—	—	30-40	7	5-10	0.7	0.6-1.2	—	—
4-8 yr	19	10-30	130	45-65	25	—	—	25-35	10	5-10	0.9	0.6-1.2	—	—
MALES														
9-13 yr	34	10-30	130	45-65	31	—	—	25-35	12	5-10	1.2	0.6-1.2	—	—
14-18 yr	52	10-30	130	45-65	38	—	—	25-35	16	5-10	1.6	0.6-1.2	—	—
19-30 yr	56	10-35	130	45-65	38	—	—	20-35	17	5-10	1.6	0.6-1.2	—	—
31-50 yr	56	10-35	130	45-65	38	—	—	20-35	17	5-10	1.6	0.6-1.2	—	—
50-70 yr	56	10-35	130	45-65	30	—	—	20-35	14	5-10	1.6	0.6-1.2	—	—
>70 yr	56	10-35	130	45-65	30	—	—	20-35	14	5-10	1.6	0.6-1.2	—	—
FEMALES														
9-13 yr	34	10-30	130	45-65	26	—	—	25-35	10	5-10	1.0	0.6-1.2	—	—
14-18 yr	46	10-30	130	45-65	26	—	—	25-35	11	5-10	1.1	0.6-1.2	—	—
19-30 yr	46	10-35	130	45-65	25	—	—	20-35	12	5-10	1.1	0.6-1.2	—	—
31-50 yr	46	10-35	130	45-65	25	—	—	20-35	12	5-10	1.1	0.6-1.2	—	—
50-70 yr	46	10-35	130	45-65	21	—	—	20-35	11	5-10	1.1	0.6-1.2	—	—
>70 yr	46	10-35	130	45-65	21	—	—	20-35	11	5-10	1.1	0.6-1.2	—	—
PREGNANT														
≤18 yr	71	10-35	175	45-65	28	—	—	20-35	13	5-10	1.4	0.6-1.2	—	—
19-30 yr	71	10-35	175	45-65	28	—	—	20-35	13	5-10	1.4	0.6-1.2	—	—
31-50 yr	71	10-35	175	45-65	28	—	—	20-35	13	5-10	1.4	0.6-1.2	—	—
LACTATING														
≤18 yr	71	10-35	210	45-65	29	—	—	20-35	13	5-10	1.3	0.6-1.2	—	—
19-30 yr	71	10-35	210	45-65	29	—	—	20-35	13	5-10	1.3	0.6-1.2	—	—
31-50 yr	71	10-35	210	45-65	29	—	—	20-35	13	5-10	1.3	0.6-1.2	—	—

Data from *Dietary Reference Intakes for energy, carbohydrate, fiber, fat, fatty acids, cholesterol, protein, and amino acids*, Washington, DC, 2002, National Academies Press.

Note: This table presents Recommended Dietary Allowances (RDAs) in **bold type** and Adequate Intakes (AIs) in ordinary type. RDAs and AIs may both be used as goals for individual intake. RDAs are set to meet the needs of almost all (97%-98%) individuals in a group. For healthy breastfed infants, the AI is the mean intake. The AI for other life-stage and gender groups is believed to cover the needs of all individuals in the group, but lack of data prevents being able to specify with confidence the percentage of individuals covered by this intake.

[a] Based on 1.5 g/kg per day for infants, 1.1 g/kg per day for 1 to 3 years, 0.95 g/kg per day for 4 to 13 years, 0.85 g/kg per day for 14 to 18 years, 0.8 g/kg per day for adults, and 1.1 g/kg per day for pregnant (using prepregnancy weight) and lactating women.

[b] Acceptable Macronutrient Distribution Range (AMDR) is the range of intake for a particular energy source that is associated with reduced risk of chronic disease while providing intakes of essential nutrients. If an individual has consumed in excess of the AMDR, there is a potential of increasing the risk of chronic diseases and insufficient intakes of essential nutrients.

[c] ND = Not determinable because of lack of data of adverse effects in this age group and concern with regard to lack of ability to handle excess amounts. Source of intake should be from food only to prevent high levels of intake.

[d] Approximately 10% of the total can come from longer-chain, *n-3* fatty acids.

Williams'
Basic Nutrition
& Diet Therapy

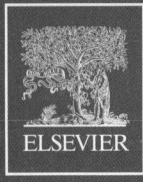

ELSEVIER

evolve

The Latest *Evolution* in *Learning*

Evolve provides online access to free learning resources and activities designed specifically for the textbook you are using in your class. The resources will provide you with information that enhances the material covered in the book and much more.

Visit the Web address listed below to start your learning evolution today!

▶▶ *LOGIN: http://evolve.elsevier.com/Williams/basic/*

Evolve Student Learning Resources for Nix: *Williams' Basic Nutrition & Diet Therapy*, Twelfth Edition, offers the following features:

- **Test Questions**
  Multiple-choice questions organized by chapter test your knowledge of key content and provide instant scoring and feedback.

- **Suggestions for Additional Study**
  These activities provide opportunities to apply the nutrition information presented in the textbook in real-life situations to broaden the learning experience.

- **Crossword Puzzles**
  These fun and effective exercises are a great way to reinforce key terms from each section of the textbook.

- **WebLinks**
  This exciting resource allows you to link to hundreds of web sites carefully chosen to supplement the content of the textbook. The WebLinks are regularly updated, with new ones added as they develop.

Think outside the book... evolve.

Williams'
Basic Nutrition & Diet Therapy

TWELFTH EDITION

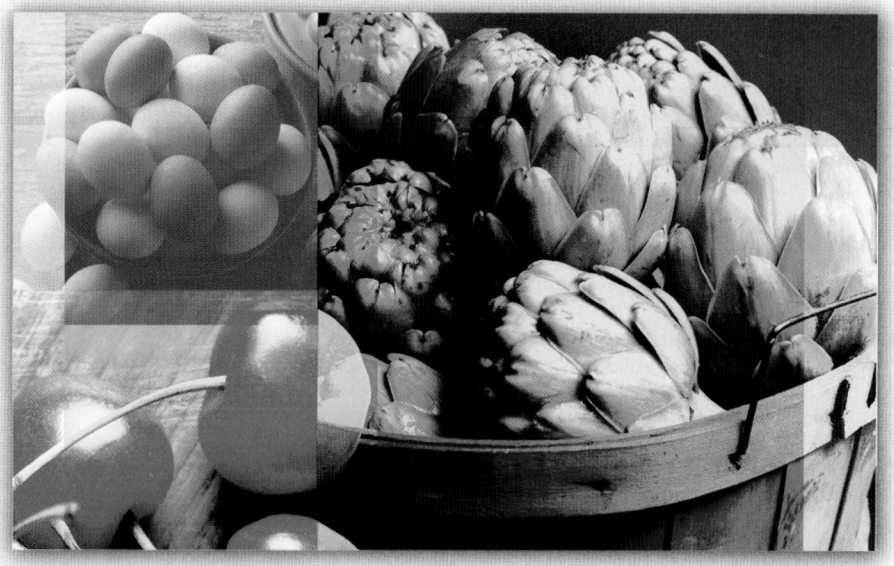

Staci Nix, MS, RD, CD

Instructor
Division of Nutrition
College of Health
University of Utah
Salt Lake City, Utah

with 150 illustrations

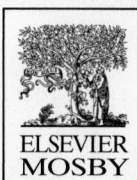

ELSEVIER
MOSBY

ELSEVIER
MOSBY

11830 Westline Industrial Drive
St. Louis, Missouri 63146

WILLIAMS' BASIC NUTRITION & DIET THERAPY

Copyright © 2005, Mosby, Inc. All rights reserved.

No part of this publication may be reproduced or transmitted in any form or by any means, electronic or mechanical, including photocopying, recording, or any information storage and retrieval system, without permission in writing from the publisher.

Permissions may be sought directly from Elsevier's Health Sciences Rights Department in Philadelphia, PA, USA: phone: (+1) 215 239 3804, fax: (+1) 215 239 3805, e-mail: healthpermissions@elsevier.com. You may also complete your request on-line via the Elsevier homepage (http://www.elsevier.com), by selecting 'Customer Support' and then 'Obtaining Permissions'.

NOTICE

Nutrition is an ever-changing field. Standard safety precautions must be followed, but as new research and clinical experience broaden our knowledge, changes in treatment and drug therapy may become necessary or appropriate. Readers are advised to check the most current product information provided by the manufacturer of each drug to be administered to verify the recommended dose, the method and duration of administration, and contraindications. It is the responsibility of the licensed prescriber, relying on experience and knowledge of the patient, to determine dosages and the best treatment for each individual patient. Neither the publisher nor the author assumes any liability for any injury and/or damage to persons or property arising from this publication.

Previous editions copyrighted 1958, 1962, 1966, 1969, 1975, 1980, 1984, 1988, 1992 1995, and 2001.

Library of Congress Cataloging-in-Publication Data
Williams' basic nutrition and diet therapy / [edited by] Staci Nix.
   p. cm.
  Includes bibliographical references and index.
  ISBN-13: 978–0–323–02602–4   ISBN-10: 0–323–02602–8

  1. Diet therapy. 2. Nutrition. 3. Nursing. I. Nix, Staci.

RM216. W6865 2004
615.8′54–dc22   2004053241

Senior Editor: Yvonne Alexopoulos
Associate Developmental Editor: Kristin Hebberd
Publishing Services Manager: Catherine Jackson
Project Manager: Anne Konopka
Design Coordinator: Teresa McBryan

ISBN-13: 978–0–323–02602–4
ISBN-10: 0–323–02602–8

Printed in China
Last digit is print number: 9 8 7 6 5 4 3

REVIEWERS

Mary Babcock, MS, RD
Medical Nutrition Therapist
Veteran's Hospital
Adjunct Faculty
Wilkes University
Wilkes-Barre, Pennsylvania;
Part-Time Instructor
Marywood University
Scranton, Pennsylvania;
Adjunct Faculty
College Misericordia
Dallas, Pennsylvania

Dorice M. Czajka-Narins, PhD
Retired Professor
Department of Nutrition & Food Science
College of Health Sciences
Texas Woman's University
Denton, Texas

Betty Kenyon, RD, LMNT
Consultant Dietitian
Panhandle Community Services
Gering, Nebraska;
Adjunct Faculty
Western Nebraska Community College
Scottsbluff, Nebraska

Johnnie Nichols
Instructor
Vocational Nursing Department
Panola College
Carthage, Texas

Ruth Novitt-Schumacher, RN, BSN, MSN
Clinical Instructor
Department of Maternal Child Nursing
College of Nursing
University of Illinois at Chicago
Chicago, Illinois

Anne O'Donnell, MS, MPH, RD
Nutrition Instructor
Diet Tech Program Coordinator
Consumer and Family Studies Department
Santa Rosa Junior College
Santa Rosa, California

Rena K. Quinton, MS, RD
Nutritionist
Health Promotion Council
Philadelphia, Pennsylvania

Anita K. Reed, MSN, RN
Instructor
St. Elizabeth School of Nursing
Lafayette, Indiana

Mary Ryan, RN, BSN, MEd
Instructor
Central School of Practical Nursing
Cleveland, Ohio

Patricia Hart Terry, PhD, RD, LD
Associate Professor and Chair
Department of Human Sciences and Design
School of Education
Samford University
Birmingham, Alabama

To Sue Rodwell Williams, who has dedicated
much of her life to the education of others
and
To my grandmothers with much love:
Mildred Cochran and Tommie Nix

PREFACE TO THE INSTRUCTOR

Through eleven successful editions of this book, Sue Rodwell Williams provided a sound learning resource and a handy manual in basic nutrition for support personnel in health care. As she is now enjoying retirement, I hope to carry on her work and continually provide you with texts of equal quality for many years to come.

As always we have tried to capture the excitement of nutrition knowledge and its application to human health in this edition. The field of nutrition is a dynamic human endeavor that has expanded and changed since the publication of previous editions. Three main factors continue to change the modern face of nutrition. First, the science of nutrition continues to grow rapidly with exciting research. New knowledge in any science challenges some traditional ideas and lends to the development of new ones. Instead of primarily focusing on nutrition in the treatment of disease, we are expanding the search for disease prevention and general enhancement of life through nutrition. Thus was the spirit during the establishment of the current Dietary Reference Intakes. Second, the rapidly increasing multiethnic diversity of the United States population enriches our food patterns and presents varying health care needs. Third, the public is more aware and concerned about health promotion and the role of nutrition, largely because of the media's increasing attention. Clients and patients are raising more questions and seeking intelligent answers. They want sound information to deal with common misinformation and fads, as well as with legitimate controversy. They want to be more involved in their own health care, and an integral part of that care is nutrition.

This new edition continues to reflect upon the evolving face of nutritional science. Its guiding principle is our own commitment, along with that of our publisher, to the integrity of the material. Our basic goal is to produce a new book for today's needs, with updated content, and to meet the expectations and changing needs of students, faculty, and practitioners of basic health care.

BASIC OBJECTIVES

This text is primarily designed for students in licensed practical or vocational nursing (LPN/LVN) programs, as well as for diet technicians or aides. It is also appropriate for programs in various health-related professions.

The general purpose is to introduce basic principles of nutrition and present their applications in person-centered care. As in previous editions, basic concepts are carefully explained when introduced. In addition, our personal concerns are ever-present, as follows: (1) that this introduction to the science and practice we love will continue to lead students and readers to enjoy learning about nutrition in the lives of people and stimulate further reading in areas of personal interest; (2) that caretakers will be alert to nutrition news and questions raised by their increasingly diverse clients and patients; and (3) that contact and communication with professionals in the field of nutrition will help to build a strong team approach to clinical nutritional problems in all patient care.

FEATURES

Sue Rodwell Williams established a very user-friendly, clearly understood writing style through the previous editions of this text. In keeping with her format, I have updated content areas to meet the needs of a rapidly developing science and society.

■ *Current chapter materials.* All chapters continue to include materials to help meet practice needs. In Part 1, *Introduction to Basic Principles of Nutritional Science*, Chapter 1 focuses on the directions of health care and health promotion, risk reduction for disease prevention, and community health care delivery systems, with emphasis on team care and the active role of clients in educated self-care. A description and illustration accompanies the familiar Food Guide Pyramid. The Dietary Reference Intakes (DRIs), the most current dietary recommendations, are introduced and incorporated throughout chapter discussions in Part 1, as well as throughout the rest of the text. Current research updates all of the basic nutrient/energy chapters in the remainder of Part 1. In Part 2, *Nutrition throughout the Life Cycle*, Chapters 10, 11, and 12 reflect current material on human growth and development needs in different parts of the life cycle. Current National Academy of Science guidelines for positive weight gain to meet the metabolic demands of pregnancy and lactation are reinforced. Positive growth support for infancy, childhood, and adolescence is emphasized. The expanding health-maintenance needs of a growing adult population through the aging process focus on building a healthy lifestyle to reduce disease risks.

In Part 3, *Community Nutrition and Health Care*, a strong focus on community nutritional needs is coordinated with a strong emphasis on weight management and physical fitness as health care benefits and risk reduction. The Nutrition Labeling and Education Act is discussed in terms of its current regulations and helpful label format, as well as its effects on food marketing. Highlights of food-borne diseases reinforce concerns about food safety in a changing marketplace. Chapter 14 and Appendix J reinforce information on America's multiethnic cultural food patterns and various religious dietary practices. New information on the topics of obesity and genetics, along with the use of diet drugs, is included in Chapter 15. Chapter 16 discusses aspects of athletics to clarify the ongoing practice of glycogen loading for endurance events, the proliferation of sports drinks, and the dangerous illegal use of steroids by athletes and body builders.

In Part 4, *Clinical Nutrition*, chapters are updated to reflect current medical treatment and approaches to nutrition management. Special areas include developments in gastrointestinal disease, heart disease, diabetes mellitus, renal disease, surgery, cancer, and AIDS.

- *Book format and design.* The chapter format and use of color continue to enhance the book's appeal. Basic chapter concepts and overview, illustrations, tables, boxes, definitions, headings, and subheadings make the content easier and more interesting to read.
- *Learning supplements.* Educational aids have been developed to assist both students and instructors in the teaching/learning process. Please see the *Ancillaries* section on the next page for more detailed information.
- *Illustrations.* Color illustrations, including artwork, graphs, charts, and photographs, help students and

practitioners better understand the concepts and clinical practices presented.
- *Content threads.* This book shares a number of features—reading level; cover design; Key Concepts; Key Terms; Critical Thinking Questions; Chapter Challenge Questions; References; Further Reading and Resources; Glossary; and Cultural Considerations, For Further Focus, and Clinical Applications boxes—with other Elsevier books intended for students in demanding and fast-paced nursing curricula. These common threads help promote and hone the skills these students must master. (See the Content Threads page after this preface for more detailed information on these learning features.)

LEARNING AIDS

As indicated, this new edition is especially significant because of its use of many learning aids throughout the text.

- *Part openers.* To provide the "big picture" of the book's overall focus on nutrition and health, the four main sections are introduced as successive developing parts of that unifying theme.
- *Chapter openers.* To immediately draw students into the topic for study, each chapter opens with a short list of the basic concepts involved and a brief chapter overview leading into the topic to "set the stage."
- *Chapter headings.* Throughout each chapter, the major headings and subheadings in special type or color indicate the organization of the chapter material, making for easy reading and understanding of the key ideas. Main concepts and terms are also brought out with color or bold type and italics.
- *Special boxes.* The inclusion of *For Further Focus*, *Cultural Considerations*, and *Clinical Applications* boxes leads students a step further on a given topic or presents a case study for analysis. These boxes enhance understanding of concepts through further exploration or application.
- *Case studies.* In clinical care chapters, case studies are provided in *Clinical Applications* boxes to focus students' attention to related patient care problems. Each case is accompanied by questions for case analysis. Students can use these examples for similar patient care needs in their own clinical assignments.
- *Diet therapy guides.* In clinical chapters, various diet therapy guides provide practical help in patient care and education.
- *Definitions of terms.* Key terms important to students' understanding and application of the material in pa-

tient care are presented in two ways. They are identified in the body of the text, often with interesting word derivations to accompany term descriptions, and also are listed in a glossary at the back of the book for quick reference.

■ *Summaries.* A brief summary at the end of each chapter reviews chapter highlights and helps students see how the chapter contributes to the book's "big picture." Students then can return to any part of the material for repeated study and clarification of details as needed.

■ *Critical Thinking Questions.* To help students understand key parts of the chapter or apply it to patient care problems, critical thinking questions are posed after each chapter summary for review and analysis of the material presented.

■ *Chapter Challenge Questions.* In addition, self-test questions in true-false, multiple choice, and matching formats are provided at the end of each chapter to allow students to test their basic knowledge of the chapter's contents.

■ *References.* Background references throughout the text provide resources used throughout the chapter for students who may want to probe a particular topic of interest.

■ *Further Reading and Resources.* To encourage further reading of useful materials, expand students' knowledge of key concepts, and help students apply material in practical ways for patient care and education, a brief list of annotated resources—including books, journals, and web sites—is provided at the end of each chapter.

■ *Appendixes.* The numerous appendixes include an extensive table of food nutrient values from *Mosby's Nutritrac Nutrition Analysis CD-ROM*, a copy of which is included in this text, along with information on the cholesterol content of foods, dietary fiber, and sodium and potassium. The *Exchange Lists for Meal Planning* are included, along with *Canada's Food Guide to Healthy Eating* and the growth charts published by the Centers for Disease Control and Prevention (CDC). These, and all of the appendixes provided, serve as valuable reference tools and guides in learning and practice.

ANCILLARIES

■ *Instructor's Manual and Test Bank.* This valuable ancillary, which contains an *Instructor's Manual*, a *Test Bank*, and *Transparency Masters*, is available in **print, CD-ROM** (Win/Mac), and **online** formats. The *Instructor's Manual* portion includes detailed chapter outlines; essay questions; and extensive print, audiovisual, software, and web site resources that can be used for activities, projects, or further study. The *Test Bank* includes approximately 700 questions in NCLEX, multiple-choice format. In addition, 34 *Transparency Masters* are provided at the back of the print ancillary and made available on the CD-ROM and web site as a full-color electronic *Image Collection*.

■ *Mosby's Nutritrac Nutrition Analysis CD-ROM.* A FREE nutrition analysis CD-ROM with a database of more than 3000 food items is included with every text. This software allows users to analyze nutrition and calculate food intake and energy expenditure for effective diet analysis.

■ *Evolve web site.* A web site created specifically for this book is accessible at *http://evolve.elsevier.com/ Williams/basic/*. (See the Evolve page at the beginning of the text for more information.) In addition to the *Instructor's Manual* and *Test Bank*, which are located in the *Instructor's Resource* portion of the web site, a *Students' Resource* is also available online to give students the opportunity to reinforce the book's key terms and concepts and provide sources for further study. *Crossword Puzzles* highlight the book's key definitions and terms in a fun and engaging way. *Suggestions for Additional Study* give students the opportunity to apply the knowledge they have learned in real-life situations. *Test Questions* provide students with practice questions and immediate feedback to help them prepare for exams. *WebLinks* offer direct links to a wealth of web sites on nutrition-related topics above and beyond information covered in the book.

■ *Nutrition Resource Center web site.* This informative web site is available at *www3.us.elsevierhealth.com/ Nutrition/* to provide the reader with access to information about all Elsevier nutrition texts in one convenient location.

ACKNOWLEDGMENTS

I am ever thankful for the opportunity to come on board with Elsevier. Much appreciation and respect goes to Mrs. Sue Rodwell Williams for her establishment of such a highly successful text. There have been many people involved in the production of this book, but it certainly would not be what it is without the previous eleven editions, along with all the support staff involved in each of those.

Without the encouragement and recommendation from Klaus Gurgel, Senior Educational Publisher's Representative, I would not be the current author of this text; thank you for your foresight and kind words. Throughout this entire process, various staff members from Elsevier have kindly provided guidance and assistance,˙to all of whom I am grateful. I would like to especially acknowledge the patience, thoroughness, and professionalism of Yvonne Alexopoulos, Senior Editor; Melissa Boyle and Kristin Hebberd, Developmental Editors; and Anne Konopka, Project Manager. Your work on this text has been integral to its success.

I would like to acknowledge the hard work and dedication of Elsevier's Nursing Marketing Department for supporting this book through its many editions and bridging the gap between an idea and the many students who will hopefully learn from and enjoy this text. In addition, I am grateful to the many reviewers who have critiqued this edition. Your involvement provides the strength and thoroughness that no author can accomplish alone.

Finally, I want to thank my family and friends who have compassionately dealt with me and *the book*. Your abundant support sustains me.

Staci Nix

CONTENT THREADS

The twelfth edition of *Williams' Basic Nutrition & Diet Therapy* shares a number of learning features with other Elsevier titles used in nursing programs. These user-friendly "Content Threads" are designed to streamline the learning process among the variety of books and content areas included in this fast-paced and demanding curriculum.

Shared elements included in *Williams' Basic Nutrition & Diet Therapy*, twelfth edition, include the following:

- **Reading level:** The easy-to-read and user-friendly format, as well as the often personal writing style, engage the reader and help unfold the information simply and effectively.
- **Cover design:** Graphic similarities help readers to instantly recognize the book as containing content and features relevant to today's nursing curricula.
- Bulleted lists of **Key Concepts** on each chapter opening page help focus the student on the "big picture" content presented.
- **Key Terms** presented in color are readily apparent throughout the book. In addition, key terms boxes presented on the book pages in which the terms are discussed provide complete definitions and often word origins to help with memory association.
- **Critical Thinking Questions** presented after each chapter's summary encourage the student not only to recall the information but also to analyze its implications and uses.
- **Chapter Challenge Questions** presented in true-false, multiple-choice, and matching formats help students to test their comprehension of various content areas. Answers are provided in the back of the book.
- A complete list of **References** is accompanied by **Further Reading and Resources,** a section that includes a wealth of resources—books, journal articles, and web sites—that supplement the information provided in the textbook.
- The **Glossary** is an alphabetical listing of the key terms presented throughout the textbook.
- Three types of boxes—**Cultural Considerations, For Further Focus,** and **Clinical Applications**—explore current "hot" topics in nutrition today and provide insight beyond the information presented in the chapter text.

PREFACE TO THE STUDENT

Basic Nutrition & Diet Therapy is a market leader in nutrition textbooks for support personnel in health care. It provides careful explanations of the basic principles of scientific nutrition and presents their applications in person-centered care in health and disease.

The author, Staci Nix, provides this important information in an easy-to-read, user-friendly format by including helpful learning tools throughout the text. Check out the following features to familiarize yourself with the book and help you get the most value out of this text:

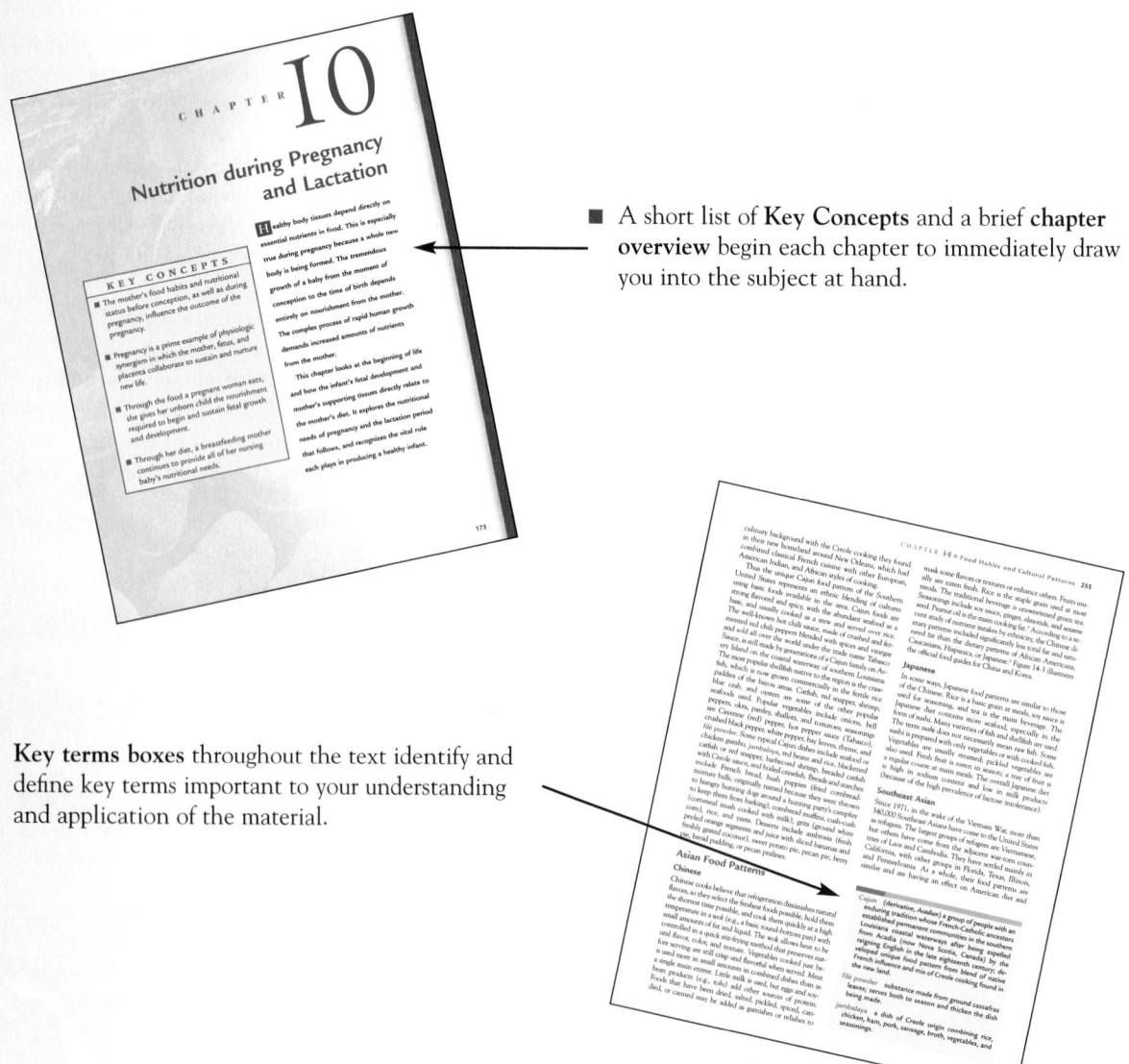

■ A short list of **Key Concepts** and a brief **chapter overview** begin each chapter to immediately draw you into the subject at hand.

■ **Key terms boxes** throughout the text identify and define key terms important to your understanding and application of the material.

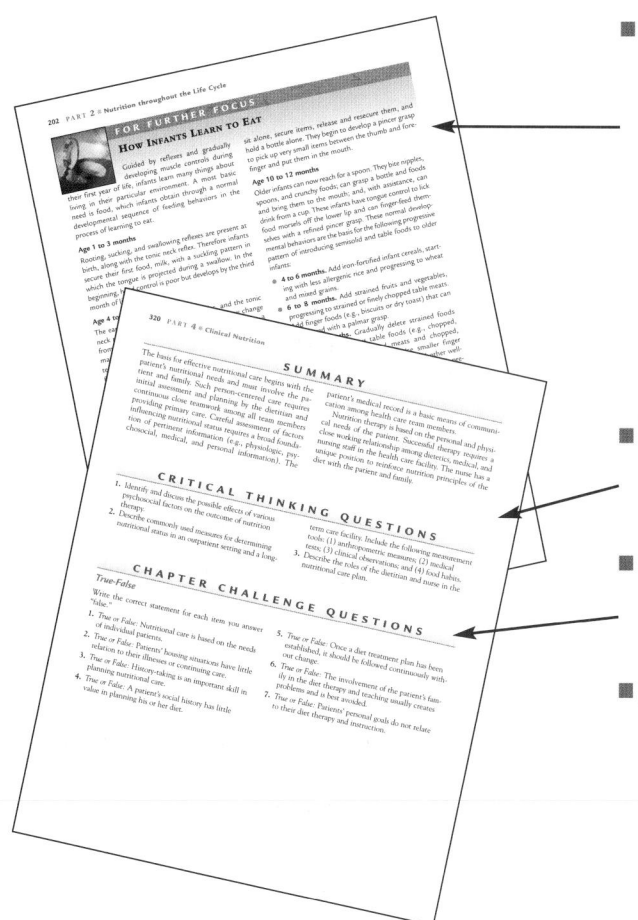

■ **For Further Focus, Cultural Considerations,** and **Clinical Applications** boxes take you one step further in the discussion of a given topic, enhancing your understanding of concepts through further exploration or application.

■ A brief **Summary** is included at the end of every chapter to review content highlights and help you see how particular chapters contribute to the book's overall focus.

■ **Critical Thinking Questions** and **Chapter Challenge Questions** are presented after each chapter summary for review and analysis and allow you to apply key concepts to patient care problems.

■ **References** and **Further Reading and Resources** complete the chapter with lists of relevant citations that provide a wealth of nutrition-related information above and beyond the book's content.

Your free copy of the latest version of the **Nutritrac Nutrition Analysis CD-ROM** is also included in the back of this text. *Nutritrac* provides the easiest way to analyze nutrition and calculate food intake and energy expenditure for effective diet analysis. Here is what you will find: an updated food database with more than 3000 foods, 18 food categories, and an updated *Detailed Energy Expenditure* section that includes more than 150 common/daily, sporting, recreational, and occupational activities.

Be sure to visit our two web sites of interest.

1. A brand new **Evolve** web site has been created specifically for this book at *http://evolve.elsevier.com/Williams/basic/*. (See the Evolve page at the beginning of this text for more information.) The following exciting features are available:

   ■ *Crossword Puzzles* are a fun way to reinforce your understanding of key terms presented throughout the text.

   ■ *Test Questions* give you a chance to practice for your exams and receive immediate feedback.

   ■ *Suggestions for Additional Study* encourage you to go that extra step to apply the knowledge you've learned in real-life situations.

   ■ *WebLinks* offer direct links to a wealth of nutrition-related web sites and allow you to take your learning a step further.

2. A **Nutrition Resource Center** web site is available at *www3.us.elsevierhealth.com/Nutrition/* to provide you access to all the Elsevier nutrition texts in one convenient location.

We are pleased that you have included *Basic Nutrition & Diet Therapy* as a part of your nutrition education. Be sure to check out our web site at *www.elsevierhealth.com* for all your health science educational needs!

CONTENTS

Williams'
Basic Nutrition
& Diet Therapy

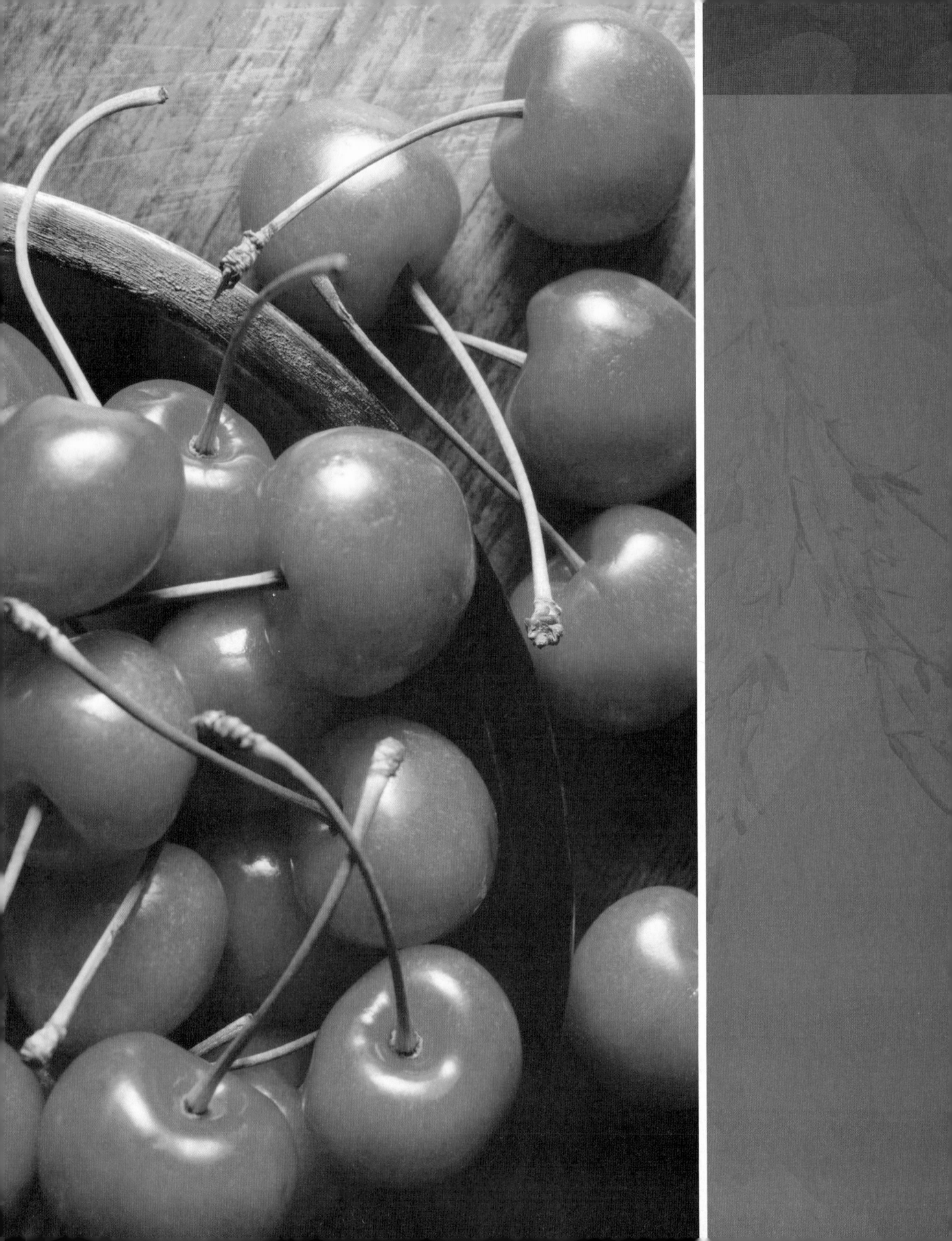

Food, Nutrition, and Health

We live in a world with rapidly changing elements—our environment, food supply, population, and scientific knowledge. Within different environments, our bodies, personalities, needs, and goals change. These constant changes of life must be in some kind of positive balance to produce healthy living. Therefore to be realistic within these concepts of change and balance, our study of food, nutrition, and health care must focus upon health promotion. Although we may view and define health and disease in different ways, a primary basis for promoting health and preventing disease must always start with good food and the sound nutrition it provides. This basic study of nutrition has primary importance in the following two ways: it is fundamental for our own health, and it is essential for the health and well-being of our patients and clients.

KEY CONCEPTS

■ Optimal personal and community nutrition is a major component of health promotion.

■ Certain nutrients in food are essential to our health and well-being.

■ Food and nutrient guides help us to plan a balanced diet according to individual needs and goals.

HEALTH PROMOTION

Basic Definitions

Nutrition and Dietetics

Nutrition concerns the food people eat and how their bodies use it. Nutritional science comprises the body of scientific knowledge governing humans' food requirements for maintenance, growth, activity, reproduction, and lactation. Dietetics is the health profession responsible for applying nutritional science to promote human health and treat disease. The registered dietitian (RD), also referred to as the *clinical nutrition specialist* or *public health nutritionist* in the community, is the nutrition authority on the health care team. These health care professionals carry the major responsibility of nutritional care in patients and clients.

Health and Wellness

Good nutrition is essential to good health throughout life, beginning with prenatal life and extending through old age. In its simplest terms, health is defined as the absence of disease; but this definition is too narrow. Life experience shows that the definition of health is much more. It must include extensive attention to the roots of health in meeting basic human needs (i.e., physical, mental, psychological, and social well-being). This approach recognizes the individual as a whole and relates health to both internal and external environments. The concept of *wellness* broadens this approach one step further. Wellness seeks the full development of potential for all persons, within whatever environment they may find themselves. It implies a balance between activities and goals: work vs. leisure, lifestyle choices vs. health risks, and personal needs vs. others' expectations. Wellness implies a positive dynamic state motivating a person to seek a higher level of functioning.

Wellness Movement and National Health Goals

The current wellness or fitness movement, which is rooted in the 1970s, continues to be a fundamental response to the medical care system's emphasis on illness and disease and the rising costs of medical care. Since the 1970s, "holistic" health and health promotion have focused on lifestyle and personal choice in helping persons and families develop plans for maintaining health and wellness. The U.S. national health goals continue to reflect this wellness philosophy. People are also becoming more comfortable with our rapidly developing modern biotechnology. The pivotal report, *Healthy People 2000*, published in 1990 by the U.S. Department of Health and Human Services, had wide influence.[1] The most recent report in this series, *Healthy People 2010*, continues to focus on the nation's main objective of positive health promotion and disease prevention. This report outlines specific objectives for meeting the following three broad public health goals:[2]

1. An increase in the span of healthy life
2. Reduction of health disparities
3. Access to preventive health care services

A major theme throughout the report is the encouragement of healthy choices in diet, weight control, and other risk factors for disease—especially in the report's specific nutritional objectives. Community health agencies continue to implement these goals and objectives in local and state public and private health programs, especially in areas where malnutrition and poverty exist. All of these efforts recognize personal nutrition as an integral component of health and health care for all persons.

Traditional and Preventive Approaches to Health

The *preventive* approach to health involves identifying risk factors that increase a person's chances of developing a particular health problem. By knowing these factors, people can then choose behaviors that will prevent or minimize their risks for disease. On the other hand, the *traditional* approach to health only attempts change when symptoms of illness or disease already exist, at which point those who are ill seek out a physician to diagnose, treat, and "cure" the condition. The traditional approach has little value for lifelong positive health. Major chronic problems (e.g., heart disease or cancer) may be developing long before overt signs become apparent.

Importance of a Balanced Diet

Food and Health

Food is a necessity of life. However many people are only concerned with food insofar as it relieves their hunger or satisfies their appetites, not with whether it supplies their bodies with all the components of good nutrition. The core practitioners of the health care team (i.e., physician, dietitian, and nurse) are all aware of the important part that food plays in maintaining good health and recovering from illness. To identify possible contributing factors, food habits, choices, and sources should be evaluated in individuals suffering from chronic illness. Therefore assessing a patient's nutritional status and identifying nutritional needs are primary activities in the development of a health care plan.

Signs of Good Nutrition

A lifetime of good nutrition is evidenced by a well-developed body, the ideal weight for body composition (i.e., ratio of muscle mass to fat mass) and height, and good muscle development. In addition, skin is smooth and clear, hair is glossy, and eyes are clear and bright. Signs of good nutrition can extend to good posture and alert facial expression. Appetite, digestion, and elimination are normal. Well-nourished persons are more likely to be mentally and physically alert and have a positive outlook on life. They are also more able to resist infectious diseases than undernourished persons. Within wide varieties of cultural food habits, a wise diet not only creates healthier persons but also extends their years of normal functioning. This is particularly important with our current trends of population growth and ever-increasing life expectancy. In 2000, life expectancy reached a high of 74.1 years for men and 79.5 for women.[3]

FUNCTIONS OF NUTRIENTS IN FOOD

To sustain life, the nutrients in foods must perform the following three basic functions within the body:

1. Provide energy
2. Build tissue
3. Regulate metabolic processes

Metabolism refers to the sum of all body processes that accomplish these three basic life-sustaining tasks.

An important nutritional-metabolic fact emerges in the following outline of these three basic nutrient functions. This fact is the fundamental principle of *nutrient interaction*, which means two things: (1) individual nutrients have many specific metabolic functions, including primary and supporting roles; and (2) no nutrient ever works alone. The human body is a fascinating whole made up of many parts and processes. Intimate metabolic relationships exist among all the basic nutrients and their metabolic products. This key principle of nutrient interaction is demonstrated more clearly in the following chapters. Although the various nutrients may be separated for study purposes, remember that they do not exist that way in the human body. They always interact as a dynamic whole to produce and maintain the body.

Energy Sources

Carbohydrates

Dietary carbohydrates (e.g., starches and sugars) provide the body's primary source of fuel for heat and energy. They also maintain the body's back-up store of quick energy as **glycogen,** which is sometimes called "animal starch" (see Chapter 2). Human energy is measured in heat units called **kilocalories** (abbreviated *kcalories* or *kcal*; see Chapter 6). Each gram of carbohydrate consumed yields 4 kcal of body energy. This number is called the "fuel factor" for carbohydrates. In a well-balanced diet, carbohydrates should provide about 45% to 65% of the total kcalories.

---

health promotion (A.S. *hal,* hale, sound; L. *promovere,* to move forward) active involvement in behaviors or programs that advance positive well-being.

nutrition (L. *nutritic,* nourishment) the sum of the processes involved in taking in nutrients and assimilating and using them to maintain body tissue and provide energy; a foundation for life and health.

nutritional science the body of science, developed through controlled research, that relates to the processes involved in nutrition: international, community, and clinical.

dietetics management of diet and the use of food; the science concerned with the nutritional planning and preparation of foods.

registered dietitian (RD) a professional dietitian, accredited with an academic degree of undergraduate or graduate study program who has passed required registration examinations administered by the American Dietetic Association.

health a state of optimal physical, mental, and social well-being; relative freedom from disease or disability.

metabolism (Gr. *metaballein,* to turn about, change, or alter) the sum of all chemical changes that take place in the body by which it maintains itself and produces energy for its functioning. Products of the various reactions are called *metabolites.*

glycogen (Gr. *glykys,* sweet; *gennan,* to produce) a polysaccharide, the main storage form of carbohydrate, largely stored in the liver and to a lesser extent in muscle tissue.

kilocalorie (Gr. *chilioi,* thousand; L. *calor,* heat) the general term *calorie* refers to a unit of heat measure and is used alone to designate the small calorie. The calorie used in nutritional science and the study of metabolism is the large calorie, 1000 calories, or kilocalorie, to be more accurate and avoid the use of very large numbers in calculations. A kilocalorie is the measure of heat necessary to raise the temperature of 1000 g (1 L) of water 1° C.

Fats

Dietary fats, from both animal and plant sources, provide the body's secondary, or storage, form of heat and energy. This form is more concentrated, yielding 9 kcal for each gram consumed and thus having a fuel factor of 9. In a well-balanced diet, fats should provide no more than 20% to 35% of the total kcalories, with most of this amount (approximately two thirds) being unsaturated fats from plant sources (see Chapter 3).

Proteins

The body may draw from dietary or tissue protein to obtain necessary energy when the supply of fuel from carbohydrates and fats is insufficient. When this occurs, protein can yield 4 kcal/g, making its fuel factor 4. In a well-balanced diet, protein should provide about 10% to 35% of the total kcalories (see Chapter 4). Although the primary function of protein is tissue building, some of it may be used for energy if necessary.

Tissue Building

Proteins

The primary function of protein is tissue building. Dietary protein provides **amino acids,** which are the building units necessary for constructing and repairing body tissues. Tissue building is a constant process that ensures growth and maintenance of a strong body structure and vital substances for its tissue functions.

Other Nutrients

Several other nutrients that contribute to building and maintaining tissues are described in the following paragraphs.

Vitamins and Minerals. An example of the use of a vitamin in tissue building is that of vitamin C in developing the cementing intercellular ground substance. This substance, collagen, helps build strong tissue and prevents tissue bleeding. Two major minerals, calcium and phosphorus, function in building and maintaining bone tissue. Another key mineral is iron, which contributes to building the oxygen carrier hemoglobin in red blood cells (RBCs). Several other vitamins and minerals are discussed in greater detail in Chapters 7 and 8 with regard to their function, including tissue building.

Fatty Acids. Fatty acids, derived from fat metabolism, help build the central fat substance of cell walls and promote the transport of fat-soluble materials across the cell wall.

Regulation and Control

The multiple chemical processes in the body necessary for providing energy and building tissue are carefully regulated and controlled to maintain a smooth, balanced operation. Otherwise, there would be chaos within the body systems, and death would result. Life and health result from a constant dynamic balance among all body parts and processes. Vitamins and minerals are nutrients that help regulate many body processes.

Vitamins

Many vitamins function as coenzyme factors, which are components of cell enzymes, in governing chemical reactions during cell metabolism. For example, this is true for most of the B-complex vitamins.

Minerals

Many minerals also serve as coenzyme factors with enzymes in cell metabolism. For example, cobalt, which is a central constituent of vitamin B_{12} (cobalamin), functions with this vitamin to combat pernicious anemia.

Other Nutrients

Water and fiber also function as regulatory agents. In fact, water is *the* fundamental agent for life itself, providing the essential base for all metabolic processes. Dietary fiber helps regulate the passage of food material through the gastrointestinal tract and influences the absorption of various nutrients.

GOOD NUTRITION

Optimal Nutrition

Optimal nutrition means that a person receives and uses substances that are obtained from a *varied* diet of carbohydrates, fats, proteins, minerals, vitamins, water, and dietary fiber in ideal amounts for that specific individual. The desired amounts of these nutrients should be balanced to cover variations in health and disease and provide reserve supplies without unnecessary excesses.

Undernutrition

Dietary surveys have shown that approximately one third of the U.S. population lives on suboptimal diets. That does not necessarily mean that these Americans are undernourished. Some persons can maintain health on somewhat less than the optimal amounts of various nutrients in a state of borderline nutrition. However, on average someone re-

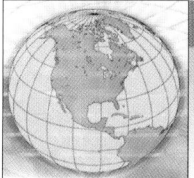

CULTURAL CONSIDERATIONS

FOOD INSECURITY

Food insecurity is defined by the U.S. Department of Agriculture (USDA) as limited or uncertain availability of nutritious and adequate food. Using this definition, the Food Security Institute reported that 10.5 million households, 10.2% of all U.S. households, suffered from food insecurity in 1998.[a] Many studies document widespread hunger and malnutrition among the poor, especially in the growing number of homeless—including mothers with young children. America's Second Harvest, the nation's largest organization of emergency food providers, estimated that 9 million children in the United States receive emergency food services each year.[b] Malnourished children have stunted growth and episodes of infection and disease, which often have lasting effects on intellectual development.[c,d] In 2000, food insecurity rates were two and three times more prevalent, respectively, among non-metro Hispanics and African Americans than non-metro Caucasians.[e] Worldwide, about 40,000 to 50,000 people die *each day* from malnutrition, whereas an estimated 450 million to 1.3 billion people do not have enough to eat.[f]

[a]Food Security Institute: *USDA releases new national data on household food security: Hunger and food security remain stubbornly high despite strong economy* (Food Security Institute Bulletin). Medford, Mass, August 1999, Tufts University, Center on Hunger and Poverty, School of Nutrition Science & Policy.
[b]America's Second Harvest: *Hunger in America 2001,* Chicago, November 2001, America's Second Harvest.
[c]Brekey WR: It's time for the public health community to declare war on homelessness, *Am J Pub Health* 87(2):153, 1997.
[d]Brown JL, Pollitt E: Malnutrition, poverty, and intellectual development, *Sci Am* 274(2):38, 1996.
[e]Nord M, for the USDA/Economic Research Service: Rates of food insecurity and hunger unchanged in rural households, *Rural America,* 16(4):42, 2002.
[f]Staff report, Public Policy News: Translating the science behind the Dietary Reference Intakes, *J Am Diet Assoc* 98(7):756, 1998.

ceiving less than the desired amounts of nutrients has a greater risk for physical illness than someone receiving the appropriate amounts. Such nutritionally deficient people are limited in their physical work capacity, immune system function, and mental activity. They lack the nutritional reserves to meet any added physiologic or metabolic demands from injury or illness or to sustain fetal development during pregnancy or proper growth in childhood. This state may result from poor eating habits or a continuously stressful environment with little or no income.

Malnutrition

Signs of more serious malnutrition appear when nutritional reserves are depleted and nutrient and energy intake is not sufficient to meet day-to-day needs or added metabolic stress. Many malnourished people live in conditions of poverty. Such conditions influence the health of all involved, but especially that of the most vulnerable persons (i.e., pregnant women, infants, children, and elderly adults). In the United States, one of the wealthiest countries on earth, many studies document widespread hunger and malnutrition among the poor, indicating that food-security problems involve urban development issues, economic policy, and more general poverty issues. (See the Cultural Considerations box, "Food Insecurity," for more information.)

Malnutrition also occurs in our hospitals sometimes. For example, acute trauma or chronic illness, especially among older persons, places added stress on the body, and the daily nutrient and energy intake of these persons is insufficient to meet their needs.

Overnutrition

Some persons may be in a state of overnutrition that results from excess nutrient and energy intake over time. In a sense, overnutrition can be another form of malnutrition, especially when excess caloric intake produces harmful gross body weight (i.e., morbid obesity; see Chapter 15). Harmful overnutrition can also occur in persons who use excessive (e.g., "megadose") amounts of nutrient supplements over time; producing damaging tissue effects (see Chapter 7).

amino acids nitrogen-bearing compounds that form the structural units of protein. The various food proteins, when digested, yield their specific constituent amino acids, which are then available for use by the cells to synthesize specific tissue proteins.

NUTRIENT AND FOOD GUIDES FOR HEALTH PROMOTION

Nutrient Standards

Most of the developed countries of the world have established standards for the major nutrients to serve as a guideline for maintaining healthy populations. These standards are not intended to indicate individual requirements or therapeutic needs but rather, on the basis of current scientific knowledge, to serve as a reference for intake levels of the essential nutrients to adequately meet the known nutritional needs of most healthy population groups. Although these standards are similar in most countries, they may vary somewhat according to the philosophy of the scientists and practitioners in a particular country on the purpose and use of such standards. In the United States, these standards have been updated and reorganized and are now called the **Dietary Reference Intakes (DRIs)**.[4] With the growing population of elderly persons, the optimal allowances for older adults are an increasing concern because of poor diets or eating problems (see Chapter 12).

Dietary Reference Intakes (DRIs) a system of reference values that can be used for assessing and planning diets for healthy populations and many other purposes. These values revise and enlarge the Recommended Dietary Allowances (RDAs), which have been published by the National Academy of Sciences since 1941.

Recommended Dietary Allowances (RDAs) recommended daily allowances of nutrients and energy intake for population groups according to age and sex, with defined weight and height. They are established and reviewed periodically by a representative group of nutritional scientists, in relation to current research. These standards vary little among the developed countries.

MyPyramid a visual pattern of the current basic five food groups, arranged in a pyramid shape to indicate proportionate amounts of daily food choices. The largest food group, bread/cereal, forms the entire foundation. The next two narrowing tiers indicate relatively fewer daily portions of vegetables and fruits, and then of the milk/cheese and meat/dry beans/egg groups. The small tip at the pyramid top indicates sparing use of fats, oils, and sweets.

United States Standards: Dietary Reference Intakes

Since 1941, the **Recommended Dietary Allowances (RDAs)**, published by the National Academy of Sciences, has been the authoritative source setting standards for the minimum amounts of nutrients necessary to protect almost all persons against the risk for nutrient deficiency. The U.S. RDA standard was first published during World War II as a guide for planning and obtaining food supplies for national defense and providing average population standards as a goal for good nutrition. Over the years, these standards have been revised and expanded about every 5 to 10 years to reflect increasing scientific knowledge and social concerns about nutrition and health.

Since the last edition of the RDAs was published in 1989, both public awareness and research attention have shifted to reflect an increasing emphasis on nutrient requirements for maintaining optimum health for individuals and groups within the general population. This change of emphasis resulted in the DRIs project. The creation of the new DRIs involved hundreds of distinguished U.S. and Canadian scientists, divided into seven functional panels who have examined hundreds of nutritional studies on both the health benefits of nutrients and the hazards of taking too much of a nutrient. The Academy has numerous divisions of councils and is supported by the National Institutes of Health (Figure 1-1). The working group of nutrition scientists responsible for these standards comprises the Food and Nutrition Board of the Institute of Medicine. The new DRI recommendations were published over several years in a series of seven volumes.[5-8]

The DRIs include recommendations for each gender and age group, as well as recommendations for pregnancy and lactation. For the first time, excessive amounts of nutrients are identified as tolerable upper intakes. The new DRIs incorporate and expand on the well-established RDAs. The DRIs encompass four interconnected categories of nutrient recommendations, as follow:

1. *Recommended Dietary Allowance (RDA)*. This is the daily intake of a nutrient that meets the needs of almost all healthy individuals of specific age and gender. Individuals should use the RDA as a guide to achieve adequate nutrient intake to decrease the risk of chronic disease. RDAs are only established when there is enough scientific evidence about a specific nutrient.
2. *Estimated Average Requirement (EAR)*. This is the intake level that meets the needs of half of the individuals in a specific group. This quantity is used as the basis for developing the RDA.
3. *Adequate Intake (AI)*. The AI is used as a guide when there is not enough scientific evidence avail-

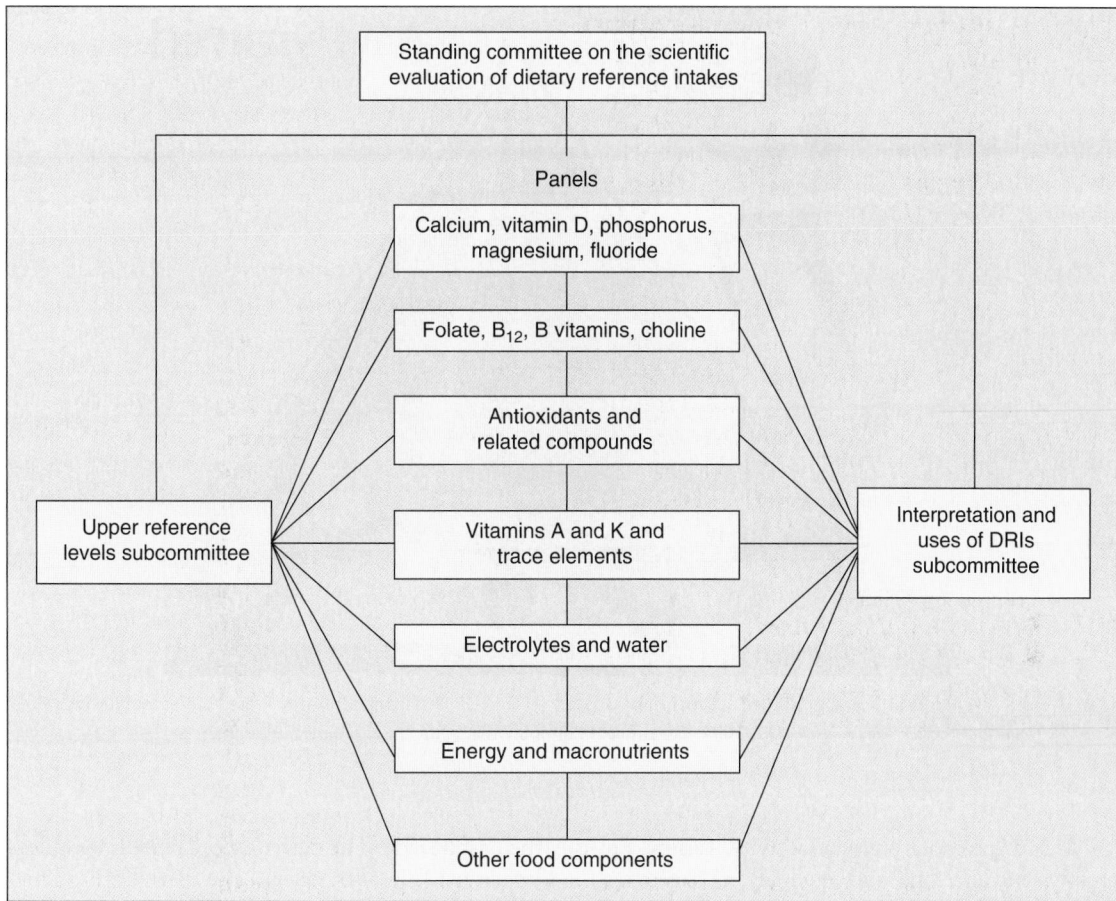

Figure 1–1 Dietary Reference Intakes (DRIs) panels of the Institute of Medicine of the National Academy of Sciences. (From Food and Nutrition Board, Institute of Medicine, National Academy of Sciences: *Dietary reference intakes for thiamin, riboflavin, niacin, vitamin B₆, folate, vitamin B₁₂, pantothenic acid, biotin, and choline,* Washington, DC, 1998, National Academies Press.)

able to establish the RDA figure. Both the RDA and the AI may be used as goals for individual intake.

4. *Tolerable Upper Intake Level (UL).* This indicator is not a recommended intake, but sets the maximum intake that is unlikely to pose adverse health risks in almost all healthy individuals. For most nutrients, the UL refers to the total daily intake from food, fortified food, and nutrient supplements.

Other Standards

Over the years, Canadian and British standards have been similar to the U.S. standards. The current U.S. DRIs were developed with Canadian nutritional science associates and is similar to British standards. In less developed countries, where factors such as the quality of available protein foods must be considered, individuals look to standards such as those set by the Food and Agriculture Organization (FAO) and World Health Organization (WHO). Nonetheless, all of these standards provide a guideline to help health care workers in a variety of population groups promote good health and prevent disease through sound nutrition.

Food Guides and Recommendations

To interpret and apply sound nutrient standards, health care workers need practical food guides to use in nutrition education and food planning with persons and families. Such tools include the U.S. Department of Agriculture (USDA) Food Guide Pyramid and the U.S. Dietary Guidelines.

MyPyramid

The new MyPyramid food guidance system (Figure 1-2), released in early 2005 by the USDA, provides the public with a valuable nutrition education tool. The goal of this

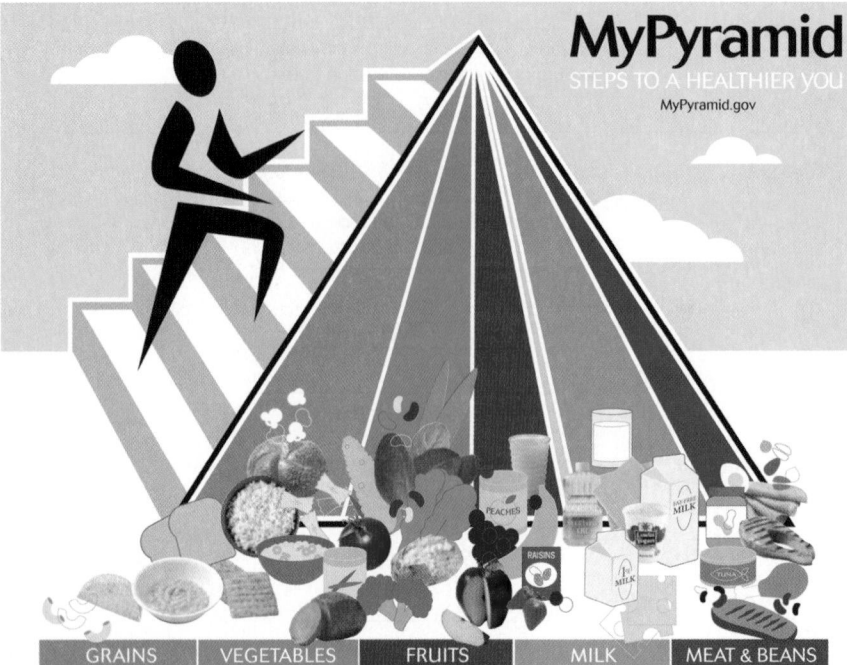

Figure 1–2   MyPyramid food guidance system mini-poster. (From U.S. Department of Agriculture, Center for Nutrition Policy and Promotion: *MyPyramid mini-poster,* Washington, DC, 2005, Government Printing Office [*http://www.mypyramid.gov/downloads/MiniPoster.pdf*].)

food guide is to promote physical activity, variety, proportionality, moderation, and gradual improvements. Consumers are encouraged to personalize their own plans through the public web site (*www.mypyramid.gov*) by entering the individual's age, gender, and activity level. The system will create a plan with individualized calorie levels and specific recommendations for serving amounts from each food group. The current recommendations reflect the DRIs and *Dietary Guidelines for Americans 2005* (see Figure 1-3). In addition, the MyPyramid site will provide consumers with individualized Meal Tracking Worksheets and access to the MyPyramid Tracker, an online dietary and physical activity assessment tool.

Dietary Guidelines for Americans

The *Dietary Guidelines for Americans* were issued as a result of growing public concerns beginning in the 1960s and the subsequent Senate investigations studying hunger and nutrition in the United States. These guidelines are based on our developing alarm about chronic health problems in an aging population and changing food environment. They relate current scientific thinking to America's leading health problems. A new updated statement is issued every 5 years. Recent review by expert committees has only led to minimal changes over

the past decade. The current set of guidelines, released in January 2005, also reflects the new DRIs. This issue reflects a comprehensive evaluation of the scientific evidence between diet and health, based on findings in a current U.S. report issued jointly by the USDA and the Department of Health and Human Services (DHHS).

The guidelines promote 9 focus areas, 23 general recommendations, and 18 specific population recommendations. The nine focus areas are (1) adequate nutrients within calorie needs, (2) weight management, (3) physical activity, (4) food groups to encourage, (5) fats, (6) carbohydrates, (7) sodium and potassium, (8) alcoholic beverages, and (9) food safety (Figure 1-3). The current guidelines continue to serve as a useful general guide for promoting dietary and lifestyle choices that reduce the risk for chronic disease. Although no guidelines can guarantee health or well-being, and people differ widely in their food needs, these general statements can lead persons to evaluate their food habits and move toward general improvements. Good food habits based on moderation and variety can help to build sound healthy bodies.

Other Recommendations

Other organizations, such as the American Cancer Society (*www.cancer.org*) and American Heart Association (*www.americanheart.org*) also have their own inde-

GRAINS Make half your grains whole	VEGETABLES Vary your veggies	FRUITS Focus on fruits	MILK Get your calcium-rich foods	MEAT & BEANS Go lean with protein
Eat at least 3 oz. of whole-grain cereals, breads, crackers, rice, or pasta every day 1 oz. is about 1 slice of bread, about 1 cup of breakfast cereal, or ½ cup of cooked rice, cereal, or pasta	Eat more dark-green veggies like broccoli, spinach, and other dark leafy greens Eat more orange vegetables like carrots and sweetpotatoes Eat more dry beans and peas like pinto beans, kidney beans, and lentils	Eat a variety of fruit Choose fresh, frozen, canned, or dried fruit Go easy on fruit juices	Go low-fat or fat-free when you choose milk, yogurt, and other milk products If you don't or can't consume milk, choose lactose-free products or other calcium sources such as fortified foods and beverages	Choose low-fat or lean meats and poultry Bake it, broil it, or grill it Vary your protein routine — choose more fish, beans, peas, nuts, and seeds

For a 2,000-calorie diet, you need the amounts below from each food group. To find the amounts that are right for you, go to MyPyramid.gov.

| Eat 6 oz. every day | Eat 2½ cups every day | Eat 2 cups every day | Get 3 cups every day;
for kids aged 2 to 8, it's 2 | Eat 5½ oz. every day |

Find your balance between food and physical activity
- Be sure to stay within your daily calorie needs.
- Be physically active for at least 30 minutes most days of the week.
- About 60 minutes a day of physical activity may be needed to prevent weight gain.
- For sustaining weight loss, at least 60 to 90 minutes a day of physical activity may be required.
- Children and teenagers should be physically active for 60 minutes every day, or most days.

Know the limits on fats, sugars, and salt (sodium)
- Make most of your fat sources from fish, nuts, and vegetable oils.
- Limit solid fats like butter, stick margarine, shortening, and lard, as well as foods that contain these.
- Check the Nutrition Facts label to keep saturated fats, *trans* fats, and sodium low.
- Choose food and beverages low in added sugars. Added sugars contribute calories with few, if any, nutrients.

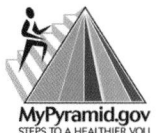

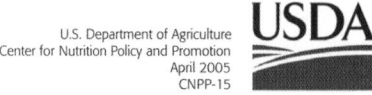

U.S. Department of Agriculture
Center for Nutrition Policy and Promotion
April 2005
CNPP-15

Figure 1–2 cont'd   MyPyramid food guidance system mini-poster. (From U.S. Department of Agriculture, Center for Nutrition Policy and Promotion: *MyPyramid mini-poster,* Washington, DC, 2005, Government Printing Office [*http://www.mypyramid.gov/downloads/MiniPoster.pdf*].)

pendent dietary guidelines. That does not mean that these guidelines are in conflict with the U.S. Dietary Guidelines. In most cases, the guidelines set by various national organizations are modeled after the U.S. Dietary Guidelines. This may seem a bit confusing and redundant, but the difference is the emphasis on prevention of certain chronic diseases, such as heart disease and cancer.

Individual Needs

Person-Centered Care

Regardless of the type of food guide or recommendations used, health care professionals must remember that food patterns vary with individual needs, tastes, habits, living situations, and energy demands. Persons who eat nutri-

tionally balanced meals, spread fairly evenly throughout the day, can usually work more efficiently and sustain a more even energy supply.

Changing Food Environment

Our food environment has been changing rapidly in recent years. There are more processed food items of variable or unknown nutrient quality. American food habits may have deteriorated in some ways. Despite a plentiful food supply, surveys give evidence of malnutrition, even among hospitalized patients. Nurses and other health care professionals have an important responsibility to observe patients' food intake carefully (Figure 1-4). However, in general it is encouraging to note that Americans are gradually learning that what

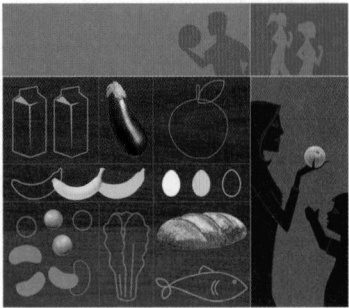

Dietary Guidelines
for Americans
2005

U.S. Department of Health and Human Services
U.S. Department of Agriculture
www.healthierus.gov/dietaryguidelines

ADEQUATE NUTRIENTS WITHIN CALORIE NEEDS

- Consume a variety of nutrient-dense foods and beverages within and among the basic food groups while choosing foods that limit the intake of saturated and *trans* fats, cholesterol, added sugars, salt, and alcohol.
- Meet recommended intakes within energy needs by adopting a balanced eating pattern, such as the USDA Food Guide or the DASH Eating Plan.

WEIGHT MANAGEMENT

- To maintain body weight in a healthy range, balance calories from foods and beverages with calories expended.
- To prevent gradual weight gain over time, make small decreases in food and beverage calories and increase physical activity.

PHYSICAL ACTIVITY

- Engage in regular physical activity and reduce sedentary activities to promote health, psychological well-being, and a healthy body weight.
  - To reduce the risk of chronic disease in adulthood: Engage in at least 30 minutes of moderate-intensity physical activity, above usual activity, at work or home on most days of the week.
  - For most people, greater health benefits can be obtained by engaging in physical activity of more vigorous intensity or longer duration.
  - To help manage body weight and prevent gradual, unhealthy body weight gain in adulthood: Engage in approximately 60 minutes of moderate- to vigorous-intensity activity on most days of the week while not exceeding caloric intake requirements.
  - To sustain weight loss in adulthood: Participate in at least 60 to 90 minutes of daily moderate-intensity physical activity while not exceeding caloric intake requirements. Some people may need to consult with a healthcare provider before participating in this level of activity.
- Achieve physical fitness by including cardiovascular conditioning, stretching exercises for flexibility, and resistance exercises or calisthenics for muscle strength and endurance.

FOOD GROUPS TO ENCOURAGE

- Consume a sufficient amount of fruits and vegetables while staying within energy needs. Two cups of fruit and 2½ cups of vegetables per day are recommended for a reference 2,000-calorie intake, with higher or lower amounts depending on the calorie level.

- Choose a variety of fruits and vegetables each day. In particular, select from all five vegetable subgroups (dark green, orange, legumes, starchy vegetables, and other vegetables) several times a week.
- Consume 3 or more ounce-equivalents of whole-grain products per day, with the rest of the recommended grains coming from enriched or whole-grain products. In general, at least half the grains should come from whole grains.
- Consume 3 cups per day of fat-free or low-fat milk or equivalent milk products.

FATS

- Consume less than 10 percent of calories from saturated fatty acids and less than 300 mg/day of cholesterol, and keep *trans* fatty acid consumption as low as possible.
- Keep total fat intake between 20 to 35 percent of calories, with most fats coming from sources of polyunsaturated and monounsaturated fatty acids, such as fish, nuts, and vegetable oils.
- When selecting and preparing meat, poultry, dry beans, and milk or milk products, make choices that are lean, low-fat, or fat-free.
- Limit intake of fats and oils high in saturated and/or *trans* fatty acids, and choose products low in such fats and oils.

CARBOHYDRATES

- Choose fiber-rich fruits, vegetables, and whole grains often.
- Choose and prepare foods and beverages with little added sugars or caloric sweeteners, such as amounts suggested by the USDA Food Guide and the DASH Eating Plan.
- Reduce the incidence of dental caries by practicing good oral hygiene and consuming sugar- and starch-containing foods and beverages less frequently.

SODIUM AND POTASSIUM

- Consume less than 2,300 mg (approximately 1 tsp of salt) of sodium per day.
- Choose and prepare foods with little salt. At the same time, consume potassium-rich foods, such as fruits and vegetables.

ALCOHOLIC BEVERAGES

- Those who choose to drink alcoholic beverages should do so sensibly and in moderation—defined as the consumption of up to one drink per day for women and up to two drinks per day for men.
- Alcoholic beverages should not be consumed by some individuals, including those who cannot restrict their alcohol intake, women of childbearing age who may become pregnant, pregnant and lactating women, children and adolescents, individuals taking medications that can interact with alcohol, and those with specific medical conditions.
- Alcoholic beverages should be avoided by individuals engaging in activities that require attention, skill, or coordination, such as driving or operating machinery.

FOOD SAFETY

- To avoid microbial food-borne illness:
  - Clean hands, food contact surfaces, and fruits and vegetables. Meat and poultry should not be washed or rinsed.
  - Separate raw, cooked, and ready-to-eat foods while shopping, preparing, or storing foods.
  - Cook foods to a safe temperature to kill microorganisms.
  - Chill (refrigerate) perishable food promptly and defrost foods properly.
  - Avoid raw (unpasteurized) milk or any products made from unpasteurized milk, raw or partially cooked eggs or foods containing raw eggs, raw or undercooked meat and poultry, unpasteurized juices, and raw sprouts.

Figure 1–3 Summary of the nine focus areas included in the *Dietary Guidelines for Americans 2005*. (Image from U.S. Department of Health and Human Services: *Dietary Guidelines for Americans 2005*, Washington, DC, 2005, Government Printing Office [*http://www.health.gov/dietaryguidelines/dga2005/document/media/dgacover.pdf*]. Text from U.S. Department of Health and Human Services, U.S. Department of Agriculture: *Dietary Guidelines for Americans 2005: Key recommendations*, Washington, DC, 2005, USDHHS, USDA [*http://www.health.gov/dietaryguidelines/dga2005/recommendations.htm*].)

Figure 1–4   Nutrition education in the health care setting. (Credit: PhotoDisc.)

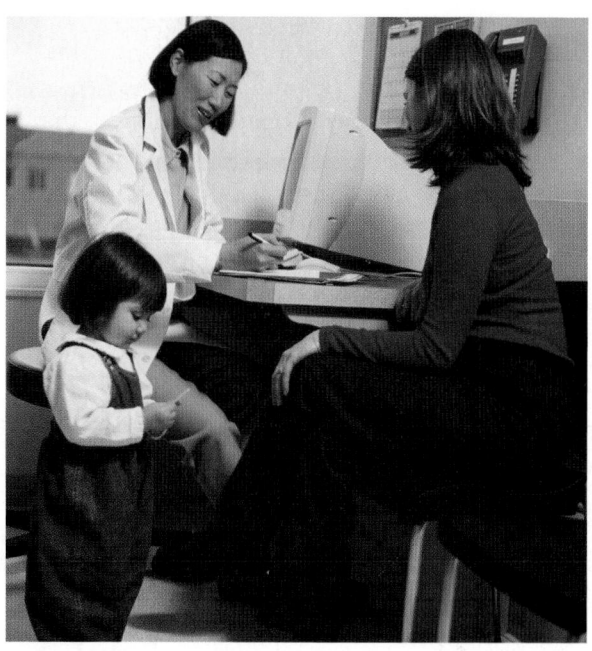

they eat does influence their health. Even fast food restaurants, where Americans often eat, are beginning to respond to their customers' desires for less fat, and some have also added self-help salad bars. Other chain, family, and university restaurants are developing and testing similar patterns in new menu items. More than ever, Americans are being selective about what they eat. Guided by the FDA nutrition labels on processed food items, shoppers' choices indicate an increased awareness of nutritional values. Details of these marketing regulations are given in Chapter 14.

SUMMARY

Good food and key nutrients are essential to life and health. In our changing world, an emphasis on health promotion and disease prevention through reducing health risks has become our primary health goal. The importance of a balanced diet in meeting this health goal through the functioning of its component nutrients is fundamental. Food guides that help persons plan such a healthy diet include the DRIs, the Food Guide Pyramid, the *Dietary Guidelines for Americans*, and others.

CRITICAL THINKING QUESTIONS

1. What is the current U.S. national health goal? Define this goal in terms of health, wellness, and the differences between traditional and preventive approaches to health.
2. Why is a balanced diet important? List and describe some signs of good nutrition.
3. What are the three basic functions of foods and their nutrients? Describe the general roles of nutri-

ents in relation to the following: (1) main nutrient(s) for each function; and (2) other contributing nutrients.
4. With regard to both purpose and use, compare the DRIs with the Food Guide Pyramid.
5. Using the Food Guide Pyramid, plan a day's food pattern for a selected person with modifications according to the *Dietary Guidelines for Americans*.

CHAPTER CHALLENGE QUESTIONS

True-False

Write the correct statement for each item you answer "false."

1. *True or False:* The diet-planning tool *Dietary Guidelines for Americans* stresses the two basic concepts of variety and moderation in food habits.

2. *True or False:* Food processing has little influence on food taste, appearance, safety, or nutrient values.

3. *True or False:* Malnutrition is not a problem in the United States.

Multiple Choice

1. Nutrients are
   a. chemical elements or compounds in foods that have specific metabolic functions.
   b. foods that are necessary for good health.
   c. metabolic control substances, such as enzymes.
   d. nourishing foods used to cure certain illnesses.

2. All nutrients needed by the body
   a. must be obtained by specific food combinations.
   b. must be obtained by vitamin or mineral supplements.
   c. have only one function and use in the body.
   d. are supplied by a variety of foods in many different combinations.

3. All persons throughout life, as indicated by the DRIs, need
   a. the same nutrients in varying amounts.
   b. the same amount of nutrients in any state of health.
   c. the same nutrients at any age in the same amounts.
   d. different nutrients in varying amounts.

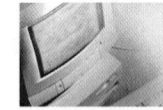

Please refer to the Students' Resource section of this text's Evolve web site for "Suggestions for Additional Study."

REFERENCES

1. U.S. Department of Health and Human Services, Public Health Service: *Healthy People 2000:* National health promotion and disease prevention objectives—nutrition priority area, *Nutr Today* 25(6):29, 1990.
2. U.S. Department of Health and Human Services: *Healthy People 2010: understanding and improving health,* Washington, DC, 2000, Government Printing Office.
3. Miniño AM and others: *Deaths: final data for 2000.* National vital statistics reports 50(15), Hyattsville, MD, 2002, National Center for Health Statistics.
4. Yates AA, Schlicker SA, Suitor CW: Dietary Reference Intakes: the new basis for recommendation for calcium and related B vitamins, and choline, *J Am Diet Assoc* 98(6):699, 1998.
5. Food and Nutrition Board, Institute of Medicine: *Dietary reference intakes for calcium, phosphorous, magnesium, vitamin D, and fluoride,* Washington, DC, 1998, National Academies Press.
6. Food and Nutrition Board, Institute of Medicine: *Dietary reference intakes for thiamin, riboflavin, niacin, vitamin B₆, folate, vitamin B₁₂, pantothenic acid, biotin, and choline,* Washington, DC, 1999, National Academies Press.
7. Food and Nutrition Board, Institute of Medicine: *Dietary reference intakes for vitamin C, vitamin E, selenium, and carotenoids,* Washington, DC, 2000, National Academies Press.
8. Food and Nutrition Board, Institute of Medicine: *Dietary reference intakes for energy, carbohydrate, fiber, fat, fatty acids, cholesterol, protein, and amino acids,* Washington, DC, 2002, National Academies Press.
9. Center for Nutrition Policy and Promotion. U.S. Department of Agriculture, The Food Guide Pyramid Update (accessed April 2004), http://www.cnpp.usda.gov/pyramid-update/index.html.

FURTHER READING AND RESOURCES

- American Dietetic Association (ADA): *www.eatright.org*
- American Society for Clinical Nutrition: *www.faseb.org/ascn*
- National Academy of Sciences/National Research Council (NAS/NRC): *www.nationalacademies.org/nrc*
- Society for Nutrition Education: *www.sne.org*

   The organizations listed in the preceding are key sources of up-to-date information and research about nutrition. Each site has a unique focus and may be helpful in keeping abreast on current topics.

- Biggerstaff MA and others: Living on the edge: examination of people attending food pantries and soup kitchens, *Social Work* 47(3):267, 2002.

This article explores the prevalence of food insecurity, hunger, and poverty. The authors describe the different types of food service programs available and the individuals who are most likely to use them.

- Painter J and others: Comparison of international food guide pictorial representations, *J Am Diet Assoc* 102(4):483, 2002.

   Around the world, various countries have created food guide pictorial representations similar to the Food Guide Pyramid in America. This article compares the shapes chosen by a variety of countries and explores the way in which each representation is tailored to their individual cultural needs.

2

Carbohydrates

A s discussed in Chapter 1, key nutrients in food sustain life and promote health. These tremendous results are possible because the human body's unique use of these nutrients provides three essential life and health needs: (1) energy to do its work; (2) building materials to maintain its form and functions; and (3) control agents to regulate these processes efficiently.

These three basic life and health functions of nutrients are closely related; no nutrient ever works alone. This chapter, as indicated in the previous chapter, looks at each of the nutrients separately, remembering that in our bodies they do not exist or work that way; and considers the body's primary fuel for its energy system—carbohydrates.

KEY CONCEPTS

- Carbohydrate foods provide practical energy (calorie) sources because of their availability, relatively low cost, and storage capacity.

- Carbohydrate structures vary from simple to complex, so they can provide both quick and extended energy for the body.

- Dietary fiber, an indigestible carbohydrate, serves separately as a body regulatory agent.

NATURE OF CARBOHYDRATES

Relation to Energy

Basic Fuel Source

Energy is a necessity for life. It is the power an organism requires to do work. Any energy system must first have a basic fuel supply. In the earth's energy system, vast energy resources from the sun enable plants, through their internal system of photosynthesis, to transform solar energy into carbohydrates, the stored fuel form of plants.[1] Because the human body can rapidly break down these stores of quick and sustaining energy foods (sugars and starches), they provide the major source of energy, in the form of calories.

Throughout this text the term *energy* often is used synergistically with the terms *calorie, kilocalorie,* and *kcalorie* (see definition of kilocalorie in Chapter 1). Our bodies need energy to survive. Both involuntary (heart pumping and lungs breathing) and voluntary actions (walking and talking) require energy. That energy is derived from calories supplied by food.

---

photosynthesis   (Gr. *photos,* light; synthesis, putting together) process by which plants containing chlorophyll are able to manufacture carbohydrate by combining CO_2 from air and water from soil. Sunlight is used as energy; chlorophyll is a catalyst.

$$6\ CO_2 + 6\ H_2O + Energy \rightarrow Chlorophyll \rightarrow$$
$$C_6H_{12}O_6 + 6\ O_2$$

saccharide   (L. *saccharum,* sugar) chemical name for sugar molecules. May occur as single molecules in monosaccharides (glucose, fructose, galactose), two molecules in disaccharides (sucrose, lactose, maltose), or multiple molecules in polysaccharides (starch, dietary fiber, glycogen).

simple carbohydrates   sugars with a simple structure of one or two single-sugar (saccharide) units. A monosaccharide is composed of one sugar unit; a disaccharide is composed of two sugar units.

complex carbohydrates   large, complex molecules of carbohydrates composed of many sugar units (polysaccharides). Complex forms of dietary carbohydrates are starch, which is digestible and provides a major energy source, and dietary fiber, which is indigestible (humans lack the necessary enzymes) and thus provides important bulk in the diet.

Energy-Production System

To produce energy from a basic fuel supply, a successful energy system must be able to do the following three things:

1. Change the basic fuel to a refined fuel that the machine is designed to use
2. Carry this refined fuel to the places that need it
3. Burn this refined fuel in the special equipment set up at these places

Far more efficient than any man-made machine, the body easily does these three things. It digests its basic fuel, carbohydrate, changing it to glucose. The body then absorbs and, through blood circulation, carries this refined fuel to cells that need glucose. Glucose is burned in the specific and intricate equipment in these cells, and energy is released through the process of cell metabolism. Because the human body can rapidly break down the starches and sugars that are eaten to yield energy, carbohydrates are called "quick energy" foods.

Dietary Importance

There are also practical reasons for the large quantities of carbohydrates in diets all over the world. First, carbohydrates are widely available and easily grown (e.g., grains, legumes, vegetables, and fruits). In some countries, carbohydrate foods make up almost the entire diet. In the typical American diet, about half of the total kcalories is in the form of carbohydrates. Second, carbohydrates are relatively low in cost when compared with many other food items. Third, carbohydrates may be easily stored. They can be kept in dry storage for relatively long periods without spoilage. Modern processing and packaging extend the shelf-life of carbohydrate products almost indefinitely.

The U.S. Department of Agriculture (USDA) regularly surveys individual food intakes. These reports usually indicate that about half of the total kcalories in the American diet come from carbohydrates, with children consuming somewhat more than adults. Daily intake of sugars by Americans accounts for about 20% of total kcalories and may range as high as 40% in individuals consuming increased amounts of sweets and foods processed with high-fructose corn syrup. As a result, the typical American sugar consumption is always considerably higher than the FDA guidelines for a healthy diet, which states that added sugars should comprise no more than 25% of total kcalories. The remainder of the total carbohydrate kcalories comes from starches.

Chemical class name	Class members	Sources
TABLE 2-1 Summary of Carbohydrate Classes		
Monosaccharides Single sugars, simple carbohydrates	Glucose (dextrose)	Corn syrup (large use in processed foods)
	Fructose	Fruits, honey
	Galactose	Lactose (milk)
Disaccharides Double sugars, simple carbohydrates	Sucrose	"Table" sugar: sugar cane, sugar beets Molasses
	Lactose	Milk
	Maltose	Starch digestion, intermediate Sweetener in food products Starch digestion, final

Polysaccharides
Multiple sugars, complex carbohydrates
	Starch	Grains and grain products
		  Cereal, bread, crackers, and other baked
		    goods
		  Rice, corn, bulgur
		Legumes
		Potatoes and other vegetables

	Glycogen	Storage form of carbohydrate in animal tissue

Illustrations from Mahan LK, Escott-Stump S: *Krause's food, nutrition, & diet therapy,* ed 11, Philadelphia, 2004, Saunders.

Classes of Carbohydrates

The name *carbohydrate* comes from its chemical nature. A carbohydrate is composed of carbon (C), hydrogen (H), and oxygen (O), with the hydrogen:oxygen ratio usually that of water: H_2O. Its abbreviated name, CHO, which is the combination of the chemical symbols of its three components, is often used in medical charts or various notations. The term **saccharide** is used as a carbohydrate class name and comes from the Latin word *saccharum,* meaning "sugar." Thus a saccharide unit is a single sugar unit. Carbohydrates are classified according to the number of sugar, or saccharide, units making up their structure: *mono*saccharides have one sugar unit; *di*saccharides have two sugar units; and *poly*saccharides have many sugar units. Monosaccharides and disaccharides are small, simple structures of only one- and two-sugar units, so they are called **simple carbohydrates.** However, polysaccharides are large, complex compounds of many saccharide units in long chains, so they are called **complex carbohydrates.** For example, starch, the most significant polysaccharide in human nutrition, is made up of many coiled and branching chains in a tree-like structure. Each of the multiple branching chains is composed of 24 to 30 sugar units of glucose, which gradually split off in digestion to supply a steady source of energy over a period of time. Table 2-1 summarizes these classes of carbohydrates.

Monosaccharides

The three important simple single sugars in nutrition are glucose, fructose, and galactose. Monosaccharides, the building blocks for all carbohydrates, require no further digestion. They are quickly absorbed from the intestine into the blood stream and carried to the liver. In the liver, they are converted by enzymes into glycogen for a constant back-up energy supply or used for immediate energy needs.

Glucose. The basic single sugar in body metabolism is glucose, which is the form of sugar circulating in the blood and is the primary fuel to the cells. It is not usually found as such in the diet, except for in corn syrup used alone or in processed food items. The body supply comes mainly from the digestion of starch. Glucose is a moderately sweet sugar. Glucose is also sometimes called *dextrose,* to denote the structure of the molecule.

Fructose. Fructose is found mainly in fruits, from which it gets its name, or in honey. Although honey is sometimes thought of as a sugar substitute, it is actually a sugar itself; therefore it cannot be considered a substitute. The amount of fructose in fruits depends on the degree of ripeness. As a fruit ripens, some of its stored starch turns to sugar. High-fructose corn syrups are increasingly being used in processed food products and are a major factor of increased sugar intake. Fructose is the sweetest of the simple sugars.

Galactose. Galactose is not usually found as such in the diet but comes mainly from the digestion of milk sugar, or lactose.

Disaccharides

Disaccharides are simple double sugars, comprised of two single-sugar units linked together. The three disaccharides important in nutrition are sucrose, lactose, and maltose.

Sucrose = Glucose + Fructose
Lactose = Glucose + Galactose
Maltose = Glucose + Glucose

Sucrose. Sucrose is common table sugar. Its two single-sugar units are glucose and fructose. Sucrose is used in the form of granulated, powdered, or brown sugar and is made from sugar cane or sugar beets. Molasses, a by-product of sugar production, is also a form of sucrose. When people speak of sugar in the diet, they usually mean sucrose.

Lactose. The sugar in milk, formed in mammary glands, is lactose. Its two single-sugar units are glucose and galactose. Lactose is the only common sugar not found in plants and is less soluble and sweet than sucrose. Lactose remains in the intestine longer than other sugars and encourages the growth of certain useful bacteria. Cow's milk contains 4.8% lactose, and human milk contains 7% lactose. Because lactose aids in the absorption of calcium and phosphorus, the presence of all three nutrients in milk is a fortunate circumstance, as well as an example of why milk is one of nature's best "package" foods.

Maltose. Maltose is not usually found as such in the diet. It is derived in the body from the intermediate digestive breakdown of starch. Because starch is made up entirely of many single-glucose units, the two single-sugar units that compose maltose are both glucose. Synthetically derived maltose is used as a sweetener in various processed foods.

Polysaccharides

Polysaccharides are complex carbohydrates composed of many single sugar units. The important polysaccharides in nutrition include starch, glycogen, and dietary fiber.

Starch. Starches are by far the most significant polysaccharides in the diet. They are found in grains, legumes and other vegetables, and some fruits in minute amounts. Starches are more complex in structure than simple sugars. Thus they break down more slowly and supply energy over a longer period of time. For starch to be used more promptly by the body, the outer membrane can be broken down by grinding or cooking. Cooking of starch not only improves its flavor but also softens and ruptures the starch cells, making digestion easier. Starch mixtures thicken when cooked because the portion that encases the starch granules has a gel-like quality, thickening the starch mixture in the same way that pectin causes jelly to set.

Starch is the most important dietary carbohydrate worldwide. The value of starch in human nutrition and health has recently received a great deal of recognition. The U.S. Dietary Reference Intakes (DRIs; see Chapter 1) recommend that 45% to 65% of our total kcalories come from carbohydrates, with a greater portion of that intake coming from complex carbohydrates.[2] In many other countries, where starch is a staple food, it makes up an even higher portion of the diet. The major food sources of starch (Figure 2-1) include grains in the form of cereal, pasta, crackers, bread, and other baked goods; legumes in the form of beans and peas; potatoes, rice, corn, and bulgur; and other vegetables, especially of the root variety.

The term *whole grain* is used for food products such as flours, breads, or cereals that are produced from unrefined grain, which is grain that still retains its outer bran layers and inner germ endosperm (Figure 2-2) and their nutrients (i.e., dietary fiber, minerals, and vitamins). *Enriched grains* are refined grain products to which key nutrients— usually minerals (e.g., iron) and vitamins (e.g., A, C, D, thiamin, riboflavin, and niacin)—have been added. Ready-to-eat breakfast cereals usually contain additional nutrients such as vitamins D, E, B_6, and folic acid, as well as the minerals phosphorus, magnesium, and zinc. These cereals, which are a favorite breakfast item for children, have become a major source of their vitamin and mineral intake.

Glycogen. Glycogen, found in animal muscle tissue, is similar in structure to starch, so it is sometimes called *animal starch.* Glycogen is not a significant source of

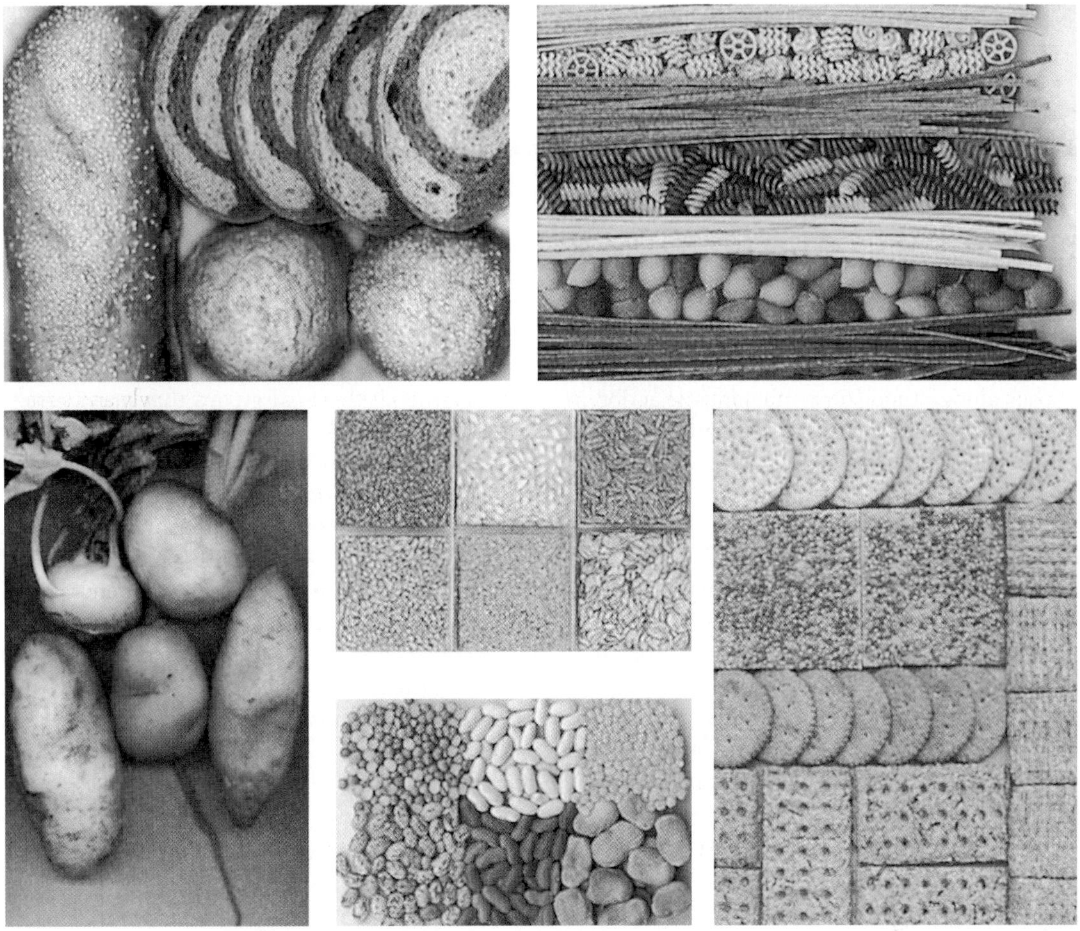

Figure 2–1   Complex carbohydrate foods. (Credit: Amy Buxton.)

carbohydrate in the diet. Rather, it is a carbohydrate formed within the body's tissues and is crucial to the body's metabolism and energy balance. Glycogen is found in the liver and muscles, where it is constantly recycled (i.e., broken down to form glucose for immediate energy needs and synthesized for storage in the liver and muscles). These small stores of glycogen help sustain normal blood glucose during short-term fasting periods (e.g., sleep) and provide immediate fuel for muscle action. These reserves also protect cells from depressed metabolic function and injury. The process of blood glucose regulation, with regard to glycogen breakdown, is discussed in greater detail in Chapter 20.

Dietary Fiber. Several types of dietary fiber are polysaccharides. Because humans lack the necessary enzymes to digest dietary fiber, these substances do not have a direct

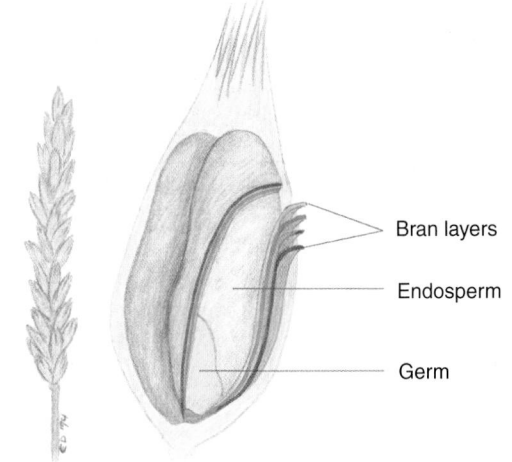

Figure 2–2   Kernel of wheat, showing bran layers, endosperm, and germ. (Credit: Eileen Draper.)

Bran layers

Endosperm

Germ

energy value like other carbohydrates. However, their inability to be digested makes these materials important dietary assets. Increasing attention has focused on the relation of fiber to health promotion and disease prevention, especially to gastrointestinal (GI) problems and management of diabetes.[3] The types of dietary fiber important in human nutrition are described in the following paragraphs.

Cellulose. Cellulose is the chief part of the framework of plants. It remains undigested in the GI tract and provides important bulk to the diet. This bulk helps move the food mass along, stimulates normal muscle action in the intestine, and forms feces for elimination of waste products. The main sources of cellulose are the stems and leaves of vegetables and the coverings of seeds and grains.

Noncellulose Polysaccharides. Hemicellulose, pectins, gums and mucilages, and algal substances are noncellulose polysaccharides. They absorb water and swell to a larger bulk, thus slowing the emptying of the food mass from the stomach, binding bile acids (including cholesterol)[4] in the intestine, and preventing spastic colon pressure by providing bulk for normal muscle action. Noncellulose polysaccharides also provide fermentation material on which colon bacteria can work.

Lignin. Lignin, the only noncarbohydrate type of dietary fiber, is a large compound that forms the woody part of certain plants. It binds the cellulose fibers in plants, giving added strength and stiffness to plant cell walls. It also combines with bile acids and cholesterol in the human intestine, preventing their absorption.

Table 2-2 provides a summary of these dietary fiber classes, along with the sources and functions of each.

As a means of simplification, dietary fiber is usually divided into two groups based on solubility. Cellulose, lignin, and most hemicelluloses are not soluble in water. The rest of the dietary fibers (e.g., most pectins and other polysaccharides such as gums and mucilages), however, are water soluble. These two classes of dietary fiber based on solubility are summarized in Box 2-1. The looser physical structure and greater water-holding capacity of gums, mucilages, pectins, and algal polysaccharides (e.g., those derived from seaweed) partly account for their greater water solubility.

In general, the food groups that provide needed dietary fiber include whole grains, legumes, vegetables, and fruits in their many food forms (i.e., legumes, vegetables, and fruits with as much of their skin remaining as possible). Whole grains provide a special natural "package" of both the complex carbohydrate starch and the fiber in its coating. In addition, whole grains contain an abundance of vitamins and minerals.[5]

Many health organizations have recommended increasing the intake of complex carbohydrates in general or dietary fiber in particular.[6,7] The Food and Nutrition

---

BOX 2–1 Summary of Soluble and Insoluble Fibers in Total Dietary Fiber

Insoluble	Soluble
Cellulose	Gums
Most hemicelluloses	Mucilages
Lignin	Algal polysaccharides
	Most pectins

TABLE 2–2 Summary of Dietary Fiber Classes

Dietary fiber class	Source	Function
Cellulose	Main cell wall constituent of plants	Holds water; reduces elevated colonic intraluminal pressure
Noncellulose polysaccharides		Slow gastric emptying; provides fermentable material for colonic bacteria with production of gas and volatile fatty acids; binds bile acids and cholesterol
Gums	Secretions of plants	
Mucilages	Plant secretions and seeds	
Algal polysaccharides	Algae, seaweed	
Pectin substances	Intercellular cement plant material	
Hemicellulose	Cell wall plant material	Holds water and increases stool bulk; reduces elevated colonic pressure; binds bile acids
Lignin	Woody part of plants	Antioxidant; binds bile acids, cholesterol, and metals

Board has always indicated that a desirable fiber intake should not be achieved by adding concentrated fiber supplements to the diet, but by eating a higher fiber diet of whole grains, fruits, vegetables, and legumes, which also provide vitamins and minerals. The recommended daily intake of fiber for men and women 50 years and younger is 38 and 25 g per day, respectively. The DRIs are reduced to 30 and 21 g per day for men and women over the age of 50.[2] This intake requires consistent use of whole grains, legumes, vegetables, fruits, seeds, and nuts. Unfortunately, Americans do not meet the recommended servings of grains, vegetables, and fruit on a daily basis. On average, only 27% of individuals meet the recommended servings of grains, 36% meet the vegetable recommendations, and a mere 20% consume the recommended fruit servings per day.[8] A table of

the dietary fiber content of some commonly used foods is provided in Table 2-3 and Appendix C (see the For Further Focus box, "Fiber . . . What's All the Fuss About?").

As with many things in nutrition, too much fiber can be problematic as well. Sudden increases in fiber intake can result in gas, bloating, and constipation.[9] Fiber intake should be increased gradually, along with water intake, to an appropriate amount for the individual. Also, excessive amounts of dietary fiber can trap small amounts of minerals and prevent their absorption into the GI tract. This function of fiber is beneficial when "trapping" or binding bile acids, such as cholesterol, but it may compromise nutritional status if fiber intake greatly exceeds the recommendations to the point of reducing mineral absorption.

TABLE 2–3	Dietary Fiber and Caloric Value for Selected Foods		
Food	**Serving size**	**Dietary fiber (g)**	**Kcalories**
BREADS AND CEREALS			
All Bran	⅓ cup	13	75
Complete Oat Bran	¾ cup	4	105
Complete Wheat Bran	¾ cup	5	92
Cracklin' Oat Bran	¾ cup	6.4	225
Fiber One	½ cup	14.4	60
Oatmeal	1 cup	4	138
Popcorn, air-popped	1 cup	1.2	30
Raisin Bran	½ cup	3.5	94
100% Bran	⅓ cup	8.3	83
Shredded Wheat n' Bran	⅔ cup	4	98
Whole wheat bread	1 slice	2	69
FRUIT			
Apple, raw with skin	1 medium (2¾" diameter)	3.7	81
Apricot	1 medium	0.7	17
Banana	1 medium (7-7⅞" long)	2.8	108
Blueberries	½ cup	2	40
Cherries	½ cup	0.8	26
Dates, dried	1	0.6	23
Grapefruit	½ cup pieces	1.25	38
Orange	1 medium (2⅝" diameter)	3.1	61
Peach	1 medium (2½" diameter)	2	42
Prune, dried	1	0.6	20
Raisins, seedless	½ cup (not packed)	3	217
Strawberries	½ cup sliced	1.9	25

Continued.

TABLE 2–3	Dietary Fiber and Caloric Value for Selected Foods—*cont'd*		
Food	**Serving size**	**Dietary fiber (g)**	**Kcalories**
LEGUMES			
Black beans	½ cup	7.5	113
Garbanzo beans	½ cup	6.2	134
Kidney beans	½ cup	5.6	112
Lima beans	½ cup	6.5	108
VEGETABLES			
Asparagus, cooked	½ cup	1.4	21
Black-eyed peas	½ cup	4.1	80
Broccoli, cooked	½ cup	2.3	22
Carrots, raw strips	½ cup	1.8	26
Cauliflower, cooked	½ cup	1.7	14
Corn	½ cup	2.2	88
Green beans (snap beans), cooked	½ cup	2	22
Green peas	½ cup	4.4	67
Potato, baked, with skin	1 medium (2¼"-3¼" diameter)	3.8	160
Sweet potato, baked in skin	1 medium (2" × 5")	3.4	117
Tomato, raw, chopped	½ cup	1	19

Data from U.S. Department of Agriculture, Agricultural Research Service, Nutrient Data Laboratory: *USDA Nutrient Database for Standard Reference, Release 15,* Washington, DC, 2002, USDA/AGS, Nutrient Data Laboratory Home Page: *www.nal.usda.gov/fnic/foodcomp.*

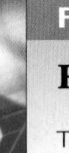

FOR FURTHER FOCUS

FIBER . . . WHAT'S ALL THE FUSS ABOUT?

The National Institutes of Health and World Health Organization, along with most all other health-related agencies in the world, have been promoting the intake of fiber for years. The benefits have been clearly defined in clinical trial after trial.[4-8] Scientists are confident that some of the health benefits of consuming adequate amounts of fiber are as follows:

- Lowers blood cholesterol levels
- Promotes normal bowel function and movements and prevents constipation
- Increases satiety, which aids in obesity prevention
- Protects against colon cancer
- Slows glucose absorption, thereby reducing blood glucose spikes and reducing insulin secretion
- Prevents and helps manage diverticulosis

However, the average fiber intake in American diets remains at less than half of the recommendation. Americans are not alone, however. Kromhout and colleagues* evaluated physical activity, body mass index, subscapular skin-

fold (a measurement of body fat percentage), fat intake, and fiber intake in men ages 40 to 59 in seven countries. The recommendation of fiber intake (38-50 g/day of fiber) for this age group was met by only two countries, Finland and Greece. Although Japan reported the lowest daily intake of fiber, they were only slightly lower than the average U.S. dietary fiber intake. In addition, the researchers found physical activity and dietary fiber to be the most important environmental determinants of body fat within the parameters measured.

What will it ultimately take for Americans to heed the warning signs? At what point will Americans value their lives enough to stop looking for that magic pill to make them thin and free from risk factors of chronic disease, and, instead, start making the small lifestyle changes that have proved effective time and again? What lifestyle factors in your life could use a makeover? What lifestyle choices can you be proud of and share with others?

---

*Kromhout D and others: Physical activity and dietary fiber determine population body fat levels: the Seven Countries Study, *Int J Obes Relat Metab Disord* 25(3):301, 2001.

Other Sweeteners

Sugar alcohols and alternative sweeteners are often used as sugar replacers. Sweeteners, such as sugar alcohols, that contribute to total calorie intake are considered nutritive sweeteners. Nonnutritive sweeteners, or alternative sweeteners, are sugar substitutes that do not have any caloric value.

Nutritive Sweeteners. The sugar alcohols (sorbitol, mannitol, and xylitol) are the alcohol forms of sucrose, mannose, and xylose. Sugar alcohols provide 2 to 3 kcalories per gram, the same as other carbohydrates. Probably the most well known of these compounds is sorbitol, which has been widely used as a sucrose substitute in various foods, candies, chewing gum, and beverages. Sugar alcohols share absorption with glucose in the small intestine. However, they are absorbed more slowly and do not increase the blood sugar as rapidly as glucose. Therefore sugar alcohols are often used in products intended for individuals who cannot tolerate a high blood sugar level, such as individuals with diabetes. The downside of using excessive amounts of sugar alcohols in food products is that the slowed digestion may result in diarrhea. The advantage of using a sugar alcohol to replace sugar is lowered risk of dental caries because oral bacteria cannot use the alcohol for fuel.

Nonnutritive Sweeteners. Nonnutritive sweeteners are manufactured specifically to be used as alternative, or artificial, sweeteners in food products. Because nonnutritive sweeteners do not supply any kcalories, they provide the sweet taste without contributing to total energy intake. People typically associate these sweeteners with "diet" foods. Alternative sweeteners most commonly used in the United States are aspartame and saccharin. Nonnutritive sweeteners are several hundred times sweeter than sucrose, or table sugar. Therefore very small quantities can be used to produce the same sweet taste. Table 2-4 provides a summary of artificial sweeteners and their relative sweetness value compared with table sugar.

FUNCTIONS OF CARBOHYDRATES

Primary Energy Function

Basic Fuel Supply

The main function of carbohydrates is to provide the primary fuel for the body. To meet energy needs, carbohydrates burn in the body at the rate of 4 kcal/g. Thus the fuel factor for carbohydrates is 4. Carbohydrates fur-

TABLE 2–4	Sweetness of Sugars and Artificial Sweeteners	
Substance		**Sweetness value**
SUGAR OR SUGAR PRODUCT		
Levulose, fructose		173
Invert sugar		130
Sucrose		100
Glucose		74
Sorbitol		60
Mannitol		50
Galactose		32
Maltose		32
Lactose		16
ARTIFICIAL SWEETENERS		
Cyclamate (banned in United States)		30
Aspartame (Nutra-Sweet)*		180
Acesulfame-K (Sunette)		200
Saccharin (Sweet 'N Low)		300
Sucralose		600
Alitame (approval pending)		2000

From Mahan LK, Escott-Stump S: *Krause's food, nutrition, & diet therapy,* ed 11, Philadelphia, 2004, Saunders.
*Nutritive (has calories).

nish readily available energy that is needed not only for physical activities but also for all the work of the body cells. Fat is also a fuel, but the body only needs a small amount of dietary fat, mainly to supply the essential fatty acids (see Chapter 3).

Reserve Fuel Supply

Glycogen reserves supply vital backup fuel. The total amount of carbohydrate in the body, including both glycogen and blood sugar, is relatively small. Without constant supply, however, this total amount of available

sugar alcohols nutritive sweeteners that provide 2 to 3 kcal per gram; sorbitol, mannitol, and xylitol. Produced in food industry laboratories for use as sweeteners in candies, chewing gum, beverages, and other foodstuffs; side effect of diarrhea limits use.

sorbitol a sugar alcohol formed in mammals from glucose and converted to fructose. Named for its initial discovery in nature, it is found in ripe berries of the tree *Sorbus acuparia* and also occurs in small quantities in various other berries, cherries, plums, and pears.

glucose only provides enough energy for about a half-day of moderate activity. Therefore to maintain a normal blood glucose level and prevent a breakdown of fat and protein in tissue, individuals must eat carbohydrate foods regularly to meet energy demands.

Special Tissue Functions

Carbohydrates also serve special functions in many body tissues and organs.

Liver

Glycogen reserves in the liver and muscles provide a constant exchange with the body's overall energy-balance system. These reserves, especially in the liver, protect cells from depressed metabolic function and resulting injury.

Protein and Fat

Carbohydrates help regulate both protein and fat metabolism. If there is sufficient dietary carbohydrate to meet general body energy needs, protein does not have to be broken down to supply energy. This *protein-sparing action* of carbohydrate protects protein, allowing it to be used for its major role in tissue growth and maintenance. Likewise, with sufficient carbohydrate for energy, fat is not needed to supply large amounts of energy. Such a rapid breakdown of fat would produce excess materials called *ketones,* which result from incomplete fat oxidation in the cells. Ketones are strong acids. The condition of acidosis, or *ketosis,* upsets the normal acid-base balance of the body and can become serious. This protective action of carbohydrate is called its *antiketogenic* effect.

Heart

The constant action of the heart muscle sustains life. Although fatty acids are the preferred regular fuel for the heart muscle, glycogen is a vital emergency fuel. In a damaged heart, low glycogen stores or inadequate carbohydrate intake may cause symptoms of cardiac disorder and angina.

Central Nervous System

Constant carbohydrate intake and reserves are necessary for proper functioning of the central nervous system (CNS). The master center of the CNS, the brain, has no stored supply of glucose; therefore it is especially dependent on a minute-to-minute supply of glucose from the blood. Sustained and profound shock from low blood sugar may cause brain damage and can result in death.

FOOD SOURCES OF CARBOHYDRATES

Starches

As indicated, starches provide fundamental complex carbohydrate foods for slowly available glucose (SAG), thus sustaining the energy sources of primary rapidly available glucose (RAG).[1] Starches are the central type of food for a balanced diet. In unrefined forms, they also provide important sources of fiber and other nutrients. Table 2-5 outlines the carbohydrate content of commonly consumed foods.

Sugars

Sugar per se is not the villain in the story of health. The problem lies in the large quantities of sugar that many people consume, often to the exclusion of other important foods; although high-sugar diets do carry health risks, such as dental caries and obesity. The average American consumes about one-third pound of sugar per day, which may lead to problems. So, as with many things, moderation is the key.

DIGESTION OF CARBOHYDRATES

Mouth

The digestion of carbohydrate foods, starches and sugars, begins in the mouth and progresses through the successive parts of the GI tract, accomplished by two types of actions: (1) mechanical or muscle functions that break the food mass into smaller particles; and (2) chemical processes in which specific **enzymes** break down the food nutrients into still smaller usable metabolic products.[10] The chewing of the food, a process called *mastication,* breaks food into fine particles and mixes it with saliva. During this process, the salivary enzyme *salivary amylase* (commonly referred to as *ptyalin*) is secreted by the *parotid* glands, which lie under each ear at the back of the jaw. Salivary amylase acts on starch to begin its breakdown into dextrins (i.e., intermediate starch breakdown products) and disaccharides (primarily maltose). Carbohydrates that are eaten in the form of monosaccharides travel to the stomach and small intestines for absorption without further digestion.

Stomach

Wavelike contractions of the muscle fibers of the stomach wall continue the mechanical digestive process. This action, which is called *peristalsis,* further mixes food particles with gastric secretions to facilitate chemical digestion. The gastric secretions contain no specific enzyme for the breakdown of carbohydrates. The hydrochloric acid in the stomach stops the action of the salivary amylase in the food mass. Before the food mixes completely with the acidic stomach secretions, however, up to 20% to 30% of the starch may have been changed to maltose. Muscle action continues to mix the food mass and move it to the lower part of the stomach. Here the food mass is a thick creamy *chyme*, ready for its controlled emptying through the *pyloric valve* into the *duodenum*, the first portion of the small intestine.

Small Intestine

Peristalsis continues to aid digestion in the small intestine by mixing and moving the chyme along the length of the tube. Chemical digestion of carbohydrate is completed in the small intestine by specific enzymes from both the pancreas and intestine.

Pancreatic Secretions

Secretions from the *pancreas* enter the duodenum through the common bile duct. These secretions contain the starch enzyme *pancreatic amylase*. This enzyme continues the breakdown of starch to disaccharides and monosaccharides.

Intestinal Secretions

Enzymes attached to the **brush border** (microvilli) of the intestinal tract contain three disaccharidases: *sucrase*, *lactase*, and *maltase*. These specific enzymes act on their respective disaccharides to render the monosaccharides—glucose, galactose, and fructose—

TABLE 2–5	Carbohydrate Content of Foods (Percent of Weight)
Sugar	**Carbohydrate (%)**
CONCENTRATED SWEETS	
Sugar: cane, beet, powdered,	99.5
brown, maple	90-96
Candies	70-95
Honey (extracted)	82
Syrup: table blends, molasses	55-75
Jams, jellies, marmalades	70
Carbonated, sweetened beverages	10-12
FRUITS	
Prunes, apricots, figs (cooked, unsweetened)	12-31
Bananas, grapes, cherries, apples, pears	15-23
Fresh: pineapple, grapefruit, oranges, apricots, strawberries	8-14
MILK	
Skim	6
Whole	5
Starch	**Carbohydrate (%)**
GRAIN PRODUCTS	
Starches: corn, tapioca, arrowroot	86-88
Cereals (dry): corn, wheat, oat, bran	68-85
Flour: corn, wheat (sifted)	70-80
Popcorn (popped)	77
Cookies: plain, assorted	71
Crackers, saltines	72
Cakes: plain, without icing	56
Bread: white, rye, whole wheat	48-52
Macaroni, spaghetti, noodles, rice (cooked)	23-30
Cereals (cooked): oat, wheat, grits	10-16
VEGETABLES	
Boiled: corn, white and sweet potatoes, lima and dried beans, peas	15-26
Beets, carrots, onions, tomatoes	5-7
Leafy: lettuce, asparagus, cabbage, greens, spinach	3-4

From Mahan LK, Escott-Stump S: *Krause's food, nutrition, & diet therapy*, ed 11, Philadelphia, 2004, Saunders.

enzyme   (Gr. *en,* in; *zyme,* leaven) specific proteins produced in cells that digest or change specific nutrients in specific chemical reactions without being changed themselves in the process. Their action is therefore that of a catalyst. Digestive enzymes in the GI secretions act on food substances to break them down into simpler compounds. An enzyme is usually named according to the substance (substrate) on which it acts, with common word ending of -ase; for example, sucrase is the specific enzyme for sucrose, which it breaks down into glucose and fructose.

brush border   cells that are located on the microvilli within the lining of the intestinal tract. The microvilli are tiny hairlike projections that protrude from the mucosal cells that help increase surface area for the digestion and absorption of nutrients.

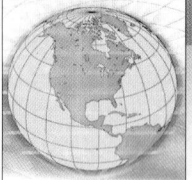

CULTURAL CONSIDERATIONS

ETHNICITY AND LACTOSE INTOLERANCE

In the United States, African Americans and Native Americans suffer from lactose intolerance significantly more than Caucasian Americans. Almost 100% of Native Americans endure some level of lactose intolerance compared with 95% of African Americans and 12% of Caucasian Americans.* In other countries, individuals most commonly experiencing discomfort caused by the lack of lactase are the Chinese (93% intolerant), Thais (98% intolerant), Africans (20% to 89% intolerant), and Australian Aborigines (85% intolerant). The Swiss, Swedish, and Europeans have significantly less trouble with lactose digestion: less than 10% of their populations report any discomfort.

These individuals are lactose-intolerant but usually can tolerate some low-lactose milk products such as cheese. Lactose intolerance is not an allergy. Most affected individuals can handle varying levels of lactose in their diet. The amount well tolerated is individual and should be explored by gradually introducing small amounts of lactose-containing foods into the diet while keeping note of any side effects. The strong genetic link to lactose intolerance indicates there is little chance for a drastic change in response to dietary lactose over a lifetime. However, many individuals do experience slight changes. Some people become even more intolerant with age, whereas others are able to gradually accept more.

*National Digestive Diseases Clearinghouse, National Institute of Diabetes and Digestive and Kidney Diseases, National Institutes of Health: *Lactose intolerance,* Bethesda, MD, (accessed December 2002), NDDC/NIDDK/NIH [*www.niddk.nih.gov/health/digest/pubs/lactose/lactose.htm*]

---

ready for absorption directly into the **portal** blood circulation.

Lactose intolerance, the inability to break lactose down into its monosaccharide units (glucose and galactose), results from a lack of the enzyme lactase. Symptoms include bloating, gas, abdominal pain, and diarrhea. Lactose intolerance affects about 75% of adults worldwide, with a much higher prevalence in some countries and ethnic groups (see the Cultural Considerations box, "Ethnicity and Lactose Intolerance").

A summary of the major aspects of carbohydrate digestion through the successive parts of the GI tract is shown in Table 2-6. The overall processes of absorption and metabolism of all of the energy-yielding nutrients together (carbohydrate, fat, and protein) are discussed in Chapter 5.

BODY NEEDS FOR CARBOHYDRATES

Dietary Reference Intakes

In the nutrient standards, energy needs are listed as total kcalories, which includes caloric intake from fat and protein, as well as carbohydrate. According to the 2002 published DRIs, 45% to 65% of an adult's total caloric intake should come from carbohydrate foods.[2] This translates to 225 to 325 g of carbohydrates for a 2,000-kcal/day diet. The recommended fiber intake can be achieved by choosing carbohydrate foods consisting of whole grain cereals, legumes, vegetables, and fruits, which also provide minerals and

TABLE 2–6	Summary of Carbohydrate Digestion	
Organ	**Enzyme**	**Action**
Mouth	Salivary amylase	Starch → Dextrins → Disaccharides (maltose)
Stomach	None	(Above action continued to minor degree)
Small intestine	Pancreatic amylase	Starch → Dextrins → Disaccharides (maltose)
	Intestinal:	
	Sucrase	Sucrose → Glucose + Fructose
	Lactase	Lactose → Glucose + Galactose
	Maltase	Maltose → Glucose + Glucose

CLINICAL APPLICATIONS

WHAT IS YOUR DIETARY REFERENCE INTAKE FOR CARBOHYDRATES, SUGAR, AND FIBER?

Based on the current DRIs, let us calculate the amount of calories and grams of carbohydrates recommended for you to consume on a daily basis. This requires you to know how many total calories you consume on a daily basis.

Step 1: Keep track of everything you eat for one day. You can use the CD-ROM included with this book to calculate your daily food intake. This is your *total energy intake.* (Chapter 6 discusses the evaluation of total energy intake relative to weight).

Step 2: Total energy intake = ___ kcalories.

Step 3: Multiply your total energy intake by 45% (0.45) and 65% (0.65) to get the recommended number of *kcalories from carbohydrates (CHO).*
___ total kcal × 0.45 = ___ kcal
___ total kcal × 0.65 = ___ kcal

Example:
2200 total kcal × 0.45 = 990 kcal
2200 total kcal × 0.65 = 1430 kcal
Recommended range of total kcalories from CHO =
990 − 1430 kcal/day

How many *grams of CHO* do you need based on these recommendations?

Step 4: Divide your recommended range of kcalories from CHO by 4. There are 4 kcalories per gram of CHO.
___ kcal/day from CHO ÷ 4 =
___ g of CHO/day

Example:
990 − 1430 kcal/day from CHO ÷ 4 =
247.5 − 357.5 g of CHO/day
Recommended range of total grams of CHO =
247.5 − 357.5 g of CHO/day

What is the maximum amount of total kcalorie consumption that can come from *added sugars,* according to the DRIs? Added sugars are added to food and beverages during production. The majority of added sugars in American diets come from candy, soft drinks, fruit drinks, pastries, and other sweets. The DRIs recommend limiting added sugar intake to no more than 25% of total kcalories consumed.

Step 5: Multiply your total energy intake by 25% (0.25) to get the maximum number of *kcalories from added sugars.*
___ total kcal × 0.25 = ___ kcal

Example:
2200 total kcal × 0.25 = 550 kcal
Maximum amount of total kcalories from added sugar = 550 kcal/day

Step 6: Determine how many grams of added sugar by dividing the maximum kcal/day of added sugar by 4.
___ kcal/day from added sugar ÷ 4 =
___ g of added sugar/day

Example:
550 kcal/day from added sugar ÷ 4 =
137.5 g of added sugar/day
Therefore the 137.5 g of added sugar is the recommended *limit* per day.

---

vitamins. In addition, the DRIs recommend limiting added sugar to no more than 25% of total calories consumed. (See the Clinical Applications box, "What Is Your Dietary Reference Intake for Carbohydrates, Sugar, and Fiber?" to calculate your specific carbohydrate recommendations.)

Dietary Guidelines for Americans

The *Dietary Guidelines for Americans* are general guidelines to promote health; therefore they do not outline specifics in terms of caloric consumption or where those kcalories should come from. Instead, the *Guide-*lines advise individuals to "let the Pyramid guide your food choices,"[11] indicating that grains, fruits, and vegetables should be the foundation of a healthy diet.

---

portal (L. *porta,* a portal or doorway) an entrance or gateway; for example, the portal blood circulation designates the entry of blood vessels from the intestines into the liver, carrying nutrients for major liver metabolism, then draining into the body's main systemic circulation to deliver metabolic products to body cells.

SUMMARY

The primary source of energy for most of the world's population comes from carbohydrate foods. These foods are from widely distributed plant sources, such as grains, legumes, vegetables, and fruits. For the most part, these food products store easily and are relatively low in cost.

Two basic types of carbohydrates supply energy: simple and complex. Simple carbohydrates are made up of single- and double-sugar units (monosaccharides and disaccharides). Because simple carbohydrates are easy to digest and absorb, they provide quick energy. Complex carbohydrates, or polysaccharides, are made up of many sugar units. They break down more slowly and thus provide sustained energy over a longer period of time.

Dietary fiber in most of its forms is a complex carbohydrate that is not digestible. It occurs mainly as the structural parts of plants and provides important bulk in the diet, affects nutrient absorption, and benefits health.

Carbohydrate digestion starts briefly in the mouth with the initial action of the salivary amylase to begin breaking down starch into smaller units. There is no enzyme for starch breakdown in the stomach, but muscle action continues to mix the food mass and move it on to enter the small intestine, where pancreatic amylase continues the chemical digestion. Final starch and disaccharide digestion occurs in the small intestine with the action of specific enzymes (sucrase, lactase, and maltase) to produce the single-sugar units glucose, fructose, and galactose, which are then absorbed directly into the portal blood circulation to the liver.

CRITICAL THINKING QUESTIONS

1. Why is carbohydrate the predominant type of food in the world's diets? Give some basic examples of these carbohydrate foods.
2. What are the main classes of carbohydrates? Describe each in terms of general nature, functions, and main food sources.
3. Compare starches and sugars as a basic fuel. Why are complex carbohydrates a significant part of a healthy diet? What is the recommendation about the use of sugars in such a diet? Why?
4. Describe the types and functions of dietary fiber. What are the main food sources? What amount of fiber is generally recommended in a healthy diet?
5. What is glycogen? Why is it a vital tissue carbohydrate?

CHAPTER CHALLENGE QUESTIONS

True-False

Write the correct statement for each item answered "false."

1. *True or False:* Carbohydrates are composed of carbon, hydrogen, oxygen, and nitrogen.
2. *True or False:* Starch is the main source of carbohydrate in the diet.
3. *True or False:* Lactose is a very sweet, simple, monosaccharide found in a number of foods.
4. *True or False:* Glucose is the form of sugar circulating in the blood.
5. *True or False:* Glycogen is an important long-term storage form of energy because relatively large amounts are stored in the liver and muscles.
6. *True or False:* Modern food processing and refinement have reduced dietary fiber.

Multiple Choice

1. Which of the following carbohydrate foods provides energy the *quickest*?
   a. Slice of bread
   b. Oat bran muffin
   c. Milk
   d. Orange juice
2. A quickly available but limited form of energy is stored in the liver by conversion of glucose to
   a. glycerol.
   b. glycogen.
   c. protein.
   d. fat.

3. The current DRIs recommend ____% of a person's total daily caloric intake to come from carbohydrate sources.

a. 5% to 15%

b. 20% to 35%

c. 35% to 50%

d. 45% to 65%

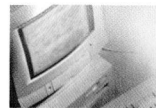

Please refer to the Students' Resource section of this text's Evolve web site for "Suggestions for Additional Study."

REFERENCES

1. Nevins DJ: Sugars: their photosynthesis and subsequent biological interconversions, *Am J Clin Nutr* 6(suppl 55): 996S, 1995.
2. Food and Nutrition Board, Institute of Medicine: *Dietary reference intakes for energy, carbohydrate, fiber, fat, fatty acids, cholesterol, protein, and amino acids,* Washington, DC, 2002, National Academies Press.
3. Marlett JA and others: Position of the American Dietetic Association: health implications of dietary fiber, *J Am Diet Assoc* 102(7):993, 2002.
4. Davy BM and others: High-fiber oat cereal compared with wheat cereal consumption favorably alters LDL-cholesterol subclass and particle numbers in middle-aged and older men, *Am J Clin Nutr* 76(2):351, 2002.
5. Slavin JL and others: The role of whole grains in disease prevention, *J Am Diet Assoc* 101(7):780, 2001.
6. Leonetti F and others: Clinical, physiopathological and dietetic aspects of metabolic syndrome, *Dig Liver Dis* 34(suppl 2):134S, 2002.
7. McKeown NM and others: Whole-grain intake is favorably associated with metabolic risk factors for type 2 diabetes and cardiovascular disease in the Framingham Offspring Study, *Am J Clin Nutr* 76(2):390, 2002.
8. Nielsen SJ and others: Trends in energy intake in U.S. between 1977 and 1996: similar shifts seen across age groups, *Obes Res* 10(5):370, 2002.
9. Health tip: Reducing excess gas, *Mayo Clin Health Lett* Oct 19(10):3, 2001.
10. Marsh MN, Riley SA: Digestion and absorption of the nutrients and vitamins. In Feldman M, Scharschmidt BF, Sleisenger MH, editors: *Gastrointestinal and liver disease,* ed 6, vol 2, Philadelphia, 1998, Saunders.
11. U.S. Department of Health and Human Services: *Healthy People 2010: understanding and improving health,* Washington, DC, 2000, Government Printing Office.

FURTHER READING AND RESOURCES

- U.S. Department of Health and Human Services: *www.dhhs.gov*
- Centers for Disease Control and Prevention: *www.cdc.gov*
- International Food Information Council Foundation: *www.ific.org*

  The preceding organizations are valuable resources of nutrition and health-related information. Take advantage of their easily accessed web sites.

- Nielsen SJ and others: Trends in energy intake in U.S. between 1977 and 1996: similar shifts seen across age groups, *Obes Res* 10(5):370, 2002.

  Are Americans eating more calories? Where are the majority of the calories coming from? Where are Americans eating? These are all questions that the authors evaluate in this interesting look at America's food consumption patterns.

- Raben A and others: Sucrose compared with artificial sweeteners: different effects on ad libitum food intake and body weight after 10 wk of supplementation in overweight subjects, *Am J Clin Nutr* 76(4):721, 2003.

  The authors explore the role of artificial sweeteners in body-weight regulation in overweight subjects. For 10 weeks subjects consumed supplemental drinks and foods with either sucrose or artificial sweeteners. Results were determined by comparing total energy intake, body weight, fat mass, and blood pressure. Do artificial sweeteners work?

- Schefrin R: Good carbs, bad carbs, *Today's Dietitian* 5(4):36, 2003.

  Carbohydrates are the topic of much debate in weight loss programs. This article gives a brief overview of carbohydrates and their role in insulin resistance, the glycemic index, and how human bodies respond.

CHAPTER 3

Fats

KEY CONCEPTS

- Dietary fat supplies essential body tissue needs, both as an energy fuel and a structural material.

- Foods from animal and plant sources supply distinct forms of fat that affect health in different ways.

- Excess dietary fat, especially from animal food sources, is a health risk factor.

Americans, and people in most other developed countries, have traditionally eaten a diet relatively high in fat. People in the United States have maintained a rich food pattern, with about 34% of the total caloric intake coming from fat. Now, however, health concerns are well established and Americans are beginning to eat less fat, especially animal fats.

This chapter considers fat as not only an essential nutrient, concentrated storage fuel, and tissue need, but also a health hazard when excessive, keeping attitudes and habits about fat and health realistic.

THE NATURE OF FATS

Dietary Importance

Fats are a storage form of concentrated fuel for the human energy system. As such, they back up carbohydrates, the primary fuel, as an available energy source. In food, fats may be in the form of either solid fat or liquid oil. Fats are not soluble in water and are greasy.

Classes of Fats

Lipids

The overall name for the chemical group of fats and fat-related compounds is **lipids,** which comes from the Greek word *lipos,* meaning "fat." The word *lipid* appears in combination words used for fat-related health problems. For example, the condition of an elevated level of blood fats is called *hyperlipidemia.*

Triglycerides

Fats are made up of the same basic chemical elements that compose carbohydrates: carbon, hydrogen, and oxygen. As a group, fats are called **glycerides** because they are composed of *glycerol* with *fatty acids* attached. Whether in food or body tissue, fatty acids combine with glycerol to form glycerides. Most natural fats, whether in animal or plant sources, have three fatty acids attached to their glycerol base, so their chemical name is **triglyceride.** When encountering the word *triglycerides,* think of it as the chemical name for fat.

Fatty Acids

The main building blocks of fats are **fatty acids.** Fatty acids can be classified by their chain length as short-, medium-, or long-chain fatty acids. The chains are made up of carbon atoms with a methyl group ($-CH_3$) on one end and a carboxyl group ($-COOH$) on the other end. Short-chain fatty acids have two to four carbons, whereas medium- and long-chains have 6 to 10 and more than 12 carbons, respectively. Fatty acids have two significant characteristics, one of which relates to the concept of saturation and the other to essentiality.

Saturated Fatty Acid. When a substance is described as **saturated,** it contains all the material it is capable of holding. For example, a sponge is saturated with water when it holds all the water it can hold. Similarly, fatty acids are "saturated" or "unsaturated" according to whether or not they are filled with hydrogen. Thus a saturated fatty acid is one whose structure is filled with all of the hydrogen bonds it can hold and, as a result, is heavier, denser, and more solid (e.g., meat fats). If most of the fatty acids mak-

ing up a fat are saturated, that fat is said to be a *saturated fat.* Most saturated fats are of animal origin. Figure 3-1 shows a variety of food sources of fat, including saturated fat from meat, dairy, and eggs.

Unsaturated Fatty Acid. A fatty acid that is not completely filled with all the hydrogen it can hold is unsaturated, and as a result is less heavy and less dense (e.g., a liquid oil). If most of the fatty acids making up a given fat are unsaturated, that fat is said to be an *unsaturated fat.* If the component fatty acids have *one* unfilled spot, the fat is called a *mono*unsaturated fat. For example, olives and olive oil, peanuts and peanut oil, canola oil (rapeseed), almonds, pecans, and avocados supply monounsaturated fats. If the component fatty acids have two or more unfilled spots, the fat is called a *poly*unsaturated fat. Examples of such fats, in order of their degree of unsaturation, are the vegetable oils: safflower, corn, cottonseed, and soybean. Fats from plant sources usually are unsaturated (Figure 3-2). However, notable exceptions are coconut and palm oils, which are saturated. Although world production of saturated tropical oils (e.g., palm, palm kernel, and coconut) has increased rapidly since the 1970s, use of these oils in the United States has not followed suit. These saturated oils generally have contributed less than 4% of Americans' total daily fat intake and only about 8% of their daily saturated fat intake.

---

lipids   (Gr. *lipos,* fat) the chemical group name for organic substances of a fatty nature. The lipids include fats, oils, waxes, and other fat-related compounds such as cholesterol.

glycerides   chemical group name for fats, from their base substance glycerol; formed from the glycerol base with one, two, or three fatty acids attached to make monoglycerides, diglycerides, and triglycerides. Glycerides are the principal constituents of adipose tissue and are found in animal and vegetable fats and oils.

triglycerides   chemical name for fats in the body or in food; compound of three fatty acids attached to a glycerol base.

fatty acids   the major structural components of fats.

saturated   (L. *saturare,* to fill) state of being filled; state of fatty acid components of fats being filled in all their available carbon bonds with hydrogen, making the fat harder and more solid. Such solid food fats are generally from animal sources.

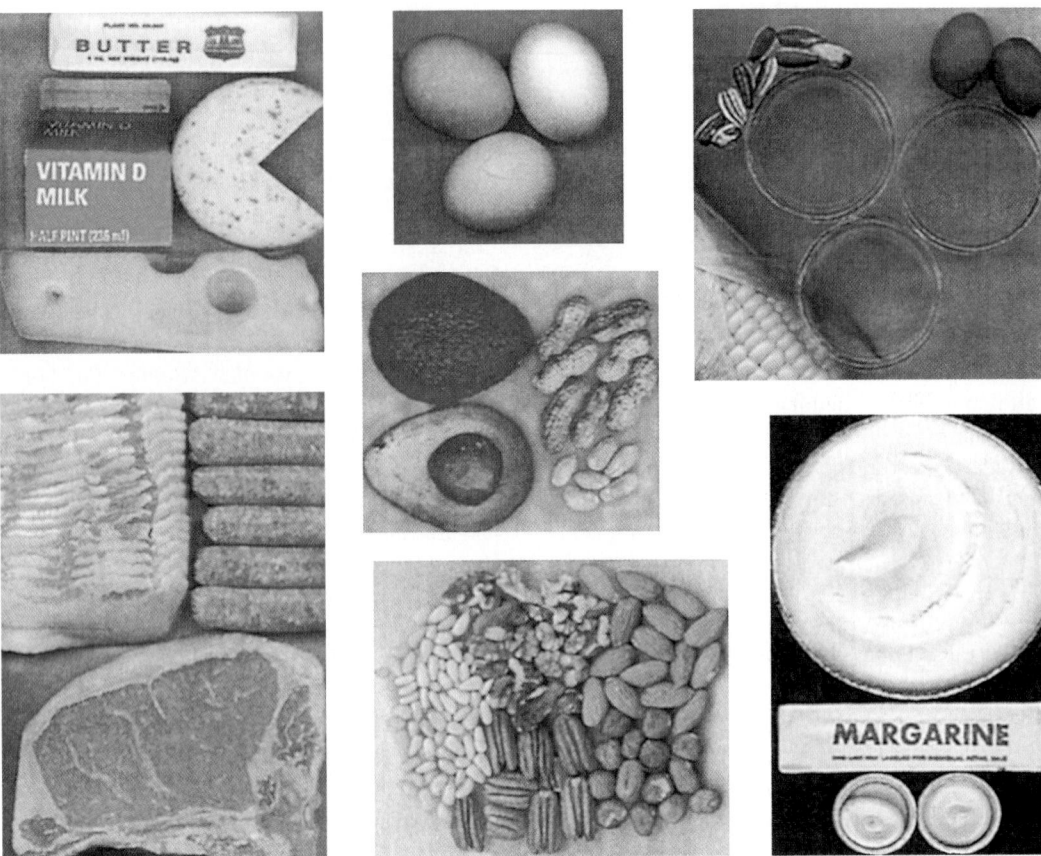

Figure 3–1   Food sources of fat. (Credit: Amy Buxton.)

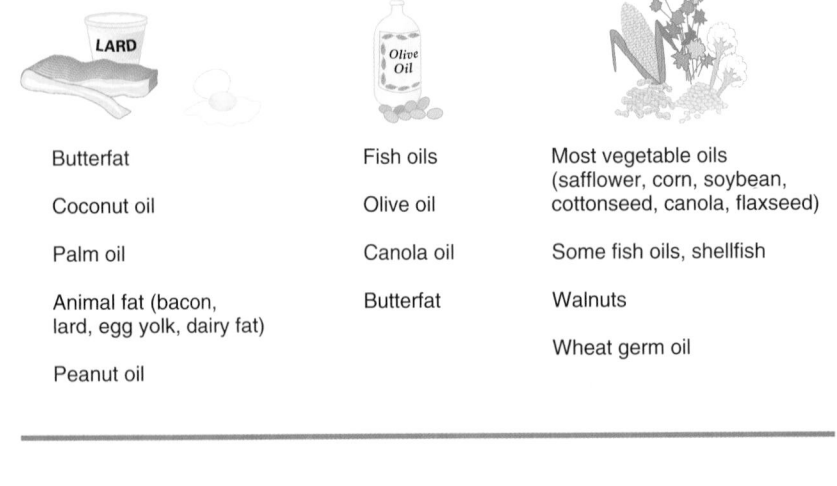

Butterfat	Fish oils	Most vegetable oils (safflower, corn, soybean, cottonseed, canola, flaxseed)
Coconut oil	Olive oil	
Palm oil	Canola oil	Some fish oils, shellfish
Animal fat (bacon, lard, egg yolk, dairy fat)	Butterfat	Walnuts
Peanut oil		Wheat germ oil

Saturated   Monounsaturated   Polyunsaturated

Figure 3–2   Spectrum of food fats according to the degree of saturation of component fatty acid. Fats within foods can contain saturated and unsaturated fatty acids and therefore fit into more than one place along the spectrum of saturation. (Credit [drawings]: Eileen Draper.)

Essential Fatty Acid. The term *essential* or *nonessential* is applied to a nutrient according to its relative necessity in the diet. A nutrient is essential if either of the following is true: (1) its absence will create a specific deficiency disease; or (2) the body cannot manufacture it and must obtain it from the diet. A diet with 10% or less of its total kcalories from fat cannot supply adequate amounts of essential fatty acids. The only fatty acids known to be essential for complete human nutrition are the polyunsaturated fatty acids **linoleic** and **linolenic.** Essential fatty acids must come from the foods we eat. The body is capable of producing saturated fatty acids, monounsaturated fatty acids, and cholesterol. Therefore there are no set recommendations of daily intake for these. The Dietary Reference Intakes (DRIs) for linoleic acid, found in polyunsaturated vegetable oils, are set at 17 grams per day for men and 12 grams per day for women. Linolenic acid is primarily found in milk, soybeans, and flaxseed oil and is necessary in much lesser quantities than linoleic acid. The recommendations for linolenic acid intake are 1.6 and 1.1 grams per day for men and women, respectively.[1] Both of these fatty acids serve important functions related to tissue strength, cholesterol metabolism, muscle tone, blood clotting, and heart action.

Lipoproteins

Lipoproteins are combinations of fat (lipids), protein (the protein part is called an *apoprotein*), and other fat-related substances, which are the major vehicles for transport in the blood stream. Because fat is insoluble in water and blood is mainly water, fat cannot travel freely in the blood stream; it needs a water-soluble carrier. The body solves this problem by wrapping small particles of fat in a covering of protein, which is soluble in water. The blood then carries these little packages of fat to and from the cells to supply needed nutrients. Lipoproteins contain triglycerides, cholesterol, and other materials (e.g., fat-soluble vitamins). A lipoprotein's relative load of fat and protein determines its density. The higher the protein load, the higher the lipoprotein's density. The higher the fat load, the lower the lipoprotein's density. Groups of *low-density lipoproteins* (LDLs) carry fat and cholesterol to cells. Groups of *high-density lipoproteins* (HDLs) carry free cholesterol from body tissue to the liver for breakdown and excretion. All lipoproteins are closely associated with lipid disorders and the underlying blood vessel disease in heart attacks, *atherosclerosis*. These relationships are discussed in greater detail in Chapter 19.

Cholesterol

Although cholesterol is often discussed in connection with dietary fat, it is not a fat itself. Many people confuse it with saturated fats, but **cholesterol** belongs to a group of chemical substances called *sterols*. Its name comes from the body material where it was first identified, gallstones. Hence, *chole-* refers to the gallbladder or bile, and *-sterol* refers to the family group name. Cholesterol is a vital substance in human metabolism that occurs naturally in all animal foods. Because it is only synthesized in animal tissue, there is no cholesterol in plant foods. The main food sources of cholesterol are egg yolks and organ meats, such as liver and kidney, as well as other meats (see Appendix B). To ensure that it always has the relatively small amount of cholesterol necessary for sustaining life, the human body synthesizes the *endogenous* cholesterol in many body tissues, particularly in the liver, which is a major source, as well as small amounts in the adrenal cortex, skin, intestines, testes, and ovaries. Consequently there is no biological requirement for dietary cholesterol and no DRI set for cholesterol consumption. The *Dietary Guidelines for Americans* recommend consuming a diet low in cholesterol. Epidemiologic studies have found links between cholesterol intake and increased risk for coronary heart disease.[1]

linoleic acid   essential fatty acid consisting of 18 carbons and two double bonds. Found in vegetable oils.

linolenic acid   essential fatty acid with 18 carbon atoms and three double bonds. Found in soybean, canola, and flaxseed oil.

lipoproteins   chemical complex of fat and protein that serve as the major carriers of lipids in the plasma. They vary in density according to the size of the fat load being carried; the lower the density, the higher the fat load. The combination package with water-soluble protein makes possible the transport of non–water-soluble fatty substances in the water-based blood circulation.

cholesterol   (Gr. *chole,* bile; *steros,* solid) a fat-related compound, a sterol, synthesized only in animal tissues; a normal constituent of bile and a principal constituent of gallstones. In the body, cholesterol is synthesized mainly in the liver. In the diet, it is found only in animal food sources. In human body metabolism, cholesterol is important as a precursor of various steroid hormones such as sex hormones and adrenal corticoids. In disordered lipid metabolism, however, it is a major factor in atherosclerosis, the underlying disease process in coronary arteries that leads to heart attacks.

FUNCTIONS OF FAT

Fat in Foods

Energy

In addition to carbohydrates, fats serve as a fuel for energy production. Fat is also an important storage form of body fuel because excess carbohydrate intake is easily converted into stored fat. Fat is a much more concentrated form of fuel, yielding 9 kcal/g when burned by the body, compared with carbohydrate's yield of 4 kcal/g.

Essential Nutrients

Food fats supply the body with essential fatty acids. As long as an adequate amount of essential fatty acids are consumed, the body is capable of endogenously producing other fats and cholesterol as needed. Food fats also carry fat-soluble vitamins (see Chapter 7) and aid in their absorption.

Flavor and Satisfaction

Some fat in the diet adds flavor to foods and contributes to a feeling of *satiety* or satisfaction after a meal. These effects are partly caused by the slower rate of digestion of fats compared with that of carbohydrate. This satiety also results from the fuller texture and body that fat gives to food mixtures and the slower emptying time of the stomach that it necessitates. The absence of this satiation and hunger-delay experienced by some people on low-fat diets may contribute to client dissatisfaction and problems with necessary changes in food habits to establish a lowered fat and cholesterol intake.

Fat Substitutes

Several fat substitutes, compounds that are not absorbed and thus contribute little or no kcalories, are being marketed or tested to provide improved flavor and physical texture to low-fat foods and help reduce total dietary fat. Two examples of these fat substitutes are Simplesse (NutraSweet, Chicago, IL), which is made by reshaping the protein of milk whey or egg whites, and Olestra (Procter & Gamble, Cincinnati, OH), which is a nondigestible form of sucrose.

Fat in the Body

Adipose Tissue

Fat stored in various parts of the body is called **adipose** tissue, from the Latin word *adiposus*, meaning "fatty." A weblike padding of this tissue supports and protects vital organs, and a layer of fat directly under the skin is important in regulating body temperature. A special fat covering protects nerve fibers and helps relay nerve impulses.

Cell Membrane Structure

Fat forms the fatty center of cell walls, helping to transport nutrient material across cell membranes.

FOOD SOURCES OF FAT

Variety of Sources

Animal Fats

The predominant supply of saturated fats comes from animal sources. Because fats are made up of a combination of fatty acids, as building blocks, there are exceptions to this rule. The most concentrated food sources of saturated fats include meat fats (e.g., bacon and sausage), dairy fats and products (e.g., cream, ice cream, butter, and cheese), and egg yolk. The exceptions are coconut, peanut, and palm oils, which also contain saturated fatty acids. The American diet has traditionally featured meats and other foods of animal origin. Surveys have shown that animal products in particular (e.g., red meats [beef, veal, pork, lamb]; poultry, fish and shellfish; separate animal fats [lard], milk and milk products, and eggs) contribute more than half of the total fat to U.S. diets, three fourths of the saturated fat, and all of the cholesterol.

However, lean red meats, especially beef, are gaining marketing attention. Pasture-fed lean beef with little tissue marbling of fat and well-trimmed of external edge fat often contains less than 5% fat and has cholesterol-lowering effects. When regular, market beef cuts are used in the diet; however, there is little or no beneficial effect on serum cholesterol levels. These results indicate that the meat fat, not the moderate portions of very lean meat, increases cholesterol levels. Even greater cholesterol-lowering effects can be achieved from regular moderate use of polyunsaturated sunflower oil or monounsaturated olive oil in the place of saturated fat.[2]

Plant Fats

Plant foods supply mostly monounsaturated and polyunsaturated fats. Food sources for unsaturated fats include vegetable oils (e.g., safflower, corn, cottonseed, soybeans, peanuts, and olives; see Figure 3-2), but, as indicated, coconut and palm oils are exceptions. These oils are saturated fats used mainly in commercially processed food items. In addition, some animal fats contain small amounts of unsaturated fats. Specifically, fish oils are a good source of the polyunsaturated essential fatty acids.

Hydrogenated Fat

Margarine and shortenings are made from unsaturated vegetable oils when hydrogen is introduced into the fat molecule. This process is called *hydrogenation*, a word that frequently appears on the labels of such commercial fat products. To make margarine a substitute for butter, the hydrogenated product also may be churned with cultured milk, to give it a butter flavor, and fortified with vitamins A and D. Fortified margarine is the nutritional equivalent of butter and has the same caloric value. Margarine, which is economical, tasteful, and lower in saturated fat, is 80% fat and fortified with 15,000 International Units (IU) of vitamin A per pound.

Cis _and_ Trans _Fatty Acid Products._ Health professionals have been concerned about the increasing number of hydrogenated (hardened) food products being made from the _cis_ and _trans_ forms of unsaturated fatty acids.[3] These two chemical terms—_cis_ and _trans_—refer to two different shapes that a fat molecule can have as its structure. The illustration here shows the two structures in a molecule of oleic acid, which is a common monounsaturated fatty acid that has a chain of 18 carbon atoms:

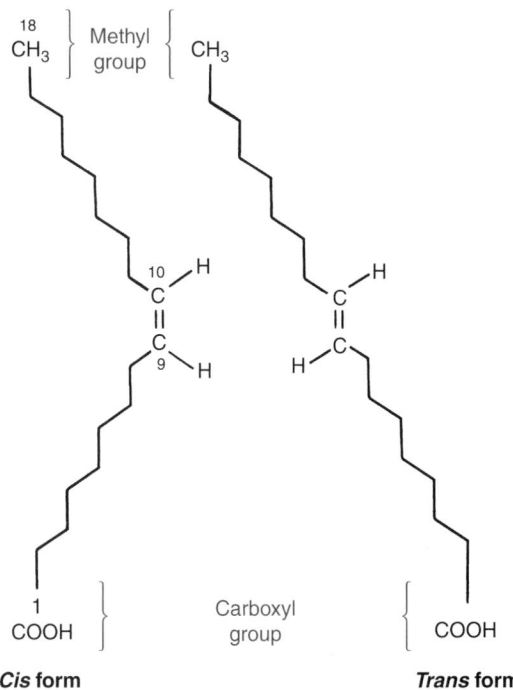

Cis form   **_Trans_ form**

All naturally occurring fatty acid molecules have a bend in the chain of atoms at the point of the chemical bond in the middle of the chain. This form is called _cis_ (same side). When vegetable oils are partially hydrogenated to make food products, however, the normal bend is changed so that the chains of atoms are on opposite sides of the central bond. This form is called _trans_ (opposite side). Commercially hydrogenated fats in margarine, fast food, and many other food products are in the _trans_ form.[4] Increased use of these products, especially margarine, has stirred debate about accumulating trans fatty acids in the body. Some of the observed effects include elevation of serum lipids, im-

proved essential fatty acid metabolism, and modification of membrane properties.[5] In response to these growing health concerns, the food industry has developed solid and soft tub _trans_-free fat products for concerned individuals.

Food Label Information

Nutrition labeling on food products provides particular information about fat. U.S. Food and Drug Administration (FDA) food-labeling regulations provide the following mandatory and voluntary (italicized) information:

Nutrition panel content:

- Calories from fat
- _Calories from saturated fat_
- Total fat
- Saturated fat
- _Polyunsaturated fat_
- _Monounsaturated fat_
- Cholesterol

In addition, the FDA will require food manufacturers to provide the amount of trans fatty acids on the nutrition facts panel by 2006.

The nature and amount of dietary fat and cholesterol are special health concerns related to some cancers, coronary heart disease, diabetes, and obesity (see the Cultural Considerations box, "Ethnic Differences in Lipid Metabolism"). The FDA has approved a series of _health claims_ that link one or more dietary components to the reduced risk of a specific disease. The following health claims are approved about fat:

- _Fat and cancer:_ A diet low in total fat may reduce the risk of some cancers.
- _Saturated fat and cholesterol and coronary heart disease:_ Diets low in saturated fat and cholesterol may reduce the risk of coronary heart disease.

See A _Food Labeling Guide_ published by the FDA's Center for Food Safety and Applied Nutrition at _http://vm.cfsan.fda.gov/~dms/flg-6c.html_ for more information on FDA-approved health claims. This site provides a table with approved claims, food requirements, and model claim statements. Food labels and health claims will be discussed further in Chapter 13.

Characteristics of Food Fat Sources

For practical purposes, food fats can be classified as _visible_ or _invisible_ fats to help individuals become aware of all food sources of fat.

adipose (L. _adeps,_ fat; _adiposus,_ fatty) fat present in cells of adipose (fatty) tissue.

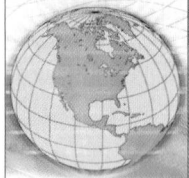

CULTURAL CONSIDERATIONS

ETHNIC DIFFERENCES IN LIPID METABOLISM

Dietary patterns and habits form at an early age as a result of both family influence and environmental factors. The dietary fat intake in some individuals is much lower than others simply because that is the way they were raised. However, since the unveiling of the human genome, we are learning that there are also biological differences that may not only affect our dietary patterns, but also determine the way in which our bodies handle the nutrients we eat. It has long since been established that the prevalence for obesity differs between ethnic and racial population, but the exact cause continues to be ambiguous.

African-American and Caucasian women are often the subjects for study in obesity research. The incidence of obesity in African-American women is significantly higher than that of their Caucasian counterparts. There is accumulating evidence suggesting biological differences in lipid metabolism between the ethnic groups may be the cause.

Bower and colleagues found that African-American women have an increased capacity to synthesize fat from glucose in adipose tissue when compared with Caucasian women.* Thus they are more efficient at converting excess kcalories into stored fat and contributing to the higher rate of obesity among African-American women.

Differences such as these will continue to unfold with continued study of the human genome. Differences such as these will also guide individuals in their dietary choices with regard to how their body will respond to specific nutrients. There are many places in the path from fat in our food to fat on our body that are subject to inspection and evaluation. The science of lipid digestion, metabolism, and utilization will remain a hot topic for debate and research for years to come.

*Bower JF and others: Ethnic differences in *in vitro* glyceride synthesis in subcutaneous and omental adipose tissue, *Am J Physiol Endocrinol Metab* 283(5):E988, 2002.

Visible Fat

The obvious fats are plain to see and include butter, margarine, separate cream, salad oils and dressings, lard, shortening, fat meat (e.g., bacon, sausage, and salt pork), and the visible fat of any meat. It is easier to control visible fats in the diet than those that are less apparent.

Invisible Fat

Some dietary fats are less visible, so individuals who want to control dietary fat also must be aware of these food sources. Invisible fats include cheese, the cream portion of homogenized milk, egg yolk, nuts, seeds, olives, avocados, and lean meat. Even when all of the visible fat has been removed from meat (e.g., the skin on poultry and the obvious fat on the lean portions), about 6% of the total fat surrounding the muscle fibers remains.

Digestibility and Market Availability of Food Fats

The digestibility of fats varies somewhat according to the food source and cooking method. Butter digests more completely than meat fat. Fried foods, especially those saturated with fat in the frying process, are digested more slowly than baked or broiled foods. When fried foods are cooked at too high of a temperature, they are more difficult

to digest because substances in the fat break down into irritating materials. Fried foods should be consumed sparingly, and the temperature of the fat should be carefully controlled during frying. Although lower fat food products are now generally more available in our food markets, there are still many high-fat products beckoning for the customer's attention. In any case, fat is an essential part of a healthy, well-balanced diet. Our overall health goal is to reduce the amount of *excessive* fat used in the diet.

BODY NEEDS FOR FAT

Dietary Fat and Health

American Diet

From reading world health reports and caring for malnourished patients, it is evident that fats make up an essential nutrient class.[6] The role of fat-modified foods in the American diet, however, has been increasing.[7] The American diet has traditionally been high in fat. Fats in the diet supply flavor to food, providing a sense of satisfaction and enhancing eating pleasure. However, people often eat more than they intend or need. The average amount of fat consumed per person in the United States, for all individuals ages 2 and older is 134% of the recommendations based on the Dietary Reference Intakes

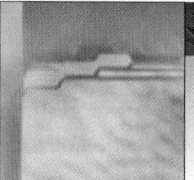

CLINICAL APPLICATIONS

HOW MUCH FAT ARE YOU EATING?

Keep an accurate record of everything you eat and drink for 1 day. Be sure to include all fat or other nutrient seasonings used with your foods (salad dressing, sugar, mayonnaise, etc.). If you want a more representative picture, use the nutrient analysis program that came with this book or another program to which you have access and keep a 3- to 7-day record.

Step 1: Calculate the total kilocalories and grams of each of the energy-yielding nutrients (carbohydrates, fat, and protein) in everything you eat. Multiply the total

grams of each energy nutrient by its respective fuel value:

$$\text{Fat} \underline{\hspace{1cm}} \text{g} \times 9 = \underline{\hspace{1cm}} \text{kcal}$$
$$\text{Protein} \underline{\hspace{1cm}} \text{g} \times 4 = \underline{\hspace{1cm}} \text{kcal}$$
$$\text{Carbohydrate} \underline{\hspace{1cm}} \text{g} \times 4 = \underline{\hspace{1cm}} \text{kcal}$$

Step 2: Next, calculate the percentage of each energy nutrient in your total diet:

$$(\text{Fat kcal} \div \text{total kcal}) \times 100 = \% \text{ fat kcal in diet}$$

Step 3: Finally, compare your diet with the fat in a typical American diet (30% to 45% fat) and with the U.S. dietary goal (20% to 35% fat).

(DRIs) for Americans.[8] This amount exceeds that needed by the average person. No more than 20% to 35% of the diet's total kcalories should come from fat. Many individuals with health problems have adjusted to lower amounts of fat, with goals such as 15% to 25% of the total kcalories. This amount could easily provide an adequate amount of the essential fatty acids, linolenic and linoleic acid, to meet the physiologic needs of the body.

Health Problems

If fat is vital to human health, what is the concern about fat in the diet? Research continues to validate results indicating that health problems from fat relate to too much dietary fat, specifically saturated fat.

Amount of Fat. Too many kcalories in the diet, regardless of the source (fat, carbohydrates, or protein), will exceed the requirement of immediate energy needs. The excess is stored as body fat. Increased body fat and weight have been associated with risk factors for health problems such as diabetes, hypertension, and heart disease. Look for more details about these relationships in the later section on clinical nutrition. How much fat is in your own diet? You might try figuring it out for a day (see the Clinical Applications box, "How Much Fat Are You Eating?").

Type of Fat. An excess of cholesterol and saturated fat in the diet, which comes from animal food sources, has been associated as a specific risk factor for atherosclerosis, the underlying blood vessel disease that contributes to heart attacks and strokes (see Chapter 19). A decrease in dietary saturated fats (e.g., using polyunsaturated and

monounsaturated fats instead) has been shown to reduce serum total cholesterol in many individuals.[2] When substituted for saturated fat in the diet, monounsaturated fats (e.g., olive oil) reduce the LDL cholesterol.

Health Promotion

The ongoing movement in American health care is toward health promotion and disease prevention through reduction of risk factors related to chronic disease. Heart disease continues to be a leading cause of death in developed countries, and much attention is given to reducing the various risk factors leading to this disease. Excess dietary fat, particularly saturated fat and cholesterol, contributes to these risk factors, which include obesity, diabetes, elevated blood fats, and elevated blood pressure. Additional lifestyle risk factors include smoking, increased stress, and lack of exercise, especially in middle-aged and older individuals.[9,10] Thus a middle-aged or older adult who eats a high-fat diet, is overweight, and has a high level of blood cholesterol and blood pressure should reduce both weight and amount of dietary fat, especially animal fat. Today there is increasing emphasis—especially for persons at least 40 years of age—on the importance of keeping the body's total daily energy use in balance with the total daily caloric intake, especially of dietary fat.[11,12] Children are learning in grade school about healthier food habits with less fat. Healthier food habits are especially important for children in high-risk families (e.g., families having identified lipid disorders and heart disease at young adult ages) who should develop moderation in fat use, as well as other aspects of a healthy lifestyle, at an early age.

In addition, changes are gradually being made in the fast-food industry to reduce the traditional high-fat content of their menu items. For example, most of the fast-food chains are shifting to leaner meat for hamburgers and more variety in food choices (e.g., grilled chicken and fish sandwiches; breakfast items such as fruit, waffles, pancakes, and hot and cold cereals; baked potatoes; chili; and fresh and packaged salads) and using vegetable oil for frying. Many fast-food restaurants are experimenting and surveying customers about use of fat substitutes.

Low-fat diets, fad diets, and other issues about weight loss are discussed in more detail in Chapter 15.

DIGESTION OF FATS

Mouth

The various animal and plant fats (triglycerides) that naturally occur in foods are taken into the body with the diet. The task is to change these basic fuel fats into a refined fuel the cells can burn for energy. Like other macronutrients (carbohydrates and proteins), fats are broken down into their basic building blocks, fatty acids, through the process of digestion. When foods are eaten, some initial chemical fat breakdown may begin in the mouth by action of a *lingual lipase*, which is secreted by Ebner's glands at the back of the tongue. However, the primary digestive action occurring in the mouth is mechanical. Foods are broken up into smaller particles through chewing and moistened for passage into the stomach.

Stomach

Little, if any, chemical fat digestion takes place in the stomach. General muscle action continues to mix the fat with the stomach contents. No significant amount of fat enzymes is present in the gastric secretions except a *gastric lipase* (tributyrinase), which acts on emulsified butterfat. As the main gastric enzymes act on other specific nutrients in the food mix, fat is separated out from them and prepared for its major, chemical-specific breakdown in the small intestine.

Small Intestine

Fat digestion occurs primarily in the small intestine. The major enzymes necessary for the chemical changes are not present until fat reaches the small intestine. These specific digestive agents come from three major sources: a preparation agent from the gallbladder and specific enzymes from the pancreas and the small intestine itself.

Bile from the Gallbladder

The fat coming into the duodenum, the first section of the small intestine, stimulates the secretion of *cholecystokinin*, a local hormone from glands in the intestinal walls. In turn, cholecystokinin causes the gallbladder to contract, relax its opening muscle, and subsequently secrete bile into the intestine by way of the common bile duct. The bile is first produced in large dilute amounts in the liver, which then sends it to the gallbladder for concentration and storage so that it is ready for use with fat, as needed. Bile is not an enzyme but functions as an emulsifier. Emulsification is not a chemical digestive process but is the important preparation of fat for chemical digestion by its specific enzymes. This preparation process accomplishes two important tasks: (1) it breaks the fat into small particles, greatly enlarging the total surface area available for action of the enzyme; and (2) it lowers the surface tension of the finely dispersed and suspended fat particles, allowing the enzymes to penetrate more easily.[13] This process is similar to the emulsification action of detergents. The bile also provides an alkaline medium necessary for the action of the fat enzyme *pancreatic lipase*.

Enzymes from the Pancreas

Pancreatic juice flowing into the small intestine contains an enzyme for fat and another one for cholesterol. First, *pancreatic lipase*, a powerful fat enzyme, breaks off one fatty acid at a time from the glycerol base of fats (triglycerides). One fatty acid plus a diglyceride, then another fatty acid plus a monoglyceride, are produced in turn. Each succeeding step of this breakdown occurs with increasing difficulty. In fact, separation of the final fatty acid from the remaining monoglyceride is such a slow process that less than a third of the total fat present actually reaches complete breakdown. The final products of fat digestion to be absorbed are fatty acids, monoglycerides, and glycerol. Some remaining fat may pass into the large intestine for fecal elimination. The enzyme *cholesterol esterase* acts on cholesterol esters to form a combination of free cholesterol and fatty acids in preparation for absorption into the lymph vessels and finally into the blood stream (see Chapter 5).

Enzyme from the Small Intestine

The small intestine secretes an enzyme in the intestinal juice called *lecithinase*, which acts on lecithin, another lipid compound, breaking it down for absorption. Table 3-1 summarizes fat digestion in the successive parts of the gastrointestinal tract.

TABLE 3-1	Summary of Fat Digestion	
Organ	**Enzyme**	**Activity**
Mouth	Small amount of lingual lipase	Some initial fat breakdown Mechanical, mastication
Stomach	No major enzyme	Mechanical separation of fats as protein and starch digested out
Small intestine	Small amount of gastric lipase tributyrinase	Tributyrin (butterfat) to fatty acids and glycerol
	Gallbladder bile salts (emulsifier)	Emulsifies fats
	Pancreatic lipase (steapsin)	Triglycerides to diglycerides and monoglycerides in turn, then fatty acids and glycerol

Absorption

Fat absorption into the gastrointestinal cells and blood stream is more involved than the absorption of either carbohydrates or protein. This is because triglycerides are not soluble in water and cannot enter into the blood stream, which is mostly water. Within the small intestines, bile salts surround the monoglycerides and fatty acids to form **micelles.** The non–water-soluble fat particles are found in the middle of the packaged micelle, whereas the water-soluble part faces outward. This structure allows for the absorption of fat into the intestinal mucosal cell. Once inside the intestinal cell, the bile acids are released from the package and recycled within the body. The monoglycerides and fatty acids re-form triglycerides, which are then packaged into a lipoprotein called **chylomicrons.** Chylomicrons are made of triglycerides, cholesterol, phospholipids, and proteins. Again, this structure allows for the products of fat digestion to enter into circulation. Chylomicrons first enter into the lymphatic circulatory system, and then eventually enter the blood stream.

DIETARY FAT REQUIREMENTS

Dietary Reference Intakes

Healthy diet guidelines stress the health benefits of a diet low in fat, saturated fat, and cholesterol. All guidelines recommend that the fat content of the diet not exceed 20% to 35% of the total kcalories, that less than 10% of the kcalories should be provided from saturated fats, and that dietary cholesterol be limited to 300 mg/day (see Chapter 1). The current average consumption of fat is about 34% of the total kcalories. As mentioned, fat is an essential part of the diet; therefore diets completely devoid of fat are equally unhealthy and can result in essential fatty acid deficiency.

Dietary Guidelines for Americans

In line with the current national health goal of health promotion through disease prevention by reducing identified risks of chronic disease, the *Dietary Guidelines for Americans* recommend general control of fat in the diet, especially saturated fat and cholesterol. Several practical ways of lowering fat in the diet are as follows:

■ *Meat:* Use only lean cuts of all meats, and use more poultry and seafood (with exception of shrimp, which is high in dietary cholesterol). Remove skin

---

bile (L. *bilis,* bile) a fluid secreted by the liver and transported to the gallbladder for concentration and storage; released into the duodenum with the entry of fat to facilitate enzymatic fat digestion by acting as an emulsifying agent.

emulsifier an agent that breaks down large fat globules into smaller, uniformly distributed particles; action accomplished in the intestine chiefly by bile acids, which lower the surface tension of the fat particles, breaking the fat into many smaller droplets, thus greatly increasing the surface area of fat and facilitating contact with the fat-digesting enzymes.

micelles packages of free fatty acids, monoglycerides, and bile salts. The non–water-soluble fat particles are found in the middle of the package, whereas the water-soluble part faces outward and allows for the absorption of fat into the intestinal mucosal cell.

chylomicron *(kye-lo-MY-cron)* lipoprotein formed in the intestinal cell composed of triglycerides, cholesterol, phospholipids, and protein. Allows for absorption of fat into the lymphatic circulatory system before entering blood circulation.

from poultry and trim fat from all meats. Avoid added fat in cooking. Use smaller portions (e.g., 2 to 4 oz) of meat. For example, a boneless chicken breast is about 3 to 4 oz.
- *Eggs:* Limit intake of eggs to approximately two or three a week. Cook and serve without added fat. Use egg whites freely.

- *Milk and milk products:* Use low-fat or fat-free milk and milk products. Use cheeses with lower fat content.
- *Food preparation:* Avoid added fat as much as possible in food preparation and cooking. Use alternative seasonings such as herbs, spices, lemon and lime juice, onion, garlic, fat-free broth, or wine. Use low-fat or fat-free salad dressings or herb-seasoned or wine vinegars.

SUMMARY

Fat is an essential body nutrient, serving important body needs as a back-up storage fuel—secondary to carbohydrate—for energy. Fat also supplies important tissue needs as a structural material for cell walls, protective padding for vital organs, insulation to maintain body temperature, and covering for nerve fibers.

Food fats have different forms and body uses. Saturated fats come primarily from animal food sources and carry health risks for the body. Plant food sources are the richest source for unsaturated fats and help reduce health risks. Cholesterol is a fat-related substance, synthesized only by animals. When consumed in excessive amounts, cholesterol also contributes to health risks for developing cardiovascular disease. Americans generally consume more fat than they need or is healthy for them. Reducing total fats and saturated fat and maintaining a low-cholesterol diet are recommended for health promotion and disease prevention.

When various foods containing fat and cholesterol are eaten, specific digestive agents including bile and pancreatic lipase prepare and break down the fats (triglycerides). Fatty acids and glycerides are incorporated into chylomicrons and absorbed via the lymphatic system into blood circulation.

CRITICAL THINKING QUESTIONS

1. Compare fat with carbohydrate as a fuel source in the body's energy system. Name several other important functions of fat in human nutrition and health.
2. Define the terms *lipids, triglycerides, fatty acids, cholesterol,* and *lipoproteins.* Distinguish between saturated and unsaturated fats, giving food sources for each.
3. Why is a controlled amount of dietary fat recommended for health promotion? How much fat should a healthy diet contain?

CHAPTER CHALLENGE QUESTIONS

True-False

Write the correct statement for each item you answer "false."

1. *True or False:* Fat has the same energy value as carbohydrate.
2. *True or False:* Fat is composed of the same basic chemical elements as carbohydrate.

3. *True or False:* Corn oil is a saturated fat.
4. *True or False:* Polyunsaturated fats predominantly come from animal food sources.
5. *True or False:* Lipoproteins, produced mainly in the liver, carry fat in the blood.

Multiple Choice

1. The fuel form of fat found in food sources is:
   - **a.** triglyceride
   - **b.** fatty acid
   - **c.** glycerol
   - **d.** lipoprotein

2. Which of the following statements about the saturation of fats is correct?
   - **a.** The degree of saturation does not depend on the amount of hydrogen in the fatty acids that make up the fat.

b. Unsaturated fats come from animal food sources.

c. The more saturated the fat, the softer it tends to be.

d. Fats composed of fatty acids with two or more "unfilled" spaces in their structure are called *polyunsaturated*.

3. If an individual implemented a low saturated fat diet to lower the risk for heart disease, which of the following foods would be used more frequently?

a. Whole milk

b. Olive oil and vinegar salad dressing

c. Butter

d. Cheddar cheese

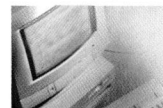

Please refer to the Students' Resource section of this text's Evolve web site for "Suggestions for Additional Study."

REFERENCES

1. Food and Nutrition Board, Institute of Medicine: *Dietary reference intakes for energy, carbohydrate, fiber, fat, fatty acids, cholesterol, protein, and amino acids,* Washington, DC, 2002, National Academies Press.
2. Montoya MT and others: Fatty acid saturation of the diet and plasma lipid concentrations, lipoprotein particle concentrations, and cholesterol efflux capacity, *Am J Clin Nutr* 75(3):484, 2002.
3. Williams SR, Schlenker E: *Essentials of nutrition and diet therapy,* ed 8, St Louis, 2003, Mosby.
4. Katz AM: Trans-fatty acids and sudden cardiac death, *Circulation* 105(6):697, 2002.
5. Lemaitre RN and others: Cell membrane *trans*-fatty acids and the risk of primary cardiac arrest, *Circulation* 105(6):669, 2002.
6. Klein S, Jeejeebhoy KN: The malnourished patient: nutrition assessment and management. In Feldman M, Scharschimedt BF, Sleisenger MH, eds: *Gastrointestinal and liver disease,* ed 6, vol 1, Philadelphia, 1998, Saunders.
7. Peterson S and others: Impact of adopting lower-fat food choices on energy and nutrient intakes of American adults, *J Am Diet Assoc* 99(2):177, 1999.
8. Economic Research Service, U.S. Department of Agriculture, Briefing Room: *Diet and health: food consumption and nutrient intake tables,* Washington, DC, (accessed December 2002), USDA [*www.ers.usda.gov/briefing/Diet AndHealth/data/nutrients/*].
9. Tanasescu M and others: Exercise type and intensity in relation to coronary heart disease in men, *JAMA* 288(16):1994, 2002.
10. Carlsson CM, Stein JH: Cardiovascular disease and the aging woman: overcoming barriers to lifestyle changes, *Curr Womens Health Rep* 2(5):366, 2002.
11. Mela DJ: Determinants of food choice: relationships with obesity and weight control, *Obes Res* 9(4):249S, 2001.
12. Lyznicki JM and others: Obesity: assessment and management in primary care, *Am Fam Physician* 63(11):2185, 2001.
13. Guyton AC, Hall JE: *Textbook of medical physiology,* ed 10, Philadelphia, 2000, Saunders.

FURTHER READING AND RESOURCES

- Eldridge AL and others: A role for olestra in body weight management, *Obes Rev* 3(1):17, 2002.
- Wylie-Rosett J: Fat substitutes and health: an advisory from the Nutrition Committee of the American Heart Association, *Circulation* 105(23):2800, 2002.

   These interesting articles describe fat substitutes that are now available in the marketplace, and their role in achieving dietary recommendations for fat intake.

- Abusabha R and others: Dietary fat reduction strategies used by a group of adults aged 50 years and older, *J Am Diet Assoc* 101(9):1024, 2001.

   The authors investigate strategies used by individuals who were successful at reducing their long-term daily fat intake. Health care professionals should explore a variety of methods for encouraging positive dietary change in patients.

CHAPTER 4

Proteins

Many different proteins in the body make human life possible. Each one of these thousands upon thousands of specific body proteins has a unique structure designed to do an assigned task. Amino acids are among the essential units of human bodies and are the building blocks of all protein. Humans obtain amino acids from the variety of food proteins eaten every day. This chapter looks at the specific nature of proteins, both in food and in human bodies; and explains why protein balance is essential to life and health and how that balance is maintained.

KEY CONCEPTS

■ Food proteins provide the amino acids necessary for building and maintaining body tissue.

■ Protein balance, both within the body and in the diet, is essential to life and health.

■ The quality of a protein food, and its ability to meet the body's needs, is determined by the composition of amino acids.

THE NATURE OF PROTEINS

Amino Acids: Basic Building Material

Role as Building Units

All protein, whether in our bodies or in the food we eat, is made up of building units known as **amino acids.** Amino acids are joined in unique, chain sequences to form specific proteins. Each amino acid is joined by a peptide bond (Figure 4-1). Two amino acids joined together are called a dipeptide. Polypeptides are chains of up to 100 amino acids. There are hundreds of amino acids linked together to form a single protein. When protein foods are eaten, the protein (e.g., casein in milk and cheese, albumin in egg white, or gluten in wheat products) is broken down into amino acids in the digestive process. Amino acids are then reassembled in the body in a *specific* order to form a variety of proteins (e.g., collagen in connective tissue; myosin in muscle tissue; hemoglobin in red blood cells; digestive enzymes or hormones) needed by the body. To maintain its solvency, each protein chain adopts a folded form, which can fold and unfold according to metabolic need.[1] Because proteins are relatively large, complex molecules, they are often subject to mutations, or malformations in structure. For example, protein-folding mistakes are involved in Alzheimer's disease, which robs many older adults of their mental capacity.[2]

Dietary Importance

Amino acids are named for their chemical nature. The word *amino* refers to compounds containing nitrogen. Like carbohydrates and fats, proteins have a basic structure of carbon, hydrogen, and oxygen. However, unlike carbohydrates and fats, which contain no nitrogen, protein is about 16% nitrogen. As such, protein is the pri-mary source of nitrogen in the diet. In addition, some proteins contain small but valuable amounts of the minerals sulfur, phosphorus, iron, and iodine.

Classes of Amino Acids

There are 20 common amino acids, all of which are vital to human life and health. These amino acids are classified as indispensable, dispensable, or **conditionally indispensable** *in the diet* according to whether the body can make them (Box 4-1). These classifications are formerly known as essential, nonessential, or conditionally essential, respectively.

Indispensable Amino Acids

Nine amino acids are classified as indispensable amino acids because the body cannot manufacture them in sufficient quantity, or at all (see Box 4-1). Thus as the word *indispensable* implies, these amino acids are necessary in the diet and cannot be left out. Under normal circumstances, the remaining 11 amino acids are easily synthesized by the body to meet continuous metabolic demands throughout the life cycle.

---

amino acids   nitrogen-bearing compounds that form the structural units of protein. When digested, the various food proteins yield their constituent amino acids, which are then available for use by the cells to synthesize specific tissue proteins.

conditionally indispensable amino acids   These are normally considered dispensable amino acids because the body can make them. However, under certain circumstances, such as illness, the body cannot make them in high enough quantities and they become indispensable in the diet.

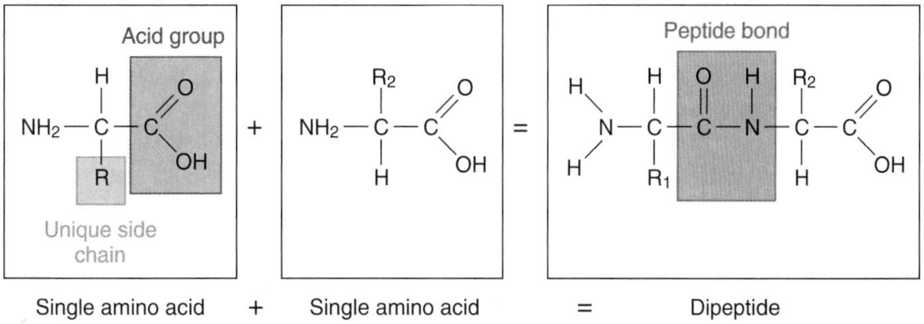

Figure 4–1   Amino acid structure. (Modified from Mahan LK, Escott-Stump S: *Krause's food, nutrition, & diet therapy,* ed 10, Philadelphia, 2000, Saunders.)

> ### BOX 4-1 Indispensable, Dispensable, and Conditionally Indispensable Amino Acids
>
> | Indispensable | Dispensable | Conditionally Indispensable |
> |---|---|---|
> | Histidine | Alanine | |
> | Isoleucine | Aspartic acid | Arginine |
> | Leucine | Asparagine | Cysteine |
> | Lysine | Glutamic acid | Glutamine |
> | Methionine | Serine | Glycine |
> | Phenylalanine | | Proline |
> | Threonine | | Tyrosine |
> | Tryptophan | | |
> | Valine | | |

Dispensable Amino Acids

The word *dispensable* can be misleading; all amino acids have essential tissue-building and metabolic functions in the body. However, as used here the term refers to five amino acids that the body can synthesize from other amino acids (provided the necessary building blocks and enzymes), and are thus not necessary in the diet (see Box 4-1). These amino acids are needed by the body for healthy life, but are dispensable in the diet.

Conditionally Indispensable Amino Acids

The remaining six amino acids are classified as *conditionally indispensable* (see Box 4-1). Under certain physiologic conditions these amino acids, which are normally synthesized in the body like the dispensable amino acids, must be consumed in the diet. Arginine, cysteine, glutamine, glycine, proline, and tyrosine are indispensable when endogenous sources cannot meet the metabolic demands. For example, the human body can make cysteine from the essential amino acid methionine. However, when the diet is deficient in methionine, cysteine must be consumed in the diet, therefore making it an indispensable amino acid under that situation. Severe physiologic stress, illness, and genetic disorders also may render an amino acid conditionally indispensable. Phenylketonuria (PKU) is a genetic disorder in which the individual lacks the enzyme needed to convert phenylalanine to tyrosine. Thus tyrosine must be supplied via the diet and is conditionally indispensable.

Balance

The term *balance* refers to the relative intake and output of substances in the body to maintain equilibrium necessary for health in various circumstances throughout life.

This concept of balance can be applied to life-sustaining protein and the nitrogen it supplies.

Protein Balance

The body's tissue proteins are constantly being broken down into amino acids, a process called *catabolism*, and then resynthesized into tissue proteins as needed, a process called *anabolism*. To maintain nitrogen balance, the part of the amino acid that contains nitrogen may be removed by *deamination*, then converted to ammonia (NH_3), and excreted as urea in the urine. The remaining non-nitrogen residue can be used to make carbohydrate or fat or reattached to make another amino acid, if necessary. The rate of this protein and nitrogen turnover varies in different tissues, according to their degree of metabolic activity.

Tissue turnover is a continuous process of reshaping, rebuilding, and adjusting as necessary to maintain overall protein balance within the body. The body also maintains a balance between tissue protein and plasma protein, which are then further balanced with dietary protein intake. With this finely balanced system, a "pool" of amino acids from both tissue protein and dietary protein is always available to meet construction needs (Figure 4-2).

Nitrogen Balance

The body's nitrogen balance indicates how well its tissues are being maintained. The intake and use of dietary protein is measured by the amount of nitrogen intake in food protein and the amount of nitrogen excreted in the urine. For example, 1 g of urinary nitrogen results from the digestion and metabolism of 6.25 g of protein. Thus if 1 g of nitrogen is excreted in the urine for every 6.25 g of protein consumed, the body is said to be in nitrogen balance. This balance is the normal pattern in adult health, but at different times of life or in states of malnutrition or illness, the balance may shift to be either positive or negative.

Positive Nitrogen Balance. A positive nitrogen balance exists when the body takes in more nitrogen than it excretes, thus storing more nitrogen by building more tissue than it is losing (by breaking down tissue). This situation occurs normally during periods of rapid growth (e.g., infancy, childhood, and adolescence) and pregnancy and lactation. A positive nitrogen balance also occurs in individuals who have been ill or malnourished and are being "built back up" with increased nourishment. In such cases, protein is stored to meet increased needs for tissue building and associated metabolic activity.

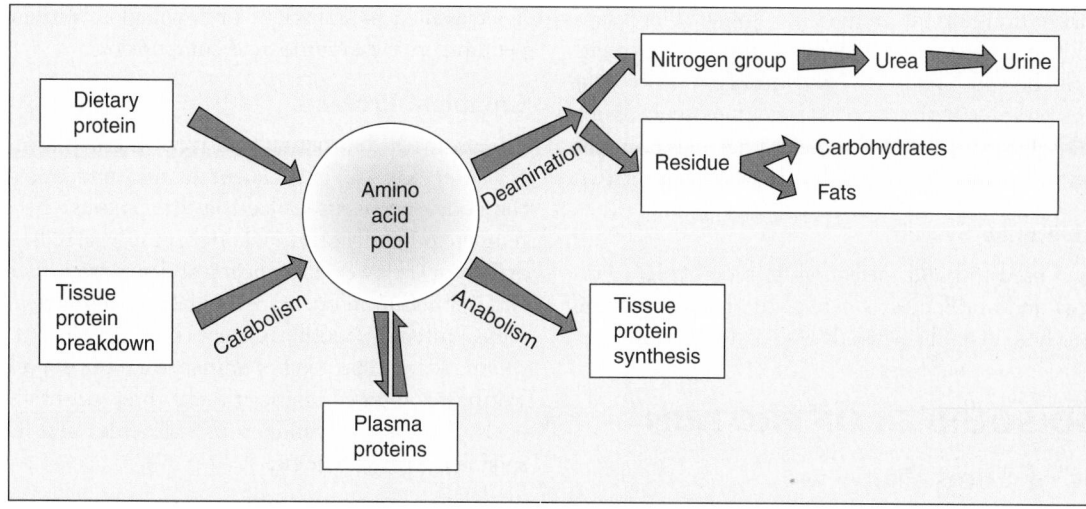

Figure 4–2   Balance between protein compartments and amino acid pool.

Negative Nitrogen Balance. A negative nitrogen balance occurs when the body takes in less nitrogen than it excretes. This means that the body has an inadequate protein intake and is losing nitrogen by breaking down more tissue than it is building up. This situation arises in states of malnutrition and illness. For example, this nitrogen imbalance is seen in individuals when protein deficiency—even when kcalories from carbohydrate and fat are adequate—causes the classic protein deficiency disease *kwashiorkor*. Failure to maintain nitrogen balance may not become apparent for some time but eventually causes loss of muscle tissue, impairment of body organs and functions, and increased susceptibility to infection. In children, negative nitrogen balance causes growth retardation.

FUNCTIONS OF PROTEIN

Primary Tissue Building

Protein is the fundamental structural material of every cell in the body. In fact, the largest portion of the body, excluding the water content, is made up of protein. Body protein, mainly the lean mass of muscles, accounts for about three fourths of the dry matter in most tissues, excluding bone and adipose fat. Protein not only makes up the bulk of the muscles, internal organs, brain, nerves, skin, hair, and nails, but also is a vital part of regulatory substances such as enzymes, hormones, and blood plasma. All of these tissues must be constantly repaired and replaced. The primary functions of protein are to repair worn-out, wasted, or damaged tissue and build up new tissue. Thus protein meets growth needs and maintains tis-

sue health during adult years. In fact, protein is central to the biochemical machinery that makes cells run.[3]

Additional Body Functions

In addition to its basic tissue-building function, protein has other body functions relating to energy, water balance, metabolism, and the body's defense system.

Energy System

As described in previous chapters, carbohydrates are the primary fuel source for the body's energy system, assisted by fat as a stored fuel. In times of need, protein may furnish additional body fuel to sustain body heat and energy, but this is a less efficient, back-up source for use only when there is an insufficient supply of carbohydrate and fat. The available fuel factor of protein is 4 kcal/g.

Water Balance

Plasma protein, especially albumin, helps to control water balance throughout the body by exerting osmotic pressure to maintain normal circulation of tissue fluids and capillary blood flow.

Metabolism

Protein aids metabolic functions through enzymes, transport agents, and hormones. Digestive and cell enzymes are proteins that control metabolic processes. Enzymes necessary for the digestion of carbohydrates (amylase), fats (lipase), and proteins (proteases) are all proteins in nature. Proteins also act as the vehicle in which nutrients are carried throughout the body. Lipoproteins are necessary to transport fats in the water-soluble blood supply. Other examples are hemoglobin, the vital oxygen-carrier in the red blood cells, and transferrin, the iron transport protein in the blood. Hormones, such as insulin and glucagon, are also proteins that play a major function in the metabolism of glucose (see Chapter 20).

Body Defense System

Protein is used to build special white blood cells (lymphocytes) and antibodies as part of the body's immune system to help defend against disease and infection.

FOOD SOURCES OF PROTEIN

Types of Food Proteins

Fortunately, most foods contain a mixture of proteins that complement one another. In a mixed diet, animal and plant foods provide a wide variety of many nutrients and proteins that supplement each other (Figure 4-3). Thus the key to a balanced diet is *variety*. Food proteins are classified as complete or incomplete proteins, depending on their amino acid composition.

Complete Proteins

Protein foods that contain all nine indispensable amino acids (see Box 4-1) in sufficient quantity and ratio to meet the body's needs are called *complete proteins*. These proteins are primarily of animal origin (e.g., egg, milk, cheese, and meat). However, soybeans and soy products are the exception. Soy products are the only plant sources of complete proteins. Another exception is gelatin. Although gelatin is a protein food of animal origin, it is a relatively worthless protein because it lacks three essential amino acids (tryptophan, valine, and isoleucine) and has only small amounts of leucine.

Incomplete Proteins

Protein foods that are deficient in one or more of the nine indispensable amino acids are called *incomplete proteins*. These proteins generally are of plant origin (e.g., grains, legumes, nuts, seeds, vegetables, and fruits) but

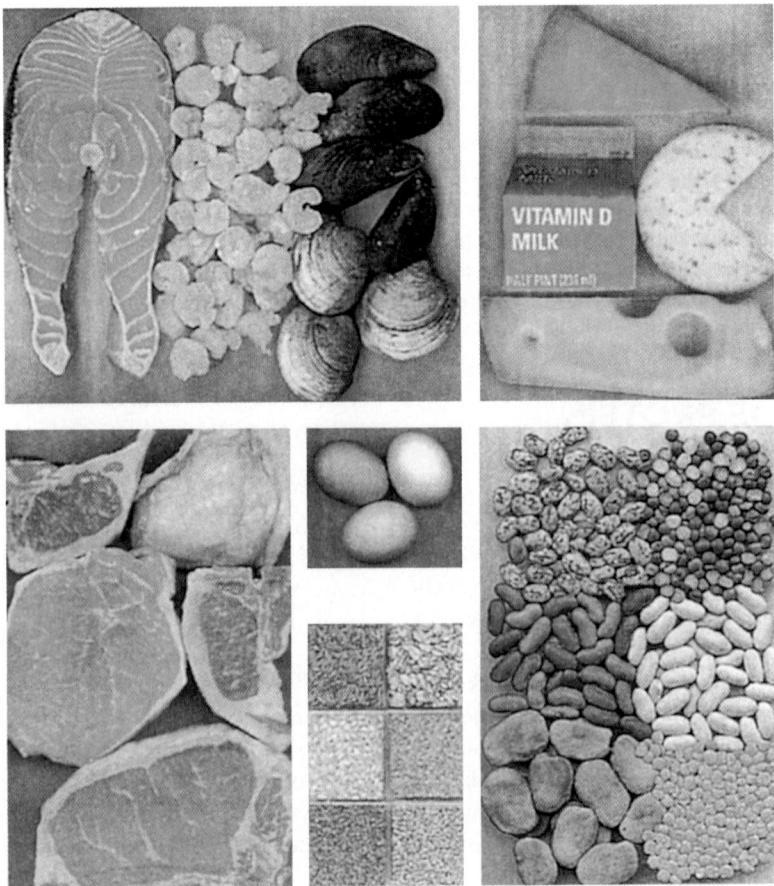

Figure 4-3   Complete and incomplete protein foods. (Credit: Amy Buxton.)

are found in foods that make valuable contributions to the total dietary protein.

Vegetarian Diets

Complementary Protein

Current knowledge of protein metabolism and the "pooling" of amino acid reserves (see Figure 4-2) indicates that a mixture of plant proteins can provide adequate amounts of amino acids when the basic use of various grains is expanded to include soy protein and other dried legume proteins (i.e., beans and peas).[4] Because most plant proteins are incomplete, lacking one or more indispensable (or essential) amino acids, match plant foods so that the amino acids missing in one food are supplied in another. This is the art of combining plant protein foods so that they "complement" one another and supply all nine indispensable amino acids.

Normal eating pattern through the day, together with the body's reserve supply of protein, usually ensures a complementary amino acid balance. The underlying requirement for vegetarians, as for all people, is to eat a sufficient amount of varied foods to meet normal nutrient and energy needs (see the Cultural Considerations box, "Indispensable Amino Acids and Their Complementary Food Proteins").

Types of Vegetarian Diets

Vegetarian diets differ according to the beliefs or needs of individuals following these food patterns. Approximately 2.5% of the total U.S. population followed a vegetarian diet in 2000.[4] There are a variety of reasons that lead people to choose a vegetarian diet: environmental or animal cruelty concerns, health reasons, religions adherence (e.g., Buddhism, Hinduism, Seventh-Day Adventists, and Zen), or aversion to consuming

CULTURAL CONSIDERATIONS

INDISPENSABLE AMINO ACIDS AND THEIR COMPLEMENTARY FOOD PROTEINS

More than 12 million Americans follow a vegetarian diet today. This trend in dietary pattern has gained significant followers in the past decade, especially female adolescents and young adults. A large percentage of the worldwide population follows various forms of vegetarian diets for religious, traditional, or economic reasons. Seventh-Day Adventists follow a lacto-ovo-vegetarian diet, whereas individuals of the Hindu and Buddhist faith are generally lacto-vegetarian. The Mediterranean diet has such a strong emphasis on grains, pastas, vegetables, and cheese that very little other animal products (beef, chicken, and fish) are consumed. In other areas of the world, the economic burden of animal products does not allow the consumption of such foods. Any form of a vegetarian diet can be healthy; however, a good understanding of how to achieve complete protein balance is necessary.

All nine indispensable, or essential, amino acids must be supplied by the diet. It is believed that protein from both animal and plant sources can meet protein requirements adequately. One concern related to a vegetarian diet is in getting a balanced amount of the indispensable amino acids to complement each other and make complete food combinations.

In making complementary food combinations to balance the needed amino acids, families of foods (e.g., grains, legumes, and dairy) must be mixed. For example, grains are low in threonine and high in methionine, whereas legumes are just the opposite—low in methionine and high in threonine. Therefore grains and legumes help balance one another in the accumulation of all indispensable amino acids. The addition of milk products and eggs enhance the amino acid adequacy for lacto-ovo-vegetarians. Here are a few sample food combination dishes to illustrate complementary protein combinations:

- *Grains and peas, beans, or lentils:* brown rice and beans, whole grain bread with pea or lentil soup, wheat or corn tortilla with beans, peanut butter on bread, Indian dishes of rice and dal (a legume), Chinese dishes of tofu and rice
- *Legumes and seeds:* falafel, soybeans and pumpkin or sesame seeds, Middle Eastern hummus (garbanzo beans and sesame seeds) or tahini
- *Grains and dairy:* whole wheat pasta and cheese, yogurt and a multi-grain muffin, cereal and milk, cheese sandwich with whole grain bread

Prepared with a variety of herbs and spices, such dishes can supply needed nutrients and good eating.

animal products. A diet void of animal products is not always a choice. In some areas in the world, vegetarianism is simply a result of the lack of resources and availability of animal products.

In general, there are four basic types:

1. *Lacto-ovo-vegetarians:* Lacto-ovo-vegetarians follow a food pattern that allows dairy products and eggs (Figure 4-4). Their mixed diet of plant and animal food sources, excluding only meat and fish, poses no nutritional problems.
2. *Lacto-vegetarians:* Lacto-vegetarians accept only dairy products from animal sources to complement their basic diet of plant foods. The use of milk and milk products (e.g., cheese) with a varied mixed diet of whole or enriched grains, legumes, nuts, seeds,

fruits, and vegetables in sufficient quantities to meet energy needs provides a balanced intake.

3. *Ovo-vegetarians:* The only animal foods included in the ovo-vegetarian diet are eggs. Because eggs are an excellent source of complete proteins, individuals following this diet do not have to be overly concerned with complementary proteins on a daily basis.
4. *Vegans:* Vegans follow a strict vegetarian diet and use no animal foods. Their food pattern is composed entirely of plant foods (e.g., whole or enriched grains, legumes, nuts, seeds, fruits, and vegetables). The use of soybeans, soy milk, soybean curd (tofu), and processed soy protein products enhances the nutritional value of the diet, and these products are well-tolerated and accepted. Careful planning and sufficient food intake ensure adequate nutrition.

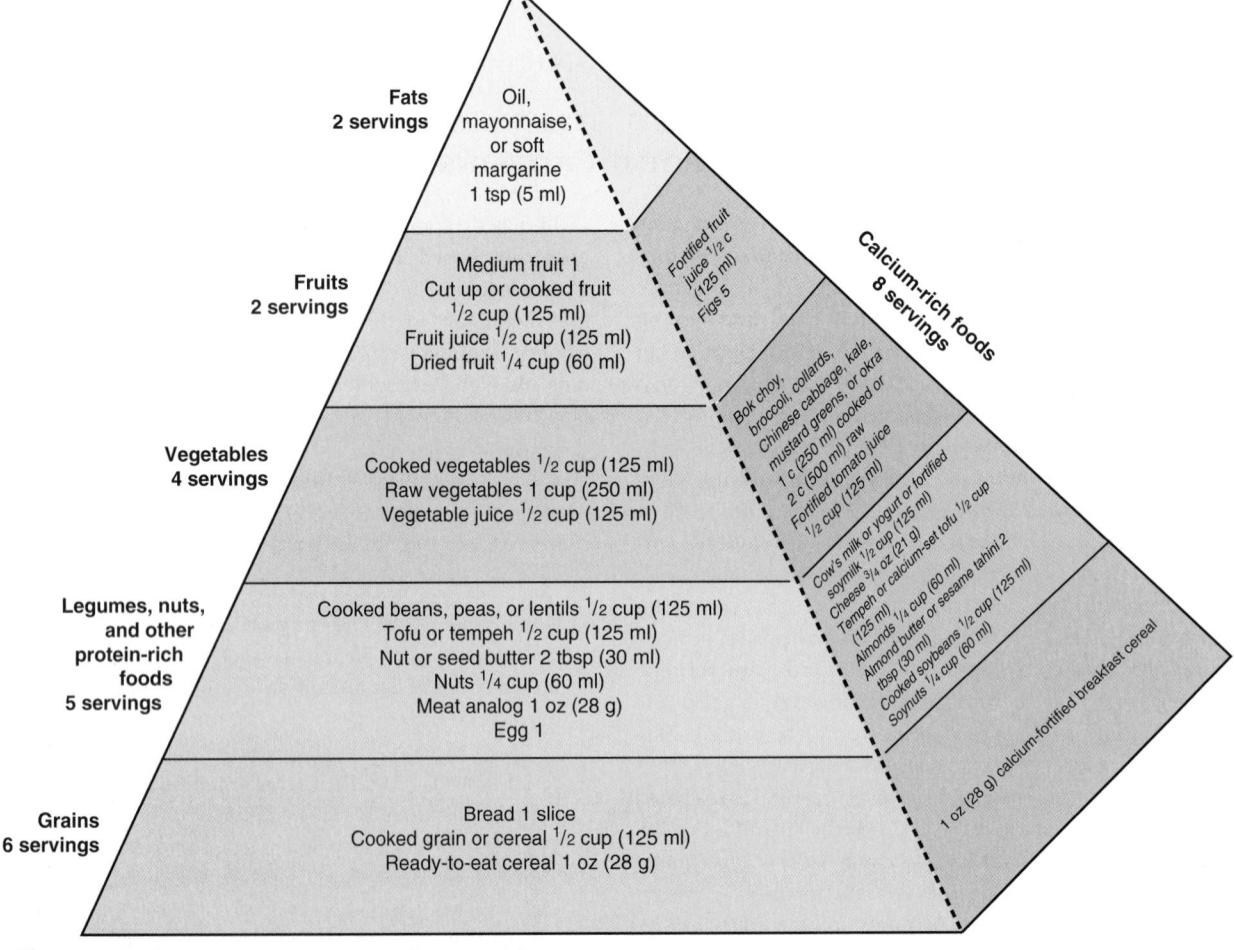

Figure 4–4   Lacto-ovo-vegetarian diet pyramid. (From Messina V and others: A new food guide for North American vegetarians, *J Am Diet Assoc* 103(6):771-775, 2003. Copyright American Dietetic Association.)

The American Dietetic Association's current position paper on vegetarian diets indicates that the former conscious combining of complementary plant proteins within every given meal is unnecessary.[4] It is more important to achieve balance throughout the day.

Health Benefits and Risk

There have been many heated debates about the adequacy of vegetarian diets. Studies have found individuals following a vegan diet to have an inadequate intake of various nutrients, including protein, calcium, phosphorus, zinc, selenium, vitamin D, vitamin B_{12}, and riboflavin.[5,6] Additional concerns are warranted in studies that find reduced albumin synthesis, an important endogenous protein, and reduced iron stores in men and women following vegetarian diets.[7,8]

However, some of the same studies document a higher intake in vegetables, legumes, and fiber and a lower intake of refined sugars, saturated fat, and cholesterol. Upon extensive review of the effects of vegetarian diets in various medical conditions, researchers concluded that "dietary intervention with a vegetarian diet seems to be a cheap, physiologic and safe approach for the prevention, and possible management of modern lifestyle diseases."[9] Diseases in which a positive association was made are diabetes, cardiovascular disease, stroke, dementia, age-related macular degeneration, gastrointestinal disease, and cancer. The preventive mechanism at work in the vegetarian diet is the rich supply of monounsaturated and polyunsaturated fatty acids, fiber, complex carbohydrates, antioxidants, and a restriction in saturated fat. To reap the benefits of a vegetarian diet, a well-balanced diet from a variety of foods is necessary. The American Dietetic Association and the Dietitians of Canada state that "well-planned vegan, lacto-vegetarian, and lacto-ovo-vegetarian diets are appropriate for all stages of the life cycle, including pregnancy and lactation."[4]

DIGESTION OF PROTEINS

Mouth

After protein is eaten, it must be changed into the necessary, ready-to-use building units, amino acids. This work is done through the successive parts of the gastrointestinal tract by the mechanical and chemical processes of digestion. The mechanical breaking down of protein foods occurs by chewing in the mouth. The food particles are mixed with saliva and passed on to the stomach as a semisolid mass.

Stomach

Because proteins are such large, complex structures, a series of enzymes is necessary to finally break them down and produce individual amino acids, the primary form of absorption. Unlike enzymes needed for carbohydrate and fat digestion, all enzymes involved in protein digestion (proteases) are stored as inactive **proenzymes** called zymogens. Zymogens are then activated upon need. Humans cannot store enzymes needed for protein digestion in an active form or else the cells and organs (made of structural proteins) that produce and store them would be digested as well.

Chemical digestion of protein begins in the stomach. In fact, the stomach's chief digestive function overall is the first stage in the enzymatic breakdown of protein. The following three agents in the gastric secretions help with this task.

Pepsin

Pepsin is the main gastric enzyme, specific to proteins. It is first produced as an inactive proenzyme, *pepsinogen,* by a single layer of cells (i.e., the chief cells) in the stomach wall. The hydrochloric acid within gastric juices then changes pepsinogen to the enzyme pepsin. The active **pepsin** begins splitting the links between the protein's amino acids, which changes the large amino acid chains that make up the protein into smaller short chains called *peptides.* If the protein were held in the stomach longer, pepsin could continue this breakdown until only the individual amino acids of the protein remained. However, with normal gastric emptying time, pepsin only completes the first stage of breakdown.

Hydrochloric Acid

Hydrochloric acid provides the acid medium necessary to convert pepsinogen to active pepsin. Hydrochloric acid also begins the unfolding and denaturing of the complex protein chains. This unfolding makes the individual amino acids more available for enzymatic action.

---

proenzyme an inactive precursor (forerunner substance from which another substance is made) that is converted to the active enzyme by the action of an *acid,* another enzyme, or other means. Also called *zymogen.*

pepsin (Gr. *pepsis,* digestion) the main gastric enzyme specific for proteins. Pepsin begins breaking large protein molecules into shorter chain polypeptides; gastric hydrochloric acid is necessary to activate.

Rennin

The gastric enzyme **rennin** is only present in infancy and childhood and is especially important in the infant's digestion of milk. Rennin and calcium act on the casein of milk to produce a curd. By coagulating milk into a more solid curd, rennin prevents the food from passing too rapidly from the infant's stomach to the small intestine.

Small Intestine

Protein digestion begins in the acidic medium of the stomach and is completed in the alkaline medium of the small intestine. Enzymes from secretions of both the pancreas and intestine take part.

---

rennin   milk-curdling enzyme of the gastric juice of human infants and young animals such as calves. Do not confuse with renin, which is an important enzyme produced by the kidney that plays a vital role in producing angiotensin, a potent vasoconstrictor and stimulant for release of the hormone aldosterone from the adjacent adrenal glands.

trypsin   (Gr. *trypein,* to rub; *pepsis,* digestion) a protein-splitting enzyme, secreted as the inactive proenzyme *trypsinogen* in the pancreas, that is activated and acts in the small intestine to reduce proteins to shorter chain polypeptides and dipeptides.

chymotrypsin   (Gr. *chymos,* semifluid food mass from digestion; *trypein,* enzyme trypsin) a protein-splitting enzyme, secreted as the inactive proenzyme *chymotrypsinogen* in the pancreas, that is activated and acts in the small intestine to continue breaking down proteins into shorter chain polypeptides and dipeptides.

carboxypeptidase   (L. *carbo-,* carbon; *oxy,* oxygen) specific protein-splitting enzyme, secreted as the inactive proenzyme procarboxypeptidase in the pancreas, that is activated by trypsin in the small intestine to break off the acid (*carboxyl,* COOH) end of the peptide chain, producing smaller chained peptides and free amino acids.

aminopeptidase   specific protein-splitting enzyme, secreted by small glands in the walls of the small intestine that breaks off the nitrogen-containing amino ($-NH_2$) end of the peptide chain, producing smaller chained peptides and free amino acids.

dipeptidase   specific final enzyme in the protein-splitting system that produces the last two free amino acids.

Pancreatic Secretions

The following three enzymes produced by the pancreas continue breaking down proteins into simpler and simpler substances:

1. **Trypsin,** secreted first as inactive trypsinogen, is activated by the enzyme enterokinase. Enterokinase is secreted from the intestinal cells upon contact with food entering the duodenum, the first section of the small intestine. The active trypsin then works on proteins and large polypeptide fragments carried from the stomach. This enzymatic action produces small polypeptides and dipeptides.
2. **Chymotrypsin,** secreted first as the inactive chymotrypsinogen, is activated by the trypsin already present. The active enzyme then continues the same protein-splitting action of trypsin.
3. **Carboxypeptidase** attacks the acid (carboxyl) end of the peptide chains, producing small peptides and some free amino acids. Carboxypeptidase is also first released as the inactive proenzyme, procarboxypeptidase, and is activated by trypsin.

Intestinal Secretions

Glands in the intestinal wall produce two more protein-splitting enzymes to complete the breakdown and free the remaining amino acids:

1. **Aminopeptidase** attacks the nitrogen-containing (amino) end of the peptide chains and releases amino acids one at a time, producing peptides and free amino acids.
2. **Dipeptidase,** the final enzyme in the protein-splitting system, completes the large task by breaking the remaining dipeptides into two free amino acids.

This finely coordinated system of protein-splitting enzymes breaks down the large, complex proteins into progressively smaller peptide chains and frees each individual amino acid, a tremendous overall task. The free amino acids are now ready to be absorbed directly into the portal blood circulation for use in building body tissues. This remarkable system of protein digestion is summarized in Table 4-1.

BODY NEEDS FOR PROTEIN

Protein Requirements: Influencing Factors

The following three factors influence our requirement for protein: (1) tissue growth needs, (2) quality of the dietary protein, and (3) additional needs owing to illness or disease.

TABLE 4–1	Summary of Protein Digestion			
	Enzyme			
Organ	**Inactive precursor**	**Activator**	**Active enzyme**	**Digestive action**
Mouth			None	Mechanical only
Stomach (acidic)	Pepsinogen	Hydrochloric acid	Pepsin	Protein → polypeptides
			Rennin (infants) (calcium necessary for activity)	Casein → coagulated curd
Intestine (alkaline) Pancreatic secretions	Trypsinogen	Enterokinase	Trypsin	Protein, polypeptides → polypeptides, dipeptides
	Chymotrypsinogen	Trypsin	Chymotrypsin	Protein, polypeptides → polypeptides, dipeptides
	Procarboxypeptidase	Trypsin	Carboxypeptidase	Polypeptides → simpler peptides, dipeptides, amino acids
Intestinal secretions			Aminopeptidase	Polypeptides → peptides, dipeptides, amino acids
			Dipeptidase	Dipeptides → amino acids

Tissue Growth

During rapid growth periods of the human life cycle, more protein per unit of body size is necessary to build new tissue, as well as maintain present tissue. Human growth is most rapid during the following periods: fetal growth during the mother's pregnancy, infant growth during the first year of life plus the lactation needs of a breastfeeding mother, and adolescent growth and development into adulthood. Young childhood is a sustained time of continued growth but at a somewhat slower rate. For adults, protein requirements level off to meet tissue-maintenance needs, but individual needs may vary.

Dietary Protein Quality

The nature of the protein foods eaten and their pattern of amino acids significantly influence the quality of the dietary protein. Sufficient kcalories or energy intake—especially from nonprotein foods—is also necessary to conserve protein for tissue building. Finally, the digestion and absorption of the protein consumed is affected by the comparative complexity of its structure, as well as its preparation and cooking. The comparative quality of protein foods has been determined by the four basic measures that follow:

1. *Chemical score (CS)* is a value derived from the amino acid pattern of the food. Using a high-quality protein food, such as egg, and giving it a value of 100, other foods are compared according to their amino acid ratios.

2. *Biological value (BV)* is based on nitrogen balance.
3. *Net protein utilization (NPU)* is based on the biological value and the degree of the food protein's digestibility.
4. *Protein efficiency ratio (PER)* is based on the weight gain of a growing test animal in relation to its protein intake.

Table 4-2 compares various protein food scores based on these measures of protein quality. As seen in the table, egg and milk proteins lead all the lists. The quality and digestibility of most plant proteins is significantly less than animal proteins; therefore the dietary protein needs of vegans who rely solely on plant foods for protein may be higher than nonvegetarians.[4] In other words, because the protein provided by whole wheat products is only about half as bioavailable as protein from eggs, twice as much protein from whole wheat products would have to be eaten to get the same amount of useable protein.

Regardless of dietary preferences for protein foods, a sound diet is the best way for a healthy person to obtain quality protein. There is no necessity for amino acid supplements.

Illness or Disease

An illness or disease, especially when accompanied by fever and increased tissue breakdown (catabolism), increases the body's need for protein and kcalories for rebuilding tissue and to meet the demands of increased metabolic rate. Traumatic injury requires extensive tissue

TABLE 4–2	Comparative Protein Quality of Selected Foods			
Food	Chemical score*	BV	NPU	PER
Egg	100	100	94	3.92
Cow's milk	95	93	82	3.09
Fish	71	76	—	3.55
Beef	69	74	67	2.30
Unpolished rice	67	86	59	—
Peanuts	65	55	55	1.65
Oats	57	65	—	2.19
Polished rice	57	64	57	2.18
Whole wheat	53	65	49	1.53
Corn	49	72	36	—
Soybeans	47	73	61	2.32
Sesame seeds	42	62	53	1.77
Peas	37	64	55	1.57

Data modified from Guthrie H: *Introductory nutrition,* ed 6, New York, 1986, McGraw-Hill; and Food and Nutrition Board, Institute of Medicine: *Recommended dietary allowances,* ed 10, Washington, DC, 1989, National Academies Press.
BV = Biologic value; *NPU* = net protein utilization; *PER* = protein efficiency ratio.
*Amino acid.

rebuilding. After surgery, extra protein is needed for wound healing and restoring losses. Extensive tissue destruction, as occurs with massive burns, requires a large protein increase for the healing and grafting processes.

Dietary Deficiency or Excess

As with any nutrient, moderation and balance are the key to health. Too much or too little dietary protein can be problematic in overall body function.

Protein-Energy Malnutrition

Protein-energy malnutrition (PEM) can occur in a variety of situations. The most severe cases are found in less industrialized countries where not only protein-rich foods are in short supply, but all foods are. Children are at the highest risk for developing PEM because of their elevated needs during rapid growth and development. However, PEM can affect anyone at any age. Persons with poor nutrient intake, such as the elderly or eating disorder patients, may suffer from PEM as well. It is not common that PEM exists without overall energy deficiency. However, individuals with high protein needs during infection or disease, such as AIDS, cancer, and liver failure, are sometimes victims of PEM, despite seemingly adequate total energy intake. As mentioned, protein has many critical functions in the body. Thus a dietary deficiency has multiple consequences directly related to these functions. Without the amino acid building blocks, the body can not synthesize needed structural (muscle) or functional (enzymes, antibodies, hormones, etc.) proteins.

Two severe forms of PEM are kwashiorkor and marasmus. Characteristics of the two forms of PEM are very different, as described below. Kwashiorkor is thought to result from an acute deficiency of protein, whereas marasmus results from a more chronic deficiency. The end result with either form is stunted growth, weakened immune system, and poor development.

Kwashiorkor. Kwashiorkor is common in children between the ages of 18 to 24 months who have been breastfed all their lives and then are rapidly weaned, usually because the arrival of a younger sibling. These children are switched from nutritionally balanced breast milk to a diluted diet of mostly carbohydrates and little protein. The term kwashiorkor is a Ghanian word that refers to the disease that takes over the first child when the second child is born. The children may receive adequate total kcalories, but lack enough kcalories from protein sources. Characteristics of kwashiorkor include edema in the feet and legs, and a bloated abdomen, both from lack of protein in the blood to maintain fluid balance and transport fat away from the liver.

Marasmus. Individuals with marasmus have a very emaciated appearance with little or no body fat. This is a chronic form of energy and protein deficiency—basic starvation. Stunted growth and development are even more severe with this form of PEM. Marasmus is more likely to affect individuals of all ages, suffering from inadequate food sources.

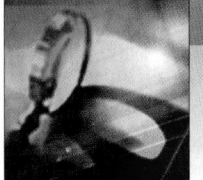

FOR FURTHER FOCUS

The Precious Price of a High-Protein Diet

The per capita consumption of protein continues to rise, right along with the total caloric intake. In the United States, the per capita per day consumption of kcalories and grams of protein rose from 3300 kcal and 96 g protein to 3800 kcal and 111 g protein, respectively, from 1970 to 1999.* Not coincidentally, significant weight gains and the health risk associated with obesity (heart disease, diabetes, hypertension, some forms of cancer, etc.) have been noted. As a result, 63.9% of men and 78% of women are actively trying to lose or maintain weight.†

Health care professionals are not only concerned about the rising rate of obesity in this country, but also of the methods in which people are trying to combat it. In a survey of more than 100,000 people, most persons trying to lose weight were not using the recommended methods to lose weight—by reducing calories and increasing physical activity.† One of the more popular diets is the high-protein, low-carbohydrate diet. Such diets may not be harmful for most people, but there are currently no long-term studies to confirm their safety either. On the other hand, there have been studies linking excessive protein intake with many health risk (increased cholesterol, increased uric acid levels, increased calcium loss, etc.).‡

High-protein diets are higher in total fat, saturated fat, and cholesterol. Initial weight loss associated with a high-protein, high-fat diet is caused by the induction of metabolic ketosis, as well as fluid loss from a lack of carbohydrates.‡ Ketosis eventually suppresses the appetite, ultimately leading to reduced caloric intake and weight loss. The debate is concerning the side effects of the diet. Is it really necessary to overconsume protein, fat, saturated fat, and cholesterol to obtain weight loss? When evaluating more than 10,000 dieting individuals, researchers found those following a *high carbohydrate* diet had the *lowest* body mass index (BMI:weight for height measurement) and those on a low-carbohydrate/*high-protein* diet had the *highest* BMI.§ Thereby, indicating that the key to weight loss is not found in the high-protein, high-fat diet.

In a statement for health care professionals from the Nutrition Committee of the Council on Nutrition, Physical Activity, and Metabolism of the American Heart Association researchers concluded that "high-protein diets are not recommended because they restrict healthful foods that provide essential nutrients and do not provide the variety of foods needed to adequately meet nutritional needs."‡

*Economic Research Service, U.S. Department of Agriculture, Briefing Room: Diet and health: food consumption and nutrient intake tables, Washington, DC, (accessed November 2002), ERS/USDA [*http://www.ers.usda.gov/briefing/DietAndHealth/data/nutrients/*].
†Serdula MK and others: Prevalence of attempting weight loss and strategies for controlling weight, *JAMA* 282:1353, 1999.
‡Sachiko T and others: Dietary protein and weight reduction, *Circulation* 104(15):1869, 2001.
§Kennedy ET and others: Popular diets: correlation to health, nutrition, and obesity, *J Am Diet Assoc* 101(4):411, 2001.

Excess Dietary Intake

Contrary to popular belief (at least in some recent fad diets in the United States), there is such a thing as too much dietary protein. (See the Further Focus box, "The Precious Price of a High-Protein Diet"). The body has a finite need for protein. In other words, once a person has met the dietary protein needs, additional protein is deaminated (the nitrogen is removed) and stored as fat or used as energy. Eating excess protein does not build muscle. Only exercising with enough protein to support growth can do that. The main problems with diets heavily laden with protein are:

1. They usually are also high in saturated fats—a known risk for cardiovascular disease.
2. If a person fills up on protein foods, there may be little room for fruits, vegetables, and other whole grains.
3. The kidneys have to work overtime to rid the body of excess nitrogen.
4. Excess protein increases calcium losses in the bone when dietary calcium is inadequate.

Although most protein and amino acid supplements are not harmful, they are unnecessary in a balanced diet.

Dietary Guides

Dietary Reference Intakes and Recommended Dietary Allowances

The Recommended Dietary Allowances (RDAs) continue to be the principal dietary guide for protein consumption and are part of the Dietary Reference Intakes (DRIs) standards. Similar to carbohydrate and fat recommendations, the National Academy of Sciences has set the DRIs for proteins as a percentage of the total kcalorie consumption. Children and adults should get 10% to 35% of their total caloric intake from protein. The RDA standards relate to the age, sex, and weight of the "average" person and are based on analysis of available nitrogen balance studies. Protein RDAs are highest at birth and slowly decline into adulthood. The RDA for both men and women is set at 0.8 g of high-quality protein per kg of desirable body weight per day (0.8 g/kg body weight per day).[10] Needs are higher for infants, pregnant and breastfeeding women, and potentially for vegans.

To calculate the protein needs of an individual consuming 2200 kcal per day based on the DRI recommendation of 10% to 35% of total kcalories, perform the following calculations:

(1) 2200 kcal × 0.10 − 0.35 = 220 − 770 kcal per day from protein
(2) 220 − 770 kcal ÷ 4 kcal/g = 55 − 192.5 g of protein per day

To calculate the protein needs of a female who is 5'4" with an ideal body weight (see Chapter 15) of 120 lbs, based on the RDA of 0.8 g protein/kg body weight per day, perform the following calculations:

(1) Convert weight in pounds to weight in kg (2.2 lbs = 1 kg), as follows:
    120 lbs ÷ 2.2 lb/kg = 54.5 kg
(2) 54.5 kg × 0.8 g/kg = 43.6 g protein per day

Therefore a 5'4" female consuming 2200 kcal per day with a minimum of 10% of her calories coming from high-quality protein will exceed her RDA for protein (43.6 g per day). It should be noted that the RDAs are set to meet the nutritional requirements of most healthy people. Severe physical stress, such as illness, disease, and surgery can increase one's needs for protein.

Dietary Guidelines for Americans

There are no known benefits in the consumption of a diet with a high animal protein content, which also carries added fat. However, there are some potential health risks. These risks relate to certain cancers, coronary heart disease associated with increased animal fat, urinary calcium loss and kidney stones, as well as chronic renal failure (see Chapter 21) associated with the increased protein. Therefore the *Dietary Guidelines for Americans* recommend that individuals choose foods from each of the five food groups according to the Food Guide Pyramid, consuming moderate amounts of foods from the meat and bean group. Moderate amounts equal two to three servings per day.

Americans generally eat more protein than necessary, especially in the form of meat, which carries considerable animal fat. Cutting down consumption of meat to leaner moderate portions would also bring the health benefits of reducing the intake of saturated animal fat. Table 4-3 provides a comparison of protein food portions.

TABLE 4–3	Foods High in Protein	
Food	**Approximate amount**	**Protein (g)**
Beef, cube steak	4 oz cooked	27.6
Chicken, fryer	½ breast (4 oz raw)	26.9
Chicken, hen, stewed	1 thigh or ½ breast	26.5
Veal, leg or shoulder	3 oz cooked	25.2
Turkey	3 oz cooked	24.9
Beef, round	3 oz cooked	24.7
Goose, roasted	3 oz cooked	24.6
Scallops	5-6 medium	23.8
Beef, chuck roast	3 oz cooked	23.4
Chicken	¼ broiler	22.4
Lamb leg	3 oz cooked	21.6
Tuna	3 oz cooked	21.6
Halibut	3 oz cooked	21
Ham	3 oz cooked	20.7
Pork loin	3 oz cooked	20.7
Beef, hamburger	3 oz cooked	20.5
Salmon	⅔ cup	20.5
Liver (beef, calf, or pork)	3 oz cooked	20.4
Haddock	3 oz cooked	20.2
Duck, roasted	3 oz cooked	20
Soy burger	1 patty	18
Lentils	1 cup	17.8
Kidney beans	1 cup	15.3
Oysters	6 medium	15.1
Cottage cheese	4 oz	14
Yogurt	1 cup	14
Roasted soynuts	3 Tbsp	10
Tofu	½ cup	10
Milk	1 cup	8.5
Peanut butter	2 Tbsp	8
American cheddar cheese	1 oz	7
Soy milk	1 cup	6.7
Egg	1 medium	6.3

SUMMARY

Proteins provide the human body with its primary tissue-building units, amino acids. Of the 20 common amino acids, nine are indispensable in the diet because the body cannot manufacture them as it can the remaining 11. Foods that supply all the indispensable amino acids are called complete proteins. These foods are mostly of animal origin (e.g., egg, milk, cheese, and meat). Plant protein foods (e.g., grains, legumes, nuts, seeds, vegetables, and fruits) are considered incomplete proteins because they lack one or more of the indispensable amino acids. The exception is soy protein, which is of plant origin and provides complete proteins. Strict vegan diets use only plant proteins; but other vegetarian diets may include dairy, egg, and sometimes fish.

Constant turnover of tissue protein occurs between tissue building (anabolism) and tissue breakdown (catabolism). Adequate dietary protein and a reserve "pool" of amino acids help to maintain this overall protein balance. Nitrogen balance is a measure of overall protein balance. A mixed diet of a variety of foods, together with sufficient nonprotein kcalories from the primary fuel foods, supplies a balance of protein and other nutrients. Only strict vegetarians (vegans) risk protein imbalance and other nutritional deficiencies in iron, zinc, calcium, and vitamin B$_{12}$.

After protein foods are eaten, a powerful digestive team of six protein-splitting enzymes frees individual unique amino acids for their vital tissue-building tasks.

Protein requirements are influenced mainly by growth needs and the nature of the diet in terms of protein quality and energy intake. Clinical influences on protein needs include fever, disease, surgery, or other trauma to body tissues.

CRITICAL THINKING QUESTIONS

1. What is the difference between indispensable and dispensable amino acids? Why is this difference important?
2. Compare complete and incomplete protein foods. Give examples of each.
3. Describe the different types of vegetarian diets. Compare each in terms of protein quality and risk for nutrient deficiencies.
4. Describe the factors that influence protein requirements.

CHAPTER CHALLENGE QUESTIONS

True-False

Write the correct statement for each item you answer "false."

1. *True or False:* Complete proteins of high biological value are found in whole grains, dried beans and peas, and nuts.
2. *True or False:* The primary function of dietary protein is to supply the necessary amino acids to build and repair body tissue.
3. *True or False:* Protein provides a main source of body heat and muscle energy.
4. *True or False:* The average American diet contains a relatively small amount of protein.
5. *True or False:* Because they are smaller, infants and young children need less protein per unit of body weight than adults.
6. *True or False:* In old age the protein requirement decreases because of decreased physical activity.
7. *True or False:* Healthy adults are in a state of nitrogen balance.
8. *True or False:* Positive nitrogen balance exists during periods of rapid growth (e.g., in infancy and adolescence).
9. *True or False:* When negative nitrogen balance exists, an individual is less able to resist infection and general health deteriorates.
10. *True or False:* Egg protein has a higher biological value than meat protein.

Multiple Choice

1. Nine of the 20 amino acids are "indispensable," meaning that
   a. the body cannot make them and must get them in the diet.
   b. they are indispensable in body processes and the rest are not.
   c. the body makes them because they are the life-essential ones.
   d. after making them, the body uses them for growth.

2. A complete protein food of high biological value contains
   a. all 20 of the amino acids in sufficient amounts to meet human requirements.
   b. the nine indispensable amino acids in any proportion because the body can always fill in the necessary differences.
   c. all of the 20 amino acids from which the body can make additional amounts of the nine indispensable ones, as necessary.
   d. all nine of the indispensable amino acids in correct proportion to meet human requirements.

3. A state of negative nitrogen balance occurs during periods of
   a. pregnancy.
   b. adolescence.
   c. injury or surgery.
   d. infancy.

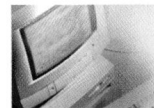

Please refer to the Students' Resource section of this text's Evolve web site for "Suggestions for Additional Study."

REFERENCES

1. Cordes MHJ and others: Evolution of a protein fold in vitro, *Science* 284(5412; Apr 9):325, 1999.
2. Peterson J: Simulations nab protein-folding mistakes, *Science News* 155(Mar 6):150, 1999.
3. Barinaga M: New clues to how proteins link up to run the cell, *Science* 283(Feb 26):1247, 1999.
4. Mangels AR, Messina V, Melina V: Position of the American Dietetic Association and Dietitians of Canada: vegetarian diets, *J Am Diet Assoc* 103(6):748, 2003.
5. Larsson CL, Johansson GK: Dietary intake and nutritional status of young vegans and omnivores in Sweden. *Am J Clin Nutr* 76(1):100, 2002.
6. Donaldson MS: Metabolic vitamin B_{12} status on mostly raw vegan diet with follow-up using tablets, nutritional yeast, or probiotic supplements, *Ann Nutr Metab* 44:229, 2000.
7. Caso G and others: Albumin synthesis is diminished in men consuming a predominantly vegetarian diet, *J Nutr* 130:528, 2000.
8. Ball MJ, Bartlett MA: Dietary intake and iron status of Australian vegetarian women, *Am J Clin Nutr* 70(3):353, 1999.
9. Segasothy M and Phillips PA: Vegetarian diet: panacea for modern lifestyle diseases? *J Med* 92:531, 1999.
10. Food and Nutrition Board, Institute of Medicine: *Dietary reference intakes for energy, carbohydrate, fiber, fat, fatty acids, cholesterol, protein, and amino acids*, Washington, DC, 2002, National Academies Press.

FURTHER READING AND RESOURCES

- Food and Nutrition Information Center: *www.nal.usda.gov/fnic/etext/000058.html*
- North American Vegetarian Society: *www.navs-online.org/*
- Vegetarian Resource Group: *www.vrg.org/*
- Vegetarian Nutrition Dietetic Practice Group: *www.vegetariannutrition.net/*

   The preceding organizations provide a good source of information about vegetarian diets.

- Messina V and others: A new food guide for North American vegetarians, *J Am Diet Assoc* 103(6):771, 2003.

   The authors design and explain a new Food Guide Pyramid appropriate for vegetarians. This article reviews the nutrient needs from each food group and the best sources for achieving nutritional balance. A great resource for vegetarians.

- Lemon PW: Beyond the zone: protein needs of active individuals. *J Am Coll Nutr* 19(5 suppl):513S, 2000.

   Lemon explores the controversy surrounding the protein needs of athletes. Are protein supplements warranted? He also examines the factors affecting dietary protein needs.

5

Digestion, Absorption, and Metabolism

As described in previous chapters, nutrients the body requires do not come ready to use, but rather packaged as foods in a variety of forms. Body cells cannot use nutrients in these forms, so whole food must be changed to simpler substances. In this process, bodies must also free the food nutrients and re-form and reroute them to meet special life needs.

This chapter explains how this marvelous process of change takes place, and views the overall process of food digestion and nutrient absorption as one continuous whole made up of a series of successive events. Throughout this chapter, the unique body structures and functions that make this process—and life—possible are reviewed.

KEY CONCEPTS

- Through a balanced system of mechanical and chemical change, food is broken down into simpler substances and the food's nutrients are released and re-formed for the body's use.

- Special organ structures and functions conduct these changes through the successive parts of the overall system.

DIGESTION

Basic Principles

Principle of Change

Body cells cannot use food as it is eaten. Food must be changed into simpler substances to be absorbed and then into other, even simpler, substances that cells can use to sustain life. Preparing food for the body's use involves many steps that make up the overall process of digestion, absorption, transport, and metabolism.

Digestion is the process in which food is broken down in the gastrointestinal tract, releasing many nutrients in forms the body can use.

Absorption is the process in which these nutrients are taken into the cells lining the gastrointestinal tract.

Transport is the movement of nutrients through the circulatory system from one area of the body to another.

Cell metabolism is the sum of the vast number of chemical changes in the cell, the functional unit of life, which finally produces the essential materials necessary for energy, tissue building, and metabolic controls.

Principle of Wholeness

The parts of this overall process of change do not exist separately but make up one continuous whole. The different parts of the gastrointestinal tract and their relative positions within the body are shown in Figure 5-1. Food components travel through this system until ultimately they are delivered to the cells or excreted as waste.

Mechanical and Chemical Changes

For nutrients to be delivered to cells, food must go through a series of mechanical and chemical changes. Together, these two types of actions make up the overall process of digestion.

The specific mechanical and chemical actions that occur during digestion of carbohydrates, proteins, and fats have been discussed in their respective chapters within this text. This chapter touches on those actions as a whole and as an interdependent process.

Mechanical Digestion: Gastrointestinal Motility

Beginning in the mouth, muscles and nerves in the walls of the gastrointestinal tract coordinate their actions to provide the necessary motility for digestion to proceed. The word motility means the ability to move spontaneously. This automatic response to the presence of food enables the system to break up the food mass and move it along the digestive pathway at the best rate. Muscles and nerves work together to produce this smoothly running motility.

Muscles. The layers of smooth muscle composing the gastrointestinal wall interact to provide two general types of movement, as follows: (1) muscle tone or tonic contraction, which ensures continuous passage of the food mass and valve control along the way; and (2) periodic muscle contraction and relaxation, which are rhythmical waves that mix the food mass and move it forward. These alternating muscular contractions and relaxations that force the contents forward are known as peristalsis, a term from two Greek words: peri, meaning "around," and stalsis, meaning "contraction."

Nerves. Specific nerves regulate muscle action along the gastrointestinal tract. A complex network of nerves in the gastrointestinal wall extends from the esophagus to the anus. This network is called the intramural nerve plexus. These nerves do three things: (1) control muscle tone in the wall, (2) regulate the rate and intensity of the alternating muscle contractions, and (3) coordinate all of the various movements. When all is well, these many, finely tuned movements flow together like those of a great symphony, and people are unaware of them. But when all is not well, the discord is felt as pain. Such problems and diseases with the gastrointestinal tract are discussed in Chapter 18.

Chemical Digestion: Gastrointestinal Secretions

A number of secretions work together to make chemical digestion possible. There are generally five types of substances involved: the basic enzymes that break down food and four other substances that help these enzymes do their specific jobs.

Enzymes. Digestive enzymes are proteins, specific in kind and quantity for breaking down specific nutrients.

Hydrochloric Acid and Buffer Ions. Hydrochloric acid and buffer ions are needed to produce the correct pH (e.g., degree of acidity or alkalinity) necessary for enzyme activity.

Mucus. Secretions of mucus lubricate and protect the mucosal tissues lining the gastrointestinal tract, as well as help to mix the food mass.

Water and Electrolytes. The products of digestion are carried and circulated through the tract and into the tissues by water and electrolytes.

Bile. Made in the liver and stored in the gallbladder, bile divides fat into smaller pieces to expose more surface area for the actions of fat enzymes.

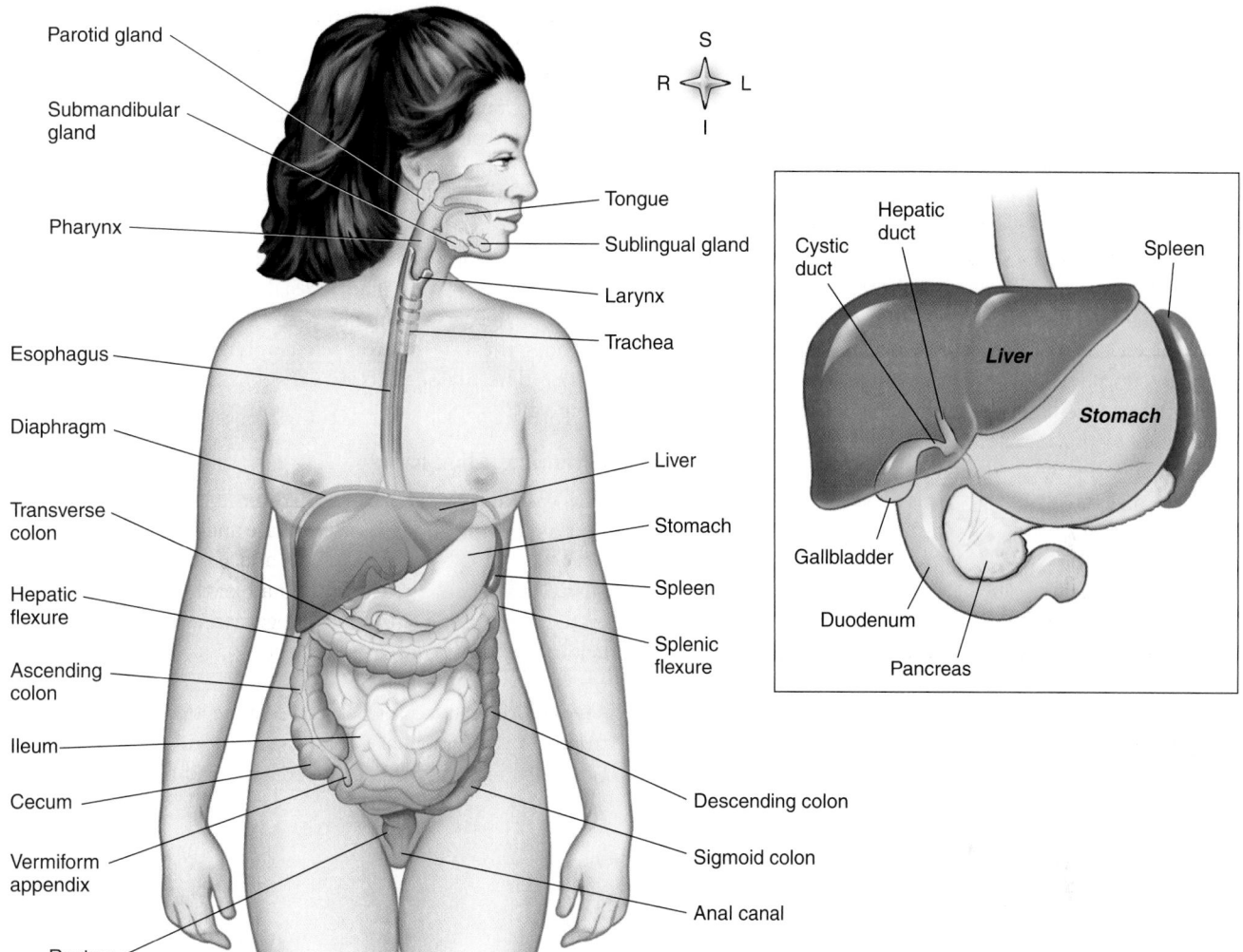

Figure 5–1   The gastrointestinal system. Through the successive parts of the system, multiple activities of digestion liberate and re-form food nutrients for our use. (From Thibodeau GA, Patton KT: *Anatomy and physiology,* ed 5, St Louis, 2003, Mosby.)

Secretory cells in the intestinal tract and nearby accessory organs (e.g., pancreas and liver) produce each of the preceding substances for specific jobs in chemical digestion. The secretory action of these cells or glands is stimulated by the following: (1) the presence of food, (2) nerve impulse, or (3) hormones specific for certain nutrients.

Digestion in the Mouth and Esophagus

Mechanical Digestion

In the mouth, the process of *mastication* (e.g., biting and chewing) begins to break down food into smaller particles. The teeth and oral structure are particularly suited for this

work. After the food is chewed, the mixed mass of food particles is swallowed and passes down the esophagus largely by peristaltic waves controlled by nerve reflexes. Muscles at the base of the tongue facilitate the swallowing process. Then, if the body is in the upright position, gravity aids the movement of food down the esophagus. At the entrance to the stomach, the gastroesophageal sphincter muscle relaxes to allow the food to enter, then constricts again to retain the food within the stomach cavity. If the sphincter is not working properly, it may allow acid-mixed food to seep back into the esophagus. The result is a discomforting feeling of heartburn.

Heartburn has nothing to do with the heart but has been called this because sensations are perceived as originating in the region of the heart. A hiatal hernia is another common cause of heartburn. This occurs when part of the stomach protrudes upward into the chest cavity (thorax).

Chemical Digestion

The salivary glands secrete material containing salivary amylase, also called *ptyalin*. *Amylase* is the general name for any starch-splitting enzyme. Small glands at the back of the tongue (Ebner's glands) secrete a *lingual lipase*. *Lipase* is the general name for any fat-splitting enzyme, but in this case the food does not remain in the mouth long enough for much chemical action to occur. The salivary glands also secrete a mucous material that lubricates and binds food particles to facilitate the swallowing of each food *bolus*, or lump of food material. Mucous glands also line the esophagus, and their secretions help move the food mass toward the stomach.

Digestion in the Stomach

Mechanical Digestion

Under sphincter muscle control from the esophagus, which joins the stomach at the cardiac notch, the food enters the *fundus*, the upper portion of the stomach, in individual bolus lumps as swallowed. In the body of the stomach, muscles gradually knead, store, mix, and propel the food mass forward in slow, controlled move-

ments. By the time the food mass reaches the *antrum*, the lower portion of the stomach, it is now a semi-liquid, acid-food mix called chyme. A constricting sphincter muscle at the end of the stomach, the *pyloric valve*, controls the flow at this point. This valve releases the acidic chyme slowly so that it can be quickly buffered by the alkaline intestinal secretions and not irritate the mucosal lining of the *duodenum*, which is the first section of the small intestine. The caloric density of a meal, which mainly results from its fat component, not just its volume or particular composition, influences the rate of stomach emptying at the pyloric valve.[1] The major parts of the stomach are shown in Figure 5-2.

Chemical Digestion

The gastric secretions contain three types of materials that aid chemical digestion in the stomach.

Acid. Parietal cells, within the lining of the stomach, secrete hydrochloric acid to create the necessary degree of acidity for gastric enzymes to work.

Mucus. Mucous secretions protect the stomach lining from the erosive effect of the hydrochloric acid. Secretions also bind and mix the food mass and help move it along.

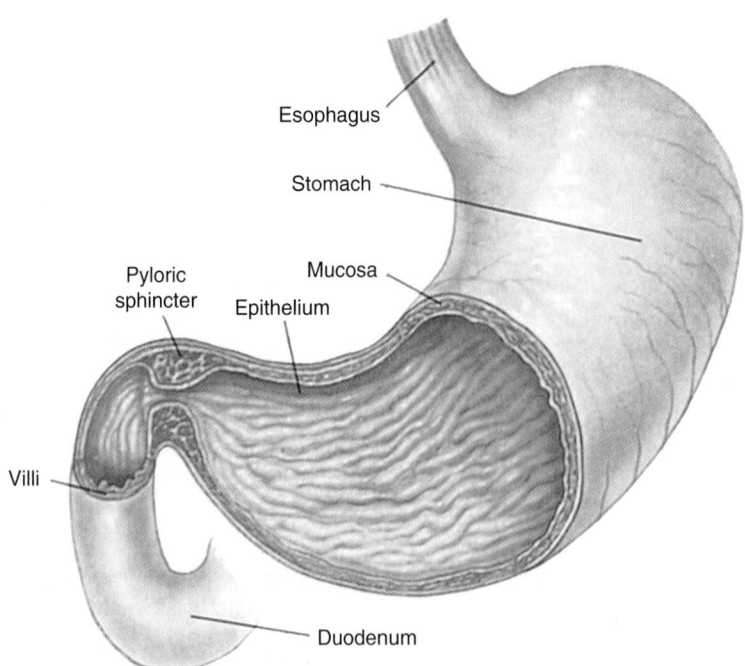

Figure 5-2   Stomach. (Credit: Bill Ober, from Raven PH, Johnson GB: *Biology*, ed 3, New York, 1992, McGraw-Hill.)

Enzymes. The inactive enzyme *pepsinogen* is secreted by stomach cells and is activated by the hydrochloric acid to become the protein-splitting enzyme **pepsin.** Other cells produce small amounts of a specific gastric lipase called *tributyrinase* because it works on tributyrin (butterfat), but this is a relatively minor activity in the stomach.

Various sensations, emotions, and foods stimulate nerve impulses that trigger these secretions. It is not without reason that the stomach is said to "mirror the person within." For example, anger and hostility increase secretions. Fear and depression decrease secretions, as well as inhibit blood flow and motility. Additional hormonal stimulus occurs when food enters the stomach.

Digestion in the Small Intestine

Up to this point, digestion of food has been largely mechanical, delivering a semifluid mixture of fine food particles and watery secretions to the small intestine. Chemical digestion has been minimal. Thus the major task of digestion, and the absorption that follows, occurs in the small intestine. The structural parts, synchronized movements, and array of specific enzymes of the small intestine are highly developed for the final task of mechanical and chemical digestion.

Mechanical Digestion

Under the control of nerve impulses, walls stretch from the food mass or hormonal stimuli, and the intestinal muscles produce several types of movement that aid digestion, as follow:[2]

- *Peristaltic waves* slowly push the food mass forward, sometimes with long, sweeping waves over the entire length of the intestine.
- *Pendular movements* from small, local muscles sweep back and forth, stirring the chyme at the mucosal surface.
- *Segmentation rings* from the alternating contraction and relaxation of circular muscles progressively chop the food mass into successive soft lumps and mix them with secretions.
- *Longitudinal rotation,* by long muscles running the length of the intestine, rolls the slowly moving food mass in a spiral motion, mixing it and exposing new surfaces for absorption.
- *Surface villi motions* stir and mix the chyme at the intestinal wall, exposing additional nutrients for absorption.

Chemical Digestion

The small intestines, together with the gastrointestinal accessory organs (pancreas, liver, and gallbladder) supply many secretory materials to meet the major burden of chemical digestion. The pancreas and intestines secrete enzymes specific for the digestion of carbohydrates, proteins, and fat.

Pancreatic Enzymes

1. *Carbohydrate:* **Pancreatic amylase** converts starch to the disaccharides maltose and sucrose.
2. *Protein:* **Trypsin** and **chymotrypsin** split large protein molecules into smaller and smaller peptide fragments, and finally into single amino acids. **Carboxypeptidase** removes end amino acids from peptide chains.
3. *Fat:* **Pancreatic lipase** converts fat to glycerides and fatty acids.

salivary amylase (Gr. *amylon,* starch) a starch-splitting enzyme in the mouth, commonly called *ptyalin* (Gr. *ptyalon,* spittle) that is secreted by the salivary glands.

chyme (Gr. *chymos,* juice) semifluid food mass in the gastrointestinal tract following gastric digestion.

pepsin (Gr. *pepsis,* digestion) the main gastric enzyme specific for proteins. Pepsin begins breaking large protein molecules into shorter chain polypeptides; gastric hydrochloric acid is necessary to activate.

pancreatic amylase major starch-splitting enzyme that is secreted by the pancreas and acts in the small intestine.

trypsin (Gr. *trypein,* to rub; *pepsis,* digestion) a protein-splitting enzyme formed in the small intestine by action of enterokinase on the inactive precursor trypsinogen.

chymotrypsin (Gr. *chymos,* semifluid food mass from digestion; *trypein,* enzyme trypsin) one of the protein-splitting and milk-curdling pancreatic enzymes activated in the small intestine from the precursor chymotrypsinogen; breaks specific amino acid peptide links of protein.

carboxypeptidase (L. *carbo-,* carbon; *oxy,* oxygen) a protein enzyme that splits off the chemical group carboxyl (–COOH) at the end of peptide chains.

pancreatic lipase (Gr. *lipos,* fat) a major fat-splitting enzyme produced by the pancreas and secreted into the small intestine to digest fat.

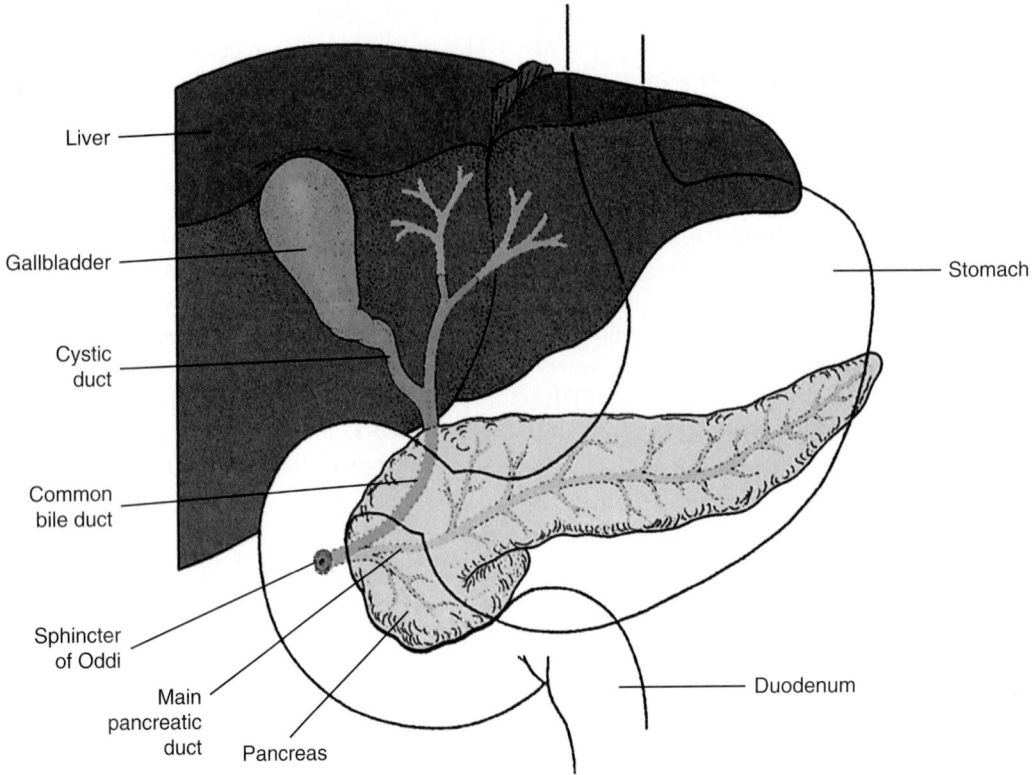

Figure 5–3   Organs of the biliary system and the pancreatic ducts.

BOX 5–1 Functions of the Liver

Major Functions

Bile production (for fat digestion)
Synthesis of proteins and blood clotting factors
Metabolism of hormones and medications
Regulation of blood glucose levels
Urea production (to remove waste products of normal
   metabolism)

**Specific Metabolic Functions
of the Energy-Yielding Nutrients**

Lipolysis: breaking down lipids to fatty acids and glycerol
Lipogenesis: building up of fatty acids and glycerol to lipids
Glycolysis: breaking down glucose to pyruvate to enter the
   tricarboxylic acid cycle (TCA) cycle
Gluconeogenesis: converting noncarbohydrate substances into
   glucose
Glycogenolysis: breaking down glycogen to individual glucose
   units
Glycogenesis: combining glucose to store as glycogen
Protein degradation: breaking down proteins to single amino acids
Protein synthesis: building complete proteins from individual
   amino acids

Intestinal Enzymes

1. *Carbohydrate:* Disaccharidases (e.g., maltase, lactase,
   and sucrase) convert their respective disaccharides
   (e.g., maltose, lactose, sucrose) to monosaccharides
   (e.g., glucose, fructose, and galactose). A large percent of the world's population does not actually produce enough lactase to digest lactose (milk sugar).
   As a result, these individuals cannot tolerate milk
   and milk products well, unless they are in some
   "predigested" form (e.g., yogurt, buttermilk, aged
   cheese, or lactase-treated milk).[3] Lactose-affected
   individuals also can take commercially available oral
   lactase capsules to help with digestion.
2. *Protein:* The intestinal enzyme enterokinase activates trypsinogen (from the pancreas) to become the
   protein-splitting enzyme trypsin. Amino peptidase removes end amino acids from polypeptides. Dipeptidase
   splits dipeptides into their two remaining amino acids.
3. *Fat:* Intestinal lipase splits fat into glycerides and
   fatty acids.

Mucus. Large quantities of mucus, secreted by intestinal
glands, protect the mucosal lining from irritation and
erosion caused by the highly acidic gastric contents entering the duodenum.

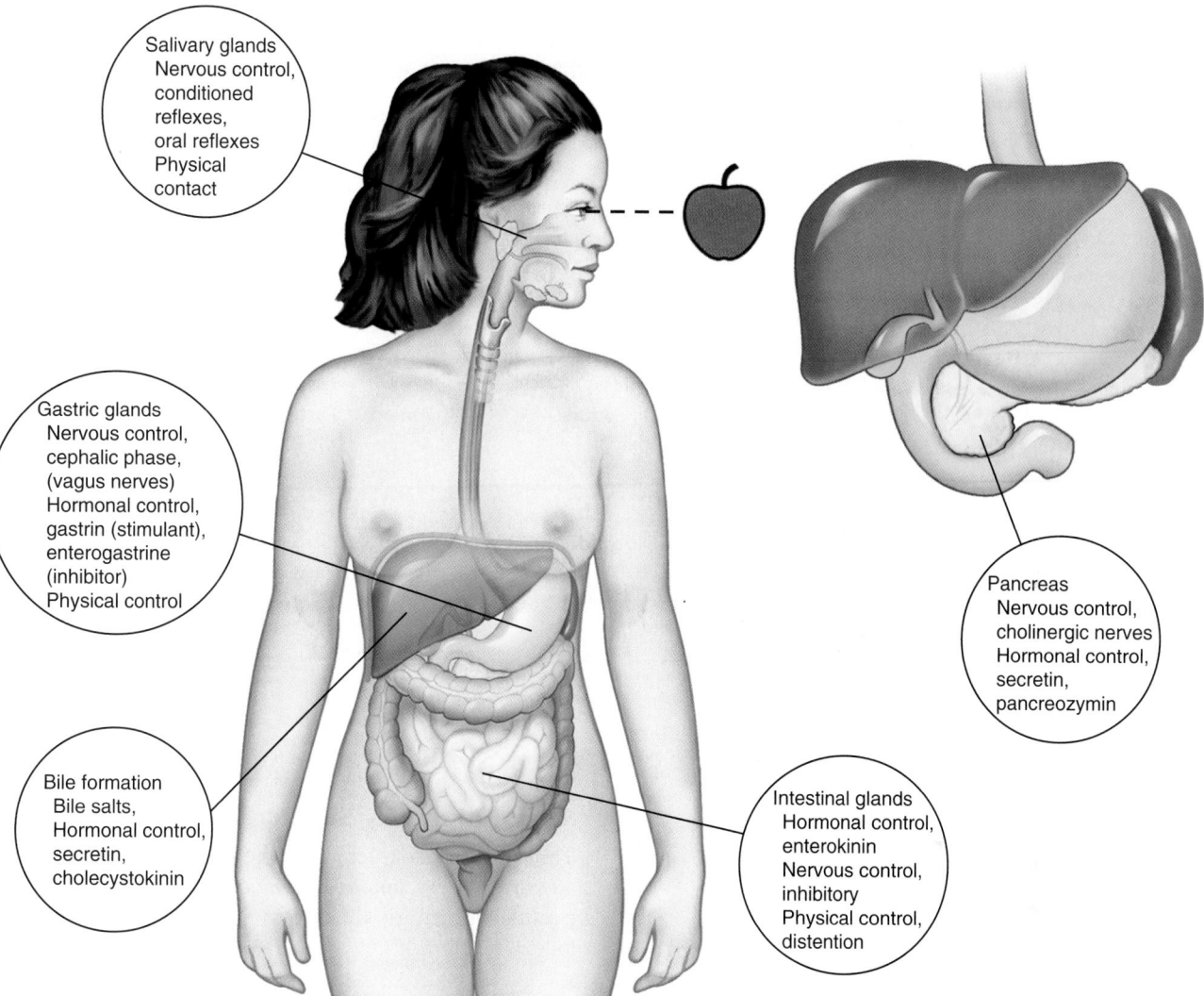

Figure 5–4   Summary of the factors influencing secretions of the gastrointestinal tract. (Illustration from Thibodeau GA, Patton KT: *Anatomy and physiology*, ed 5, St Louis, 2003, Mosby. Apple by Eileen Draper.)

Bile. The emulsifying agent bile is an important aid to fat digestion and absorption. Bile is produced by the liver and stored in the adjacent gallbladder, ready for use when fat enters the intestine.

Hormones. The hormone *secretin*, which is produced by the mucosal glands in the first part of the intestine, controls the acidity and secretion of enzymes from the pancreas. The resulting alkaline environment in the small intestine, pH 8, is necessary for the activity of the pancreatic enzymes. The hormone *cholecystokinin*, which is secreted by intestinal mucosal glands when fat is present, triggers release of bile from the gallbladder to emulsify the fat.

The arrangement of the accessory organs to the duodenum, the first section of the small intestine, is shown in Figure 5-3. These organs compose the biliary system and have vital roles in digestion and metabolism. The liver is sometimes called the "metabolic capital" of the body because it has numerous functions in the metabolism of all the converging nutrients (Box 5-1). The liver's many metabolic functions are reviewed in greater detail in Chapter 18.

The various nerve and hormone controls of digestion are illustrated in Figure 5-4. Although small individual summaries of digestion are given in each of the major nutrient chapters, a general summary of the entire digestive processes is given in Table 5-1 so that the

TABLE 5–1	Summary of Digestive Processes	
Carbohydrate	**Protein**	**Fat**
MOUTH		
Starch $\xrightarrow{\text{Salivary amylase}}$ Dextrins		Fat $\xrightarrow[\text{(limited)}]{\text{Lipase}}$ Glycerides
STOMACH		
	Protein $\xrightarrow{\text{Pepsin}_{\text{Hydrochloric acid}}}$ Polypeptides	Tributyrin (butterfat) $\xrightarrow[\text{(limited)}]{\text{Tributyrinase}}$ Glycerol Fatty acids
SMALL INTESTINE		
Pancreas	*Pancreas*	*Pancreas*
(Disaccharides)	Protein, Polypeptides $\xrightarrow{\text{Trypsin}}$ Dipeptides	Fat $\xrightarrow{\text{Lipase}}$ Glycerol
Starch $\xrightarrow{\text{Amylase}}$ Maltose and sucrose	Protein, Polypeptides $\xrightarrow{\text{Chymotrypsin}}$ Dipeptides	Glycerides ⎤ (di-, mono-)
	Polypeptides, Dipeptides $\xrightarrow{\text{Carboxypeptidase}}$ Amino acids	Fatty acids ⎦
Intestine	*Intestine*	*Intestine*
(Monosaccharides)		Fat $\xrightarrow{\text{Lipase}}$ Glycerol
Lactose $\xrightarrow{\text{Lactase}}$ Glucose and galactose	Polypeptides, Dipeptides $\xrightarrow{\text{Aminopeptidase}}$ Amino acids	Glycerides ⎤ (di-, mono-)
Sucrose $\xrightarrow{\text{Sucrase}}$ Glucose and fructose		Fatty acids ⎦
Maltose $\xrightarrow{\text{Maltase}}$ Glucose and glucose	Dipeptides $\xrightarrow{\text{Dipeptidase}}$ Amino acids	*Liver and gallbladder* Fat $\xrightarrow{\text{Bile}}$ Emulsified fat

overall process can be viewed as it is, one continuous, integrated *whole*.

ABSORPTION AND TRANSPORT

When digestion is complete, food has been changed into simple end products that are ready for cell use. Carbohydrate foods are reduced to the *simple sugars* glucose, fructose, and galactose. Fats are transformed into *fatty acids* and *glycerides*. Protein foods are changed to single *amino acids* (see Table 5-1). Vitamins and minerals also are liberated. With a water base for solution and transport, in addition to the necessary electrolytes, the whole fluid food-derived mass is now prepared for absorption as part of the large "gastrointestinal circulation." For many nutrients, especially certain vitamins and minerals, the point of absorption becomes the vital "gatekeeper" that determines how much of a given nutrient is kept for body use. Although the gastrointestinal tract is very efficient, 100% of all the nutrients consumed are not absorbed because of varying degrees of *bioavailability*. A nutrient's bioavailability is dependent on: (1) the amount of nutrient present in the gastrointestinal tract, (2) competition between nutrients for common absorptive sites, and (3) the form in which the nutrient is present. This degree of bioavailability is a factor in setting dietary intake standards.[4-6]

Absorption in the Small Intestine

Special Absorbing Structures

Three important structures of the intestinal wall surface are particularly adapted to ensure maximum absorption of essential nutrients in the digestive process (Figure 5-5), as follow:

■ *Mucosal folds:* Like the hills and valleys of a mountain range, the surface of the small intestine piles into many folds. **Mucosal folds** can easily be seen when such tissue is examined.
■ *Villi:* Closer examination under a regular light microscope reveals small, fingerlike projections, the **villi,** covering the piled-up folds of mucosal lining. These little villi further increase the area of exposed surface. Each villus has an ample supply of blood vessels to receive protein and carbohydrate materials, as well as a special lymph vessel to receive fat materials. This lymph vessel is called a *lacteal* because the fatty chyme is creamy at this point and looks like milk.
■ *Microvilli:* Even closer examination with an electron microscope reveals a multiple covering of smaller projections on the surface of each tiny villus. The covering of **microvilli** on each villus is called a *brush border* because it looks like bristles on a brush.

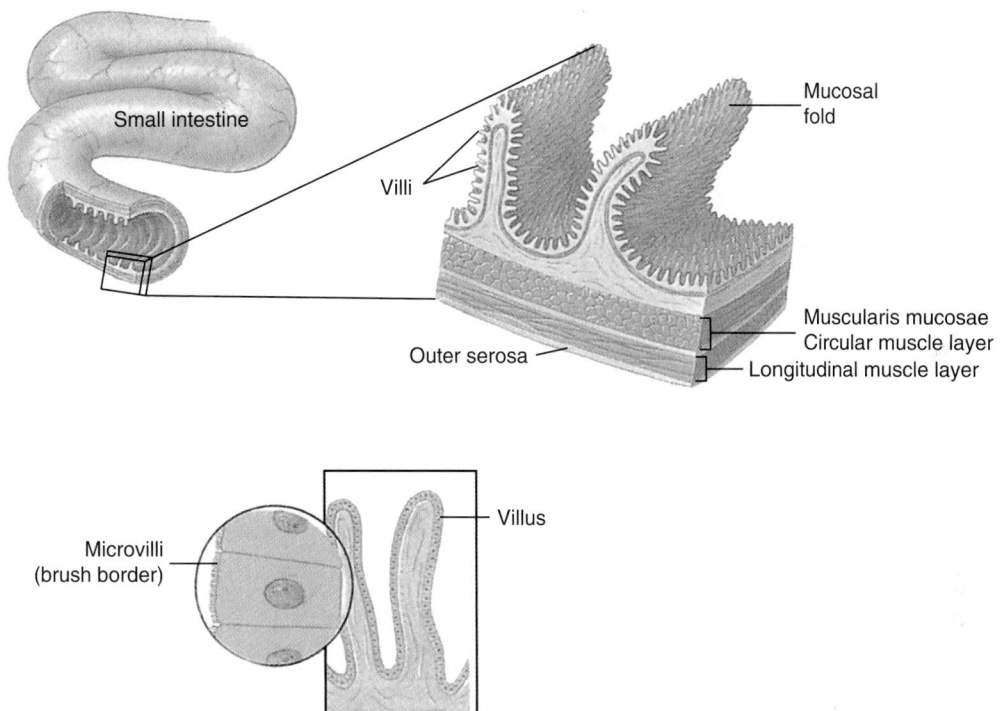

Figure 5–5   Intestinal wall. Note the arrangement of muscle layers and the structures of the mucosa that increase the surface area for absorption: mucosal folds, villi, and microvilli. (Credit: Medical and Scientific Illustration.)

These three unique structures of the inner intestinal wall—folds, villi, and microvilli—combine to make the inner surface some 600 times the area of the outer surface of the intestine. The length of the small intestine is about 660 cm (22 feet). This remarkable organ is well-adapted to deliver its precious nutrients into circulation to the body cells. In fact, the small intestine can scarcely be equaled in its feat of providing such an absorbing surface area in so compact a space. It has been estimated that if its entire surface were spread out on a flat plane, the total surface area would be as large as half a basket-ball court. Far from being the lowly "gut," the small intestine is actually one of the most highly developed, exquisitely fashioned, specialized tissues in the human body.

Absorption Processes

A number of absorbing processes complete the task of moving vital nutrients across the inner intestinal wall and into body circulation. These processes include diffusion, energy-driven active transport, and pinocytosis (Figure 5-6), as follows:

■ *Simple diffusion:* The force by which particles move outward in all directions from an area of greater concentration to an area of lesser concentration. Small materials that do not need the help of a specific protein channel to move across the mucosal cell wall use this method.

■ *Facilitated diffusion:* Similar to simple diffusion but uses a protein channel for carrier-assisted movement of larger items across the mucosal cell wall.

mucosal folds   (L. *mucus,* mucosa) large visible folds of the mucous lining of the small intestine that increase the absorbing surface area.

villi   (L. *villus,* tuft of hair) small protrusions from the surface of a membrane; fingerlike projections covering mucosal surfaces of the small intestine that further increases the absorbing surface area; visible through a regular microscope.

microvilli   (Gr. *mikros,* small; L. *villus,* tuft of hair) exceedingly small hairlike projections covering all villi on the surface of the small intestine and greatly extending the total absorbing surface area; visible through electron microscope.

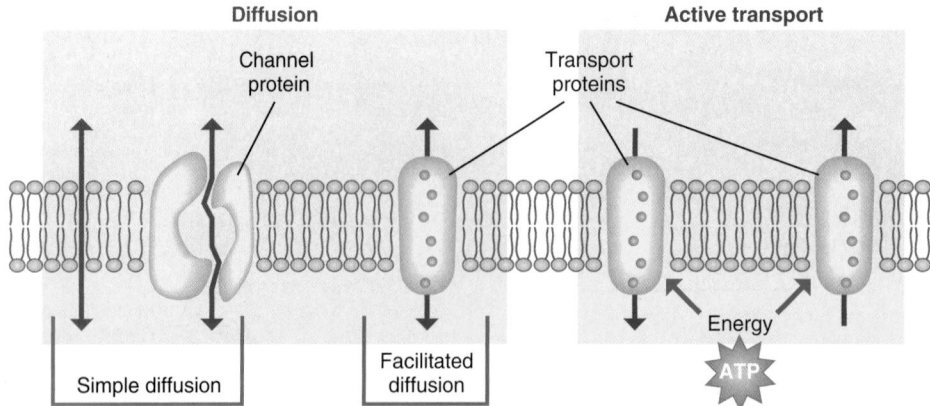

Figure 5–6   Diagram illustrating transport pathways through the cell membrane. (From Mahan LK, Escott-Stump S: *Krause's food, nutrition, & diet therapy,* ed 11, Philadelphia, 2004, Saunders.)

- *Active transport:* The force by which particles move from an area of greater concentration to an area of lesser concentration. Such active transport mechanisms usually require some sort of carrier partner to help "ferry" the particles across the membrane. For example, glucose enters absorbing cells through an active transport mechanism involving sodium (Na^+) as a "ferrying" partner.
- *Pinocytosis:* Penetration of larger materials by attaching to the thicker cell membrane and being engulfed by the cell (discussed further in Chapter 9).

Absorption in the Large Intestine

Water

The main absorptive task remaining for the large intestine is to take up needed body water. Most of the water in the chyme entering the large intestine is absorbed in the first half of the colon. Only a small amount (about 100 ml) remains to form and eliminate the feces.

---

metabolism   (Gr. *metabole,* change) sum of the chemical changes that produce the essential energy to sustain life.

catabolism   (ca-TA-bol-iz-um) metabolic process of breaking down large substances to yield the smaller building blocks.

anabolism   (an-A-bol-iz-um) metabolic process of building large substances from smaller parts.

Dietary Fiber

Food fiber is not digested because humans lack the specific enzymes required. Dietary fiber, however, contributes important bulk to the food mass throughout the process of digestion and helps to form the feces. The formation and passage of intestinal gas is a normal process but is embarrassing to some individuals (see the Clinical Applications box, "The Sometimes Embarrassing Effects of Digestion"). Table 5-2 summarizes major features of intestinal nutrient absorption.

Transport

After the breakdown of food and absorption of nutrients, they must be transported to various cells throughout the body. This transportation requires the work of both the vascular and lymphatic systems (Figure 5-7).

Vascular System

The vascular system is composed of veins and arteries and is responsible for supplying the entire body with nutrients, oxygen, and many other vital substances necessary for life. In addition, the vascular system transports waste, such as carbon dioxide and nitrogen, to the lungs and kidneys for removal.

Most of the products of digestion are water-soluble nutrients, which therefore can be absorbed into the vascular system, or blood circulatory system, directly from the intestinal cells. The nutrients travel first to the liver for immediate cell enzyme work in energy production before being dispersed to other cells throughout the body. The portion of circulation from the intestines to the liver is called *portal circulation.*

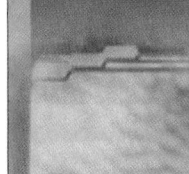

CLINICAL APPLICATIONS

THE SOMETIMES EMBARRASSING EFFECTS OF DIGESTION

After eating a meal or certain foods, some persons complain of the discomfort or embarrassment of gas. This gas is a normal by-product of digestion, but when it becomes painful or apparent to others it may become a physical and social problem.

The gastrointestinal tract normally holds about 3 oz of gas that move along with the food mass and are silently absorbed into the blood stream. Sometimes extra gas collects in the stomach or intestine, creating an embarrassing, although usually harmless, situation.

Stomach Gas

Gas in the stomach results from air bubbles trapped there and occurs when a person eats too fast, drinks through a straw, or otherwise takes in extra air while eating. Burping relieves this gas, but the following tips may help to avoid a social slip:

- Avoid carbonated beverages.
- Do not gulp.
- Chew with your mouth closed.
- Do not drink from a can or through a straw.
- Do not eat when you're nervous.

Intestinal Gas

The passing of gas from the intestine can be a social embarrassment. This gas forms in the colon, where bacteria attack undigested items, causing them to decompose and produce gas. Carbohydrates release hydrogen, carbon dioxide, and—in some people with certain types of bacteria in the gut—methane. All three of these products are odorless (although noisy) gases. Protein produces hydrogen sulfide and such volatile compounds as indole and skatole, which add a distinctive aroma to the expelled air. The following suggestions may help to control the problem:

- Cut down on simple carbohydrates (e.g., sugars). Especially observe milk's effect because lactose intolerance may be the real culprit. Substitute cultured forms such as yogurt or milk treated with a lactase product such as LactAid.
- Use a prior leaching process before cooking dry beans, to remove indigestible saccharides such as raffinose and stachyose. Although humans cannot digest these substances, they provide a feast for bacteria in the intestines. This simple procedure eliminates a major portion of these gas-forming saccharides. First, put washed dry beans into a large pot, add 4 cups of water for each pound (about 2 cups) of beans, and boil beans uncovered for 2 minutes. Then remove pot from heat, cover, and let stand for 1 hour. Finally, drain and rinse the beans, add 8 cups fresh water, bring to a boil, reduce heat, and simmer in covered pot for 1 to 2 hours, until beans are tender. Season as desired.
- Eliminate known food offenders. These vary among individuals but some of the most common offenders are beans (if not prepared for cooking as described), onions, cabbage, and high-fiber wheat products.

Once relief is achieved, slowly add more complex carbohydrates and high-fiber foods back to the diet. Once small amounts are tolerated, try moderate increases. If there is still no relief, medical help may be needed to rule out or treat an overactive gastrointestinal tract.

Lymphatic System

Because fatty materials are not water-soluble, another route must be provided. These fat molecules pass into the lymph vessels in the villi (e.g., the lacteals), flow into the larger lymph vessels of the body, and eventually enter the blood stream.

METABOLISM

Finally, the individual macronutrients in food (carbohydrates, protein, and fat) have been broken down through digestion into the basic building blocks (monosaccharides, amino acids, and fatty acids) and absorbed into the blood stream. Now it is possible for these nutrients to be converted into needed energy, or stored in the body for later use.

Energy for Fuel

Metabolism is the sum of chemical reactions occurring within a living cell to maintain life. The mitochondrion of the cell is the work center in which all metabolic reactions take place. There are two types of metabolism, **catabolism** and **anabolism.** Catabolism is the breaking down of large

TABLE 5-2	Intestinal Absorption of Some Major Nutrients			
Nutrient	**Form**	**Means of absorption**	**Control agent or required cofactor**	**Route**
Carbohydrate	Monosaccharides (glucose or galactose)	Competitive	—	Blood
		Selective	—	
		Active transport via sodium pump	Sodium	
	Fructose	Facilitated diffusion	Protein carrier	Blood
Protein	Amino acids	Selective	—	Blood
	Some dipeptides	Facilitated diffusion	Pyridoxine (pyridoxal phosphate)	Blood
	Whole protein (rare)	Pinocytosis	Protein carrier	Blood
Fat	Fatty acids	Fatty acid–bile complex (micelles)	Bile	Lymph
	Glycerides (mono-, di-)		—	Lymph
	Few triglycerides (neutral fat)	Pinocytosis	—	Lymph
Vitamins	B_{12}	Facilitated diffusion	Intrinsic factor (IF)	Blood
	A	Bile complex	Bile	Blood
	K	Bile complex	Bile	From large intestine to blood
Minerals	Sodium	Active transport via sodium pump	—	Blood
	Calcium	Active transport	Vitamin D	Blood
	Iron	Active transport	Ferritin mechanism	Blood (as transferrin)
Water	Water	Osmosis	—	Blood, lymph, interstitial fluid

substances into smaller units. The process of breaking down large carbohydrate and protein chains into their smaller building blocks, monosaccharides and amino acids—is a catabolic reaction. Anabolism is just the opposite. It is the process in which cells build large substances from smaller particles. An example is building a complex protein from single amino acids within the body.

The Krebs cycle, also known as the *citric acid cycle*, "or TCA cycle," is the hub of energy formation from food particles occurring in the mitochondria. The combined processes of metabolism ensure that the body has much needed energy, in the form of adenosine triphosphate (ATP). The rate of ATP production fluctuates. It speeds up or slows down depending on energy needs at a given time. Energy needs are minimal during sleep but increase dramatically during strenuous physical activity. Energy supply and demand are discussed further in Chapter 6. Figure 5-8 shows a brief breakdown of the macronutrients and how they enter the final step in energy production.

Because carbohydrates have 4 kcal/g and fat has 9 kcal/g, the metabolism of glucose yields less energy than the metabolism of fat, gram for gram. However, the body prefers to use glucose as its primary source of energy. Protein can be used as a source of energy as well, but this is a relatively inefficient method of creating energy and results in extra nitrogen waste. The body only breaks down protein for energy when glucose and fatty acids are in short supply.

Energy for Storage

If the amount of food consumed yields more energy than is needed, the "left-over" energy is stored for later use in the body. The human body is a very efficient organism. Energy, or kcalories, in excess of needs are not wasted. Excess glucose can be stored easily as glycogen in the liver and muscles for quick energy at a later time. The anabolic process of converting extra glucose into

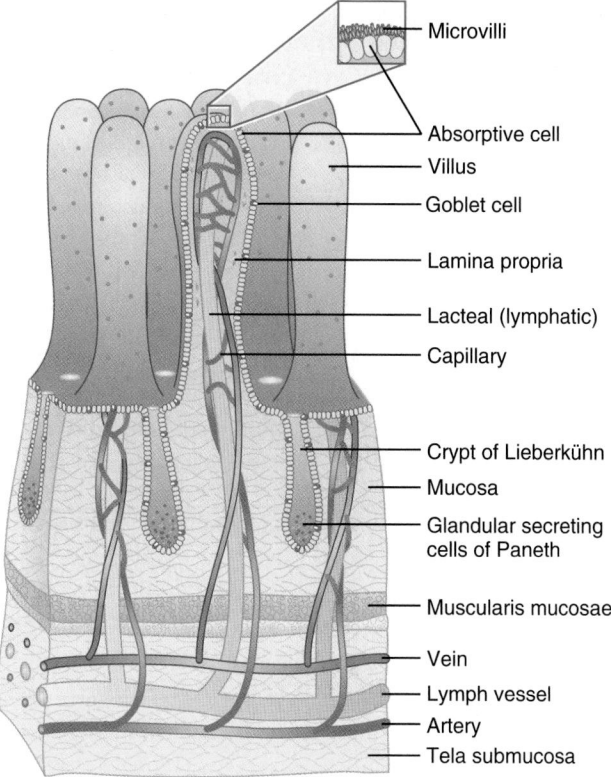

Figure 5-7   Diagram of villi of the human intestine showing the structure and blood and lymph vessels. (From Mahan LK, Escott-Stump S: *Krause's food, nutrition, & diet therapy,* ed 11, Philadelphia, 2004, Saunders.)

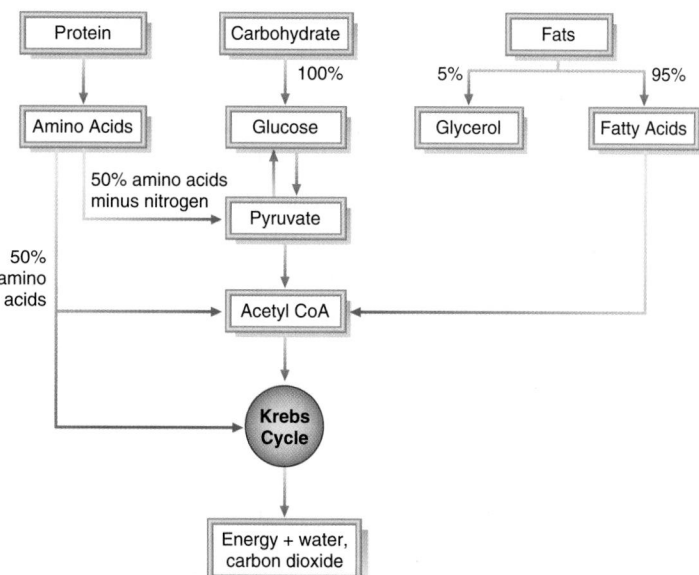

Figure 5-8   Metabolic pathways. (From Peckenpaugh NJ: *Nutrition essentials and diet therapy,* ed 9, Philadelphia, 2003, Saunders.)

FOR FURTHER FOCUS

WHAT ABOUT ALCOHOL?

Is Alcohol a Food?

Yes. Alcohol contributes to the over-all energy intake in the form of calories and, therefore is considered a food. Alcohol yields 7 kcal/g consumed, which is more than both carbohydrates and protein, yielding 4 kcal/g.

Is Alcohol a Nutrient?

Not exactly. Unlike carbohydrates, fats, proteins, vitamins, minerals, and water, alcohol performs no essential function in the body. Alcohol is not stored in the body and can be toxic in large amounts.

How Is Alcohol Digested?

The majority (85% to 95%) of alcohol is absorbed without any chemical digestion. Alcohol is one of the few substances absorbed directly into circulation from the stomach. Small amounts of alcohol can actually enter blood circulation from the mouth and esophagus. What is not absorbed in the stomach is absorbed in the small intestine and sent directly to the liver for metabolism.

Alcohol metabolism takes precedence over the metabolism of any other nutrient in the body because it is technically a toxin. The primary by-product of alcohol metabolism is acetaldehyde, the culprit for destruction of healthy tissue associated with alcohol. After detoxification, the liver uses remaining by-products to produce fatty acids. Fatty acids are converted into triglycerides and stored in the liver. A single drinking binge can result in an accumulation of fat in the liver. Repeated episodes over a period of time can lead to fatty liver disease, the first stage of alcoholic liver disease.

Alcohol metabolism is a priority for the liver, but it can only work so fast. Blood alcohol concentrations peak at approximately 30 to 45 minutes after one drink (defined as 12 oz of beer, 5 oz of wine, or 1.5 oz of 80-proof distilled spirits). The liver can only work so fast to metabolize and rid the body of alcohol, regardless of how much has been consumed, after which alcohol and its metabolites begin to accumulate in the blood.

Several factors influence an individual's ability to metabolize alcohol, such as gender, food intake, body weight, sex hormones, and medications.*

To find out more about alcohol (dangers, benefits, diseases associated with, etc.), the following web sites may prove useful:

- U.S. Department of Health and Human Services for Alcohol and Drug Information: *www.health.org*
- The National Institute on Alcohol Abuse and Alcoholism: *www.niaaa.nih.gov*
- Alcoholics Anonymous: *www.aa.org*
- National Council on Alcoholism and Drug Dependence: *www.ncadd.org*

---

*National Institute on Alcohol Abuse and Alcoholism, National Institutes of Health: *Alcohol alert: alcohol metabolism,* No. 35 PH 371, January 1997, Bethesda, MD, (accessed January 2003), NIAAA/NIH [*http://www.niaaa.nih.gov/publications/aa35.htm*].

---

glycogenesis (Gr. *glykys,* sweet; *genesis,* generation, birth) formation of stored glycogen from glucose.

lipogenesis (Gr. *lipos,* fat; *genesis,* generation, birth) formation of fat.

adipose tissue storage site for excess fat.

gluconeogenesis (Gr. *gluco,* glucose; *neos,* new; *genesis,* generation, birth; gloo-ko-nee-oh-JEN-uh-sis) formation of glucose from non-carbohydrate substances such as amino acids.

glycogen is called **glycogenesis**. Although alcohol is not considered a nutrient, it does provide 7 kcal/g. Therefore, alcohol intake adds to the overall supply of energy. See the For Further Focus box "What About Alcohol?" for more information regarding alcohol digestion.

Once the glycogen reserves are full, additional excess energy (from carbohydrates, fat, or protein) are stored as fat in adipose tissue. **Lipogenesis** is the building up of triglycerides for storage in the **adipose tissue** of the body.

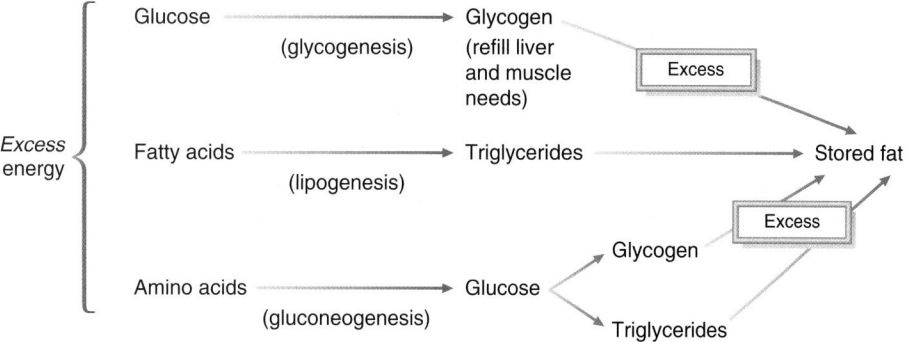

Figure 5–9   Metabolic pathways of excess energy.

Contrary to popular belief, excess protein intake is not stored as muscle. The body does use amino acids to build needed functional and structural proteins and the liver stores some free amino acids to meet rapid needs of the body. However, protein intake above and beyond the body's requirements is broken down farther so that the nitrogen unit is removed and the remaining carbon chain can be converted to glucose, if needed, or on to fat for storage. The conversion of amino acids to glucose is **gluconeogenesis.** Figure 5-9 demonstrates the pathways of excess energy from carbohydrates, fats, or protein.

Both glycogen and stored fat are available for use when energy demands require it. Energy balance and the factors that influence it are discussed in Chapter 6.

SUMMARY

Necessary nutrients as they occur in food are not available to the human body, but must be changed, released, regrouped, and rerouted into forms body cells can use. Closely related activities—digestion, absorption, and transport—ensure that key food nutrients are delivered to the cells so that the multiple metabolic tasks that sustain life can be completed.

Mechanical digestion consists of spontaneous muscular activity that is responsible for the following: (1) initial mechanical breakdown by means such as mastication and (2) movement of the food mass along the gastrointestinal tract by motions such as peristalsis. Chemical digestion involves enzymatic action that breaks food down into smaller and smaller components and releases its nutrients for absorption.

Absorption involves the passage of food nutrients from the intestines into the mucosal lining of the in-testinal wall. It occurs mainly in the small intestine by means of highly efficient intestinal wall structures that, together with a number of effective absorbing mechanisms, increase the absorbent surface area. Nutrients absorbed are then transported throughout the body by blood circulation.

Finally, the food we eat is converted into energy through the cycles of metabolism. *Metabolism* is the sum of the body processes that change our food energy from the three energy nutrients (e.g., mainly carbohydrate, some fat, and protein as backup) into various forms of energy. Throughout this cycling of our body energy, metabolism is balanced by two types of metabolic actions, as follows: (1) *anabolism,* which builds tissue and stores energy and (2) *catabolism,* which breaks down tissue and releases energy.

CRITICAL THINKING QUESTIONS

1. Describe the types of muscle movement involved in mechanical digestion. What does the word *motility* mean? How are the nerves involved?
2. Identify digestive enzymes and any related substances secreted by the following glands: salivary and mucosal glands, pancreas, and liver. What activities do they perform on carbohydrates, proteins, and fats? What stimulates the release of these enzymes? What inhibits their activity?

3. Describe four mechanisms of nutrient absorption from the small intestine. Describe the routes taken by the breakdown products of carbohydrates, pro-teins, and fats after absorption. Why must an alternate route to the blood stream be provided for fat?

4. What functions does the large intestine perform?

CHAPTER CHALLENGE QUESTIONS

True-False

Write the correct statement for each item you answer "false."

1. *True or False:* The digestive products of a large meal are difficult to absorb because the overall area of the absorbent surface of the intestines is relatively small.

2. *True or False:* Before they can work, some enzymes must be activated by hydrochloric acid or other enzymes.

3. *True or False:* Bile is an enzyme specifically used for fat breakdown.

4. *True or False:* The "gastrointestinal circulation" provides a constant supply of water and electrolytes to carry digestive secretions and substances being produced.

5. *True or False:* Secretions from the gastrointestinal accessory organs, the gallbladder and the pancreas, mix with gastric secretions in the stomach to aid digestion.

6. *True or False:* One enzyme may work on both carbohydrate and fat breakdown.

7. *True or False:* Bile is released from the gallbladder in response to a hormonal stimulus.

Multiple Choice

1. During digestion, the major muscle action that moves the food mass forward in regular rhythmic waves is called
   a. valve contraction.
   b. segmentation ring motion.
   c. muscle tone.
   d. peristalsis.

2. Gastrointestinal secretory action is affected by which of the following? (*Circle all that apply.*)
   a. Blood pressure
   b. Temperature of food
   c. Speed of eating
   d. Emotions such as anger and fear

3. Mucus is an important gastrointestinal secretion because it
   a. causes chemical changes in substances to prepare for enzyme action.
   b. helps create proper degree of acidity for enzymes to act.
   c. lubricates and protects the gastrointestinal lining.
   d. helps to emulsify fats for enzyme action.

4. Pepsin is
   a. produced in the small intestine to act on protein.
   b. a gastric enzyme that acts on protein.
   c. produced in the pancreas to act on fat.
   d. produced in the small intestine to act on fat.

5. Bile is an important secretion that is
   a. produced by the gallbladder.
   b. stored in the liver.
   c. an aid to protein digestion.
   d. a fat-emulsifying agent.

6. The route of fat absorption is
   a. the lymphatic system via the villi lacteals.
   b. directly into the portal blood circulation.
   c. with the aid of bile directly into the villi blood capillaries.
   d. with the aid of protein directly into the portal blood circulation.

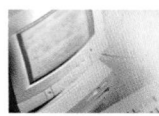

Please refer to the Students' Resource section of this text's Evolve web site for "Suggestions for Additional Study."

REFERENCES

1. Green HL, Moran JR: The gastrointestinal tract: regulator of nutrient absorption. In Shils ME, Olson JA, Shike M, eds: *Modern nutrition in health and disease,* ed 8, Philadelphia, 1994, Lea & Febiger.
2. Guyton AC, Hall JE: *Textbook of medical physiology,* ed 10, Philadelphia, 2000, Saunders.
3. National Institute of Diabetes and Digestive and Kidney Diseases, National Institutes of Health: *Lactose intolerance,* Washington, DC, (accessed December 2002), NIDDK/NIH [*http://www.niddk.nih.gov/health/digest/pubs/lactose/lactose.htm*].
4. Food and Nutrition Board, Institute of Medicine: *Dietary reference intakes for thiamin, riboflavin, niacin, vitamin B_6, folate,* vitamin B_{12}, pantothenic acid, biotin, and choline, Washington, DC, 2000, National Academies Press.
5. Food and Nutrition Board, Institute of Medicine: *Dietary reference intakes for vitamin C, vitamin E, selenium, and carotenoids,* Washington, DC, 2000, National Academies Press.
6. Food and Nutrition Board, Institute of Medicine: *Dietary reference intakes for vitamin A, vitamin K, arsenic, boron, chromium, copper, iodine, iron, manganese, molybdenum, nickel, silicon, vanadium, and zinc,* Washington, DC, 2002, National Academies Press.

FURTHER READING AND RESOURCES

- Swagerty DL and others: Lactose intolerance, *Am Fam Physician* 65(9):1845, 2002.
- McMahan S and others: Lactose intolerance: strategies for symptom management, *Adv Nurse Pract* 10(6):71, 2002.

  Lactose intolerance, the inability to digest the disaccharide lactose, affects millions of people worldwide. These articles review the pathophysiology, epidemiology, symptoms, and treatments for lactose intolerance.

- Anderson GH and others: Inverse association between the effect of carbohydrates on blood glucose and subsequent short-term food intake in young men, *Am J Clin Nutr* 76(5):1023, 2002.

  The authors explain the relationship between carbohydrate consumption, satiety, and food intake.

6

Energy Balance

E fficient human bodies constantly convert fuel energy from food into the energy used at work and play, as well as at rest. Overall, energy metabolism deals with change and balance, the constant facts of life.

Many constant changes and balances in the nutrients that food delivers to body cells produce needed energy. Fuel is "burned" and stored as necessary to provide a continuous flow of energy for the body's work.

This chapter looks at the "big picture" of energy balance among all the energy nutrients and shows how this energy intake is measured, cycled, and used to meet all the body's energy needs.

KEY CONCEPTS

■ Food energy is changed into body energy and cycled throughout the body to do work.

■ The body uses most of its energy intake for basal metabolic work needs.

■ A balance between intake of food energy and output of body-work energy maintains life and health.

■ States of being underweight and overweight reflect degrees of body energy imbalance.

HUMAN ENERGY SYSTEM

Basic Energy Needs

The body needs constant energy to do the work necessary to maintain life and health. The actions involved are both voluntary and involuntary.

Voluntary Work and Exercise

Voluntary work includes all physical actions related to a person's usual activities, as well as any additional physical exercise. Although this visible, conscious action seems to require most of the energy output, this is usually not true.

Involuntary Body Work

The greatest energy output is the result of involuntary work, which includes all activities in the body not consciously performed. These activities include such vital processes as circulation, respiration, digestion, and absorption, as well as many other internal activities that maintain life. Involuntary body functions require energy in various forms, such as: *chemical* energy (in many metabolic products), *electrical* energy (in brain and nerve activities), *mechanical* energy (in muscle contraction), and *thermal* (heat) energy to keep the body warm.

Sources of Fuel

The energy needed for voluntary and involuntary body work requires fuel, provided in the form of nutrients. As presented in previous chapters, the only three "energy nutrients" are carbohydrate, fat, and protein. Carbohydrates are the body's primary fuel, with fat assisting as a storage fuel. Protein is occasionally a back-up fuel source—and actually an inefficient one, at that—available as needed. The body must have a supply of the food fuels to provide energy for work and keep the body warm. If the sufficient primary fuel, carbohydrate, is not consumed to supply these body-energy needs, the body burns fat instead. To maintain health, the average daily food energy intake should equal the daily body energy needs, or output.

Measurement of Energy

Unit of Measure: Kilocalorie

In common usage, the word calorie refers to the amount of energy in food or expended in physical actions. However, in human nutrition the term kilocalorie (1000 calories) is used to designate the large calorie unit used in nutritional science to avoid dealing with such large numbers. A kilocalorie, abbreviated as *kcalorie* or *kcal*, is the amount of heat necessary to raise 1 kg of water 1° C (centigrade). Sometimes the international unit of measure for energy, *joule (J)*, is used. The conversion factor for changing kilocalories (kcal) to kilojoules (kJ) is 4.184; therefore 1 kcal equals 4.184 kJ.

Food Energy: Fuel Factors

As discussed, the energy nutrients (e.g., carbohydrate and fat, with protein as a back-up) have basic fuel factors. Beverage alcohol, from fermented grains and fruits, also supplies fuel. These factors reflect their relative fuel densities, as follows: (1) carbohydrate: 4 kcal/g; (2) fat: 9 kcal/g; (3) protein: 4 kcal/g; and (4) alcohol: 7 kcal/g.

Caloric and Nutrient Density

The term *density* refers to the degree of concentration of material in a given substance. More material in a smaller amount of substance gives that substance a greater density. Thus the concept of *caloric density* refers to a higher concentration of energy (kcalories) in a smaller amount of food. Therefore of the three energy nutrients, fat or foods high in fat have the highest caloric density. Similarly, foods may be evaluated in terms of their relative *nutrient density*. High nutrient density refers to a relatively high concentration of all nutrients, including vitamins and minerals, in smaller amounts of a given food. A number of food guides do not base their listed "food scores" on the concentration of nutrients in given foods but on the overall nutrient density in those foods as a general indicator of a food's contribution to health goals.

ENERGY BALANCE

Energy, like matter, cannot be "created." When energy is spoken of as being "produced," it really means that it is transformed (e.g., changed in form and cycled

---

calorie (L. *calor,* heat) a measure of heat. The energy necessary to do the work of the body is measured as the amount of heat produced by the body's work. The energy value of a food is expressed as the number of kilocalories a specified portion of the food will yield when oxidized in the body.

kilocalorie (Fr. *chilioi,* thousand; L. *calor,* heat) the general term *calorie* refers to a unit of heat measure and is used alone to designate the small calorie or as a general term in common language for the large calorie, the kilocalorie. The calorie used in nutritional science and the study of metabolism is the large calorie (1000 calories) or kilocalorie, to be more accurate and avoid the use of very large numbers in calculations.

throughout a system). Consider the human energy system as part of the total energy system on earth. In this sense, two energy systems support human life: the one within humans and the much larger one surrounding us, as follows:

1. *External energy cycle:* In the environment, the ultimate source of energy is the sun and its vast nuclear reactions. Using water and carbon dioxide as raw materials, plants transform the sun's radiation into stored chemical energy (e.g., mainly carbohydrate with some fat and protein). The food chain continues as animals, including humans, eat plants and the flesh of other animals.

2. *Internal energy cycle:* When humans eat plant and animal foods, the stored energy changes into body fuels, glucose and fatty acids, and cycles them into various other energy forms to serve body needs. These forms include the following: (1) chemical energy in the many new metabolic products made; (2) electrical energy in brain and nerve tissue;

(3) mechanical energy in muscle contraction; and (4) thermal energy in the heat to keep the body warm. As this internal energy cycle continues, water is excreted, carbon dioxide is exhaled, and heat is radiated, returning these end products to the external environment. The overall energy cycle repeats constantly, sustaining life.

Energy Intake

The total overall energy balance within the body depends on the energy intake in relation to the energy output. The main source of energy for all body work is food, backed up by stored energy in body tissues.

Sources of Food Energy

The three energy nutrients in food keep human bodies supplied with fuel. One can easily estimate personal energy intake by recording a day's actual food consumption and calculating its energy value (see Appendix A). Table 6-1 provides an example of a daily food log.

TABLE 6-1	Record of Daily Food Intake		
Time	**Food description**	**Prepared**	**Amount**
7 AM	Eggs	Fried in Pam	2 whole
	Whole wheat bread	Toasted	2 slices
	Yogurt, low-fat		6 oz
	Orange Juice	Fresh	8 oz
10 AM	Banana		1 large
	Wheat Thins		6 crackers
	Water		16 oz
12:30 PM	Salad		
	• romaine lettuce	Chopped	2 cups
	• tomato	Diced	¼ tomato
	• carrots	Sliced	¼ cup
	• croutons	Baked	¼ cup
	Thousand Island dressing		2 Tbsp
	Chicken	Grilled, chopped	5 oz
	Sweet potato	Baked	1 medium
	Water		16 oz
3 PM	Apple, Red Delicious	With skin	1 medium
	Mozzarella cheese		1.5 oz
	Water		16 oz
7:30 PM	Penne pasta	Boiled with salt	1 cup
	Salmon	Baked	4 oz
	Asparagus	Steamed	¾ cup
	Hollandaise sauce		2 Tbsp
	Tea		12 oz
	Water		16 oz

Sources of Stored Energy

When food is not available, as during sleep, longer periods of fasting, or the extreme stress of starvation, the body draws from its stores of energy.

Glycogen. A 12- to 48-hour reserve of glycogen exists in liver and muscles and is quickly depleted if not replenished by daily food intake. For example, glycogen stores maintain normal blood glucose levels for body functions during sleep hours. The first meal, breakfast (so-named because it "breaks the fast") has a significant function for energy intake.

Adipose Tissue. Although fat storage is larger than glycogen, the supply varies from person to person. Maintaining a balanced amount is important as an added energy resource.

Muscle Mass. Energy stored as protein exists in limited amounts in muscle mass, but this lean muscle mass must be maintained for health. Only during longer periods of fasting or starvation does the body turn to this tissue for energy.

Energy Output

The necessary activities to sustain life, such as normal body functions, regulation of body temperature, and the processes of tissue growth and repair, use energy from food and body reserves. The total chemical changes that occur during all of these activities are called *metabolism*. This exchange of energy in overall balance usually is expressed in kcalories. The following three demands for energy determine the body's total energy requirements: (1) resting energy expenditure; (2) physical activity; and (3) the thermic effect of food.

Resting Energy Expenditure and Basal Energy Expenditure

The term **resting energy expenditure (REE)**, or *resting metabolic rate (RMR)*, refers to the sum of all internal working activities of the body at rest and is expressed in kcalories per day. For instance, if an individual's REE were 1500 kcal, that would be the amount of energy that individual would need to consume over a 24-hour period to maintain his or her current weight while at complete rest. In general use, the terms *resting energy expenditure*, resting metabolic rate, and **basal energy expenditure (BEE)** are used interchangeably,[1] describing a vast amount of physiologic work. However, there is a technical difference between BEE and REE. Basal energy expenditure must be measured when an individual is at

complete digestive, physical, and emotional rest. Because it is often difficult to maintain the stringent conditions representing a true BEE, the measurement is most often expressed as REE. Resting energy expenditure is slightly higher than a true BEE measurement.[2,3]

Most of the body's total energy expenditure is spent maintaining necessary bodily functions in the form of BEE. The majority of that energy is used by small, but highly active tissues (e.g., liver, brain, heart, kidney, and gastrointestinal tract), which amount to less than 5% of the total body weight.[4] However, these tissues account for 60% to 75% of basal metabolic needs. Although resting muscle and adipose fat are far larger in mass, they contribute much less to the body's metabolic rate.

Measuring Resting Energy Expenditure or Basal Metabolic Rate. A measure of basal or resting metabolic rate (BMR or RMR) is sometimes made in clinical practice (e.g., on metabolic wards or research labs) using *indirect calorimetry* (Figure 6-1). This method indirectly measures the amount of energy a person uses while at rest. A portable metabolic cart allows the person to breathe into an attached mouthpiece or ventilated hood system while lying in bed and the normal exchange of oxygen and carbon dioxide is measured. From the rate of oxygen utilization, the metabolic rate can be calculated with a high degree of accuracy.

In addition, *thyroid function tests* may be used as indirect measures of BMR because the thyroid hormone regulates metabolism.[5] Thyroid function tests measure the activity of the thyroid gland and the blood levels of its hormone thyroxine. The tests also include measures of serum thyroxin levels and of serum–protein-bound iodine

---

resting energy expenditure (REE) the amount of energy needed by the body for maintenance of life at rest over a 24-hour period. Often used interchangeably with basal energy expenditure, but is actually slightly higher.

basal energy expenditure (BEE) (Gr. *basis,* base) the amount of energy needed by the body for maintenance of life when a person is at complete digestive, physical, and emotional rest (10 to 12 hours after eating, 12 to 18 hours after physical activity, and measured immediately upon waking). This basal metabolic rate (BMR) is reported as the percent of variation in the person above or below the normal number of kilocalories necessary for a person of like height, weight, sex, and age.

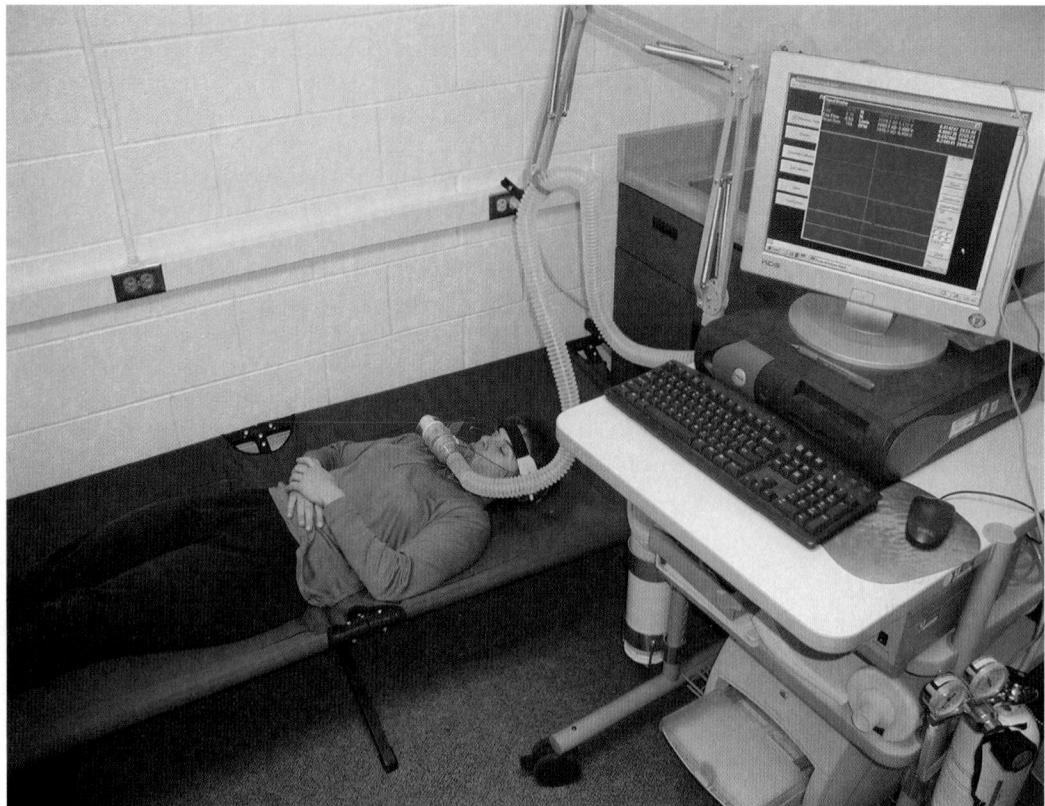

Figure 6-1   Measuring resting metabolic rate.

(PBI) and radioactive iodine uptake. Iodine's basic function is in the synthesis of thyroxine.

A general formula for calculating basal energy needs is to multiply 0.9 to 1 kcal/kg body weight (weight in pounds divided by 2.2) by the number of hours in a day. Thus the daily basal metabolic needs (in kcalories) are calculated as follows:

Men: 1 kcal × kg Body weight × 24 hours

Women: 0.9 kcal × kg Body weight × 24 hours

The classic Harris-Benedict equations provide an alternate method of estimating the basal or resting energy expenditure for adults, as follows:

Women: BEE = 655 + 9.56 × Weight (kg) + 1.85 × Height (cm) − 4.68 × Age

Men: BEE = 66.5 + 13.75 × Weight (kg) + 5 × Height (cm) − 6.78 × Age

Factors Influencing Basal Metabolic Rate. Several factors influence BMR and should be kept in mind when related test results are interpreted. The major factors affecting BMR relate to lean body mass, growth periods, body temperature, and hormonal status, as follows:[1,2]

■ *Lean body mass:* One of the greatest factors affecting BMR is the relative amount of lean body mass in the body composition. This is caused by the greater metabolic activity in lean tissues (muscles and organs) as compared with fat and bones. The BMR is higher in lean bodies, thus requiring more energy. It is lower in fat bodies, thus requiring less energy. Other factors such as surface area, sex, and age only influence BMR as they relate to the lean body mass.[4]

■ *Growth periods:* During growth periods, the growth hormone stimulates cell metabolism and raises BMR 15% to 20%. Thus the BMR slowly rises during the first few years of life,[6] levels off somewhat, rises again just before and during puberty, and then gradually declines into old age.[7,8] BMR rises significantly during pregnancy, which is a rapid growth period requiring an additional 300 kcal/day on average, because of the accelerated tissue growth and the increased work of the heart and lungs.[9] During the following period of

CULTURAL CONSIDERATIONS

HYPERMETABOLISM AND HYPOMETABOLISM: WHAT ARE THEY, AND WHO IS AT RISK?

Hypermetabolism and hypometabolism are conditions in which the metabolic rate is either significantly higher (hyper) or lower (hypo) than normal. Because the thyroid gland is responsible for producing the hormone thyroxine, which controls the metabolic rate, such conditions usually result from malformations or malfunctions of the thyroid gland. Clinically, hypermetabolism and hypometabolism are referred to as hyperthyroidism and hypothyroidism, respectively.

An individual with hyperthyroidism has a significantly higher metabolic rate, and energy needs, than normal. Such increases in energy needs are not explained by lean tissue, age, or gender. This individual has an overactive thyroid gland, producing too much thyroxine. As a result, the normal energy intake recommendations do not meet his or her needs. For example, a woman age 25, height 5'5", weight 125, normally needs around 2400 kcal per day to maintain her weight at a moderate level of activity. However, the same woman with hyperthyroidism may need 1.5 to 2.5 times as many kcalories per day to maintain her current weight.

Hypothyroidism is the opposite of hyperthyroidism. Individuals with hypothyroidism do not produce enough thyroxine and therefore require less energy than normal to maintain their current body weight. The DRIs for energy intake for a hypothyroid individual are too high and thus result in weight gain. However, there are effective medications for hypothyroidism. Typically, both hyperthyroidism and hypothyroidism are discovered in young adulthood.

Congenital hypothyroidism (CH), occurring in 1 of every 3000 to 4000 live births, is a type of hypothyroidism present at birth and can result in mental retardation if not treated. Studies have found that the risk of CH is linked with birth weight, gender, and ethnicity. Both male and female infants weighing less than 4.5 lb or greater than 10 lbs have a significantly higher risk of developing CH, whereas females of any weight have twice the prevalence of males. In a study conducted in California, African-American infants had the lowest rate of CH, whereas most ethnic groups (including Hispanics, Chinese, Filipinos, Vietnamese, Middle Easterners, Asian Indians, and Hawaiians) had an increased prevalence when compared with Caucasian infants.[*]

Another risk factor for developing abnormal thyroid function, and thus abnormal metabolism, is iodine intake. The mineral iodine is an important part of the hormone thyroxine, and one of the symptoms of iodine deficiency is abnormal thyroid function and metabolism. The incidence of hyperthyroidism and hypothyroidism has long since been linked to iodine intake.[†] Both high and low intakes of iodine are associated with thyroid disease.

Close monitoring of basal metabolism and total energy expenditure are important aspects in the treatment of thyroid disease. Medications and energy intake are then modified to control weight and prevent complications.

---

[*]Waller DK and others: Risk factors for congenital hypothyroidism: an investigation of infant's birth weight, ethnicity, and gender in California, 1990-1998, *Teratology* 62:36, 2000.
[†]Pedersen IB and others: Large differences in incidences of overt hyper- and hypothyroidism associated with a small difference in iodine intake: a prospective comparative register-based population study, *J Clin Endo Metab* 87(10):4462, 2002.

---

lactation, the breastfeeding mother's BMR increases further, and she needs extra kcalories to cover this added metabolic process of producing milk.

- *Body temperature:* Fever increases BMR approximately 7% for each 1° F (0.83° C) rise in temperature. Diseases involving increased cell activity (e.g., cancer and cardiac failure) and respiratory problems (e.g., emphysema) usually increase the BMR. In the abnormal states of starvation and malnutrition, the BMR is lowered because of the sacrifice of lean muscle mass for energy. In cold weather, especially in freezing temperatures, the BMR rises somewhat to generate more body heat to maintain normal body temperature.

- *Hormonal status:* Energy expenditure is also influenced by hormonal secretions. As mentioned, the thyroid function test is a means of measuring one's metabolism. Individuals with an underactive thyroid gland develop *hypothyroidism*, resulting in a decreased metabolic rate. Conversely, *hyperthyroidism* occurs when the thyroid gland is overactive (see the Cultural Considerations box, "Hypermetabolism and Hypometabolism: What Are They, and Who Is at Risk?"). The "fight-or-flight" reflexes increase metabolic rate because of the hormone epinephrine. Other hormones, such as growth hormone, insulin, and cortisol, are also known to increase metabolism and may fluctuate daily.

Physical Activity

Exercise involved in work or recreation (Figure 6-2) accounts for wide individual variations in energy output (see Chapter 16). Regular physical activity, balanced with adequate energy intake, is especially important to help offset the risk for heart disease and diabetes.[3,10,11] Physical activity has beneficial effects on both the body and mind throughout the adult years. Table 6-2 gives some representative kcalorie expenditures in different types of work and recreation. Mental work or study does not require additional kcalories; emotional states do not increase kcalorie needs but may require energy intake to compensate for muscle tension, restlessness, and agitated movements.

Energy expenditure used for physical activity goes above and beyond energy used for resting energy needs. It is somewhat difficult to keep track of all energy used explicitly for physical activity to calculate total energy needs. Instead, the energy used for physical activity can be estimated as a factor of RMR by categorizing physical activity level (PAL) according to standard values (1.2 to

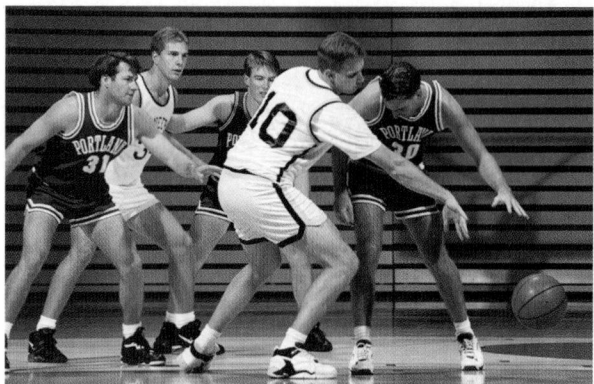

Figure 6-2   Energy output in exercise. (Credit: PhotoDisc.)

TABLE 6–2	Energy Expenditure per Pound per Hour during Various Activities*		
Activity	**Kcal/lb/hour†**	**Activity**	**Kcal/lb/hour†**
Aerobics, moderate	2.95	Sports	
Bicycling		Boxing, in ring	5.44
Light: 10-11.9 mph	2.72	Field hockey	3.63
Moderate: 12-13.9 mph	3.63	Golf	2.04
Fast: 14-15.9 mph	4.54	Rollerblading	4.42
Mountain biking	3.85	Soccer	3.85
Daily activities		Skiing, downhill, moderate	2.72
Cleaning	1.36	Skiing, cross country, moderate	3.63
Cooking	0.91	Swimming, moderate pace	3.14
Driving a car	0.91	Tennis, doubles	2.27
Eating, sitting	0.68	Tennis, singles	3.63
Gardening, general	1.81	Ultimate Frisbee	3.63
Office work	0.82	Volleyball	1.81
Reading, writing while sitting	0.70	Walking	
Sleeping	0.41	Moderate: ~3 mph (20 min/mile), level	1.50
Shoveling snow	2.72	Moderate: ~3 mph (20 min/mile), uphill	2.73
Running		Brisk: ~3.5 mph (17.14 min/mile), level	1.72
5 mph (12 min/mile)	3.63	Fast: ~4.5 mph (13.33 min/mile), level	2.86
7 mph (8.5 min/mile)	5.22	Weight training	
9 mph (6.5 min/mile)	6.80	Light or moderate	1.36
10 mph (6 min/mile)	7.26	Heavy or vigorous	2.72

Modified from Nieman DC: *Exercise testing and prescription: a health-related approach*, ed 5, New York, 2003, McGraw-Hill.

*Energy expenditure depends on the physical fitness (i.e., amount of lean body mass) of the individual and continuity of exercise.

†Multiply activity factor by weight in pounds by fraction of hour performing activity.

Example: A 150-lb person plays soccer for 45 minutes, as follows: 3.18 (Factor) × 150 (lbs) × 0.75 (Hours) = 357.75 calories burned

2.4, depending on lifestyle). This factor is then multiplied by the RMR. For example, an individual who works at a desk job and has little or no leisure activity would have a PAL of 1.4 to 1.5. Therefore multiply that person's RMR by 1.4 to 1.5 to get a range of energy expenditure involved in resting energy requirements and physical activity. (See the Clinical Applications box, "Evaluate Your Own Daily Energy Requirements," for PAL factors.)

CLINICAL APPLICATIONS

EVALUATE YOUR OWN DAILY ENERGY REQUIREMENTS

Your total energy output (in kcal) per day is the sum of your body's three uses of energy, as follows:

1. Resting metabolic rate
2. Physical activity
3. Thermic effect of food

1. Basal metabolic rate (BMR):

Use general formula:

Women: 0.9 kcal/kg/hour
Men: 1.0 kcal/kg/hour

Convert weight (lb) to kg: 1 kg = 2.2 lb
Multiply by formula:

BMR (kcal) = 1 (or 0.9) × Weight (kg) × 24 (hours in day)

2. Physical activity:

Estimate your general average level of physical activity.

The energy used by physical activity can be estimated as a factor of your **BMR** and varies with the degree of physical activity. Use this list to select your activity level:

Lifestyle and Activity	Physical Activity Level (PAL) Factor
Chair or bed-bound	1.2
Sedentary (mostly resting with little or no planned strenuous activity)	1.4-1.5
Very light (seated working environment with some movement but little or no planned strenuous activity)	1.6-1.7
Moderate (standing working environment or daily planned strenuous activity)	1.8-1.9
Heavy (strenuous working environment or daily workout routine consisting of several hours of strenuous activity)	2.0-2.4

Find the energy cost of your activity level:

Physical activity energy cost (kcal) = BMR × Your PAL

For example, if you are sedentary (mostly sitting):

BMR × 1.4 to 1.5

3. Thermic effect of food intake (TEF):

The thermic effect of food is the energy the body uses in the processes of digestion and absorption. It averages 10% of the energy in the food.

Record your food intake for one day (24 hours) and calculate estimated energy value (kcal), using either the table of food values in Appendix A or a simple computer program.

Find energy cost of thermic effect of food (TEF):

TEF (kcal) = 10% of total kcal in food consumed

4. Calculate your total energy output:

Total energy output (kcal) = BMR + Physical activity + TEF

Example 1:

A woman who weighs 130 lbs (59 kg), who eats an average of 2200 kcal per day, and who has started and maintains a regular strenuous physical exercise program:

BMR   = 0.9 kcal × 59 kg × 24 hours = 1274 kcal
Activity = BMR × 1.8   = 2293 kcal
TEF   = 2200 kcal × 10%   = 220 kcal
(using actual kcal consumed)

Total energy output = [(BMR × PAL) + TEF] = 2513 kcal

Result: This woman will lose weight. Her energy output is around 313 kcal per day greater than her food intake. Because 1 lb of body weight equals approximately 3500 kcal, she will lose about 1 lb every 10 to 12 days with the preceding eating and exercise routine.

Example 2:

A man who weighs 180 lbs (82 kg), who eats an average of 3300 kcal per day, and has a sedentary lifestyle:

BMR   = 1.0 kcal × 82 kg × 24 hours = 1968 kcal
Activity = BMR × 1.4   = 2755 kcal
TEF   = 3300 × 10%   = 330 kcal
(using actual kcal consumed)

Total energy output = [(BMR × PAL) + TEF] = 3085 kcal

Result: This man will tend to gain weight slowly over time. What would your clinical advice be to him?

Thermic Effect of Food

After eating, food stimulates metabolism and requires extra energy for digestion, absorption, and transport of the nutrients to the cells. This overall stimulating effect is called the *thermic effect of food* (TEF). About 5% to 10% of the body's total energy needs for metabolism relates to the handling of food.

Total Energy Requirement

Resting energy expenditure, physical activities, and the thermic effect of food make up a person's overall total energy requirement (Figure 6-3). To maintain daily energy balance, food-energy intake must match body-energy output. An energy imbalance, when energy intake exceeds energy output, causes obesity. Treatment should include a decrease in food kcalories and an increase in physical activity. Extreme weight loss (e.g., anorexia nervosa) results when food-energy intake does not meet body-energy requirements for extended periods of time. Treatment should include a gradual increase in food kcalories along with moderate activity and rest. Chapter 15 further discusses weight management.

Where do you stand in your own energy balance? You can estimate your energy needs by using the steps in the Clinical Applications box, "Evaluate Your Own Daily Energy Requirements." You may instead wish to record your actual food and activities for a day and calculate your energy intake (kcalories) and output (kcalorie expenditure in activities). Total your day's activity and compare it with the general type of similar activities given in Table 6-2. Estimate the total time you spent on a given activity by adding up the minutes you spent at any time on that activity, and then converting those minutes to hours (or decimal fractions of hours) for the day. For example, if you spent 10 minutes at one time and 5 minutes at another time doing the same thing, then your day's total for that activity is 15 minutes or .25 hour. Multiply this total time for a given type of activity by the average kcal/hour for that activity (see Table 6-2) and add them all up for the day's total kcalories. Use the following basic steps to estimate your energy expenditure for a day's activities:

1. Total minutes of an activity ÷ 60 = Hours of that activity
2. Total time (hr) × kcal/hour = Total kcal/day for that activity
3. Total kcal/day of all activities = Total kcal energy expenditure for day from activities

RECOMMENDATIONS FOR DIETARY ENERGY INTAKE

General Life Cycle

Growth Periods

During periods of rapid growth, extra energy per unit of body weight is necessary to build new tissue. In childhood, the most rapid growth occurs during infancy and adolescence, with continuous but slower growth in between (Table 6-3). The rapid growth of the fetus, placenta, and other maternal tissues makes increased energy intake during pregnancy and lactation a vital concern.

TABLE 6-3	Approximate Caloric Allowances from Birth to 18 Years	
Age (years)		**Kcal/lb**
INFANTS		
0-0.5		33.4
0.6-1.0		35.6
CHILDREN		
1-2		36.2
Males		
3-8		32
9-13		26.3
14-18		24
Females		
3-8		29.7
9-13		23.8
14-18		19.3

Data from Food and Nutrition Board, Institute of Medicine: *Dietary reference intakes for energy, carbohydrate, fiber, fat, fatty acids, cholesterol, protein, and amino acids,* Washington, DC, 2002, National Academies Press.

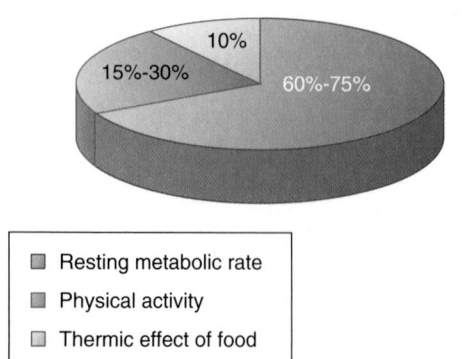

■ Resting metabolic rate
■ Physical activity
□ Thermic effect of food

Figure 6-3   Contributions of resting metabolic rate, physical activity, and the thermic effect of food to total energy expenditure.

Adulthood

With full adult growth achieved, energy needs level off, meeting requirements for tissue maintenance and usual physical activities.

<table>
<tr><td colspan="2">TABLE 6–4   Gradual Reduction of Kcalorie Needs during Adulthood</td></tr>
<tr><td>Age</td><td>Kcalorie reduction (%) for maintenance of ideal weight*</td></tr>
<tr><td>30-40</td><td>3</td></tr>
<tr><td>40-50</td><td>3</td></tr>
<tr><td>50-60</td><td>7.5</td></tr>
<tr><td>60-70</td><td>7.5</td></tr>
<tr><td>70-80</td><td>10</td></tr>
</table>

*Added percent decreases for each decade past the age of 25.

As the aging process continues, the gradual decline in BMR and physical activity decreases the total energy requirement (Table 6-4). Therefore food choices should reflect a decline in caloric density and place greater emphasis on increased nutrient density.

Dietary Reference Intakes

To determine recommendations for energy intake, the Food and Nutrition Board of the Institute of Medicine considered the average energy intake of individuals who were healthy, free-living, and maintaining a healthy body weight as determined by body mass index (BMI) measurements.[3] Table 6-5 gives the average total energy expenditure throughout life for those individuals. Note the average height, weight, BMI, and physical activity level within

TABLE 6–5   Median Height, Weight, and Recommended Energy Intake

Age (years)	Mean weight (kg [lb])	Mean height (m [in])	Mean BMI (kg/m²)	Mean basal energy expenditure (BEE) (kcal/day)	Mean physical activity level	Mean total energy expenditure (TEE) (kcal/day)
INFANTS						
0-0.5	6.9 (15)	0.64 (25)	16.86	—	—	501
0.6-1.0	9 (20)	0.72 (28)	17.20	—	—	713
CHILDREN						
1-2	11 (24)	0.82 (32)	16.19	—	—	869
MALES						
3-8	20.4 (45)	1.15 (45)	15.42	1035	1.39	1441
9-13	35.8 (79)	1.44 (57)	17.20	1320	1.56	2079
14-18	58.8 (130)	1.70 (67)	20.37	1729	1.80	3116
19-30	71 (156)	1.80 (71)	22.02	1769	1.74	3081
31-50	71.4 (157)	1.78 (70)	22.55	1675	1.81	3021
51-70	70 (154)	1.74 (69)	22.95	1524	1.63	2469
71+	68.9 (152)	1.74 (69)	22.78	1480	1.52	2238
FEMALES						
3-8	22.9 (50)	1.20 (47)	15.63	1004	1.48	1487
9-13	36.4 (80)	1.44 (57)	17.38	1186	1.60	1907
14-18	54.1 (119)	1.63 (64)	20.42	1361	1.69	2302
19-30	59.3 (131)	1.66 (65)	21.42	1361	1.80	2436
31-50	58.6 (129)	1.64 (65)	21.64	1322	1.83	2404
51-70	59.1 (130)	1.63 (63)	22.18	1226	1.70	2066
71+	54.8 (121)	1.58 (62)	21.75	1183	1.33	1564
PREGNANT						
1st trimester						+0
2nd-3rd trimester						+300/day
LACTATING						
1st 12 months						+500/day

Modified from Food and Nutrition Board, Institute of Medicine: *Dietary reference intakes for energy, carbohydrate, fiber, fat, fatty acids, cholesterol, protein, and amino acids*, Washington, DC, 2002, National Academies Press.

each age and gender group. Because a balance of energy intake and energy expenditure helps maintain a healthy weight, the Dietary Reference Intakes (DRI) for energy intake is equal to the total energy expenditure in kcalories.

Dietary Guidelines for Americans

The *Dietary Guidelines* for healthy Americans indicate energy needs by the following two recommendations: (1) maintain a healthy weight and (2) choose a diet low in fat, saturated fat, and cholesterol. Fats, the most concentrated fuel source, have the highest caloric density; and most Americans eat too much fat. A healthier energy balance also comes from using sugars only in moderation and eating a diet with plenty of vegetables, fruits, and grain products (see Chapter 1).

SUMMARY

Energy is the force or power to do work. In the human energy system, food provides energy. This energy is measured in "large calories" (e.g., every 1000 calories), or *kilocalories*. Energy from food is cycled through the body's internal energy system in balance with the external environment's energy system, powered by the sun.

Metabolism is the sum of the body processes involved in converting food into various forms of energy. These forms of energy include chemical, electrical, mechanical, and thermal energy. When food is not available, the body draws on its stored energy: glycogen, fat, and tissue protein.

Total body energy requirements are based on the following: (1) basal (e.g., maintenance) metabolism needs, which are measured by the BMR and compose the largest portion of energy needs; (2) energy for physical activities; and (3) the thermal effect of food (e.g., digesting food and absorbing and transporting nutrients). Energy requirements vary throughout life.

CRITICAL THINKING QUESTIONS

1. What are the fuel factors of the three energy nutrients? What is the fuel factor for alcohol? What do these figures mean? What is the primary energy nutrient? Why?

2. Define *resting metabolic rate*. What body tissues contribute most to resting metabolic needs? Why? What factors influence basal energy requirements? Why?

3. What factors influence nonbasal energy needs?

CHAPTER CHALLENGE QUESTIONS

True-False

Write the correct statement for each item you answer "false."

1. *True or False:* Kilocalories are nutrients in foods.

2. *True or False:* Resting metabolic rate takes into account energy used for physical activity.

3. *True or False:* The thyroid hormone, thyroxine, controls the rate of overall body metabolism.

4. *True or False:* Because children are smaller, their energy requirements are less per kilogram (or pound) of body weight than those of adults.

5. *True or False:* Physical activity level refers to the energy necessary for the digestion of food.

6. *True or False:* Different persons doing the same amount of physical activity require the same amount of energy in kcalories.

Multiple Choice

1. In human nutrition, the kilocalorie is used to
   a. provide nutrients.
   b. measure body heat energy.
   c. control energy reactions.
   d. measure electrical energy.

2. In the following family of four, who has the highest energy needs per unit of body weight?

   a. 32-year-old mother

   b. 35-year-old father

   c. 2-month-old son

   d. 70-year-old grandmother

3. An overactive thyroid causes

   a. decreased energy need.

   b. no effect on energy need.

   c. increased energy need.

   d. decreased protein needs.

4. Which of the following persons is using the most energy?

   a. Woman walking uphill

   b. Student studying for final examinations

   c. Teenager playing basketball

   d. Man driving a car

5. Which of these foods has the highest energy value per unit of weight?

   a. Bread

   b. Meat

   c. Potato

   d. Butter

6. A slice of bread contains 2 g of protein and 15 g of carbohydrate in the form of starch. What is its kcalorie value?

   a. 17 kcal

   b. 42 kcal

   c. 68 kcal

   d. 92 kcal

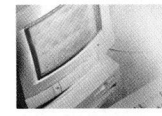

Please refer to the Students' Resource section of this text's Evolve web site for "Suggestions for Additional Study."

REFERENCES

1. Insel P, Turner RE, Ross D: *Discovering nutrition*, Boston, 2003, Jones and Bartlett.
2. Mahan LK, Escott-Stump S: *Krause's food, nutrition, & diet therapy*, ed 11, Philadelphia, 2004, Saunders.
3. Food and Nutrition Board, Institute of Medicine: *Dietary reference intakes for energy, carbohydrate, fiber, fat, fatty acids, cholesterol, protein, and amino acids*, Washington, DC, 2002, National Academies Press.
4. Wang Z and others: Resting energy expenditure-fat-free mass relationship: new insights provided by body composition modeling, *Am J Physiol Endocrinol Metab* 279(3):E539, 2000.
5. Gillam MP, Kopp P: Genetic regulation of thyroid development, *Curr Opin Pediatr* 13(4):358, 2001.
6. Butte NF and others: Energy requirements derived from total energy expenditure and energy deposition during the first 2 y of life, *Am J Clin Nutr* 72(6):1558, 2000.
7. Puggaard L and others: Age-related decrease in energy expenditure at rest parallels reductions in mass of internal organs, *Am J Human Biol* 14(4):486, 2002.
8. Poehlman ET: Menopause, energy expenditure, and body composition, *Acta Obstet Gynecol Scand* 81(7):603, 2002.
9. King JC: Physiology of pregnancy and nutrient metabolism, *Am J Clin Nutr* 71(5):1218S, 2000.
10. Liu S, Manson JE: Dietary carbohydrates, physical inactivity, obesity, and the 'metabolic syndrome' as predictors of coronary heart disease, *Curr Opin Lipidol* 12(4):395, 2001.
11. American Diabetes Association: Evidence-based nutrition principles and recommendations for the treatment and prevention of diabetes and related complications, *Diabetes Care* 25:S50, 2002.

FURTHER READING AND RESOURCES

• Pearcey SM, de Castro JM: Food intake and meal patterns of weight-stable and weight-gaining persons, *Am J Clin Nutr* 76(1):107, 2002.

  This paper discusses the importance of a healthy diet plan and physical activity that meet personal needs. The goal is to establish wise food habits and help persons develop and maintain a healthy lifestyle.

• van Marken Lichtenbelt WD and others: Individual variation in body temperature and energy expenditure in response to mild cold, *Am J Physiol Endocrinol Metab* 282(5):E1077, 2002.

  The authors take a closer look at individual differences in energy expenditure with relation to body temperature and reduced environmental temperature.

CHAPTER 7

Vitamins

More than any other group of nutrients, vitamins have captured public interest and concern. Vitamins are clearly essential nutrients; but what do they do, how much of them do human bodies need, and where do they come from? Are they better in food or in pills? From the constant attention they receive in the public press, it is known that vitamins are a concern of many people who need sound answers, not unfounded claims. The scientific study of nutrition, as reflected in the Dietary Reference Intake (DRI) guidelines, continues to expand knowledge.

This chapter looks at vitamins as a group and as individual nutrients, and explores general and specific vitamin needs and how to approach supplement use in a reasonable and realistic manner.

KEY CONCEPTS

- Vitamins are noncaloric essential nutrients that are necessary in very small amounts for specific metabolic control and disease prevention.

- Certain health problems are related to inadequate or excessive vitamin intake.

- Vitamins occur in a wide variety of foods that are packaged with the energy- and tissue-building macronutrients (e.g., carbohydrate, fat, and protein) on which vitamins work as specific catalysts to regulate body metabolism.

- Vitamin supplementation needs are individual and specific.

THE DIETARY REFERENCE INTAKES

In the study of vitamins and minerals in nutrition, one must understand the system of national recommendations for their use and how these nutrient guidelines are expanding dramatically with the introduction of DRIs.

The study of vitamins and minerals and their many functions in human nutrition continues to be a subject of intense scientific investigation and public interest. As discussed fully in Chapter 1, the DRIs are a new system of recommendations for the use of these nutrients in healthy populations. The publication of DRI reference information, under the direction of the National Academy of Sciences, took place over several years and involved numerous scientists from the United States and Canada. The DRIs, which include recommendations for each gender and age group, incorporate and expand on the well-known system of Recommended Dietary Allowances (RDAs).

Within the DRI system, there are four interconnected categories of recommendations, as follows: (1) the *Recommended Dietary Allowance* (RDA), which is the daily intake that meets the needs of almost all healthy individuals in a specified group; (2) the *Estimated Average Requirement* (EAR), which is used as the basis for developing the RDA and is the intake that meets the needs of half of the individuals in the reference population; (3) the *Adequate Intake* (AI), a guideline used when there is not enough scientific evidence available to establish an RDA; and (4) the *Tolerable Upper Intake Level* (UL), which is a new guideline that sets the maximum intake of a nutrient that is unlikely to pose a risk of toxicity in healthy individuals.

This chapter's study of vitamins and the following chapter's discussion of minerals refer to the various DRI recommendations (especially the RDAs) whenever possible. The RDAs, now established for gender and age groups, continue to be the central guides on nutrient intake for most individuals.

THE NATURE OF VITAMINS

Discovery

Early Observations

Vitamins were largely discovered during the search for cures of classic diseases that were initially thought to be associated with dietary deficiencies. As early as 1753 a British naval surgeon, Dr. James Lind, observed that on long voyages when sailors were forced to live on very limited rations because no fresh foods were available, many of them became ill and died. When Lind gave some fresh lemons and limes (which are easily stored) to the sailors on a later voyage, no one became ill. This is also how British sailors got the nickname "limeys." This vital clue then led to the discovery that *scurvy*, the curse of sailors, was caused by a dietary deficiency and was cured by adding certain fresh fruits to the diet.

Early Animal Experiments

In 1906, Dr. Frederich Hopkins of Cambridge University performed an experiment in which he fed a group of rats a diet of a synthetic mixture of protein, fat, carbohydrate, mineral salts, and water. All of the animals became ill and died. When he added milk to the purified ration, however, all of the rats grew normally. This important discovery, that there are accessory factors present in *natural* foods that are essential to life, reinforced the necessary foundation for the individual vitamin discoveries that followed.

Era of Vitamin Discovery

Most of the vitamins now known were discovered during the first half of the 1900s. The remarkable nature of these vital agents became more evident over time. A form of the name *vitamin* was first used in 1911 when Casimir Funk, a Polish chemist working at the Lister Institute in London, discovered a nitrogen-containing substance called an *amine*, which he thought was the chemical nature of these vital agents. So he called it *vitamine* ("vital-amine"). The final *e* was later dropped when other similarly vital substances turned out to be a variety of organic compounds. The name *vitamin* has been retained to designate compounds of this class of essential substances. At first, alphabet letter names were given to each vitamin discovered; however, as the number quickly increased, this practice became confusing. In recent years, more specific names based on a vitamin's chemical structure or body function have been developed and the letter names largely dropped. Today these scientific names are preferred and commonly used.

Definition

As each vitamin was discovered during the first half of the 1900s, two characteristics clearly emerged to define a compound as a vitamin, as follows:

1. It must be a vital, organic, dietary substance that is not a carbohydrate, fat, protein, or mineral and is necessary in only very *small* amounts to perform a specific metabolic function or prevent an associated deficiency disease.
2. It cannot be manufactured by the body in sufficient quantities to sustain life; therefore it must be supplied by the diet.

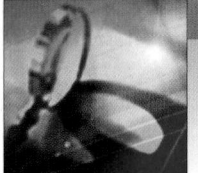

FOR FURTHER FOCUS

SMALL MEASURES FOR SMALL NEEDS

By definition, vitamins are essential nutrients necessary in small amounts for human health. But just how very small those amounts are is sometimes hard to imagine. Vitamins are measured in metric system terms such as milligram and microgram, but just how much is that? Perhaps comparing these amounts with commonly used household measures may help give you some idea.

Early in the age of scientific development, scientists realized that they needed a common language of measures that could be understood by all nations to fully exchange the rapidly developing scientific knowledge. Thus the metric system was born. Like American money, it is a simple decimal system, here applied to weights and measures. This system was developed in the mid-1800s by French scientists and named Le Système International d'Unités, which is abbreviated as SI units. Use of these more precise units is now widespread, especially because it is mandatory for all purposes in most countries besides the United States. The U.S. Congress passed the official Metric Conversion Act in 1975, but we have been slower to apply it to common use than other countries (see Appendix H). The use of this system in scientific work, however, is worldwide.

Compare the two metric measures used for vitamins in the United States. Following are the RDAs with common measures to see how small our need really is:

1. *Milligram* (mg) equals one-thousandth of a gram (28 g = 1 oz; 1 g = about ¼ tsp). RDAs are measured in milligrams for vitamins E, C, thiamin, riboflavin, niacin, B_6, pantothenic acid, and choline.
2. *Microgram* (mcg, or more often the Greek letter for "m," μ) equals one-millionth of a gram. RDAs are measured in micrograms for vitamins A (retinol equivalents), D, K, folate, B_{12}, and biotin.

Small wonder that the total amount of vitamins we need in a day would scarcely fill a teaspoon; but that small amount makes the big difference between life and death.

On the basis of these characteristics, vitamins are essential to life and health. The amount needed by the body is very small (hence the designation "micronutrients"), unless some special state or condition creates an increased need in a particular person. The total volume of vitamins a healthy person normally requires per day would barely fill a teaspoon. Thus the unit of measure for vitamins (e.g., milligrams or micrograms) is exceedingly small and difficult to visualize (see the For Further Focus box, "Small Measures for Small Needs"). However, all vitamins are essential to existence.

Classes of Vitamins

Vitamins are traditionally classified as either *fat soluble* or *water soluble*. The fat-soluble vitamins, to use their abbreviated letter names, are A, D, E, and K. The water-soluble vitamins are C and all of the B vitamins.

Functions of Vitamins

Although each vitamin has its specific metabolic task, two general functions that have been ascribed to vitamins as a group are the following: (1) control agents in cell metabolism, and (2) components of body-tissue construction. A third function, preventing specific nutritional deficiency disease, may be considered a result of their primary role in cell metabolism.

Metabolic Control Agent: Coenzyme Partner

Enzymes and coenzymes control specific chemical reactions by acting as necessary *catalysts*. This term comes from the Greek word *katalysis*, meaning "to dissolve." In chemical usage, *catalyst* refers to substances, such as enzymes, that are necessary control agents for breaking down compounds but are not themselves consumed in the process. In many cell reactions, a particular vitamin is necessary as a coenzyme partner with the regular cell enzyme to allow the reaction to proceed. Without the vitamin, the reaction cannot occur and the metabolic process involved cannot function. For example, several of the B vitamins (e.g., thiamin, niacin, and riboflavin) are essential components of the cell enzyme systems that metabolize glucose to produce energy.

Tissue Structure

Some vitamins act as tissue- or bone-building components. For example, vitamin C is essential in the synthesis of collagen, a protein needed for skin, ligament, and bone formation. In fact, the word *collagen* comes from a Greek word meaning "glue." Vitamins also act as antioxidants to protect cell structure and prevent free radical damage.

Prevention of Deficiency Diseases

If a vitamin deficiency becomes severe, a nutritional deficiency disease associated with the specific function of that vitamin becomes apparent. For example, the classic vitamin deficiency disease scurvy is caused by a lack of vitamin C. Scurvy is a hemorrhagic disease with bleeding into the joints and other internal tissues caused by fragile capillaries breaking down under normal blood pressure. Without vitamin C to produce strong capillary walls, vital internal membranes finally disintegrate and death occurs, as with British sailors 200 years ago. The name given to the vitamin, *ascorbic acid,* comes from the Latin word *scorbutus,* meaning "scurvy," so the term *ascorbic* means "without scurvy." In developed countries today, we do not often see frank scurvy, but we *do* see it— even here in America—along with other forms and degrees of malnutrition among low-income and poverty-stricken population groups.

Vitamin Metabolism

The way in which our bodies digest, absorb, and transport vitamins depends on the solubility of the vitamins, hence the classic distinction between water-soluble and fat-soluble vitamins.

Fat-Soluble Vitamins

Fat-soluble vitamins are dependent upon dietary fat for absorption and transport. They are absorbed into the gastrointestinal (GI) tract attached to fat. Once inside the mucosal lining cells, fat-soluble vitamins are incorporated into lipoproteins, right along with dietary fat, and enter the lymphatic system for circulation. The rate of absorption for fat-soluble vitamins declines when eating a meal that, although rich in fat-soluble vitamins, is low in dietary fat. For instance, skim milk has no dietary fat, but it has added fat soluble vitamin A. The vitamin A in skim milk is not as easily absorbed, when drank alone, as that of 2% or whole milk.

Unlike water-soluble vitamins, fat-soluble vitamins can be stored in the fatty compartments of the body for long periods of time. The body uses this reserve in times of inadequate intake. The ability to store fat-soluble vitamins is also the reason why excess intake can result in toxicity over time.

Water-Soluble Vitamins

Water-soluble vitamins are absorbed easily and directly into blood circulation from the GI tract. Because blood is mostly water, transport of water-soluble vitamins does not require assistance of a carrier.

With the exception of vitamin B_{12}, the body does not store water-soluble vitamins in any appreciable amount. Therefore we cannot count on a reserve supply and should incorporate foods rich in water-soluble vitamins daily. The difference in the body's ability to store vitamins dictates the toxicity effects of vitamins consumed in excess.

SECTION I
Fat-Soluble Vitamins

VITAMIN A (RETINOL)

Functions

Retinol performs the following functions in the body.

Vision

The chemical name *retinol* was given to vitamin A because of its major function in the retina of the eye. Retinol is an essential part of *rhodopsin,* which is a pigment in the eye commonly known as *visual purple.* This light-sensitive substance enables the eye to adjust to different amounts of available light. A mild deficiency of vitamin A may cause night blindness, slow adaptation to darkness, or glare blindness.

---

retinol (L. *retina,* from *rēte,* net, eye vision; suffix *-ol,* an alcohol) the chemical name of vitamin A; derived from its vision function relating to the retina of the eye, which is the back inner lining of the eyeball that "catches" the lens light refractions to form images interpreted by the optic nerve and brain and makes the necessary light-dark adaptations.

TABLE 7–1	Significant Food Sources of Vitamin A				
Food item	Quantity	Vitamin A (μg RE)	Food item	Quantity	Vitamin A (μg RE)
BREAD, CEREAL, RICE, PASTA This food group is not an important source of vitamin A.			**FRUITS** *(cont'd)*		
			Banana	1 medium	69
			Cantaloupe	¼ medium	1386
VEGETABLES			Grapefruit, pink	½ medium	162
Asparagus	½ cup	196	Orange juice	½ cup	75
Beet greens	½ cup	1110	Papaya	1 cup, cubed	735
Bok choy cabbage	½ cup	790	Peach	1 medium	399
Broccoli, fresh	1 medium stalk	1350	Prunes, dried	4	207
Broccoli, frozen	½ cup, chopped	721	Tangerine	1 medium	108
Brussels sprouts	½ cup (4 sprouts)	121	Watermelon	1 wedge (4 × 8 inches)	753
Carrots, raw	½ cup (1 medium)	2379			
Collard greens	½ cup	2223			
Corn	1 small cob	93	**MEAT, POULTRY, FISH, DRY BEANS, EGGS, NUTS**		
Dandelion greens	½ cup	1843	Clams, canned	3 oz	144
Green beans	½ cup	102	Egg, whole	1 large	78
Green peas	½ cup	144	Beef liver	3.5 oz	10,831
Kale	½ cup	1369	Chicken liver	3.5 oz	4912
Lima beans	½ cup	60			
Mustard greens	½ cup	1218	**MILK, DAIRY PRODUCTS**		
Pumpkin, canned	½ cup	2352	Cheddar cheese	1 oz	90
Romaine lettuce	½ cup, chopped	157	Milk, low-fat 2%, fortified	8 fl oz	150
Spinach	½ cup	2187	Milk, skim, fortified	8 fl oz	150
Summer squash	½ cup	123	Milk, whole, unfortified	8 fl oz	101
Sweet potato, baked, in skin	1 medium	2769	Ricotta cheese, whole milk	½ cup	182
Tomato, cooked	½ cup	325	Swiss cheese	1 oz	72
Winter squash	½ cup	1021	Yogurt, whole	8 fl oz	84
FRUITS			**FATS, OILS, SUGAR**		
Apricot, dried	4 halves	490	Butter	1 Tbsp	138
Apricot, fresh	3 medium	867	Margarine	1 Tbsp	141
Avocado	1 medium	189			

RE = Retinol equivalent.

Tissue Strength and Immunity

Retinol maintains healthy *epithelial* tissue, which is the vital protective tissue covering the body (e.g., the skin) and the inner mucous membranes in the nose, throat, eyes, GI tract, and genitourinary tract. These tissues provide our primary barrier to infection. Vitamin A is also important in the production of immune cells responsible for fighting bacterial, parasitic, and viral attacks.

Growth

Retinol is essential to the growth of skeletal and soft tissues and influences the stability of cell membranes and protein synthesis.

Requirements

Retinol requirements are influenced by factors related to its two basic forms in food sources and its storage in the body. The established RDA standard for adults is 700 μg retinol equivalents (RE) for women and 900 μg RE for men.

Food Forms and Units of Measure

Retinol occurs in two forms, as follow: (1) retinol, the fully preformed vitamin A; and (2) **carotene,** the "provitamin A," which is a pigment in yellow and green plants that the body converts to vitamin A. Because vitamin A comes in these two food forms and most of our intake is usually from *beta-carotene*, which becomes retinol in the body, vitamin A is currently measured in *retinol* equivalents. Another measure sometimes used for vitamin A is that of International Units (IU). One IU of vitamin A equals 0.3 μg retinol or 0.6 μg beta-carotene.

Body Storage

The liver can store large amounts of retinol. In healthy individuals, the storage efficiency of retinol ingested in the liver is more than 50%, and the liver contains about 90% of the body's total store. Thus when persons take large supplements of retinol in addition to dietary sources, it is possible to take a potentially toxic quantity.

Deficiency Disease

Adequate intake of retinol prevents two eye conditions, as follow: (1) *xerosis,* which is itching and burning and red inflamed lids; and (2) *xerophthalmia,* which is blindness from severe deficiency. Dietary vitamin A deficiency is the number one cause of blindness in children worldwide.

As with all vitamins, deficiency symptoms are directly related to the functions of the vitamin. Therefore a lack of vitamin A results in epithelial disorders and a compromised immune system.

Toxicity Symptoms

The condition created by excessive vitamin A intake is called *hypervitaminosis A.* Symptoms of this toxicity include joint pain, thickening of long bones, loss of hair, and jaundice. Excessive vitamin A also may cause liver injury with the following two results: (1) *portal hypertension,* which is elevated blood pressure in the blood circulation going directly to the liver from the GI tract, carrying absorbed nutrient loads after meals; and (2) *ascites,* which is fluid accumulation in the abdominal cavity.

Food Sources

Fish-liver oils, liver, egg yolk, butter, and cream are sources of preformed, natural vitamin A. Fat-soluble vitamin A only occurs naturally in the fat part of milk. Low-fat and nonfat milks and the butter substitute margarine are good sources of vitamin A because they are fortified with added vitamin A. Some good sources of beta-carotene are dark green leafy vegetables such as Swiss chard, turnip greens, kale, and spinach; and dark orange vegetables and fruits such as carrots, sweet potatoes or yams, pumpkin, mango, and apricots. Both beta-carotene and preformed vitamin A require the presence of bile salts for proper absorption from the intestine. Bile acts as an antioxidant to protect and stabilize the easily oxidized vitamin, as well as transport it through the intestinal wall. Table 7-1 provides some comparative food sources of vitamin A.

Stability

Retinol is unstable in heat and in contact with air. Cooking vegetables in an uncovered pot destroys much of their vitamin content. Quicker cooking with little water helps to preserve the vitamins. If fats are rancid or vegetables are wilted, most of the vitamin A is destroyed.

VITAMIN D (CHOLECALCIFEROL)

Vitamin D is not actually a true vitamin because it is made in our own bodies with the help of the sun's ultraviolet rays. It was mistakenly classed as a vitamin by its discoverers in 1922 because they were able to cure the childhood deficiency disease, rickets, with its only known natural form in fish liver oils. Today we know that the compound made in our skin by sunlight is actually a **prohormone.** This irradiated compound in the skin has been given the name **cholecalciferol,** often shortened to *calciferol,* because it is a fat-soluble *sterol* that controls calcium metabolism in bone-building. The initial compound in the skin is a *cholesterol* base. The irradiated cholesterol base in the skin, calciferol, is then activated by two successive enzymes, first in the liver and then in the kidney, to become the active

---

carotene a group name of three red and yellow pigments (alpha-, beta-, and gamma-carotene) found in dark green and yellow vegetables and fruits. The one most important to human nutrition is beta-carotene because the body can convert it to vitamin A, thus making it a primary source of the vitamin.

prohormone a precursor substance that the body converts to a hormone. For example, a cholesterol compound in the skin is first irradiated by sunlight and then converted through successive enzyme actions in the liver and kidney into the vitamin D hormone, which then regulates calcium absorption and bone development. Only a few food sources of vitamin D are found in food fats (e.g., cream, butter, and egg yolks), but vitamin D occurs in other processed foods (e.g., breakfast cereals and milk) through enrichment.

cholecalciferol the chemical name for vitamin D in its inactive dietary form; often shortened to calciferol.

vitamin D hormone form called calcitriol that functions in the body.

Functions

Calcitriol performs the following functions in the body.

Absorption of Calcium and Phosphorus

The hormone form calcitriol acts physiologically with two other hormones, the *parathyroid hormone* (PTH) and the thyroid hormone *calcitonin*. In balance with these two hormones, the vitamin D hormone stimulates absorption of calcium and phosphorus in the small intestine.

Bone Mineralization

Calcitriol also works with calcium and phosphorus to form bone tissue by directly regulating the rate of deposit and resorption of these minerals in bone. This balancing process builds and maintains bone tissue. Thus calcitriol has been clinically used to treat *osteoporosis*, which is a type of bone loss that leads to brittle bones and spontaneous fractures.

Requirements

A number of factors influence our requirements for vitamin D, and excessive intake is possible, especially in young infants. It is difficult to set requirements for this nutrient because of its unique hormonelike nature, its synthesis in the skin by the sun's irradiation of cholesterol there, and its limited food sources. The amount needed may vary between winter and summer, and with individual exposure to sunlight. People regularly exposed to sunlight (e.g., under appropriate conditions) have no dietary requirement for vitamin D. A substantial proportion of the U.S. population, however, is exposed to very little sunlight, especially during certain seasons, so a dietary supply is needed. The DRI research does not establish an RDA figure for vitamin D. Instead, adequate intake (AI) levels are given as guidelines. For example, the AI is 5 μg per day (200 IU) for both women and men from birth to age 50. The DRIs also set the upper limit (UL) for vitamin D for persons over age 1 at 50 μg per day.

Deficiency Disease

A deficiency of calcitriol causes rickets, a condition characterized by malformation of skeletal tissue in growing children (Figure 7-1). Children with rickets have soft long bones that bend under the weight of the child.

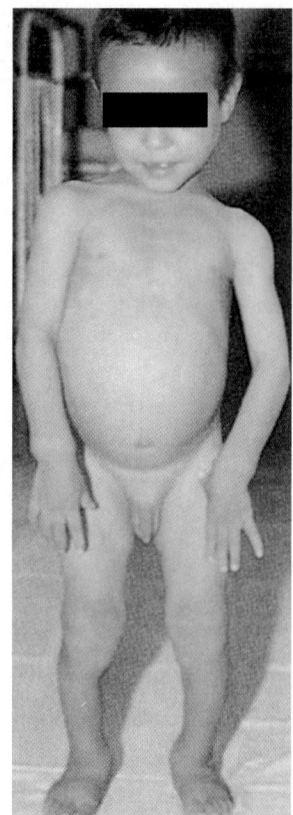

Figure 7-1   Child with rickets. Note his bowlegs.
(From McLaren DS: *A colour atlas and text of diet-related disorders,* ed 2, London, 1992, Mosby Year Book Europe Limited.)

Toxicity Symptoms

Excess intake of vitamin D, especially in infants, can be toxic. Symptoms of toxicity, or *hypervitaminosis D,* include calcification of soft tissues such as kidneys and lungs, as well as fragile bones. Prolonged intake of cholecalciferol (e.g., above 50 μg/day [2000 IU], which is 10 times the AI guideline) can produce elevated levels of calcium in the blood in infants and calcium deposits in the kidney nephrons in both infants and adults, affecting overall kidney function. For example, infant feeding may provide an excess (e.g., as much as 100 μg [4000 IU] or more) of cholecalciferol when fortified milk and fortified cereal are used in addition to variable vitamin supplements. An infant (from birth to 1 year) only needs 5 μg (200 IU) of cholecalciferol daily.[1]

Food Sources

Only yeast and fish liver oils are natural sources of vitamin D. Therefore the only regular food sources of vitamin D are those that have been fortified with the

TABLE 7–2	Significant Food Sources of Vitamin D	
Food item	**Quantity**	**Vitamin D (μg)**
BREAD, CEREAL, RICE, PASTA		
Corn flake cereal	1 cup (1 oz)/28 g	1
Granola	¼ cup (1 oz)/28 g	1.23
Raisin and bran cereal	½ cup (1 oz)/28 g	1.23
VEGETABLES		
This food group is not an important source of vitamin D.		
FRUITS		
This food group is not an important source of vitamin D.		
MEAT, POULTRY, FISH, DRY BEANS, NUTS		
This food group is not an important source of vitamin D.		
EGGS		
Egg, whole	1 large/50 g	0.68
Egg yolk	Yolk of 1 large egg/17 g	0.68
MILK, DAIRY PRODUCTS		
Evaporated milk, vitamin D–fortified	½ cup (4 fl oz)/126 g	2.50
Milk, whole or nonfat, vitamin D–fortified	1 quart/960 g	10
Milk, whole or nonfat, vitamin D–fortified	1 cup (8 fl oz)/240 g	2.50
FATS, OILS, SUGAR		
Margarine	1 Tbsp	1.50
Fish oil	1 Tbsp	34

vitamin (Table 7-2). Because it is a common food and also contains calcium and phosphorus, milk is the most practical carrier. The standard commercial practice is to add 10 μg (400 IU)/quart. But dairies and other producers must be closely regulated to ensure that this practice is consistently accurate (see the For Further Focus box "Vitamin D Toxicity: Too Much of a Good Thing"). Butter substitutes, such as margarines, are also fortified. Children on vitamin D-deficient diets (e.g., a rigid macrobiotic pattern with no milk products) are especially vulnerable to stunted bone development and rickets.

Stability

Vitamin D is stable to heat, aging, and storage.

VITAMIN E (TOCOPHEROL)

Early vitamin studies identified a substance necessary for animal reproduction that was chemically an alcohol. This substance was named **tocopherol,** from two Greek words: *tophos,* meaning "childbirth," and *phero,* meaning "to bring," with the *-ol* ending for alcohol. Tocopherol soon became known as the antisterility vitamin, but it

was soon demonstrated to have this effect only in rats and a few other animals, not in humans; all advertising claims for its contribution to sexual powers notwithstanding. A number of related compounds have since been discovered. Tocopherol (vitamin E) is actually the generic name for a group of similar fat-soluble nutrients. Three of these, designated alpha (α)-, beta (β)-, and gamma (γ)-tocopherol, display the most biological

calcitriol   the activated hormone form of vitamin D.

rickets   (Gr. *rhachitis,* a spinal complaint) a disease of childhood characterized by softening of the bones from an inadequate intake of vitamin D and insufficient exposure to sunlight; also associated with impaired calcium and phosphorus metabolism.

tocopherol   (Gr. *tokos,* childbirth; *pherein,* to carry) the chemical name for vitamin E, which was so named by early investigators because their initial work with rats indicated a reproductive function, which is not true with humans. In humans, vitamin E functions as a strong antioxidant that preserves structural membranes such as cell walls.

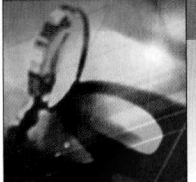

FOR FURTHER FOCUS

VITAMIN D TOXICITY: TOO MUCH OF A GOOD THING

In the United States, milk has been fortified with vitamin D since the early 1930s. As a result, rickets largely has been eradicated. From the beginning, U.S. federal regulations have specified that each quart of milk contain 10 μg (400 IU) of vitamin D. The previous measure of International Units (IU) is passing from use in relation to vitamin needs because it is a less useful measure than the metric unit micrograms (μg), which can be measured and regulated directly.

Toxic amounts of vitamin D, however, can build up in the body easily because this vitamin is stored in fat tissue and released slowly. Even today, cases of toxicity occur, usually from excessively fortified milk. For example, a

U.S. outbreak was traced to a local dairy's sporadic addition, ranging from 20 μg to nearly 6000 μg/quart, of excessive vitamin D to milk during the fortification process, even though the regulation calls for only 10 μg. Young children who drank this dairy's milk for several years did not grow normally in height and developed kidney function problems because of excess calcium in their kidney tissues. Adults suffered progressive weakness, elevated blood levels of calcium, and bone pain.

For the most part, the American dairy industry is diligent about using correct procedures for fortifying milk, but this case demonstrated that too much of an essential vitamin can cause illness.

---

activity. Of these three, α-tocopherol is the most significant in human nutrition and thus is used for measuring dietary needs.[2]

Functions

The most vital function of tocopherol is its action as an antioxidant in many tissues. An antioxidant is an agent that prevents cellular structure from being broken down by oxygen (e.g., the process of oxidation).

Antioxidant Function

Tocopherol acts as nature's most potent fat-soluble antioxidant. The polyunsaturated fatty acids (see Chapter 3) in lipid membranes of body tissues are particularly easy for oxygen to break down. Tocopherol can interrupt this oxidation process, protecting the fatty acids of the cell membrane from damage. For example, vitamin E can protect fragile red blood cell walls in premature infants from breaking down, causing anemia (see the Clinical Applications box, "Vitamin E and Premature Infants"). Vitamin E helps protect both red blood cells and muscle tissue cells.

Relation to Selenium Metabolism

Selenium is a trace mineral that works as a partner with tocopherol as an antioxidant. A selenium-containing enzyme, glutathione peroxidase, is the second line of defense in preventing oxidative damage to cell membranes. Selenium spares tocopherol by reducing its requirement, just as tocopherol does for selenium.

Requirements

Tocopherol requirements are expressed in terms of *alpha-tocopherol* in mg/day. The DRI recommendations state that the RDA standard for men and women age 14 and older is 15 mg/day, with lesser amounts necessary during childhood. Needs during the first year of infancy do not have an RDA figure, but an AI amount of 4 to 6 mg/day is used. The UL for all adults is set at 1000 mg/day.

Deficiency Disease

Young infants, especially premature infants who miss the final 1 to 2 months of gestation when tocopherol stores are normally built up, are particularly vulnerable to the tocopherol deficiency disease called hemolytic anemia. In this disease, the lipid membranes of red blood cells are easily oxidized by oxygen, and the continued loss of red blood cells leads to anemia. In older children and adults, a deficiency of tocopherol disrupts normal synthesis of *myelin*, the protective fat covering of nerve cells that helps them pass messages along to specific tissues. The main nerves involved are the following: (1) spinal cord fibers that affect physical activity (e.g., walking), and (2) the retina of the eye that affects vision.

Toxicity Symptoms

Tocopherol from food sources has no known toxic effect in humans. Supplemental intakes exceeding the UL of 1000 mg/day may interfere with vitamin K activity and blood clotting.

CLINICAL APPLICATIONS

VITAMIN E AND PREMATURE INFANTS

A medical problem found in infants, especially premature ones, has responded positively to vitamin E therapy. This problem is hemolytic anemia.

Anemia is a blood condition characterized by loss of mature, functioning red blood cells. Different types of anemia are usually named according to cause or to the nature of an abnormal nonfunctioning cell produced. The name of this type of anemia comes from its cause. The word hemolysis comes from two roots: *hemo*, referring to blood, and *lysis*, meaning dissolving or breaking. Therefore hemolysis means the bursting or dissolving of red blood cells, and the resulting condition is hemolytic anemia. Vitamin E can help prevent this destruction of red blood cells and the loss of their vital oxygen-carrying hemoglobin because it is one of the body's foremost antioxidants.

An oxidant is a compound or oxygen itself that oxidizes other compounds, thereby breaking them down or changing them. Vitamin E is readily oxidized. When there is plenty of vitamin E among the other compounds exposed to an oxidant, vitamin E can, by its nature, take on the oxidative attack, thus protecting the others. Vitamin E is fat soluble, so it is found among the polyunsaturated fatty acids that compose the core of the cell membranes in body tissues that are rich in fat. The cell membranes of red blood cells are particularly rich in these polyunsaturated lipids and are exposed to concentrated oxygen because they constantly circulate through the lungs. This situation would be destructive to the red blood cells if vitamin E was not present. Vitamin E takes the oxygen itself, protecting the polyunsaturated fatty acids and keeping the red blood cells intact to continue their life-sustaining journey throughout the body. Thus vitamin E acts as nature's most potent fat-soluble antioxidant. It interrupts the oxidative breakdown by free radicals (e.g., parts of compounds broken off by cell metabolism) in the cell, protecting the cell membrane fatty acids from the oxidative damage.

The protective need of vitamin E is especially great in small, premature infants fed formulas containing iron, which acts as an oxidant, and high concentrations of polyunsaturated fatty acids, which are vulnerable to oxidative breakdown. To avoid this problem and comply with American Academy of Pediatrics recommendations, manufacturers have increased the amount of vitamin E and lowered the iron in formulas for premature infants. The proportions of vitamin E, polyunsaturated fatty acids, and iron in today's improved formulas usually supply enough necessary nutrients, so in most cases supplements are no longer necessary to prevent hemolytic anemia in premature infants.

Food Sources

The richest sources of tocopherol are vegetable oils (wheat germ, soybean, and safflower oil). Note that vegetable oils are also the richest sources of polyunsaturated fatty acids, which vitamin E protects. Other food sources of tocopherol include nuts, fortified cereals, and avocado. Table 7-3 provides a list of vitamin E food sources.

Stability

Tocopherol is stable to heat and acids but not to alkalis.

VITAMIN K

In the early era of vitamin research Henrik Dam, a biochemist at the University of Copenhagen, discovered a hemorrhagic disease in chicks that were fed a fat-free diet and determined that the factor responsible was the absence of a fat-soluble, blood-clotting vitamin. He called it "koagulationsvitamin," or vitamin K, and the letter name has stuck. Dam later succeeded in isolating and identifying the agent from alfalfa, for which he received the Nobel prize for physiology and medicine. As with a number of vitamins, not one but several forms of vitamin K compose a group of substances with similar biologic activity in blood clotting. The major form found in plants, and initially isolated from alfalfa by Dam, is named phylloquinone because of its chemical structure. Phylloquinone is our dietary form of

---

phylloquinone   a fat-soluble vitamin of the K group found in green plants or prepared synthetically.

TABLE 7–3 Significant Food Sources of Vitamin E as Alpha-Tocopherol		
Food item	**Quantity**	**Vitamin E (mg α-TE)**
BREAD, CEREAL, RICE, PASTA		
This food group is not an important source of vitamin E.		
VEGETABLES		
Asparagus, raw	4 spears/58 g	1.15
Avocado, raw	1 medium/173 g	2.32
Brussels sprouts, boiled	½ cup (4 sprouts)/78 g	0.66
Cabbage, green, raw	½ cup, shredded/35 g	0.58
Carrot, raw	1 medium/72 g	0.32
Lettuce, iceberg, raw	¼ head/135 g	0.54
Spinach, raw	½ cup, chopped/28 g	0.53
Sweet potato, raw	1 medium/130 g	5.93
FRUITS		
Apple, raw, with skin	1 medium/138 g	0.81
Apricot, canned	4 halves/90 g	0.80
Avocado	½ medium/86.5 g	1.70
Banana, raw	1 medium/114 g	0.31
Mango, raw	1 medium/207 g	2.32
Pear, raw	1 medium/166 g	0.83
MEAT, POULTRY, FISH, DRY BEANS, EGGS		
This food group is not an important source of vitamin E.		
NUTS		
Almonds, dried	1 oz (24 nuts)/28 g	6.72
Hazelnuts, dried	1 oz/28 g	6.70
Peanut butter	1 Tbsp/16 g	3
Peanuts, dried	1 oz/28 g	2.56
Walnuts, dried	1 oz (14 halves)/28 g	0.73
MILK, DAIRY PRODUCTS		
This food group is not an important source of vitamin E.		
FATS, OILS, SUGAR		
Corn oil	1 Tbsp/14 g	1.90
Cottonseed oil	1 Tbsp/14 g	4.80
Olive oil	1 Tbsp/14 g	1.60
Palm oil	1 Tbsp/14 g	2.60
Peanut oil	1 Tbsp/14 g	1.60
Safflower oil	1 Tbsp/14 g	4.60
Soybean oil	1 Tbsp/14 g	1.50

α-TE, α-Tocopherol equivalents.

vitamin K, while menaquinone, a second form, is synthesized by intestinal bacteria. Menaquinone contributes about half of our daily supply of vitamin K.

Functions

Vitamin K is known to have two metabolic functions in the body: blood clotting and bone development.

Blood Clotting

The basic function of vitamin K is in the blood-clotting process. Vitamin K is essential for maintaining normal levels of four of the 11 blood-clotting factors. The most familiar of these vitamin K-dependent blood factors is *prothrombin* (number II). Thus phylloquinone can serve as an antidote for the excess effects of anticoagulant drugs. Phylloquinone is often used in the control and prevention of certain types of hemorrhages. Because this fat-soluble vitamin is absorbed more completely if bile is present, conditions that hinder bile flow to the small intestine reduce blood-clotting ability. If bile salts are given with vitamin K concentrate, the blood-clotting time returns to normal.

Bone Development

A more recently discovered function of vitamin K relates to bone development. Specific proteins found in bone and bone matrix are dependent on vitamin K for their synthesis and are involved with calcium in bone development. Like the blood-clotting proteins, these bone proteins bind calcium but function here to form bone crystals.

Requirements

Because intestinal bacteria synthesize a form of vitamin K, a constant supply is normally available to support dietary sources. Currently, there is not enough scientific evidence available to establish an RDA.[3] Therefore the DRIs for vitamin K are represented by an AI value. Values gradually increase from birth to adulthood. The AI standard for men is 120 μg/day and 90 μg/day for women. A recent study indicates that men and women in the 18- to 44-year-old age group reported dietary intakes below the current recommended intakes.[4]

Deficiency Disease

Deficiency disease relating to vitamin K is not usually found in humans. A deficiency is unlikely except in clinical conditions related to blood clotting, malabsorption, or lack of intestinal bacteria to synthesize the vitamin. For example, because the intestinal tract of a newborn is sterile, phylloquinone is routinely given to prevent hemorrhage when the umbilical cord is cut. The "vitamin K shot" giving at birth is commonly called AquaMephyton, Mephyton, or Phytonadione. Patients with severe malabsorption disorders, such as Crohn's disease, or who are placed on poor diets after surgery and treated with antibiotics that kill intestinal bacteria, are susceptible to vitamin K deficiency with resulting blood loss and poor wound healing.

Toxicity Symptoms

Toxicity from vitamin K—even when large amounts are taken over extended periods—has not been observed.

Food Sources

Green leafy vegetables, which provide 50 to 800 μg of phylloquinone per 100 g of food, are clearly the best dietary sources. Small amounts of phylloquinone are contributed by milk and dairy products, meats, fortified cereals, fruits, and vegetables (Table 7-4).

Stability

Vitamin K as phylloquinone is fairly stable, although it is sensitive to light and irradiation. Therefore clinical preparations are kept in dark bottles.

Table 7-5 provides a summary of the fat-soluble vitamins.

Water-Soluble Vitamins

SECTION

2

VITAMIN C (ASCORBIC ACID)

Functions

Vitamin C has several critical functions in the body. It acts as a protective agent (antioxidant), enzyme cofactor, and plays a role in many metabolic and immunologic activities.

Connective Tissue

Ascorbic acid is necessary to build and maintain strong tissues in general, but is especially important for connective tissues such as bone, cartilage, tooth

---

ascorbic acid   chemical name for vitamin C, from ability of the vitamin to cure scurvy.

TABLE 7-4	Significant Food Sources of Vitamin K	
Food item	**Quantity**	**Vitamin K (μg)**
BREAD, CEREAL, RICE, PASTA		
Oats, dry	100 g	63
Wheat bran	100 g	83
Whole wheat flour	100 g	30
VEGETABLES		
Broccoli, raw	100 g	132
Cabbage, raw	100 g	149
Cauliflower, raw	100 g	191
Lentils, dry	100 g	223
Lettuce, iceberg, raw	100 g	112
Spinach, raw	100 g	266
Turnip greens, raw	100 g	650
FRUITS		
This food group is not an important source of vitamin K.		
MEAT, POULTRY, FISH, DRY BEANS, EGGS, NUTS		
Beef liver	100 g	104
Chicken liver	100 g	80
Pork liver	100 g	88
MILK, DAIRY PRODUCTS		
This food group is not an important source of vitamin K.		
FATS, OILS, SUGAR		
Corn oil	100 g	60
Soybean oil	100 g	540

dentin, tendon, and capillary walls. The major protein involved in fibrous connective tissue is collagen. For the body to synthesis collagen, the amino acid proline must undergo a hydroxylation reaction yielding hydroxyproline. This hydroxylation reaction is dependent upon ascorbic acid. When ascorbic acid is in adequate supply, collagen, and the connective tissue it builds, develops quickly. Blood vessel tissue particularly depends upon ascorbic acid to form strong capillary walls.

General Body Metabolism

The more metabolically active body tissues (e.g., adrenal glands, brain, kidney, liver, pancreas, thymus, and spleen) have greater concentrations of ascorbic acid. The high concentration of ascorbic acid in the adrenal glands is depleted when the gland is stimulated. This depletion suggests an increased need for the vitamin during stress. There is also more ascorbic acid in a child's actively growing tissue than in adult tissue.

Ascorbic acid is an essential partner of protein for tissue building. Specifically, ascorbic acid is involved in the metabolism and conversion of certain amino acids (tyrosine, lysine, proline, phenylalanine, and tryptophan). The biosynthesis of some hormones and neurotransmitters (norepinephrine and serotonin) is also dependent on adequate supplies of ascorbic acid. Furthermore, ascorbic acid helps the body absorb iron and makes it available for hemoglobin production, thereby helping to prevent anemia. The general clinical needs of ascorbic acid relate to wound healing, fevers and infections, and growth periods.

Antioxidant Function

Similar to vitamin E, ascorbic acid is an antioxidant working to protect the body from free radical damage. Free radicals are associated with increased risk of cancer and heart disease. However, higher intakes of antioxidants, including vitamin C, may prevent the development of chronic disease.[2]

TABLE 7–5 A Summary of Fat-Soluble Vitamins

Vitamin	Functions	Recommended intake (adults)	Deficiency	UL and toxicity	Sources
Vitamin A (retinol, retinal, and retinoic acid) Provitamin A (carotene)	Vision cycle—adaptation to light and dark; tissue growth, especially skin and mucous membranes, reproduction, immune function	RDA Men: 900 μg Women: 700 μg	Night blindness, xerosis, xerophthalmia, susceptibility to epithelial infection, dry skin, impaired immunity, growth, and reproduction	UL: 3000 μg Hair loss, irritated skin, bone pain, liver damage, birth defects	Retinol (animal foods): liver, egg yolk, cream, butter or fortified margarine, fortified milk Provitamin A (plant foods): dark-green and yellow vegetables (spinach, collards, broccoli, pumpkin, sweet potatoes, carrots)
Vitamin D (cholecalciferol, ergocalciferol)	Absorption of calcium and phosphorus, calcification of bones and teeth, growth	AI Ages 19-50 yr: 5 μg 51-70 yr: 10 μg 70+: 15 μg	Rickets and growth retardation in children Osteomalacia (soft bones) in adults	UL: 50 μg Calcification of soft tissue, kidney damage, growth retardation	Synthesized in skin with exposure to sunlight, fortified milk, fish oils
Vitamin E (alpha-tocopherol)	Antioxidant—protection of materials that oxidize easily	RDA Adults: 15 mg	Breakdown of red blood cells, anemia, nerve damage, retinopathy	UL: 1000 mg (from supplements) Inhibition of vitamin K activity in blood clotting	Vegetable oils, vegetable greens, wheat germ, nuts, and seeds
Vitamin K (phylloquinone, menaquinone)	Normal blood clotting and bone development	AI Men: 120 μg Women: 90 μg	Bleeding tendencies, hemorrhagic disease, poor bone growth	UL: Not set Interference with anti-coagulation drugs	Synthesis by intestinal bacteria, dark green leafy vegetables, soybean oil, liver, milk

AI = adequate intake; *UL* = Tolerable Upper Intake Level.

CLINICAL APPLICATIONS

ASCORBIC ACID NEEDS IN SMOKERS

Free radicals are reactive molecules that can disrupt normal structure of DNA, proteins, carbohydrates, and fatty acids. Such damage is linked to an increased risk of cancer and cardiovascular disease. Cigarette smoke is one environmental source of free radicals. Our bodies fight these free radicals with antioxidants, such as vitamins E and C. Antioxidants destroy free radicals and work to protect the body from free radical damage.

As free radical production increases, antioxidant needs also increase. Cigarette smokers deplete their supply of ascorbic acid more rapidly than nonsmokers because of increased free radical exposure. The vitamin is needed to break down toxic compounds in cigarette smoke. Therefore cigarette smokers are recommended to consume an additional 35 mg of vitamin C per day to meet the increased needs.

Requirements

Ascorbic acid provides antioxidant protection. To achieve this, the DRI guidelines for adults over 18 establish an RDA of 75 mg/day for females and 90 mg/day for males, with increases for women during pregnancy and lactation. Because smokers suffer increased stress to their body tissues, the DRIs recommend that their intake be 35 mg/day higher (see the Clinical Applications box, "Ascorbic Acid Needs in Smokers"). The UL for vitamin C is 2000 mg/day for adults.

Deficiency Disease

Signs of ascorbic acid deficiency are; tissue bleeding (e.g., easy bruising, pinpoint skin hemorrhages), bone and joint bleeding, easy bone fracture, poor wound healing, and soft bleeding gums with loosened teeth. Extreme deficiency produces the disease scurvy.

Toxicity Symptoms

The UL for ascorbic acid is 2000 mg/day. Although most excess intake of water-soluble vitamins is efficiently excreted in the urine, levels above 2000 mg/day are more difficult to clear and may result in GI disturbances and osmotic diarrhea in some populations. The Institute of Medicine states that further research is warranted on toxicity effects of ascorbic acid due to the popularity of high intakes of the vitamin in the United States.[2]

Food Sources

The best food sources of ascorbic acid are citrus fruits (Figure 7-2). Additional sources include tomatoes, cabbage and other leafy vegetables, berries, melons, peppers, broccoli, potatoes (white and sweet), and other green and yellow vegetables (Table 7-6).

Stability

Ascorbic acid is easily oxidized upon exposure to air and heat. Therefore care must be taken in handling its food sources. Ascorbic acid is not stable to alkaline substances, thus baking soda—often added to cooked foods to retain pristine color—destroys the ascorbic acid content. Acidic fruits and vegetables retain their ascorbic acid content better than nonacid ones. The vitamin is also very soluble in water. The more water added while cooking, the more ascorbic acid leaches out of the fruit or vegetable into the cooking water.

THIAMIN (VITAMIN B₁)

Functions

The vitamin name thiamin comes from its chemical-ringlike structure. The basic function of thiamin as a coenzyme factor relates to the production of energy from glucose and the storage of energy as fat, making energy available to support normal growth. Thiamin is especially necessary for maintaining good function of three body systems discussed in the following text.

Gastrointestinal System

Lack of thiamin causes poor appetite, indigestion, constipation and poor stomach action from lack of muscle tone, as well as deficient gastric hydrochloric acid secretion. The cells of smooth muscles and secretory glands must have energy to do their work; thiamin is a necessary agent for producing that energy.

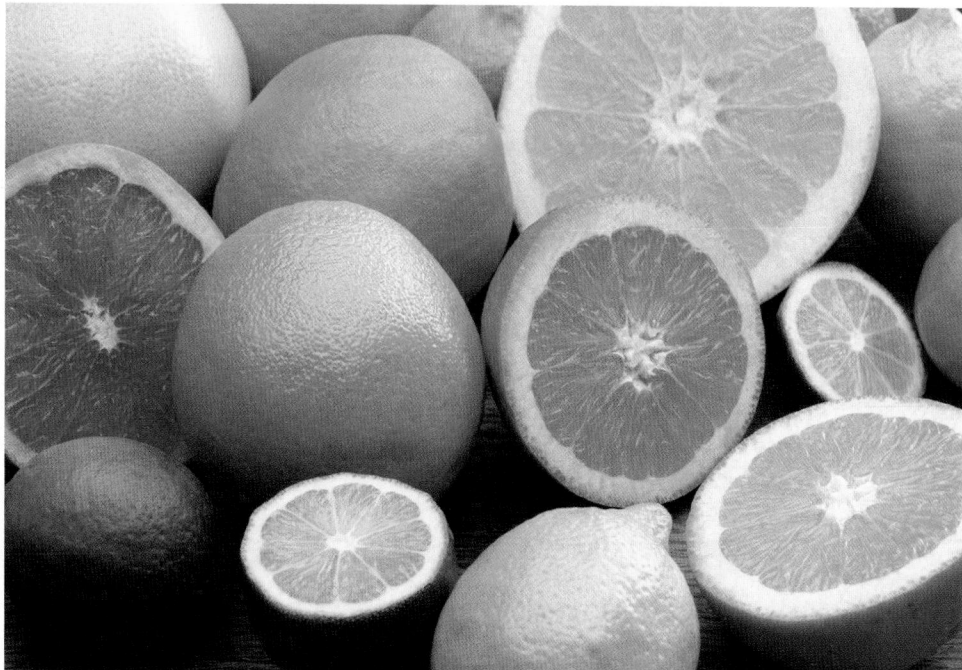

Figure 7–2   Foods high in Vitamin C. (Credit: PhotoDisc.)

Nervous System

The central nervous system depends on glucose for energy. Without sufficient thiamin, this energy is not produced and the nerves cannot conduct their work. Alertness and reflex responses decrease; apathy, fatigue, and irritability result. If the thiamin deficit continues, nerve tissue damage causes nerve irritation, pain, prickly or deadening sensations, and, finally, paralysis.

Cardiovascular System

Without constant energy, the heart muscle weakens and heart failure results. Blood circulation becomes problematic when the muscles in vessel walls also weaken. Weakened vessels dilate, leading to fluid accumulation in the lower part of the legs.

Requirements

Thiamin is directly related to the metabolic need for energy and carbohydrate. For healthy persons, the DRI guidelines establish RDAs for adults over age 18, based on average energy needs, as 1.2 mg/day for men and 1.1 mg/day for women. Children require less. For infants up to 12 months, there is no RDA; the AI figure is 0.2 to 0.3 mg/day. Increased amounts are needed during pregnancy and lactation, as well as in the treatment of infectious diseases and alcoholism. There is no UL for thiamin.

Deficiency Disease

Thiamin was first discovered as the control agent relating to the classic deficiency disease beriberi, a paralyzing disease known since antiquity that was especially prevalent in Asian countries. The name describes the disease well; it is Singhalese for "I can't, I can't," because afflicted persons were always too ill to do anything. In industrialized

---

scurvy   a vitamin-deficiency disease caused by a lack of vitamin C. It is a hemorrhagic disease with diffuse tissue bleeding, painful limbs and joints, thickened bones, and skin discoloration from tissue bleeding; bones fracture easily, wounds do not heal, gums are swollen and bleed, and teeth loosen.

thiamin   chemical name of a major B-complex vitamin; also called vitamin B_1, discovered in relation to the classic deficiency disease beriberi; important in body metabolism as a coenzyme factor in many cell reactions related to energy metabolism.

beriberi   (Singhalese for "I can't, I can't") a disease of the peripheral nerves caused by a deficiency of thiamin (vitamin B_1); characterized by pain (neuritis) and paralysis of legs and arms, cardiovascular changes, and edema.

TABLE 7–6   Significant Food Sources of Vitamin C

Food item	Quantity	Vitamin C (mg)
BREAD, CEREAL, RICE, PASTA		
This food group is not an important source of vitamin C.		
VEGETABLES		
Asparagus, boiled	½ cup (6 spears)	18
Avocado, raw	1 medium	14
Broccoli, raw	½ cup	41
Brussels sprouts, boiled	½ cup (4 sprouts)	48
Cauliflower, raw	½ cup, pieces	36
Green pepper, raw	½ cup, chopped	64
Kale, boiled	½ cup	27
Potato, baked, with skin	1 medium	26
Sweet potato, baked	1 medium	28
Tomato, raw	1 medium	22
FRUITS		
Cantaloupe, raw	½ cup, pieces	34
Grapefruit, white	½ medium	39
Kiwi, raw	1 medium	75
Lemon	1 medium	31
Lemon juice, fresh	8 fl oz	112
Orange juice, fresh	8 fl oz	124
Orange, navel	1 medium	80
Papaya, raw	1 medium	188
Pineapple, raw	½ cup	12
Raspberries, raw	½ cup	15
Strawberries, raw	½ cup	44
Tangerine, raw	1 medium	26
MEAT, POULTRY, FISH, DRY BEANS, EGGS, NUTS		
Beef liver, fried	3.5 oz	23
Ham, lean, canned; vitamin C added	3.5 oz	27
MILK, DAIRY PRODUCTS		
This food group is not an important source of vitamin C.		
FATS, OILS, SUGAR		
This food group is not an important source of vitamin C.		

societies, thiamin deficiency is largely associated with chronic alcoholism and individuals with a poor diet. Alcohol inhibits the absorption of thiamin. Alcohol-induced thiamin deficiency presents as Wernicke's encephalopathy, a disease affecting mental alertness and coordination.

Toxicity Symptoms

Because the kidneys clear excess thiamin, there is no evidence of toxicity from oral intake.

Food Sources

Although thiamin is widespread in almost all plant and animal tissues, its content is usually small. Thus thiamin deficiency is a distinct possibility when kcalories are markedly curtailed (e.g., in alcoholism or when a person is following a highly inadequate diet). Good food sources of thiamin include wheat germ, lean pork, beef, liver, whole or enriched grains (e.g., flour, bread, cereals), and legumes (Table 7-7). Eggs, fish, and a few vegetables are fair sources.

TABLE 7-7	Significant Food Sources of Thiamin	
Food item	**Quantity**	**Thiamin (mg)**
BREAD, CEREAL, RICE, PASTA		
Bran Flakes cereal	1 cup	0.46
Bread, whole wheat	1 slice	0.10
Corn muffin	1 muffin	0.10
Egg noodles, enriched	1 cup	0.20
Pasta/rice, enriched	1 cup	0.23
Wheat Flakes cereal	1 cup	0.40
VEGETABLES		
Avocado, raw	1 medium	0.19
Corn, yellow, boiled	½ cup	0.18
Green peas, boiled	½ cup	0.21
Potato, baked, with skin	1 medium	0.22
FRUITS		
Figs, dried	10	0.13
Orange juice, fresh	8 fl oz	0.22
Orange, navel, raw	1 medium	0.13
Raisins, seedless	⅔ cup	0.16
MEAT, POULTRY, FISH, DRY BEANS, EGGS, NUTS		
Beef liver, fried	3.5 oz	0.21
Black-eyed peas, boiled	1 cup	0.35
Cashews, roasted	1 oz	0.12
Chicken liver, simmered	3.5 oz	0.15
Ham, canned	3.5 oz	0.85
Kidney beans, boiled	1 cup	0.28
Lentils, boiled	1 cup	0.34
Lima beans, boiled	1 cup	0.30
Navy beans, boiled	1 cup	0.37
Peanuts, roasted	1 oz	0.12
Pecans, dried	1 oz	0.24
Pinto beans, boiled	1 cup	0.32
Sirloin steak, broiled	3.5 oz	0.13
Soybeans, boiled	1 cup	0.27
Top round, broiled	3.5 oz	0.12
Tuna, baked	3 oz	0.24

MILK, DAIRY PRODUCTS
This food group is not an important source of thiamin.

FATS, OILS, SUGAR
This food group is not an important source of thiamin.

Stability

Thiamin is a fairly stable vitamin but is destroyed by alkalis and prolonged heat at high cooking temperatures. Because it is water-soluble, little cooking water should be used. As with other water-soluble vitamins, when cooking water is retained in the dish being prepared, the vitamin is preserved.

RIBOFLAVIN (VITAMIN B₂)

Functions

The name *riboflavin* comes from the chemical nature of the vitamin. It is a yellow-green fluorescent pigment (the Latin word *flavus* means "yellow") containing a sugar named *ribose*, hence the name *riboflavin*. Riboflavin operates as a vital coenzyme factor in both energy production and tissue-protein building, so it is essential to tissue health and growth. Riboflavin is also an essential factor for glutathione peroxidase, an antioxidative enzyme.

Requirements

Riboflavin needs are related to total energy requirements for age, level of exercise, body size, metabolic rate, and rate of growth. The DRI guidelines establish an RDA for daily riboflavin intake for adults age 18 and older of 1.3 mg/day and 1.1 mg/day for men and women, respectively. The RDA is higher for women during pregnancy (1.4 mg/day) and during lactation (1.6 mg/day). There is no RDA for infants up to 12 months old; the AI figure is 0.3 to 0.4 mg/day. There is no UL for riboflavin.

Deficiency Disease

Signs of riboflavin deficiency include cracked lips and mouth corners; a swollen red tongue; eyes burning, itching, or tearing from extra blood vessels in the cornea; and a scaly greasy dermatitis in skin folds. Because nutritional deficiencies are usually multiple, riboflavin deficiencies seldom occur alone. They are most likely to occur with deficiencies of other B vitamins and protein. There is no specific deficiency disease comparable to beriberi. A rare deficiency condition of riboflavin has been given the general name ariboflavinosis. Its symptoms relate to tissue inflammation and breakdown and poor wound healing; even minor injuries easily become aggravated and do not heal well.

Toxicity Symptoms

No adverse effects from riboflavin intake from food or supplements have been reported.

Food Sources

The most important food source of riboflavin is milk. Each serving of milk and milk products contains from 0.3 to 0.5 mg of riboflavin. Other good sources include enriched grains and animal protein sources, such as meats (especially beef liver), poultry, and fish. Vegetables such as mushrooms, spinach, and avocados are good natural sources. Table 7-8 gives a summary of riboflavin food sources.

Stability

Riboflavin is destroyed by light; therefore milk is now sold and stored in plastic or cardboard cartons, instead of glass containers, to preserve the vitamin.

NIACIN (VITAMIN B₃)

Functions

The coenzyme role of niacin is that of a partner with riboflavin and thiamin in the cell-metabolism system that produces energy. In addition, niacin is a necessary part of important chemical reactions involved in DNA repair and calcium mobilization within the body.

Requirements

Factors such as age, growth, pregnancy and lactation, illness, tissue trauma, body size, and physical activity—all of which affect energy needs—influence niacin requirements. Because the body can make some of its niacin from the essential amino acid *tryptophan*, the total niacin requirement is stated in terms of niacin equivalents to account for both sources. About 60 mg of tryptophan can produce 1 mg of niacin, so this amount is designated as a *niacin equivalent* (NE). The DRI guidelines include an RDA standard for adults age 14 and over at 16 mg NE/day for men and 14 mg NE/day for women. The RDA is higher during pregnancy (18 mg NE/day) and lactation (17 mg NE/day). There is no RDA for infants up to 12 months old, but the AI amount is 2 to 4 mg NE/day. Niacin intake generally is

---

riboflavin chemical name of one of the early B vitamins, discovered in relation to an early vitamin-deficiency syndrome called "ariboflavinosis" that is mainly evidenced in breakdown of skin tissues and resulting infections; role as a coenzyme factor in many cell reactions related to energy and protein metabolism.

niacin chemical name for a B vitamin discovered in relation to the deficiency disease pellagra, largely a skin disorder; important as a coenzyme factor in many cell reactions related to energy and protein metabolism.

TABLE 7–8	Significant Food Sources of Riboflavin	
Food item	**Quantity**	**Riboflavin (mg)**
BREAD, CEREAL, RICE, PASTA		
Bran Flakes cereal	1 cup	0.40
English muffin, plain	1	0.18
Noodles, enriched	1 cup	0.19
Spaghetti, enriched	1 cup	0.11
Wheat Flakes cereal	1 cup	0.42
VEGETABLES		
Asparagus, boiled	½ cup (6 spears)	0.11
Avocado, raw	1 medium	0.21
Mushrooms, boiled	½ cup, pieces	0.23
Spinach, boiled	½ cup	0.21
Sweet potato, baked	1 medium	0.15
FRUITS		
Figs, dried	10	0.17
Prunes, dried	10	0.14
Raspberries, raw	1 cup	0.11
MEAT, POULTRY, FISH, DRY BEANS, EGGS, NUTS		
Almonds, oil-roasted	1 oz	0.28
Beef liver, fried	3.5 oz	4.14
Chicken, dark meat, roasted, without skin	3.5 oz	0.23
Chicken, light meat, roasted, without skin	3.5 oz	0.12
Chicken liver, simmered	3.5 oz	1.75
Clams, baked	3 oz (9 small)	0.36
Egg, fresh	1 large	0.15
Ground beef, regular, broiled	3.5 oz	0.19
Ham loin, lean, broiled	3.5 oz	0.31
Kidney beans, boiled	1 cup	0.10
Lentils, boiled	1 cup	0.15
Lima beans, boiled	1 cup	0.10
Mackerel, baked	3 oz	0.35
Rainbow trout, baked	3 oz	0.19
Sirloin steak, broiled	3.5 oz	0.30
Soybeans, boiled	1 cup	0.49
Top round, broiled	3.5 oz	0.27
MILK, DAIRY PRODUCTS		
Brie cheese	1 oz	0.15
Buttermilk	8 fl oz	0.38
Cheddar cheese	1 oz	0.11
Cottage cheese, creamed	1 cup	0.34
Cottage cheese, 2% fat	1 cup	0.42
Milk, skim	8 fl oz	0.34
Milk, whole	8 fl oz	0.39
Ricotta cheese, whole milk	1 cup	0.48
Yogurt, whole	8 fl oz	0.32

FATS, OILS, SUGAR
This food group is not an important source of riboflavin.

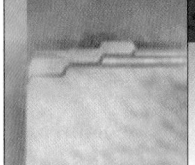

CLINICAL APPLICATIONS

NIACIN AS A TREATMENT FOR HIGH CHOLESTEROL

In addition to the many important functions of niacin, researchers have found that supplemental doses of 50 mg/day or greater may improve blood lipid profiles. At high doses, niacin decreases blood low-density lipoprotein cholesterol and triglyceride levels, both of which are linked with cardiovascular disease. In addition, pharmacologic doses of niacin improve high-density lipoprotein cholesterol, the good cholesterol. When niacin is used in this sense, it is functioning more as a drug than a vitamin and should be used only under medical supervision.

In understanding the potentially beneficial role of niacin at pharmacologic dosing, it is also critical to understand the potential side effects. The RDA for niacin in adult men and women is 16 and 14 mg niacin equivalents (NE) per day, respectively. The UL for niacin is 35 mg/day. Therefore a long-term dose of 50+ mg/day is inevitably going to have some side effects. Adverse effects from pharmacologic dosing are the same as the toxicity effects: flushing of the skin, tingling sensation in the extremities, nausea, and vomiting. Some individuals may even experience liver damage if chronic use is continued unsupervised for months or years at a time.

---

adequate in the United States; the recently reported median intake of niacin from food is 28 mg NE/day for men and 18 mg NE/day for women. The DRIs establish a UL for adults of 35 mg NE/day, based on skin flushing as the primary adverse reaction.[5]

Deficiency Disease

Symptoms of general niacin deficiency are weakness, poor appetite, indigestion, and various disorders of the skin and nervous system. Skin areas exposed to sunlight develop a dark scaly dermatitis. Extended deficiency may result in central nervous system damage with resulting confusion, apathy, disorientation, and neuritis. Such signs of nervous system damage are seen in chronic alcoholism. The deficiency disease associated with niacin is **pellagra,** which is characterized by the four Ds: dermatitis, diarrhea, dementia, and death. When therapeutic doses of niacin are given, pellagra symptoms cease. Pellagra was common in the United States and parts of Europe in the early twentieth century in regions where corn (which is low in niacin) was the primary staple food. Although pellagra has virtually disappeared in industrialized countries, it still occurs in India and parts of China and Africa.

Toxicity Symptoms

Excess intake of niacin can produce adverse physical effects, unlike thiamin and riboflavin, so a UL has been established (35 mg/day). Although there is no evidence of adverse effects from niacin naturally occurring in foods, such effects have been observed as a result of excess niacin consumption from nonprescription vitamin supplements and fortified foods. The primary reaction is a reddened flush on the skin of the face, arms, and chest that is accompanied by burning, tingling, and itching. This reaction also occurs in many patients therapeutically treated with niacin (see the Clinical Applications box, "Niacin as a Treatment for High Cholesterol").

Food Sources

Meat is a major source of niacin. The greatest intake of niacin in the United States comes from mixed dishes high in meat, poultry, or fish. In addition, niacin is ample in enriched and whole grain breads and bread products, and

---

pellagra (L. *pelle,* skin; Gr. *agra,* seizure) deficiency disease caused by a lack of dietary niacin, and an inadequate amount of protein containing the amino acid tryptophan, a precursor of niacin. Pellagra is characterized by skin lesions that are aggravated by sunlight and by GI, mucosal, neurologic, and mental symptoms. The four Ds often associated with pellagra are dermatitis, diarrhea, dementia, and death.

TABLE 7-9	Significant Food Sources of Niacin	
Food item	**Quantity**	**Niacin (mg NE)**
BREAD, CEREAL, RICE, PASTA		
Bread, whole wheat	1 slice	1
Corn meal, yellow, enriched	1 cup	4.8
Cream of Wheat cereal, regular, cooked	¾ cup	1.1
Oatmeal, cooked	¾ cup (⅓ cup dry)	0.2
Rice, white, enriched, cooked	½ cup	1.1
Wheat flour, all-purpose, enriched	1 cup	4.8
VEGETABLES		
Asparagus, boiled	½ cup (6 spears)	0.9
Avocado, raw	1 medium	3.3
Carrot, raw	1 medium	0.7
Corn, yellow, boiled	½ cup	1.3
Mushrooms, raw	½ cup, pieces	1.4
Peas, green, boiled	½ cup	1.6
Potato, baked, with skin	1 medium	3.3
Tomato, boiled	½ cup	0.9
Tomato juice	6 fl oz	1.2
FRUITS		
Banana, raw	1 medium	0.6
Figs, dried	10	1.3
Mango, raw	1 medium	1.2
Raspberries, raw	1 cup	1.1
MEAT, POULTRY, FISH, DRY BEANS, EGGS, NUTS		
Beef liver, fried	3.5 oz	14.4
Chicken liver, simmered	3.5 oz	4.5
Ground beef, regular, broiled	3.5 oz	5.8
Ham, cured, regular	3.5 oz	4.8
Peanut butter	1 Tbsp	2.2
Peanuts, dry-roasted	1 oz	3.8
Salmon, baked	3 oz	5.7
Sirloin steak, lean, broiled	3.5 oz	4.3
Swordfish, baked	3 oz	10
Top round, lean, broiled	3.5 oz	6

MILK, DAIRY PRODUCTS
This food group is not an important source of niacin.

FATS, OILS, SUGAR
This food group is not an important source of niacin.

NE = Niacin equivalent.

fortified ready-to-eat cereals. Other good sources include legumes (e.g., peanuts, dried beans, and peas). Fruits and vegetables are relatively poor sources. Table 7-9 gives the food sources of niacin.

Stability

Niacin is stable to acid and heat but is lost when cooked with excess water, unless the cooking water is retained and consumed, as in soup.

VITAMIN B₆

Functions

Vitamin B₆ is the collective name of a group of six related compounds (pyridoxine, pyridoxal, pyridoxamine, and their respective activated phosphate forms). The name *pyridoxine* comes from the vitamin's ringlike chemical structure, which is called a *pyridine ring*. Vitamin B₆ has an essential role in protein metabolism and function in many cell reactions involving amino acids. It aids neurotransmitter synthesis for brain activity and normal function of the central nervous system. Vitamin B₆ is stored in tissues throughout the body and participates in amino acid absorption, energy production, synthesis of the heme portion of hemoglobin, and niacin formation from tryptophan. In its coenzyme role, vitamin B₆ is also active in carbohydrate and fat metabolism.

Requirements

Because vitamin B₆ is involved in amino acid metabolism, its need varies directly with protein intake. The DRI guidelines set the RDA standard for healthy adults up to age 50 at 1.3 mg/day for both men and women. For older adults, the RDA is slightly higher at 1.7 mg/day for men and 1.5 mg/day for women. The RDA is also higher during pregnancy (1.9 mg/day) and lactation (2.0 mg/day). The AI figure for infants up to 12 months is 0.1 to 0.3 mg/day. The UL for adults is 100 mg/day, based on nerve-damage studies.[5]

Deficiency Disease

A deficiency of vitamin B₆ is unlikely because amounts in the general diet are large, relative to the requirement. A deficiency of vitamin B₆ causes abnormal central nervous system function with hyperirritability, neuritis, and possible convulsions. Certain types of anemia (microcytic hypochromic anemia), necessary to the formation of healthy hemoglobin, relate to a deficiency of vitamin B₆.

Toxicity Symptoms

High intake of vitamin B₆ from food sources does not result in adverse effects, but when taken in large oral-supplement doses, vitamin B₆ can be associated with lack of muscular coordination and potential nerve damage. Symptoms disappear when use of large supplements is discontinued.

Food Sources

Vitamin B₆ is widespread in foods, but many sources provide only very small amounts. Good sources include grains, enriched cereals, liver and kidney, and other meats. There are limited amounts in milk, eggs, and vegetables. Table 7-10 gives food sources of vitamin B₆.

Stability

Vitamin B₆ is stable to heat but sensitive to light and alkalis.

FOLATE

Functions

The name *folate* comes from the Latin word *folium*, meaning "leaf," and was used because a major source of its original discovery was in dark green leafy vegetables. The term *folate* is now used as the common, generic name for this vitamin, which exists in many chemical forms. The most stable form of folate is folic acid, which is rarely found in food but is the form usually used in vitamin supplements and fortified food products. In its basic coenzyme role, folate is essential to the formation of all body cells because it takes part in the creation of DNA, the important cell nucleus material that transmits genetic characteristics. Folate is also essential to the formation of hemoglobin and synthesis of amino acids.

Requirements

The DRI standards give a general RDA for folate for both men and women age 14 and over of 400 µg of dietary folate equivalent (DFE) per day. The DFE measure is used because food folate is about 50% less bioavailable to the body compared with synthetic folic acid. One µg of DFE equals 1 µg of food folate, 0.5 µg of folic acid taken on an empty stomach, or 0.6 µg of folic acid taken with food. In recognition of the role of folate in reducing the risk of neural tube defects, the DRIs include a new special recommendation that all women who can become pregnant take 400 µg daily of synthetic folic acid from fortified foods or supplements, in addition to natural folate from a varied diet. During pregnancy, the RDA is increased to 600 µg DFE/day to meet the elevated needs of fetal growth. A lactating mother needs 500 µg DFE/day. For infants, the observed AI is 65 µg DFE/day during the first 6 months, and 80 µg DFE/day from 7 to 12 months. The UL for adults has been set at 1000 µg/day of supplemental folic acid, not of DFE. The DRI recommendations are

TABLE 7–10 Significant Food Sources of Vitamin B₆ (Pyridoxine)		
Food item	**Quantity**	**Pyridoxine (mg)**
BREAD, CEREAL, RICE, PASTA		
Wheat germ, toasted	¼ cup (1 oz)	0.28
VEGETABLES		
Asparagus, boiled	1 medium	0.13
Avocado, raw	1 medium	0.48
Broccoli, boiled	½ cup	0.15
Carrot, raw	1 medium	0.11
Potato, baked, with skin	1 medium	0.70
FRUITS		
Apple, raw, with skin	1 medium	0.07
Banana, raw	1 medium	0.66
Figs, dried	10	0.42
Grape juice, bottled	8 fl oz	0.16
MEAT, POULTRY, FISH, DRY BEANS, EGGS, NUTS		
Beef liver, fried	3.5 oz	0.27
Chicken, light meat, roasted, without skin	3.5 oz	0.60
Chicken liver, simmered	3.5 oz	0.58
Ground beef, regular, broiled	3.5 oz	0.27
Ham, canned	3.5 oz	0.48
Kidney beans, boiled	1 cup	0.21
Lentils, boiled	1 cup	0.35
Lima beans, boiled	1 cup	0.30
Navy beans, boiled	1 cup	0.30
Peanut butter, chunky-style	1 Tbsp	0.14
Pinto beans, boiled	1 cup	0.27
Sirloin steak, broiled	3.5 oz	0.45
Soybeans, boiled	1 cup	0.40
Swordfish, baked	3 oz	0.32
Top round, broiled	3.5 oz	0.56
Walnuts, dried	1 oz	0.16
MILK, DAIRY PRODUCTS		
Milk, skim	8 fl oz	0.10
Milk, whole	8 fl oz	0.10
FATS, OILS, SUGAR		
This food group is not an important source of vitamin B₆.		

aimed at providing adequate safety allowances that include specific population groups at risk for deficiency, such as pregnant women, adolescents, and older adults.

Deficiency Disease

A direct deficiency of folate causes a special type of anemia, *megaloblastic anemia*, which is a particular risk during pregnancy because of increased fetal growth demands. Rapidly

pyridoxine the chemical name of vitamin B₆. In its activated phosphate form, B₂-PO₄, pyridoxine functions as an important coenzyme factor in many reactions in cell metabolism related to amino acids, glucose, and fatty acids. Clinically, pyridoxine deficiency produces a specific anemia and disturbances of the central nervous system.

growing adolescents, especially ones following fad diets and those who smoke, develop low levels of folate in the blood and risk anemia.

The role of adequate folate in reducing the serious public health problem of *neural tube defects* during preg-

nancy has received increasing study and public awareness in recent years. Neural tube defects, such as spina bifida and anencephaly, are the most common birth defects involving the brain and spinal cord. Incidences vary from 1 to 9 cases per 1000 births worldwide, with

TABLE 7–11	Significant Food Sources of Folate	
Food item	**Quantity**	**Folate (µg)**
BREAD, CEREAL, RICE, PASTA		
C.W. Post cereal	1 cup	342
Grits, corn, enriched	1 cup	75
Life cereal	1 cup	147
Mueslix Fine Grain cereal	1 cup	197
Oatmeal, fortified	¾ cup	97
Total Wheat cereal	¾ cup	400
Wheat germ, toasted	¼ cup (1 oz)	100
VEGETABLES		
Asparagus, boiled	½ cup (6 spears)	88
Avocado, raw	1 medium	113
Collard greens, boiled	1 cup	177
Mustard greens, boiled	1 cup	103
Okra pods, frozen, boiled	½ cup	134
Peas, green, boiled	1 cup	51
Romaine lettuce, chopped	1 cup	76
Spinach, boiled	1 cup	262
Turnip greens, boiled	1 cup	170
FRUITS		
Banana, raw	1 medium	22
Orange, raw	1 medium	47
Strawberries, raw	1 cup	26
MEAT, POULTRY, FISH, DRY BEANS, EGGS, NUTS		
Beef liver, fried	3.5 oz	220
Black beans, boiled	1 cup	256
Black-eyed peas, boiled	1 cup	356
Chicken liver, simmered	3.5 oz	770
Chickpeas (garbanzo beans)	1 cup	282
Egg, whole	1 large	32
Green beans, boiled	1 cup	42
Kidney beans, boiled	1 cup	229
Lima beans, boiled	1 cup	273
Navy beans, boiled	1 cup	255
Peanuts, dry-roasted	1 oz	41
Pinto beans, boiled	1 cup	294
Soybeans	1 cup	93
MILK, DAIRY PRODUCTS		
This food group is not an important source of folate.		
FATS, OILS, SUGAR		
This food group is not an important source of folate.		

the highest rates occurring in Great Britain and Ireland. This defect occurs 21 to 28 days after conception, before a woman may realize she is pregnant. Additional folic acid intake can significantly improve the folate status of women.[6,7] Thus increased folic acid intake is recommended for all women who are capable of becoming pregnant.

Toxicity Symptoms

No negative effects have been observed from the excess consumption of folate from foods. There is some evidence, however, that excess intake of folic acid from supplements or fortified food products may have toxic effects, especially in persons deficient in vitamin B_{12}, which is reflected in the UL levels.

Food Sources

Folate is found naturally in a wide distribution of foods (Table 7-11). Rich sources include chicken and beef liver, green leafy vegetables, yeast, and legumes (Figure 7-3). Natural folate from food sources is important in a varied healthy diet.[8] As part of efforts to reduce the public health problem of neural tube defects in babies, the U.S. Food and Drug Administration (FDA) has required all manufacturers to add folic acid to certain grain products (e.g., enriched white flour, white rice, corn grits, cornmeal, noodles, fortified breakfast cereals, bread, rolls, and buns) since January 1998. This fortification process has successfully reduced the incidence of neural tube defects in the United States by 19%.[9] The special DRI recommendation that women capable of becoming pregnant consume folic acid from supplements or fortified foods is one of only two current RDAs that specifically recommend vitamin sources besides those readily available in a varied diet of natural foods. (The other such recommendation concerns vitamin B_{12} and older persons.)

Stability

Folate is a relatively stable vitamin, but storage and cooking losses can be high, especially when cooked in excess water. As much as 50% of food folate may be destroyed during household preparation, food processing, and storage.

COBALAMIN (VITAMIN B_{12})

Functions

Vitamin B_{12} refers to **cobalamin**, the general term for a group of biologically active compounds whose name derives from its unique structure with a single red atom of the trace element cobalt at its center. Vitamin B_{12} is essential for normal blood formation as a coenzyme in the synthesis of the nonprotein *heme* portion of hemoglobin. Vitamin B_{12} is also essential for proper nervous system function.

Requirements

Although it is essential, the amount of dietary vitamin B_{12} needed for normal human metabolism is very small, consisting of only a few micrograms per day. The usual mixed diet easily provides this much and more. The DRI guidelines establish an RDA for men and women ages 19 and up at 2.4 μg/day. The RDA during pregnancy is 2.6 μg/day; and during lactation is 2.8 μg/day. There is no RDA for infants up to 12 months old. An observed AI during the first year is 0.4 to 0.5 μg/day. There is evidence that

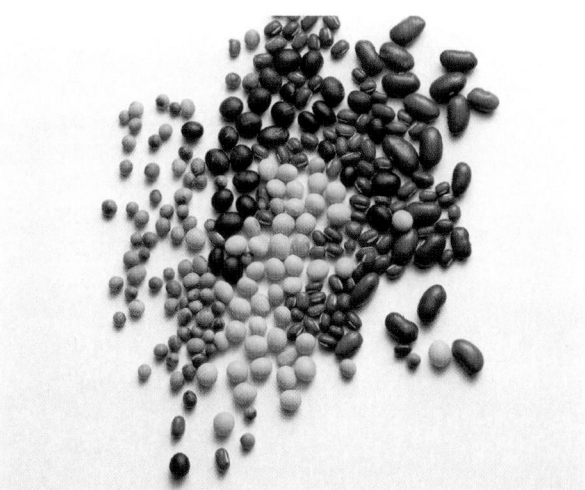

Figure 7–3 Foods high in folate. (Copyright 2004 JupiterImages Corporation.)

cobalamin the chemical name for the B-complex vitamin B_{12}; found mainly in animal protein food sources, so deficiencies are seen mostly among strict vegetarians (vegans). It is closely related to amino acid metabolism and formation of the heme portion of hemoglobin. Absence of its necessary absorbing agent in the gastric secretions, intrinsic factor, leads to pernicious anemia and degenerative effects on the nervous system, which require monthly cobalamin injections, bypassing the intestinal absorption defect.

10% to 30% of people over age 50 may poorly absorb vitamin B_{12} from food sources. Therefore the DRIs include a special recommendation that both men and women over 50 should meet their RDA primarily from foods fortified by vitamin B_{12} or from supplements.

Deficiency Disease

The search for the controlling agent responsible for *pernicious anemia* led to the discovery of vitamin B_{12}. A component of the digestive gastric secretions called *intrinsic factor* is necessary for absorption of vitamin B_{12} into the blood stream. Gastrointestinal disorders that destroy the cells lining the stomach can disrupt the secretion of intrinsic factor and thus inhibit vitamin B_{12} absorption. If the vitamin cannot be absorbed to make hemoglobin, pernicious anemia ensues. In such cases, vitamin B_{12} must be given by injection to bypass the absorption defect. Natural dietary deficiency in a mixed diet is unknown. Deficiency is much more common in elderly individuals because of lack of intrinsic factor or hydrocholoric acid, not lack of dietary intake.

TABLE 7–12	Significant Food Sources of Vitamin B_{12} (Cobalamin)	
Food item	**Quantity**	**Vitamin B_{12} (μg)**
BREAD, CEREAL, RICE, PASTA		
Total Wheat cereal	¾ cup	7.7
VEGETABLES		
This food group is not an important source of vitamin B_{12}.		
FRUITS		
This food group is not an important source of vitamin B_{12}.		
MEAT, POULTRY, FISH, DRY BEANS, EGGS, NUTS		
Beef liver, fried	3.5 oz	111.80
Chicken liver, simmered	3.5 oz	19.39
Chicken, white meat, roasted	3.5 oz	0.34
Clams, canned, drained	1 cup	158
Clams, steamed	3 oz (9 small)	84.06
Crab legs, Alaskan King	1	15.4
Egg	1 large	0.77
Ground beef, regular, broiled	3.5 oz	2.93
Ham, cured, regular	3.5 oz	0.80
Herring fillet, baked	5 oz	18.8
Lobster, baked	1 cup	4.4
Mackerel, baked	3 oz	16.15
Mussels, steamed	3 oz	20.4
Oysters, steamed	3 oz (12 medium)	32.53
Salmon, baked	3 oz	4.93
Sirloin steak, lean, broiled	3.5 oz	2.85
Swordfish, baked	3 oz	1.72
Top round, lean, broiled	3.5 oz	2.48
Tuna, baked	3 oz	9.2
MILK, DAIRY PRODUCTS		
Cheddar cheese	3.5 oz	0.83
Milk, skim	8 fl oz	0.93
Milk, whole	8 fl oz	0.87
Swiss cheese	3.5 oz	1.68
Yogurt, whole	8 fl oz	0.84
FATS, OILS, SUGAR		
This food group is not an important source of vitamin B_{12}.		

The only reported cases of dietary deficiency have been in some vegans (see Chapter 4), for whom cobalamin supplements are recommended to prevent such deficiency.[10] The general symptoms of such a deficiency include nervous disorders, sore mouth and tongue, amenorrhea, and neuritis.

Toxicity Symptoms

Vitamin B_{12} does not produce adverse effects in healthy individuals when its intake from food or supplements exceeds body needs; therefore no UL has been established.

Food Sources

Because vitamin B_{12} occurs as a protein complex in foods, its food sources are mostly from animals. The initial source, however, is synthesized from bacteria in the GI tract of herbivorous animals. Human intestinal bacteria synthesize some B_{12}, but our major source is animal foods. The richest sources are beef and chicken liver, lean meat, clams, oysters, herring, and crab (Table 7-12).

Stability

Vitamin B_{12} is stable in ordinary cooking processes.

PANTOTHENIC ACID

Functions

The name **pantothenic acid** refers to the vitamin's widespread functions in the body and sources in food. It is based on the Greek word *pantothen*, which means "from every side." Pantothenic acid is present in all forms of living things and is essential to all forms of life. In its coenzyme role, it is essential to the synthesis and functioning of the body's key activating agent, *coenzyme A*, which controls many cell metabolic reactions involving fat and cholesterol, heme formation, and amino acid activation.

Requirements

No specific RDA for pantothenic acid is given in the DRI guidelines. The usual intake range of the American diet is 4 to 7 mg/day. The DRIs set an AI amount for persons age 14 and older of 5 mg/day. The AI is slightly higher during pregnancy (6 mg/day) and lactation (7 mg/day). For infants during the first year, the observed AI is 1.7 to 1.8 mg/day.

Deficiency Disease

Given its widespread natural occurrence, deficiencies of pantothenic acid are unlikely. The only cases of deficiency are in individuals fed synthetic diets with virtually no pantothenic acid.

Toxicity Symptoms

There have been no observed adverse effects associated with pantothenic acid in humans or animals. Therefore the DRI guidelines have not established a UL for this vitamin.

Food Sources

Pantothenic acid occurs as widely in foods as in body tissues. It is found in all animal and plant cells and is especially abundant in animal tissues, whole grain cereals, and legumes (Table 7-13). Smaller amounts are found in milk, vegetables, and fruits.

Stability

Pantothenic acid is stable to acid and heat but is sensitive to alkalis.

BIOTIN

Functions

The minute traces of biotin in the body perform multiple metabolic tasks. In its coenzyme role, biotin serves as a partner with coenzyme A, of which pantothenic acid is an essential part. Biotin is also involved in the synthesis of both fatty acids and amino acids.

Requirements

The amount of biotin needed for metabolism is extremely small, measured in micrograms. The DRI guidelines do not establish an RDA for biotin. An AI

---

pantothenic acid (Gr. *pantothen,* from all sides, in every corner) a B-complex vitamin found widely distributed in nature and occurring throughout the body tissues. Its one role, which is a major one, is as an essential constituent of the body's main activating agent, coenzyme A. This special compound has extensive metabolic responsibility in activating a number of compounds in many tissues; it is a key energy metabolism substance in every cell.

TABLE 7–13	Significant Food Sources of Pantothenic Acid	
Food item	**Quantity**	**Pantothenic acid (mg)**
BREAD, CEREAL, RICE, PASTA		
All-Bran cereal	⅓ cup (1 oz)	0.49
Oatmeal, regular, quick-cooking	¾ cup (1 oz)	0.35
Soybean flour, defatted	½ cup	1
Wheat germ, toasted	¼ cup (1 oz)	0.39
VEGETABLES		
Avocado, raw	1 medium	1.68
Corn, yellow, boiled	½ cup	0.72
Potato, baked, with skin	1 medium	1.12
Squash, winter, all varieties, baked	½ cup	0.36
Sweet potato, boiled	½ cup, mashed	0.87
Tomato, boiled	½ cup	0.35
FRUITS		
Banana, raw	1 medium	0.30
Figs, dried	10	0.81
Orange juice, fresh	8 fl oz	0.47
Orange, navel, raw	1 medium	0.35
Papaya, raw	1 medium	0.66
Pomegranate, raw	1 medium	0.92
MEAT, POULTRY, FISH, DRY BEANS, EGGS, NUTS		
Beef liver, fried	3.5 oz	5.92
Black-eyed peas, boiled	½ cup	0.35
Cashews, roasted	1 oz (18 medium nuts)	0.34
Chicken, dark meat, roasted, without skin	3.5 oz	1.21
Chicken, light meat, roasted, without skin	3.5 oz	0.97
Chicken liver, simmered	3.5 oz	5.41
Egg	1 large	0.86
Egg yolk	Yolk of 1 large	0.75
Ground beef, regular, broiled	3.5 oz	0.33
Ham, cured, regular	3.5 oz	0.50
Lentils, boiled	½ cup	0.63
Lima beans, boiled	½ cup	0.35
Peanut butter, chunky-style	2 Tbsp	0.31
Peanuts, roasted	1 oz	0.39
Salmon, smoked	3 oz	0.74
Sirloin steak, broiled	3.5 oz	0.35
Top round, broiled	3.5 oz	0.48
Turkey, light meat, roasted, without skin	3.5 oz	0.68
MILK, DAIRY PRODUCTS		
Blue cheese	1 oz	0.49
Milk, skim	8 fl oz	0.81
Milk, whole	8 fl oz	0.76
Yogurt, whole	8 fl oz	0.88

FATS, OILS, SUGAR
This food group is not an important source of pantothenic acid.

figure has been set based on intakes of healthy individuals. The AI for adults age 18 and older is 30 μg/day. For infants during the first 12 months, the observed AI is 5 to 6 μg/day. The AI during pregnancy is also 30 μg/day; during lactation, it is 35 μg/day. The body also receives a supply of biotin synthesized by normal intestinal bacteria.

Deficiency Disease

Because the potency of biotin is great, even in its tiny microgram amounts in the body, there is no known natural deficiency. The only induced deficiencies have occurred in patients on long-term total parenteral nutrition (TPN) without biotin supplementation. Occasional cases of inborn errors of biotin metabolism have been observed.

Toxicity Symptoms

There is no known biotin toxicity or adverse effects from its consumption in humans or animals. No data currently support setting a UL for biotin.

Food Sources

Biotin is widely distributed in natural foods but is not equally available to the body from various foods. For example, the biotin of corn and soy meals is completely bioavailable (e.g., able to be digested and absorbed by the body). However, the biotin in wheat is almost completely unavailable to the body. The best food sources of biotin are liver, egg yolk, soy flour, cereals (except bound forms in wheat), meats, tomatoes, and yeast. Fruits are poor sources.

Stability

Biotin is a stable vitamin, but it is water soluble. A summary of these water-soluble vitamins is given in Table 7-14.

CHOLINE

Functions

Choline is a water-soluble nutrient associated with the B-complex vitamins. Choline has been insufficiently studied thus far. The DRI guidelines include choline but state that there are insufficient human data to determine whether choline is essential in the human diet.[5] The human body may be able to synthesize internally adequate choline at some stages of life. As a nutrient, choline is important in maintaining the structural integrity of cell membranes. Choline is also active in the synthesis of *acetylcholine*, which is a neurotransmitter involved in memory storage, muscle control, and other functions.

Requirements

There are insufficient data on which to establish an RDA for choline. Therefore the DRI guidelines provide an AI level for adults of 550 mg/day for men over age 14 and 425 mg/day for women over age 18. During pregnancy, the AI is 450 mg/day; during lactation it is 550 mg/day because an ample amount of choline is secreted into human milk. For infants, the observed AI figure is 125 to 150 mg/day during the first year.

Deficiency Disease

A deficiency of choline from food sources appears to be associated with liver damage. In clinical settings, patients fed with TPN solutions that did not include choline also developed liver damage, which was resolved with choline supplementation.

Toxicity Symptoms

Choline has a low level of toxicity. Adverse effects have only been observed in cases where the choline intake was several times greater than normal intake from food. Very high doses of choline have been associated with lowered blood pressure, fishy body odor, sweating, excessive salivation, and reduced growth rate.

Food Sources

Choline is found naturally in a wide variety of foods. Milk, eggs, liver, and peanuts are especially rich sources of choline. A normal, varied diet can deliver 1 g of choline per day, and typical dietary intake for adults in the United States has been estimated to be 700 to 1000 mg/day.

Stability

Choline is a stable vitamin and is water soluble like all of the B-complex vitamins.

TABLE 7–14	Summary of Vitamin C and the B-Complex Vitamins			
Vitamins	**Functions**	**Recommended intake (adults)**	**Deficiency**	**UL and toxicity**	**Sources**
Vitamin C (ascorbic acid)	Antioxidant; collagen synthesis; helps prepare iron for absorption and release to tissues for red blood cell formation, metabolism	RDA Men: 90 mg Women: 75 mg Smokers: additional 35 mg/day	Scurvy (deficiency disease), sore gums, hemorrhages, especially around bones and joints, anemia, tendency to bruise easily, impaired wound healing and tissue formation, weakened bones	UL: 2000 mg Diarrhea	Citrus fruits, kiwi, tomatoes, melons, strawberries, dark leafy vegetables, chili peppers, cabbage, broccoli, chard, green peppers, potatoes
Thiamin (vitamin B$_1$)	Normal growth; coenzyme in carbohydrate metabolism; normal function of heart, nerves, and muscle	RDA Men: 1.2 mg Women: 1.1 mg	Beriberi (deficiency disease); GI: loss of appetite, gastric distress, indigestion, deficient hydrochloric acid; CNS: fatigue, nerve damage, paralysis; CV: heart failure, edema of legs especially	UL: Not set Unknown	Pork, beef, liver, whole or enriched grains, legumes, wheat germ
Riboflavin (vitamin B$_2$)	Normal growth and energy; coenzyme in protein and energy metabolism	RDA Men: 1.3 mg Women: 1.1 mg	Ariboflavinosis; wound aggravation, cracks at corners of mouth, swollen red tongue, eye irritation, skin eruptions	UL: Not set Unknown	Milk, meats, enriched cereals, green vegetables

Vitamin	Function	RDA/AI	Deficiency	UL/Toxicity	Sources
Niacin (vitamin B$_3$, nicotinamide, nicotinic acid)	Coenzyme in energy production; normal growth, health of skin	RDA Men: 16 mg NE Women: 14 mg NE	Pellagra (deficiency disease); weakness, loss of appetite, diarrhea, scaly dermatitis, neuritis, confusion	UL: 35 mg (from supplements) Flushing, nausea, itching, liver damage at doses ≥3 g/day long term	Meat, peanuts, legumes, enriched grains
Vitamin B$_6$ (pyridoxine)	Coenzyme in amino acid metabolism: protein synthesis, heme formation, brain activity; carrier for amino acid absorption	RDA Ages 19-50 yr: 1.3 mg Men >51: 1.7 mg Women >51: 1.5 mg	Anemia, hyperirritability, convulsions, neuritis	UL: 100 mg Nerve damage	Grains, seeds, meats, poultry, seafood
Folate (folic acid, folacin)	Coenzyme in DNA and RNA synthesis, amino acid metabolism, red blood cell maturation	RDA 400 µg DFE	Megaloblastic anemia (large, immature red blood cells), poor growth, neural tube defects	UL: 1000 µg (from supplements) Masking of vitamin B$_{12}$ deficiency	Liver, green leafy vegetables, legumes, yeast, orange juice, fortified grains
Cobalamin (vitamin B$_{12}$)	Coenzyme in synthesis of heme for hemoglobin, myelin sheath formation to protect nerves	RDA 2.4 µg	Pernicious anemia, poor nerve function	UL: Not set Unknown	Liver, lean meats, fish, seafood
Pantothenic acid	Formation of coenzyme A; fat, cholesterol, protein, and heme formation	AI 5 mg	Unlikely because of widespread distribution in most foods	UL: Not set Unknown	Meats, eggs, milk, whole grains, legumes, vegetables
Biotin	Coenzyme A partner; synthesis of fatty acids, amino acids, purines	AI 30 µg	Natural deficiency unknown	UL: Not set Unknown	Liver, egg yolk, soy flour, (except bound form in wheat), nuts

AI = Adequate intake; CNS = central nervous system; CV = cardiovascular; DFE = dietary folate equivalent; GI = gastrointestinal; NE = niacin equivalent; RDA = Recommended Dietary Allowance; UL = Tolerable Upper Intake Level.

Phytochemicals

Certain plant compounds called *phytochemicals* have been identified in relation to health benefits. Phytochemicals are technically not vitamins or minerals; however, these newly discovered nutrients are similar in functions and importance. The term *phytochemical* comes from the Greek word *phyton*, meaning "plant," which indicates its chemical nature. This term describes a wide variety of chemical compounds produced by plants that act as either antioxidants or hormones in the originating plant or the person eating it. Researchers believe that fruits and vegetables provide more than 25,000 phytochemicals, many of which have yet to be identified.

FUNCTION

Multiple studies are exploring the link between phytochemical intake and reduced risk of chronic disease. What led researchers to discover phytochemicals was the difference in response to eating whole fruits and vegetables versus simply taking a vitamin or mineral supplement. Individuals relying on a diet rich in whole grains, fruits, vegetables, legumes, nuts, and seeds to obtain their vitamins and minerals benefited far more in health status than those eating mostly refined foods with supplemental vitamins and minerals.

The beneficial effects of phytochemicals are thought to result from synergistic actions of multiple nutrients, as opposed to acting as an isolated compound. It has been well documented that diets high in phytochemicals induce a protective lipid profile to protect against coronary heart disease, improve overall colon function, help prevent age-related macular degeneration and cancer, and increase antioxidant status.[11-13]

RECOMMENDED INTAKE

The National Cancer Institute expanded upon the 5-A-Day for Better Health program by using color to highlight phytochemical content of fruits and vegetables in their "Sample the Spectrum" program. Certain phytochemicals give fruits and vegetables their specific color and provide an easy distinction between the sources of different compounds. The National Cancer Institute and American Institute for Cancer Research recommend consuming a total of five to nine servings of fruits and vegetables (combined) daily. This recommendation is based on findings that dietary intake of 400 to 600 g/day of fruits and vegetables reduces one's risk of various forms of cancer.

FOOD SOURCES

Animal foods and processed, refined foods are virtually void of phytochemicals. Phytochemicals are found in whole and unrefined foods such as vegetables, fruits, legumes, nuts, seeds, whole grains, and some oils such as olive oil.[14,15]

The following list outlines the seven primary categories of phytochemicals, based on color:[14]

- *Red* foods provide lycopene
- *Yellow-green* foods provide zeaxanthin
- *Red-purple* foods provide anthocyanins
- *Orange* foods provide beta-carotene
- *Orange-yellow* foods provide flavonoids
- *Green* foods provide glucosinolates
- *White-green* foods provide allyl sulfides

By consuming one fruit or vegetable from each of the seven color categories daily, individuals can meet their daily recommendation and are provided with a variety of phytochemicals. There are also thousands of other phytochemicals not categorized in the preceding list but found distributed throughout a variety of fruits, vegetables, grains, soybeans, legumes, and nuts.

Vitamin Supplementation

ONGOING DEBATE

The debate between users and producers of vitamin supplements and those who think they have no place in health maintenance continues, fueled by extremists on both sides. On one hand, conservative health workers may dismiss anyone who suggests a need for vitamin supplements. On the other hand, self-proclaimed and noncredentialed nutrition "experts" may push megadoses of everything from **A** to **Z**. Who is right? Probably someone with sound knowledge in addition to *wisdom*, who suggests a course between these two extremes. Some people think that all persons should meet the precise RDA standards for all essential nutrients. But, as the DRI guidelines emphasize, the RDA amounts have been designed to meet the average needs of healthy population groups—not individual needs, which can vary widely in different circumstances. For individual needs, wise practitioners take an individual approach based on personal assessment of need. Not all of the ideas expressed in the ongoing debate over vitamins are equal or have scientific basis. However, it is and will remain a hot topic, because multivitamin and multimineral supplements are the most commonly bought over-the-counter item in America.

BIOCHEMICAL INDIVIDUALITY

The term *biochemical individuality* is important. It means that the body's chemical composition is not the same for every individual, and that this pattern changes within a given person at different times under various circumstances, during the normal life cycle and in disease. The concept of biochemical individuality cannot be overlooked when individual nutritional needs are assessed, because it is influenced by things such as age, sex, personal habits, work environment, living situation, and health status. Consider some of the following factors.

Life Cycle Needs

Vitamin needs fluctuate with age and situation throughout the life cycle.

Pregnancy and Lactation

The DRI guidelines explicitly establish separate recommendations for women during pregnancy and lactation that take into account the increased nutrient requirements at these times. To prevent possible birth defect damage early in pregnancy, the DRIs recommend that women capable of becoming pregnant take additional folic acid (folate) from supplements. Women may find it difficult to meet the increased nutrient needs of pregnancy by diet alone because of nutrient bioavailability, tolerances, food preferences, or other factors that can lead to a marginal diet. Supplements then may become a necessary way of ensuring adequate intake to meet the increased nutrient demands.

Infancy

Supplementation of vitamin K at birth is recommended by the American Academy of Pediatrics to prevent a rare but fatal bleeding disorder called *haemorrhagic disease of the newborn*. Vitamin D is the only other vitamin that infants may need in supplemental form if they do not receive sufficient sunlight exposure to produce enough endogenous vitamin D in their skin. (See Chapter 11.)

Children and Adolescents

Rapid growth spurts during childhood and adolescence utilize more total nutrients, including all vitamins, than during adulthood when growth has slowed or stopped. Full growth potential, specifically in height, can be hindered if adequate supplies of dietary vitamins are not provided during these times of rapid growth.

Aging

The aging process may increase the need for some nutrients because of decreased food intake and impaired nutrient absorption, storage, and usage (see Chapter 12). Marginal deficiencies of ascorbic acid, thiamin, riboflavin, pyridoxine, and cobalamin are common in the geriatric population, even in some individuals using supplements.

Lifestyle

Personal lifestyle choices and habits also may influence individual needs for nutrient supplementation.

Oral Contraceptive Use

Women using oral contraceptive agents (e.g., "the pill") find that this practice lowers serum levels of several B vitamins, including pyridoxine and niacin, as well as vitamin C. If coupled with marginal nutrient-intake levels, supplements may be necessary to maintain optimal vitamin status. However, one must first address poor dietary habits and improve that before relying on supplemental intake.

Restricted Diets

Persons who are always "dieting" may find it difficult to meet many of the nutrient standards, particularly if their meals provide less than 1200 kcal/day. Very restrictive diets are not recommended because of their link with multiple nutrient deficiencies. A wise weight-reduction program should meet all nutrient needs. Persons on strict vegetarian diets need supplements of vitamin B_{12} (cobalamin) because its only food source is that of animal origin.

Exercise Programs

Women on extensive exercise programs (e.g., training for a marathon or endurance bike race) may increase their requirement for riboflavin. Combining a restrictive diet with heavy exercise increases this need even more. This combination may indicate the need for a B-complex supplement, especially in women who do not tolerate milk, the major food source of riboflavin.

Smoking

This unhealthy habit, especially among women during their childbearing years, affects health and can reduce vitamin C levels by as much as 30%. If dietary intake is marginal and the smoker chooses not to stop, a small supplement of vitamin C (e.g., 100 mg/day) may help compensate.

Alcohol

Chronic or abusive use of alcohol can interfere with absorption of B-complex vitamins, especially thiamin, and even destroy folate. Again, multivitamin supplements rich in B vitamins help. However, a change in alcohol use must accompany this nutrition therapy to prevent deficiency effects from recurring.

Caffeine

In large quantities (e.g., the amount in four to six cups of coffee a day), caffeine flushes water-soluble vitamins out of the body faster than usual. Small supplements of B vitamins and ascorbic acid may help, but reduced caffeine intake is recommended.

Disease

In states of disease, malnutrition, debilitation, or hypermetabolic demand, each patient requires careful nutrition assessment. In cases of need, nutritional support, including therapeutic supplementation as indicated, becomes part of the total medical therapy. Diet and supplementation needs for nutrition therapy are planned to meet individual clinical requirements. Increased nutrient needs are particularly evident in cases of long-term illness.[16]

MEGADOSES

Persons taking megadoses of vitamins are using them as drugs. At such high pharmacologic levels, vitamins no longer operate as nutritional agents. The body uses both nutrients and drugs in specific amounts to do the following: (1) control or improve a physiologic condition or illness; (2) prevent a disease; or (3) relieve symptoms. The similarity of nutrients and drugs, however, ends there for many people. Most people realize that too much of any drug can be harmful or even fatal, and take care to avoid overdosing. However, too many people do not apply this same logic to nutrients and learn the dangers of vitamin megadosing only when toxic side effects occur.

Toxic Effects

Fat-soluble vitamins, especially vitamin A, can be stored in large amounts in the liver. Therefore the potential toxicity of megadoses, including liver and brain damage in extreme cases, is well known. Many people take megadoses of water-soluble vitamins, believing them to be safe because they are not stored in the body. However, the toxic effects of at least two such megadoses have been observed. For example, megadoses of vitamin B_6 at up to 5 g/day for long periods of time as therapy for premenstrual syndrome (PMS) caused lack of muscular coordination and in some cases severe nerve damage. Megadoses of ascorbic acid (e.g., more than 2 g/day) have caused GI pain, raised the risk for kidney stone formation, and reduced the action of leukocytes (white blood cells) against bacteria. Meanwhile, scientific research has failed to confirm that such megadoses cure colds or lower cholesterol or cancer risk, which are the reasons why these large amounts were used in the first place.

'Artificially Induced' Deficiencies

Megadoses of one nutrient can not only produce toxic effects of that vitamin, but can also lead to a deficiency of another vitamin. Above-normal blood levels of one nutrient may increase the need for the other nutrients

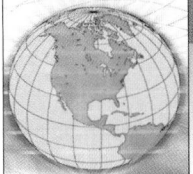

THE AMERICAN DIET

According to the Economic Research Service of the U.S. Department of Agriculture, Americans are still not meeting the recommended intake for any of the five food groups. The five food groups, according to MyPyramid guidelines, are: grains, vegetables, fruit, dairy or dairy substitute, and meat or meat substitute. Believe it or not, Americans come closer to meeting the recommended daily intake of vegetable servings than any other food group.

By consuming the recommended servings from each group, vitamin and mineral needs should be met. In looking at all individuals ages 2 and over, 84% of the population consumes the recommended grain servings per day, 89% reach the vegetable recommendations, a mere 59% of the population eat at least two servings of fruit per day, 65% and 82% meet the dairy and meat servings per day, respectively. When looking at the statistics by gender, females do better on the fruit category, but do considerably worse on all other food groups, especially the dairy and meat groups.

Women ages 60 and over do considerably well on getting in the recommended servings from each food group with exception of dairy products. Of this subgroup, 65% are not meeting their daily needs of dairy products, the best source of calcium!

How do you measure up? What about your family and friends? Prevention of deficiency, or any diseases associated with nutrient deficiency, is always better than treatment.

---

with which it works in the body, thus creating deficiency symptoms. Deficiencies also occur when a person suddenly stops taking the large amounts and a "rebound effect" results. For example, infants born to mothers who took megadoses of ascorbic acid during pregnancy have developed scurvy when their high nutrient supply was cut off at birth.

SUPPLEMENTATION PRINCIPLES

To summarize, the following basic principles may help guide nutrient supplementation decisions:

■ *Read the labels carefully.* As labels on dietary supplements come more in line with the Nutrition Labeling and Education Act of 1990, which reformed current labels on food products, consumers can have access to safe products without unfounded health claims. Professional health associations support such improved labeling on food supplements, as well as on foods. Consumers want to know that a product's ingredients, toxicity levels, potential side effects, and health claims are based on significant scientific agreement.

■ *Vitamins, like drugs, can be harmful in large amounts.* The only time larger doses may be helpful is when the body already has a severe deficiency or is unable to absorb or metabolize the nutrient efficiently.

■ *Identified individual needs govern specific supplement use.* Each person's need should be the basis for determining which nutrients and amounts are used. This helps prevent problems of excess, which may increase with a cumulative effect over time. The "blanket insurance" approach may well put more money in the multipackage manufacturer's pocket, not desired health in the buyer's body.

■ *All nutrients work together to promote good health.* Adding large amounts of one vitamin only makes the body think it is not getting enough of the others and increases the risk for developing deficiency symptoms.

■ *Food remains the best source of nutrients.* Most foods are the best "package deals" in nutrition. They provide a wide variety of nutrients in every bite, as compared with the dozen or so found in a vitamin bottle. And, *by itself*, a vitamin can do nothing. Its action is catalytic, so it must have substrate material (e.g., carbohydrate, protein, fat, and their metabolites) on which to work. With careful selection of a wide variety of foods and storage techniques and meal planning and preparation, most people can secure an ample amount of essential nutrients (see the Cultural Considerations box, "The American Diet").

■ *Evaluate the information.* The following web sites offer more detailed information about the safety and efficacy of nutrition supplementation:
Quackwatch: *www.quackwatch.com*

National Institute of Health Office of Dietary Supplements: *http://dietary-supplements.info.nih.gov*
Supplement Watch: *www.supplementwatch.com*
National Center for Complementary and Alternative Medicine: *http://nccam.nih.gov*

SUMMARY

Vitamins are organic, noncaloric food substances that are necessary in very small amounts for certain metabolic tasks. The body cannot make vitamins, but a balanced diet usually supplies sufficient vitamin intake. In individually identified situations, however, a designated supplemental amount may be needed. Megadoses carry significant risk and are on the level of drug abuse.

The fat-soluble vitamins are A, D, E, and K. Their metabolic tasks are mainly structural. The water-soluble vitamins are vitamin C (ascorbic acid), the eight B-complex vitamins (e.g., thiamin, riboflavin, niacin, vitamin B_6, folate, vitamin B_{12}, pantothenic acid, and biotin), and choline. Their major metabolic tasks relate to their roles as coenzyme factors, except for vitamin C, which helps protein build strong tissue. Little toxicity has been associated with these vitamins because they are water soluble and excess is excreted in the urine. Megadose habits with two water-soluble vitamins have brought the following results on the level of drug abuse: (1) large amounts of pyridoxine (B_6) have caused severe nerve damage; and (2) large amounts of vitamin C have been associated with GI problems and kidney stones. The possibility of toxicity is increased for fat-soluble vitamins because the body can store them. Such toxicity is no longer rare because of the current popularity of large vitamin A (retinol) supplements. All water-soluble vitamins, especially vitamin C, are easily oxidized, so care must be taken in food storage and preparation.

Phytochemicals are compounds found in whole and unrefined plant foods. A diet high in phytochemicals from a variety of sources is associated with a decreased risk of chronic disease.

Nutrition supplementation continues to be a controversial subject in today's society. With little exception, all nutrients consumed in the form of food are more bioavailable and beneficial to the body.

CRITICAL THINKING QUESTIONS

1. What is a vitamin? Describe three general functions of vitamins and give examples of each.
2. How would you advise a friend who was taking self-prescribed vitamin supplements? Give reasons and examples to support your answer.
3. Describe the effects of three vitamins that some persons take in large amounts. What are the risks involved in such megadoses?
4. Describe four situations in which vitamin supplements should be used. Give reasons and examples in each case.
5. What are phytochemicals? And how can you incorporate them into your diet?

CHAPTER CHALLENGE QUESTIONS

True-False

Write the correct statement for each item you answer "false."

1. *True or False:* A coenzyme acts alone to control a number of different types of reactions.

2. *True or False:* Carotene is preformed vitamin A found in animal food sources.

3. *True or False:* Exposure to sunlight produces vitamin D from cholesterol in the skin.

4. *True or False:* Extra vitamin C is stored in the liver to meet tissue-infection demands.

5. *True or False:* Vitamin D and sufficient calcium and phosphorus can prevent rickets.

6. *True or False:* Vitamin K is found in meat, especially liver, and in leafy vegetables.

Multiple Choice

1. Vitamin A is fat soluble and produced by humans from carotene in plant foods or consumed as the fully formed vitamin in animal foods. Which of the following supplies the greatest amount of this vitamin?

    a. Oranges

    b. Collard greens

    c. Carrots

    d. Tomatoes

2. If you wanted to increase the vitamin C content of your diet, which of the following foods would you choose in larger amounts?

    a. Liver, other organ meats, and seafood

    b. Potatoes, enriched cereals, and fortified margarine

    c. Green peppers, tomatoes, and oranges

    d. Milk, cheese, and eggs

3. Which of the following statements is true about the sources of vitamin K?

    a. Vitamin K is found in a wide variety of foods, so no deficiency can occur.

    b. Vitamin K is easily absorbed without assistance, so we can get all we absorb into our systems.

    c. Vitamin K is rarely found in foods, so a natural deficiency can occur.

    d. Most of our vitamin K for metabolic needs is produced by internal bacteria.

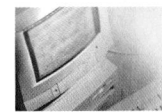 **Please refer to the Students' Resource section of this text's Evolve web site for "Suggestions for Additional Study."**

REFERENCES

1. Food and Nutrition Board, Institute of Medicine: *Dietary reference intakes for calcium, phosphorous, magnesium, vitamin D, and fluoride,* Washington, DC, 1998, National Academies Press.
2. Food and Nutrition Board, Institute of Medicine: *Dietary reference intakes for vitamin C, vitamin E, selenium, and carotenoids,* Washington, DC, 2000, National Academies Press.
3. Food and Nutrition Board, Institute of Medicine: *Dietary reference intakes for vitamin A, vitamin K, arsenic, boron, chromium, copper, iodine, iron, manganese, molybdenum, nickel, silicon, vanadium, and zinc,* Washington, DC, 2002, National Academies Press.
4. Booth SL and others: Assessment of phylloquinone and dihydrophylloquinone dietary intakes among a nationally representative sample of U.S. consumers using 14-day food diaries, *J Am Diet Assoc* 99(9):1072, 1999.
5. Food and Nutrition Board, Institute of Medicine: *Dietary reference intakes for thiamin, riboflavin, niacin, vitamin B_6, folate, vitamin B_{12}, pantothenic acid, biotin, and choline,* Washington, DC, 1999, National Academies Press.
6. Cuskelly GJ and others: Fortification with low amounts of folic acid makes a significant difference in folate status in young women: implications for the prevention of neural tube defects, *Am J Clin Nutr* 70(2):234, 1999.
7. Green NS: Folic acid supplementation and prevention of birth defects, *J Nutr* 132(8 Suppl):2356S, 2002.
8. Brouwer IA and others: Dietary folate from vegetables and citrus fruits decrease plasma homocysteine concentration in humans in a dietary controlled trial, *J Nutr* 129(4):1135, 1999.
9. Honein MA and others: Impact of folic acid fortification of the U.S. food supply on the occurrence of neural tube defects, *JAMA* 285(23):2981, 2001.
10. Donaldson MS: Metabolic vitamin B_{12} status on a mostly raw vegan diet with follow-up using tablets, nutritional yeast, or probiotic supplements, *Ann Nutr Metab* 44:229, 200.
11. Visioli F and others: Diet and prevention of coronary heart disease: the potential role of phytochemicals, *Cardiovasc Res* 47(3):419, 200.
12. Murillo G, Mehta RG: Cruciferous vegetables and cancer prevention, *Nutr Cancer* 41:17, 2001.
13. Bruce B and others: A diet high in whole and unrefined foods favorably alters lipids, antioxidant defenses, and colon function, *J Am Coll Nutr* 19(1):61, 200.
14. Heber D, Bowerman S: Applying science to changing dietary patterns, *J Nutr* 131(11 Suppl):3078S, 2001.
15. Stark AH, Madar Z: Olive oil as a functional food: epidemiology and nutritional approaches, *Nutr Rev* 60(6):170, 2002.
16. Meydani M: Nutrition interventions in aging and age-associated disease, *Ann NY Acad Sci* 928:226, 2001.

FURTHER READING AND RESOURCES

- Spina Bifida Association of America: *http://www.sbaa.org/*

  An excellent site for more information on the role of folic acid and neural tube defects.

- American Academy of Pediatrics, Committee on Genetics: Folic acid for the prevention of neural tube defects, *Pediatrics* 104(2):325, 1999.

- Kloeblen AS: Folate knowledge, intake from fortified grain products, and periconceptional supplementation patterns of a sample of low-income pregnant women according to the Health Belief Model, *J Am Diet Assoc* 99(1):33, 1999.

Here the six physicians forming the Committee on Genetics of the American Academy of Pediatrics, with the full support of all Academy members, endorse the U.S. Public Health Service recommendation that all women capable of becoming pregnant consume additional folic acid to prevent having a baby born with neural tube defects. This vital need is illustrated in a follow-up study in a high-risk population that included teaching the subjects how they may easily attain this daily goal of folate intake through the use of fortified grain products.

Minerals

When the earth was forming, shifting oceans and mountains deposited a large number of minerals into earth materials. Over time these minerals moved from rocks to soil to plants to animals and humans. As a result, the mineral content of the human body is quite similar to that of the earth.

Minerals, which are single, inert elements, may seem simple when compared with vitamins, which are large, complex, organic compounds. However, mineral micronutrients perform a fascinating variety of metabolic tasks essential to human life.

This chapter looks at this array of minerals to see how they differ from vitamins in the variety of their tasks and in the amounts, ranging from relatively large to exceedingly small, necessary to do these jobs.

KEY CONCEPTS

- The human body requires a variety of minerals in different amounts to perform numerous metabolic tasks.

- A mixed diet of varied foods and adequate energy value is the best source of the minerals necessary for health.

- Of the total amount of minerals a person consumes, only a relatively limited amount is available to the body.

THE NATURE OF BODY MINERALS

Most living matter is made up of four fundamental elements: hydrogen, carbon, nitrogen, and oxygen, the building blocks of life. The minerals necessary in human nutrition are single, inorganic elements that are widely distributed in nature. Of the 54 known earth elements in the periodic table, 25 are essential to human life. These 25 elements, in varying amounts, perform a variety of metabolic functions in the body.

Classes of Body Minerals

As described in the previous chapter, all vitamins are necessary in very small amounts to do their jobs. However, minerals occur in varying amounts in the body. For example, calcium forms a relatively large amount (e.g., about 2%) of the total body weight, with most of this amount being bone tissue. An adult who weighs 150 pounds has about 3 pounds of calcium in the body. On the other hand, iron occurs in very small amounts. The same adult has only about 3 g (about one tenth of an ounce) of iron in the body. In both cases, the amount of each mineral is essential for its specific task.

This varying amount of individual minerals in the body provides the basis for classifying them into two main groups.

Major Minerals

Elements are not called major minerals because they are more important, but because they occur in larger amounts in the body. The major minerals are defined as those requiring an intake of more than 100 mg/day. The seven major minerals are calcium, phosphorus, sodium, potassium, magnesium, chloride, and sulfur.

Trace Elements

The remaining 18 elements make up the group of trace elements. These minerals are not less important, they just occur in very small amounts in the body. Trace elements are generally defined as those having a required intake of less than 100 mg/day. Trace elements are equally essential for their specific vital tasks. Box 8-1 provides a helpful study guide.

Functions of Minerals

These seemingly simple, single elements perform an impressive variety of metabolic jobs for the body. They build, activate, regulate, transmit, and control. For example, sodium and potassium control water balance. Calcium and phosphorus build the body framework. Iron

helps build the vital oxygen carrier hemoglobin. Cobalt is the central core of vitamin B_{12}. Iodine builds thyroid hormone, which in turn regulates the overall rate of body metabolism. Thus far from being static and inert, minerals are active essential participants, helping to control many of the body's overall metabolic processes.

Mineral Metabolism

The correct amount of minerals for body needs is usually controlled at either the point of absorption or the points of tissue uptake.

Digestion

Minerals are absorbed and used in the body in their activated *ionic* (e.g., carrying an electric charge [+ or −]) form. Unlike carbohydrates, proteins, and fat, minerals do not require a great deal of mechanical or chemical digestion before absorption.

Absorption

The following general factors influence how much of a mineral actually is absorbed into the body system from the gastrointestinal (GI) tract: (1) *food form*—minerals

---

BOX 8–1 Major Minerals and Trace Elements in Human Nutrition

Major Minerals*

Calcium (Ca)	Magnesium (Mg)
Phosphorus (P)	Chloride (Cl)
Sodium (Na)	Sulfur (S)
Potassium (K)	

Trace Elements

Essential†	Essentially Unclear
Iron (Fe)	Silicon (Si)
Iodine (I)	Tin (Sn)
Zinc (Zn)	Cadmium (Cd)
Selenium (Se)	Arsenic (As)
Fluoride (Fl)	Aluminum (Al)
Copper (Cu)	
Manganese (Mn)	
Chromium (Cr)	
Molybdenum (Mo)	
Cobalt (Co)	
Boron (B)	
Vanadium (V)	
Nickel (Ni)	

*Required intake more than 100 mg/day.
†Required intake less than 100 mg/day.

in animal foods are usually more readily absorbed than those in plant foods; (2) *body need*—if the body is deficient, more is absorbed than if the body has enough; and (3) *tissue health*—if the absorbing tissue surface is affected by disease, its absorptive capacity is greatly diminished.

The absorptive method for each mineral varies depending on its characteristics. Some minerals require active transport for absorption, whereas others enter the GI tract via diffusion. Compounds found in foods also may affect the absorption efficiency of minerals. For example, the presence of fiber, phytates, or oxalates (found in a variety of whole grains, fruits, and vegetables) can bind minerals in the GI tract and inhibit or limit the mineral absorption.

Transport

Minerals are absorbed directly into blood circulation and travel throughout the body bound to plasma proteins or mineral-specific transport proteins.

Tissue Uptake

Some minerals are controlled by regulating hormones at the point of their "target" tissue uptake, with the excess excreted in urine. For example, the thyroid-stimulating hormone (TSH) controls the uptake of iodine from the blood according to the amount needed to make the thyroid hormone *thyroxine*. When more thyroxine is needed, more iodine is taken up by the thyroid gland under TSH stimulation and less is excreted. At other times, when blood levels of thyroxine are normal, less iodine is taken up by the thyroid gland and more is excreted.

Occurrence in the Body

Body minerals are found in several forms in places related to their functions. The two basic forms in which minerals occur in the body are as follows: (1) *free*—mineral atoms or molecules may be free as *ions* (meaning that they carry an electric charge) in body fluids (e.g., sodium in tissue fluids, which helps to control water balance); and (2) *combined*—minerals may be combined with other minerals (e.g., calcium with phosphorus to form bone) or organic substances (e.g., iron with heme and globin to form the organic compound hemoglobin).

MAJOR MINERALS

Calcium

Functions

Most of the U.S. food and nutrition surveys, such as those conducted regularly by the U.S. Department of Agriculture (USDA) and the National Center for Health Statistics, indicate that calcium is one of the minerals most likely to be deficient in a typical diet.[1] Men and boys consume about 25% more calcium than women and girls on average, simply because men and boys usually eat larger amounts of food. The absorption of dietary calcium depends on the following: (1) the food form (e.g., plant forms are sometimes bound with oxalates or phytates and not readily available); and (2) the interaction of three hormones (e.g., vitamin D hormone, parathyroid hormone [PTH], and calcitonin [from the thyroid gland]) that directly control absorption, along with indirect metabolic stimuli from the estrogen hormones (e.g., sex hormones produced in the ovaries and testes). Once absorbed, calcium has four basic functions in the body.

Bone and Tooth Formation. Most of the body's calcium, more than 99%, is found in bones and teeth. Approximately 1% to 2% of normal adult body weight is calcium. When calcium phosphate is removed from bone, the remaining tissue is flexible cartilage. If dietary calcium is insufficient during childhood growth, especially during initial formation of the fetal skeleton and rapid growth of long bones during adolescence, the production of healthy bone tissue is hindered. Teeth are calcified before they erupt from the gums, so dietary calcium later in life does not affect tooth structure as it does the continuing balance of calcium in bone tissue.

Blood Clotting. Calcium is essential for the formation of fibrin to compose the blood clot.

Muscle and Nerve Action. Calcium ions stimulate muscle contraction and transmit impulses along nerve fibers.

Metabolic Reactions. Calcium is necessary for many general metabolic functions in the body. Such functions include absorption of vitamin B_{12}, activation of the fat-splitting enzyme pancreatic lipase, and secretion of insulin from special cells in the pancreas where it is synthesized. Calcium also occurs in cell membranes, where it governs how permeable the membrane is to nutrients.

major minerals the group of minerals that are required by the body in amounts of more than 100 mg/day. The seven major minerals in the body are calcium, phosphorus, sodium, potassium, magnesium, chloride, and sulfur.

trace elements the group of elements, also called *micronutrients*, which are required by the body in smaller amounts of less than 100 mg/day.

Requirements

As part of the Dietary Reference Intakes (DRIs) project, the scientific panel on calcium reviewed all current research and concluded that there is not enough scientific knowledge of this nutrient's requirements through life to establish new specific Recommended Dietary Allowances (RDAs) for calcium. Although calcium is an area of active research, the DRI panel reports that the following are still areas of concern: uncertainties about the nutritional significance of some research data; a lack of firm agreement between observed survey information and experimental laboratory data; and a lack of long-term longitudinal data connecting calcium intake with long-term bone density loss. Therefore the DRI panel set Adequate Intake (AI) levels for calcium instead of a new RDA. The AI amounts should provide sufficient calcium nourishment for the body, while recognizing that a lower intake may be adequate for many individuals. Although there is currently no RDA for calcium, the Tolerable Upper Intake Level (UL) has been established, based on the maximum calcium intake above which there is a risk of adverse effects—primarily kidney stone formation (which affects 12% of the U. S. population), kidney failure, and metabolic action inhibiting the body's absorption of other minerals (e.g., iron, zinc, magnesium, and phosphorus).[2]

The DRI guidelines give AI levels by age group. For all infants up to 6 months old, the AI level is 210 mg/day; for infants 7 through 12 months, the AI is 270 mg/day. The need increases during the growth years of childhood and adolescence, during which the AIs are as follows: 1 to 3 years, 500 mg/day; 4 to 8 years, 800 mg/day; and 9 to 18 years, 1300 mg/day. For both men and women aged 19 to 50 years, the AI for desirable calcium retention is 1000 mg/day, with a rise to 1200 mg/day for those over 50 years old. During pregnancy and lactation, the AI amount is currently set equal to the level for the general age group, as follows: 1300 mg/day for up to age 18, and 1000 mg/day for ages 19 years and older. Excess calcium intake is usually associated with excessive use of high-dose supplements. The new UL is set at 2500 mg/day for individuals aged 1 year and older.

Deficiency States

Various bone deformities may occur if available calcium is insufficient during growth years. The deficiency disease *rickets* is related to inadequate vitamin D to support sufficient calcium absorption. A decrease of calcium in the blood, in relation to its serum partner phosphorus, results in *tetany*, a condition characterized by abnormal muscle spasms. The major calcium-related clinical condition today is **osteoporosis,** which is an abnormal thinning of the bones, especially in postmenopausal women, charac-

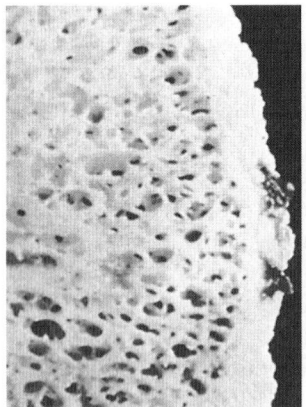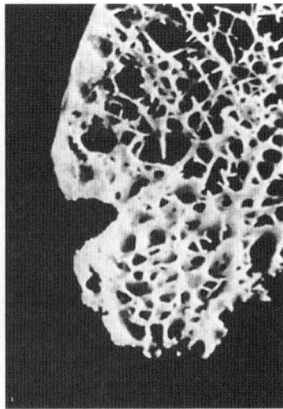

Figure 8–1 Osteoporosis. Normal bone *(left)* versus osteoporotic bone *(right)*. (From Mahan LK, Escott-Stump S: *Krause's food, nutrition, & diet therapy,* ed 11, Philadelphia, 2004, Saunders.)

terized by reduced bone mass, increased bone fragility, and a greater risk for fracture (Figure 8-1). Such fractures are becoming more and more common in elderly men as well. Each year in the United States, more than 1.5 million bone fractures, including 300,000 hip fractures, are linked to osteoporosis.

Osteoporosis is not a primary calcium deficiency disease as such, but results from a combination of factors that create chronic calcium deficiency. These factors include inadequate intake, poor intestinal absorption connected with hormones controlling calcium absorption and metabolism, and lack of physical exercise that stimulates muscle insertion action on bones and determines the strength, shape, and mass of bone. Insufficient physical exercise contributes to the development of osteoporosis; and immobility after injury or disease can cause serious loss of bone tissue. Bone is a dynamic tissue, with both new bone formation and resorption constantly occurring. A portion of the skeleton is reabsorbed and replaced by new bone each year; this bone remodeling can affect up to 50% of the total amount of bone per year in young children and about 5% in adults. Unfortunately, bone resorption often exceeds formation after menopause in women and with aging in both men and women. The precise cause of the imbalance in bone calcium deposit and resorption in osteoporosis is unknown. Thus increased calcium *alone*, in diet or supplements, neither prevents osteoporosis in susceptible adults nor successfully treats diagnosed cases. Therapies that reduce bone loss in osteoporosis include combinations of the various factors involved: dietary calcium, the active hormonal form of vitamin D, estrogens, and weight-bearing physical activity (see the Cultural Considerations box, "Bone Health in Gender and Ethnic Groups").

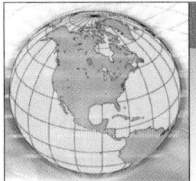

CULTURAL CONSIDERATIONS

BONE HEALTH IN GENDER AND ETHNIC GROUPS

Osteoporosis is often thought of as exclusively a problem for older white women. However, this debilitating bone disease is becoming more and more prevalent in other gender and ethnic groups as well. Approximately 20% of men over the age of 50 have osteoporosis.* Among postmenopausal American women, the incidence of osteoporosis is 21% for Caucasians and Asians, 16% for Hispanics, and 10% for African Americans.† The reasons for these observed differences by race are unclear. In addition, a recent study found dietary sources of calcium varied greatly between Euro-American and African-American athletes. Researchers reported that male Euro-Americans mostly consumed calcium in the form of dairy products whereas African-American males acquired calcium predominantly from mixed dishes and calcium-fortified foods.‡ The significance of these differences and their relationship to osteoporosis are currently under investigation.

Many factors are involved in bone mineral density and the relative risk for developing fragile bones, including: body weight, physical activity, hormonal influences, and dietary intakes of several vitamins and minerals, not just calcium. Nutrition affects bone health by providing the materials needed for tissue deposition, maintenance, and repair. Overall bone strength is determined by both bone mineral density *and* the collagen matrix formation. Collagen, a structural protein, accounts for more than 20% of the dry weight of total bone mass and

90% of the organic bone matrix. Collagen degradation is associated with osteoporosis. As such, the vitamins and minerals critical for strong collagen and bone matrix are also integral to overall bone health. A delicate balance of several nutrients is important for healthy bone building, such as protein; vitamins C, D, and K; calcium; phosphorus; copper; magnesium; manganese; potassium; and zinc.

Osteoporosis is currently costing Americans more than $10 billion annually in direct medical costs. Coupled with the general trend of an aging population, this bone disease is a serious national concern. Because bone mineral density reaches a peak mass by the average age of 30, the years before this are vital for developing healthy bones and preventing the onset of osteoporosis. Establishing peak bone mass ensures a greater reserve of bone mineral and collagen so that as age-associated degradation ensues, effects are essentially postponed or abated altogether. A healthy diet, following MyPyramid guidelines, should provide all essential nutrients and is imperative during the first three decades of life to establish healthy bones.

---

*Melton JL: The prevalence of osteoporosis: gender and racial comparison, *Epidemiology* 69:179, 2001.

†Food and Nutrition Board, Institute of Medicine: *Dietary reference intakes for calcium, phosphorus, magnesium, vitamin D, and fluoride,* Washington, DC, 1998, National Academies Press.

‡Leachman SD and others: Food sources of calcium in a sample of African-American and Euro-American collegiate athletes, *Int J Sport Nutr Exerc Metab* 11(2):199, 2001.

Toxicity Symptoms

Toxicity of calcium from food sources is highly unlikely. However, a UL for calcium has been set at 2500 mg/day because of negative effects of high calcium supplementation over time. Too much calcium is associated with an increased risk of kidney stones and decreased absorption of several other minerals. Calcium may interfere with the absorption of iron, zinc, magnesium, and phosphorus, thus increasing the requirement for these minerals.

Food Sources

Milk and milk products are the most important sources of readily available calcium (Figure 8-2). Milk used in cooking (e.g., in soups, sauces, or puddings) or in milk products such as yogurt, cheese, and ice cream are excellent sources of dietary calcium. Calcium-fortified tofu, fruit

juices, and other food products (e.g., cereals, bars, etc.) provide an equally high bioavailable source of calcium. Several plant foods also provide a natural source of this important mineral. Calcium found in low-oxalate greens such as bok choy, broccoli, collards, kale, and turnip greens is well absorbed and provides an important source of calcium for vegetarians. Oxalic acid is a compound found in some plants such as spinach, rhubarb, Swiss chard, and beet greens and certain other vegetables and

---

osteoporosis (Gr. *osteon,* bone; *poros,* passage, pore) abnormal thinning of the bone, producing a porous, fragile, latticelike bone tissue of enlarged spaces that is prone to fracture or deformity.

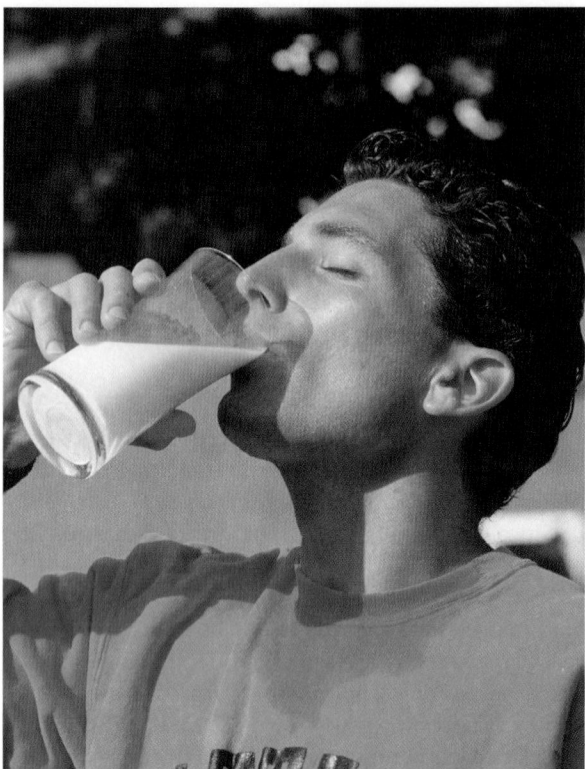

Figure 8–2   Milk is the major food source of calcium. (Credit: PhotoDisc.)

nuts that forms insoluble salts (oxalates) with calcium, interfering with calcium absorption. Secondary sources of calcium include grains, legumes, and nuts. Phytate, another plant compound in grains such as wheat, can bind calcium and interfere with its absorption. Table 8-1 lists calcium food sources.

In addition to food sources, calcium intake from supplements is widespread. Surveys show that almost 25% of women in the United States take supplements containing calcium.[2] The bioavailability of calcium from supplements depends on the dose and whether it is taken in the preferred manner with a meal. Calcium is best absorbed in doses of 500 mg or less (see the For Further Focus box, "Calcium from Food or Supplements: Which Is Better?").

Phosphorus

Functions

The phosphorus atom in nature is most commonly found combined with four oxygen atoms to form the phosphate molecule. Phosphorus serves as a partner with calcium in the major task of bone formation, but also functions in the following metabolic processes.

Bone and Tooth Formation. The calcification of bones and teeth depends on the fixing of phosphorus as calcium phosphate in the bone-forming tissue. The ratio of calcium to phosphorus in typical bone tissue is about 1.5:1.

Energy Metabolism. Phosphorus, in the form of phosphate, is necessary for the controlled oxidation of carbohydrate, fat, and protein in producing and storing available energy for the body. Phosphate contributes to energy and protein metabolism, and to cell function and genetic inheritance as an essential component of cell enzymes, thiamin, and the critical cell compounds DNA and RNA, which control cell reproduction.

Acid-Base Balance. Phosphate is an important buffer material that prevents changes in the acidity of body fluids.

Requirements

The typical American diet contains enough phosphorus to meet body needs. Surveys indicate that for those over age 6, the mean daily phosphorus intake is around 1500 mg/day for men and 1200 mg/day for women.[1] The AI level during the first 6 months is 100 mg/day, and from 7 to 12 months is 275 mg/day. Healthy infants fed human milk receive adequate phosphorus. For children, the RDA varies with the stage of growth. For ages 1 to 3 years, the RDA is 460 mg/day; for ages 4 to 8 years, it is 500 mg/day. For ages 9 to 18 years, a period of very rapid bone growth, the RDA is 1250 mg/day. The DRI guidelines have established RDAs for both men and women aged 19 and older at 700 mg phosphorus per day. For women during pregnancy and lactation, there is no additional phosphorus intake recommended above the RDA for any age group.

Deficiency States

Because phosphorus is widely distributed in foods, a deficiency is rare. A state of nearly total starvation would be needed to create a dietary phosphorus deficiency. The only evidence of deficiency has been among persons who for weeks or months habitually consume large amounts of antacids containing aluminum hydroxide. Aluminum hydroxide binds phosphorus, making it unavailable for absorption. Phosphorus deficiency results in bone loss and is characterized by weakness, loss of appetite, fatigue, and pain.

Toxicity Symptoms

It is equally rare to develop a toxicity of phosphorus from food intake. However, if phosphorus intake is significantly higher than calcium intake for a long period of time, bone resorption may occur. The DRI guidelines establish the UL for phosphorus of 4000 mg/day for persons aged 9 to 70 years.

TABLE 8–1	Significant Food Sources of Calcium	
Food item	**Quantity**	**Calcium (mg)**
BREAD, CEREAL, RICE, PASTA		
Bran muffin, homemade	1	54
Bread, whole wheat	1 slice	18
Corn muffin, from mix	1	96
Cream of Wheat cereal, cooked	¾ cup	38
Pasta, enriched, cooked	1 cup	16
Rice, enriched	1 cup	21
Wheat Flakes cereal	1 cup	43
VEGETABLES		
Artichoke, boiled	1 medium	47
Asparagus, boiled	½ cup (6 spears)	22
Avocado, raw	1 medium	19
Broccoli, raw	½ cup	21
Brussels sprouts, boiled	½ cup (4 sprouts)	28
Carrots, raw	1 medium	19
Collards, boiled	1 cup	148
Kale, chopped	½ cup	47
Peas, green, boiled	½ cup	19
Potato, baked, with skin	1 medium	115
FRUITS		
Apricots, raw	3 medium	15
Figs, dried	10	269
Orange juice, fresh	8 fl oz	27
Orange, navel, raw	1 medium	56
Papaya, raw	1 medium	72
Raspberries, raw	½ cup	14
Strawberries, raw	½ cup	11
Tangerine, raw	1 medium	12
MEAT, POULTRY, FISH, DRY BEANS, EGGS, NUTS		
Almonds, roasted	1 oz	148
Beef liver, fried	3.5 oz	11
Cashews, roasted	1 oz	13
Chicken, dark meat, roasted, without skin	3.5 oz	179
Chicken, light meat, roasted, without skin	3.5 oz	216
Egg, whole	1 large	90
Kidney beans, boiled	1 cup	50
Lentils, boiled	1 cup	37
Lima beans, boiled	1 cup	32
Peanuts, roasted	1 oz	15
Soybeans, boiled	1 cup	175
Tofu, regular	½ cup	434
MILK, DAIRY PRODUCTS OR SUBSTITUTE		
Cultured soy yogurt, fortified	½ cup	88
Milk, skim	8 fl oz	302
Milk, whole	8 fl oz	290
Yogurt, whole	8 fl oz	355
FATS, OILS		
This food group is not an important source of calcium.		
SUGAR		
Molasses, Barbados	1 Tbsp	49
Sugar, brown	1 cup	123

FOR FURTHER FOCUS

CALCIUM FROM FOOD OR SUPPLEMENTS: WHICH IS BETTER?

If only we could take a supplement to meet all our nutritional needs, then we would not have to bother with eating healthy! Unfortunately, that is the type of thinking that fuels the continued search for the "magic pill." Good health is not a simple matter and our bodies are no simple machines. They require lots of nutrients to function properly, which must be provided by the diet. One of the major minerals needed by our body is calcium. According to previous studies of average nutrient intake in the United States, such as the Continuing Survey of Food Intakes by Individuals (CSFII), relatively few Americans meet the AI for calcium through their diet.* Men consume more dietary sources of calcium throughout the life span than women, but still fall short of meeting 100% of the AI. A very small percentage of women, who are at higher risk for developing osteoporosis, meet 100% of their AI for calcium. According to the most recent CSFII, the following represents the percentages of females meeting the 1997 AI for calcium by age group: 12% of females 12 to 19, 16% of women 20 to 29, 14% of women 30 to 39, 11.5% of women 40 to 49, 5% of women 50 to 59, and 4% of women 60 and older.* Have you considered your calcium intake lately?

There are a variety of factors influencing our dietary intake of calcium. Over the past decade, Americans' food consumption patterns have changed in ways that directly affect calcium-rich food consumption. For instance, Americans: (1) are replacing milk with soft drinks; (2) are eating out more often at restaurants, where the overall calcium density is lower than meals at home; (3) seem to be perpetually dieting (and dairy products are often one of the first foods to go); and (4) are largely unaware of the healthy link between calcium-rich foods and health.†

Health organizations, such as the National Institute of Health, American Dietetic Association, American Medical Association, and National Academy of Sciences, are in agreement that the best source of calcium is from dairy products. The primary reason for this is because, unlike calcium supplements, calcium-rich foods supply the body with other beneficial nutrients as well, including protein, vitamins A, B_{12}, and D (if fortified), magnesium, potassium, riboflavin, niacin, and phosphorus.† There are also a selection of nondairy foods that naturally contain calcium, such as salmon with bones, dried beans, turnip greens, mustard greens, kale, tofu, and broccoli. It is difficult for most individuals to meet their recommended calcium intake exclusively from nondairy foods because the relative amount of calcium in these foods is significantly less than in dairy products. For example, ½ cup of fresh turnip greens has 53 mg calcium, whereas 8 oz of skim milk contains 302 mg. Also, many vegetables contain phytates and oxalates that form insoluble complexes with calcium and decrease their bioavailability to the body.

Calcium-fortified foods are excellent sources of calcium, especially for vegans or individuals who are lactose intolerant. However, as with calcium supplements, the benefits of consuming dairy products rich in many vitamins and minerals may be lost in fortified foods such as orange juice or cereal.

Keller and colleagues analyzed the consumer cost and bioavailability of calcium from all sources. They found Total cereal as the least expensive food source of calcium, with fluid milk and calcium-fortified orange juice coming in next.‡ Calcium from supplements may be found in a variety of forms including calcium carbonate, citrate, phosphate, lactate, and gluconate. The amount of calcium actually absorbed into the body from these different sources varies considerably.§ Of the calcium supplements, calcium carbonate, in a chewable form (Tums) or supplement, provides the least expensive and most bioavailable source of calcium, with a 34% absorption fraction.‡

The best way to improve overall diet is to consume a variety of foods high in calcium, preferably from dairy sources. However, calcium-fortified foods and supplements may be necessary for some individuals to meet their recommended intake of calcium. An individual consuming calcium supplements should be aware of potential side effects such as constipation and drug-nutrient interactions. Also, calcium is best absorbed in doses of 500 mg or less at a single time.

Regardless of where your calcium is coming from, take a moment to consider the overall value of your diet and assess if improvements are warranted.

---

*U.S. Department of Agriculture, Agricultural Research Service: *USDA's 1994-96 continuing survey of food intakes by individuals and 1994-96 diet and knowledge survey,* Riverdale, MD, 1999, ARS/USDA.

†Miller GD and others: The importance of meeting calcium needs with foods, *J Am Coll Nutr* 20(2):168S, 2001.

‡Keller JL and others: The consumer cost of calcium from food and supplements, *J Am Diet Assoc* 102(11):1669, 2002.

§Marcason W: How much calcium is really in that supplement? *J Am Diet Assoc* 102(11):1647, 2002.

Food Sources

Phosphorus is an essential part of all living tissue and is found in all animal and plant cells; therefore sufficient phosphorus is found in the natural food supply of virtually all animals. High-protein foods are rich in phosphorus, so milk and milk products, meat, fish, and eggs are the primary sources of phosphorus in the average diet. For humans, the bioavailability of phosphorus from plant seeds (e.g., cereal grains, beans, peas, other legumes, and nuts) is much lower because they contain *phytic acid*, which is a storage form of phosphorus that humans cannot digest directly. However, intestinal bacteria can help the body receive up to 50% of its phosphorus from these sources. Table 8-2 outlines some main food sources of phosphorus.

TABLE 8–2 Significant Food Sources of Phosphorus		
Food item	**Quantity**	**Phosphorus (mg)**
BREAD, CEREAL, RICE, PASTA		
Bran Flakes cereal	¾ cup	158
Bran muffin, homemade	1	111
Bread, whole wheat	1 slice	65
English muffin, plain	1	64
Oatmeal, cooked	¾ cup	133
Pasta, enriched, cooked	1 cup	70
Rice, enriched, cooked	1 cup	57
Wheat Flakes cereal	1 cup	98
VEGETABLES		
Artichoke, boiled	1 medium	72
Avocado, raw	1 medium	73
Brussels sprouts, boiled	½ cup (4 sprouts)	44
Corn, yellow, boiled	½ cup	84
Peas, green, boiled	½ cup	94
Potato, baked, with skin	1 medium	115
Spinach, boiled	½ cup	50
Sweet potato, baked	1 medium	62
FRUITS		
Figs, dried	10	128
Orange juice, fresh	8 fl oz	42
Raisins, seedless	⅔ cup	97
MEAT, POULTRY, FISH, DRY BEANS, EGGS, NUTS		
Almonds, roasted	1 oz (22 nuts)	156
Bacon, fried	3 medium slices	64
Beef liver, fried	3.5 oz	461
Beef top round, lean, broiled	3.5 oz	246
Black-eyed peas, boiled	1 cup	266
Chicken, dark meat, roasted, without skin	3.5 oz	179
Chicken, light meat, roasted, without skin	3.5 oz	216
Chickpeas (garbanzo beans), boiled	1 cup	275
Clams, canned	3 oz	287
Cod, baked	3 oz	117
Crab, Alaskan king, steamed	3 oz	238
Egg, whole	1 large	90
Ground beef, regular, broiled	3.5 oz	170
Halibut, baked	3 oz	242
Ham, canned, lean	3.5 oz	224

Continued

TABLE 8-2	Significant Food Sources of Phosphorus—*cont'd*	
Food item	**Quantity**	**Phosphorus (mg)**
MEAT, POULTRY, FISH, DRY BEANS, EGGS, NUTS—*cont'd*		
Lentils, boiled	1 cup	356
Lobster, steamed	3 oz	157
Oysters, steamed	3 oz (12 medium)	236
Peanut butter, creamy style	1 Tbsp	60
Peanuts, roasted	1 oz	100
Pinto beans, boiled	1 cup	273
Sirloin steak, lean, broiled	3.5 oz	244
Sole, baked	3.5 oz	344
Soybeans, boiled	1 cup	421
Tofu, regular	½ cup	120
Trout, rainbow, baked	3 oz	272
Tuna, light, canned in water	3 oz	158
Walnuts, dried	1 oz	132
MILK, DAIRY PRODUCTS		
Cheddar cheese	1 oz	145
Cottage cheese, creamed	1 cup	277
Milk, skim	8 fl oz	247
Milk, whole	8 fl oz	227
Swiss cheese	1 oz	171
Yogurt, whole	8 fl oz	215

FATS, OILS, SUGAR
This food group is not an important source of phosphorus.

Sodium

Functions

Sodium is one of the most plentiful minerals in the body. About 120 mg (4 oz) is present in an adult body. The main function of sodium is body-water balance, which is further discussed in Chapter 9. Sodium also has important tasks in acid-base balance and muscle action.

Water Balance. Ionized sodium is the major guardian of the body's water *outside* the cells (extracellular), which helps to prevent dehydration. Variation in sodium concentration largely controls the movement of water from one body part to another via *osmosis*. Sodium is also an integral part of the digestive juices secreted into the GI tract, most of which are then reabsorbed.

Acid-Base Balance. Sodium accounts for about 90% of the alkalinity of extracellular fluids and helps to balance acid-forming elements. Excess alkalinity, a condition called *alkalosis*, may result from the continued use of antacid drugs containing sodium.

Muscle Action. Sodium ions, in partnership with potassium, are necessary for the normal response of stimulated nerves, the transmission of nerve impulses to muscles, and the contraction of muscle fibers.

Nutrient Absorption. Sodium, an essential part of the cell membrane system, transports glucose and galactose across membranes in the small intestine.

Requirements

The body is able to function on various amounts of dietary sodium through mechanisms designed to conserve or excrete the mineral as needed. As a result, there is no specific RDA for sodium within the DRI guidelines. Individual sodium needs vary greatly depending on growth stages, sweat loss, and medical conditions (e.g., diarrhea). The DRI standards include an adequate intake of the three major electrolytes needed for body fluid balance: sodium, chloride, and potassium. A sodium intake of 1.5 g/day for healthy persons, who are not losing excess sodium through extended exercise and sweating, should adequately meet needs. Adults ages 50 to 70 have a slightly reduced AI (1.3 g/day) corresponding to decreased energy intake. The AI for individuals over age 71 is 1.2 g/day.[3]

Deficiency States

Deficiencies of sodium rarely happen because the body's need is low and intake is high. Exceptions occur during heavy body sweating, as may be the case with those engaged in heavy labor or athletes doing strenuous physical exercise in a hot environment for extended periods of time. Such persons may need additional salt to replace these heavy sodium losses. Deficiencies may result in acid-base balance problems and muscle cramping.

Commercial sports drinks, which replace sodium, glucose, and fluid, may be useful for athletes in endurance events. Most persons do not require these beverages for nonendurance activities.

Toxicity Symptoms

The sodium content of the average American diet, which contains a high amount of processed foods, usually far exceeds the recommended intake range, with an average of 8.5 g of table salt daily, or 3400 mg of sodium.[1] Excess sodium intake has been linked to hypertension in some individuals who are salt sensitive. However, for most people with healthy kidneys and adequate water intake, the body excretes excess sodium in the urine. Acute excessive intakes of sodium chloride (table salt) accumulate in the extracellular spaces. To balance the concentration, water is pulled into the extracellular space and can result in edema. The current DRIs set the UL for sodium intake at 2.3 g/day but state that some individuals may have a much lower tolerance.[3]

Food Sources

Common table salt, as used in cooking, seasoning, and processing foods, is the main dietary source of sodium. Sodium occurs naturally in foods and, in general, is most prevalent in foods of animal origin. There is enough sodium in natural food sources to meet the body's needs. When food manufacturers add salt and other sodium compounds to processed foods, sodium intake levels increase dramatically. For example, cured ham has about 20 times more sodium than raw pork. Natural food sources include animal products such as milk, meat, and eggs, and vegetables such as carrots, beets, leafy greens, and celery. (See Appendix D for sodium and potassium content of foods and Appendix E for salt-free seasoning guides.)

Potassium

Functions

The adult body contains about 270 mg (9 oz) of potassium, nearly twice the amount of sodium. Potassium is not only a partner with sodium in the body's water balance; it also has many metabolic functions.

Water Balance. Potassium is the major electrolyte controlling the water *inside* cells (intracellular). It balances with the sodium concentration in the extracellular fluid.

Metabolic Reactions. Potassium plays a role in the conversion of blood glucose to stored glycogen, storage of nitrogen in muscle protein, and production of energy.

Muscle Action. Potassium ions also contribute to nerve-impulse transmission to stimulate muscle action. Along with magnesium and sodium, potassium acts as a muscle relaxant in balance with calcium, which causes muscle contraction. The heart muscle is very sensitive to potassium levels; therefore proper concentration of potassium in the blood is particularly important.

Insulin Release. Potassium is necessary for the release of insulin from pancreatic cells in response to a rise in blood-glucose levels.

Blood Pressure. Sodium is one of the main dietary factors linked to elevated blood pressure; however, elevated blood pressure may be more related to the sodium:potassium ratio than the amount of dietary sodium alone. A potassium intake equal to that of sodium may be the preventive factor; such is the basis for the Dietary Approaches to Stop Hypertension (DASH) diet. (See *www.nhlbi.nih.gov/health/public/heart* for more information.)

Requirements

As with sodium, the present DRI guidelines do not establish an RDA for potassium, although potassium is a dietary essential. An AI of potassium appears to be approximately 4.7 g/day for all adults.[3] The National Research Council recommends an increase in potassium intake through increased consumption of fruits and vegetables. The average American and Canadian diet provides significantly less than the established AI, with a median daily intake of 2 to 3 g/day.[3]

Deficiency States

Symptoms of potassium deficiency are well defined but seldom related to inadequate dietary intake. Potassium deficiency is more likely to develop during such clinical situations as prolonged vomiting or diarrhea, use of diuretic drugs, severe malnutrition, or surgery. Deficiency is also a concern during the use of hypertension drugs, because diuretics cause a reduction in potassium. Those who couple diuretics with the excessive use of drugs that replace potassium also may experience a potassium imbalance. Characteristic symptoms of deficiency include heart muscle problems with possible cardiac arrest, weakness of respiratory muscles with breathing difficulties, poor intestinal muscle tone with resulting bloating, and overall muscle weakness.

Toxicity Symptoms

As with sodium, the kidney normally excretes excess potassium so that toxicity does not occur. However, if an extremely high potassium level were to accumulate in the blood because of excessive oral or intravenous intake, the heart could weaken to the point of stopping.

Food Sources

Because potassium is an essential part of all living cells, it is abundant in natural foods. The richest dietary sources of potassium are unprocessed foods: fruits such as oranges and bananas, vegetables such as broccoli and leafy green vegetables, fresh meats, whole grains, and milk products. Those who eat large amounts of fruits and vegetables have a high potassium intake. The plant form of potassium is very soluble; therefore much of the potassium content may be lost when cooked with excessive water (unless the water is retained). Table 8-3 lists food sources of potassium.

Chloride

Functions

Chloride is the chemical form of chlorine as it appears in the human body. Chloride accounts for about 3% of the body's total mineral content and is widely distributed throughout body tissues. Predominantly, chloride is found in the extracellular fluid compartments where it helps control the water and acid-base balances. Its two significant functions involve digestion and respiration.

Digestion. Chloride is a key element in the hydrochloric acid secreted in gastric juices. The action of gastric enzymes requires the proper acidity level of stomach fluids. This acid secretion also helps maintain the acid-base balance in body fluids.

Respiration. Chloride ions help red blood cells transport large amounts of carbon dioxide to the lungs for release in breathing. The chloride ions move easily in and out of

red blood cells in balance with the carbon dioxide to counteract any potential changes in the acid-base balance. This movement of chloride in and out of red blood cells is called the *chloride shift*.

Requirements

The AI for chloride for young adults is set at 2.3 g/day, based on a molecular equivalence to sodium.[3] Similar to sodium AIs, the need for chloride gradually declines with age after 50 years.

Deficiency States

A dietary deficiency of chloride does not occur under normal circumstances. Because the normal intake and output of chloride from the body parallels that of sodium, conditions leading to a sodium deficiency also can lead to a chloride deficiency. The primary reason for chloride deficiency is from excessive losses through vomiting, which leads to metabolic alkalosis from disturbances in acid-base balance.

Toxicity Symptoms

The only known dietary cause of chloride toxicity is from severe dehydration where the concentration of chloride is too great. There are no DRI established ULs for chloride.

Food Sources

Dietary chloride is provided almost entirely by sodium chloride, which is the chemical name for ordinary table salt. The kidneys are very efficient in reabsorbing chloride when the dietary intake is low.

Magnesium

Functions

Magnesium has widespread metabolic functions and is found in all body cells. An adult body contains about 25 g of magnesium (a little less than 1 oz). About 60% of this magnesium is present in the bones.

General Metabolism. Magnesium is a necessary catalyst for more than 300 reactions in cells that produce energy, synthesize body compounds, or absorb and transport nutrients.

Protein Synthesis. Magnesium activates amino acids for protein synthesis and facilitates the synthesis and maintenance of the cell genetic material, DNA. When cells replicate, they must produce new protein. This replication process requires a precise amount of magnesium to function correctly.

TABLE 8–3	Significant Food Sources of Potassium	
Food item	**Quantity**	**Potassium (mg)**
BREAD, CEREAL, RICE, PASTA		
Bran Flakes cereal	¾ cup	184
Bran muffin, homemade	1	99
Oatmeal, cooked	¾ cup	99
Pasta, enriched, cooked	1 cup	85
Wheat Flakes cereal	1 cup	110
Wheat germ, toasted	¼ cup (1 oz)	268
VEGETABLES		
Artichoke, boiled	1 medium	316
Asparagus, boiled	½ cup (6 spears)	279
Avocado, raw	1 medium	1097
Broccoli, raw	½ cup, chopped	143
Brussels sprouts, boiled	½ cup (4 sprouts)	247
Carrots, raw	1 medium	233
Corn, yellow, boiled	½ cup	204
Mushrooms, boiled	½ cup, pieces	277
Potato, baked, with skin	1 medium	844
Spinach, boiled	½ cup	419
Sweet potato, baked	1 medium	397
Tomato, raw	1 medium	254
FRUITS		
Apple, raw, with skin	1 medium	159
Banana	1 medium	451
Cantaloupe	1 cup, pieces	494
Dates, dried	10	541
Figs, dried	10	1332
Orange juice, fresh	8 fl oz	486
Orange, navel	1 medium	250
Prunes, dried	10	626
Prune juice, canned	8 fl oz	706
Raisins, seedless	⅔ cup	751
MEAT, POULTRY, FISH, DRY BEANS, EGGS, NUTS		
Almonds, dry-roasted	1 oz (22 nuts)	219
Beef liver, fried	3.5 oz	364
Beef top round, lean, broiled	3.5 oz	442
Black-eyed peas, boiled	1 cup	476
Chicken, dark meat, roasted, without skin	3.5 oz	240
Chicken, light meat, roasted, without skin	3.5 oz	247
Clams, steamed	3 oz (9 small)	534
Crab, blue, steamed	3 oz	275
Ground beef, regular, broiled	3.5 oz	292
Halibut, baked	3 oz	490
Ham, canned, lean	3.5 oz	364
Lentils, boiled	1 cup	731
Lima beans, boiled	1 cup	955
Lobster, steamed	3 oz	299
Mackerel, baked	3 oz	341

Continued.

TABLE 8–3	Significant Food Sources of Potassium—*cont'd*	
Food item	**Quantity**	**Potassium (mg)**
MEAT, POULTRY, FISH, DRY BEANS, EGGS, NUTS—*cont'd*		
Oysters, steamed	3 oz (12 medium)	389
Peanut butter, creamy style	1 Tbsp	110
Peanuts, dry-roasted	1 oz	184
Pinto beans, boiled	1 cup	800
Salmon, baked	3 oz	319
Sirloin steak, lean, broiled	3.5 oz	403
Soybeans, boiled	1 cup	886
Trout, rainbow, baked	3 oz	539
Tuna, light, canned in water, with salt	3 oz	267
MILK, DAIRY PRODUCTS		
Cottage cheese, creamed	1 cup	177
Milk, skim	8 fl oz	406
Milk, whole	8 fl oz	368
Yogurt, whole	8 fl oz	351
FATS, OILS		
This food group is not an important source of potassium.		
SUGAR		
Molasses, black	1 Tbsp	585
Sugar, brown	1 cup	499

Muscle Action. Magnesium ions help conduct the nerve impulses that stimulate muscle contraction. Magnesium, in balance with calcium, acts as a relaxant during muscle activity, after contraction.

Basal Metabolic Rate. Magnesium influences the secretion of the thyroid hormone thyroxine, thus helping the body maintain a normal metabolic rate and adapt to cold temperatures.

Requirements

The DRI guidelines establish RDA amounts by age group and gender. For infants, the AI level is 30 mg/day during the first 6 months and 75 mg/day from 7 to 12 months. The RDA is the same for both boys and girls during childhood and early adolescence: 80 mg/day for ages 1 to 3 years; 130 mg/day for ages 4 to 8 years; and 240 mg/day for ages 9 to 13 years. For the age group 14 to 18 years, the RDA is 410 mg/day for boys and 360 mg/day for girls. For those 19 to 30 years old, the RDA is 400 mg/day for men and 310 mg/day for women. For persons 31 years of age and older, the RDA is 420 mg/day for men and 320 mg/day for women. The RDA is somewhat higher during pregnancy: 400 mg/day for women 18 and younger and 350 to 360 mg/day

for women 19 and older. There is not an increased magnesium recommendation during lactation.[2]

Deficiency States

A magnesium deficiency that is purely dietary is very rare in persons consuming natural diets. Symptoms of magnesium deficiency have been observed in clinical situations such as starvation, persistent vomiting or diarrhea with loss of magnesium-rich GI fluids, and surgical trauma. Magnesium depletion is also found in various diseases involving cardiovascular and neuromuscular function, in diabetes mellitus, kidney disease, and alcoholism. Deficiency symptoms include muscle weakness and cramps, hypertension, and blood vessel constriction in the heart and brain.

Toxicity Symptoms

Magnesium consumed as a natural component of food has not been observed to have any adverse effects at high intake levels.[2] Therefore, the DRI standards establish the UL only for magnesium intake from supplements and pharmaceutical preparations. The UL from such sources is 350 mg/day for persons aged 9 and older, with lesser amounts for children.[2] Individuals with renal insufficiency are at greater risk for developing toxicity if they are taking dietary supplements. Those individuals consuming excessive amounts from supplements may experience nausea, vomiting, and diarrhea.

Food Sources

Although magnesium is relatively common in foods, the content level is variable. Unprocessed foods have the highest concentrations of magnesium. Major food sources include nuts, soybeans, cocoa, seafood, whole grains, dried beans and peas, and green vegetables. Relatively poor sources include most fruits (other than bananas), milk, meat, and fish. More than 80% of the magnesium content in cereal grains is lost with the removal of the germ and outer layers. Significant amounts of magnesium also may be present in drinking water in regions that have hard water with a fairly high mineral content.

Sulfur

Functions

An essential part of protein structure, sulfur is present in all body cells and participates in widespread metabolic and structural functions.

Hair, Skin, and Nails. Sulfur is involved in the structure of hair, skin, and nails through its presence in two amino acids, methionine and cystine, that are concentrated in the tissue protein keratin.

General Metabolic Functions. Combined with hydrogen, sulfur is important as a high-energy bond in building many tissue compounds. Sulfur helps transfer energy as needed in various tissues.

Vitamin Structure. Sulfur is a part of several vitamins (e.g., thiamin, pantothenic acid, and biotin) that in turn act as coenzymes in cell metabolism.

Collagen Structure. Sulfur is necessary for collagen synthesis and thus is important in building connective tissue.

Requirements

Dietary requirements for sulfur are not stated as such because sulfur is supplied by protein foods containing the amino acids methionine and cystine.

Deficiency States

Deficiency states have not been reported. Such conditions only relate to general protein malnutrition and the absence of the sulfur-carrying amino acids.

Toxicity Symptoms

Dietary intake is unlikely to reach toxic levels of sulfur.

Food Sources

A diet with adequate protein contains adequate sulfur. Sulfur is primarily available to the body as part of the organic sulfur compounds in its two amino acid carriers, methionine and cystine. Thus animal protein foods are the main dietary sources of sulfur. Sulfur is widely available in meat, eggs, milk, cheese, legumes, and nuts.

Table 8-4 provides a summary of the major minerals.

TRACE ELEMENTS

Iron

Functions

Iron has the longest and best described history of all the micronutrients. Iron is essential for life but toxic in excess. Thus the body has developed exquisite systems for balancing iron intake and excretion and for efficiently transporting iron in and out of cells to maintain health.[4-6] Iron functions both in the synthesis of hemoglobin and the body's general metabolism. The human body contains about 45 mg iron/kg body weight.

Hemoglobin Synthesis. Most of the body's iron, about 70%, occurs in red blood cells. Iron is an essential component of heme, the nonprotein part of the hemoglobin structure. Hemoglobin in red blood cells carries oxygen to the cells for oxidation and metabolism. Iron is also a necessary part of myoglobin, which is a similar compound in muscle tissue.

General Metabolism. Iron is necessary for proper glucose metabolism in the cell, antibody production, drug detoxification in the liver, collagen and purine synthesis, and conversion of carotene to vitamin A. To accomplish these vital functions, precise mechanisms regulate the amount of iron in the body, according to the body's need.

Requirements

Iron needs vary throughout life relative to growth and development. The DRIs establish recommended intakes of iron for children as follows: the AI for infants up to 6 months of age is 0.27 mg/day; for 7 to 12 months the RDA is 11 mg/day; 7 mg/day for ages 1 to 3 years; and 10 mg/day for ages 4 to 8 years. Recommended Dietary Allowances for iron from ages 9 and up are between 8 and 11 mg/day for males to accommodate for growth spurts and 8 to 18 mg/day for females.[7] Women require more iron to cover the losses during menstruation and

TABLE 8-4 Summary of Major Minerals

Mineral	Functions	Recommended intakes (adults)	Deficiency	UL and toxicity	Sources
Calcium (Ca)	Bone and teeth formation, blood clotting, muscle contraction and relaxation, nerve transmission	AI Ages 19-50 yrs: 1000 mg >51 yrs: 1200 mg	Tetany, rickets, osteoporosis	UL: 2500 mg Increases risk of kidney stones, constipation; interferes with absorption of other nutrients	Dairy products, fish bones, fortified orange juice and cereals, legumes, green leafy vegetables
Phosphorus (P)	Bone and tooth formation, energy metabolism, DNA and RNA, acid-base balance	RDA 700 mg	Unlikely, but can cause bone loss, loss of appetite, weakness	UL: 4000 mg Bone resorption (loss of calcium)	High-protein foods (meat, dairy) and soft drinks
Sodium (Na)	Major extracellular fluid control, water balance, acid-base balance, muscle action, transmission of nerve impulse and resulting contraction	AI Ages 19-50 yrs: 1.5 g 51-70 yrs: 1.3 g >71 yrs: 1.2 g	Fluid shifts, acid-base imbalance, cramping	UL: 2.3 g Hypertension in salt-sensitive people, edema	Table salt, processed foods (luncheon meats, salty snacks)
Potassium (K)	Major intracellular fluid control, acid-base balance, regulation of nerve impulse and muscle contraction, blood pressure regulation	AI Ages >14 yrs: 4.7 g	Irregular heartbeat, difficulty breathing, muscle weakness	UL: Not set Cardiac arrest	Fresh fruits, vegetables, meats, whole grains
Chloride (Cl)	Acid-base balance (chloride shift), hydrochloric acid (digestion)	AI Ages 19-50 yrs: 2.3 g 51-70 yrs: 2.0 g >71 yrs: 1.8 g	Hypochloremic alkalosis in prolonged vomiting, diarrhea	UL: Not set Unlikely	Table salt, processed foods
Magnesium (Mg)	Coenzyme in metabolism, muscle and nerve action, aids thyroid hormone secretion	RDA Men: 400-420 mg Women: 310-320 mg	Tremor, spasm, low serum level following gastrointestinal losses or renal losses from alcoholism, convulsions	UL: 350 mg (from supplements) Nausea, vomiting, diarrhea	Whole grains, nuts, legumes, green vegetables, seafood, cocoa
Sulfur (S)	Essential constituent of cell protein, hair, skin, nails, vitamin, and collagen structure; high-energy sulfur bonds in energy metabolism	Diets adequate in protein contain adequate sulfur	Unlikely	UL: Not set Unlikely	Meat, eggs, cheese, milk, nuts, legumes

UL = Tolerable Upper Intake Level; RDA = Recommended Dietary Allowance.

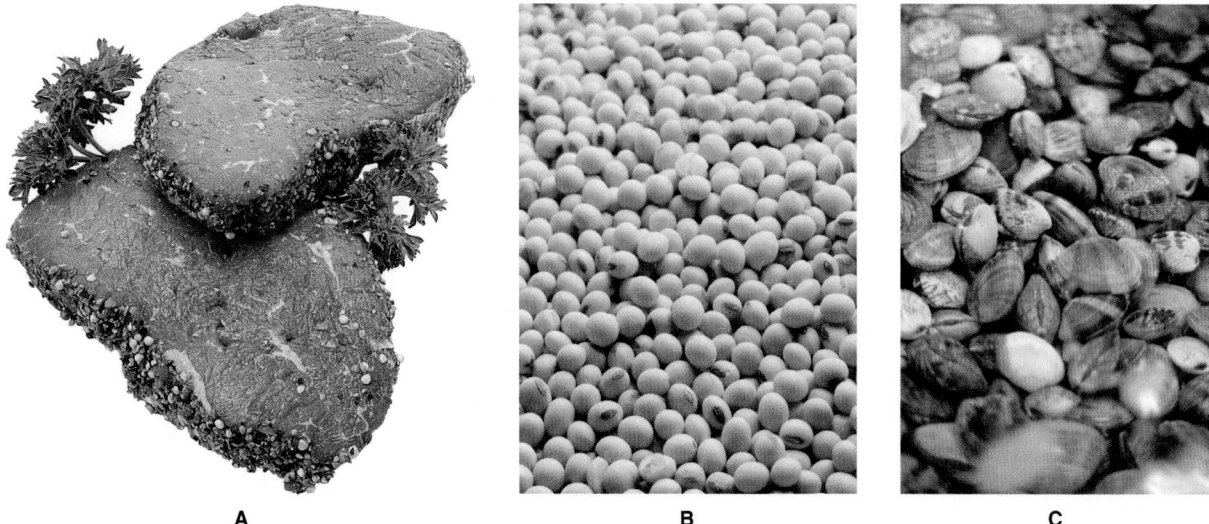

A   B   C

Figure 8–3 Food sources of dietary iron: **A,** beef; **B,** black-eyed peas; and **C,** oysters and clams. (Copyright 2004 JupiterImages Corporation.)

pregnancy. During pregnancy, a woman's RDA for iron increases to 27 mg/day. This increase usually requires an iron supplement because neither the usual American diet nor the iron stores of many women can meet the increased iron demands.

Deficiency States

The major condition indicating a deficiency of iron is anemia, which is characterized by a decrease in the number of red blood cells, a drop in the amount of cell hemoglobin, or both. Iron deficiency anemia is the most prevalent nutritional problem in the world today. More than 2 billion people worldwide are iron deficient; women and children are affected more than others. This lack of iron and the inability to use it may result from several causes, as follows: (1) inadequate supply of dietary iron; (2) excessive blood loss; (3) inability to form hemoglobin in the absence of other necessary factors such as vitamin B_{12} (e.g., pernicious anemia); (4) lack of gastric hydrochloric acid necessary to help liberate iron for absorption; (5) presence of various inhibitors of iron absorption (e.g., phosphate or phytate); or (6) mucosal lesions affecting the absorbent surface area.

Toxicity Symptoms

Iron toxicity from a single large dose (20 to 60 mg/kg) can be fatal. In the United States, iron overdose from supplements is the leading cause of poisoning among young children. Symptoms include nausea, vomiting, and diarrhea. If not treated immediately, several organ systems may be adversely affected, including the cardio-vascular system, central nervous system, kidney, liver, and hematologic system.[7]

Chronically elevated iron intake may impair the absorption of zinc, cause GI upset, and increase the risk for developing heart disease and cancer.[7] The congenital disease, *hemochromatosis* is an autosomal recessive disorder that results in iron overload, even though iron intake is within the normal range. This disorder affects 1 in 300 individuals of northern European descent. Individuals absorb excessive amounts of iron from food, and over time, usually 40 to 60 years, the accumulated iron causes widespread organ damage. Treatment involves reduced iron intake and regular blood withdrawal.

Food Sources

The typical Western diet provides an average of 6 mg of iron per 1000 kcal of energy intake. Iron is widely distributed in the U.S. food supply, mainly in meat, eggs, vegetables, and cereals (Figure 8-3). Iron is especially present in liver and fortified cereal products. The body absorbs iron more easily in conjunction with vitamin C. Iron occurs in food in two forms, *heme* and *nonheme*, a factor that affects its absorption and hence its avail-

---

anemia (Gr. *an-*, negative prefix; *haima*, blood) blood condition characterized by a decreased number of circulating red blood cells, hemoglobin, or both.

TABLE 8–5   Characteristics of Heme and Nonheme Portions of Dietary Iron

Heme (smallest portion)	Nonheme (largest portion)
FOOD SOURCES	
None in plant sources; 40% of iron in animal sources	All iron in plant sources; 60% of iron in animal sources
ABSORPTION RATE	
Rapid; transported and absorbed intact	Slow; tightly bound in organic molecules

ability to the body. Heme iron is the most easily absorbed form of dietary iron, but it contributes the smallest amount of the total iron intake. Heme iron is found in only 40% of the animal food sources and no plant foods (Table 8-5). Nonheme iron is less easily absorbed because it occurs in a more tightly bound form in foods, yet the majority of our food sources—60% of the animal food sources and all of the plant food sources—contain this form. To help enhance the absorption and availability of nonheme iron, food sources of vitamin C, moderate amounts of lean meats, and enriched cereal products must be included in the diet. Table 8-6 lists food sources of iron.

TABLE 8–6   Significant Food Sources of Iron

Food item	Quantity	Iron (mg)
BREAD, CEREAL, RICE, PASTA		
Bran Flakes cereal	¾ cup	4.50
Bran muffin, homemade	1	1.26
Bread, whole wheat	1 slice	0.86
Cream of Wheat, regular, cooked	¾ cup	7.70
Oatmeal, cooked	¾ cup	1.19
Pasta, enriched, cooked	1 cup	2.40
Rice, white, enriched, cooked	1 cup	1.80
Wheat Flakes cereal	1 cup	4.45
VEGETABLES		
Artichoke, boiled	1 medium	1.62
Avocado, raw	1 medium	2.04
Broccoli, boiled	½ cup	0.89
Brussels sprouts, boiled	½ cup	0.94
Peas, green, boiled	½ cup	1.24
Potato, baked, with skin	1 medium	2.75
Spinach, boiled	½ cup	3.21
FRUITS		
Dates, dried	10	0.96
Figs, dried	10	4.18
Prune juice, canned	8 fl oz	3.03
Prunes, dried	10	2.08
Raisins, seedless	⅔ cup	2.08
MEAT, POULTRY, FISH, DRY BEANS, EGGS, NUTS		
Almonds, roasted	1 oz (22 nuts)	1.08
Beef liver, fried	3.5 oz	6.28
Beef top round, lean, broiled	3.5 oz	2.88
Black-eyed peas, boiled	1 cup	4.29
Cashews, roasted	1 oz	1.70

Iodine

Functions

Iodine, like iron, has a long history of study. The average adult body contains only 20 to 50 mg of iodine. In human nutrition, iodine's basic function is to participate in the thyroid gland's synthesis of the hormone thyroxine. The pituitary gland releases TSH, which controls the thyroid gland's uptake of iodine, in direct response to the level of thyroxine circulating in the blood. When the blood level of thyroxine decreases below normal, the pituitary gland releases more TSH, thus stimulating the thyroid gland to take up more iodine for thyroxine synthesis. The trans-port form of iodine in the blood is called serum *protein-bound iodine* (PBI). After thyroxine (e.g., in its two hor-monal forms, T3 and T4) is used to stimulate metabolic processes in cells, it is broken down in the liver and the iodine portion is excreted in bile as inorganic iodine. Therefore the basic overall function of iodine relates to the control of the body's basal metabolic rate (BMR) by its role in synthesizing thyroxine.

Requirements

The body's need for iodine has undergone extensive study. To maintain desirable tissue levels of iodine, the adult body's minimum requirement is 50 to 75 μg/day; therefore

TABLE 8–6 Significant Food Sources of Iron—*cont'd*		
Food item	**Quantity**	**Iron (mg)**
MEAT, POULTRY, FISH, DRY BEANS, EGGS, NUTS—*cont'd*		
Chicken, dark meat, roasted, without skin	3.5 oz	1.33
Chicken, light meat, roasted, without skin	3.5 oz	1.06
Chickpeas (garbanzo beans), boiled	1 cup	4.74
Clams, steamed	3 oz (9 small)	23.76
Crab, blue, steamed	3 oz	0.77
Egg, whole	1 large	1.04
Ground beef, regular, broiled	3.5 oz	2.44
Halibut, baked	3 oz	0.91
Ham, canned, lean	3.5 oz	0.94
Lentils, boiled	1 cup	6.59
Lima beans, boiled	1 cup	4.50
Mackerel, baked	3 oz	1.33
Oysters, steamed	3 oz (12 medium)	11.39
Pinto beans, boiled	1 cup	4.47
Shrimp, steamed	3 oz (15 large)	2.62
Sirloin steak, lean, broiled	3.5 oz	3.36
Sole, baked	3.5 oz	1.40
Soybeans, boiled	1 cup	8.84
Tofu, regular	½ cup	6.60
Trout, rainbow, baked	3 oz	2.07
Tuna, light, canned in water	3 oz	2.72
MILK, DAIRY PRODUCTS		
This food group is not an important source of iron.		
FATS, OILS		
This food group is not an important source of iron.		
SUGAR		
Molasses, black	1 Tbsp	3.20
Sugar, brown	1 cup	4.90

to provide an extra margin of safety, the RDAs recommend an intake of 150 μg/day for all persons 14 and older. Lesser amounts are indicated for infants and children. During pregnancy, the need increases to 220 μg/day and during lactation it increases to 290 μg/day.[7]

Deficiency States

A lack of iodine in the diet contributes to several deficiency diseases, as discussed in the following sections.

Goiter. A lack of iodine in the diet causes the classic condition of goiter, which often occurs in areas where the water and soil contain little iodine (Figure 8-4). Some 800 million people live in these iodine deficient areas of underdeveloped countries where goiter is a large health problem. An enlargement of the thyroid gland, sometimes to a tremendous size, characterizes goiter. When the thyroid gland is starved for iodine, it cannot produce a normal amount of thyroxine. With this low level of thyroxine in the blood, the pituitary gland continues to produce more and more TSH. These large amounts of TSH continually stimulate the nonproductive thyroid gland, causing it to increase greatly in size. Such an iodine-starved thyroid gland may weigh 0.45 to 0.67 kg (1 to 1.5 lbs) or more.

Cretinism. Cretinism is characterized by physical deformity, dwarfism, and mental retardation. This serious condition occurs in children born to mothers who had limited iodine intake during adolescence and pregnancy. During pregnancy, the mother's iodine need takes prece-

dence over that of the developing child. Thus the fetus suffers from iodine deficiency, and continues to do so after birth. These children are retarded in both physical and mental development.

Hypothyroidism. An adult form of hypothyroidism, called *myxedema*, occurs when a poorly functioning thyroid gland cannot make enough thyroxine and the BMR is greatly reduced. The symptoms of this condition are thin, coarse hair, dry skin, poor cold tolerance, weight gain, and a low, husky voice.

Hyperthyroidism. An opposite condition, hyperthyroidism, in which the accelerated thyroid gland produces excessive thyroxine and the BMR is greatly increased, also may occur in adults. Hyperthyroidism is known as Graves' disease, or *exophthalmic* goiter, from the general symptom of protruding eyeballs. Other symptoms include weight loss, hand tremors and general nervousness, increased appetite, and intolerance of heat.

Toxicity Symptoms

Incidental intake of iodine through supplementation may result in toxicity for some persons. Excess iodine may result in acnelike skin lesions or may worsen the preexisting acne of adolescents or young adults. Excessive amounts also may cause "iodine goiter," which could be misdiagnosed as goiter caused by insufficient iodine.

Research has found that: (1) moderately excessive iodine is relatively harmless;[8] (2) persons living in certain

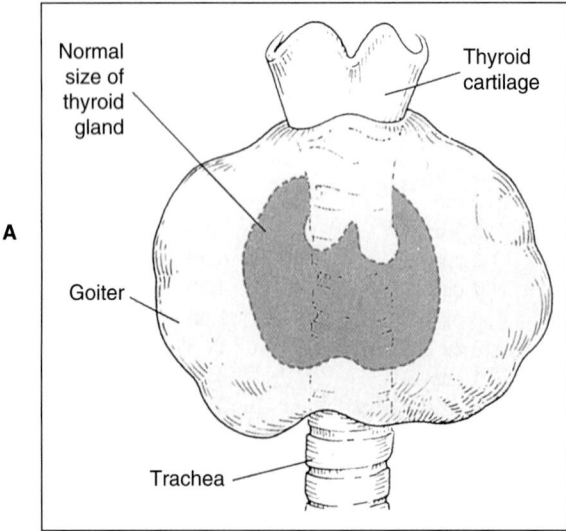

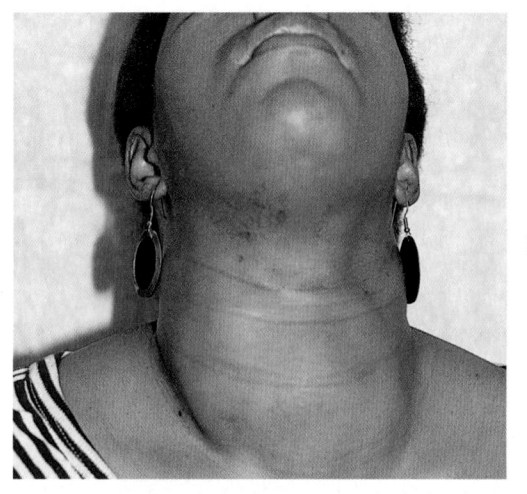

Figure 8–4 A, Illustration of a goiter. B, The extreme enlargement is a result of extended duration of iodine deficiency. (**B,** From Swartz MH: *Textbook of physical diagnosis history and examination,* ed 3, Philadelphia, 1999, Saunders.)

regions may be at greater risk of goiter; and (3) individual iodine intake is highly variable and may be insufficient (e.g., depending on geographic location and food supply). Therefore although the risk of toxicity exists, continued use of iodized salt is still widely practiced in several countries, including the United States.

Food Sources

The amount of iodine in natural food sources varies considerably depending on the iodine content of the soil. Seafood provides a good amount of iodine. The major reliable source, however, is iodized table salt, with each gram containing 76 μg of iodine. The presence of salt in processed foods supplies iodine even for those persons who do not use table salt.

Zinc

Functions

Zinc is an essential trace element with wide clinical significance. Zinc is especially important during growth periods such as pregnancy, lactation, infancy, childhood, and adolescence. The amount of zinc in the adult body is about 1.5 g in women and 2.5 g in men. Zinc is present in minute quantities in all body organs, tissues, fluids, and secretions. In these tissues, zinc participates in three different types of metabolic functions, as outlined in the following text.

Enzyme Constituent. Zinc's wide tissue distribution reflects its broad metabolic activity as an essential part of cell enzyme systems. Close to 100 such zinc enzymes have been identified. In its role in protein metabolism, zinc is associated with wound healing and healthy skin. It has great influence on any rapidly growing tissues, so its effect on reproduction is highly significant.

Immune System. A considerable amount of zinc bound to protein is present in the leukocytes (e.g., white blood cells), which are a major component of the body's immune system. Zinc affects the immune system through its essential role in the synthesis of nucleic acids (e.g., DNA and RNA) and protein. Zinc also is needed for lymphocyte transformation. Lymphoid tissue, which gives rise to lymphocytes, contains a large amount of zinc. The leukocytes of patients with leukemia, for example, contain about 10% less zinc than normal.

Other Functions. Zinc interacts with insulin in the pancreas, serving as a storage form of the hormone. It is also involved in the function of hemoglobin and taste and smell acuity.

Requirements

The DRIs establish an AI for infants during the first 3 years of life at 2 to 3 mg/day and 5 mg/day for children 4 to 8 years of age. Needs continue to rise until adulthood for both genders. Males 14 and older require 11 mg/day zinc, whereas females need 8 mg/day, with the exception of 14- to 18-year-old girls whose needs are slightly higher. Pregnant women require 11 mg/day to meet fetal growth needs and 12 mg/day for lactation. Pregnant or lactating females under the age of 18 require 2 mg/day more than older women. The zinc content of the typical mixed diet of adults in the United States averages 13 mg/day.[9]

Deficiency States

Zinc is imperative during periods of rapid tissue growth such as childhood and adolescence. Retarded physical growth (e.g., dwarfism) and retarded sexual maturation, especially in males, have been observed in some populations where dietary intake of zinc is low. Impaired taste and smell (e.g., hypogeusia and hyposmia) are improved with increased zinc intake if previous dietary intakes were inadequate. Zinc deficiency commonly causes poor wound healing, hair loss, diarrhea, and skin irritation. Patients with poor appetites, subsisting on marginal diets in the face of chronic wounds and illnesses and tissue breakdown, may be particularly vulnerable to developing a zinc deficiency (see the For Further Focus box, "Zinc Barriers"). Children 1 to 3, adolescent females, and persons over 71 reported the lowest zinc intake on the third National Health and Nutrition Examination Survey and are at greater risk for deficiency than other age or gender groups.[9]

Toxicity Symptoms

As with several other minerals, zinc toxicity from food sources is uncommon. However, prolonged supplementation in excess of recommendations can cause adverse effects such as nausea, vomiting, and decreased immune function. The UL for zinc (40 mg/day) was established based on the negative effect of excess zinc supplementation on copper metabolism. Excess zinc inhibits the absorption of copper, thus resulting in a copper deficiency.[7]

---

goiter (L. *gutter,* throat) an enlarged thyroid gland caused by lack of enough available iodine to produce the thyroid hormone thyroxine.

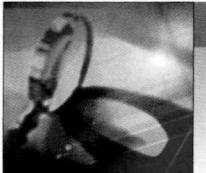

FOR FURTHER FOCUS

ZINC BARRIERS

Are people eating more zinc but absorbing it less? Current trends toward a "heart-healthy" diet may be the reason why. Some Americans may be at risk for developing zinc deficiency, not because they are avoiding zinc-rich foods, but because they are choosing foods and supplements that reduce its availability for absorption. The following provide examples:

● Animal foods, rich in readily available zinc, are consumed less by an increasingly cholesterol-conscious public.
● Dietary fiber, which is being promoted by some persons as a cardiovascular panacea, may hinder absorption and create a negative zinc balance.
● Food processing may make zinc less available.
● Vitamin-mineral supplements may contain iron:zinc ratios greater than 3:1 and provide enough iron to inhibit zinc absorption.

The risk for zinc deficiency is greatest among pregnant and breastfeeding women. Low levels of zinc can reduce the amount of protein available to carry iron and vitamin A to the target tissues and can reduce the mother's appetite and taste for foods. As a result, the fetus is at even greater risk for inadequate growth and development.

The following suggestions may help increase dietary zinc:

● Include some form of animal food (e.g., meat, milk, and eggs) or vegetarian acceptable fortified food in the diet each day to ensure a minimal intake of zinc.
● Avoid extensive use of alcohol.
● Avoid "crash" diets.

Signs of zinc deficiency are fairly rare in the United States but are becoming more apparent among at-risk persons (e.g., older adults hospitalized with long-term chronic illness). There is no need, however, for the general public to try to overprotect themselves with massive supplement doses. These large doses may compete with other elements, such as iron, and create other deficiency problems. Excess zinc can lead to nausea, abdominal pain, anemia, and immune system impairment. As with all other nutrients, too much of a good thing can sometimes be as bad as, or even worse than, too little.

Food Sources

The greatest source of dietary zinc in the United States is meat, which supplies about 70% of the zinc consumed. Seafood, particularly oysters, is another excellent source of zinc. Legumes and whole grains are additional sources, but they are less available to the body. A balanced diet usually meets adult needs for zinc, but considerable evidence shows that diets high in processed foods may be low in zinc. Animal food sources supply a major portion of dietary zinc. Strict vegetarians, especially women, may be at risk for developing marginal zinc deficiency. Table 8-7 gives food sources of zinc.

Selenium

Functions

Selenium is present in all body tissues except fat. The highest concentrations of selenium appear in the liver, kidney, heart, and spleen. Selenium functions with specific proteins as an essential part of an antioxidant enzyme, glutathione peroxidase, which protects cells and their lipid membranes from oxidative damage. An abundance of selenium can help spare the use of vitamin E, because they both protect against free radical damage. Selenium also functions as a part of the protein center of teeth and participates in the regulation of thyroid hormone action and vitamin C activity.

Recent human studies suggest that selenium's antioxidant function may have a protective role in the development of certain cancers.[10] The DRI panel on antioxidants reviewed the current scientific research on selenium. The panel concluded that although selenium intakes higher than the RDA level may have an anticancer effect in humans, more large-scale research is necessary to establish such an effect.[11]

Requirements

The DRI reference volume on antioxidants includes the revised RDAs for selenium. The recommendations are by age group, without a gender difference. For both men and women 14 and older, the RDA amount is 55 μg/day. The RDA is progressively reduced for children: 40 μg/day

TABLE 8-7 Significant Food Sources of Zinc

Food item	Quantity	Zinc (mg)
BREAD, CEREAL, RICE, PASTA		
Bran muffin, homemade	1	1.08
Bread, whole wheat	1 slice	0.42
Cream of Wheat, cooked	¾ cup	0.24
English muffin, plain	1	0.41
Oatmeal, cooked	¾ cup	0.86
Pasta, enriched, cooked	1 cup	0.70
Wheat Flakes cereal	1 cup	0.63
VEGETABLES		
Artichoke, boiled	1 medium	0.43
Asparagus, boiled	½ cup (6 spears)	0.43
Avocado, raw	1 medium	0.73
Brussels sprouts, boiled	½ cup (4 sprouts)	0.25
Collards, boiled	½ cup	0.23
Peas, green, boiled	½ cup	0.95
Potato, baked, with skin	1 medium	0.65
FRUITS		
Apricots, raw	3 medium	0.28
Cantaloupe, raw	½ cup	0.25
Figs, dried	10	0.94
MEAT, POULTRY, FISH, DRY BEANS, EGGS, NUTS		
Almonds, roasted	1 oz (22 nuts)	1.39
Beef liver, fried	3.5 oz	6.07
Cashews, roasted	1 oz	1.59
Chicken, dark meat, roasted, without skin	3.5 oz	2.80
Chicken, light meat, roasted, without skin	3.5 oz	1.23
Chickpeas (garbanzo beans), boiled	1 cup	2.51
Clams, canned	3 oz	2.32
Crab, Alaskan king, steamed	3 oz	6.48
Egg, whole	1 large	0.72
Ham, canned, lean	3.5 oz	1.93
Kidney beans, boiled	1 cup	1.89
Lentils, boiled	1 cup	2.50
Lima beans, boiled	1 cup	1.79
Lobster, steamed	3 oz	2.48
Oysters, cooked	3 oz	35
Peanuts, roasted	1 oz	0.93
Soybeans, boiled	1 cup	1.98
Tofu, regular	½ cup	0.99
MILK, DAIRY PRODUCTS		
Milk, skim	8 fl oz	0.98
Milk, whole	8 fl oz	0.93
Yogurt, whole	8 fl oz	1.34

FATS, OILS, SUGAR
This food group is not an important source of zinc.

for children 9 to 13 years of age; 30 μg/day for children 4 to 8 years of age; and 20 μg/day for children 1 to 3 years of age. The DRI does not establish an RDA for infants. Based on mean intakes of human milk, an infant's observed AI level is 15 μg/day for the first 6 months and 20 μg/day for 7 to 12 months. The recommended intake during pregnancy is 60 μg/day and 70 μg/day during lactation.[11] Recent studies have found that the selenium compounds in breast milk are more biologically available to infants than the selenium in formulas.[12]

Deficiency States

Selenium deficiency can significantly compromise the immune function. Mild deficiency may decrease the ability to fight infection, whereas severe deficiency may put individuals at risk for certain types of cancer. Research indicates that an adequate intake of selenium plays a role in preventing Keshan disease. Keshan disease, named after the area in China where it was discovered, is a heart muscle disease. It primarily affects young children and women of childbearing age and can lead to heart failure from cardiomyopathy (e.g., degeneration of the heart muscle).

Toxicity Symptoms

The most common symptom of selenium toxicity is brittleness in the hair and nails. Other problems include GI upset, skin rash, garlic odor, and nervous system abnormalities.[11] Most known dietary cases of toxicity are in isolated regions of the world where the soil has extremely high levels of selenium, such as China. The UL for selenium is 400 μg/day for persons 14 and older.

Food Sources

Most selenium in food is highly available to the body. The amount of selenium in food is dependent upon the quantity of selenium in the soil used to graze animals and grow plants. Unlike plants, animals require selenium. Seafood, kidney, and liver are consistently good sources of selenium. To a lesser extent, other meats also provide selenium. Grains and other seeds are more variable, depending on the selenium content of the soil in which they are grown. Fruits and vegetables generally contain little selenium. In the United States and Canada, the dietary intake of selenium varies by geographic region, but these local differences are reduced by the national food distribution system.

The following sections briefly review the remaining essential trace elements.

Fluoride

Fluoride forms a strong bond with calcium, which means that fluoride accumulates in calcified body tissues, such as bones and teeth. Fluoride's main function in human nutrition is to prevent dental caries. Fluoride strengthens the ability of the tooth structure to withstand the erosive effect of bacterial acids. The continuous intake of fluoride throughout life maximizes the protective effect of fluoride on teeth and maintains an adequate level of fluoride in tooth enamel. To a great extent, the fluoridation of the public water supply (for which the optimal level is 1 mg/L) is responsible for the remarkable decline in dental caries in recent decades. The use of fluoridated toothpaste (0.1%) and improved dental hygiene habits also benefit dental health.

Because fluoride stimulates new bone formation, it became an experimental drug in the treatment of osteoporosis. Presently, no evidence supports fluoride's ability to prevent osteoporosis. According to the DRI guidelines, there is an insufficient amount of knowledge about fluoride; therefore specific RDAs are currently unattainable. Alternatively, the DRI lists observed AI amounts by age group. For adults 19 and older, the AI is 4 mg/day for men and 3 mg/day for women, with smaller amounts for children. There is not a recommended increase in fluoride intake during pregnancy and lactation. The DRI guidelines set the UL for fluoride at 10 mg/day for persons 9 and older. Fish, fish products, and tea contain the highest concentrations of fluoride in foods. Cooking in fluoridated water raises the fluoride levels in many foods.

Copper

This trace element has frequently been called the "iron twin" because the two are metabolized in much the same way and share functions as components of cell enzymes. Both are also related to energy production and hemoglobin synthesis. Severe copper deficiency is rare, attributable to individual adaptation to somewhat lower intakes. However, copper depletion, sufficient enough to cause low blood levels, has been observed during total parenteral nutrition (TPN) and in cases of anemia. For adults, the DRI guidelines establish RDAs for dietary copper intake at 900 μg/day for all adults. There is a recommended increase in copper intake for pregnant or lactating women to meet increased needs (pregnant, 1 mg/day; lactating, 1.3 mg/day). Wilson's disease is a genetic disorder causing abnormal storage of copper in the body. Without treatment, Wilson's disease can result in liver and nerve damage. Natural foods contain a wide distribution of copper. Its richest food sources are organ meats, especially liver, followed by seafood, nuts, and seeds, including legumes and grains.

Manganese

The adult body contains about 20 mg of manganese, found mainly in the liver, pancreas, pituitary gland, and bone. Although it is considered a dietary essential, manganese is also toxic at high levels.[7] Manganese functions like other trace elements as an essential part of cell enzymes that catalyze many important metabolic reactions. Absorption and retention of manganese are associated with serum ferritin concentration.[13] Manganese deficiency is rare, but it has been reported in cases of diabetes and pancreatic insufficiency and in protein-energy malnutrition states such as *kwashiorkor*. Manganese toxicity occurs as an industrial disease, *inhalation toxicity*, in miners and other workers with prolonged exposure to manganese dust. The excess manganese accumulates in the liver and central nervous system, producing severe neuromuscular symptoms similar to those of Parkinson's disease.

The DRIs estimate an AI of 2.3 mg/day for adult males and 1.8 mg/day for adult females over the age of 19. Needs gradually increase from childhood and there is an additional need for pregnant and lactating women at 2.0 mg/day and 2.6 mg/day, respectively. The best food sources of manganese are of plant origin. Whole grains, cereal products, and teas are the richest food sources, and fruits and vegetables are somewhat less rich. Dairy products, meat, fish, and poultry are poor sources of manganese.

Chromium

The precise amount of chromium present in body tissues is uncertain because analysis is difficult. Although large geographic variations occur, the total body content is less than 6 mg. Chromium functions as an essential component of the organic complex *glucose tolerance factor* (GTF), which stimulates the action of insulin. Insulin resistance shown by impaired glucose tolerance has responded positively to chromium supplements, restoring normal blood glucose levels. Chromium supplements also are effective in the treatment of elevated serum cholesterol, lowering LDL cholesterol and increasing HDL cholesterol. For adults, the AI of chromium intake is 35 μg/day for men and 25 μg/day for women. Chromium needs gradually rise

from infancy to adulthood and then decline after the age of 50. Pregnant and lactating women have an increased need of 30 μg/day and 45 μg/day, respectively. Brewer's yeast is a rich source of chromium, and most grains and cereal products contain significant amounts.

Molybdenum

Absorption studies indicate that molybdenum is better absorbed than many minerals, and inadequate dietary intake is unlikely.[14] The amount of molybdenum in the body is exceedingly small; it ranges from 0.1 to 1 μg per gram of body tissue. Molybdenum functions as a catalyst component in several cell enzyme systems and is essential for a number of metabolic reactions. For adults, the RDA of molybdenum is 45 μg/day. Pregnant and lactating women need an additional 5 μg/day. The amounts of molybdenum in foods vary considerably, depending on the growth environment. Food sources include legumes, whole grains, milk, leafy vegetables, and organ meats. Table 8-8 provides a summary of selected trace elements.

Other Essential Trace Elements

An RDA or AI was not set for the remaining trace elements: aluminum, arsenic, boron, nickel, silicon, tin or vanadium. At the time of the 2002 DRI published for these nutrients, there were not enough data to establish such recommendations.[7] Most of them are deemed essential to the nutrition of specific animals and probably are essential in human nutrition, as well, although how they are metabolized in humans is not yet fully understood. Because these elements occur in such small amounts, they are more difficult to study, and dietary deficiency is highly unlikely.

Boron, nickel, and vanadium are the only ones that have enough information to establish a tolerable upper intake level. The UL for both boron and vanadium were set based on data gathered from animal studies. They are as follows: boron 20 mg/day and vanadium 1.8 mg/day for adults. The UL for arsenic was set at 1 mg/day.

MINERAL SUPPLEMENTATION

The same principles in the previous chapter relating to vitamin supplements guide the use of mineral supplements. Special needs during growth periods and in clinical situations may require individual supplements of specific major minerals or trace elements.

TABLE 8-8   Summary of Selected Trace Elements

Element	Functions	Recommended intakes (adults)	Deficiency	UL and toxicity	Sources
Iron (Fe)	Hemoglobin and myoglobin formation, cellular oxidation of glucose, antibody production	RDA Men: 8 mg Women: 19-50 yrs: 18 mg >50 yrs: 8 mg	Anemia, pale skin, impaired immune function	UL: 45 mg Nausea, vomiting, diarrhea, liver, kidney, heart, and CNS damage Hemochromatosis: iron overload disease	Liver, meats, egg yolk, whole grains, enriched bread and cereal, dark green vegetables, legumes, nuts
Iodine (I)	Synthesis of thyroxine, which regulates cell oxidation and BMR	RDA 150 µg	Goiter, cretinism, hypothyroidism, hyperthyroidism	UL: 1100 µg Goiter	Iodized salt, seafood
Zinc (Zn)	Essential enzyme constituent, protein metabolism, storage of insulin, immune system, sexual maturation	RDA Men: 11 mg Women: 8 mg	Impaired wound healing and taste and smell acuity, retarded sexual and physical development	UL: 40 mg Nausea, vomiting, decreased immune function, impaired copper absorption	Meat, seafood (especially oysters), eggs, milk, whole grains, legumes
Selenium (Se)	Forms glutathione peroxidase, spares vitamin E as an antioxidant; protects lipids in cell membrane	RDA 55 µg	Impaired immune function, Keshan disease, heart muscle failure	UL: 400 µg Brittleness of hair and nails, GI upset	Seafood, kidney, liver, meats, whole grains
Fluoride (Fl)	Constituent of bone and teeth; prevents dental caries	AI Men: 4 mg Women: 3 mg	Increased dental caries	UL: 10 mg Dental fluorosis	Fluoridated water, toothpaste
Copper (Cu)	Associated with iron in energy production, hemoglobin synthesis, absorption and transport of iron, nerve and immune function	RDA 900 µg	Anemia, bone abnormalities	UL: 10 mg Toxicity disease: Wilson's disease resulting in liver and nerve conduction damage	Liver, seafood, whole grains, legumes, nuts
Manganese (Mn)	Activates reactions in urea synthesis, energy metabolism, lipoprotein clearance, and synthesis of fatty acids	AI Men: 2.3 mg Women: 1.8 mg	Clinical deficiency present only in protein-energy malnutrition	UL: 11 mg Inhalation toxicity in miners: neuromuscular disturbances	Cereals, whole grains, soybeans, legumes, nuts, tea, vegetables, fruits
Chromium (Cr)	Associated with glucose metabolism	AI Men: 35 µg Women: 25 µg	Impaired glucose metabolism	UL: Not set Unlikely	Whole grains, cereal products, brewer's yeast
Molybdenum (Mo)	Constituent of many enzymes	RDA 45 µg	Unlikely	UL: 2 mg Unlikely	Organ meats, milk, whole grains, leafy vegetables, legumes

AI = Adequate Intake; BMR = basal metabolic rate; CNS = central nervous system; GI = gastrointestinal; RDA = Recommended Dietary Allowances; UL = Tolerable Upper Intake Level.

Life Cycle Needs

Added minerals may be needed during rapid growth periods throughout the life cycle.

Pregnancy and Lactation

Women require added magnesium, iron, zinc, selenium, iodine, copper, manganese, chromium, and molybdenum to meet the demands of rapid fetal growth during pregnancy. Recommended Dietary Allowances remain elevated for several minerals throughout lactation to meet both mother and infant needs.

Adolescence

Rapid growth during adolescence requires increased calcium and phosphorus for growth of long bones. If an adolescent's diet provides insufficient calcium, the risk for bone density problems (e.g., osteoporosis) in later adult years is increased. Too much dietary phosphorus and not enough calcium can result in bone resorption of calcium to maintain an appropriate blood ratio. With the major increases in per capita consumption of soda drinks (high in phosphorus) in the United States, coupled with a decrease in milk consumption, there is an increased concern for poor bone growth during these critical years.

Supplements combining iron with folate may be indicated for adolescent girls who may soon begin to menstruate and enter the child-bearing years.[15,16]

Adulthood

Healthy adults do not need mineral supplementation, but questions have been raised in media and advertising about the need for calcium to prevent and treat osteoporosis. Although currently marketed to prevent osteoporosis, calcium supplements alone have little effect, especially when the overall diet is poor. A well-rounded, varied diet combined with adequate physical exercise maintains optimal bone health in most adults. In addition, an idiopathic (e.g., cause unknown) form of osteoporosis that occurs in young adults does not respond to calcium supplements. At any adult age, calcium supplements alone neither prevent nor successfully treat osteoporosis, the cause of which is not clear and involves multiple factors. Calcium may be used as part of a treatment program together with vitamin D hormone, estrogen, and increased physical activity.

Clinical Needs

Persons with certain clinical problems or those at high risk for developing such problems may require mineral supplements.

Iron-Deficiency Anemia

One of the most prevalent health problems encountered in population surveys is iron-deficiency anemia. The need for increased iron has long been established for pregnant and breastfeeding women.[7] The following high-risk groups also may need to supplement their diets: adolescent girls on poor diets, low-income adolescent boys, athletes, vegetarians, and elderly persons on poor diets.

Weight-Loss Programs

The Women's Healthy Lifestyle Project was a recent study of the association between body weight and bone mineral density (BMD); 236 healthy women aged 44 to 50 participated with a goal of modest weight loss or preventing weight gain.[17] All of these women were randomly assigned to a control group or to a lifestyle-intervention group of behavior modification designed to reduce dietary fat and caloric intake. The women in the weight-loss group who modified their lifestyles to lose weight, however, lost more BMD than those in the weight-stable control group. Therefore programs for weight loss must consider the possible results of BMD loss and iron status, and should be planned accordingly.

Zinc Deficiency

Movement toward a plant-based vegetarian diet has amplified concern about possible zinc deficiency because of the low zinc content of such diets (see the Clinical Applications box, "Case Study: A Vegan Child and Her Family"). The American Dietetic Association and Dietitians of Canada Position Statement about vegetarian diets indicates that zinc requirements for individuals with high phytate diets may exceed the current DRIs.[18] Concern is greatest in children and elderly persons, whose needs are highest or are already consuming less zinc than recommended.[9] Signs of deficiency are slow growth, impaired taste and smell, poor wound healing, and skin problems, but it takes 3 to 24 weeks for symptoms to appear. Others at risk include alcoholics, persons on long-term low-calorie diets, and elderly persons in long-term institutional care.

Potassium-Losing Drugs

Persons requiring long-term use of potassium-losing diuretic drugs for treatment of hypertension may need potassium-replacement supplements. Increased intake of foods high in potassium also is necessary.

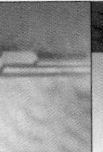

CLINICAL APPLICATIONS

CASE STUDY: A VEGAN CHILD AND HER FAMILY

A vegan couple decided to raise their 2-year-old daughter on their strict vegan diet. Often the child did not finish her meals and ate snacks of fruits and cookies. The parents eventually began to notice that she was not growing at the same rate as the other children and was becoming thin.

Consider what you have learned about all macronutrients (carbohydrates, protein, and fat) and micronutrients (vitamins and minerals) and the needs of children following a vegan diet.

Questions for Analysis

1. What food patterns would you expect in this family (e.g., what food groups are included or excluded)? What dietary factor may have been involved in the child's poor growth? Consider vitamins and minerals as well as protein and total energy.

2. What advice would you offer these parents to improve their child's nutritional status?

3. Plan 1 day's food for this family that would meet their nutritional needs within their vegan pattern. Indicate any added foods to specifically meet the child's needs.

4. Would nutrient supplementation be indicated for this family, especially for the child? Why or why not? What would you suggest to them?

See the following references for additional help:
Mangels AR, Messina V: Considerations in planning vegan diets: infants, *J Am Diet Assoc* 101(6):670, 2001.
Messina V, Mangels AR: Considerations in planning vegan diets: children, *J Am Diet Assoc* 101(6):661, 2001.
Mangels AR, Messina V, Melina V: Position of the American Dietetic Association and Dietitians of Canada: vegetarian diets, *J Am Diet Assoc* 103:748, 2003.

SUMMARY

Minerals are single, inorganic elements that are widely distributed in nature. They are absorbed in the body and used in their activated ionic form to build body tissue; activate, regulate, and control metabolic processes; and transmit neurologic messages.

Minerals are classified according to their relative amounts in the body. Major minerals are necessary in larger quantities and make up 60% to 80% of all the inorganic material in the body. *Trace elements*, which are necessary in quantities as small as a microgram (μg), make up less than 1% of the body's inorganic material.

Recommended Dietary Allowances have not been set for all minerals because of the lack of scientific data. However, AI or UL have been set for most all essential minerals without RDAs.

Mineral supplementation, as vitamin supplementation, continues to be on the forefront of many hot topic debates. There are periods throughout the life cycle, and specific disease states, that render supplements an important part of the diet. However, in most situations a balanced diet consisting of foods from each food group provides an adequate supply of all essential nutrients.

CRITICAL THINKING QUESTIONS

1. List the seven major minerals and describe their functions and the problems created by dietary deficiency or excess.

2. List the trace elements proved to be essential in human nutrition. Which ones have established RDAs, either within the DRI system or previously? Which ones have "safe and adequate intakes" suggested? Why is it difficult to establish RDAs and DRIs for everyone?

3. Considering the normal dietary supply of essential minerals, would you recommend taking a multimineral dietary supplement? If so, to whom and for what reasons?

CHAPTER CHALLENGE QUESTIONS

True-False

Write the correct statement for each item you answer "false."

1. *True or False:* Most of the phosphorus in the diet is absorbed and used by the body for bone formation.

2. *True or False:* Typical adult use of sodium is about 10 times the amount the body actually requires for metabolic balance.

3. *True or False:* Potassium is the major electrolyte controlling the water outside cells.

4. *True or False:* Chloride is a necessary component of stomach fluids.

5. *True or False:* Copper has many metabolic functions, the most important of which is its role in thyroxine synthesis.

6. *True or False:* A high intake of selenium has definitely been proved to prevent cancer in almost everyone.

7. *True or False:* Iodine is associated with iron functions in the body and is called the "iron twin."

Multiple Choice

1. Overall calcium balance is mostly maintained by which two interbalanced regulatory agents?
   a. Vitamin A and thyroid hormone
   b. Ascorbic acid and growth hormone
   c. Vitamin D and parathyroid hormone
   d. Phosphorus and TSH

2. Optimum levels of body iron are controlled at the point of absorption, interrelated with a system of transport and storage. Which of the following statements correctly describes this iron-regulating process?
   a. The iron form in foods requires an acid medium to reduce it to the form necessary for absorption.
   b. Most of the iron ingested in food, about 70% to 90%, is absorbed.
   c. Vitamin C acts as a binding and carrying agent to transport and store iron.
   d. When red blood cells are destroyed, the iron used in making the hemoglobin is excreted.

3. The only known function of fluoride in human nutrition is for dental health. Which of the following statements correctly describes this relation?
   a. Small amounts of fluoride produce mottled, discolored teeth.
   b. Fluoridation of the public water supply in very small amounts helps prevent dental caries.
   c. Topical application of fluoride is not effective on young teeth.
   d. Fluoride works with calcium to build strong teeth.

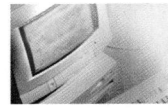

Please refer to the Students' Resource section of this text's Evolve web site for "Suggestions for Additional Study."

REFERENCES

1. Bialostosky K and others: *Dietary intake of macronutrients micronutrients and other dietary constituents: United States 1988-94,* Vital Health Stat 11(245), Hyattsville, MD, 2002, National Center for Health Statistics, Centers for Disease Control and Prevention, U.S. Department of Health and Human Services.

2. Food and Nutrition Board, Institute of Medicine: *Dietary reference intakes for calcium, phosphorus, magnesium, vitamin D, and fluoride,* Washington, DC, 1988, National Academies Press.

3. Food and Nutrition Board, Institute of Medicine: *Dietary reference intakes for water, potassium, sodium, chloride, and sulfate,* Washington, DC, 2004, National Academies Press.

4. Monsen ER: The ironies of iron, *Am J Clin Nutr* 69(2):831, 1999.

5. Hunt JR, Roughead ZK: Nonheme-iron absorption, fecal ferritin excretion, and blood indexes of iron status in women consuming controlled lactoovovegetarian diets for 8 weeks, *Am J Clin Nutr* 69(3):944, 1999.

6. Andrews and others: Iron transport across biologic membranes, *Nutr Rev* 57(4):114, 1999.

7. Food and Nutrition Board, Institute of Medicine: *Dietary reference intakes for vitamin A, vitamin K, arsenic, boron, chromium, copper, iodine, iron, manganese, molybdenum, nickel, silicon, vanadium, and zinc*, Washington, DC, 2002, National Academies Press.

8. Yang F and others: Epidemiological survey on the relationship between different iodine intakes and the prevalence of hyperthyroidism, *Eur J Endocrinol* 146(5):613, 2002.

9. Briefel RR and others: Zinc intake of the U.S. population: findings from the third National Health and Nutrition Examination Survey, 1988-1994, *J Nutr* 130(Suppl): 1367S, 2000.

10. Bialy TL and others: Dietary factors in the prevention and treatment of nonmelanoma skin cancer and melanoma, *Dermatol Surg* 28(12):1143, 2002.

11. Food and Nutrition Board, Institute of Medicine: *Dietary reference intakes for vitamin C, vitamin E, selenium, and carotenoids*, Washington, DC, 2000, National Academies Press.

12. Dorea JG: Selenium and breast-feeding, *Br J Nutr* 88(5):443, 2002.

13. Finley JW: Manganese absorption and retention by young women is associated with serum ferritin concentration, *Am J Clin Nutr* 70(1):37, 1999.

14. Turnlund JR and others: Molybdenum absorption and utilization in humans from soy and kale intrinsically labeled with stable isotopes of molybdenum, *Am J Clin Nutr* 69(8):1217, 1999.

15. Tee E-S and others: School administered weekly iron-folate supplements improve hemoglobin and ferritin concentrations in Malaysian adolescent females, *Am J Clin Nutr* 69(6):1249, 1999.

16. Picciano MF: Iron and folate supplementation in adolescent females, *Am J Clin Nutr* 69(6):1069, 1999.

17. Salamone LM and others: Effect of a lifestyle intervention on bone mineral density (BMD) in premenopausal women: a randomized trial, *Am J Clin Nutr* 70(1):97, 1999.

18. Mangels AR, Messina V, and Melina V: Position of the American Dietetic Association and Dietitians of Canada: vegetarian diets, *J Am Diet Assoc* 103:748, 2003.

FURTHER READING AND RESOURCES

- Medline Plus Health Information. A service of the U.S. National Library of Medicine and the National Institutes of Health: *www.nlm.nih.gov/medlineplus/vitaminandmineralsupplements. html*

  This web site provides the most current information about vitamins and minerals. The site provides an encyclopedia, drug information, dictionaries, and articles about research and clinical applications of vitamins and minerals.

- The National Heart, Lung, and Blood Institute: *www.nhlbi.nih.gov/health/public/heart/*

- American Dental Association: *www.ada.org/public/topics/ index.asp*

  The preceding web sites are good sources for information on certain minerals in the diets and their role in general health. Go to The National Heart, Lung, and Blood Institute web site to learn about the role of sodium and heart disease, such as hypertension, and how to follow a low-sodium diet. Examine the American Dental Association Oral Health Topics for more information on the protective role of fluoride in dental hygiene.

CHAPTER 9

Water Balance

Water is the most vital nutrient to human existence. In fact, the majority of the earth's surface is covered by water. Human life, and all other life forms sharing this planet, depends on a constant supply of water from the earth's ever-moving cycle. Humans can survive far longer without food than water. Only the constant need for air is more demanding.

One of the most basic nutritional tasks is meeting this need for a continuous supply of water. Ensuring a balanced distribution of this precious water to all the body cells is a primary physiologic function.

This chapter briefly looks at the finely developed water-balance system in the body, how this system works, and the various parts and processes that sustain it, thereby sustaining life itself.

KEY CONCEPTS

■ Throughout the body, water exists as a unified whole with constant ebb and flow among its interfacing parts.

■ Collective water compartments, inside and outside of cells, maintain a balanced distribution of total body water.

■ The concentration of various solute particles in the body's water solution determines internal shifts and balances of water.

■ A state of dynamic equilibrium (e.g., homeostasis) among all parts of the body's water-balance system sustains life.

BODY WATER FUNCTIONS AND REQUIREMENTS

Water: The Fundamental Nutrient

Basic Principles

Three basic principles are essential to an understanding of the balance and uses of water in the human body, as outlined in the following text.

A Unified Whole. The human body forms one continuous body of water. The "sea within" is contained by a protective envelope of skin. Enclosed within the skin, water moves freely to all parts, controlled only by water's chemical nature.[1] Virtually every space inside and outside of cells is filled with water-based body fluids. Therefore in this warm, watery, chemical environment, all the processes necessary to life are sustained. Water is indeed an essential nutrient necessary for life.

Body Water Compartments. Water does not simply slosh around in the body. The key word *compartment* is generally used in human physiology to refer to the dynamic systems within the body. The body's water can be treated as a whole, encompassing all the water in the body, as well as in separate individual locations throughout the body (e.g., intracellular or extracellular compartments) where the body stores and uses water. At the cellular level, *membranes* separate compartments of water. The body's dynamic mechanisms are constantly shifting water to places of the greatest need and maintaining equilibrium among all parts.

Particles in the Water Solution. The concentration and distribution of *particles* in the water solution (in various places throughout the body) determine all of the internal shifts and balances between compartments within the total body water.

Homeostasis

Picture body water as a unified whole, sustained in critical balance to protect life. The body's state of dynamic balance is called **homeostasis.** Many years previously a thoughtful physiologist, W.B. Cannon, viewed these balance principles as "body wisdom."[2] He applied the term *homeostasis* to the capacity built into the body to maintain its life systems, despite what enters the system from the outside. The first part of the word, *homeo-*, is from a Greek word meaning "similar." The second half of the word, *-stasis*, is from another Greek root, meaning "balance." The body has a great capacity to employ numerous, finely balanced, *homeostatic mechanisms* to protect its vital water supply.

Body Water Functions

To serve life-sustaining functions, the body water supply (1) acts as a solvent, (2) serves as a means of transport, (3) provides form and structure, (4) regulates temperature control, and (5) provides lubrication for the body.

Solvent. Water provides the basic liquid solvent for all chemical processes within the body. The word *hydrolysis* is used to describe this water-based chemical activity. The first part of the word, *hydro-*, means "water," and the second part, *-lysis*, means "to break apart." Thus with water as the basic solvent, multiple water solutions may be formed as needed throughout the body to allow life-sustaining metabolic activities (e.g., energy production and tissue building) to proceed.

Transport. Water circulates throughout the body in the form of blood and various other secretions and tissue fluids. In this circulating fluid, the many nutrients, secretions, metabolites (e.g., products formed from metabolism), and other materials can be carried freely about to meet the needs of all the body cells. The cell is the functional unit of life. Its fundamental needs for oxygen and nourishment, as well as needs for all its chemical activities, must be met at all times.

Body form and structure. Water also helps to give structure and form to the body by filling in spaces within body tissues. For example, striated (from the Latin for "furrow" or "line") muscle contains more water than any other body tissue, except blood.

Body temperature. Water is necessary to help maintain a stable body temperature. As the temperature rises, sweat increases and evaporates, thus cooling the body.

Body lubricant. Water also has a lubricating effect on moving parts of the body. For example, fluid within joints (e.g., *synovial* fluid) helps to provide smooth movement.

Body Water Requirements

The body's requirement for water varies according to several factors: temperature, activity level, functional losses, metabolic needs, age, and other dietary factors.

Surrounding temperature. As the temperature rises in the surrounding environment, body water is lost as sweat in an effort to maintain body temperature. Water intake must accommodate such losses in sweat. This increasing temperature may be caused by the natural climate or the heat produced by physical work.

Activity level. Heavy work or extensive physical activity, such as in sports, increases the water requirement for two reasons: (1) more water is lost as sweat, and (2) more water is necessary for the increased metabolic demand involved in physical activity.

Functional losses. When any disease process interferes with the normal functioning of the body, water requirements are affected. For example, in gastrointestinal (GI) problems such as prolonged diarrhea, large amounts of water may be lost. In such cases, replacement of this lost water is vital to prevent dehydration.

Metabolic needs. The work of body metabolism requires water. A general rule is that about 1000 ml of water—as pure water and other water-based beverages—is necessary for every 1000 kcal in the diet. On average, beverages supply about two thirds of the body's water intake. Solid foods supply the remaining one third.

Age. Age plays an important role in determining water needs, especially in the case of an infant. An infant needs about 1500 ml of water per day. Water intake is critical for an infant because of the following: (1) an infant's body content of water is large (e.g., approximately 70% to 75% of the total body weight), and (2) a relatively large amount of this total body water is outside of the cells, and thus more easily lost.

To meet adult fluid needs, and thus be well hydrated, the average sedentary woman should consume about 2200 ml (9 cups) of liquids per day. A sedentary man should consume about 2900 ml (12 cups) of fluid per day.[1] However, very active persons require more fluid to offset losses. Dehydration presents special concerns in elderly adults. Moderate to severe dehydration is associated with delirium, urinary tract infections, respiratory infections, skin breakdown, and constipation. Research has found decreased fluid intake and dehydration positively linked with the development of coronary heart disease.[3] In addition, in a recent review of the literature, elderly individuals exhibited an overall decreased thirst sensation and reduced fluid intake when experiencing dehydration, as compared with younger adults.[4]

Other dietary factors. Certain dietary additives and medications can affect water requirements because of their natural diuretic effect. A *diuretic* is any substance that induces urination and subsequent fluid loss. Two diuretics that are common in our society are alcohol and caffeine. Several medications contain diuretics specifically for the purpose of reducing overall body fluid, as in the case of hypertension, or as a side effect. Individuals on medications promoting water loss should be monitored for dehydration and electrolyte balance.

THE HUMAN WATER BALANCE SYSTEM

Body Water: The Solvent

Amount and Distribution

In a man's body, 55% to 65% of the total body weight is water; in a woman's body, 45% to 55% is water.[1] The higher water content of men generally results from their greater muscle mass, because muscle contains a relatively large amount of water. This total body water is divided into two major categories or *compartments*, depending on its placement in the body.

Total Water Outside Cells. The total body water outside of the cells is called the *extracellular fluid* (ECF). This water collectively makes up approximately 15% to 20% of the total body weight. About one fourth of the ECF (e.g., 4% to 5% of the total body weight) is contained in the blood plasma. The remaining three fourths (e.g., 15% of the total body weight) is composed of the following: (1) water surrounding the cells and bathing the tissues; (2) water in dense tissue such as bone; and (3) water moving through the body in various tissue secretions. The water in the blood plasma includes the total fluid in the heart and all the blood vessels. The fluid surrounding the cells in the tissues is called *interstitial fluid*. This tissue circulation helps to move materials in and out of body cells to sustain life. Fluid in transit includes all the water in various body fluids and secretions, such as those of the salivary glands, thyroid gland, liver, pancreas, gallbladder, GI tract, gonads, various mucous membranes, skin, kidneys, and eye spaces.

Total Water Inside Cells. Total body water inside the cells is called the *intracellular fluid* (ICF). This water collectively amounts to about twice of that outside the cells, making up about 30% to 40% of the total body weight. This is not surprising, however, because the cell is the basic unit of life and all life-sustaining work (e.g., metabolism) is done within the cells.

The relative amounts of water in the different body water compartments are compared in Table 9-1.

---

homeostasis (Gr. *homoios,* like, unchanging; *stasis,* standing, stable) the state of relative dynamic equilibrium within the body's internal environment; a balance achieved through the operation of various interrelated physiologic mechanisms.

TABLE 9-1	Volumes of Body Fluid Compartments*		
Body fluid	Infant	Adult male	Adult female
EXTRACELLULAR FLUID			
Plasma	4	4	4
Interstitial fluid	26	15	10
INTRACELLULAR FLUID	45	38	33
TOTAL	75	57	47

From Thibodeau GA, Patton KT: *Anatomy & physiology,* ed 3, St Louis, 1996, Mosby. Art credit: Rolin Graphics.
*Percentage of body weight.

Overall Water Balance. Water enters and leaves the body by various routes, controlled by basic mechanisms such as thirst and hormones. The average adult metabolizes 2.5 to 3 L of water per day in a balance between intake and output.

Water Intake. Water enters the body in three main forms, as follows: (1) as preformed water in liquids that are drunk; (2) as preformed water in foods that are eaten; and (3) as a product of cell oxidation when nutrients are burned in the body for energy (e.g., metabolic water or "water of oxidation"). The estimated water intake of an average adult is 2600 ml/day.

The vital need for water in older adults, however, is too often overlooked. The normal thirst mechanism usually diminishes with age, so dehydration can easily occur. Many older persons suffer from dry mouth caused by severe reduction in the flow of saliva, which in turn affects their food intake. This condition may be associated with the use of certain medications, disease, or radiation therapy to the head and neck. Conscious attention to adequate fluid intake (e.g., not less than the recommended minimum of 1500 to 2000 ml daily and not dependent on normal thirst) is an important part of health maintenance and care.[5,6]

Water Output. Water leaves the body through the kidneys, skin, lungs, and feces. Of these output routes, the largest amount of water exits through the kidneys. A cer-

tain amount of water must be excreted as urine to carry out various waste products of metabolism. This is called *obligatory* water loss because it is compulsory for survival and must occur daily for health. The kidneys also may put out an additional amount of water each day, depending on body activities and needs. This additional, or *optional*, water loss varies according to the climate and physical activity. For example, athletes require a large increase in water intake, especially in hot weather. The American College of Sports Medicine recommends drinking 400 to 600 ml of fluid 2 to 3 hours before exercise, with an additional 150 to 350 ml (6 to 12 oz) of fluid at 15- to 20-minute intervals throughout the duration of exercise.[7] Some athletes hyperhydrate with glycerol because of its osmotic properties, but more research is necessary before this action can be recommended.[8] Fluid needs of athletes will be discussed further in Chapter 16. On average, the daily water output from the body totals about 2600 ml, which balances the average intake of water.

Table 9-2 summarizes the comparative intake and output of body water balance.

Solute Particles in Solution

The solutes in body water are a variety of particles in varying concentrations. Two main types of particles control water balance in the body: electrolytes and plasma protein.

TABLE 9–2	Approximate Daily Adult Intake and Output of Water			
			Output (loss) ml/day	
Form of water	Intake (replacement) ml/day	Body part	Obligatory (insensible) ml/d	Optional (according to need) ml/d
Preformed		Lungs	350	
Liquids	1200-1500	Skin		
In foods	700-1000	Diffusion	350	
Metabolism	200-300	Sweat	100	±250
(oxidation		Kidneys	900	±500
of food)		Feces	150	
TOTAL	2100-2800	TOTAL	1850	750
	(approx. 2600 ml/day)		(approx. 2600 ml/day)	

Electrolytes

Electrolytes are small, inorganic substances (e.g., either single-mineral elements or small compounds) that can dissociate or break apart in a solution and carry an electrical charge. These charged particles are called *ions*, from the Greek word meaning "wanderer." Thus these particles are free to wander throughout a solution to maintain its chemical balance. In any chemical solution, the separate particles are constantly in balance between cations and anions.

Cations. Cations are ions carrying a positive charge (e.g., sodium $[Na^+]$, potassium $[K^+]$, calcium $[Ca^{2+}]$, and magnesium $[Mg^{2+}]$).

Anions. Anions are ions carrying a negative charge (e.g., chloride $[Cl^-]$, carbonate $[CO_3^{2-}]$, phosphate $[PO_4^{3-}]$, and sulfate $[SO_4^{2-}]$).

The constant balance between the two major electrolytes—sodium $[Na^+]$ outside the cell and potassium $[K^+]$ inside the cell—maintains water balance between these two water compartments. Because of their small size, electrolytes can diffuse freely across most membranes of the body, thereby maintaining a constant balance between the intracellular and extracellular water.

The balance between cation and anion concentration maintains a state of chemical neutrality necessary for life. Electrolyte concentration in body fluids is measured in terms of *milliequivalents* (mEq). The number of electrolytes per unit of fluid in a solution is expressed as mEq/L. Table 9-3 outlines the balance between cations and anions in the intracellular and extracellular fluid compartments. The number of total anion and cation particles in each compartment is exactly balanced.

Plasma Proteins

Plasma proteins, mainly in the form of albumin and globulin, are organic compounds of large molecular size. They do not move as freely across membranes as electrolytes, which are much smaller. Thus plasma protein molecules are retained in blood vessels, controlling water movement in the body and guarding blood volume by influencing the shift of water in and out of capillaries in balance with the surrounding water. In this function, plasma proteins are called *colloids*, from the

TABLE 9–3	Balance of Cation and Anion Concentrations in Extracellular and Intracellular Fluids*	
Electrolyte	ECF (mEq/L)	ICF (mEq/L)
CATION		
Sodium (Na^+)	142	35
Potassium (K^+)	5	123
Calcium (Ca^{2+})	5	15
Magnesium (Mg^{2+})	3	2
TOTAL	155	175
ANION		
Chloride (Cl^-)	104	5
Phosphate (PO_4^{3-})	2	80
Sulfate (SO_4^{2-})	1	10
Protein	16	70
Carbonate (CO_3^{2-})	27	10
Organic acids	5	
TOTAL	155	175

ECF = Extracellular fluid; *ICF* = intracellular fluid.
*This balance maintains electroneutrality within each compartment.

Greek word *kolla*, meaning "glue," and exert **colloidal osmotic pressure (COP)** to maintain the integrity of the blood volume. Cellular proteins help guard cell water in a similar manner.

Small Organic Compounds

In addition to electrolytes and plasma protein, other small organic compounds are dissolved in body water. However, their concentration is too small to ordinarily influence shifts of water. Although in some instances, they are found in abnormally large concentrations and do influence water movement. For example, glucose is a small particle circulating in body fluids, but it can influence water loss from the body when it is in abnormally high concentrations (e.g., in uncontrolled diabetes).

Separating Membranes

Two quite different types of membranes separate and contain body water throughout the body. These membranes are the capillary membrane and the cell membrane.

Capillary Membrane

The walls of the capillaries are fairly free membranes because they are thin and porous. Therefore water molecules and small particles can move freely across them. Such small particles, having free passage across capillary walls, include electrolytes and various nutrient materials. As indicated, however, larger particles such as plasma protein molecules cannot pass through the small pores in the capillary membrane. These larger molecules remain in the capillary vessel and exert an important pressure control (e.g., COP) to keep the water circulating from capillaries and surrounding tissue cells.

Cell Membrane

Cell walls are thicker membranes specially constructed to protect and nourish the cell contents. To accomplish these tasks, cell membranes are structured almost in sandwich fashion, with outer layers and penetrating channels of protein and an inner structure of fat material. Special transport mechanisms are necessary to carry substances across cell membranes.

Forces Moving Water and Solutes across Membranes

The presence of separating membranes (e.g., the capillary membrane and the cell membrane) requires certain physical and chemical forces to control the movement of body water and particles in solution across them.

Osmosis

The term **osmosis** comes from the Greek word *osmos*, which means "a driving or pushing force, an impulse." Osmosis describes nature's fundamental impulse to balance or equalize opposing forces. In human physiology, the term *osmosis* is used to describe the process or force (e.g., "osmotic pressure") that impels water molecules to move throughout the body. When solutions of different concentrations exist on either side of semipermeable body membranes, the pressure of the crowded molecules moves them across the membrane to help equalize the solutions on both sides. Therefore osmosis can be defined as the force that moves water molecules from an area of greater concentration of water molecules (e.g., with fewer particles in solution) to an area of lesser concentration of water molecules (e.g., with more particles in solution). Osmosis distributes water molecules more evenly throughout the body (e.g., water balance) and thus provides a solvent base for materials the water must carry.

Diffusion

As osmosis applies to water molecules, diffusion applies to the particles in solution. Diffusion is the force by which these particles move outward in all directions from an area of greater concentration of particles to an area of lesser concentration of particles (discussed in Chapter 5). The relative movement of water molecules and solute particles by osmosis and diffusion effectively balance solution concentrations, and hence pressures, on both sides of the separating membrane. The two balancing forces of osmosis and diffusion are shown in Figure 9-1.

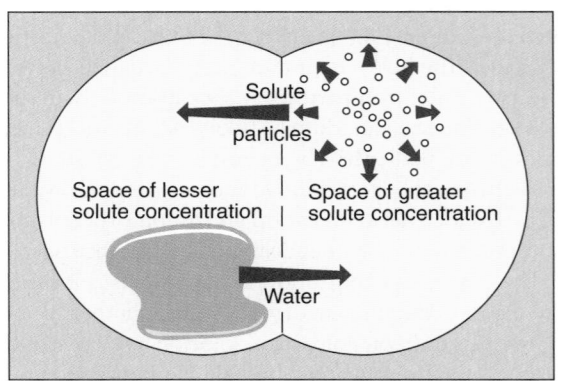

Figure 9–1   Movement of molecules, water, and solutes by osmosis and diffusion.

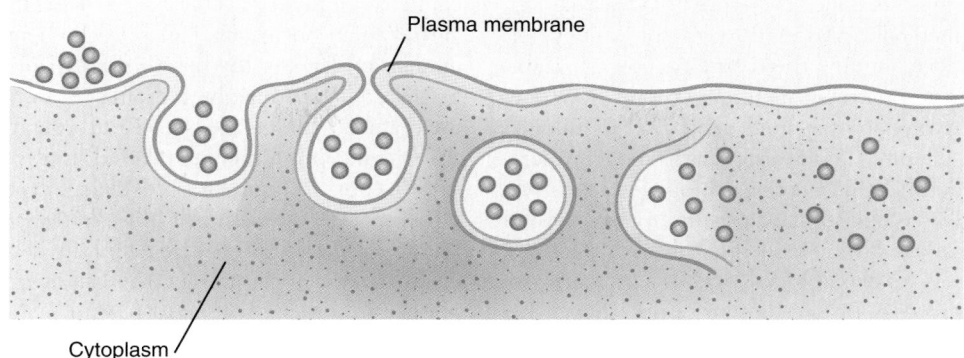

Plasma membrane

Cytoplasm

Figure 9–2   Pinocytosis, which describes engulfing of large molecules by the cell.

Filtration

Water is forced, or filtered, through the pores of membranes when the pressure outside the membrane is different. This difference in pressure results from the differences in the particle concentrations of the two solutions, causing water and small particles to move back and forth between capillaries and cells according to shifting pressures.

Active Transport

Particles in solution that are vital to body processes must move across membranes throughout the body at all times, even when the pressures are against their flow. Thus some type of energy-driven *active transport* is necessary to carry these particles "upstream" across separating membranes. Such active transport mechanisms usually require some sort of carrier partner to help "ferry" the particles across the membrane (also discussed in Chapter 5).

Pinocytosis

Sometimes larger particles, such as proteins and fats, enter absorbing cells by the process of *pinocytosis* (Figure 9-2), which means "cell drinking." In this process, larger molecules attach themselves to the thicker cell membrane and are then engulfed by the cell. In this way, they are encased in a *vacuole* (L. *vacuus*, meaning "empty"; plus ending *-ole*, meaning "small"), which is a small space or cavity formed in the protoplasm of the cell. In this small cavity, nutrient particles are carried across the cell membrane and into the cell. Once inside the cell, the vacuole opens and the cell enzymes metabolize the particles. Pinocytosis is one of the basic mechanisms by which fat is absorbed from the small intestine.

Tissue Water Circulation: The Capillary Fluid Shift Mechanism

One of the body's most important controls in maintaining overall water balance is the *capillary fluid shift mechanism*. This mechanism operates a balancing act between opposing fluid pressures to nourish the life of the cell.

Purpose

Water and other nutrients are constantly circulating through the body tissues via blood vessels. However, to nourish cells the water and nutrients must get out of the blood vessels—the capillaries—and into the cells. Water and cell metabolites, products of metabolism leaving the cell, must then get back into the capillaries to circulate throughout the body. In other words, essential water, nutrients, and oxygen must be pushed out of blood circulation into tissue circulation to distribute their goods throughout the body; then water, cell metabolites, and

colloidal osmotic pressure (COP)   fluid pressure produced by protein molecules in the plasma and cell. Because proteins are large molecules, they do not pass through the separating membranes of the capillary walls. Thus they remain in their respective compartments, exerting a constant osmotic pull that protects vital plasma and cell fluid volumes in these areas.

osmosis   (Gr. *osmos*, a thrusting) passage of a solvent, such as water, through a membrane that separates solutions of different concentrations, tending to equalize the concentration pressures of the solutions on either side of the membrane.

carbon dioxide must be pulled back into blood circulation to dispose of metabolic wastes through the kidneys or lungs. The body maintains this constant flow of water through the tissues, carrying materials to and from the cells, by means of opposing fluid pressures, as follows: (1) *hydrostatic pressure,* an intracapillary blood pressure from the contracting heart muscle pushing blood into circulation; and (2) *colloidal osmotic pressure,* pressure from the plasma proteins drawing tissue fluids back into ongoing circulation. A *filtration* process operates according to the differences in osmotic pressure on either side of the capillary membrane.

Process

When blood first enters the capillary system from the larger vessels coming from the heart—the arterioles, the greater blood pressure from the pumping heart muscle forces water and small particles (e.g., glucose) into the tissues to bathe and nourish the cells. This force of blood pressure is an example of *hydrostatic* pressure (*hydro-* meaning "water" and *-static* meaning "balance"). Plasma protein particles, however, are too large to go through the pores of capillary membranes. When the circulating tissue fluids are ready to reenter the blood capillaries, the initial blood pressure has diminished. The COP of the concentrated protein particles remaining in the capillary vessel is now the greater influence. Colloidal osmotic pressure draws water and its metabolites back into the

capillary circulation after having served the cells and carries them on to larger vessels, the venules, for blood circulation back to the heart. A small amount of normal turgor pressure from the resisting tissue of the capillary membrane remains the same and operates throughout the system. This fundamental fluid shift mechanism constantly controls water balance through its capillary-tissue circulation to nourish cells all over the body. This vital fluid flow through tissue is maintained by the balance between blood pressure and the osmotic pressure of the plasma protein particles (Figure 9-3).

Organ Systems Involved

In addition to blood circulation, the human water-balance system uses two other major organ systems to control the overall water balance of the body. The other systems involved are the GI circulation, which supports digestion and absorption of nutrients, and the renal circulation, which maintains normal blood levels of various nutrients and metabolites.

Gastrointestinal Circulation

Water from the blood plasma, containing vital electrolytes, is continually secreted into the GI tract to aid the processes of food digestion and nutrient absorption. In the latter portion of the intestine, most of the water and electrolytes are then reabsorbed into the blood to

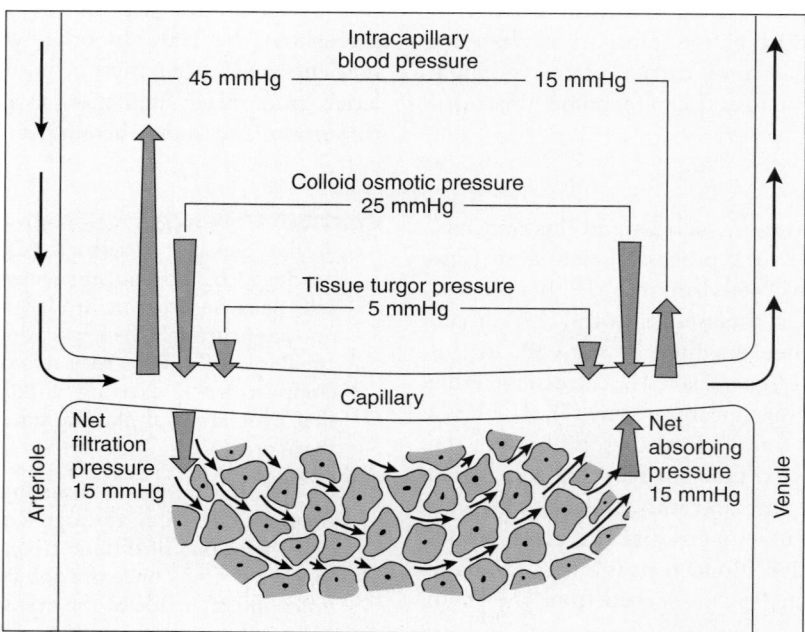

Figure 9–3   The fluid shift mechanism. Note the balance of pressures that controls the flow of fluid.

circulate over and over again. This constant movement of a large volume of water and its electrolytes among the blood, secreting cells, and GI tract is called *GI circulation*. The sheer magnitude of this vital GI circulation, as shown in Table 9-4, indicates the seriousness of fluid loss from the upper or lower portion of the GI tract. This circulation is maintained in *isotonicity* with the surrounding water outside of cells (e.g., including the blood) and carries risk for clinical imbalances, as follows.

Law of Isotonicity. The GI fluids are part of the extracellular fluid compartments, which also includes blood. All of these fluids are held in isotonicity, meaning a state of equal osmotic pressure resulting from equal concentrations of electrolytes and other solute particles. For example, when a person drinks water (e.g., plain water without any solutes or accompanying food), electrolytes and salts enter the intestine from the surrounding blood supply to equalize pressures. If a concentrated solution of food is ingested, additional water is then drawn into the intestine from the surrounding blood to dilute the intestinal contents. In each instance, water and electrolytes move among the parts of the extracellular fluid compartment to maintain solutions that are *isotonic* (e.g., have an equal concentration of particles) in the GI tract with the surrounding fluid. If an imbalance of the pressures involved goes unchecked, it will eventually draw on the intracellular fluid compartment in an effort to restore balance, creating a risk for critical cell dehydration (see the Clinical Applications box, "Principles of Oral Rehydration Therapy").

Clinical Applications. The law of isotonicity has many clinical implications. For example, what would happen if a patient undergoing gastric suctioning drank water? Or if a patient being fed by tube were given the formula too rapidly at too concentrated a dilution? In the first case,

the water would cause the stomach to produce more secretions containing electrolytes. Then the electrolytes would be lost in the suctioning. In turn the plasma, from which the electrolytes were supplied, would be gradually depleted of these electrolytes and unable to supply them to tissue cells. In the second case, the concentrated (e.g., *hypertonic*) solution given by tube would cause water to shift into the intestine to dilute the solution, thus rapidly shrinking the surrounding blood volume. This condition would then produce symptoms of shock, reflecting the body's effort to restore blood volume.

Because of the large amounts of water and electrolytes involved, upper and lower GI losses are the most common cause of clinical fluid and electrolyte problems. Such problems exist, for example, in cases of persistent vomiting or prolonged diarrhea, in which large amounts of precious water and electrolytes are lost (see the Clinical Applications box, "Adverse Effects of Progressive Dehydration"). The large concentration of electrolytes involved in GI circulation is shown in Table 9-5 on p. 166.

Renal Circulation

The kidneys maintain the appropriate levels of all constituents of blood by filtering it and then selectively reabsorbing water and needed materials to be carried throughout the body. Through this continual "laundering" of the blood by the millions of nephrons in the kidneys, water balance and the proper solution of blood are maintained. When disease occurs in the kidneys and this filtration process does not operate normally, water imbalances occur (see Chapter 21).

Hormonal Controls

Two basic hormonal controls operate in the kidneys to help maintain constant body water balance, as discussed in the following sections.

Antidiuretic Hormone Mechanism. Antidiuretic hormone (ADH), also called *vasopressin,* is produced by the pituitary gland. Antidiuretic hormone is a water-conserving mechanism that works on the kidneys' nephrons to induce reabsorption of water. In any stressful situation with threatened or real loss of body water, this hormone is released to conserve vital body water.

Aldosterone Mechanism. The hormone *aldosterone* is produced by the adrenal glands, which are located on top of each kidney, in response to a reduced renal filtration rate or decreased sodium level. Aldosterone triggers the kidneys' nephrons to reabsorb sodium. Therefore it is primarily a sodium-conserving mechanism but it also exerts a secondary control over water reabsorption (because

TABLE 9–4	Approximate Total Volume of Digestive Secretions*	
Secretion	**Volume (ml)**
Saliva	1500
Gastric	2500
Bile	500
Pancreatic	700
Intestinal	3000
TOTAL	8200

*Produced in 24 hours by an adult of average size.

PRINCIPLES OF ORAL REHYDRATION THERAPY

The principles of electrolyte absorption dictate rehydration methods for children suffering from diarrhea. Although diarrhea usually is considered a trivial problem in developed countries, it is responsible for the deaths of one fourth to one half of all children under 4 years of age worldwide. Although 90% of the mortality from diarrhea is associated with fluid loss, the mere provision of water alone can be dangerous.

Intravenous (IV) therapy, developed by Darrow in the 1940s, provided sodium chloride—a base—and potassium in water and proved very successful. Unfortunately, however, IV therapy is not readily available to those who need it most. A large number of isolated, poor rural families, in both developed and developing countries do not have access to health care facilities because of their lack of trans-portation or money. Fortunately, though, the World Health Organization (WHO) has developed an oral rehydration therapy (ORT) that is much less expensive and is being used in the United States, as well as in undeveloped countries. If safe drinking water is available, the ORT solution can easily be mixed at home under the guidance of a public health worker and administered by a family member (see figure). The ingredients are 1 L safe water, 3.5 g table salt (e.g., sodium chloride), 2.5 g baking soda (e.g., sodium bicarbonate), 1.5 g potassium chloride, and 20 g glucose. This ORT is based upon principles of sodium absorption in the small intestine.

Transport of Metabolic Compounds

A number of metabolic compounds—principally glucose but also certain amino acids, dipeptides, and disaccharides—depend on sodium to cross the intestinal wall.

Additive Effects

The rate at which sodium is absorbed depends on the presence of substances such as glucose or other protein metabolic products. The more substances present, the better the absorption of sodium.

Water Absorption

The rate of water absorption is enhanced as sodium absorption improves. Thus a solution of sodium and potassium salts plus glucose can be given orally.

In addition to the ORT, infants and older children with acute diarrhea also should be fed so that the added burden of malnutrition from fasting is avoided. Such fasting practices were based on the former belief that recovery is more effective if the bowel is allowed to rest and heal. To the contrary, children should be fed their regular age diets (e.g., breast milk, formula, or solid foods), allowed to determine the amount of food they need, and given extra food as the diarrhea subsides to recover nutritional deficits. Food choices should be guided by individual tolerances. Use of the old so-called BRAT diet (e.g., bananas, rice, applesauce, and tea or toast) is not recommended because it does not include typical foods consumed by infants and small children and only compounds the energy-nutrient decline.

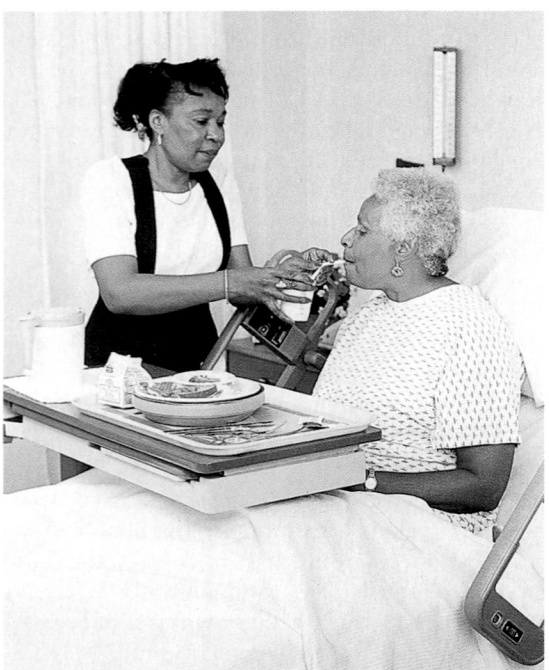

Patient receiving oral rehydration. (From Christensen BL, Kockrow EO: *Foundations of nursing*, ed 4, St Louis, 2004, Mosby.)

CLINICAL APPLICATIONS

ADVERSE EFFECTS OF PROGRESSIVE DEHYDRATION

As little as a 3% loss of total body weight from dehydration can result in impaired physical performance. Physical performance is relative to the individual in question. A runner who is progressively losing body water in the form of sweat, without appropriate fluid replacements, will likely suffer from decreased speed or endurance. However, an elderly person who has also lost 3% of his or her body weight may suffer dramatically more complicated side effects. For example, if this elderly individual has lost body fluids from excessive vomiting or diarrhea, or simply from lack of water intake, the physical performance at hand may be navigating a flight of stairs. Impairment in "physical performance" for this individual may lead to a fall. That, in turn, could present a series of medical complications.

Individuals suffering from fever, diarrhea, and vomiting can lose body weight in the form of fluids very rapidly. Likewise, the risk of dehydration increases in hot, humid environments and at altitudes greater than 8200 feet.* The figure shown in this box demonstrates progressive complications associated with total body water loss. Note that the thirst response is not present until approximately 0.5% total body weight loss. Such is the reason why relying solely on thirst for an indication of fluid needs is not always the most sensitive indicator. By the time you are thirsty, you have already lost precious body water.

*Manore MM, Barr SI, Butterfield GE: American College of Sports Medicine, American Dietetic Association, Dietitians of Canada Joint position statement: nutrition and athletic performance, *Med Sci Sports Exerc* 32(12):2130, 2000.

PERCENTAGE OF BODY WEIGHT LOST

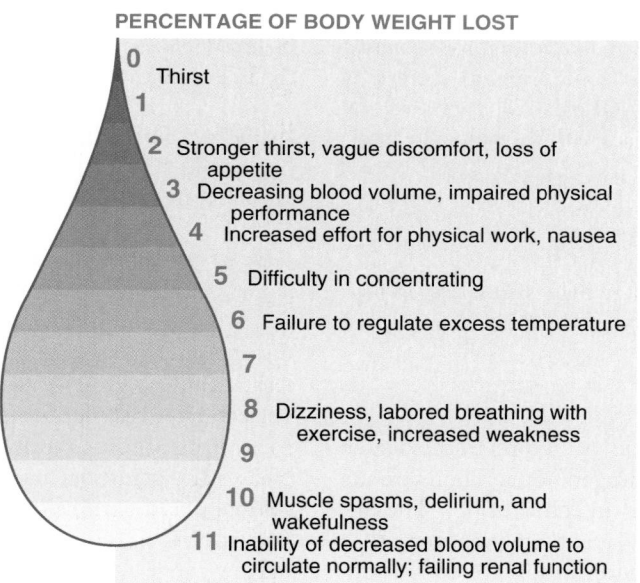

0 Thirst
1
2 Stronger thirst, vague discomfort, loss of appetite
3 Decreasing blood volume, impaired physical performance
4 Increased effort for physical work, nausea
5 Difficulty in concentrating
6 Failure to regulate excess temperature
7
8 Dizziness, labored breathing with exercise, increased weakness
9
10 Muscle spasms, delirium, and wakefulness
11 Inability of decreased blood volume to circulate normally; failing renal function

Adverse effects of dehydration. (From Mahan LK, Escott-Stump S: *Krause's food, nutrition, & diet therapy,* ed 11, Philadelphia, 2004, Saunders.)

TABLE 9–5	Approximate Concentration of Certain Electrolytes in Digestive Fluids*			
Secretion	Na⁺	K⁺	Cl⁻	HCO
Saliva	10	25	10	15
Gastric	40	10	145	0
Pancreatic	140	5	40	110
Jejunal	135	5	110	30
Bile	140	10	110	40

*In mEq/L.

water follows sodium). Both ADH and aldosterone may be activated by stressful situations, such as body injury or surgery.

HUMAN ACID-BASE BALANCE SYSTEM

The optimal degree of acidity or alkalinity must be maintained in various body water solutions and secretions to support human life. This vital balance is achieved by solutions of both acids and bases with the help of a buffer system.

Acids and Bases

The concept of acids and bases relates to *hydrogen* ions both in its measurement symbol, pH, and its definition of the terms *acid* and *base*.

Measurement

A substance is *more or less* acid, according to the degree of its concentration of hydrogen ions. Therefore its degree of acidity is expressed in terms of pH. The abbreviation *pH* is derived from a mathematical term that refers to the **p**ower of the **h**ydrogen ion concentration. A pH of 7 is the neutral point between an acid and a base. Because pH is in effect a negative mathematical factor, the higher the hydrogen ion concentration (e.g., more acid), the lower the pH number; similarly, the lower the hydrogen ion concentration (e.g., less acid), the higher the pH number. Because a pH of 7 is the neutral point, substances with a pH *below* 7 are *acid*. Substances with a pH *above* 7 are *alkaline*.

Acids. An acid is defined as a compound that has more hydrogen ions; enough to releases extra hydrogen ions when in solution.

Bases. A base is a compound that has fewer hydrogen ions. Thus in solution it takes up hydrogen ions, effectively reducing the solution's acidity.

Acid-Base Buffer System

The body deals with degrees of acidity by maintaining buffer systems to handle an excess of either acid or base. A buffer system is a mixture of acidic and alkaline components, an acid and a base partner, that together protect a solution from wide variations in its pH, even when strong bases or acids are added to it. For example, if a strong acid is added to a buffered solution, the base partner reacts with the acid to form a weaker acid. If a strong base is added to the solution, the acid partner combines with the intruder to form a weaker base.

Main Buffer System

The human body contains many buffer systems because only a relatively narrow range of pH is compatible with life. The carbonic acid (H_2CO_3)/base bicarbonate ($NaHCO_3$) buffer system, however, is the body's main buffer system for the following three reasons.

Available Materials. The raw materials for producing carbonic acid (H_2CO_3) are readily available. Water (H_2O) and carbon dioxide (CO_2) are always accessible.

Ease of Adjustment. The lungs and kidneys can easily adjust to changes in acidity, quickly returning body fluids to normal pH level. Hyperventilation (increasing the depth and rate of breathing) increases the release of CO_2, an acid, thus combating acidosis. Conversely, hypoventilation (slowing down the depth and pace of breathing) retains CO_2, which ultimately increases the acidity of blood to alleviate alkalosis. The normal pH of extracellular fluid is 7.4, with a range of 7.35 to 7.45. The pH must be maintained within this narrow range to sustain life. Lungs and kidneys work closely together to prevent metabolic or respiratory acidosis or alkalosis.

Base-to-Acid Ratio. The bicarbonate buffer system is able to maintain this essential degree of acidity in the body fluids because bicarbonate (basic) is about 20 times more abundant than carbonic acid. This *20:1 ratio* is maintained even though the absolute amounts of the two partners may fluctuate during adjustment periods. Whether or not added base or acid enters the system, as long as the 20:1 ratio is maintained, over time the extracellular fluid (ECF) pH is held constant.

SUMMARY

The human body is approximately 50% to 60% water. The primary functions of body water are to give form and structure to the body tissue, provide the water environment necessary for cell work, and control body temperature. Body water is distributed in two collective body water compartments: intracellular and extracellular. The water inside cells is the larger portion, accounting for about 35% of the total body weight. The water outside cells consists of the fluid in spaces between cells (e.g., interstitial and lymph fluid), blood plasma, secretions in transit (e.g., GI circulation), and smaller amount of fluid in cartilage and bone.

The overall water balance of the body is maintained by fluid intake and output. Two types of solute particles control the distribution of body water, as follows: (1) electrolytes, mainly charged mineral elements; and (2) plasma protein, mainly albumin. These solute particles influence the movement of water across cell or capillary membranes, allowing tissue circulation to nourish cells.

The acid-base buffer system, which is mainly controlled by the lungs and kidneys, uses electrolytes and hydrogen ions to maintain a normal ECF pH of about 7.4. This pH level is necessary to sustain cell life.

CRITICAL THINKING QUESTIONS

1. Why is total body water considered a "unified whole?" What does the term *body compartment* mean? How does this term apply to body water balance?
2. Define the term *homeostasis*. Give examples of how this state is maintained in the body.
3. Describe five factors that influence water requirements. List and describe five functions of body water.
4. Apply your knowledge of the capillary fluid shift mechanism to account for the gross body edema seen in children suffering from protein energy malnutrition.

CHAPTER CHALLENGE QUESTIONS

Matching

Match the terms provided with the corresponding items listed in the following.

DEFINITIONS

1. Chief electrolyte guarding the water outside of cells
2. An ion carrying a negative electrical charge
3. Sodium-conserving mechanism or control agent
4. Simple passage of water molecules through a membrane separating solutions of different concentrations from the side of lower concentration of solute particles to that of higher concentration of particles, thus tending to equalize the solutions

TERMS

a. Osmosis
b. Solutes
c. Diffusion
d. Cation
e. Interstitial fluid
f. Homeostasis

Continued

5. A substance (element or compound) that, in solution, conducts an electrical current and is dissociated into cations and anions

6. Particles in solution, such as electrolytes and protein

7. State of dynamic equilibrium maintained by an organism among all its parts and controlled by many finely balanced mechanisms

8. Chief electrolyte guarding the water inside of cells

9. Major plasma protein that guards and maintains the blood volume

10. Fluid located inside the cell walls

11. An ion carrying a positive electrical charge

12. The body's method of maintaining tissue water circulation via opposing fluid pressures

13. Force exerted by a contained fluid (e.g., blood pressure)

14. Movement of particles throughout a solution and across membranes outward from the area of denser concentration of particles to all surrounding spaces

15. A type of fluid outside of cells

16. Movement of particles in solution across cell membranes and against normal osmotic pressures, involving a carrier and energy for the work

g. Anion

h. Potassium

i. Albumin

j. Hydrostatic pressure

k. Sodium

l. Electrolyte

m. Active transport

n. Aldosterone

o. Capillary fluid shift mechanism

p. Intracellular fluid

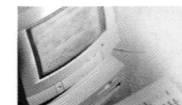

Please refer to the Students' Resource section of this text's Evolve web site for "Suggestions for Additional Study."

REFERENCES

1. Kleiner SM: Water: an essential but overlooked nutrient, *J Am Diet Assoc* 99(2):200, 1999.
2. Cannon WB: *The wisdom of the body*, New York, 1932, W.W. Norton and Co.
3. Chan J and others: Water, other fluids, and fatal coronary heart disease: the Adventist health study, *Am J Epidemiol* 155(9):827, 2002.
4. Kenny WL, Chiu P: Influence of age on thirst and fluid intake, *Med Sci Sports Exerc* 33(9):1524, 2001.
5. Harrell R and others: How geriatricians identify elder abuse and neglect, *Am Med Sci* 323(1):34, 2002.
6. Wakefield B and others: Monitoring hydration status in elderly veterans, *West J Nurs Res* 24(2):132, 2002.
7. Manore MM, Barr SI, Butterfield GE: American College of Sports Medicine, American Dietetic Association, Dietitians of Canada Joint position statement: nutrition and athletic performance, *Med Sci Sports Exerc* 32(12):2130, 2000.
8. Wagner DR: Hyperhydrating with glycerol: implications for athletic performance, *J Am Diet Assoc* 99(2):207, 1999.

FURTHER READING AND RESOURCES

- American College of Sports Medicine: *www.acsm.org*
- Sports, Cardiovascular, and Wellness Nutritionists (SCAN): *www.nutrifit.org*

    The preceding organizations provide up-to-date recommendations for water and electrolyte balance, specifically for athletes, in addition to a plethora of other health information.

- Speedy DB and others: Exercise-associated hyponatremia: a review, *Emerg Med* 13(1):17, 2001.
- Gardner JW: Death by water intoxication, *Mil Med* 167(5):432, 2002.

    Both articles explore the dangers associated with excess water intake. As with most things, there is always a limit at which point too much is not always a good thing, water included.
    Although dehydration is a much more common problem, overhydration can be very dangerous. Thus distinguishing the signs and symptoms of the two hydration extremes is critical.

- Robinson JR: Water, the indispensable nutrient, *Nutr Today* 5(1):16, 1970.

    This classic but still current article by a New Zealand physician who is a world authority clearly describes the processes involved in body water balance. This article is filled with excellent charts and diagrams to illustrate key principles.

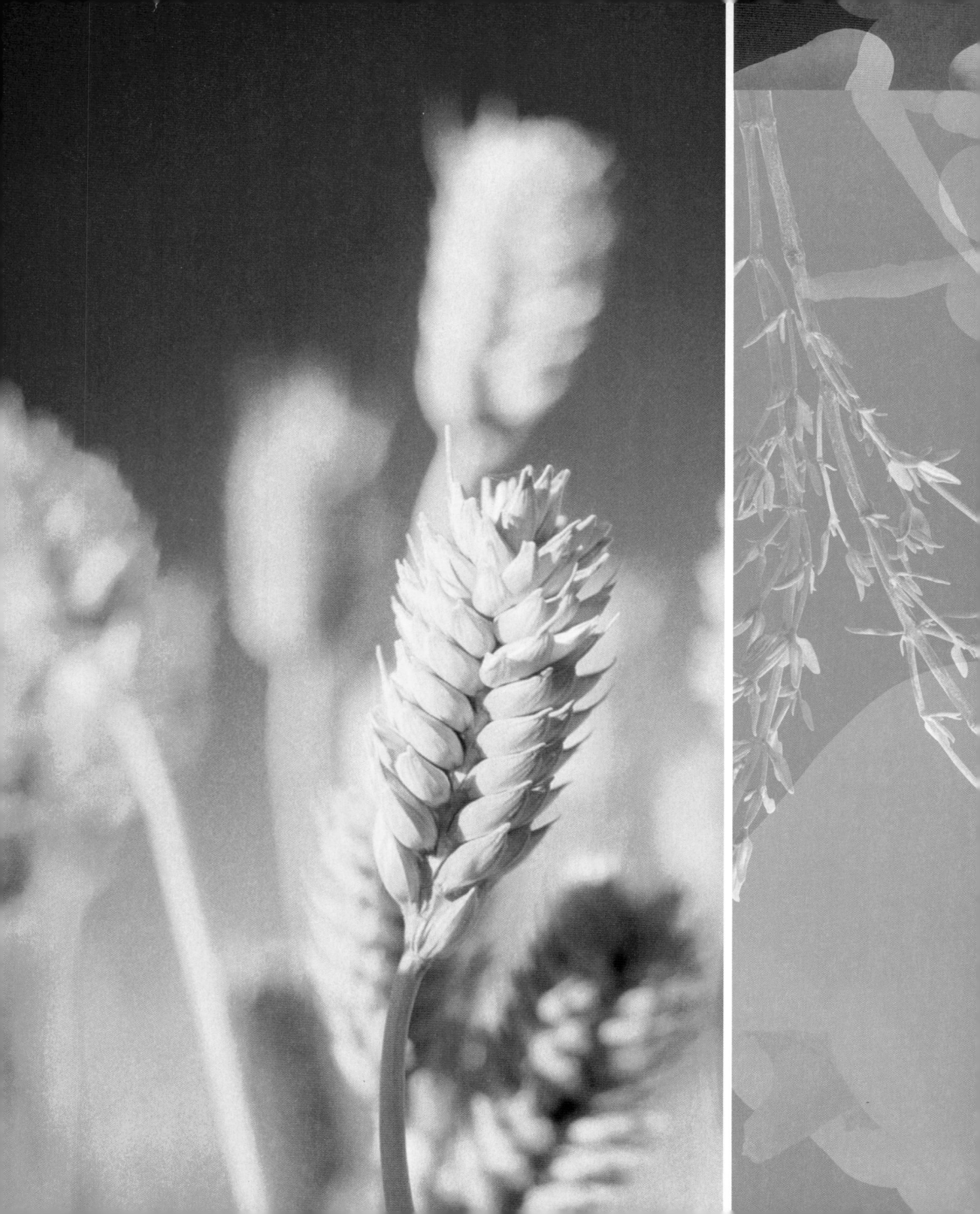

Nutrition throughout the Life Cycle

CHAPTER 10

Nutrition during Pregnancy and Lactation

KEY CONCEPTS

- The mother's food habits and nutritional status before conception, as well as during pregnancy, influence the outcome of the pregnancy.

- Pregnancy is a prime example of physiologic synergism in which the mother, fetus, and placenta collaborate to sustain and nurture new life.

- Through the food a pregnant woman eats, she gives her unborn child the nourishment required to begin and sustain fetal growth and development.

- Through her diet, a breastfeeding mother continues to provide all of her nursing baby's nutritional needs.

Healthy body tissues depend directly on essential nutrients in food. This is especially true during pregnancy because a whole new body is being formed. The tremendous growth of a baby from the moment of conception to the time of birth depends entirely on nourishment from the mother. The complex process of rapid human growth demands increased amounts of nutrients from the mother.

This chapter looks at the beginning of life and how the infant's fetal development and mother's supporting tissues directly relate to the mother's diet. It explores the nutritional needs of pregnancy and the lactation period that follows, and recognizes the vital role each plays in producing a healthy infant.

NUTRITIONAL DEMANDS OF PREGNANCY

Not many years ago, traditional practices and diet during pregnancy were highly restrictive in nature, built upon assumptions and folklore of the past and having little or no basis in scientific fact. Early obstetricians even developed the notion that semistarvation of the mother during pregnancy was a blessing in disguise because it produced a small, lightweight baby who was easy to deliver. To this end, they used a diet restricted in kcalories, protein, water, and salt for pregnant women.

Developments in both nutritional and medical science have refuted these ideas and laid a sound base for positive nutrition in current maternal care. However, old dogma dies hard. Shreds of old beliefs are sometimes still evidenced, but it is now known that it is very important to both the mother's and child's health that a pregnant woman eat a well-balanced diet with increased amounts of all the essential nutrients. In fact, women who have always eaten a well-balanced diet are in a good state of nutrition at conception, even before they know they are pregnant. Such women have a better chance of having a healthy baby and remaining in good health than women who have been undernourished.

The 9 months between the time of conception and the birth of a fully formed baby is a marvelous period of rapid growth and intricate functional development. All of these tremendous activities require increased energy and nutrient support to produce a positive, healthy outcome. General guidelines for these increases are provided in the comprehensive Dietary Reference Intakes (DRI) standards by the National Academy of Sciences, Committee on Nutritional Status During Pregnancy and Lactation.[1-5]

The DRI guidelines are based on general needs for healthy populations. Some women (e.g., those who are poorly nourished when becoming pregnant or those carrying additional risks) demand more nutritional support. Within this chapter, the basic nutritional needs for positive support of a normal pregnancy are reviewed, with emphasis on critical energy and protein requirements, as well as key vitamin and mineral needs. In each case, there are reasons for the increased demand, general amount of increase, and food sources to supply it. The following section underscores the importance of sufficient weight gain and the problems facing high-risk mothers and infants.

Energy Needs

Reasons for Increased Need

During pregnancy, the mother needs more energy, in the form of kcalories, for two important reasons: (1) to supply the increased fuel demanded by the enlarged metabolic workload of both mother and fetus, and (2) to spare protein for the added tissue-building requirements. For these reasons, the mother must have more nutrient-dense food.

Amount of Energy Increase

The national standard recommends an increase of about 300 kcal per day (e.g., for a total of about 2200 to 2500 kcal for most women) starting with the second trimester of pregnancy, which is approximately a 15% to 20% increase over the energy need of nonpregnant women. Active, large, or nutritionally deficient women—who may require as much as 2700 to 3000 kcal per day—require even more energy. The emphasis always should be on ample kcalories to secure nutrient and energy needs of a rapidly growing fetus. Sufficient weight gain is vital to a successful pregnancy. Increased complex carbohydrates and protein in the diet are the preferred sources of energy, especially during late pregnancy and lactation.

Protein Needs

Reasons for Increased Need

Protein serves as the building blocks for the tremendous growth of body tissues during pregnancy.

Rapid Growth of the Fetus. The mere increase in size of the fetus from one cell to millions of cells in a 3.2-kg (7-lb) infant in only 9 months indicates the relatively large amount of protein required for such rapid growth.

Development of the Placenta. The placenta is the fetus's lifeline to the mother. The mature placenta requires sufficient protein for its complete development as a vital and unique organ to sustain, support, and nourish the fetus during growth.

---

hemoglobin   (Gr. *haima,* blood; L. *globus,* globe) a conjugated protein in red blood cells that is composed of a compact, rounded mass of polypeptide chains forming globin, the protein portion, and attached to an iron-containing red pigment called heme. Carries oxygen in the blood to cells.

plasma protein   any of a number of protein substances carried in the circulating blood. A major one is *albumin,* which maintains the fluid volume of the blood through its colloidal osmotic pressure.

Growth of Maternal Tissues. To support the pregnancy and lactation to follow, increased development of uterine and breast tissue is required.

Increased Maternal Blood Volume. The mother's blood volume increases 20% to 50% during pregnancy. More circulating blood is necessary to nourish the child and support most of the increased metabolic workload. However, with extra blood volume comes a need for more synthesis of blood components, especially hemoglobin and plasma protein, which are proteins vital to the pregnancy. An increase in hemoglobin helps supply oxygen to the growing number of cells. Meanwhile, plasma protein (albumin) production increases relative to the growing blood supply to regulate circulation between capillaries and cells. Albumin in the blood provides the osmotic force constantly needed to pull the tissue fluids back into circulation after they have bathed and nourished the cells. Thus albumin prevents an abnormal accumulation of water in the tissues, beyond the normal edema of pregnancy.

Amniotic Fluid. Amniotic fluid, which contains various proteins, surrounds the fetus during growth and guards it against shock or injury.

Storage Reserves. Increased storage reserves of tissue are needed in the mother's body to prepare for the large amount of energy required during labor, delivery, immediate postpartum period, and lactation.

Amount of Increase

Protein intake should increase 25 g per day during pregnancy, on top of nonpregnancy needs.[6] This increase is approximately 50% more than the average adult requirement. However, a large number of high-risk or active pregnant women require even more protein.

Food Sources

The only *complete* protein foods of high biologic value are milk, egg, cheese, soy products, and meat (e.g., beef, poultry, fish, pork). Certain other *incomplete* proteins from plant sources such as legumes and grains contribute additional secondary amounts. Protein-rich foods also contribute other nutrients, such as calcium, iron, and B vitamins. The amount of food from each food group that supplies the needed protein is indicated in the daily core food plan given in Table 10-1.

Key Mineral and Vitamin Needs

Increases in most all minerals and vitamins are needed during pregnancy to meet the greater structural and metabolic requirements. These increases are indicated in the DRI tables inside this book's front cover. Several of

TABLE 10–1	Daily Food Guide for Women				
			Recommended minimum servings		
			Nonpregnant		
Food group	Single serving		11-24 years	25+ years	Pregnant/ lactating
PROTEIN FOODS Provide protein, iron, zinc, and B vitamins for growth of muscles, bone, blood, and nerves. Vegetable protein provides fiber to prevent constipation	*Animal protein:* 1 oz cooked chicken or turkey 1 oz cooked lean beef, lamb, or pork 1 oz or ¼ cup fish or other seafood 1 egg 2 fish sticks or hot dogs 2 slices luncheon meat		4.5	4.5	6
	Vegetable protein: ½ cup cooked dry beans, lentils, or split peas 3 oz tofu 1 oz or ¼ cup peanuts or pumpkin or sunflower seeds 1½ oz or ⅓ cup other nuts 2 Tbsp peanut butter		0.5	0.5	1

Modified from California Department of Health Services, Maternal and Child Health: *Nutrition during pregnancy and postpartum period: a manual for health care professionals,* Sacramento, CA, 1990, CDHS.

Continued.

TABLE 10-1   Daily Food Guide for Women—*cont'd*

Food group	Single serving	Recommended minimum servings Nonpregnant 11-24 years	Recommended minimum servings Nonpregnant 25+ years	Pregnant/ lactating
MILK PRODUCTS Provide protein and calcium to build strong bones and teeth, and healthy nerves and muscles; and promote normal blood clotting	8 oz milk 8 oz yogurt 1 cup milk shake 1½ cups cream soup (made with milk) 1½ oz or ⅓ cup grated cheese (e.g., cheddar, Monterey Jack, mozzarella, or Swiss) 1½ to 2 slices presliced American cheese 4 Tbsp Parmesan cheese 2 cups cottage cheese 1 cup pudding 1 cup custard or flan 1½ cups ice milk, ice cream, or frozen yogurt	3	2	3
BREADS, CEREALS, GRAINS Provide carbohydrates and B vitamins for energy and healthy nerves; also provide iron for healthy blood. Whole grains provide fiber to prevent constipation	1 slice bread 1 dinner roll ½ bun or bagel ½ English muffin or pita 1 small tortilla ¾ cup dry cereal ½ cup granola ½ cup cooked cereal ½ cup rice ½ cup noodles or spaghetti ¼ cup wheat germ 1 4-inch pancake or waffle 1 small muffin 8 medium crackers 4 graham cracker squares 3 cups popcorn	7‡	6‡	7‡
VITAMIN C–RICH FRUITS AND VEGETABLES Provide vitamin C to prevent infection and promote healing and iron absorption; also provide fiber to prevent constipation	6 oz orange, grapefruit, or fruit juice enriched with vitamin C 6 oz tomato juice or vegetable juice cocktail 1 orange, kiwi, or mango ½ grapefruit or cantaloupe ½ cup papaya 2 tangerines ½ cup strawberries	1	1	1

‡Four servings of whole grain products daily.

TABLE 10-1	Daily Food Guide for Women—*cont'd*			
		Recommended minimum servings		
		Nonpregnant		Pregnant/ lactating
Food group	Single serving	11-24 years	25+ years	
VITAMIN C–RICH FRUITS AND VEGETABLES—cont'd	½ cup cooked or 1 cup raw cabbage			
	½ cup broccoli, Brussels sprouts, or cauliflower			
	½ cup snow peas, sweet peppers, or tomato puree			
	2 tomatoes			
VITAMIN A–RICH FRUITS AND VEGETABLES				
Provide beta-carotene and vitamin A to prevent infection and promote wound healing and night vision; also provide fiber to prevent constipation	6 oz apricot nectar or vegetable juice cocktail	1	1	1
	3 raw or ¼ cup dried apricots, ¼ cantaloupe, or ¼ mango			
	1 small or ½ cup sliced carrots			
	2 tomatoes			
	½ cup cooked or 1 cup raw spinach			
	½ cup cooked greens (beet, chard, collards, dandelion, kale, mustard)			
	½ cup pumpkin, sweet potato, winter squash, or yams			
OTHER FRUITS AND VEGETABLES				
Provide carbohydrates for energy and fiber to prevent constipation	6 oz fruit juice (if not listed above)	3	3	3
	1 medium or ½ cup sliced fruit (apple, banana, peach, pear)			
	½ cup berries (other than strawberries)			
	½ cup cherries or grapes			
	½ cup pineapple			
	½ cup watermelon			
	¼ cup dried fruit			
	½ cup sliced vegetable (asparagus, beets, green beans, celery, corn, eggplant, mushrooms, onion, peas, potato, summer squash, zucchini)			
	½ artichoke			
	1 cup lettuce			
UNSATURATED FATS				
Provide vitamin E to protect tissue	⅛ medium avocado	3	3	3
	1 tsp margarine			
	1 tsp mayonnaise			
	1 tsp vegetable oil			
	2 tsp salad dressing (mayonnaise-based)			
	1 Tbsp salad dressing (oil-based)			

Note: The Daily Food Guide for Women may not provide all the kilocalories each woman requires. The best way to increase intake is to include more than the minimum servings recommended.

these essential substances have key roles in pregnancy and require special attention.

Minerals

Calcium. A good supply of calcium, along with phosphorus, magnesium, and vitamin D, is essential for fetal development of bones and teeth, as well as the mother's own body needs. Calcium is also necessary for proper clotting of blood. A diet that includes 3 to 4 cups of vitamin A– and D–fortified milk daily, plus dairy or dairy-substitute products (e.g., cheese, yogurt) and generous amounts of green vegetables and enriched/whole grains usually supplies enough calcium. During pregnancy, physiologic changes occur in the mother's absorption capacity to help meet the needs of some nutrients, specifically calcium, zinc, and selenium.[7] The body's enhanced capability to absorb and retain these nutrients from the diet during pregnancy helps the mother meet her nutrient needs and those of the growing fetus. Calcium supplements may be needed in cases of poor maternal stores or pregnancies involving more than one fetus. Because food sources of the two major minerals (calcium and phosphorus) are almost the same, a diet sufficient in calcium also provides enough phosphorus.

Iron and Iodine. Particular attention is given to iron and iodine intake during pregnancy. Iron is essential for the increased hemoglobin synthesis required for the greater maternal blood volume, as well as for the baby's necessary prenatal storage of iron. Because iron occurs in small amounts in food sources, and much of this intake is not in a readily absorbable form, the maternal diet alone can rarely meet needs. The current standards recommend a daily iron intake of 27 mg/day, which is significantly more than a woman's normal need of 18 mg/day.[4] Consuming foods high in vitamin C along with dietary sources of iron enhances the body's ability to absorb and utilize low bioavailable sources of iron. Because the increased pregnancy requirement is difficult to meet with the iron content of a typical U.S. diet or the iron stores of some women, daily iron supplements often are recommended.[5] Adequate iodine intake is essential for producing more thyroxine, which is the thyroid hormone needed in greater amounts to control the increased basal metabolic rate during pregnancy. This increased iodine need is easily ensured by the use of iodized salt.

Vitamins

Increased attention to most all vitamins is needed to support a healthy pregnancy. Vitamins A and C are needed in higher amounts during pregnancy because they are

both important elements in tissue growth. The B vitamins are needed in increased amounts because of their vital roles as coenzyme factors in energy production and protein metabolism. Vitamin B_{12} supplements are mandatory at DRI levels of 2.6 μg/day during pregnancy and 2.8 μg/day during lactation.[2]

Folate. Folate builds mature red blood cells throughout pregnancy and is also particularly needed during the early periconceptional period (e.g., from about 2 months before conception to week 6 of gestation) to ensure healthy embryonic tissue development and prevent malformation of the neural tube.[8,9] This tissue forms during the critical period from 17 to 30 days gestation and grows into the mature infant's spinal column and its network of nerves. A neural tube defect is any malformation of the embryonic brain or spinal cord. **Spina bifida** and **anencephaly** are the two most common forms of neural tube defects. Spina bifida, which affects about 2000 newborns in the United States each year, occurs when the lower end of the neural tube fails to close.[10] As a result, the spinal cord and backbones do not develop properly. The severity of spina bifida varies with the size and location of the opening in the spine with disability ranging from mild to severe, with limited movement and function.

Anencephaly occurs when the upper end of the neural tube fails to close. In these cases, the brain fails to develop or is absent entirely. Pregnancies affected by anencephaly often end in miscarriages or death soon after delivery.

The current DRIs recommend a daily folate intake of 600 μg during pregnancy and 400 μg/day for nonpregnant females during child-bearing years. Women who are unable to achieve such dietary recommendations via foods fortified with folate need a folate supplement. All enriched flour and grain products, as well as fortified cereals, contain a well-absorbed form of dietary folic acid. Other natural sources of folate include: liver, dark green leafy vegetables, legumes (e.g., pinto beans, black beans, and kidney beans), soybeans, wheat germ, orange juice, asparagus, and broccoli.

Vitamin D. Increased vitamin D needs, to ensure absorption and utilization of calcium and phosphorus for fetal bone growth, can be met by the mother's intake of 3 to 4 cups of fortified milk in her daily food plan. Fortified milk contains 10 μg (400 IU) of cholecalciferol (vitamin D) per quart, which is twice the AI amount. The mother's exposure to sunlight increases endogenous synthesis of vitamin D as well.

Weight Gain during Pregnancy

Amount and Quality

The mother's optimal weight gain during pregnancy, sufficient to support and nurture her and the fetus, is essential. Weight gain should not be viewed negatively. It is a positive reflection of good nutritional status and contributes to a successful course and outcome of pregnancy and should be assessed individually. The average weight gained is about 11 to 13 kg (24 to 28 lbs), as indicated in Table 10-2. A report of the National Academy of Sciences, *Nutrition During Pregnancy*, recommends setting weight gain goals together with the pregnant woman according to her prepregnancy nutritional status and body mass index (BMI), as follows:[5]

- Underweight women (BMI <19.8): 28 to 40 lbs
- Normal-weight women (BMI 19.8 to 26): 25 to 35 lbs
- Overweight women (BMI 26 to 29): 15 to 25 lbs
- Obese women (BMI >29): ~15 lbs
- Teenage girls: 35 to 40 lbs (upper end of the recommended range)
- Women carrying twins: 35 to 45 lbs (total target)

The important consideration in each case is not only the quantity of weight gain but also the *quality* of the gain and the foods consumed to bring it about. There is a definite connection between high-risk, low-birth-weight babies and inadequate maternal weight gain during the pregnancy.[5] Severe caloric restriction during pregnancy is potentially harmful to the developing fetus and the mother. Such a restricted diet cannot supply all the energy and nutrients essential to the growth process. Thus weight reduction *never* should be undertaken during pregnancy. To the contrary, adequate weight gain, relative to prepregnancy weight recommendations, should be supported with the use of a nourishing, well-balanced diet.

Rate of Weight Gain

Approximately 1 to 2 kg (2 to 4 lbs) is the average amount of weight gain during the first trimester (e.g., first 3 months) of pregnancy. Thereafter, approximately 0.5 kg (1 lb) a week during the remainder of the pregnancy is usual, although some women should gain more. Only unusual patterns of gain (e.g., a sudden sharp increase in weight after the 20th week of pregnancy, possibly indicating excessive and abnormal water retention) must be watched. On the other hand, an insufficient or low maternal weight gain in the

TABLE 10–2	Approximate Weight Gain during a Normal Pregnancy
Product	**Weight**
Fetus	3400 g (7.5 lbs)
Placenta	450 g (1 lb)
Amniotic fluid	900 g (2 lbs)
Uterus (weight increase)	1100 g (2.5 lbs)
Breast tissue (weight increase)	1400 g (3 lbs)
Blood volume (weight increase)	1800 g (4 lbs; 1500 ml)
Maternal stores	1800-3600 g (4-8 lbs)
TOTAL	11,000-13,000 g (11-13 kg; 24-28 lbs)

second or third trimester increases the risk for intrauterine growth retardation.[11] Increased energy demand is normal during late pregnancy and prepares for full infant growth needs and the mother's approaching delivery and lactation. As always, carbohydrates, selected from enriched or whole grain breads and cereals, fruits, vegetables, and legumes, are the preferred energy sources.

Role of Sodium

Just as with restriction of kcalories, routine restriction of sodium during pregnancy is physiologically unsound. Maintenance of the increased volume of maternal blood, which is normal during pregnancy to support the increased metabolic work, requires adequate amounts of sodium and protein. A moderate amount (e.g., approximately 2 to 3 g/day) of dietary sodium is needed and can be achieved through the general use of salt in cooking and seasoning. Extra use of table salt, or excessive consumption of salty processed foods, is

---

spina bifida   (L. *spina,* spine; *bifidus,* cleft into two parts or branches) congenital defects in the embryonic fetal closing of the neural tube to form a portion of the lower spine, leaving the spine unclosed and the spinal cord open in various degrees of exposure and damage.

anencephaly   (Gr. *an,* not; *enkephalos,* the brain) congenital absence of the brain resulting from the incomplete closure of the upper end of the neural tube.

not necessary. The typical American diet already contains 3 to 6 g/day, predominantly supplied from processed foods.

Daily Food Plan

General Plan

Ideally, some form of a food plan is developed for the pregnant woman on an individual basis to meet her increased nutritional needs. Such a core plan (see Table 10-1) can serve as a guideline, with additional amounts of foods used as needed to meet caloric needs. This core food plan is built upon basic foods available in American markets and designed to supply necessary nutrient increases. Energy needs increase as the pregnancy progresses, and the recommended increment of 300 kcal/day applies to the second and third trimesters. However, adolescent, underweight, or malnourished women need special attention to increased energy needs from the outset of the pregnancy.

Alternative Food Patterns

The core food plan provided here might be only a starting point for women with alternate food patterns. Such food patterns exist among women from different ethnic backgrounds, belief systems, and lifestyles, making individual diet counseling important. *Specific nutrients*, not necessarily specific foods, are required for successful pregnancies and may be found in a variety of foods. Wise health care workers encourage pregnant women to use foods that serve both their personal and nutritional needs, whatever such foods may be. Many resources have been developed to serve as guides for a variety of alternative food patterns (e.g., ethnic and vegetarian). If the mother's vegetarian pattern includes dairy products and eggs (lacto-ovo), there is no problem in achieving a sound diet to meet pregnancy needs by increasing the use of animal proteins. Strict vegans can meet dietary protein needs through the use of soy foods (e.g., tofu, soy milk, soy yogurt, and soy beans) and complementary proteins (see Chapter 4).

Specific counseling on avoidance of alcohol, caffeine, tobacco, and drugs during pregnancy is also important. Information about the direct effects of poor nutrition on the fetus—especially as related to brain development, learning problems, and developmental delays—helps to motivate many pregnant women to choose a well-selected diet of optimal nutritional value. Fetal alcohol syndrome, a series of mental and physical abnormalities suffered by infants of mothers who abused alcohol during pregnancy, is one of the major causes of mental retardation in the United States.

Basic Principles

Whatever the food pattern, two important principles govern the prenatal diet, as follow: (1) pregnant women should eat a sufficient *quantity* of food, and (2) pregnant women should eat *regular meals and snacks*, avoiding any habit of fasting or skipping meals, especially breakfast.

GENERAL CONCERNS

Functional Gastrointestinal Problems

Nausea and Vomiting

"Morning sickness" in early pregnancy (which actually has nothing to with the morning and can happen at any time throughout the day), is usually mild, only occurring briefly during the first trimester. It is caused by hormonal adaptations in the first weeks and may be increased by stress or anxieties about the pregnancy itself. The following simple treatment usually helps relieve symptoms: small frequent meals and snacks that are fairly dry and consist mostly of easily digested energy foods (e.g., carbohydrates) with liquids between—not with—meals. If this sickness becomes severe and prolonged, a condition called *hyperemesis gravidarum*, medical treatment is required.

Constipation

Although usually a minor complaint, constipation may occur in the latter part of pregnancy as a result of the increasing pressure of the enlarging uterus and the muscle-relaxing effect of placental hormones on the gastrointestinal tract, reducing normal peristalsis. Helpful remedies include adequate exercise, increased fluid intake, and high-fiber foods such as whole grains, vegetables, dried fruits (especially prunes and figs), and other fruits and juices. Pregnant women should avoid artificial laxatives.

Hemorrhoids

Hemorrhoids (e.g., enlarged veins in the anus, often protruding through the anal sphincter) are a fairly common complaint during the latter part of pregnancy. This vein enlargement usually is caused by the increased weight of the baby and the downward pressure it produces. Hemorrhoids may cause considerable discomfort, burning, and itching and may even rupture and bleed under the pressure of a bowel movement, causing the mother more anxiety. Hemorrhoids usually are controlled by the dietary suggestions given for constipation. Sufficient rest during the latter part of the day also may help relieve some of the downward pressure of the uterus on the lower intestine.

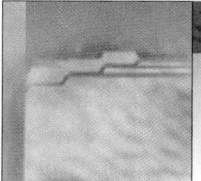

CLINICAL APPLICATIONS

NUTRITIONAL RISK FACTORS IN PREGNANCY

Risk Factors at the Onset of Pregnancy

- Age: 18 years or younger; 35 years or older
- Frequent pregnancies: three or more during a 2-year period
- Poor obstetric history or poor fetal performance
- Poverty
- Bizarre or trendy food habits
- Abuse of nicotine, alcohol, or drugs
- Therapeutic diet required for a chronic disorder
- Weight: <85% or >120% of standard weight

Risk Factors during Pregnancy

- Low hemoglobin or hematocrit: Hgb <12.0 g; Hct <34.0 mg/dl
- Inadequate weight gain: Any weight loss or weight gain of <1 kg (2 lbs) per month after the first trimester
- Excessive weight gain: >1 kg (2 lbs) per week after the first trimester

Heartburn

Pregnant women sometimes voice the related complaints of heartburn or a "full" feeling. These discomforts occur especially after meals and are caused by the pressure of the enlarging uterus crowding the stomach. Gastric reflux of food (e.g., now a liquid food mass mixed with stomach acid) may occur in the lower esophagus, causing irritation and a burning sensation. This common complaint has nothing to do with heart action but is called heartburn because of the close proximity of the lower esophagus to the heart. The full feeling comes from general gastric pressure, lack of normal space in the area, a large meal, or gas formation. Dividing the day's food intake into a series of small meals and avoiding large meals at any time usually helps relieve these complaints. Comfort sometimes is improved by wearing loose-fitting clothing.

Effects of Iron Supplements

An iron supplement usually is given during pregnancy to meet the increased iron needs. Effects of added iron include gray or black stools and sometimes nausea, constipation, or diarrhea. To help avoid food-related effects, iron supplements should be taken 1 hour before or 2 hours after a meal with a liquid such as water or orange juice, not milk or tea. Iron absorption in the body is increased with foods high in vitamin C (e.g., orange juice, tomato juice, strawberries, cantaloupe, and broccoli) and decreased with milk, other dairy foods, eggs, tea, coffee, whole grain bread, and cereal. Individuals taking iron supplements also should be educated on good food sources of zinc. High iron intake, from supplements, can reduce the body's ability

to absorb zinc and may result in suboptimal zinc status. Good sources of zinc include crab meat, beef, turkey, and fortified cereals.

High-Risk Mothers and Infants

Identifying Risk Factors

Pregnancy-related deaths claim 300 to 500 women in the United States each year. And, according to the Centers for Disease Control and Prevention (CDC), an additional 500 to 800 deaths are most likely pregnancy related. Furthermore, it is estimated that up to one half of these pregnancy-related deaths could be prevented.[12] Identifying risk factors and addressing them early are critical in promoting a healthy pregnancy. Such risk factors are listed in the Clinical Applications box, "Nutritional Risk Factors in Pregnancy."

To avoid the compounding results of poor nutrition during pregnancy, mothers at risk for complications should be identified as soon as possible. These nutrition-related factors are based on clinical evidence of inadequate nutrition. Do not wait for clinical symptoms of poor nutrition to appear. The best approach is to identify poor food patterns and prevent nutritional problems from developing. Three types of dietary patterns that do not support optimal maternal and fetal nutrition are as

fetal alcohol syndrome combination of physical and mental birth defects in infants born to mothers who abused alcohol during pregnancy.

follows: (1) insufficient food intake, (2) poor food selection, and (3) poor food distribution throughout the day.

Teenage Pregnancy

According to the CDC, the United States has the highest teenage pregnancy rate of all developed countries. An estimated 1 million teenagers become pregnant each year, with about one third of these pregnancies ending in abortion and 95% of them unintended.[13] Not only is pregnancy at this early age physically and emotionally difficult for the teen, it is also a substantial financial burden. The CDC estimates that the public cost from teenage childbearing totaled $120 billion between 1985 and 1990.[14] From a nutritional standpoint, special care must be given to support adequate growth of both mother and fetus. The current DRIs distinguish specific vitamin and mineral needs for pregnant females less than 18 years old. See the Cultural Considerations box, "Pregnant Teenagers," for more information on health and nutrition for adolescent mothers.

Planning Personal Care

Every pregnant woman needs personalized care and support during pregnancy. However, women with risk factors such as those listed here have special counseling needs. In each case, one must work with the mother in a sensitive and supportive manner to help her develop a healthy food plan that is both practical and nourishing. Dangerous practices, such as fad dieting, extreme macrobiotic diets, or pica, should be identified. *Pica* is the name given to a craving for and consumption of nonfood items (e.g., chalk, laundry starch, or clay), a practice sometimes seen in pregnant or malnourished individuals.[15,16]

Recognizing Special Counseling Needs

In addition to avoiding dangerous practices, several special needs require sensitive counseling—including those related to age and parity (e.g., number of pregnancies and time in between), detrimental lifestyle habits, and socioeconomic problems.

Age and Parity. Pregnancies at either age extreme of the reproductive cycle carry special risks. Adolescent pregnancy adds many social and nutritional risks as its social upheaval and physical demands are imposed on an immature, teenage girl (see the Cultural Considerations box, "Pregnant Teenagers"). Sensitive counseling must involve both information and emotional support with good prenatal care throughout. On the other hand, pregnant women who are more than 35 years of age and having their first child also require special attention.

These women may be more at risk for high blood pressure (e.g., either preexisting or pregnancy-induced) and need guidance about the rate of weight gain and use of dietary sodium. In addition, women with a high parity rate (e.g., who have had several pregnancies within a limited number of years) may benefit from family planning guidance because they enter each successive pregnancy at a higher risk, drained of nutrition resources and usually facing the increasing physical and economic pressures of child care. Such counseling may include discussions of acceptable means of contraception and nutrition information and support.

Social Habits: Alcohol, Cigarettes, and Drugs. These three personal lifestyle habits can cause fetal damage and are contraindicated during pregnancy. Extensive, habitual alcohol use leads to the well-documented *fetal alcohol syndrome* (FAS), which has become a leading cause of mental retardation and other birth defects.[17] Cigarette smoking, or exposure to environmental tobacco smoke during pregnancy causes placental abnormalities and fetal damage, including prematurity and low birth weight, largely resulting from impaired oxygen transport[18,19] (see the Clinical Applications box, "Who Will Have the Low-Birth-Weight Baby?").

Drug use, medicinal or recreational, poses many problems for both mother and fetus, especially the use of illegal drugs. Self-medication with over-the-counter drugs also may present adverse effects. Drugs cross the placenta and enter the baby's circulation, thus creating a potential addiction in the unborn child. Dangers come not only from the drug or contaminated needles, but also from the impurities contained in street drugs.

Vitamin abuse from megadosing with basic nutrients such as vitamin A during pregnancy also may bring fetal damage. Drugs made from vitamin A compounds (e.g., retinoids such as tretinoin [Accutane], prescribed for severe acne) have caused spontaneous abortion of malformed fetuses by women who conceived during such acne treatment. Thus the use of these drugs without contraception is contraindicated.

Caffeine. Caffeine is widely used and can cross the placenta and enter fetal circulation. Average adult consumption of caffeine is 4 mg/kg body weight per day, with pregnant women consuming much less, 1 mg/kg per day. Caffeine stays in the blood stream significantly longer in pregnant women during the third trimester than other adults (average half-life of 10 to 20 hours versus 2 to 6 hours).[20] Studies have found conflicting results over the years in regard to the effects of caffeine on outcome of pregnancies, primarily because the majority of females who

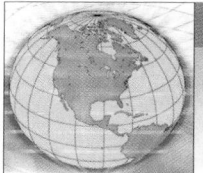

CULTURAL CONSIDERATIONS

PREGNANT TEENAGERS

Few situations are as life-changing for a single teenage girl and her family as an unintended pregnancy. Depending on how she and her family, as well as her partner, deal with the situation, there may be lifelong consequences not only for them but also for the broader community. Adolescent pregnancy rates have historically been higher for African Americans than for Caucasians in the United States, but rates are gradually declining in all ethnic groups.* Birth rates for teenagers ages 15 to 19 are highest in the southern states.

Pregnant teenagers are at high risk for pregnancy complications and poor outcome with increased rates of low birth weight and infant mortality. The following two problems contribute to these complications: (1) the physiologic demands of the pregnancy compromise the teenager's needs for her own unfinished growth and development; and (2) the psychosocial influences of low income; inadequate diet; and the teenage peer culture's experimentation with alcohol, smoking, and other drugs. Little or no access to appropriate prenatal care also may significantly contribute to a lack of nutritional support for the pregnancy. Early nutrition intervention is essential and can change the course of events and the pregnancy outcome, but is not an easy task. Changes from the inconsistent, often poor food pattern of teenagers are difficult to achieve, and their care is challenging. Experienced, sensitive health workers in teen clinics emphasize the need for supportive individual and group nutrition counseling. The following suggestions may help to secure a positive and healthy environment for the teen.

Know Each Client Personally

All nutrition services must be tailored to the unique needs and characteristics of each pregnant teenager. Many have lower educational levels and even limited reading skills to which educational material must be adapted. Low-income teens lack the financial resources to maintain an adequate diet, and those living at home may have little control over the food available to them. Personal stress over the pregnancy is paramount and nutrition concerns often are not a priority. Skipping meals and snacking are common; even dieting is frequent.

Seek Ways to Motivate Clients

Schedule appointments on days that clients are coming in to pick up their Women, Infants, and Children (WIC) food packages. Invite the teen's mother and friends to accompany her to group counseling sessions so they can support the recommendations that are made. Make each recommendation concrete and reasonable. Avoid scare tactics.

Make Appropriate Assessments

Use simple, concrete forms for evaluating dietary intake. This traditional model can be used, with increased amounts indicated for pregnancy, as both an educational and assessment tool.

Make Practical Interventions

Plan short, enjoyable, active learning sessions. Use positive reinforcement liberally. Provide specific suggestions for carrying out changes at home. Review progress in follow-up sessions. Always maintain a positive, supportive atmosphere.

Support the Teenager's Responsibility

Help the teenager learn to be responsible. In the final analysis, pregnant teenagers must take on responsibility, often for the first time, for their own nourishment and the nourishment of others. Helping them in a supportive manner to understand and carry out this responsibility, which ultimately only they can do, is a primary objective of nutrition counseling. Nutrition consultants must be skillful in establishing the kind of rapport and relationship where these responsibilities can develop and grow.

*Martin JA and others: *Births: final data for 2000,* National Vital Statistics Reports 50(5), Hyattsville, MD, 2002, National Center for Health Statistics, Centers for Disease Control and Prevention, US Department of Health and Human Services.

---

consume excess caffeine also smoke and use alcohol, both of which are known **teratogens.** Upon extensive review of the reproductive and developmental risks associated with caffeine consumption, researchers have concluded that when used in extreme excess, caffeine may result in injury to the fetus.[20] Such injuries include low birth weight,

teratogen   (Gr. *teratos,* monster; *gennan,* to produce) drug or substance causing birth defect.

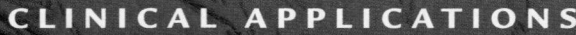

CLINICAL APPLICATIONS

WHO WILL HAVE THE LOW-BIRTH-WEIGHT BABY?

The number of babies weighing less than 2500 g (5 lbs) at birth is still problematic. Perinatal dietitians are aware of the dietary factors, especially poor weight gain during pregnancy, that contribute to this problem. The prevalence of the turn-of-the-century adage to "grow the baby to fit the pelvis" continues to influence some physicians, nurses, and expectant mothers to limit prenatal weight gain to 9 kg (20 lbs) or less to avoid obstetric problems at delivery. This practice is harmful and is refuted by current evidence that a weight gain of 25 to 35 lbs for average-weight women and 28 to 40 lbs for underweight women correlates with a healthy birth weight of more than 2500 g (5 lbs).

The obsession with weight control during pregnancy can lead to harmful restrictions of vital energy and nutrients. Weight reduction should never be attempted during pregnancy. Such diets are extremely dangerous to the fetus. Even the common habit of skipping breakfast, especially late in pregnancy, may impair intellectual development by quickly producing a state of pseudostarvation. Increased ketoacidosis from fat breakdown can cause neurologic damage to the fetus.

Nondietary Factors Influencing the Trend toward More Low-Birth-Weight Babies

- Rise in number of older first-time mothers (e.g., more than 35 years of age)

- Number of teenage pregnancies
- Previous induced abortions
- Technologic advances in neonatal care, which keeps premature infants alive longer
- Race: nonCaucasians have higher rates of low birth weight infants than Caucasians.

Reducing the Risk of Low-Birth-Weight Infants

- Explain the reasons for gaining sufficient weight as recommended.
- Help mothers who smoke or drink to stop using cigarettes or alcohol.
- Monitor excessive weight gain and sodium intake in older first-time mothers, who are at risk for prenatal essential hypertension and obesity.
- Explore the eating habits of teenagers, working with the mother and father, if possible, to include nutrient-dense foods in meals and snacks.
- Stay informed of federal, state, and local supplemental food programs (e.g., the Women, Infants, and Children (WIC) program [see Chapter 13]) that ensure an adequate intake of nutrients in low-income women.
- Encourage regular eating patterns throughout pregnancy.

---

smaller head circumference, and congenital malformations. However, toxic doses are not likely to occur under normal conditions. The overall conclusion is that moderate amounts of caffeine (5 to 6 mg/kg per day) throughout the day do not have negative effects on reproduction or fetal health. This is not true when caffeine is used in conjunction with other teratogens, such as alcohol and cigarette smoke. One cup of coffee contains approximately 100 mg of caffeine and caffeinated soft drinks range between 10 and 50 mg/12 oz serving. Thus a 60-kg (132-lb) woman should limit caffeine intake to about 300 mg/day, or 3 cups of coffee. Mothers should be aware that caffeine stays in the blood stream of a newborn much longer than an adult, with a half-life of 4 days.

Socioeconomic Problems. Special counseling often is needed for women and young girls living in low-income situations. Poverty especially puts pregnant women in

grave danger because they need resources for financial assistance and food supplements. Dietitians and social workers on the health care team can provide special counseling and referrals. Community resources include programs such as the special Supplemental Food Program for Women, Infants, and Children (WIC), which has helped many low-income mothers have healthy babies (Figure 10-1).

Complications of Pregnancy

Anemia

Iron deficiency anemia is common during pregnancy. About 10% of the women in large U.S. prenatal clinics have low hemoglobin and hematocrit levels (measurements of iron status). Anemia is more prevalent among poor women, many of whom live on marginal diets barely adequate for subsistence, but is by no means

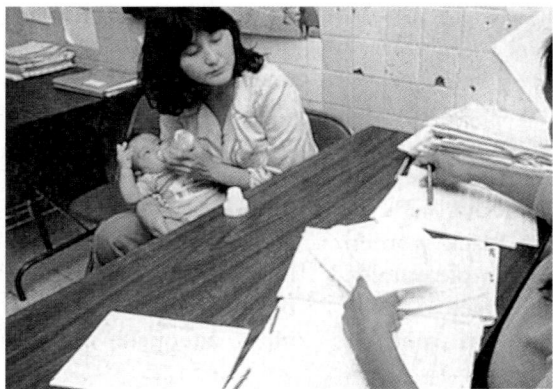

Figure 10–1 This mother is a participant in the U.S. government's Women, Infants, and Children (WIC) program. (Credit: U.S. Department of Agriculture, Washington, DC.)

restricted to lower economic groups. A deficiency of iron or folate in the mother's diet can cause nutritional anemia. Dietary intake must be determined and supplements used as indicated. During the second and third trimesters of pregnancy, a low-dose iron supplement of 30 mg of ferrous iron daily can provide the amount of extra iron needed.

Neural Tube Defect

The DRI recommendation of 400 μg/day of folate for women who are capable of becoming pregnant is increased to 600 μg/day during pregnancy.[2] This is especially important when individual dietary adequacy is doubtful or there is a genetic high risk for neural tube defect in the family. Women who do not frequently eat fruit, juices, whole grain or fortified cereals, green leafy vegetables, or take folate supplements are likely to have below optimal folate intake.

Intrauterine Growth Failure

Many studies have shown what good sense and experience clearly indicate: children born with intrauterine growth retardation (IUGR) have multiple survival and growth problems.[11] Many factors may contribute to IUGR, but low prepregnancy weight, inadequate weight gain during pregnancy, and smoking are strong factors. In adolescents, low weight gain by 20 weeks into the pregnancy has been shown to carry a twofold risk.[11]

Pregnancy-Induced Hypertension

Formerly called *toxemia*, pregnancy-induced hypertension (PIH) is especially related to diets low in protein, kcalories, calcium, and salt. Such malnutrition affects the liver and its metabolic activities. PIH classically has been associated with poverty and most often found in women subsisting on inadequate diets with little or no prenatal care, although it can happen to anyone. Symptoms of PIH, which occur in late pregnancy, are elevated blood pressure, abnormal and excessive water retention, albumin in the urine, and—in severe cases—convulsions, a condition called *eclampsia*. Specific treatment varies according to individual symptoms and needs, but in any case optimal nutrition is important and medical attention is required.

Gestational Diabetes

During pregnancy, glucose (sugar) in the urine (e.g., *glycosuria*) is not uncommon. In susceptible women, it results from the increased metabolic workload during pregnancy and the increased volume of blood with its load of metabolites, including glucose. Some of this extra glucose then "spills over" into the urine. For this reason, prenatal clinics routinely screen each pregnant woman and provide careful follow-up for those who show glycosuria or have blood glucose levels above 110 mg (6.1 mmol/L) within 2 hours after a meal. Particular attention is given to women at higher risk for developing *gestational* (e.g., pregnancy-induced) diabetes, including those age 30 and over who are overweight (BMI >26) and have a history of any of the following predisposing factors:

- Family history of diabetes or ethnicity associated with high incidence of diabetes
- Previously unexplained stillbirths
- Large babies weighing 4 kg (9 lbs) or more
- Habitual abortions
- Birth of babies with multiple congenital defects
- Obesity

Gestational diabetes occurs more frequently among African Americans, Hispanic/Latino Americans, and Native Americans. Twenty to fifty percent of these women subsequently develop type 2 diabetes. Therefore it is important to identify them and provide close follow-up testing and treatment with special diet and insulin, as needed. These women are at higher risk for fetal damage, prematurity, or delivery of a very large baby, a complicating condition called *macrosomia* that is associated with survival dangers. Current studies of pregnant women also have shown elevated blood lipid levels where there had been no previous history.[21]

Preexisting Disease

Preexisting clinical conditions, such as hypertension, diabetes, phenylketonuria (PKU), or other diseases, complicate pregnancy. In each case, a woman's pregnancy is managed, usually by a team of specialists, according to the principles of care related to pregnancy and the particular disease involved.

LACTATION

Trends

The number of mothers choosing to breastfeed has been on the rise since the 1960s, with 83% of North American mothers currently initiating breastfeeding.[22] The following factors have contributed to this choice: (1) more mothers are informed about the benefits of breastfeeding; (2) practitioners recognize that human milk can meet unique infant needs, as shown in Table 10-3; (3) maternity wards and alternative birth centers are being modified to support successful lactation; and (4) community support is more available, even in some workplaces.[23-25] Breastfeeding initiation and continuation is higher among Caucasian, well educated, married, older, nonsmoking women of a higher socioeconomic status. The American Academy of Pediatrics recommends breastfeeding for at least the first

	Human milk			
TABLE 10–3 Nutritional Composition of Human Milk versus Cow's Milk*				
Nutrient	**Colostrum (1-5 days)**	**Transitional (6-10 days)**	**Mature**	**Mature cow's milk**
Kcalories	67	72	74	70
Protein (g)	2.7	1.6	0.9	3.3
Carbohydrate (g)†	5.3	6.6	7.2	4.8
Fat (g)	2.9	3.6	4.5	3.7
Lactalbumin (g)		0.8	0.3	0.4
FAT-SOLUBLE VITAMINS				
A (IU)	296	283	240	303
D (IU)			5	4
E (mg)	0.8	1.32	0.2	0.06
K (μg)			2.3	
WATER-SOLUBLE VITAMINS				
Thiamin (mg)	0.015	0.006	0.014	0.042
Riboflavin (mg)	0.029	0.033	0.035	0.16
Niacin (mg)	0.075	0.15	0.20	0.085
Pantothenic acid (mg)	0.183	0.288	0.18	0.30
Vitamin C (mg)	4.4	5.4	4.3	0.9
Folate (μg)	0.05	0.02	0.52	0.23
MINERALS				
Calcium (mg)	31	34	30	125
Phosphorus (mg)	14	17	15	96
Iron (mg)	0.09	0.04	0.03	0.04
Zinc (mg)	0.5	0.4	0.16	0.37
Magnesium (mg)	4.2	3.5	4	13
Iodine (μg)	6		6	11
ELECTROLYTES				
Sodium (mg)	5	19	17	76
Potassium (mg)	74	63	53	152
Chloride (mg)	58	30	37	108

Modified from Mitchell MK: *Nutrition Across the Life Span,* ed 2, Philadelphia, 2003, Saunders. Based on data from *Geigy scientific tables,* ed 7, Basel, Switzerland, Ciba-Geigy, Ltd.
*Per 100 ml.
†Lactose.

12 months postpartum.[26] However, only 29% of American mothers continue any form of breastfeeding until 6 months postpartum.[22] Most women report to having discontinued breastfeeding because of perceived difficulties, such as sore nipples, infant spitting up, engorged breast, and so on. With proper instruction and a caring environment, many of these difficulties can be overcome. Almost all women who choose to breastfeed their infants can do so. Well-nourished mothers who breastfeed exclusively provide adequate nutrition, with solid foods usually added to the baby's diet at about 6 months of age.

Physiologic Process of Lactation

The female breasts, or mammary glands, are highly specialized secretory organs (Figure 10-2). Throughout pregnancy the mammary glands are preparing for lactation. The mammary glands are capable of extracting certain nutrients from the maternal blood, in addition to synthesizing other compounds. The combined effort results in the nutrient-complete breast milk. Upon delivery, milk production and secretion is stimulated by the two hormones *prolactin* and *oxytocin*.

Stimulation of the nipple from infant suckling sends nerve signals to the brain of the mother (Figure 10-3). This nerve signal then causes the release of prolactin and oxytocin. Prolactin is the "milk-producing" hormone and oxytocin is the hormone responsible for the *let-down*

reflex. Let-down is the process of the milk moving from the upper milk-producing cells down to the nipple for infant suckling. Milk production is a supply-and-demand procedure. The mammary glands are stimulated to produce milk each time the infant feeds. Therefore the more the mother breastfeeds, the more milk she produces, thus always meeting the infant's needs.

Nutritional Needs

The basic diet followed during pregnancy, as well as the prenatal nutrient supplement used, can be continued through the lactation period. In general, attention to three areas of lactation support is needed.

Diet

Energy and Nutrients. Milk production requires energy (e.g., about 800 kcal/day) for both the process and the product. Thus more food is needed to meet energy demands. Because some of this energy need may be met by extra fat stored during pregnancy, the national standard is 500 kcal/day throughout lactation more than a woman's normal need of about 2200 kcal, for a total of

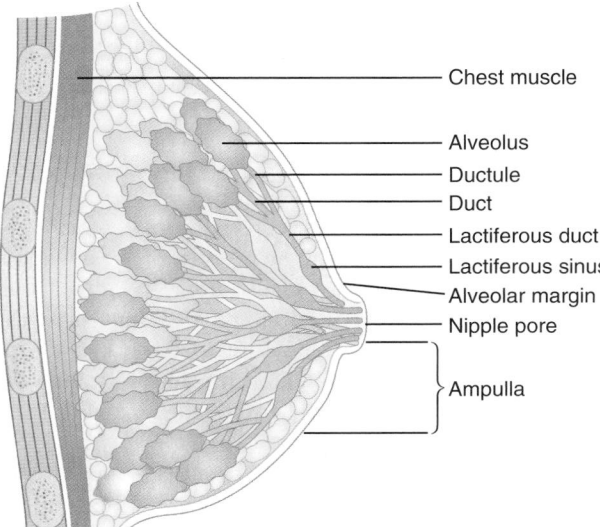

Figure 10–2 Anatomy of the breast. (From Mahan LK, Escott-Stump S: *Krause's food, nutrition, & diet therapy,* ed 11, Philadelphia, 2004, Saunders.)

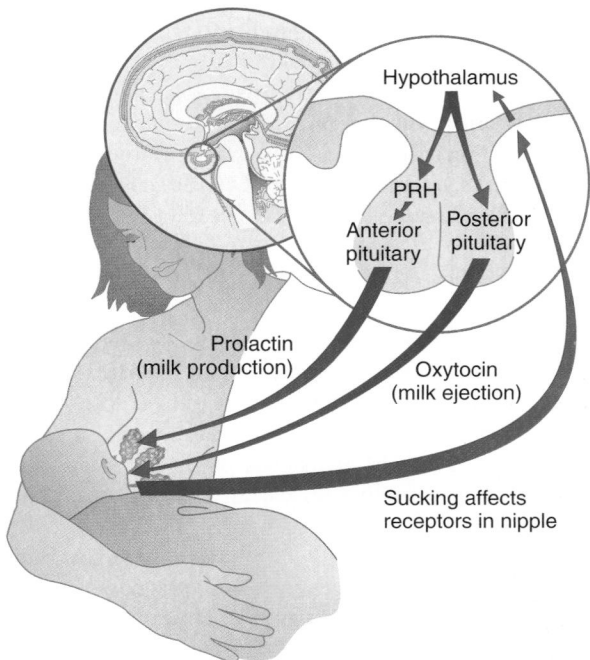

Figure 10–3 Physiology of milk production and the let-down reflex. *PRH,* Prolactin-releasing hormone. (From Mahan LK, Escott-Stump S: *Krause's food, nutrition, & diet therapy,* ed 11, Philadelphia, 2004, Saunders.)

2700 kcal/day. The need for protein during lactation is 25 g/day more than a woman's average need of 46 g/day (0.8 g/kg body weight per day), for a total of 71 g/day (or 1.1 g/kg body weight per day).[6] These lactation energy and nutrient increases are shown in the DRI standards (see this book's inside front cover). The core food plan for meeting these lactation needs (see Table 10-1) includes three servings of milk products (or vegetarian substitute); six to eight servings of protein foods; one to two servings of dark-green or yellow vegetables; one to two servings of vitamin C-rich fruits and vegetables; two to three servings of other vegetables, fruits, and juices; seven to eight servings of whole grain or enriched breads and cereals; and moderate amounts of butter or fortified margarine.

Fluids. Because milk is a fluid, breastfeeding mothers need ample fluids for adequate milk production (~3 L/day). Water and other sources of fluid such as juices, milk, and soup contribute to the fluid necessary to produce milk. Beverages containing alcohol and caffeine should be limited or avoided because they are secreted to some extent in the mother's milk.

Rest and Relaxation

In addition to the increased diet and adequate fluids, breastfeeding mothers require rest, moderate exercise, and relaxation. Because the production and let-down reflexes of breastfeeding are hormonally controlled, some negative environmental and psychological factors can adversely affect the amount of milk a mother can produce. Such factors are called "prolactin-inhibitors" and include stress, fatigue, prolonged bed rest, complications, or irregular breastfeeding. The nurse and dietitian often help by counseling mothers about their new family situations and may help them to develop plans to meet their personal needs.

Advantages of Breastfeeding

There are many physiologic and practical advantages to breastfeeding, including the following:[26,27]

1. *Fewer infections* because the mother transfers certain antibodies or immune properties in human milk to her nursing infant
2. *Fewer allergies and intolerances*, especially in allergy-prone infants (cow's milk contains a number of potentially allergy-causing proteins that human milk does not have); mothers with a family history of allergies are encouraged to breastfeed
3. *Ease of digestion* because human milk forms a softer curd in the gastrointestinal tract that is easier for the infant to digest
4. *Convenience and economy* because the mother is freed from the time and expense involved in buying and preparing formula, and her breast milk is always ready, sterile, and provides a cost-effective method of feeding
5. *Improved cognitive development* in childhood, with a positive relationship between the duration of breastfeeding and IQ in the child

The American Dietetic Association and American Academy of Pediatrics encourages and strongly supports breastfeeding for all able mothers for the first 12 months of life and continued thereafter for as long as mutually desired.[26,28]

SUMMARY

Pregnancy involves the fundamental interaction of the following three distinct yet unified biologic entities: the fetus, placenta, and mother. Maternal needs also reflect the increasing nutritional needs of the fetus and placenta. Optimal weight gain varies with the normal nutritional status and weight of the woman, with a goal of about 25 to 35 lbs for a woman of average weight. Sufficient weight gain is important during pregnancy to support the rapid growth taking place. However, the nutritional quality of the diet is as significant as the actual weight gain.

Common problems during pregnancy include first-trimester nausea and vomiting associated with hormonal adaptations and later constipation, hemorrhoids, or heartburn resulting from the pressure of the enlarging uterus. These problems usually are relieved without medication by simple, often temporary, changes in the diet. Unusual or irregular eating habits, age, parity, prepartum weight status, and low income are among the many related conditions that put pregnant women at risk for complications.

The ultimate goal of prenatal care is a healthy infant and a healthy mother who can breastfeed her child if she chooses to do so. Human milk provides essential nutrients in quantities that are uniquely suited for optimal infant growth and development.

CRITICAL THINKING QUESTIONS

1. Which six nutrients are required in larger amounts during pregnancy? Describe their special roles, and identify four food sources of each.
2. Identify two common gastrointestinal problems associated with pregnancy and describe the diet management of each.

3. Discuss the major nutritional factors needed to support lactation. What additional, nonnutritional needs does the breastfeeding mother have, and what suggestions can you give to help her meet them?
4. Why is additional fluid needed for lactation?

CHAPTER CHALLENGE QUESTIONS

True-False

Write the correct statement for each item you answer "false."

1. *True or False:* The development of the fetus is directly related to the diet of the mother.
2. *True or False:* Strict weight control during pregnancy is necessary to avoid complications.
3. *True or False:* Salt should be removed from the pregnant woman's diet to prevent edema.
4. *True or False:* A higher risk for pregnancy complications occurs in teenage and older women.
5. *True or False:* A woman's diet before pregnancy has little effect on the outcome of her pregnancy.

6. *True or False:* No woman should ever gain more than 15 to 20 lbs during pregnancy.
7. *True or False:* Rapid growth of the fetal skeleton requires increased calcium in the mother's diet.
8. *True or False:* Inadequate vitamin D during pregnancy contributes to faulty skeletal development in the fetus.
9. *True or False:* Anemia is common during pregnancy.
10. *True or False:* Additional kcalories and fluids are needed during lactation.

Multiple Choice

1. Blood volume during pregnancy
   a. increases.
   b. decreases.
   c. remains unchanged.
   d. fluctuates widely.
2. Pregnant mothers taking high doses of iron supplements are potentially at risk for deficiencies of which of the following minerals because of nutrient interactions?
   a. Calcium
   b. Phosphorus
   c. Selenium
   d. Zinc
3. Which of the following foods has the highest iron content to help meet the need for increased iron during pregnancy?
   a. Lean beef
   b. Liver

   c. Orange juice
   d. Milk
4. The increased need for vitamin A during pregnancy may be met by increased use of foods such as
   a. chicken.
   b. extra egg whites.
   c. citrus fruits.
   d. carrots.
5. Which of the following hormones is responsible for milk let-down during lactation?
   a. Prolactin
   b. Estrogen
   c. Oxytocin
   d. Human growth hormone

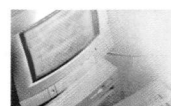

Please refer to the Students' Resource section of this text's Evolve web site for "Suggestions for Additional Study."

REFERENCES

1. Food and Nutrition Board, Institute of Medicine: *Dietary reference intakes for calcium, phosphorous, magnesium, vitamin D, and fluoride*, Washington, DC, 1998, National Academies Press.
2. Food and Nutrition Board, Institute of Medicine: *Dietary reference intakes for thiamin, riboflavin, niacin, vitamin B$_6$, folate, vitamin B$_{12}$, pantothenic acid, biotin, and choline*, Washington, DC, 1999, National Academies Press.
3. Food and Nutrition Board, Institute of Medicine: *Dietary reference intakes for vitamin C, vitamin E, selenium, and carotenoids*, Washington, DC, 2000, National Academies Press.
4. Food and Nutrition Board, Institute of Medicine: *Dietary reference intakes for vitamin A, vitamin K, arsenic, boron, chromium, copper, iodine, iron, manganese, molybdenum, nickel, silicon, vanadium, and zinc*, Washington, DC, 2002, National Academies Press.
5. National Academy of Sciences, Committee on Nutritional Status During Pregnancy and Lactation, Food and Nutrition Board: *Nutrition during pregnancy*, Washington, DC, 1990, National Academies Press.
6. Food and Nutrition Board, Institute of Medicine: *Dietary reference intakes for energy, carbohydrate, fiber, fat, fatty acids, cholesterol, protein, and amino acids*, Washington, DC, 2002, National Academies Press.
7. King JC: Effect of reproduction on the bioavailability of calcium, zinc, and selenium, *J Nutr* 131:1355S, 2001.
8. Green NS: Folic acid supplementation and prevention of birth defects, *J Nutr* 132(8 suppl):2356S, 2002.
9. Mackey AD, Picciano MF: Maternal folate status during extended lactation and the effect of supplemental folic acid, *Am J Clin Nutr* 69(1):285, 1999.
10. Honein MA and others: Impact of folic acid fortification of the U.S. food supply on the occurrence of neural tube defects, *JAMA* 285(23):2981, 2001.
11. Strauss RS, Dietz WH: Low maternal weight gain in the second or third trimester increases the risk for intrauterine growth retardation, *J Nutr* 129(5):988, 1999.
12. National Center for Chronic Disease Prevention and Health Promotion, Division of Reproductive Health, Centers for Disease Control and Prevention: *Safe motherhood. Fact sheet: pregnancy-related deaths in the United States, 1987-1990*, Atlanta, (accessed February 2003), U.S. Department of Health and Human Services/CDC [*www.cdc.gov/nccdphp/drh/mh_prgdeath.htm*].
13. Martin JA and others: *Births: final data for 2000*, National Vital Statistics Reports 50(5), Hyattsville, MD, 2002, National Center for Health Statistics, Centers for Disease Control and Prevention, U.S. Department of Health and Human Services.
14. National Center for Chronic Disease Prevention and Health Promotion, Centers for Disease Control and Prevention: *Teen pregnancy*, Atlanta, (accessed July 2002), U.S. Department of Health and Human Services/CDC [*www.cdc.gov/* keyword "teen pregnancy"].
15. Rose EA and others: Pica: common but commonly missed, *J Am Board Fam Pract* 13(5):353, 2000.
16. Simpson E and others: Pica during pregnancy in low-income women born in Mexico, *West J Med* 173:20, 2000.
17. Ornoy A: The effects of alcohol and illicit drugs on the human embryo and fetus, *Isr J Psychiatry Relat Sci* 39(2):120, 2002.
18. Dejmek J and others: The exposure of nonsmoking and smoking mothers to environmental tobacco smoke during different gestational phases and fetal growth, *Environ Health Perspect* 110(6):601, 2002.
19. Lindbohm ML and others: Effects of exposure to environmental tobacco smoke on reproductive health, *Scand J Work Environ Health* 28(2 suppl):84, 2002.
20. Christian MS, Brent RL: Teratogen update: evaluation of the reproductive and developmental risks of caffeine, *Teratology* 64:51, 2001.
21. Jovanovic L: Time to reassess the optimal dietary prescription for women with gestational diabetes, *Am J Clin Nutr* 70(1):3, 1999.
22. Dennis CL: Breastfeeding initiation and duration: a 1990-2000 literature review, *JOGNN* 31:12, 2002.
23. Beshgetor D and others: Attitudes toward breast-feeding among WIC employees in San Diego County, *J Am Diet Assoc* 99(1):86, 1999.
24. Chezem J, Friesen C: Attendance at breast-feeding support meetings: relationship to demographic characteristics and duration of lactation in women planning postpartum employment, *J Am Diet Assoc* 99(1):83, 1999.
25. Kannan S and others: Cultural influences on infant feeding beliefs of mothers, *J Am Diet Assoc* 99(1):88, 1999.
26. American Academy of Pediatrics: Breastfeeding and the use of human milk, *Pediatrics* 100(6):1035, 1997.
27. Oddy WH and others: Breast feeding and cognitive development in childhood: a prospective birth cohort study, *Paediatr Perinat Epidemiol* 17:81, 2003.
28. Position of The American Dietetic Association: Promotion of breast-feeding, *J Am Diet Assoc* 97(6):662, 1997.

FURTHER READING AND RESOURCES

- American Academy of Pediatrics: *www.aap.org*
- Canadian Paediatric Society: *www.cps.ca*
- March of Dimes Birth Defects Foundation: *www.modimes.org*
- Birth Defect Research for Children, Inc.: *www.birthdefects.org*
- La Leche League International, Inc.: *www.lalecheleauge.org*
- U.S. Department of Agriculture Women, Infants, and Children Program: *www.fns.usda.gov/wic*

    The preceding organizations can all be reached via the web sites provided. Each organization has an earnest interest in the health care of pregnant women and their children. For information on a variety of topics about pregnancy and lactation, explore the preceding sites.

- Vozenilek GP: What they don't know could hurt them: increasing public awareness of folic acid and neural tube defects, *J Am Diet Assoc* 99(1):20, 1999.

    This brief article draws a clear picture of the cloud of ignorance that still hangs over the general population about the devastating results of neural tube defects in an affected child from birth, because of the mother's folic acid deficiency early in pregnancy.

- Martin JA and others: *Births: final data for 2000*, National Vital Statistics Reports 50(5), Hyattsville, MD, 2002, National Center for Health Statistics, Centers for Disease Control and Prevention, U.S. Department of Health and Human Services [*www.cdc.gov/nchs/data/nvsr/nvsr50/nvsr50_05.pdf*].

    The National Vital Statistics Reports, provided in part by the CDC, can be fully accessed via the Internet. This report gives an in-depth look at teen pregnancy, risk factors, and general health care of births in the United States.

Nutrition in Infancy, Childhood, and Adolescence

In any culture, food nurtures both the physical and emotional process of "growing up" for each infant, child, or adolescent. Food, feeding, and eating during these significant years of childhood do not exist apart from the broader overall process of growth and development. The entire process ultimately has a hand in creating and designing the whole person.

This chapter considers food and feeding in an individual and unique manner, as a basic part of "growing up" for each person. It then relates the various age-group nutritional needs and food patterns to individual psychosocial development, as well as physical growth.

KEY CONCEPTS

- Normal growth of individual children varies within a relatively wide range of measures.

- Human growth and development require both nutritional and psychosocial support.

- A variety of food patterns and habits supply the energy and nutrient requirements of normal growth and development, although basic nutritional needs change with each growth period.

NUTRITION FOR GROWTH AND DEVELOPMENT

Life Cycle Growth Pattern

The normal human life cycle follows four general stages of overall growth, with individual variances along the way.

Infancy

Growth is rapid during the first year of life, with the rate tapering off somewhat in the latter half of the year. Most infants double their birth weight by the time they are 6 months of age and triple it by 1 year of age. Growth in length is not quite as rapid, but on average, infants increase birth length by 50% in the first year and double it by age 4.

Childhood

Between infancy and adolescence, the childhood growth rate slows and becomes irregular. Growth occurs in small spurts, during which children have increased appetites and eat accordingly. Appetites usually taper off during periodic plateaus. Parents who recognize the ebb and flow of normal growth patterns in the "latent period of childhood" will relax and enjoy their child. On the other hand, inexperience or lack of knowledge of this normal flux in growth and appetite can result in stress and battles over food between parents and children.

Adolescence

The onset of puberty begins the second stage of rapid growth, which continues until adult maturity. The flooding sex hormones and increased growth hormone bring multiple and often bewildering body changes to young adolescents. During this period, long bones grow rapidly, sex characteristics develop, and fat and muscle mass increase.

Adulthood

With physical maturity comes the final phase of a normal life cycle. Physical growth levels off during adulthood and then gradually declines during old age. However, mental and psychosocial development lasts a lifetime.

Measuring Childhood Growth

Individual Growth Rates

Children grow at widely varying rates. Therefore the best counsel for parents is that children are *individuals.* Growth is not inadequate because its rate does not equal that of another child. General measures of growth in children relate not only to physical development but also to mental, emotional, social, and cultural growth.

Physical Growth

Growth charts, such as those developed by the National Center for Health Statistics (NCHS) and the Centers for Disease Control and Prevention (CDC), provide an assessment tool for measuring normal growth patterns in infants, children, and adolescents. These charts are based on large numbers of well-nourished children representing the national population. They are used as guides to follow an individual child's pattern of physical growth in relation to the general percentile growth curves of the population. The current charts, published in May of 2000, allow the practitioner to plot the growth patterns for height (or length), weight, and head circumference. New to the growth charts are the body mass index (BMI)-for-age charts for children ages 2 to 20 years. This addition is the first of its kind that can be used continuously from 2 years of age into adulthood. Because BMI in childhood is a determinant of adulthood BMI, the risk of obesity can be identified early.[1] There are specific growth charts for males and females and for infants from birth to 36 months (Figure 11-1) and then a separate set of growth charts for children and adolescents from age 2 to 20 years (see Appendix I). It is critical to select the appropriate chart to get an accurate reading (see the Cultural Considerations box, "Growth Charts: Can You Use Them for All Children?" for more information).

Individual measures of physical growth for children include weight and height, head circumference, general signs of health, laboratory tests, and nutritional study of general eating habits. Accurately measuring length (for infants and toddlers), height, weight, and head circumference is critical to the assessment process. Small errors in measurement can easily lead to false alarm about a child's growth pattern.

Psychosocial Development

Tests are used to measure mental, emotional, social, and cultural growth and development. Food is intimately related to these aspects of psychosocial development, as well as to physical growth. The growing child does not learn food attitudes and habits in a vacuum but in close personal and social relationships.

---

body mass index (BMI) body weight in kilograms divided by the square of height in meters (kg/m^2). Correlates with body fatness and health risk associated with obesity.

CDC Growth Charts: United States

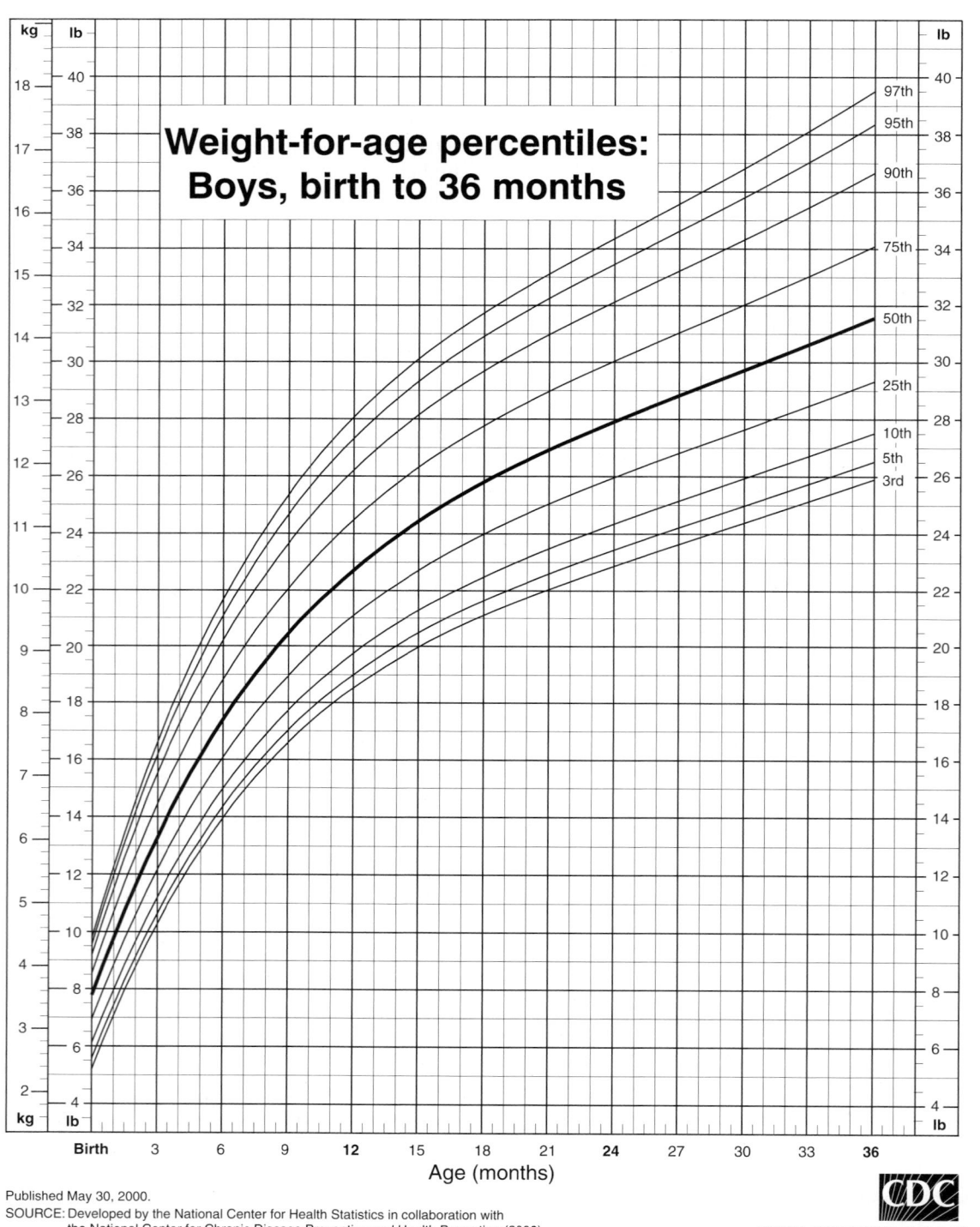

Weight-for-age percentiles: Boys, birth to 36 months

Published May 30, 2000.
SOURCE: Developed by the National Center for Health Statistics in collaboration with
the National Center for Chronic Disease Prevention and Health Promotion (2000).

SAFER · HEALTHIER · PEOPLE™

Figure 11–1   Example of one growth chart produced by the Centers for Disease Control and Prevention: United States.
(Source: Developed by the National Center for Health Statistics in collaboration with the National Center for Chronic Disease Prevention and Health Promotion [2000], Hyattsville, MD.)

CULTURAL CONSIDERATIONS

GROWTH CHARTS: CAN YOU USE THEM FOR ALL CHILDREN?

The new CDC growth charts, released in May 2000, replaced the previously used charts from 1977. The current set of charts have a new addition, the body mass index (BMI)-for-age charts for both girls and boys aged 2 to 20 years. The new charts also include breastfed infants and are racially and ethnically diverse.

To accurately assess a child's growth, three things are critical: (1) an appropriate growth reference, (2) an accurate measurement, and (3) an accurate calculation of a child's age. Growth charts are not used to identify "short" or "tall" children. They are used as a means of continuous assessment of a child's growth rate. Children are identified with a certain percentile of the population in terms of a specific anthropometric measurement. For example, if a child has a height-for-age at the 70th percentile, then 30% of the children of the same age and gender are taller and 69% are shorter. With adequate nutrition, and in the absence of disease, this child should continue to grow on the 70th percentile curve.

Health professionals use the 5th and 95th percentiles as a cutoff point at which children falling outside of this range are screened for potential health- or nutrition-related problems. Children and adolescents with a BMI-for-age above the 85th percentile are at risk for being overweight as adults. The cutoff point of the 95th percentile on the BMI-for-age charts correlates to a BMI of 30 in young adults, which is considered obese. Because the BMI-for-age charts correlate with the adult BMI index, it can be used continuously from childhood into adulthood, providing a lifelong assessment tool that indicates risk factors for chronic disease associated with obesity.

Breastfed infants have a slightly different growth curve than formula-fed infants. Breastfed infants grow slightly more rapidly than formula-fed infants in the first 2 months of life and then the rate of growth declines to a rate slower than formula-fed infants.* The previous growth charts were predominantly based on formula-fed infants. The new charts use a combined population of both formula-fed and breastfed infants. However, only about one third of the total population was breastfed for more than 3 months. Thus normal growth patterns of breastfed infants may still vary from standardized growth charts.

The World Health Organization (WHO) is currently in the process of publishing a set of international growth charts based on their feeding recommendations, which are: breastfed for at least 12 months with solid foods introduced between 4 and 6 months. These growth charts, from birth to 5 years, are specific and appropriate for infants and children who have been exclusively breastfed.

In regard to charting growth patterns of an adolescent, practitioners should be aware of the racial differences about timing of sexual maturation and how that relates to overall weight and body fatness. According to a recent study analyzing data from the Third National Health and Nutrition Examination Survey, non-Hispanic African-American girls and boys begin the process of sexual maturity before Mexican American or non-Hispanic Caucasian children.† Such differences are specifically important when assessing growth on a growth chart because more mature children are likely to be taller and heavier than their less mature peers.

There were not enough individuals participating in the data collection for the current growth charts to create charts specific to racial or ethnic groups. Therefore the CDC promotes the use of the standard growth charts for all racial and ethnic groups. Future studies will determine if significant differences exist and warrant the development of charts specific to cultural backgrounds.

Excellent information and step-by-step instructions on how to accurately plot a child's growth chart are provided on the CDC web site at: *www.cdc.gov/growthcharts/.*

---

*Dewey KG: Nutrition, growth, and complementary feeding of the breastfed infant, *Pediatr Clin North Am* 48(1):87, 2001.
†Sun SS and others: National estimates of the timing of sexual maturation and racial differences among U.S. children, *Pediatrics* 110(5):911, 2001.

NUTRITIONAL REQUIREMENTS FOR GROWTH

Energy Needs

Kilocalories

The demand for energy, as measured in kcalories from food, is relatively large during childhood. During the first 3 years of life, children need an average of 90 to 110 kcal/kg body weight per day to support rapid growth. This is significantly higher than adult needs of 30 to 40 kcal/kg per day. Energy needs of premature infants are even greater, ranging from 105 to 130 kcal/kg per day. The Dietary Reference Intake (DRI) values in Table 6-5 present general recommendations for energy and nutrient needs at different ages. However, specific individual needs vary with age and condition. For example, the total daily caloric intake of an average 5-year-old is spent in the following way:

■ Basal metabolism: 50%
■ Physical activities: 25%
■ Tissue growth: 12%
■ Fecal loss: 8%
■ Metabolic effect of food: 5%

However, some children are much more physically active than others and have a higher kcal/kg per day expenditure. Likewise, a child who is experiencing rapid growth has higher specific individual needs than a similar child who has not yet reached his or her growth spurt.

Energy Nutrients

Of the total kilocalories, carbohydrates are the main energy source. Carbohydrates also act as a protein-sparer so that the protein vital for building tissue during childhood growth is not diverted for energy needs. Fat is a back-up energy source and supplies *linoleic acid*, which is an essential fatty acid necessary for growth.

Protein Needs

Protein is the fundamental *tissue-building* substance of the body. It supplies the essential, specific building materials, amino acids, for tissue growth and maintenance. As a child grows, the protein requirements per unit of body weight gradually decrease. For example, for the first 6 months of life, the protein requirements of an infant are 2.2 g/kg of body weight; but the protein needs of a fully grown adult are only 0.8 g/kg. A healthy, active, growing child usually eats enough of a variety of foods to supply the necessary protein and kcalories for overall growth.

Water Requirements

Water is an essential nutrient, second only to oxygen for life. Metabolic needs, especially during periods of rapid growth, demand adequate fluid intake. For example, compare infant and adult water needs. Infants require more water per unit of body weight than adults for two important reasons, as follows: (1) a greater percentage of the infant's total body weight is made up of water; and (2) a larger proportion of the infant's total body water is outside the cells and hence more easily available for loss, potentially resulting in dehydration. In 1 day, an infant generally consumes an amount of water equivalent to 10% to 15% of body weight, whereas an adult consumes a daily amount equivalent to 2% to 4% of body weight. Table 11-1 provides a summary of the estimated daily fluid needs during growth years.

Mineral and Vitamin Needs

Although yielding no energy themselves, minerals and vitamins have important roles in tissue growth and maintenance, as well as in overall energy metabolism. Positive childhood growth depends on adequate amounts of all essential substances. Several of these materials are specifically important during the rapid growth years.

Calcium

Calcium needs are critical during the most rapid growth periods of infancy and adolescence. In infancy, mineralization of the skeleton is taking place, while bones are growing larger and teeth are forming from initial buds. In adolescence, the skeleton grows most rapidly to its adult size. Bone density, particularly in long bones and vertebrae, demands adequate calcium, along with phosphorus and vitamin D. In fact, as a preventive measure to reduce the risk for osteoporosis in older adults, both research and clinical experience indicate that calcium must be emphasized during adolescence. Calcium intake during rapid adolescent bone

TABLE 11–1	Approximate Daily Fluid Needs during Growth Years		
Age	**ml/kg**	**Age**	**ml/kg**
0-3 months	120	4-7 years	95
3-6 months	115	7-11 years	90
6-12 months	110	11-19 years	50
1-4 years	100	>19 years	30

growth (e.g., both in size and density) is far more effective than the use of more poorly absorbed calcium supplements in older adult years.[2] Furthermore, adolescents taking prednisone or other prescribed steroid therapy have particularly high needs for adequate calcium intake because this line of medication can cause growth stunting and lowered bone density, especially if taken before puberty.

Iron

Iron is essential for hemoglobin formation and cognitive development in the early years. The iron content of breast milk is highly absorbable and fully meets the needs of an infant for the first 6 months of life.[3] At that point, the infant's nutritional needs for iron typically exceed that provided exclusively by breast milk, and the addition of solid foods (e.g., enriched cereal, egg yolk, and meat) at about 6 months of age helps supply additional iron. Infants who are not breastfed need iron-fortified formula. Cow's milk, which is very low in iron, should be avoided completely for the first year of life.

Vitamin Supplements

Although there has been much debate over the years about dietary supplement of vitamins and minerals in breastfed infants, the American Academy of Pediatrics recognizes only two vitamins that are potentially needed in supplemental form: vitamins K and D.[4] Nearly all infants born in the United States and Canada receive a prophylactic shot of 1 mg vitamin K and no further supplementation is recommended for breast- or formula-fed infants. Oral supplementation of vitamin D is still controversial because most infants are exposed to sunlight and therefore can produce vitamin D in their own skin. The amount of vitamin D in breast milk is dependent on the mother's intake and exposure to sunlight.[5] Therefore for infants with inadequate sunlight exposure (e.g., infants living in extremely northern latitudes such as Alaska, where there is very little sunlight for 6 months of the year) or whose mothers are vitamin D deficient, an oral supplement of 5 to 10 μg/day (200 to 400 IU/day) is recommended.[5,6] Formula-fed infants do not need an additional supplement of vitamin D because the formula is already fortified.

Excessive supplementation in infants is not unheard of and, as with adults, there are dangers of toxicity. Excess amounts of vitamins A and D, *hypervitaminosis,* are of special concern in feeding children (see Chapter 7). Excess intake may occur over prolonged periods as a result of ignorance, carelessness, or misunderstanding. Parents should only provide the amount directed and no more.

AGE GROUP NEEDS

Infancy

At birth, the development as a unique human being begins. This process continues throughout life. Food is intimately related at each stage of development because physical growth and personal psychosocial development go hand in hand.

Immature Infants

Special care is crucial for tiny, immature babies. There are two primary categories of immature babies, defined by weight or gestational age.

Weight. Defined by birth weight, low-birth-weight (LBW) babies weigh less than 2500 g (5 lbs); very-low-birth-weight (VLBW) babies weigh less than 1500 g (3 lbs); extremely low-birth-weight (ELBW) babies weigh less than 990 g (2 lbs).

Gestational Age. Defined by gestational age, premature babies are born preterm (e.g., at under 270 days of gestation) and weigh less than 2500 g (5 lbs). Small-for-gestational-age (SGA) babies are born at full term but have suffered some degree of intrauterine growth failure before birth and have general growth retardation and low weight. Note that growth retardation does not necessarily affect mental development.

All immature infants are subject to problems with growth and nutrition. Because their bodies are not fully formed, they differ from full-term infants of normal weight. Immature infants have the following: (1) more body water, less protein, and fewer minerals; (2) little subcutaneous fat to maintain body temperature; (3) poorly calcified bones; (4) incomplete nerve and muscle development, making their sucking reflexes weak; (5) limited ability for digestion-absorption and renal function; and (6) an immature liver, lacking developed metabolic enzyme systems or adequate iron stores. To survive, these "tiny babies" require special feeding.

Type of Milk. Immature babies have grown well on both breast milk (with an added human milk fortifier) and special formulas. Table 11-2 compares these special formulas with standard, full-term infant formulas and human milk.

Methods of Feeding. Tube feeding and peripheral vein feeding are used in special cases, but both carry hazards and are avoided if possible. For most immature infants, bottle feeding or nursing can be successful with much

TABLE 11–2 Nutritional Value of Special Formulas and Human Milk for the Preterm Infant								
	Advisable intake by birth weight		Human milk		Standard formulas	Special premature formulas		
Nutritional component	1.0 kg (2.2 lbs)	1.5 kg (3.3 lbs)	Preterm	Mature	Enfamil* Similac† SMA‡	Enfamil Premature with Whey*	Similac Special Care†	"Preemie" SMA‡
Kilocalories/deciliter			73	73	67	81	81	81
Protein (g/100 kcal)	3.1	2.7	2.3§	1.5	2.2	3	2.7	2.5
VITAMINS, FAT-SOLUBLE								
D (IU/120 kcal/kg/day)	600	600	—	4	70-75	75	180	76
E (IU/120 kcal/kg/day)	30	30	—	0.3	2-3	2	4	2
VITAMINS, WATER-SOLUBLE								
Folic acid (µg/120 kcal/kg/day)	60	60	—	8	9-19	36	45	14
Vitamin C (mg/120 kcal/kg/day)	60	60	—	7	10	10	45	10
MINERALS								
Calcium (mg/100 kcal)	160	140	40	43	66-78	117	178	92
Phosphorus (mg/100 kcal)	108	95	18	20	49-66	58	89	49
Sodium (mEq/100 kcal)	2.7	2.3	1.5¶	0.8	1-1.8	1.7	1.9	1.7

*Mead Johnson Nutritionals, Evansville, IN.
†Ross Products, Columbus, OH.
‡Wyeth Laboratories, PA.
§Range: 1.9-2.8 g/100 kcal.
¶Range: 0.9-2.3 mEq/100 kcal.

care and support. Infants who have not yet developed the sucking reflex (acquired around 32 weeks' gestation) can still benefit from breast milk, provided the mother is willing and able to pump her breast milk to be delivered to the baby via tube feeding.

Full-Term Infants

Mature newborns have more finely developed body systems and grow rapidly, gaining about 168 g (6 oz) per week during the first 6 months. The feeding process is an important component of the bonding relationship between parent and child. The mother may choose to breastfeed or use a formula and add solid foods later (e.g., at about 6 months of age) when the baby can handle them.

Breastfeeding

Human milk is the ideal first food for infants and is the primary recommendation of pediatricians and nutritionists.[6-8] The nutrients in human milk are uniquely adapted to meet the growth needs of the infant, in forms more easily digested, absorbed, and used. Breastfeeding supports early immunity for the baby, helps the mother's uterus quickly return to normal size, and facilitates the important mother-child bonding process. Breastfeeding can be successfully started and maintained by most women who try, have support, and consume an appropriate diet for lactation (see Chapter 10). During pregnancy the breasts prepare for lactation and, toward term, produce a thin fluid called **colostrum**. As the infant grows, the breast milk develops and adapts in composition to match the needs of the developing child. The fat content of breast milk, the major energy source, changes from the beginning to the end of a single feeding. Fore milk, the first milk to let down, is the lowest in fat content. Mid-milk has progressively more fat content; and hind-milk, the milk coming at the end of the feeding, has the highest fat content. Thus fully emptying each breast at every feeding is important to provide the infant with the energy-dense hind-milk.

The newborn's rooting reflex, oral needs for sucking, and basic hunger usually make breastfeeding simple for healthy, relaxed mothers (Figure 11-2). Working mothers who want to breastfeed their babies can do so by using manual expression or a breast pump while at work, as well as freezing and storing milk in sealed plastic baby bottle liners for later use. Childcare facilities provided in some business and industry settings support breastfeeding by employed mothers. Breastfeeding mothers can find support and guidance through local groups of the national La Leche League or professional certified lactation counselors.

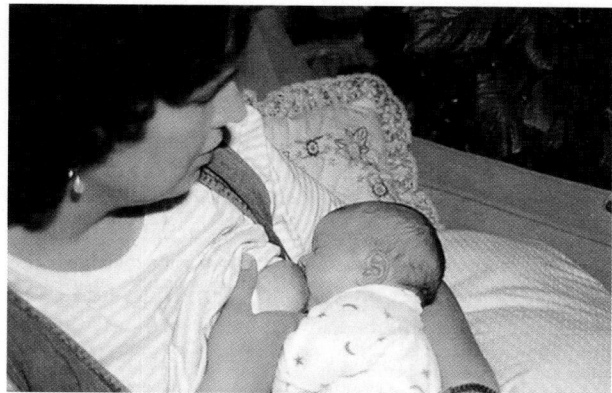

Figure 11–2   Breastfeeding the newborn infant. Note that the mother avoids touching the infant's outer cheek so as not to counteract the infant's natural rooting reflex at the touch of the breast. (Courtesy Marjorie Pyle, RNC, *Lifecircle,* Costa Mesa, CA. From Dickason EJ, Silverman BL, Schult MO: *Maternal-infant nursing care,* ed 3, St Louis, 1998, Mosby.)

Bottle Feeding

If a mother chooses not to breastfeed, or some condition in either the mother or baby prevents it, bottle feeding of an appropriate formula is an acceptable alternative. Sterile procedures in formula preparation, the amount of formula consumed, and weaning from the bottle are some of the concerns mothers have voiced.

Cleaning Bottles and Nipples. Rinse bottles and nipples after each feeding, using special bottle and nipple brushes and forcing water through nipple holes to prevent milk from crusting in them.

Preparing the Formula. Whether preparing a single bottle for each feeding or a day's batch, scrub, rinse, and sterilize all equipment by the *terminal sterilization* method. Most mothers who bottle feed their infants use a standard commercial formula (see Table 11-2). In some cases of potential milk allergy or intolerance, a soy-based formula (not soy milk) is used. For infants who are allergic to both cow's milk and soy-based formulas, a special predigested

colostrum   (L. *colostrum,* premilk) a thin, yellow fluid first secreted by the mammary gland a few days after childbirth, preceding the mature breast milk. It contains up to 20% protein including a large amount of lactalbumin, more minerals, and less lactose and fat than mature milk, as well as immunoglobulins that represent the antibodies found in maternal blood.

formula such as Pregestimil or Nutramigen (both from Mead Johnson Nutritionals, Evansville, IN) or Alimentum (Ross Products, Columbus, OH) may be medically advised. With any commercial formula, manufacturer's instructions for mixing concentrated or powdered formula with water should be precisely and consistently followed; and the formula should be refrigerated until use. Throughout the process, scrupulous cleanliness and accurate dilution are essential to prevent infection and illness. Most babies who are hospitalized for vomiting and diarrhea are bottle fed. A ready-to-feed formula only requires a sterile nipple and bypasses many problems, but is more expensive.

Feeding the Formula. Babies drink formula either cold or warm, they just like it to be consistent. Tilt the bottle to keep the nipple full of milk to prevent air swallowing and hold the baby's head somewhat elevated during feeding to facilitate the passage of milk into the stomach. Never prop the bottle and leave the baby alone to feed, especially as a pacifier at sleep time. This practice deprives

the infant of the cuddling that is a vital part of nurturing and also allows milk to pool in the mouth, causing choking, earache, or *bottle mouth* with early tooth decay. Never put a child to sleep with a bottle of milk or fruit juice or other caloric liquid capable of pooling in the mouth. Natural bacteria found in the mouth feeds on carbohydrates, producing enamel-damaging acid. Baby bottle tooth decay is a serious, but completely avoidable, problem resulting from this practice.

Weaning

Throughout the feeding process, observant parents learn early to recognize their baby's signs of hunger and satiety and follow the baby's leads. Babies are individuals and set their own particular needs according to age, activity level, growth rate, and metabolic efficiency. A newborn has a very small stomach, holding only 1 to 2 fluid ounces, but gradually takes more as the stomach capacity enlarges relative to overall body growth. The amounts of increased intake during the first 6 months vary and reflect

TABLE 11–3	Guideline for Adding Solid Foods to Infant's Diet during the First Year
Foods added*	**Feeding**
6 TO 7 MONTHS	
Cereal and strained cooked fruit	10 AM and 6 PM
Egg yolk (at first, hard-boiled and sieved; soft-boiled or poached later)	
Strained cooked vegetable and strained meat	2 PM
Zweiback or hard toast	At any feeding
7 TO 9 MONTHS	
Meat: beef, lamb, or liver (broiled or baked and finely chopped)	10 AM and 6 PM
Potato: baked or boiled and mashed or sieved	
9 MONTHS TO 1 YEAR OR OLDER (SUGGESTED MEAL PLAN)	
Milk: 240 ml (8 oz)	7 AM
Cereal: 2-3 Tbsp	
Strained fruit: 2-3 Tbsp	
Zweiback or dry toast	
Milk: 240 ml (8 oz)	NOON
Vegetables: 2-3 Tbsp	
Chopped meat or meat substitute: 2 Tbsp	
Cooked fruit: 2-3 Tbsp	
Milk: 240 ml (8 oz)	3 PM
Toast or Zweiback	
Milk: 240 ml (8 oz)	6 PM
Chopped meat or meat substitute: 2 Tbsp	
Potato: baked or mashed, 2-3 Tbsp	
Cooked fruit	
Zweiback or toast	

*Semisolid foods should be given immediately before milk feeding. First, 1 or 2 tsp should be given. If food is accepted and tolerated well, the amount should be increased 1 to 2 Tbsp per feeding.

individual growth patterns. The following quantities are averages:

- *1 month*: 2 to 3 oz, six to eight feedings, 20 oz total
- *2 months*: 4 to 5 oz, six to seven feedings, 28 oz total
- *3 months*: 6 to 7 oz, five to six feedings, 30 oz total
- *4 months*: 6 to 8 oz, four to five feedings, 30 oz total
- *5 months*: 7 to 8 oz, four to five feedings, 34 oz total
- *6 months*: 7 to 8 oz, four to five feedings, 38 oz total

By 6 to 8 months of age, as increasing amounts of other foods are used, **weaning** from bottle feeding takes place. For some children, growing physical capacities and the desire for independence lead to self-weaning, but many children need a little added encouragement from parents.

Cow's Milk

An infant should never be fed cow's milk during the first year of life. Unmodified cow's milk is not suitable for infants; its concentration may cause gastrointestinal bleeding and provides too heavy a load of solutes for the infant's renal system. Infants and toddlers under age 2 also should not be fed reduced fat cow's milk (e.g., skim or low-fat milk) for the following reasons: (1) *insufficient energy* is provided, and (2) *linoleic acid*, the essential fatty acid for growth in the fat portion, is lacking. To meet infant needs during the first year of life, the American Academy of Pediatrics recommends breast milk, supplemented by vitamin D (if the mother is deficient and the child has inadequate exposure to sunlight), with the gradual addition of iron-fortified foods beginning at

about 6 months.[6] An alternative formula is appropriate, in place of breast milk, if the mother chooses.

Solid Food Additions

In some ethnic groups, there is a traditional pattern of starting solid foods early.[9] However, the recommended practice is to introduce solid foods at about 6 months of age. Because the infant's system cannot use solid foods well before 6 months, they are not yet needed. When solid foods are started, there is no one specific sequence of food additions that must be followed. However, some organizations promote the introduction to vegetables before fruits. The root of this recommendation is that fruits are much sweeter than vegetables and infants may take a preference for the sweet taste first and then not take kindly to the more bitter taste of vegetables. A general guide is given in Table 11-3, but individual needs and responses vary and suggestions of individual practitioners are the guide. Foods usually are introduced one at a time, starting with iron-fortified cereal, and in small amounts so that if there is an adverse reaction the offending food is easily identified. Over time, the child is introduced to a variety of foods and comes to enjoy many of them (Figure 11-3). Children's eating behaviors are complex and continue to change with age.[10,11]

A variety of commercial baby foods are available and are now prepared without added sugar, salt, or monosodium glutamate. Some mothers prefer to prepare their own baby food. Baby food can be prepared at home easily by cooking and straining vegetables and fruits, freezing a batch at a time in ice cube trays, and storing the cubes in plastic bags in the freezer. A single cube can later be reheated for feeding. Throughout the early feeding period, whatever plan is followed, the following basic principles should guide the feeding process: (1) *necessary* nutrients, not any specific food or sequence, are needed; (2) food is a basis of *learning*, and (3) *normal physical development* guides the feeding behavior (see the For Further Focus box, "How Infants Learn to Eat"). Good food habits begin early in life and continue as the child grows. By 8 or 9 months of age, infants should be able to eat so-called table foods (e.g., cooked, chopped, and simply seasoned foods) without needing special infant foods.

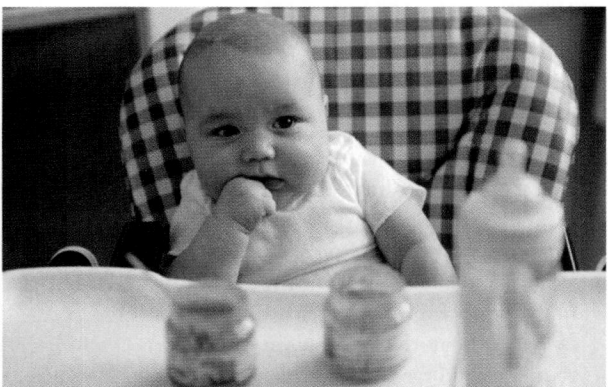

Figure 11–3 This child is taking a variety of solid food additions and developing wide tastes. Here, feeding serves as a source not only of physical growth but also of psychosocial development. Optimal physical development and security are evident, the result of sound nutrition and loving care. (Credit: PhotoDisc.)

wean (Middle English, 1000 AD, *wenen,* to accustom) to gradually accustom a young child to food other than the mother's milk or a bottle-fed substitute formula as the child's natural need to suckle wanes.

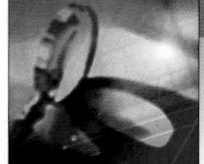

FOR FURTHER FOCUS

HOW INFANTS LEARN TO EAT

Guided by reflexes and gradually developing muscle controls during their first year of life, infants learn many things about living in their particular environment. A most basic need is food, which infants obtain through a normal developmental sequence of feeding behaviors in the process of learning to eat.

Age 1 to 3 months

Rooting, sucking, and swallowing reflexes are present at birth, along with the tonic neck reflex. Therefore infants secure their first food, milk, with a suckling pattern in which the tongue is projected during a swallow. In the beginning, head control is poor but develops by the third month of life.

Age 4 to 6 months

The early rooting and biting reflex fades, and the tonic neck reflex has faded by 16 weeks. Infants now change from a suckling pattern with a protruded tongue to a mature, stronger suck with liquids, and a munching pattern begins. Infants are now able to grasp objects with a fistlike palmar grip, bringing them to the mouth and biting them.

Age 7 to 9 months

The gag reflex weakens as infants begin chewing solid foods and develop a normal controlled gag along with control of the choking reflex. Munching movements now develop as older infants increase their intake of solid foods and chew with a rotary motion. These infants can sit alone, secure items, release and resecure them, and hold a bottle alone. They begin to develop a pincer grasp to pick up very small items between the thumb and forefinger and put them in the mouth.

Age 10 to 12 months

Older infants can now reach for a spoon. They bite nipples, spoons, and crunchy foods; can grasp a bottle and foods and bring them to the mouth; and, with assistance, can drink from a cup. These infants have tongue control to lick food morsels off the lower lip and can finger-feed themselves with a refined pincer grasp. These normal developmental behaviors are the basis for the following progressive pattern of introducing semisolid and table foods to older infants:

- **4 to 6 months.** Add iron-fortified infant cereals, starting with less allergenic rice and progressing to wheat and mixed grains.
- **6 to 8 months.** Add strained fruits and vegetables, progressing to strained or finely chopped table meats. Add finger foods (e.g., biscuits or dry toast) that can be secured with a palmar grasp.
- **9 to 12 months.** Gradually delete strained foods and introduce various table foods (e.g., chopped, well-cooked vegetables and meats and chopped, well-cooked or canned fruits). Use smaller finger foods as the pincer grasp develops. Add other well-cooked mashed or chopped table foods, all prepared without added salt or sugar, and help the child to drink moderate amounts of juice by cup.

Summary Guidelines

The Nutrition Committee of the American Academy of Pediatrics (AAP) has provided the following recommendations to guide infant feeding:

- *Breastfeeding* provides the ideal first food for the infant, continued for at least the first full year of life, supplemented with a vitamin K shot at birth, vitamin D (if lifestyle factors indicate a need), and iron-fortified foods after 6 months of age.
- *Commercial formulas* provide an alternative to breastfeeding during the first year of life; fluoride supplements may be mixed in if the local water supply is not fluoridated (after 6 months of age).

- *Solid foods* may be introduced at approximately 4 to 6 months of age, after the extrusion reflex of early infancy disappears and the ability to swallow solid food is established.
- *Whole cow's milk* may be introduced at the end of the first year if the infant is consuming one third of his or her kilocalories as a balanced mixture of solid foods, including cereals, vegetables, fruits, and other foods to supply adequate sources of vitamin C and iron. Reduced fat or fat-free cow's milk is not recommended until after the age of 2.
- *Iron-fortified formula* should be used for any infant not breastfeeding or for an older infant (e.g., more than 6 months of age) who does not consume a sig-

nificant portion of his or her kcalories from added solid foods.

- **Allergens** such as wheat, egg white, citrus juice, nuts, and chocolate should not be introduced as early solid foods but added later, after tolerance has been established through their gradual use.
- *Honey* should not be given to an infant under 1 year of age because botulism spores have been reported in honey and the immune system capacity of the young infant cannot resist this infection.
- *Food with high risk for choking* and aspiration, such as hot dogs, nuts, grapes, carrots, popcorn, cherries, peanut butter, and round candy, are best delayed for careful use only with the older child and not given to an infant.

Throughout the first year of life, the requirements for physical growth and psychosocial development are met by human milk or formula, a variety of solid food additions, and a loving, trusting relationship between parents and child.

Childhood

Toddlers (1 to 3 Years)

Once children learn to walk, at about 1 year of age, these toddlers are off and away, into everything and learning new skills. This dawning sense of self, which is a fundamental foundation for ultimate maturity, carries over into many areas, including food. After parents are accustomed to the rapid growth and resulting appetite of the first year of life, they may be concerned when they see their toddler eating less food and at times having little appetite, while being easily distracted from food to another activity (see the Clinical Applications box, "Toddler and Preschooler Feeding Made Simple"). Increasing the variety of foods available helps children develop good food habits. The food preferences of young children grow directly from the frequency of a food's use in pleasant surroundings and the increased opportunity to become familiar with a number of foods. Sweets should be reserved for special occasions, and not used habitually or as bribes to get a child to eat.

Preschool Children (3 to 5 Years)

Physical growth and appetite continue in spurts. Mental capacities develop and the expanding environment is gradually explored. Children continue to form life patterns in attitudes and basic eating habits as a result of social and emotional experiences. These varying experiences frequently lead to food jags (e.g., brief sprees or binges of eating one particular food) that last a few days but are usually short-lived and of no major concern. Again, the key to

happy and healthy eating is food variety and relatively small portions. The U.S. Department of Agriculture (USDA) developed a child-friendly version of MyPyramid with dietary and physical activity recommendations and messages designed to appeal to young children (Figure 11-4).

Group eating becomes a significant means of socialization (see the Clinical Applications box, "Toddler and Preschooler Feeding Made Simple"). For example, during preschool food preferences grow according to what the group is eating. Children in kindergarten also have early learning about healthy eating. The Five a Day, Let's Eat and Play program is designed for preschoolers and allows them to participate in food preparation and then eat their creation.[12] In another program, the Growing Healthy project, kindergartners plant and tend gardens of various vegetables as part of their learning experience.[13] In such situations a child learns a variety of different food habits and forms new social relationships.

School-Age Children (5 to 12 Years)

The generally slow and irregular growth rate continues in the early school years, and body changes occur gradually. In the year or two before adolescence, in particular, reserves are being laid for the rapid growth period ahead. This is the last lull before the storm. By this time, body types are established and growth rates vary widely. Girls' development usually bypasses boys' in the latter part of this period. With the stimulus of school and a variety of learning activities, children experience increasing mental and social development, the ability to work out problems, and competitive activities. They begin moving from dependence on parental patterns to the standards of peers, in preparation for coming maturity.

Food preferences are the products of earlier years, but school-age children are increasingly exposed to new stimuli, including television, which influence food habits. The relationship between sound nutrition and intellectual learning has long been recognized, establishing breakfast as a particularly important meal for school-age children. The school lunch program provides a nourishing noon meal for many children who otherwise would lack one. The classroom also provides positive learning opportunities, particularly when parents provide support at home. An interested and motivated teacher can integrate nutrition into many other learning activities. School breakfast and lunch

allergens food proteins eliciting an immune system response, or "allergic reaction." Symptoms may include itching, swelling, hives, diarrhea, difficulty breathing, or anaphylaxis, in the worst cases.

CLINICAL APPLICATIONS

TODDLER AND PRESCHOOLER FEEDING MADE SIMPLE

Parents waste a lot of time coaxing, arguing, begging, and even threatening their 2- to 5-year-olds to eat more than one and a half peas at dinner time. You can help save parents' time, tears, and energy by developing child-feeding strategies based on the normal developmental needs of their little ones.

1. Parents should be reminded of the following:
   - **Children are not growing as fast as they did during the first year of life.** Consequently, they need less food.
   - **Children's energy needs are irregular.** Just watch their activity level. Provide food as needed to help their bodies keep up with the many activities "planned" for each day.

2. The following suggestions may make child-feeding easier:
   - **Offer a variety of foods.** After a taste, put new food aside if not taken; then try again later to help develop broad tastes.
   - **Serve small portions.** Let children ask for seconds if they are still hungry.
   - **Guide children in serving themselves small portions.** Like adults, children's eyes tend to be bigger than their stomachs. Constant, gentle reminders help them learn when to stop.
   - **Avoid over-seasoning.** Let tastes develop gradually. If a food is too spicy, no amount of cajoling will make them eat it.
   - **Do not force foods that the child dislikes.** Individual food dislikes usually do not last very long. If the child shuns one food, offer a similar one if it's available at that meal (e.g., offer a fruit if the child rejects a vegetable) so that there's little chance of deficiency signs cropping up soon.
   - **Do not put away the main meal before serving dessert.** If there is a dessert, hold on to the main meal food. Amazing but true: if they're still hungry, some children will ask for more food from the main meal after finishing dessert.
   - **Keep "quick-fix" nutritious foods around for "off-hour" meals.** The word "snack" is not appro-

priate for the amount of food some youngsters eat between regular meals. To keep parents from turning into permanent short-order chefs, keep foods such as fresh and dried fruit, 100% fruit or vegetable juice, cheese, peanut butter, whole grain bread, and crackers to serve between meals and to provide essential nutrients.
   - **Enroll the child in a nursery school or preschool program.** Because food is not always available in the classroom, little students learn to eat at regular times. They also tend to try foods they rejected at home, probably because of peer pressure or a desire to impress a new authority figure, the teacher.
   - **Be patient.** Remember that although adults may be discussing world events over broccoli, toddlers are just now learning how to pick it up with their fork.

Toddlers may take longer. They may not even eat at all. Nevertheless, with flexibility, time, patience, and a sense of humor, most parents find that they can get enough nutrients into their children to keep them alive and happy throughout the preschool years. When presented with nutritious food choices, preschoolers tend to self-regulate their intake to meet energy needs without adult intervention.

For more information on typical feeding patterns for children, the following books are good sources:

- *How to Get Your Kid to Eat . . . but Not Too Much,* Ellyn Satter, RD, MSW (1997, Bull Publishing, Boulder, CO)
- *Child of Mine: Feeding with Love and Good Sense,* Ellyn Satter, RD, MSW (ed 3, 2000, Bull Publishing, Boulder, CO)
- *The American Dietetic Association Guide to Healthy Eating for Kids: How Your Children Can Eat Smart from Five to Twelve,* Jodie Shield, MEd, RD, Marry Mullen, MS, RD (2002, Wiley Publishing, Indianapolis)
- *Healthy Foods, Healthy Kids: A Complete Guide to Nutrition for Children from Birth to Six-Year-Olds,* Elizabeth Ward, MS, RD (2002, Adams Media Corporation, Avon, MA)
- *American Academy of Pediatrics Guide to Your Child's Nutrition: Making Peace at the Table and Building Healthy Eating Habits for Life,* edited by William H. Deitz, MD, PhD, FAAP, and Loraine Stern, MD, FAAP (1999, Random House, New York)

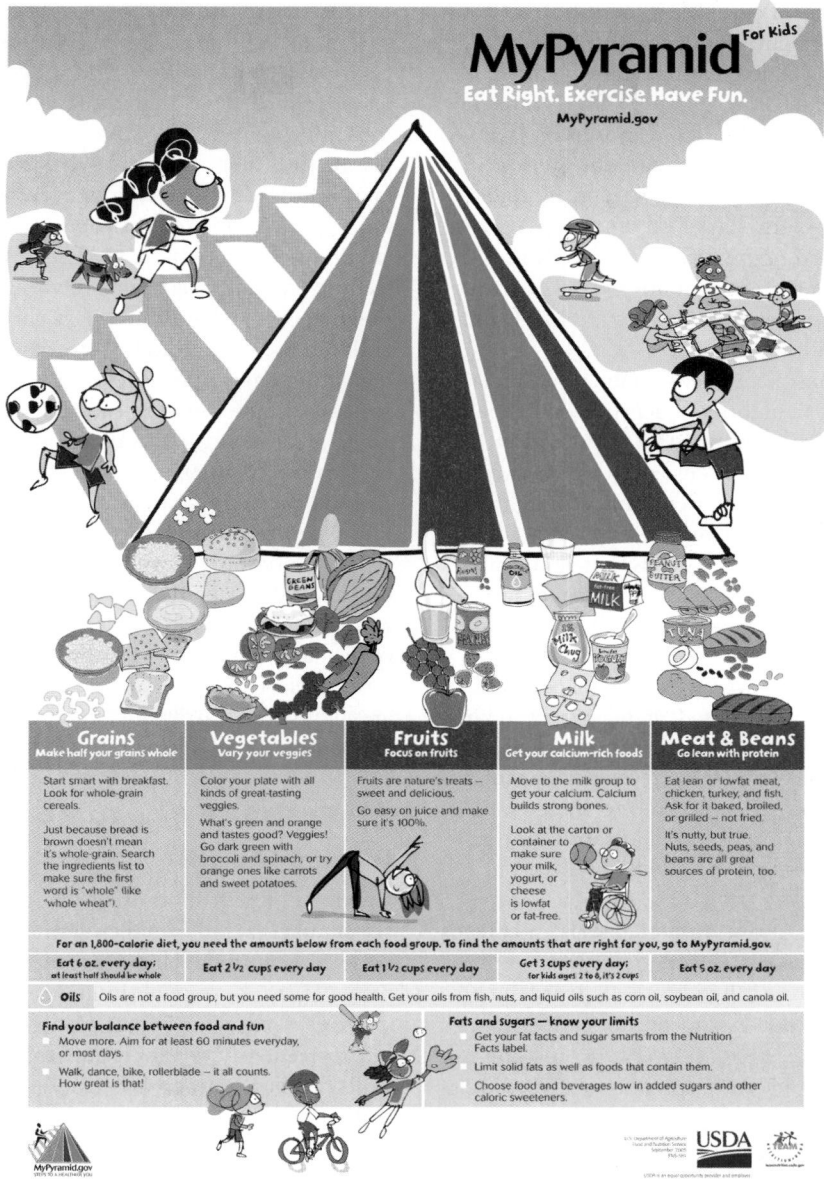

Figure 11–4   MyPyramid for Kids, targeted to meet the needs of children ages 6 through 11. (From U.S. Department of Agriculture, Team Nutrition: *MyPyramid for Kids: Advanced,* Washington, DC, 2005, Government Printing Office [*http://teamnutrition.usda.gov/Resources/mpk_poster2.pdf*].)

programs, which have a large effect on a child's health, are discussed further in Chapter 13.

Common Nutritional Problems in Childhood

Failure to Thrive. The term *failure to thrive* has been used in pediatrics to describe infants, children, or adolescents who fail to grow and develop normally. Failure to thrive most commonly affects young children (1 to 5 years) of

both sexes. Sometimes pediatricians use a brief hospital stay to classify infants who fail to thrive. Careful nutrition assessment is essential for identifying underlying causes of feeding problems. The following factors may be involved:

■ *Clinical disease.* Central nervous system disorders, endocrine disease, congenital defects, or partial intestinal obstruction.

■ *Neuromotor problems.* Poor sucking or abnormal muscle tone from the retention of primitive reflexes that should have already faded; eating, chewing, and swallowing problems.

■ *Dietary practices.* Parental misconceptions or inexperience about what constitutes a "normal" diet for infants; inappropriate formula feeding or improper dilutions in mixing formula.

■ *Unusual nutrient needs or losses.* Adequate diet for growth but inadequate nutrient absorption and thus excessive fecal loss; hypermetabolic state requiring increased dietary intake.

■ *Psychosocial problems.* Family environment and relationships resulting in emotional deprivation of the child, requiring medical-nutritional intervention; similar problems also may occur later (e.g., between 2 and 4 years of age) when parents and children have conflicts about normal changes caused by slowed childhood growth and energy needs that result in changing food patterns, food jags, erratic appetites, reduced milk intake, and disinterest in eating.

Failure to thrive is often caused by a complex of factors; and there are no easy solutions. Careful history taking, supportive nutritional guidance, and warm personal care are necessary to influence growth patterns in these infants and young children and are a big help to these families. Careful and sensitive correction of the social and environmental issues surrounding the problem is essential.

Anemia. Although the fortification of cereals and breads with iron has drastically reduced the cases of iron-deficiency anemia in the United States, it is still a common problem in children with certain eating trends. Children most often deficient in overall iron stores are those formula-fed infants who are not receiving iron-fortified formula and older infants (6 months and older) who are not consuming iron-fortified cereals and foods. *Milk anemia* is a term sometimes used for toddlers (more than age 1) who have excessive consumption of milk, which is a poor source of iron and displaces other iron-rich foods. These toddlers and parents are relying on cow's milk for the majority of their nutrient intake. Although these children also may be eating iron-fortified foods, the high calcium intake may inhibit the absorption of iron. Iron-deficiency anemia has been linked with delayed cognitive development in children.

Obesity. Childhood and adolescent obesity has been on the rise for the past 20 years and continues to climb. High blood pressure and type 2 diabetes, health concerns that have historically been associated with older, overweight adults, are increasingly becoming a problem in school-age children. Both genetics and environment play major roles in the risk for obesity; however, some researchers believe that these variables are unlikely to work independently.[14] Meaning that although overweight parents are more likely to have overweight kids, these families are also self-selecting environments that promote the development of obesity. Such environmental factors include high-fat food selection, or a restrictive feeding practice that ultimately results in overeating and binging, coupled with low physical activity. Infants and children are very capable of recognizing satiety and self-regulating energy needs. However, this innate awareness seems to decline between the ages of 3 and 5 when "super-sized" meal servings start to influence the amount of food eaten, despite satiety.[14]

Physical activity is an important part of a healthy lifestyle from birth to death. By developing an appreciation for, and an enjoyment of, regular physical activity during childhood, the risk for obesity may be reduced along with the health problems associated with it. On the other hand, long hours in front of a television, unnecessary snacking, and no involvement in physical activity are habits that start young, die hard, and set the stage for an overweight or obese childhood.

Adolescence (12 to 18 Years)

Physical Growth

The final growth spurt of childhood occurs with the onset of puberty. This rapid growth is evident in increasing body size and development of sex characteristics in response to hormonal influences. The rate of these changes varies widely among individual boys and girls, but particularly distinct growth patterns do emerge. Girls develop an increasing amount of fat deposit, especially in the abdominal area. As the bony pelvis widens in preparation for future childbearing and subcutaneous fat increases, the size of the hips also increases, causing much anxiety to many figure-conscious young girls. In boys, physical growth is seen more in increased muscle mass and long-bone growth. At first, a boy's growth spurt is slower than that of a girl, but he soon passes her in weight and height.

Researchers have found an association with the timing of sexual maturation and the risk for obesity. Females who experience sexual maturation early are more likely to become overweight or obese than females who do not mature until later.[15] However, this association is just the opposite for boys. Males who matured earlier were more likely to be thinner than their counterparts. There are also racial differences about timing of maturation; non-

Hispanic African-American girls and boys begin the process of sexual maturity before Mexican-American or non-Hispanic Caucasian children.[16] Such differences are specifically important when assessing growth on a growth chart. Age and stage of sexual maturation are associated with body fatness and overall weight (see the Cultural Considerations box, "Growth Charts: Can You Use Them for All Children?" for more information).

Eating Patterns

Teenagers' eating habits are greatly influenced by their rapid growth, as well as by their self-conscious peer pressure; hence, their acceptance of popular food fads. Teenagers tend to skip lunch more often than breakfast, derive a great deal of their energy from snacks, eat at fast-food restaurants because these are frequent "hangouts," and are likely to eat any kind of food at any time of day. Unfortunately, some teenagers begin to get a significant portion of their total caloric intake in the form of alcohol. Even a mild form of alcohol abuse, when combined with the elevated nutritional demands of adolescence, can easily affect their nutritional status. In general overall nutrition, boys usually fare better than girls. Their larger appetite and sheer volume of food consumed usually ensure an adequate intake of nutrients. On the other hand, under a greater social pressure for thinness, girls may tend to restrict their food and have inadequate nutrient intake.

Eating Disorders

Social, family, and personal pressures concerning figure control strongly influence many young girls, and an increasing number of young boys. As a result, they sometimes follow unwise, self-imposed "crash" diets for weight loss. In some cases, self-starvation occurs. Complex eating disorders such as *anorexia nervosa* and *bulimia nervosa*

may develop. Psychologists have traditionally identified mothers as the main source of family pressure to remain thin. However, fathers may also contribute to the problem if they are emotionally distant and do not provide important feedback to build self-worth and self-esteem in their young children. Parents must help their children see themselves as loved no matter what they weigh, so they are not as vulnerable to social influences that equate extreme thinness with beauty. Eating disorders can have severe effects and involve a distorted body image and a morbid, irrational pursuit of thinness. Such disordered eating often begins in the early adolescent years, when many girls see themselves as "fat" even though their average weight is often below the normal weight for their height. The longer the duration of the illness, the less likely full recovery will be achieved. Thus early detection and intervention are critical for restoration of overall health.[17] These eating disorders are discussed further in Chapter 15 on weight management.

Teenage Pregnancy

The number of teenage pregnancies continues to be a problem in the United States. With a background of inadequate diet, many of these girls are poorly prepared for the demands of pregnancy (see the Clinical Applications box "Pregnant Teenagers" in Chapter 10). They must complete their own growth and development while supplying the extra needs of the baby. A teenage girl who is not very nutritionally prepared for pregnancy is at risk for complications such as spontaneous abortion, premature labor, pregnancy-induced hypertension (PIH), and delivery of an immature, low-birth-weight baby. A girl who has maintained good nutrition has a better chance to deliver a healthy baby. These young mothers need much personal support and health care counseling to help reduce their infant mortality rate.

SUMMARY

Growth and development of healthy children depend on optimal nutritional support. In turn, this good nutrition depends on many social, psychological, cultural, and environmental influences that affect individual growth potential throughout the life cycle.

From birth, the nutritional needs of children change with each unique growth period. *Infants* experience rapid growth. Human milk is preferred as their first food, with solid foods delayed until about 6 months of age when their digestive and physiologic processes have matured. *Toddlers*, *preschoolers*, and *school-age children* experience slowed and irregular growth. During this period, their

energy demands are less, but they require a well-balanced diet for continued growth and health. Social and cultural factors influence their developing food habits.

Adolescents experience a large growth spurt before adulthood. This rapid growth involves both physical and sexual maturation. Boys usually obtain their increased caloric and nutrient demands because they eat larger amounts of food. Girls more often feel social and peer pressure to restrict their food to control their weight, causing some to develop severe eating disorders. This pressure may also prevent them from forming the nutritional reserves necessary for future childbearing.

CRITICAL THINKING QUESTIONS

1. Preterm and full-term infants have different nutritional needs. Explain why immature infants have special dietary needs.
2. Why is breastfeeding the preferred method of feeding infants? Compare breastfeeding with the commercial formulas available for bottle-fed babies.
3. Outline an appropriate schedule for a new parent to use as a guide for adding solid foods to his or her baby's diet during the first year of life. What foods are not appropriate at this age?

4. Compare the changes in growth and development of toddlers, preschoolers, and school-age children. What factors influence their nutritional needs and eating habits?
5. Consider the factors that influence the changing nutritional needs and eating habits of adolescents. Who is usually at greater nutritional risk during this period, boys or girls? Why? What suggestions do you have for reducing the nutritional risk at this vulnerable age?

CHAPTER CHALLENGE QUESTIONS

True-False

Write the correct statement for each item you answer "false."

1. *True or False:* A good way to keep infants and toddlers (birth to age 2) from being overweight is to use nonfat milk in their diets.
2. *True or False:* A variety of carbohydrate foods in a child's diet helps provide all the essential amino acids for growth.
3. *True or False: Failure to thrive* is a condition in pregnant women who fail to grow and develop normally throughout the pregnancy.

4. *True or False:* The rooting and sucking reflexes must be learned before a newborn infant can obtain milk from the breast.
5. *True or False:* A toddler needs the same food variety as an adult, according to the Food Guide Pyramid, but with larger serving sizes.

Multiple Choice

1. Fat is needed in the child's diet to supply
   a. minerals.
   b. water-soluble vitamins.
   c. essential amino acids.
   d. essential fatty acids.
2. An iron deficiency in childhood is associated with which of the following diseases?
   a. Scurvy
   b. Rickets
   c. Anemia
   d. Pellagra

3. Growth and development of a school-age child are characterized by
   a. a rapid increase in physical growth with increased food requirements.
   b. more rapid growth of girls in the latter part of the period.
   c. body changes associated with sexual maturity.
   d. increased dependence on parental standards or habits.

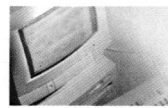

Please refer to the Students' Resource section of this text's Evolve web site for "Suggestions for Additional Study."

REFERENCES

1. Centers for Disease Control and Prevention, National Center for Health Statistics: *CDC growth charts: United States*, Atlanta, 2000, CDC [*www.cdc.gov/growthcharts/*].
2. Krebs NF: Bioavailability of dietary supplements and impact of physiologic state: infants, children and adolescents, *J Nutr* 131:1351S, 2001.
3. Grifin IJ, Abrams SA: Iron and breastfeeding, *Pediatr Clin North Am* 48(2):401, 2001.
4. Committee on Nutrition, American Academy of Pediatrics: Vitamins. In Kleinman RD, editor: *Pediatric nutrition handbook*, ed 4, pp 275-277, Elk Grove Village, IL, 1998, AAP.
5. Greer FR: Do breastfed infants need supplemental vitamins? *Pediatr Clin North Am* 48(2):415, 2001.
6. American Academy of Pediatrics Work Group on Breast-Feeding: Policy statement on breast-feeding, *Pediatrics* 100:1035, 1997.
7. Dewey KG: Nutrition, growth, and complementary feeding of the breastfed infant, *Pediatr Clin North Am* 48(1):87, 2001.
8. Dewey KG and others: Effects of exclusive breastfeeding for four versus six months on maternal nutritional status and infant motor development: results of two randomized trials in Honduras, *J Nutr* 131:262, 2001.
9. Browner YL and others: Early introduction of solid foods among urban African-American participants in WIC, *J Am Diet Assoc* 99(4):457, 1999.
10. Hill AJ: Developmental issues in attitudes to food and diet, *Proc Nutr Soc* 61(2):259, 2002.
11. Johnson SL: Children's food acceptance patterns: the interface of ontogeny and nutrition needs, *Nutr Rev* 60(5 pt 2):S91, 2002.
12. Levy PM, Cooper J: Five a day, let's eat and play: a nutrition education program for preschool children, *J Nutr Ed* 31:235B, 1999.
13. Casen KL: Children are "growing healthy" in South Carolina, *J Nutr Ed* 31:235A, 1999.
14. Birch LL, Davison KK: Family environmental factors influencing the developing behavioral controls of food intake and childhood overweight, *Pediatr Clin North Am* 48(4):893, 2001.
15. Wang Y: Is obesity associated with early sexual maturation? A comparison of the associations in American boys versus girls, *Pediatrics* 110(5):903, 2002.
16. Sun SS and others: National estimates of the timing of sexual maturation and racial differences among U.S. children, *Pediatrics* 110(5):911, 2002.
17. Rome ES and others: Children and adolescents with eating disorders: the state of the art, *Pediatrics* 111(1):98, 2003.

FURTHER READING AND RESOURCES

- KidsHealth: *www.kidshealth.org*
- National Center for Education in Maternal & Child Health: *www.ncemch.org*
- Tips for Using the Food Guide Pyramid for Young Children: *www.usda.gov/cnpp/KidsPyra/PyrBook.pdf*
- Using the Food Guide Pyramid: A Resource for Nutrition Educators: *www.nalusda.gov/fnic/Fpyr/guide.pdf*
- Kinetic: *www.kidnetic.com*

  The preceding web sites are excellent resources for childhood nutrition information. One of the most important parts of working with parents and children on feeding and health issues is to have access to up-to-date information and ideas. Explore the web sites above to discover current topics on health and nutrition issues facing youth today.

- Johnson RK, Nicklas TA: Position of The American Dietetic Association: dietary guidance for healthy children aged 2 to 11 years, *J Am Diet Assoc* 99(1):93, 1999.

  This position paper from The American Dietetic Association states the association's current position on the nutritional guidance for young children up to age 11. This paper also indicates the need for regular exercise.

- Li R, Grummer-Strawn L: Racial and ethnic disparities in breastfeeding among United States infants: Third National Health and Nutrition Examination Survey, 1988-1994, *Birth* 29(4):251, 2002.
- Davis SP and others: Childhood obesity reduction by school based programs, *ABNF J* 13(6):145, 2002.

  The two papers above explore racial and ethnic diversity in feeding practices and prevalence of obesity in the United States.

12

Nutrition for Adults: The Early, Middle, and Later Years

KEY CONCEPTS

■ Gradual aging throughout the adult years is an individual process based on genetic heritage and life experience.

■ Aging is a total life process, with biological, nutritional, social, economical, psychological, and spiritual aspects.

The rapid growth and development of the adolescent years bring humans to physical maturity as adults. Physical growth in size levels off but continues in the constant cell growth and reproduction necessary to maintain human bodies. Other aspects of growth and development (e.g., mental, social, psychological, and spiritual) continue for a lifetime.

Food and nutrition continue to provide essential support during the adult aging process. Life expectancy is lengthening, so health promotion and disease prevention are even more important as quality of life is ensured throughout the extended years.

This chapter explores the ways in which positive nutrition can help adults lead healthier and happier lives.

ADULTHOOD: CONTINUING HUMAN GROWTH AND DEVELOPMENT

Coming of Age in America

As the pace of modern life becomes faster in the twenty-first century, adults in America are experiencing tremendous change in the composition of the population and the impact of technology on the economy. The report from the U.S. Department of Health and Human Services, *Healthy People 2010: Understanding and Improving Health*, presents national goals for helping all people make informed decisions about their health.[1] The work of the U.S. Census Bureau and the President's Council of Economic Advisors also report on important changes in the population and the economy.[2,3]

Population and Age Distribution

By the year 2010, according to the U.S. Census Bureau, the U.S. population will have grown to 300 million people, up 9% from the year 2000 total of 275 million. The average size of American households will continue to decline, from 2.59 to 2.53 persons. The U.S. population will continue to become older for the next several decades, with its median age increasing from 36 years in 2000 to 37 years in 2010. The older segments of the population will grow significantly during this period; people over age 65 will increase from 35 to 40 million, and those over 85 will increase from 4.3 to 5.8 million (Figure 12-1).

Life Expectancy and Quality of Life

Life expectancy has increased dramatically over the past century, from only 47 years in 1900 to 77 years in 2000. By 2010, the average life expectancy will rise to 78 years. By gender, life expectancy in 2010 will be 74 for men and 81 for women. However, there are substantial differences in life expectancy among various population groups and household incomes (see the Cultural Considerations box, "Racial and Ethnic Composition of America's Population"). Women outlive men by an average of 6 years. Americans consistently value the health-related quality of life—one's personal sense of physical and mental health and ability to act within the environment—to be extremely important, and the quality of life is a major focus of the Healthy People initiative.[1]

Economic Expansion

During the second half of the 1990s, the United States economy experienced dramatic sustained growth.[3] By

> **life expectancy** the number of years a person of a given age may expect to live. Life expectancy is affected by environment, gender, and race.

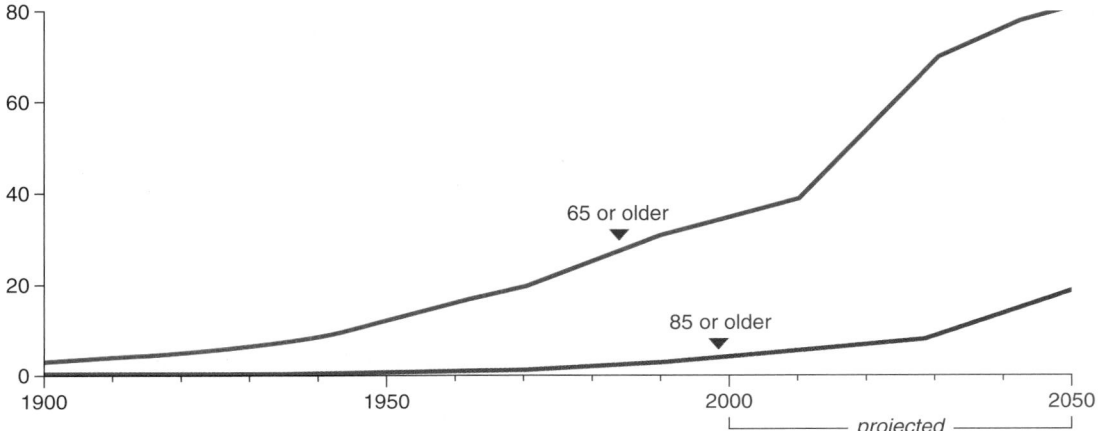

Total number of persons age 65 or older, by age group, 1900 to 2050, in millions

65 or older

85 or older

Note: Data for the years 2000 to 2050 are middle-series projections of the population.
Reference population: These data refer to the resident population.
Source: U.S. Census Bureau, Decennial Census Data and Population Projections.

Figure 12-1 Projections of the population for persons age 65 or older in the United States. (Data from Federal Interagency Forum on Aging-Related Statistics: *Older Americans 2000: key indicators of well-being*, Hyattsville, MD, (accessed October 2003), Federal Interagency Forum on Aging-Related Statistics [*www.agingstats.gov/chartbook2000/default.htm*].

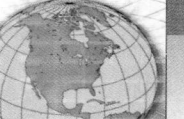

CULTURAL CONSIDERATIONS

RACIAL AND ETHNIC COMPOSITION OF AMERICA'S POPULATION

By the year 2010, a shifting racial and ethnic pattern will continue to reshape the American population as a whole. The U.S. Census Bureau projects that the proportion of Caucasians in the population, not including Hispanic Americans, will decline from 72% in 2000 to 68% in 2010. Hispanic Americans, the fastest-growing group in the country, will grow to 43 million people (14%), becoming the second largest segment of the population. By 2010, African Americans will number 37 million (12%). The racial and ethnic composition of the elderly population is also projected to change dramatically over the next half century.

Projected distribution of the population age 65 and older, by race and Hispanic origin, 2000 and 2050

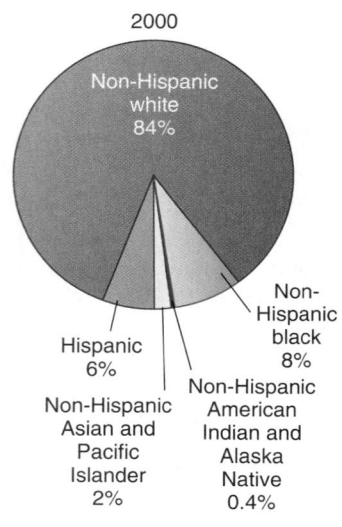

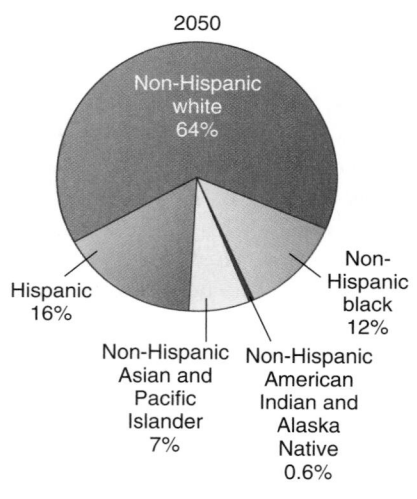

Note: Data are middle-series projections of the population. Hispanics may be of any race.
Reference population: These data refer to the resident population.
Source: U.S. Census Bureau, Population Projections.

Data from Federal Interagency Forum on Aging-Related Statistics, *Older Americans 2000: key indicators of well-being*, Hyattsville, MD, (accessed October 2003), Federal Interagency Forum on Aging-Related Statistics [*www.agingstats.gov/chartbook2000/default.htm*).

---

the year 2010, more than 50% of all jobs will be in information industries or require technical skills. The largest group of new entrants into the labor force will continue to be women.

Shaping Influences on Adult Growth and Development

Today's adults are growing and developing within this broader, rapidly changing world. The overall process of human aging begins at birth and lasts a lifetime. Each stage has unique potential for growth and fulfillment. The peri-

ods of adulthood—young, middle, and older years—are no exception. Many individual and group events mark the course; but at each stage, four basic areas of adult life— physical, psychosocial, socioeconomic, and nutritional— shape its general growth and development.

Physical Growth

Because physical maturity is reached in the late teen years, overall physical growth of the human body, governed by its genetic potential, levels off in the early adult years. Physical growth is no longer a process of increasing numbers of cells and body size but is the vital growth of new cells to replace old ones. This process maintains vigor and wholeness of body structure and function, increases learning, and strengthens mental capacities. Then at older ages, physical growth gradually declines and individual vigor reflects the health status of preceding years.

Psychosocial Development

Human personality development continues through the adult years. Three unique stages of personal psychosocial growth progress through the young, middle, and older years.

Young Adults (20 to 44 Years). With physical maturity, young adults are increasingly independent. They form many new relationships, adopt new roles, and make many choices concerning continued education, career, jobs, marriage, and family. Young adults experience considerable stress but also significant personal growth. These are years of career beginnings, establishing one's own home, and starting young children on their way through the same life stages, all part of early personal struggles to make one's way in the world. Sometimes health problems relate to these early stress periods.

Middle Adults (45 to 64 Years). The middle years often present an opportunity to expand personal growth. In most cases, children have grown and gone to make their own lives, and parents may have a sense of "it's my turn now." This is also a time of coming to terms with what life has offered, a "regrouping" of ideas, life directions, and activities. There is also a sort of regeneration of one's own life in the lives of young people following along a similar path. Early evidence of chronic disease appears in some middle adults. Wellness, health promotion, and reduction of disease risks are becoming the focus of health care.

Older Adults (65 Years and Older). Adults vary widely in their personal and physical resources to deal with older age. They may have a sense of wholeness and completeness, or they may increasingly withdraw from life. If the outcome of their life experiences is positive, they arrive at older ages as rich persons—rich in the wisdom of their years—and enjoy life and health, enriching the lives of those around them. But some elderly people arrive at these years poorly equipped to deal with adjustments of aging and the health problems that may arise. As this population continues to grow, the subdivision of young old (65 to 74), elderly (75 to 84), and old old (85+) has become increasingly popular and important as the general health and quality of life is ever improving.

Socioeconomic Status

We all grow up and live our lives in a social and cultural context. Now our rapidly changing world is experiencing major social and economic shifts. Most adults and their families are feeling the strain in some way. These pressures directly influence food security and health. As they age, many older persons find themselves under increasing financial pressure. Economic insecurity creates added stress and often leads to the need for food assistance (Figure 12-2). Sometimes social and financial pressures, along with a decreasing sense of acceptance and productivity, cause many elderly persons to feel unwanted and unworthy. Depression is a clinical syndrome, not part of normal aging, and is more common in women than men. Hospitalized elderly patients are particularly susceptible to depression, the leading cause of unintended weight loss in this population. One study identified 17% to 37% of elderly patients in a primary care facility as having depression.[4] All people need a sense of belonging, achievement, and self-esteem. Instead many elderly people are often lonely, restless, unhappy, and uncertain.[5]

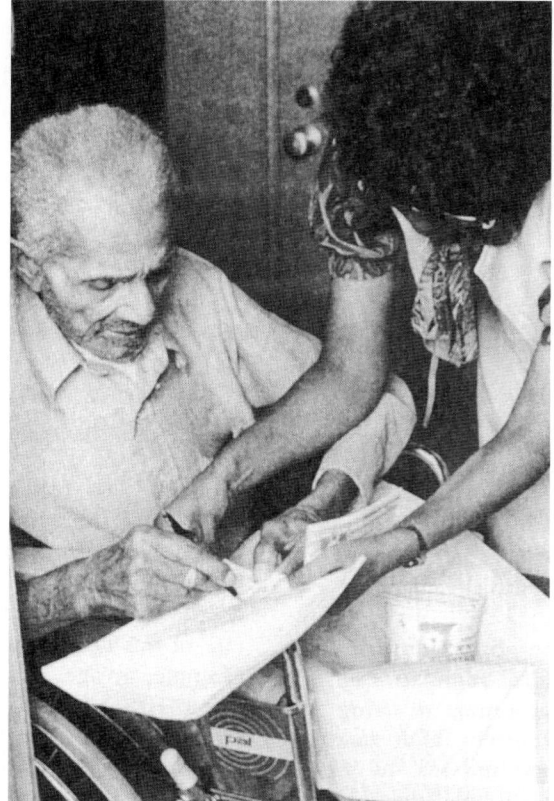

Figure 12-2 Elderly disabled man assisted by the Food Stamp Program to obtain needed food. (Credit: U.S. Department of Agriculture, Washington, DC.)

Basic needs common to older persons are economic security, personal effectiveness, suitable housing, constructive and enjoyable activities, satisfying social relationships, and spiritual values. An increasing number of very healthy, motivated, "young old" adults are contributing to the productive work force and are redefining what it means to be a senior citizen.

Nutritional Needs

The basic energy and nutrient needs of individual adults in each age group vary according to living and working situations. The Dietary Reference Intake (DRI) standards for healthy adults by age and sex supply most needs, but the aging process influences individual nutritional needs. Only in the most recent DRIs have scientists distinguished the nutrient needs of the 50- to 70-year-olds from the 71+ age group. One reason for this was a lack of a large enough population of healthy elderly adults to study their nutrient requirements and determine if their needs continue to change throughout the life span.

THE AGING PROCESS AND NUTRITIONAL NEEDS

General Physiologic Changes

Biological Changes

Human biological growth, and then decline, extends over the entire life span. Throughout life, all experiences make their imprint on individual genetic heritage. Everyone ages in different ways, depending on individual make-up and resources.

During middle and older adulthood, however, there is generally a gradual loss of functioning cells with reduced cell metabolism starting at approximately age 30. As a result, body organ systems gradually lose some capacity to do their jobs and maintain their reserves. The rate of this decline accelerates in later life. For example, by age 70 the kidneys and lungs lose about 10% of their former weight, the liver loses 18% of its weight, and skeletal muscle is reduced by 40%. Not all skeletal muscle mass loss is mandatory though. A major contributing factor in this loss is the lack of exercise. According to the Centers for Disease Control and Prevention (CDC), more than 60% of U.S. adults do not get the recommended amount of daily activity.[6] The Institute of Medicine, part of the National Academy of Sciences, recommends 60 minutes of moderate exercise every day to maintain a healthy weight.[7] (See Chapter 16 for more information on physical activity.)

Hormonal changes during the aging process have many repercussions in general health. The common de-

cline in insulin production often results in elevated blood glucose levels and diabetes. Decreases in melatonin, the hormone responsible for regulating body rhythms, may interfere with normal cycles of wakefulness and sleep. Part of the normal changes in body composition is attributed to decreases in growth hormone, and the sex hormones estrogen and testosterone. **Menopause,** the end of a woman's child-bearing years, is marked by the cessation of estrogen and progesterone production by the ovaries. This dramatic change in a woman's life, usually occurring between the ages of 35 and 58, represents the most significant hormonal change associated with age. The period of decline in estrogen and progesterone production is accompanied by an increase in body fat, a decrease in lean tissue, and an increase in the risk of chronic disease (specifically heart disease and osteoporosis). Despite these changes, women today are better equipped than ever before, with both social and medical support, to embrace this period of life and maintain health for many decades to come.

Effect on Food Patterns

Some of the physical changes of aging affect food patterns. For example, secretion of digestive juices and motility of gastrointestinal muscles gradually diminish, causing decreased absorption and use of nutrients. Decreased taste, smell, and vision also affect appetite and reduce food intake. Several other conditions commonly afflicting the elderly are not so obviously related to food intake but should be considered. For example, decreased hand function, which is especially common in the elderly,[8] can reduce one's hand-eye coordination and ability to cook and prepare food. Older persons often experience increased concern about body functions, more social stress, personal losses, and fewer social opportunities to maintain self-esteem. All of these concerns affect food intake. Much of what is considered "just aging" in older people is really the result of poor nutrition. Lack of sufficient nourishment is the primary nutrition problem of older adults.

Individuality of the Aging Process

The general process of **senescence** affects all older adults, although the biological changes in aging are general, each person is unique, and older persons show a wide variety of individual responses. Individuals get old at different rates and in different ways, depending on their genetic heritage and their health and nutrition resources of past years. Each older adult has specific needs. Some individuals are in the best shape of their lives *after* retirement! There are men and women completing marathons in the 80- to 85-year-old age group today.[9]

Nutritional Needs

Kilocalories: Energy

Because of gradual loss of functioning body cells and reduced physical activity, adults generally require less energy intake as they grow older. Basal metabolic rate (BMR) declines an average of 1% to 2% per decade with a more rapid decline occurring around age 40 for men and 50 for women.[7] The current national standard is based on estimates of 5% decreased metabolic activity in middle and older years. The mean energy expenditure for women (with a BMI of 18.5 to 25) ages 51 to 70 is 2066 kcal/day and for women over age 71 is 1564 kcal/day. For men of the same age and BMI, energy expenditure averages 2469 kcal/day and 2238 kcal/day, respectively.[7] These recommendations are based on averages of the population and may vary greatly between individuals. Physical and health status, as well as living situations, influence overall energy and nutrient requirements. Knowledge of the energy and nutrient needs of elderly persons also has many gaps. For example, there is doubt about traditional standards of "ideal" weight based on BMI tables. Ongoing review of these tables indicates that the weight ranges associated with longer lives are not necessarily the "desirable" weights given but weights 10% to 25% greater. Thus thin older adults, rather than those of moderate weight, have a reduced life expectancy. The basic fuels necessary to supply these energy needs are primarily carbohydrate, along with moderate fat.

Carbohydrate. About 45% to 65% of the total diet kilocalories should come from carbohydrate foods, with the majority being mostly complex carbohydrates (e.g., whole grains). The National Academy of Sciences has determined that an absolute minimum of 130 g of carbohydrates per day is necessary to maintain normal brain function for children and adults.[7] Easily absorbed sugars (simple sugars in soft drinks, candy, and sweets) also may be used for energy but should be used in limited amounts, no more than 10% of total kcalorie intake. There is a tendency for decreased glucose tolerance with aging. Decreased glucose tolerance is the "prediabetes" syndrome in which insulin response to glucose in the blood stream is inadequate to maintain blood glucose levels within a normal range. Although fasting blood glucose is elevated in individuals with glucose intolerance, it is not high enough for a diagnosis of diabetes. Balanced meals and snacks including carbohydrates, fat, and protein can help avoid excessively high blood glucose concentrations and help delay or avoid the onset of diabetes.

Fat. Fats usually contribute approximately 30% of total kcalories and provide a back-up energy source, important fat-soluble vitamins, and essential fatty acids. A reasonable goal is to avoid large quantities of fat and emphasize the quality of the fat used. Fat digestion and absorption may be delayed in elderly persons, but these functions are not greatly disturbed. Sufficient fat for helping food taste better aids appetite and in some cases provides needed kcalories to prevent excessive weight loss.

Protein. The current national standard recommends an adult protein intake of 0.8 g/kg of body weight, making the total protein need 56 g/day for an average-weight man and 46 g/day for an average-weight woman. Protein should provide approximately 10% to 35% of the total kcalories (see Chapter 4).[7] There may be an increased need for protein during illness, convalescence, or a wasting disease. In any case, protein needs are related to two basic factors, as follows: (1) the protein quality (the quantity and ratio of its amino acids), and (2) adequate total kcalories in the diet. Healthy adults consuming a balanced diet do not need supplemental amino acid preparations, which are an expensive and inefficient source of available nitrogen.

Vitamins and Minerals

A diet with a variety of foods should supply most vitamins and minerals in the amounts needed for healthy adults. Although, several of these essential nutrients may need special attention in relation to a few possible health problems in aging.[10]

Osteoporosis. Vitamin D and calcium are essential nutrients for growth and maintenance of healthy bone tissue. Osteoporosis is a disorder in which bone mineral density is low and bones become brittle with a high risk of breaking. Currently, 56% of women and 18% of men over the age of 50 have reduced bone mineral density.[11] The prevalence of low bone density and subsequent risk of developing osteoporosis increases significantly with age. Osteoporosis is 10 times more common in women over the age of 80 than that of women 50 to 59 years old.[11] Race and ethnicity are also determining factors in overall bone health in the elderly. According to the most

---

menopause (Gr. *men,* month; *pauses,* cessation) the end of menstrual activity and capacity to bear children.

senescence (L. *senescere,* to grow old) the process or condition of growing old.

recent National Health and Nutrition Examination Survey (NHANES III), low bone density is most common among Caucasian women, with Mexican-American women next and African-American women the least likely to develop osteoporosis.[11] Contributing factors include the following: (1) less use of calcium-rich food such as milk and other dairy products; (2) loss of appetite and lack of adequate body fat; (3) less outdoor physical exercise; and (4) decreased capacity of the skin to produce vitamin D with exposure to sunlight.[12,13] The DRI standards recommend an Adequate Intake (AI) level for vitamin D of 10 μg/day (200 IU) for both men and women age 51 to 70 and 15 μg/day (400 IU) for ages 70 and up (up from the 5 μg/day recommendation in earlier years).[14] To meet the dietary recommendation for vitamin D, elderly individuals should consume foods fortified with vitamin D or take a dietary supplement. Chapter 7 discusses food sources of calcium and vitamin D.

Anemia. The poor diet of many older adults lacks sufficient iron to prevent iron-deficiency *anemia*. These individuals need attention and encouragement to help them eat more iron-rich foods, along with vitamin C-rich foods for added iron absorption (see Chapter 8).

Nutrient Supplementation

Surveys indicate that 44% of women and 35% of men take vitamin supplements regularly, with higher use in non-Hispanic whites than either non-Hispanic blacks or Mexican Americans.[15] The use of nutrition supplements by elderly adults, usually on a self-prescribed basis, is common. Among all age and gender categories, supplement use is the highest in women over the age of 80 (55%)![15] Although such routine use may not be necessary, supplements are often recommended for persons in debilitated states or malabsorption. This is especially true for the malnutrition often seen in homebound elderly persons, for example, as was shown in a comprehensive study in Texas of a rural Hispanic population who were at serious nutritional risk.[16] In addition, the DRIs specify that individuals over the age of 50 should consume vitamin B_{12} in supplemental form *or* through fortified foods because of the high risk of deficiency resulting from decreased gastric acidity.[10] Hydrochloric acid is secreted from the gastric mucosal cells and is necessary for vitamin B_{12} digestion, along with intrinsic factor. However, as people age, production and secretion of this acid often decreases and results in inadequate vitamin B_{12} status. Such persons need a nourishing diet to help restore tissue strength and health.

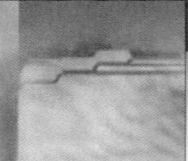

CLINICAL APPLICATIONS

FEEDING OLDER ADULTS WITH SENSITIVITY

Many older adults have eating problems and may easily become malnourished. Each person is a unique individual with particular needs and requires sensitive support to meet both nutritional and personal requirements. A personal approach, providing assistance for eating when needed, can help meet these needs.

Basic Guidelines

- *Analyze food habits carefully.* Learn about the attitudes, situations, and desires of the older person. Nutritional needs can be met with a variety of foods, so make suggestions in a practical, realistic, and supportive manner.
- *Never moralize.* Never say, "Eat this because it's good for you." This approach has little value for anyone, especially for those struggling to maintain their personal integrity and self-esteem in a youth-oriented, age-fearing culture that largely alienates its aged.
- *Encourage food variety.* Mix new foods with familiar "comfort foods." New tastes and seasonings often

encourage appetite and increase interest in eating. Many people think that a bland diet is best for all elderly persons, but it is not. The decreased taste sensitivity of aging necessitates added attention to variety and seasoning. Smaller amounts of food and more frequent meals also may encourage better nutrition.

Assisted Feeding Suggestions

- Make no negative remarks about the food served.
- Identify the food being served.
- Allow the person at least three bites of the same food before going on to another food to allow time for the taste buds to become accustomed to the food.
- Give sufficient time for the person to chew and swallow.
- If using a syringe to feed, never feed more than 30 ml (1 oz) at a time to allow enough time for the person to swallow and always remove the syringe from the mouth during swallowing.
- Give liquids throughout the meal, not just at the beginning and end.

CLINICAL NEEDS

Health Promotion and Disease Prevention

Reduction of Risk for Chronic Disease

The emphasis of adult health care is on reducing individual risks for developing chronic disease as persons grow older. This approach has always been used in development of the *Dietary Guidelines for Americans* and the national health objectives. These guidelines outline lifestyle changes that people can make to live healthier lives (see Figure 1-3, *Dietary Guidelines for Americans 2005*). The guidelines emphasize individual needs and good eating habits based on moderation and variety.

Nutritional Status

Many of the health problems of older adults not only result from general aging but also from states of malnutrition (see the Clinical Applications box, "Feeding Older Adults with Sensitivity"). This undernourishment may develop for several reasons, as follows: (1) poor food habits, often from lack of appetite or loneliness and not wanting to eat alone, as well as lack of sufficient money to buy needed food; (2) oral problems, such as poor teeth or poorly fitting dentures; (3) general gastrointestinal problems, such as declining salivary secretions and dry mouth with diminished thirst and taste sensations, less hydrochloric acid secretion in the stomach, decreased enzyme and mucus secretion in the intestines, and general decline in gastrointestinal motility. Older adults may voice concerns about adequate dietary fiber. Individual medical complaints range from vague indigestion or "irritable colon" to specific diseases such as *peptic ulcer* or *diverticulitis* (see Chapter 18). Box 12-1 outlines the DETERMINE signs of malnutrition.

A recent study published in the *Journal of American Dietetic Association* focused on the nutritional status of older adults and their dentition status (number of teeth). Researchers found a positive association between the number of teeth an individual had and his or her overall nutritional status as determined by both dietary intake and blood levels of certain nutrients.[17] They concluded that dental status should be a consideration during nutrition counseling and assessment.

Dehydration, a problem in any age group, is common in the elderly population. Reduced thirst sensation, coupled with declining function of the kidneys, can lead to an overall decline in body water status. Water needs, relative to total energy needs, do not decline with age.

Weight Management

Both excessive weight loss and excessive weight gain can be signs of malnutrition. Many of the same depressed living situations and emotional factors that result in unhealthy weight loss may also lead to excessive weight gain. Overeating or undereating becomes a compensation for the conditions encountered by some individuals in older age. Obesity among adults has been on the rise in all subgroups of the elderly population. The prevalence of obesity in men 45 to 54 increased from 12.5% to more than 30% between 1960 and 2000. Likewise, obesity in men in the age groups 55 to 64 and 65 to 74 more than tripled during that 40-year span. Women are not immune to this trend. Obesity among women increased as follows: women 45 to 54 experienced an increase from 20.3% to 38.1%; in women 55 to 64, obesity increased from 24.4% to 43.1%; and in women 65 to 74, obesity increased from 23.2% to 38.8% during the same time span.[18]

BOX **12–1** DETERMINE Your Nutritional Health: Warning Signs of Malnutrition

D Disease, illness, or chronic condition that causes you to change the way you eat, makes it hard for you to eat, or puts your nutritional health at risk.

E Eating poorly, either too little or too much, or avoiding whole food groups can lead to poor health.

T Tooth loss/mouth pain makes it difficult to eat.

E Economic hardship makes it very hard to purchase the foods you need to stay healthy.

R Reduced social contact may negatively affect morale, well-being, and appetite.

M Multiple medicines increase the chance for side effects such as increased or decreased appetite, constipation, change in taste acuity, weakness, diarrhea, nausea, etc.

I Involuntary weight loss/gain is an important warning sign of poor health.

N Needs assistance in self-care, such as walking, shopping, and cooking, may limit your ability to provide for yourself and increase your dependence on others who may or may not be around often enough to help meet your needs.

E Elder years above age 80 increases the risk of frailty and health problems.

From The Nutrition Screening Initiative: *Determine your nutritional health*, Washington, DC, (accessed October 2003), Nutrition Screening Initiative, a project of the American Academy of Family Physicians, and The American Dietetic Association, and funded in part by a grant from Ross Products Division, Abbott Laboratories Inc. [*www.aafp.org/x17367.xml*].

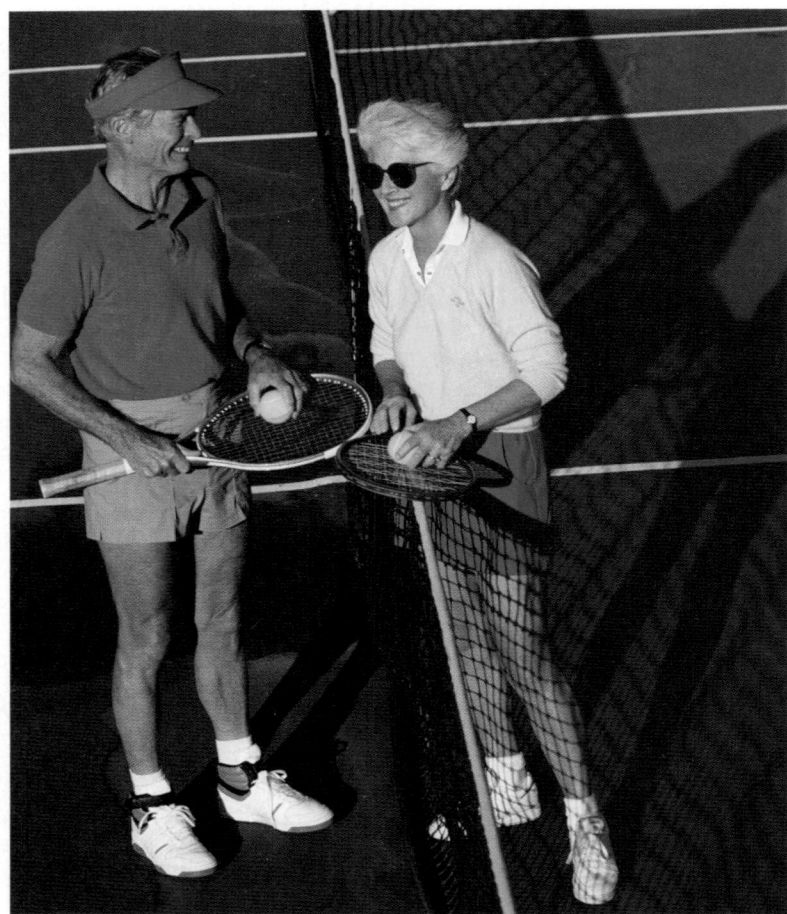

Figure 12–3 Healthy older adults enjoying physical exercise (Credit: PhotoDisc.)

BOX 12–2 Benefits of Physical Activity for Senior Adults

Physical activity has the following special benefits for older adults:

- Helps maintain the ability to live independently and reduces the risk of falling and fracturing bones
- Can help reduce blood pressure in some people with hypertension
- Helps people with chronic, disabling conditions improve stamina and muscle strength
- Reduces symptoms of anxiety and depression and fosters improved mood and feelings of well-being
- Helps maintain healthy bones, muscles, and joints
- Helps control joint swelling and pain associated with arthritis

From National Center for Chronic Disease Prevention and Health Promotion, Centers for Disease Control and Prevention: Benefits of physical activity for senior adults, *Chronic Disease Notes & Reports* 12(3):11, 1999.

As stated, physical activity is generally lacking in the American adult population. Not only is physical activity a major contributor to weight management, it can prevent many of the most debilitating conditions of old age.[19] As the population continues to age, health care facilities are adapting to the increasing need for aerobic and stretching classes aimed specifically at older adults who enjoy and benefit from daily exercise (Figure 12-3). Box 12-2 discusses the benefits of physical activity as indicated by the CDC.

Individual Approach

In all cases, personal and realistic planning with every person is essential. Individual personalities and problems are unique, and individual needs vary widely. A malnourished older person needs much personal, sensitive support to build improved eating habits (see the Clinical Applications boxes, "Feeding Older Adults with Sensitivity" and "Case Study: Situational Problem of an Elderly Woman").

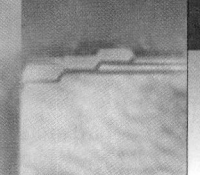

CLINICAL APPLICATIONS

CASE STUDY: SITUATIONAL PROBLEM OF AN ELDERLY WOMAN

Mrs. Johnson, a recently widowed 78-year-old, lives alone in a three-bedroom house in a large city. A fall 1 year ago resulted in a broken hip, and now she depends on a walker for limited mobility. Her only child, a daughter, lives in a distant city and does not care to bear the burden of responsibility for her mother. Mrs. Johnson's only income is a monthly Social Security check for $548. Her monthly property taxes, insurance payments, and utility bills amount to $461.

A recent medical examination revealed that Mrs. Johnson has iron-deficiency anemia and has lost 12 pounds in the past 3 months. Her current weight is 80 pounds; she is 5 feet, 2 inches tall. Mrs. Johnson states that she has not been hungry, and her daily diet is repetitious: broth, a little cottage cheese and canned fruit, saltine crackers, and hot tea. She lacks energy, rarely leaves the house, and appears emaciated and generally distraught.

Questions for Analysis

1. Identify Mrs. Johnson's personal problems and describe how they might have influenced her eating habits. How has her physical problem influenced her food intake?
2. What nutritional improvements could she make in her diet (include food suggestions), and how are these related to her physical needs at this stage of her life?
3. What practical suggestions do you have for helping Mrs. Johnson cope with her physical and social environment? What resources, income sources, food, and companionship can you suggest? How do you think these suggestions would benefit her nutritional status and overall health?

Chronic Diseases of Aging

Chronic diseases of aging (e.g., heart disease, cancer, arthritis, diabetes, Alzheimer's disease, and renal disease) may occur in adult years or at a younger age if given a strong family history. Approximately 80% of the elderly population suffers from at least one chronic disease and 50% have at least two. Health experts believe that chronic disease is not an inevitable consequence of aging and estimate that the majority of these cases could have been prevented by lifestyle modifications. The CDC recommends the following lifestyle changes to promote health and prevent chronic disease in adulthood: (1) stop smoking and limit alcohol intake, (2) be moderately physically active for half an hour on 5 days or more of the week, (3) maintain a healthy weight, and (4) eat a diet low in fat to control cholesterol levels.[19]

Diet Modifications

Diet modifications and nutritional support are an important part of therapy for chronic disease. Details of these modified diets are given in Chapters 17 to 23. In any situation, individual needs and food plans are essential for successful therapy.

Drugs

Because people are living longer (many with chronic diseases), older adults may be taking as many as 8 to 12 different prescription drugs for multiple health problems, in addition to over-the-counter drugs. Multiple medication use can affect overall nutritional status because many drug-nutrient interactions can occur (see Chapter 17 for more detail). Many of the medications often used by the elderly (blood pressure medication, antacids, anticoagulation medications, laxatives, diuretics, and decongestants) can directly affect appetite or absorption and use of nutrients, possibly contributing to malnutrition. Each person needs careful evaluation of all drugs used and instruction on how to take these medications in relation to food intake.

COMMUNITY RESOURCES

Government Programs for Older Americans

Older Americans Act

The Administration on Aging of the U.S. Department of Health and Human Services administers programs for older adults under the Older Americans Act Amendments of 1987. Nutrition programs are promoted through Title III—Grants for State and Community Programs on Aging, Part C—Nutrition Services. These services include both congregate and home-delivered meals, with related nutrition education and food-service components.

Congregate Meals. This program provides older Americans, particularly those with low incomes, with low-cost, nutritionally sound meals in senior centers and other public or private community facilities. In these settings, older adults can gather for a hot noon meal and have access to both good food and social support.

Home-Delivered Meals. For those who are ill or disabled and cannot attend the congregate meals, meals are delivered by couriers to their homes. This service meets nutritional needs and provides human contact and support. The couriers are usually volunteers concerned about the people and their needs. A courier is often the only person a homebound individual may contact during the day.

United States Department of Agriculture

The U.S. Department of Agriculture (USDA) provides both research and services for older adults.

Research Centers. Research centers for studies on aging are being established in various areas of the United States. For example, a Human Nutrition Research Center on Aging has been built at Tufts University in Boston and is the largest research facility in the United States specifically authorized by Congress to study the role of nutrition in aging. Studies there involve research on topics such as the protein needs of the aged, the nutritional status of elderly men and women, and the prevention and slowing of osteoporosis through nutritional support. Much more knowledge about the nutritional requirements of older adults is needed to provide better care.

Extension Services. The USDA operates agricultural extension services in state "land grant" universities, including food- and nutrition-education services. County home advisors help communities with practical materials and counsel for elderly persons and community workers.

Public Health Service

The Public Health Service (PHS) is a major division of the U.S. Department of Health and Human Services. Skilled health professionals work in the community through local and state public health departments. Public health nutritionists are important members of this health care team, providing nutrition counseling and education and helping with various food-assistance programs.

Professional Organizations and Resources

National Groups

The American Geriatric Society and the Gerontological Society are national professional organizations of physicians, nurses, dietitians, and other interested health care workers. These societies publish journals and promote community and government efforts to meet the needs of aging persons.

Community Groups

Local medical societies, nursing organizations, and dietetic associations sponsor various programs to help meet the needs of elderly people. An increasing number of qualified registered dietitians are also in private practice in most communities and can supply a variety of individual and group services. Senior centers in local communities are also valuable resources.

Volunteer Organizations

Many activities of volunteer health organizations (e.g., the American Heart Association and the American Diabetes Association) relate to the needs of older persons and may serve as both a rewarding opportunity for young old adults and an important source of health sustaining activities/information/resource for old old adults.

SUMMARY

Meeting the nutritional needs of adults—especially older adults—is a challenge for several reasons. We have lacked sufficient research on which to base the determination of energy and nutrient needs as persons grow older. Current and past social, economic, and psychological factors influence needs, and the biological process of aging differs widely in individuals. As the life expectancy continues to increase, research and recommendations on needs of an aging population are slowly uncovered.

Much of the illness in older adults results from malnutrition, not from the effects of aging. Thus in working with older people, food habits must be carefully analyzed and approached with encouragement to make any positive changes. Individual supportive guidance and patience are necessary, using available nutrition resources as needed.

CRITICAL THINKING QUESTIONS

1. Mr. Jones is a healthy, active 82-year-old man. He exercises regularly and enjoys a variety of foods. Recently he has started putting on weight. He says he eats exactly the same amount of food he ate when he was 30 years younger. How would you explain to Mr. Jones his weight gain and what suggestions would you make to prevent any additional unwanted weight gain?

2. Identify and describe three major factors contributing to malnutrition in older adults. How do these factors influence the nutrition-counseling process?

3. Your patient/client is on a limited budget and has poor vision with shaky hands. Knowing that fresh fruit and vegetables are often expensive and require washing and cutting, what suggestions would you make for your client to meet the suggested servings of five fruits and vegetables per day?

CHAPTER CHALLENGE QUESTIONS

True-False

Write the correct statement for each item you answer "false."

1. *True or False:* Older persons in American society generally are given much value and made to feel needed and productive.

2. *True or False:* Total energy needs slowly decline as we age, but water needs decline very rapidly.

3. *True or False:* Beginning at about the age of 30, a gradual increase occurs in the performance capacity of most organ systems that lasts throughout adulthood.

4. *True or False:* We have an extensive research base of knowledge about the nutritional needs of elderly persons and can state their specific energy and nutrient requirements.

5. *True or False:* The simplest basis for judging the adequacy of kcalorie intake is the maintenance of normal weight.

6. *True or False:* The protein requirement increases with age.

7. *True or False:* Exercise is not recommended for elderly individuals.

Multiple Choice

1. The basic biological changes of old age include:
   a. an increase in the number of cells.
   b. a decreasing need for water.
   c. an increased basal metabolic rate.
   d. a gradual loss of functioning cells and reduced cell metabolism.

2. The DETERMINE questionnaire is designed to identify signs of
   a. physical fitness.
   b. emotional stability.
   c. malnutrition.
   d. specific vitamin deficiencies.

3. Which of the following is an example of a physiologic change in aging? *(Circle all that apply.)*
   a. Increased cell metabolism to meet increased aging needs
   b. Decreased gastrointestinal motility
   c. A gradual increase in the body's muscle mass
   d. Decreased digestive secretions

4. Which of the following actions would help elderly persons in finding solutions to health problems? *(Circle all that apply.)*
   a. Analyze the individual living situation and food habits carefully.
   b. Reinforce good habits, leave harmless ones alone, and suggest needed changes that are practical within the living situation.
   c. Encourage variety in foods and seasonings.
   d. Explore and use available community resources for assistance.

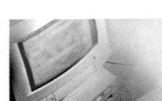

Please refer to the Students' Resource section of this text's Evolve web site for "Suggestions for Additional Study."

REFERENCES

1. U.S. Department of Health and Human Services: *Healthy people 2010: understanding and improving health*, Washington, DC, 2000, USDHHS/Government Printing Office.

2. U.S. Census Bureau, U.S. Department of Commerce: *Statistical abstract of the United States 1999*, ed 119, Washington, DC, 1999, U.S. Department of Commerce/Government Printing Office.

3. Council of Economic Advisors: *Economic report of the President*, Washington, DC, 2000, Council of Economic Advisors/Government Printing Office.

4. Alexopoulous GS: Depression and other mood disorders, *Clin Geriatr* 8(11):69, 2000.

5. Serby M, Yu M: Overview: depression in the elderly, *Mt Sinai J Med* 70(1):38, 2003.

6. National Center for Chronic Disease Prevention and Health Promotion, Centers for Disease Control and Prevention: *Physical activity and health: a report of the surgeon general, adults*, Atlanta, (accessed March 2003), NCCDPHP/CDC [*www.cdc.gov/nccdphp/sgr/adults.htm*].

7. Food and Nutrition Board, Institute of Medicine: *Dietary reference intakes for energy, carbohydrate, fiber, fat, fatty acids, cholesterol, protein, and amino acids*, Washington, DC, 2002, National Academies Press.

8. Carmeli E and others: The aging hand, *J Gerontol A Biol Sci Med Sci* 58(2):M146, 2003.

9. New York Road Runners: *New York City Marathon 2002 results: age group and team awards*, New York, (accessed March 2003), New York Road Runners [*www.nyrrc.org/race/2001/malawr.htm*].

10. Food and Nutrition Board, Institute of Medicine: *Dietary reference intakes for thiamin, riboflavin, niacin, vitamin B_6, folate, vitamin B_{12}, pantothenic acid, biotin, and choline*, Washington, DC, 1999, National Academies Press.

11. National Center for Health Statistics, Centers for Disease Control and Prevention: *National Health and Nutrition Examination Survey: osteoporosis*, Hyattsville, MD, (accessed March 2003), NCHS/CDC/USDHHS [*www.cdc.gov/nchs/data/nhanes/databriefs/osteoporosis.pdf*].

12. Packard PT, Heaney RP: Medical nutrition therapy for patients with osteoporosis, *J Am Diet Assoc* 97:414, 1997.

13. Ullom-Minnich P: Prevention of osteoporosis and fractures, *Am Fam Phys* 60(1):194, 1999.

14. Food and Nutrition Board, Institute of Medicine: *Dietary reference intakes for calcium, phosphorus, magnesium, vitamin D, and fluoride*, Washington, DC, 1997, National Academies Press.

15. National Center for Health Statistics, Centers for Disease Control and Prevention, U.S. Department of Health and Human Services: *National Health and Nutrition Examination Survey: use of dietary supplements*, Hyattsville, MD, (accessed March 2003), NCHS/CDC/USDHHS [*www.cdc.gov/nchs/data/nhanes/databriefs/dietary.pdf*].

16. Marshall JA and others: Indicators of nutritional risk in a rural elderly Hispanic and non-Hispanic white population: the San Luis Valley health and aging study, *J Am Diet Assoc* 99(3):315, 1999.

17. Sahyoun NR and others: Nutritional status of the older adult is associated with dentition status, *J Am Diet Assoc* 103:61, 2003.

18. National Center for Health Statistics, Centers for Disease Control and Prevention, U.S. Department of Health and Human Services: *Healthy weight, overweight, and obesity among persons 20 years of age and over, according to sex, age, race, and Hispanic origin: United States, 1960-1962, 1971-1974, 1976-1980, 1988-1994, and 1999-2000*, Hyattsville, MD, (accessed March 2003), NCHS/CDC/USDHHS [*www.cdc.gov/nchs/data/hus/tables/2002/02hus070.pdf*].

19. National Center for Chronic Disease Prevention and Health Promotion: *Preventing the diseases of aging, Chronic Disease Notes & Reports* 12(3):1, 1999 [*www.cdc.gov/nccdphp/cdfall99.pdf*].

FURTHER READING AND RESOURCES

- Administration on Aging: *www.aoa.dhhs.gov*
- Centers for Medicare & Medicaid Services: *http://cms.hhs.gov*
- National Institute on Aging: *www.nia.nih.gov/*
- American Society on Aging: *www.asaging.org*
- Gerontological Society of America: *www.geron.org*
- National Council on the Aging: *www.ncoa.org*
- Eldercare Locator: *www.eldercare.gov*

  The organizations listed above are excellent sources of information on elderly nutrition, health, and community services for the elderly.

- Kamel HK: Sarcopenia and aging, *Nutr Rev* 61(5):157, 2003.

  This article discusses the preventable, and unavoidable, loss of muscle mass (sarcopenia) associated with age. Causes (malnutrition, decreased physical activity, and reduced hormone production) and effects (physical disability, frailty, hormonal irregularity) of sarcopenia are explored.

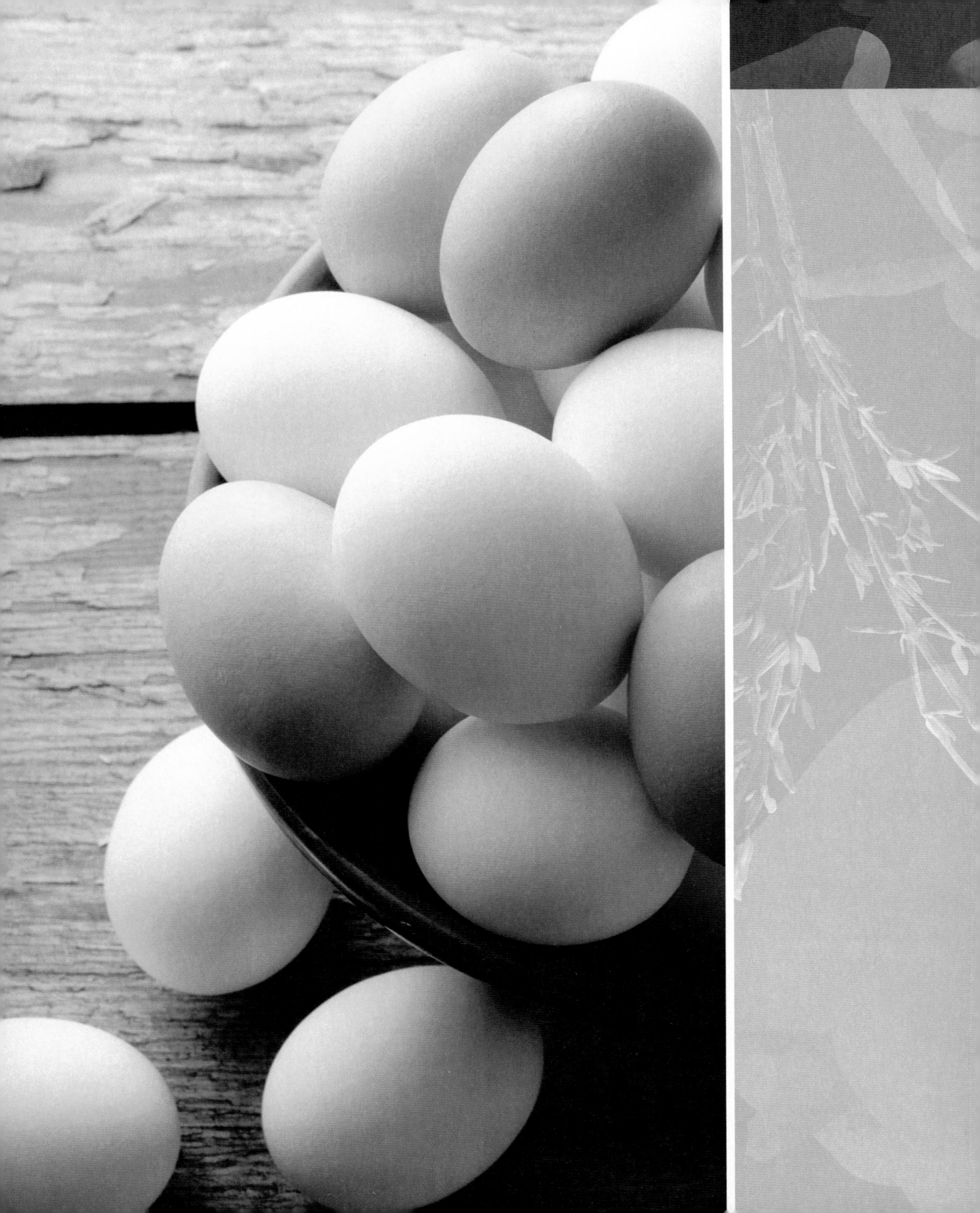

Community Nutrition and Health Care

13

Community Food Supply and Health

T he health of a community largely depends on the safety of its available food and water supply. The American system of government control agencies and regulations, along with local and state public health officials, works diligently at maintaining a safe food supply and is generally, but not always, successful. The food supply in the United States has undergone dramatic changes over the past few decades.

This chapter explores factors that influence the safety of the food. America's bountiful food supply is accompanied by certain hazards. Potential health problems related to the food supply can arise from several sources, such as lack of sanitation, food-borne disease, and poverty.

KEY CONCEPTS

■ Modern food production, processing, and marketing have both positive and negative influences on food safety.

■ Many organisms in contaminated food transmit disease.

■ Poverty often prevents individuals and families from having adequate access to their surrounding community food supply.

FOOD TECHNOLOGY

The character of America's food supply has changed radically over the years. These changes, which have swept the food-marketing system, are rooted in widespread social changes and scientific advances. The agricultural and food processing industries have developed various chemicals to increase and preserve the food supply. However, critics voice concerns about how these changes have affected food safety and the overall environment. Such concerns are usually focused on pesticide use and food additives.

Agricultural Pesticides

Reasons for Use

Large American agricultural corporations, as well as individual farmers, use a number of chemicals to improve their crop yields. These materials have made the advances in food production necessary to feed a growing population possible. For example, farmers use certain chemicals to control a wide variety of destructive insects that reduce crop yield (Figure 13-1).

Problems

Concerns and confusion continue about the use and effects of these chemicals. Problems have developed in four main areas, as follows: (1) the pesticide residues on foods; (2) the gradual leaching of the chemicals into ground water and surrounding wells; (3) the increased exposure of farm workers to these strong chemicals; and (4) the increased amount of chemicals necessary as insects develop a tolerance. Over time, use of these chemicals has created a pesticide dilemma: What do we do in the face of conflicting interests? Thousands of pesticides are in use, and assessing the risks of specific pesticides in use is a very important, but difficult, task.

Alternative Agriculture

An increasing number of concerned farmers, with help from soil scientists, are turning to alternative agricultural methods instead of heavy reliance on pesticide use.

Organic Farming. Organic plant foods are grown without synthetic pesticides, fertilizers, sewage sludge, bioengineering, or ionizing radiation. Organic meat, poul-

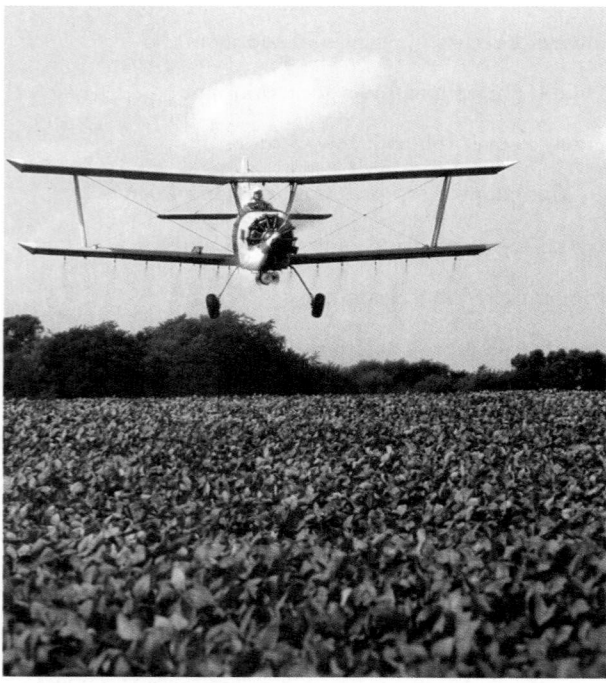

Figure 13–1   Farmer applies insecticide to corn crop. (Credit: Ken Hammond, Agricultural Research Service, U.S. Department of Agriculture, Washington, DC.)

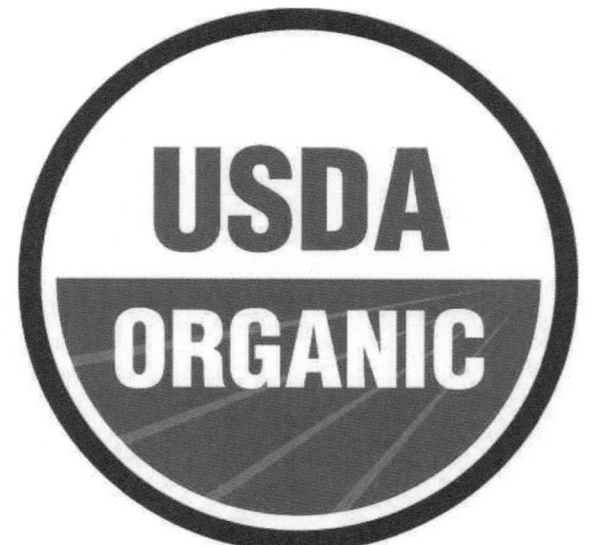

Figure 13–2   Official U.S. Department of Agriculture (USDA) organic seal, available at *www.ams.usda.gov/nop/ Consumers/Seal.htm.* (From The National Organic Program, Agricultural Marketing Service, U.S. Department of Agriculture, Washington, DC.)

try, eggs and dairy products are from animals raised without antibiotics or growth hormones. As of October 2002, the U.S. Department of Agriculture enacted a set of nationally recognized standards to identify certified "organic" food. For a food to carry the U.S. Department of Agriculture (USDA) Organic Seal (Figure 13-2), the farm and processing plant where the food was grown and packaged must have undergone government inspections and have met the strict USDA organic standards (see the For Further Focus, "Organic Food Standards"). All foods produced organically are not required to use the organic label; it is a voluntary program. However, companies using the label on their food without certification face a fine of up to $10,000.[1] Sales of organic foods are rapidly growing and an increasing number of farmers, especially in California, the major supplier of U.S. fruits and vegetables, are using **organic farming.**

Certified organic foods are not recognized as being more safe or nutritious than conventionally produced foods. Organic farmers can still use natural pesticides and fertilizers and therefore are not pesticide-free foods. Other common points of confusion are in the use of the following terms: natural, hormone free, and free range. These terms are not synonymous with "organic." Truthful terms

organic farming farming methods that use natural means of pest control and meet the standards set by the USDA National Organic Program. Organic foods are grown or produced without the use of synthetic pesticides or fertilizers, sewage sludge, or ionizing radiation.

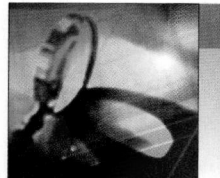

FOR FURTHER FOCUS

ORGANIC FOOD STANDARDS

The National Organic Program, a constituent of the USDA, was established to ensure standards of "organic" foods. In response to the growing market for organic foods, the National Organic Program has set strict standards for the growth, production, and labeling of organic foods. Although many methods prohibited by the organic standards, such as irradiation and genetic modifications, are deemed safe by the USDA, these methods of farming have been banned in certified organic foods because of public concern.

There are four labeling categories for organic foods with specific guidelines for each, as follows:

- *100% Organic:* Products carrying this label must be made or produced exclusively with certified organic ingredients and must have passed a government inspection. These products may use the USDA Organic Seal on their label and advertisements.
- *Organic:* Products labeled as "organic" must contain 95% to 100% organic ingredients and also must have passed a government inspection. The National Organic Program must approve all other ingredients for use as nonagricultural substances or products not commercially available in organic form. These products may also use the USDA Organic Seal with the percent of organic ingredients listed.

- *70% Organic ingredients:* Products made with at least 70% certified organic ingredients may state on the product label: "made with organic ingredients," and list up to three ingredients or food groups. These foods must also meet the National Organic Program guidelines for growth or production without synthetic pesticides, fertilizers, sewage sludge, or ionizing radiation. The USDA Organic Seal may not be displayed on these products or used in advertising.
- *Less than 70% organic ingredients:* Foods made with less than 70% certified organic ingredients may not use the USDA Organic Seal or make any organic claims on the front panel of the package. They can list the specific organic ingredients on the side panel of the package.

All food products with at least 70% organic ingredients must also supply the name and address of the government-approved certifying agent on the product.

For more information on the USDA organic standards, visit the National Organic Program web site at *www.ams. usda.gov/nop/,* call the National Organic Program at 202-720-3252, or write to USDA-AMS-TM-NOP, Room 4008 S. Bldg., Ag Stop 0268, 1400 Independence SW, Washington, DC 20250.

about the production of a food can appear on the food label but do not mean that the product is organic. The term "natural" may be used on products that contain no artificial ingredients, coloring ingredients, or chemical preservatives; and the product and its ingredients are not more than minimally processed. The Food Safety and Inspection Service of the USDA do not approve the terms *hormone free* or *antibiotic free*. Instead, the phrases *raised without added hormones* and *raised without added antibiotics* are allowed, provided that the producer is able to supply an affidavit attesting to the production practices employed that support the claim. One important note about the use of hormones is that they are only approved for use in beef cattle and lamb production. Therefore any such claim on a chicken product would be allowed only if it were followed immediately with the statement, "Federal regulations prohibit the use of hormones in poultry."

Genetic Modification. Plant physiologists are developing strains of genetically modified (GM) foods that reduce the need for toxic pesticides and herbicides. Genetic manipulation, in various forms, has been used to improve crops for thousands of years, but most U.S. consumers are unaware of the extent to which these foods have entered the marketplace.[2] More than 60% of processed foods contain some form of genetically modified ingredients; therefore most all people in the United States have consumed some form of GM foods at some point, such as a seedless orange or watermelon! An example of biotechnology in today's agriculture is the use of genetically modified corn that expresses a specific protein that ultimately serves as an insecticide. Organic farmers have used this type of biotechnology for more than 40 years. Approved genetic modifications currently are used to protect against virus infections and insects on tomatoes, potatoes, squash, and papaya, among others.[2] Genetically engineered crops are tested extensively on composition, safety, and environmental effects. The National Institute of Health (NIH), Animal Plant Health Inspection Service of the USDA, Food and Drug Administration (FDA), and the Environmental Protection Agency (EPA) are all involved in the strict regulation of genetically modified foods in commercial use, which are the most heavily regulated new foods.

The benefits of genetic modifications are not limited to benefits to the producer. Technology is advancing to the point of engineering food to increase its nutritional value, medicinal properties, taste, and esthetic appeal.[2] Plants are produced with increased fiber, antioxidants, and essential amino acids, all of which are beneficial to the consumer and may have positive effects on human nutrition worldwide.[3] More than 50 biotechnology crop products are approved for commercialization in the United States (Figure 13-3).

Irradiation. Irradiation can kill bacteria and parasites on the food after harvest. Irradiation helps prevent foodborne illness caused by *E. coli, Salmonella, Campylobacter, Listeria, Cyclospora, Shigella,* and *Salmonella.*[4] There are three different methods of irradiation, all of which are approved by the World Health Organization (WHO), Centers for Disease Control and Prevention (CDC), USDA, and FDA. The use of irradiation is not a *new* science; wheat flour and white potatoes were approved for irradiation in the early 1960s. In addition to reducing or eliminating disease-causing germs, irradiation can be used to increase the shelf-life of produce. Foods that are irradiated: (1) have essentially unaltered nutritional value, (2) are not radioactive, (3) have no harmful substances introduced as a result of irradiation, but (4) may taste slightly different.[4] A variety of foods have been approved for irradiation in the United States, including meat, poultry, grains, some seafood, fruits, vegetables,

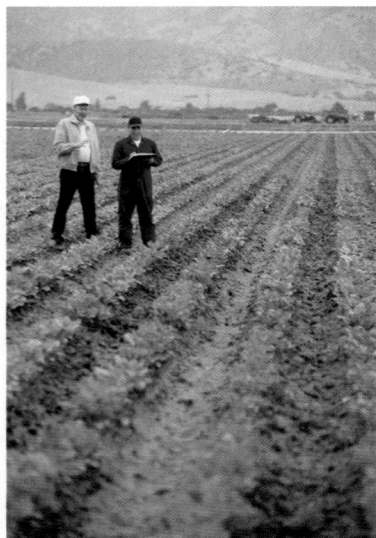

Figure 13-3 Geneticist and technician evaluate sugar beet breeding in California. (Credit: Scott Bauer, Agricultural Research Service, U.S. Department of Agriculture, Washington, DC.)

Figure 13-4 Radura symbol of irradiation, available at *www.fsis. usda.gov/OA/pubs/image_library/index. htm.* (From Food Safety and Inspection Service, U.S. Department of Agriculture, Washington, DC.)

herbs, and spices. The FDA requires all irradiated foods be appropriately labeled with either the radura symbol for irradiation (Figure 13-4) or by a written description stating the food has been exposed to irradiation.

Food Additives

The use of *food additives* (e.g., chemicals intentionally added to foods to prevent spoilage and extend shelf-life) is not new to the food industry either. The two most common additives are sugar and salt, although people often forget to include these basic ingredients as "food additives." Some additives have been used for centuries as preservatives, especially salt in cured meats.

Over the past few decades, the number and variety of food additives have increased in the food supply. The current variety of food market items would be impossible without them. Scientific advances have created these processed food products, and the changing society has created the market for them. The expanding population, greater work force, and more complex family life have increased the desire for more variety and convenience in foods, as well as better safety and quality. Food additives help achieve these needs and serve many purposes. For example, additives do the following: (1) enrich foods with added nutrients; (2) produce uniform qualities (e.g., color, flavor, aroma, texture, and general appearance); (3) standardize many functional factors (e.g., thickening or stabilization [keeping parts from separating]); (4) preserve foods by preventing oxidation; and (5) control acidity or alkalinity to improve flavor, texture, and the cooked product. Table 13-1 lists some examples of food additives. A number of micronutrients and antioxidants are used as additives in processed foods, not for their ability to increase nutrient content but for their technical effects either during processing or in the final product.

FOOD SAFETY AND HEALTH PROMOTION
Government Control Agencies

The food supply in the Unites States has exploded in recent years. Keeping the food supply safe is no small task. Several federal agencies now help control the safety and quality of our food. The *FDA* is the primary governing body of American food supply, with exception of meat and poultry. The *USDA Food Safety and Inspection Service* (FSIS) is responsible for food safety of both domestic and imported meat and poultry (Figure 13-5). The *National Marine Fisheries Service* (NMFS) is responsible for the safety of seafood and fisheries. The *Environmental*

Protection Agency (EPA) regulates the use of pesticides and other chemicals, in addition to ensuring the safety of public drinking water. Regulation of advertising and truthful marketing of food products is in itself a large job and is the duty of the *Federal Trade Commission* (FTC). The *Centers for Disease Control and Prevention* (CDC) monitors and investigates cases of food-borne illness and is proactive in education and prevention against it. There are multiple other federal, state, and local agencies participating in education and research to promote safety in the food supply.

Food and Drug Administration
Enforcement of Federal Food-Safety Regulations. The FDA is a law enforcement agency charged by the U.S. Congress to ensure, among other things, that America's food supply is safe, pure, and wholesome. The agency enforces federal food-safety regulations through various activities, including the following: (1) enforcing food sanitation and quality control; (2) controlling food additives; (3) regulating the movement of foods across state lines; (4) maintaining the nutrition labeling of foods; (5) ensuring the safety of public food service; and (6) ensuring the safety of most food products. The agency's methods of enforcement are recall, seizure, injunction, and prosecution. The use of recalls is the most common method, followed by seizures of contaminated food.

Consumer Education. The FDA's division of consumer education conducts an active program of protection through consumer education and general public information. Special attention is given to nutrition misinformation. Materials are prepared and distributed to individuals, students, and community groups. Consumer specialists work through all FDA district offices.

Research. Along with the USDA's Agricultural Research Service, FDA scientists continually evaluate foods and food components through their own research. For a more health-conscious public and a changed marketplace, the FDA is developing nutrition guidelines for a variety of food products, including main dishes, meat substitutes, fruit juices and fruit drinks, and snack foods.

Development of Food Labels
Early Development of Label Regulations

In the mid-1960s, the FDA established "truth in packaging" regulations that dealt mainly with food standards. As food processing developed and the number of items grew, the labels also needed to have more nutrition information added. Both types of label information are important to consumers.

TABLE 13–1	Examples of Food Additives	
Function	**Chemical compound**	**Common food uses**
Acid, alkalis, buffers	Sodium bicarbonate	Baking powder
	Tartaric acid	Fruit sherbets
		Cheese spread
Antibiotics	Chlortetracycline	Dip for dressed poultry
Anticaking agents	Aluminum calcium silicate	Table salt
Antimycotics	Calcium propionate	Bread
	Sodium propionate	Bread
	Sorbic acid	Cheese
Antioxidants	Butylated hydroxyanisole (BHA)	Fats
	Butylated hydroxytoluene (BHT)	Fats
Bleaching agents	Benzoyl peroxide	Wheat flour
	Chlorine dioxide	
	Oxides of nitrogen	
Color preservative	Sodium benzoate	Green peas
		Maraschino cherries
Coloring agents	Annatto	Butter, margarine
	Carotene	
Emulsifiers	Lecithin	Bakery goods
	Monoglycerides and diglycerides	Dairy products
		Confections
	Propylene glycol alginate	
Flavoring agents	Amyl acetate	Soft drinks
	Benzaldehyde	Bakery goods
	Methyl salicylate	Candy, ice cream
	Essential oils, natural extractives	Canned meats
	Monosodium glutamate	Meat, vegetables, and sauces
Nonnutritive sweeteners	Saccharin	Diet canned fruit
	Aspartame	Low-calorie soft drinks
Nutrient supplements	Potassium iodide	Iodized salt
	Vitamin C	Fruit juices
	Vitamin D	Milk
	Vitamin A	Margarine
	B vitamins, iron	Bread and cereal
Sequestrants	Sodium citrate	Dairy products
	Calcium pyrophosphoric acid	
Stabilizers and thickeners	Pectin	Jellies
	Vegetable gums (carob bean, carrageenan, guar)	Dairy desserts, chocolate milk
	Gelatin	Confections
	Agar-agar	"Low-calorie" salad dressings
Yeast foods and dough conditioners	Ammonium chloride	Bread, rolls
	Calcium sulfate	
	Calcium phosphate	

Food Standards. The basic *standard of identity* requires that labels on foods not having an established reference standard must list all the ingredients in the order of amount found in the product. Other food standard information on labels relates to food quality, fill of container, and enrichment.

Nutrition Information. Under regulations adopted in 1973, the FDA began developing a labeling system that describes a food item's nutritional value to meet the increasing interest and concern of consumers. Some producers began to add limited information on their own to meet this increasing market demand. Many persons be-

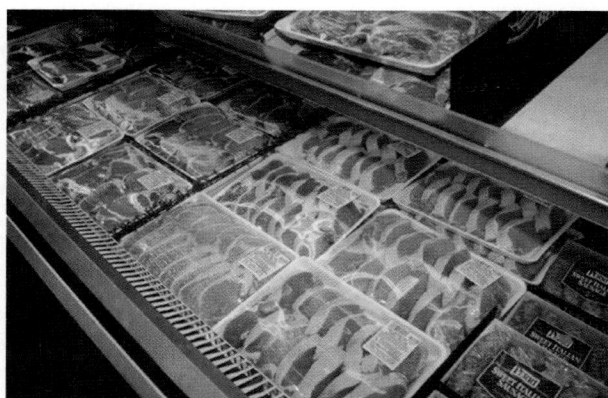

Figure 13–5   Food safety of pork and other meat products is the responsibility of the U.S. Department of Agriculture (USDA) Food Safety and Inspection Service (FSIS). (Credit: Ken Hammond, Agricultural Research Service, U.S. Department of Agriculture, Washington, DC.)

came concerned that nutrition labeling was inadequate, but the real problem was what, how much, and in what format. Information about nutrients and food constituents that consumer groups believed should be listed on labels included the amount of macronutrients (e.g., carbohydrate, protein, fat) and their total energy value (e.g., calories), key micronutrients (e.g., vitamins, minerals), sodium, cholesterol, and saturated fat. Concerned public and professional groups also wanted nutrients to be identified in terms of percentages of the current DRI or RDA standard per defined portion.[5,6]

Background of Present Food and Drug Administration Label Regulations

Over the past 10 years, two factors fueled rapid progress toward better food labels. These factors were the following: (1) increase in the variety of food products entering the U.S. marketplace, and (2) changing patterns of American food habits. Both factors led many health-conscious consumers and professionals alike to increasingly rely on nutrition labeling on foods to help meet health goals.[5,6] A number of labeling problems, including lack of uniformity, misleading health claims, and indefinite terms such as "natural" and "light," persisted.

These problems indicated a need to reorganize and coordinate the entire food-labeling system. This need had been reinforced by three previous landmark reports relating nutrition and diet to national health goals: *The Surgeon General's Report on Nutrition and Health*, the National Research Council's *Diet and Health*, and the Public Health Service's national health goals and objectives to be reached by the year 2000, *Healthy People 2000*.

Based on these reports, the Institute of Medicine of the National Academy of Sciences established a Committee on the Nutrition Components of Food Labeling to study and report on the scientific issues and practical needs involved in food-labeling reform. The report of this committee provided basic guidelines for the rule-making process conducted by the FDA and U.S. Departments of Agriculture and Health and Human Services, for submission to the U.S. Congress to achieve the needed reforms (see the For Further Focus box, "Nutrition Labeling: Recommendations for a New Century"). Three areas of concern formed the basis of recommendations from the Institute of Medicine, National Research Council, as follows: (1) foods for mandatory regulations; (2) the format of label information; and (3) education of consumers. This report became the basic guideline for the final law and regulations enacted by the U.S. Congress in 1994.

Current Food Label Format

Nutrition Facts Label. The food label format that is so familiar to us now is very different from the one used in the 1970s and 1980s. The title *Nutrition Facts* is printed in bold eye-catching letters. An example of the current food-label format is given in Figure 13-6. Manufacturers of processed foods may choose to include additional information, such as calories from saturated fat, polyunsaturated fat, monounsaturated fat, potassium, soluble and insoluble fiber, sugar alcohol (e.g., sorbitol), other carbohydrates, or other vitamins and minerals.

Another key term is *percent daily value* (%DV). The FDA set 2000 calories as the reference amount for calculating the %DV, although individuals may vary greatly in their specific needs. As a reference tool, the %DVs can be used to determine the overall value for a specific nutrient in the food (see the For Further Focus Box, "A Glossary of Terms for Current Labels"). For example, if the %DV for total fat in one serving of potato chips were 25%, that means that by eating the chips, you would have eaten one quarter of your total fat allowance for the entire day.

In addition, the serving size (e.g., the amount of the food customarily consumed) must be given and expressed in household measures, followed by the metric weight in parentheses and the total number of servings per container.[7]

Health Claims. Health claims that link nutrients or food groups with risk for disease are strictly regulated. To make an association between a food product and a specific disease, the FDA must approve the claim, the food must meet the criteria set forth for that specific claim, and the wording used on the package must be approved.

FOR FURTHER FOCUS

NUTRITION LABELING: RECOMMENDATIONS FOR A NEW CENTURY

The U.S. government is now committed by law to the food labeling reform mandated by a health-conscious public, a proliferation of new health-related food products marketplace, and concerned health professionals. It is apparent that nutrition "sells" in today's consumer market.

As part of the rule-making process and final regulations to administer the Nutrition Labeling and Education Act (NLEA) at the FDA and USDA, the initial report and recommendations of the Institute of Medicine's Committee on the Nutrition Components of Food Labeling, National Academy of Sciences, formed the foundation for final implementation of the law. This baseline focus resulted from a 1-year study requested by the U.S. Departments of Health and Human Services (HHS) and Agriculture (USDA). The study committee made the following recommendations, which are embodied in NLEA law:

Foods Covered by Nutrition Labeling

- Nutrition labeling should be mandatory on most packaged foods.
- Nutrition labeling should be provided at the point of purchase for produce, seafood, meats, and poultry.
- Restaurants should make the nutrient content of menu items available to customers on request.

Label Presentation

- The FDA and USDA should set standardized serving sizes.
- More complete ingredient listings should be provided on all foods.
- A modified regulatory scheme should be established for the development and approval of lower-fat alternative foods that currently have standards of identity.

Educating Consumers

- A well-designed nutrition labeling program should be fashioned as one part of a comprehensive education program, concurrent with the adoption of regulations on the labeling of nutrition content and format, to help consumers make wise dietary choices.

From the beginning of the process, the U.S. Congress wanted to develop legislative proposals to clarify the legal basis for reforms. The food industry, health professionals, and consumer groups wanted to promote changes in nutrition labeling that reflect the actual current dietary guidelines (RDAs) and related product development. These recommendations of the committee have provided a helpful foundation for all concerned.

A list of foods or nutrients currently approved for use in the United States and the specific disease they are associated with is listed in the For Further Focus Box, "A Glossary of Terms for Current Labels." An example of such a health claim would be the link between a diet low in dietary saturated fat and cholesterol and a reduced risk of coronary heart disease. For a food to carry this label it must be low in saturated fat, low in cholesterol, and low in total fat. If the food is fish or game meats, it must be deemed "extra lean." The specific wording of the claim must include the following: *saturated fat and cholesterol, coronary heart disease,* or *heart disease,* and a physician statement of the claim defines high or normal total cholesterol. The FDA also provides model claim statements that food producers may choose from. For this specific claim, the model statement is, "although many factors affect heart disease, diets low in saturated fat and cholesterol may reduce the risk of this disease."[8]

FOOD-BORNE DISEASE

Costs of Food-Borne Disease

Many disease-bearing organisms inhabit our environment and can contaminate the food and water. The Public Health Service estimates 76 million people become sick because of food-borne illness with 325,000 hospitalizations annually in the United States alone.[9] Much has been learned in the past decade about the pathogens that commonly contaminate food and water and the ways in which to prevent food-borne illness outbreaks. However, lapses in control still occur, resulting in high incidences of illness and death, as well as economic burden. Costs for medical care and personal salary losses quickly add up, totaling approximately $83 billion per year for the United States.[9] A recent report of *Salmonella* infection in California included accounts of real economic costs that effect government public health facilities, private health

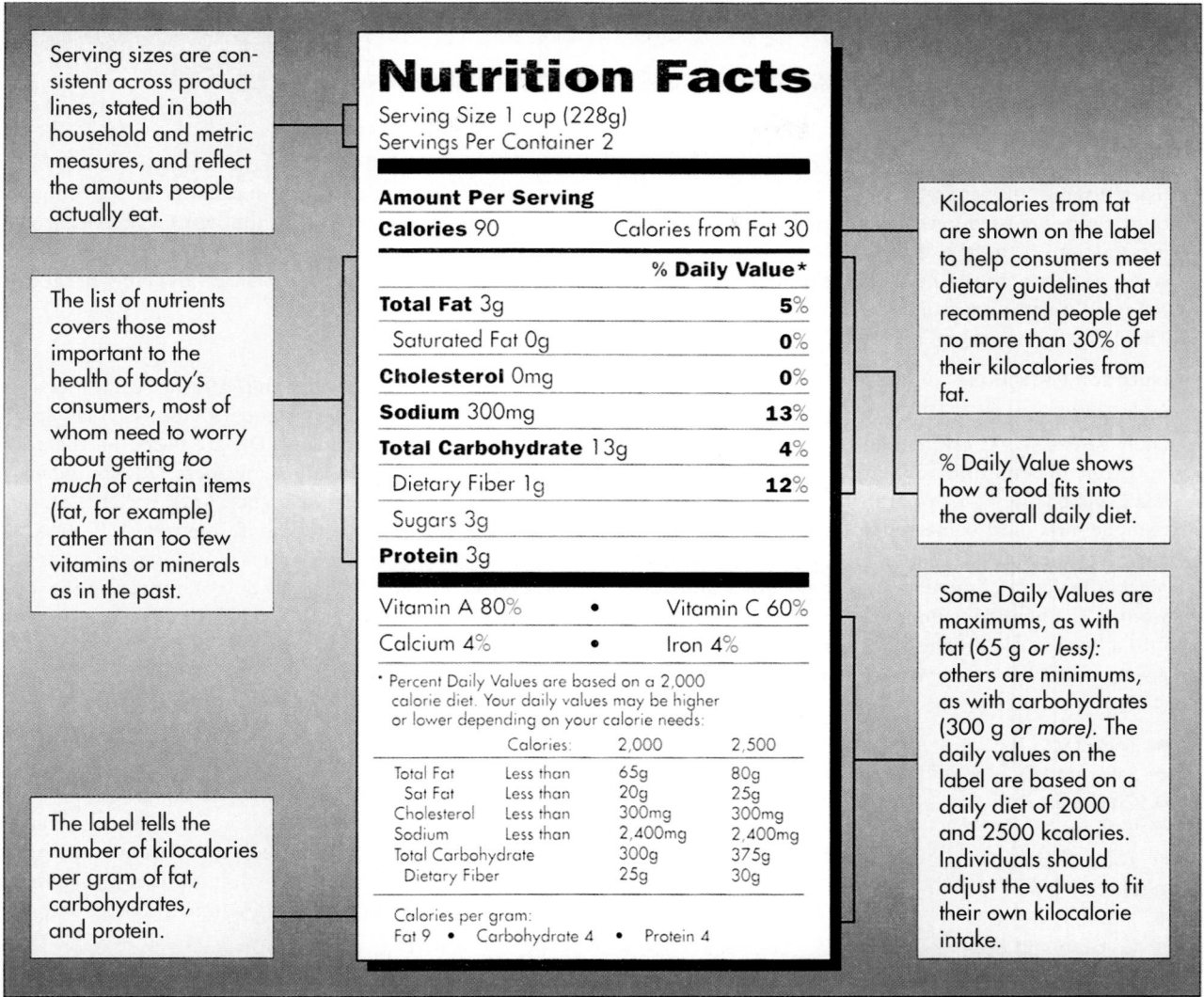

Serving sizes are consistent across product lines, stated in both household and metric measures, and reflect the amounts people actually eat.

The list of nutrients covers those most important to the health of today's consumers, most of whom need to worry about getting *too much* of certain items (fat, for example) rather than too few vitamins or minerals as in the past.

The label tells the number of kilocalories per gram of fat, carbohydrates, and protein.

Nutrition Facts
Serving Size 1 cup (228g)
Servings Per Container 2

Amount Per Serving

Calories 90	Calories from Fat 30
	% Daily Value*
Total Fat 3g	**5**%
Saturated Fat 0g	**0**%
Cholesterol 0mg	**0**%
Sodium 300mg	**13**%
Total Carbohydrate 13g	**4**%
Dietary Fiber 1g	**12**%
Sugars 3g	
Protein 3g	

Vitamin A 80%	•	Vitamin C 60%
Calcium 4%	•	Iron 4%

* Percent Daily Values are based on a 2,000 calorie diet. Your daily values may be higher or lower depending on your calorie needs:

	Calories:	2,000	2,500
Total Fat	Less than	65g	80g
Sat Fat	Less than	20g	25g
Cholesterol	Less than	300mg	300mg
Sodium	Less than	2,400mg	2,400mg
Total Carbohydrate		300g	375g
Dietary Fiber		25g	30g

Calories per gram:
Fat 9 • Carbohydrate 4 • Protein 4

Kilocalories from fat are shown on the label to help consumers meet dietary guidelines that recommend people get no more than 30% of their kilocalories from fat.

% Daily Value shows how a food fits into the overall daily diet.

Some Daily Values are maximums, as with fat (65 g *or less):* others are minimums, as with carbohydrates (300 g *or more).* The daily values on the label are based on a daily diet of 2000 and 2500 kcalories. Individuals should adjust the values to fit their own kilocalorie intake.

Figure 13–6   Example of a food product label showing the detailed Nutrition Facts box of nutrition information mandated by the U.S. Food and Drug Administration (FDA) under the Nutrition Labeling and Education Act. (From the U.S. Food and Drug Administration, Washington, DC.)

care centers, nursing care centers, as well as patients' personal earnings from inability to work. The authors estimated cost of hospitalizations for salmonellosis in the state of California from 1990 to 1999 was more than $200 million, with a disproportionately high incidence occurring in elderly persons and young children.[10] Microbiologic diseases (bacterial and viral) represent the majority of these outbreaks nationwide, with a large range of cost associated with each type of infection. *Listeria, Salmonella, E. coli,* and *Campylobacter jejuni* are the most common infections in home and community breakouts.[9] Recent sources of infections include water from

public drinking water at a county fair, ice cream from a widespread distributor, and raw milk or soft cheeses.[11,12]

Food Sanitation

Buying and Storing Food

Control of food-borne disease focuses on strict sanitation measures and rigid personal hygiene. First, the food itself should be of good quality and not defective or diseased. Second, its dry or cold storage should protect it from deterioration or decay, which is especially important for such products as refrigerated convenience foods, the fastest-

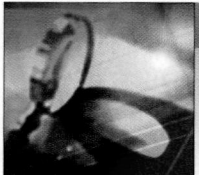

FOR FURTHER FOCUS

A GLOSSARY OF TERMS FOR CURRENT LABELS

To improve communication between producers and consumers, all must use the same "dictionary" supplied by the FDA. Whether these terms are used in the common format of nutrition information in the box titled "Nutrition Facts" or elsewhere as part of the manufacturer's product description, everyone must work from the same FDA "dictionary." The following is a sampling:

Nutrition Facts Box

Daily Values

Daily values (DVs) are reference values that relate the nutrition information to a total daily diet of 2,000 kcal, which is appropriate for most women and teenage girls, and some sedentary men. The footnote indicates the daily values for a 2,500-kcal diet, which meets the needs of most men, teenage boys, and active women. To help consumers determine how a food fits into a healthy diet, the following nutrients, in the order given, must be listed as percent of the daily value (DV%):

- Total fat
- Saturated fat
- Cholesterol
- Sodium
- Total carbohydrate
- Dietary fiber
- Vitamins A and C
- Calcium and iron

Daily Reference Value

As part of the DVs listed here, the Daily Reference Values (DRVs) are a set of dietary standards for the following eight nutrients: total fat, saturated fat, cholesterol, total carbohydrate, dietary fiber, protein, potassium, and sodium. DRVs do not appear on the label because they are part of a food's DV.

Reference Daily Intake

As part of the DVs listed here, the Reference Daily Intakes (RDIs) are a set of dietary standards for essential vitamins, minerals, and protein. RDIs are based on the actual Recommended Dietary Allowances (RDAs), which are part of the Dietary Reference Intakes (DRI) standards. This replaced the old confusing term "US RDA," which was developed by food manufacturers as an estimate based on old RDAs. RDIs do not appear on the label because they are part of a food's DV.

Descriptive Terms on Products

The FDA has specifically defined many terms that manufacturers must follow if they wish to use the term on their product. The following are some examples:

- *Fat free:* Less than 0.5 g of fat per serving.
- *Low cholesterol:* 20 mg of cholesterol or less per serving and per 100 g; 2 g saturated fat or less per serving. Any label claim about low cholesterol is prohibited for all foods that contain more than 2 g of saturated fat per serving.

---

growing segment of the convenience food market and potentially the most dangerous because they are not sterile. These vacuum-packaged or modified-atmosphere chilled food products are only minimally processed, not sterilized, and risk temperature abuse. Home refrigerator temperatures should be held at 40° F or lower. At temperatures above 45° F, any precooked or leftover foods are potential reservoirs for bacteria that survive the cooking and can recontaminate the cooked food. For food safety, it pays to be careful at all critical points (Figure 13-7), as follows:[13-15]

- *Clean:* Wash hands and surfaces often.
- *Separate:* Do not cross-contaminate.
- *Cook:* Cook to proper temperatures.
- *Chill:* Refrigerate promptly.

All food preparation areas must be scrupulously clean, and foods must be washed or cleaned well. Cooking procedures and temperatures must be followed as directed. All utensils, dishes, and anything else coming in contact with food must be clean. Leftover food should be stored and reused appropriately or discarded. Garbage must be contained and disposed of in a sanitary manner. Safe methods of food handling, cooking, and storage are easy to do and are mostly common sense, but are also often neglected and the cause of food-borne illness.

Food safety publications for all types of foods and populations can be found at the Food Safety and Inspection Service web site at *www.fsis.usda.gov/OA/pubs/consumerpubs.htm.*

- *Light* or *Lite:* At least a one-third reduction in kcalories (e.g., 40 kcal with minimum fat reduction of 3 g; if fat contributes 50% or more of total kcalories, fat content must be reduced by 50% compared with the reference food).
- *Less sodium:* At least a 25% reduction; 140 mg or less per reference amount per serving.
- *High:* 20% or more of the DV per serving.
- *Reduced saturated fat:* At least 25% less saturated fat than an appropriate reference food.
- *Lean:* Applied to meat, poultry, and seafood; less than 10 g of fat, 4 g of saturated fat, and 95 mg of cholesterol per reference amount, and 100 g for individual foods.
- *Extra lean:* Applied to meat, poultry, and seafood; less than 5 g of fat, 2 g of saturated fat, and 95 mg of cholesterol per reference amounts and/or 100 g for individual foods.

For more information, refer to *A Food Labeling Guide, Appendix A,* from the Center for Food Safety and Applied Nutrition, U.S. Food and Drug Administration, at *www. cfsan.fda.gov/~dms/flg-6a.html.*

Health Claims

The FDA guidelines indicate that any health claim on a label must be supported by substantial scientific evidence and has found that the following claims meet this test and are appropriate for:

- Low sodium and the prevention of hypertension
- Calcium and the prevention of osteoporosis
- Low dietary fat and a reduced risk of cancer
- Low dietary cholesterol and saturated fat and reduced coronary heart disease risk
- Fiber-containing grain products, fruits, and vegetables and a reduced cancer risk
- Grain products and fruits and vegetables that contain fiber, especially soluble fiber and the prevention of coronary heart disease
- Fruits and vegetables rich in vitamins A or C and lowered cancer risk
- Folate and the prevention of neural tube defects
- Dietary sugar alcohol and the prevention of dental caries
- Soy protein and reduced risk of coronary heart disease
- Plant sterol/stanol esters and reduced risk of coronary heart disease
- Potassium and a lowered risk of high blood pressure and stroke

For more information, refer to *A Food Labeling Guide, Appendix C,* from the Center for Food Safety and Applied Nutrition, U.S. Food and Drug Administration at *www. cfsan.fda.gov/~dms/flg-6c.html.*

Preparing and Serving Food

All persons handling food, especially those working with public food services, should follow strict measures to prevent contamination. For example, simple hand washing, along with clean clothing and aprons, is imperative. Basic rules of hygiene should apply to all persons handling food, whether they work in food processing and packaging plants, process and package foods in markets, or prepare and serve food in restaurants. In addition, persons with an infectious disease should have limited access to direct food handling. The Hazard Analysis and Critical Control Point (HACCP) food safety system focuses on preventing food-borne illness through identifying critical points and eliminating hazards. Many organizations, including the USDA and FDA, utilize HACCP standards. The USDA has developed specific standards for a variety of food products. For more information on HACCP, go to the official web site at:*www.cfsan.fda.gov/~lrd/haccp.html.*

Food Contamination

Food-borne illness usually presents itself as flulike symptoms but can advance to a lethal illness. Not all bacteria found in foods are harmful to humans; some are even beneficial, such as the bacteria in yogurt. Bacteria that are harmful to humans are referred to as *pathogens.* Certain subgroups of the population are at higher risk for developing food-borne illness because of age and physical condition. Groups at the highest risk are young

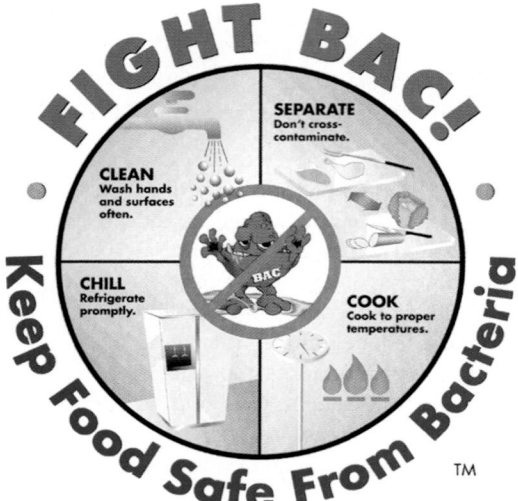

Figure 13–7　The Partnership for Food Safety Education developed the Fight BAC! campaign to prevent food-borne illness. Campaign graphics are available at *www.fightbac.org.* (From Partnership for Food Safety Education, Washington, DC.)

children, pregnant women, elderly individuals, and people with compromised immune systems.[15]

Bacterial Food Infections

Bacterial food infections result from eating food contaminated by large colonies of different types of bacteria. Specific diseases result from specific bacteria (e.g., *salmonellosis, shigellosis,* and *listeriosis*).

Salmonellosis. Salmonellosis is caused by *Salmonella,* a bacterium named for the American veterinarian-pathologist Daniel Salmon (1850 to 1914), who first isolated and identified the species commonly causing human food-borne infections: *S. typhi* and *S. paratyphi.* Approximately 40,000 cases of salmonellosis are reported in the United States each year, although thousands of other cases are suspected to go unreported.[16] These organisms grow readily in common foods such as milk, custard, egg dishes, salad dressing, and sandwich fillings. Seafood from polluted waters, especially shellfish such as oysters and clams, also may be a source of infection. Unsanitary handling of foods and utensils can spread the bacteria. Resulting cases of gastroenteritis may vary from mild diarrhea to severe attacks. Practices of immunization, pasteurization, and sanitary regulations involving community water and food supplies, as well as food handlers, help to control such outbreaks. Because incubation and multiplication of the bacteria take time (after the food is

eaten), symptoms of food infection develop relatively slowly (e.g., usually at least 12 to 24 hours later). The illness usually lasts 4 to 7 days with affected individuals recovering completely.

Shigellosis. Shigellosis is caused by the bacteria *Shigella,* named for the Japanese physician Kiyoshi Shiga (1870 to 1957), who first discovered a main species of the organism, *S. dysenteriae,* during a dysentery epidemic in Japan in 1898. About 18,000 cases are reported annually, but because many cases are not diagnosed, the CDC estimates the actual number of cases may be as much as 20 times higher.[17] Shigellosis usually is confined to the large intestine and may vary from a mild transient intestinal disturbance in adults to fatal dysentery in young children. The bacteria grow easily in foods, especially in milk, which is a common vehicle of transmission to infants and children. The boiling of water or pasteurization of milk kills the organisms, but the food or milk may easily be reinfected through unsanitary handling. The disease is spread similarly to how salmonella is transmitted (e.g., by feces, fingers, flies, milk, and food and articles handled by unsanitary carriers). Shigellosis, similar to salmonellosis, is more common in the summer and is most common in young children.[17]

Listeriosis. Listeriosis is caused by the bacteria *Listeria,* which was named for the English surgeon Baron Joseph Lister (1827 to 1912), who first applied knowledge of bacterial infection to the principles of antiseptic surgery in a benchmark 1867 publication that led to "clean" operations and the development of modern surgery. However, only within the past 20 years has knowledge of bacteria's role in directly causing food-borne disease in humans (e.g., both occasional illness and disease epidemics) increased and the major species causing human illness, *L. monocytogenes,* been identified. Before 1981, *Listeria* was thought to be only an organism of animal disease transmitted to humans by direct contact with infected animals. However, now it is clear that this organism widely occurs in the environment and in high-risk individuals such as elderly persons, pregnant women, infants, or patients with suppressed immune systems and can produce rare but often fatal illness, with severe symptoms such as diarrhea, flulike fever and headache, pneumonia, sepsis, meningitis, and endocarditis. About one third of all listeriosis cases occur in pregnant women.[18] Food-borne disease has been traced to a variety of foods including soft cheese, poultry, seafood, raw milk, commercially broken and refrigerated raw liquid whole eggs, and meat products (e.g., pâté).

Bacterial Food Poisoning

Food poisoning is caused by the ingestion of bacterial toxins that have been produced in the food by the growth of specific kinds of bacteria before the food is eaten. The powerful toxin is ingested directly, so symptoms of the food poisoning develop rapidly. Two types of bacterial food poisoning, *staphylococcal* and *clostridial*, are most commonly responsible.

Staphylococcal food poisoning was named for the shape of the causative organism, which is mainly *Staphylococcus aureus*, round bacteria forming masses of cells (Gr. *staphyle*, bunch of grapes; *kokkus*, berry). *S. aureus* is the most common form of bacterial food poisoning in the United States. Powerful preformed toxins in the contaminated food produce illness rapidly (e.g., 1 to 6 hours after ingestion). The symptoms appear suddenly and include severe cramping and abdominal pain with nausea, vomiting, and diarrhea, usually accompanied by sweating, headache, fever, and sometimes prostration and shock. However, recovery is fairly rapid and symptoms subside within 24 hours (see the Clinical Applications box, "Case Study: A Community Food Poisoning Incident"). The amount of toxin ingested and the susceptibility of the individual eating it determine the degree of severity. The source of the contamination is usually a staphylococcal infection on the hand of a worker preparing the food. This infection is often minor and considered harmless or even unnoticed by the food handler. Foods that are particularly effective carriers for staphylococci and their toxins include custard or cream-filled bakery goods, processed meats, ham, tongue, cheese, ice cream, potato salad, sauces, chicken and ham salads, and combination dishes such as spaghetti and casseroles. The toxin causes no change in the normal appearance, odor, or taste of the food, so the victim has no warning. A careful food history helps determine the source of the poisoning, and portions of the food are obtained for bacterial examination, if possible. Few bacteria may be found because heating kills the organisms but does not destroy the toxins produced.

Clostridial food poisoning was named for the spore-forming rod-shaped bacteria (Gr. *kloster*, spindle), mainly *Clostridium perfringens* and *Clostridium botulinum*, which can also form powerful toxins in infected foods. *C. perfringens* spores are widespread in the environment (e.g., in soil, water, dust, refuse, and everywhere else). This organism multiplies in cooked meat and meat dishes and develops its toxin in foods held at warm or room temperatures for extended periods of time. A number of outbreaks from food eaten in restaurants, college dining rooms, and school cafeterias have been reported. In most cases, cooked meat was improperly prepared or refriger-

ated. Control rests principally on careful preparation and adequate cooking of meats, prompt service, and immediate refrigeration at sufficiently low temperatures. The bacteria *C. botulinum* causes far more serious, often fatal food poisoning, *botulism*, from ingestion of food containing its powerful toxin. Depending on the dose of toxin taken and the individual response, the illness may vary from mild discomfort to death within 24 hours. Mortality rates are high. Nausea, vomiting, weakness, and dizziness are initial complaints. The toxin progressively irritates motor nerve cells and blocks transmission of neural impulses at the nerve terminals, causing gradual paralysis. Sudden respiratory paralysis with airway obstruction is the major cause of death. *C. botulinum* spores are widespread in soil throughout the world and may be carried on harvested food to the canning process. Like all *clostridia*, this species is **anaerobic** or nearly so. The relatively air-free can and the canning temperatures (above 27° C [80° F]) provide good conditions for toxin production. The development of high standards in the commercial canning industry has eliminated this source of botulism, but cases still result each year, mainly from ingestion of carelessly home-canned foods. Because boiling for 10 minutes destroys the toxin (not the spore), all home-canned food, no matter how well preserved it is considered to be, should be boiled for at least 10 minutes before it is eaten. Within the United States, Alaska and Washington have the highest incidence of botulism, with Alaska having by far the greater number of cases because of native habits of eating uncooked or partially cooked meat that has been fermented, dried, or frozen. Table 13-2 summarizes examples of bacterial sources of food contamination.

Viruses

Illnesses produced by viral contamination of food are few when compared with those produced by bacterial sources. These include upper respiratory infections (e.g., colds and influenza) and viral infectious hepatitis. Explosive epidemics of infectious hepatitis have occurred in schools, towns, and other communities after fecal contamination of water, milk, or food. Contaminated shellfish from polluted waters also have caused several outbreaks. Again, stringent control of community water and food supplies, as well as personal hygiene and sanitary practices of food handlers, is essential for prevention of disease.

---

anaerobic (Gr. *an-*, without; *aer*, air; *bios*, life) a microorganism that can live and grow in an oxygen-free environment.

CASE STUDY: A COMMUNITY FOOD POISONING INCIDENT

John and Eva Wesson agreed that their lodge dinner had been the best they had ever had, especially the dessert, custard-filled cream puffs, John's favorite. He had eaten two of them, despite Eva's protests. Maybe that was why he began to feel ill shortly after they arrived home. Eva's stomach felt a little upset too, so they both took some antacid pills, thinking their "stomachaches" were from eating more rich food than they were accustomed to. They went to bed early.

However, by 11:00 PM Eva woke up alarmed. John was vomiting and having diarrhea and increasingly severe stomach cramps. He complained of a headache, and his pajamas were wet with sweat. He had a fever and appeared to be in shock. Eva began to have similar pains and symptoms, although they were not as severe as John's.

The phone rang. It was one of their friends who had been at the lodge dinner. She and her husband were also experiencing the same reactions.

By now John was prostrate, unable to move. Eva immediately called their physician, who arranged for John to be taken to the hospital. After treatment in the emergency room for shock, followed by observational care and rest the following day, John's symptoms had subsided and he was allowed to go home. The doctor advised them to eat lightly for a few days and get more rest and said that he would investigate the cause in the meantime. During the next few days, John and Eva learned that almost all their friends who had been at the lodge dinner had had an experience similar to theirs.

The doctor contacted the public health department to report the incident. His was one of several similar calls, a public health officer said, and the department was already investigating.

The following week, the officer returned the doctor's call to report his findings. The cream puffs that the lodge restaurant served that evening had been purchased from a local bakery. At the bakery, health officials had located a worker with an infected cut on his little finger: "a small thing," the worker said. He couldn't understand what all the fuss was about.

The health officials also located the delivery truck driver, who had started out at midmorning to make his rounds and take the cream puffs to the restaurant. On questioning the driver, however, they learned that the truck had broken down during the afternoon deliveries before he reached the restaurant. The driver said that he had been irritated by a 3-hour wait at the garage while the truck was being fixed. But he still got the order to the restaurant in time for the dinner, he said, so what was the problem?

At the restaurant, the chef said that everyone was so busy with the dinner that when the cream puffs finally arrived, no one had time to give much notice to them. They had decided that there was no point in putting the cream puffs in the refrigerator at the time because they were to be served in a short while.

When John and Eva's doctor called them afterward to report the story, John and Eva decided they would not eat at that restaurant again. Besides, by then John had lost his taste for cream puffs.

Questions for Analysis

1. Why is control of the community's food supply an important responsibility of the health department?
2. Which disease agents may be carried by food or water?
3. What was the agent causing John and Eva's illness? Was this a food infection or a food poisoning? How do you know?
4. While the investigation was going on and before John and Eva learned the real cause of their illness, John thought it must have been caused by "those things farmers and food processors put into food these days." What substances did John mean? Can you give some examples?
5. Why are these materials used for growing and processing food?
6. What controls are there for their use?
7. What are some ways in which food is protected from its point of production to the table? How can food be preserved for later use?
8. Which agency controls food safety and quality? How does it do so?

TABLE 13-2	Selected Examples of Bacterial Food-Borne Disease		
Food-borne disease	**Causative organisms (genus, species)**	**Food source**	**Symptoms and course**
BACTERIAL FOOD INFECTIONS			
Salmonellosis	Salmonella *S. typhi* *S. paratyphi*	Milk, custards, egg dishes, salad dressings, sandwich fillings, polluted shellfish	Mild to severe diarrhea, cramps, vomiting; appearance 12-24 hours or more after eating; duration of 1-7 days
Shigellosis	Shigella *S. dysenteriae*	Milk and milk products, seafood, salads	Mild diarrhea to fatal dysentery (especially in young children); appearance 7-36 hours after eating; duration of 3-14 days
Listeriosis	Listeria *L. monocytogenes*	Soft cheese, poultry, seafood, raw milk, meat products (pâté)	Severe diarrhea, fever, headache, pneumonia, meningitis, endocarditis; symptoms appearing after 3-21 days
BACTERIAL FOOD POISONING			
(Enterotoxins Staphylococcal)	Staphylococcus *S. aureus*	Custards, cream fillings, processed meats, ham, cheese, ice cream, potato salad, sauces, casseroles	Severe abdominal pain, cramps, vomiting, diarrhea, sweating, headache, fever, prostration; sudden appearance 1-6 hours after eating; symptoms generally subsiding within 24 hours
Clostridial Perfringens enteritis	Clostridium *C. perfringens*	Cooked meat, meat dishes held at warm temperature	Mild diarrhea, vomiting; appearance 8-24 hours after eating; duration of 1 day or less
Botulism	*C. botulinum*	Improperly home canned foods; smoked and salted fish, ham, sausage, shellfish	Symptoms ranging from mild discomfort to death within 24 hours; initial nausea, vomiting, weakness, and dizziness progressing to motor and sometimes fatal breathing paralysis
E. coli infection	Escherichia *E. coli* 0157:H7	Meats; raw vegetables; unpasteurized milk, water, apple juice, and cider; person-to-person contact	Severe diarrhea and stomach cramps, dehydration, stroke; appearance within a few days after eating; duration of ~8 days

Parasites

The following two types of worms are of serious concern in relation to food: (1) roundworms, such as the *trichina* (*Trichinella spiralis*) worm found in pork, and (2) flatworms, such as the common tapeworms of beef and pork. The following control measures are essential: (1) laws controlling hog and cattle food sources and pastures to prevent transmission of the parasites to the meat produced for market; and (2) avoidance of rare beef or undercooked pork as an added personal precaution.

Environmental Food Contaminants

Heavy metals such as lead and mercury may also contaminate food and water, as well as the air and environmental objects. Although lead poisoning in the United States has declined dramatically since the removal of

lead from gasoline, it remains to plague certain subgroups of the population. Children are especially vulnerable to lead poisoning, particularly children of poor families sheltered in urban hotels or other impoverished areas with peeling lead paint.[19] Of all sources of lead, paint is the chief source of contamination. An estimated 38 million homes in the United States have leaden paint surfaces, with young children living in a lot of them. Housing in the Northeast and Midwest United States are twice as likely to have lead paint as housing in the South or West.[20] These children face lead exposure by eating paint chips or breathing air-borne particles of paint dust from abrasive paint removal before remodeling. Drinking water may be a major source of lead in high-risk households whose water comes through leaden service pipes or plumbing joints that have been sealed with lead solder. Current EPA rules for public drinking water, however, have lowered the controlled lead exposure levels even further. Children suffering these elevated lead exposures develop permanent neurologic damage.[21] Studies also have found this same high-risk population group deficient in iron, a condition which can increase lead absorption by a four to five-fold increase, thus further complicating lead toxicity.[22]

Natural toxins produced by plants or microorganisms also contaminate the food and water supply. Mercury, found naturally in the environment in addition to human production, is converted to methyl mercury by bacteria. Methyl mercury is a toxin contaminating large bodies of water and the fish within. This contamination can pass through the food chain to humans. Aflatoxin, another natural toxin, is produced by fungi and may contaminate foods such as peanuts, tree nuts, corn, and animal feed.

Other food contaminants and pollutants that may pose a risk to human health may come from a variety of sources (e.g., factories, sewage, and fertilizers) but end up leaching out into the ground contaminating food-production areas and the water supply.

FOOD NEEDS AND COSTS

Hunger and Malnutrition

Worldwide Malnutrition

Hunger, even famine and death, exists in many countries of the world today. Lack of sanitation, cultural inequality, overpopulation, and economic and political structure that do not appropriately utilize resources are all factors that may contribute to malnutrition. Chronic food or nutrient shortages within a population perpetuates the "cycle of malnutrition," in which undernourished pregnant women give birth to low-birth-weight infants. These infants are then highly susceptible to infant mortality or growth retardation during childhood. Without meeting the high nutrient needs throughout childhood and adolescence, the incidence of malnourished or growth-stunted adults with shorter life expectancy and reduced work capacity continues to rise. Malnutrition may result from total kcalorie deficiency or single-nutrient deficiencies. The most common deficiencies in the world today are protein-energy malnutrition, vitamin A deficiency, iodine deficiency, and iron deficiency. Figure 13-8 shows the complicated interaction of many factors leading to malnutrition.

In 1996 the United Nations Committee on world food security, the World Food Summit, gathered to address the 800 million people worldwide that do not have enough food to meet basic nutritional requirements. The long-term goal of this committee is to eliminate world hunger and establish a sustainable food supply for all people. The plan of action is composed of six commitments all focused on stabilizing social, economical, and environmental production and distribution of nutritionally adequate food. The committee is responsible for monitoring, evaluating, and consulting on the international food security situation and to follow-up with a report in the year 2006. Information and updates on the progress of this committee can be accessed at: *www.fao. org/wfs/index_en.htm.*

Malnutrition in America

Hunger does not stop at the U.S. border. In the United States, one of the wealthiest countries on earth, many studies document hunger and malnutrition among the poor. In 2000, more than 11 million households in the United States were identified as food insecure. Food insecurity is defined as "limited or uncertain availability of nutritionally adequate and safe foods or limited or uncertain ability to acquire acceptable foods in socially acceptable ways."[23] Individuals at highest risk of suffering from food insecurity within the United States are African Americans, Hispanics, single mothers, and households in central city and non-metropolitan areas.[23] At both the government and personal levels of any society, food availability and use involves money and politics. Various factors are involved, such as land management practices, water distribution, food production and distribution policies, and food assistance programs for individuals and families in need. A "culture of poverty" often develops among the poor and is reinforced by society's values and attitudes.

Food Assistance Programs

In situations of economic stress and natural disasters, individuals and families need financial help. There are currently persons in the United States who experience hunger every day. It may be necessary to discuss available food assistance programs and make appropriate referrals.

Commodity Supplemental Food Program

Under the Commodity Supplemental Food Program (CSFP), the USDA purchases food items that are good sources of nutrients often lacking in the diets of the target population (low-income pregnant and breastfeeding women, other new mothers up to 1 year postpartum, infants, children up to age 5, and elderly people at least 60 years of age). The USDA then distributes the food to state agencies and tribal organizations. From there, the food is dispersed to local agencies for public allocation. Lo-

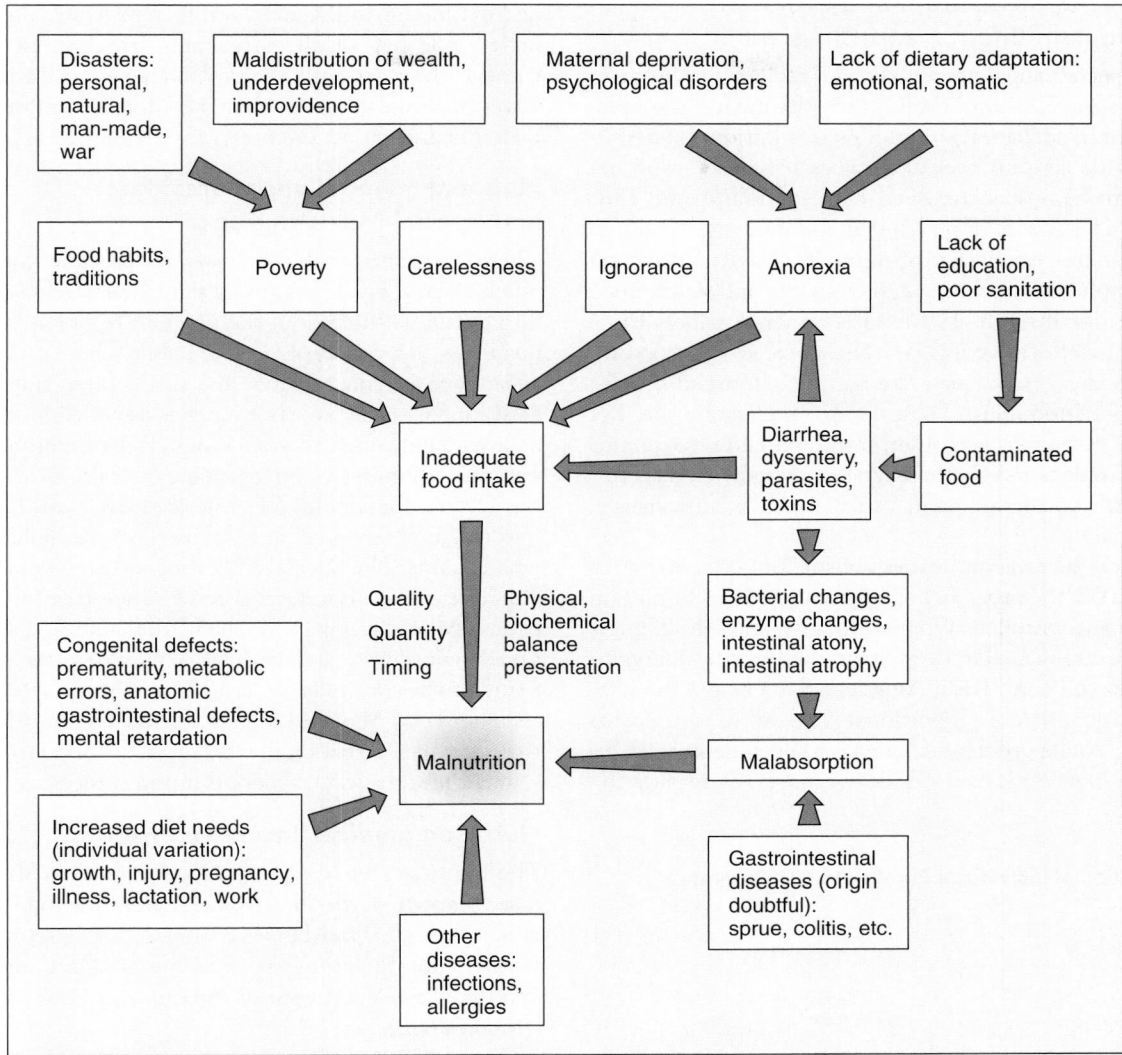

Figure 13–8   Multiple etiology of malnutrition. (Modified from Williams CD: Malnutrition, *Lancet* 2:342, 1962.)

cal agencies, such as the departments of health, social services, education, or agriculture, are responsible for evaluating eligibility, providing nutrition education, and dispersing of food. This program is not currently available in every state. Information about eligibility, availability, and foods provided can be accessed on the CSFP web site at *www.fns.usda.gov/fdd/programs/csfp/default.htm*. Congress appropriated $114 million for CSFP in fiscal year 2003.

Food Stamp Program

The Food Stamp Program began in the late depression years of the 1930s and was further developed in the 1960s and 1970s. This program has helped many poor persons purchase needed food, although federal cuts in

the 1980s curtailed its help to many persons in need. The USDA estimated that 17.3 million people received food stamps in the United States each month in 2001, the majority of which were children or elderly.[24] Under this program, the person or "household" is issued coupons, or "food stamps," which are supposed to sufficiently cover or supplement the household's food needs for 1 month. Households must have a monthly income below the program's eligible poverty limit to qualify. The Food Stamp Program is in operation in the 50 states, the District of Columbia, Guam, and the U.S. Virgin Islands and is administered at the local level. More information about this program can be found at the Food and Nutrition Service web site at *www.fns.usda.gov/fsp/*.

Special Supplemental Food Program for Women, Infants, and Children

The Special Supplemental Food Program for Women, Infants, and Children (WIC) provides nutrition supplementation, education, counseling in addition to referrals for health care and social services to women who are pregnant or postpartum, and to their infants and children under age 5. The Women, Infants, and Children program has established criteria for participation and each applicant must be income eligible and determined at nutritional risk.[25] The food is either distributed free or purchased with vouchers. The vouchers are good for such foods as milk, eggs, cheese, juice, fortified cereals, and infant formulas. These foods supplement the diet with rich sources of protein, iron, and certain vitamins to help reduce risk factors such as poor growth patterns, low birth weight or prematurity, toxemia, miscarriage, and anemia.

The WIC program was established in 1972 and as of April 2000, the program had approximately eight million participants enrolled. Women, Infants, and Children offices are established in every state, the District of Columbia, Guam, Puerto Rico, American Samoa, and the U.S. Virgin Islands. A disproportionate amount of participants (34% of total participants) are found in three states, California, New York, and Texas.[25] Figure 13-9 displays the distribution of individuals enrolled in WIC. Approximately one half of all participants are children ages 1 through 5, and non-Hispanic Caucasians make up the largest race and ethnic percentage. More information can be found at *www.fns.usda.gov/wic/DEFAULT.HTM*.

National School Lunch, Breakfast, and Special Milk Programs

These programs enable schools to provide nutritious lunches and breakfasts to low-income students. The USDA offsets the cost of the program by donating large quantities of a variety of foods to public schools. Children eat free or at reduced rates, and this is often their main food intake of the day. The lunches provided must fulfill approximately one third of a child's RDA for protein, vitamin A, vitamin C, iron, calcium, and calories and meet the Dietary Guidelines for Americans that call for diets lower in total fat and contain more fruits, vegetables, and whole grains. The Special Milk Program provides milk to children who do not have access to the other meal programs. More information about the National School Lunch, Breakfast, and Special Milk Programs can be found at *www.fns.usda.gov/cnd/*. There is also a National Summer Food Service Program for low-income children that provides nutritionally balanced meals during the summer months when school is not in session.

Nutrition Services Incentive Program

The Nutrition Services Incentive Program (NSIP), formerly known as the Nutrition Program for the Elderly, is a joint operation between the U.S. Department of Health and Human Service's Administration on Aging and the U.S. Department of Agriculture's Food and Nutrition Services.

The NSIP provides cash or commodities for the delivery of nutritious meals to elderly people. Regardless of their income, all persons over 60 can eat hot lunches at some community center under the Congregate Meals Program or, if they are ill or disabled, receive meals at home under the Home-Delivered Meals Program. The act specifies that economically and socially needy persons be given priority. Both programs accept voluntary contributions for meals. More information can be found at *www.fns.usda.gov/fdd/programs/nsip/*.

Food Buying and Handling Practices

For many American families, the problem is spending their limited food dollars wisely. Even on a low-cost plan for food purchasing, an average family of four can expect to spend approximately $507 per month on food alone.[26] Shopping for food can be complicated, especially when

Distribution of Individuals Enrolled in WIC Program

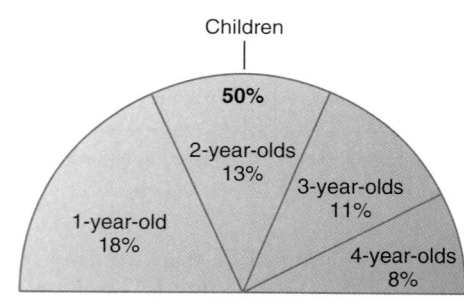
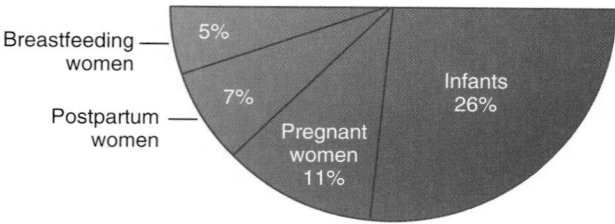

Figure 13–9   Distribution of individuals participating in the Women, Infants, and Children program. (Data from the Food and Nutrition Service, U.S. Department of Agriculture, Washington, DC, 2002.)

each marketed item in a supermarket's overabundant supply shouts, "Buy me!" Food marketing is big business, and producers compete for prize placement and shelf space. A large supermarket may stock 10,000 or more different food items, with more added daily. A single food item may be marketed a dozen different ways at as many different prices. In diet counseling, clients and families typically express their greatest need as help with buying food. The following wise shopping and handling practices help provide healthy foods, as well as control food costs.

Planning Ahead

Use market guides in newspapers, plan general menus, and keep a checklist of kitchen supplies. Make out a list ahead of time according to the location of items in a regularly used market. Such planning controls "impulse buying" and extra trips.

Buying Wisely

Know the market, market items, packaging, labels, grades, brands, portion yields, measures, and food values in various market units. Read labels carefully. Watch for sale items. Only buy in quantity if it results in real savings and the food can be adequately stored or used. Be cautious in selecting so-called convenience foods. The time saved may not be worth the added cost. For fresh foods and good buys, also try alternative food sources such as farmers' markets, consumer co-ops, and gardens.

Storing Food Safely

Control food waste and prevent illness from food spoilage or contamination. Conserve food by storing items according to the nature and use of each. Use dry storage, covered containers, and correct temperature refrigeration as needed. Keep opened and partly used food items at the front of the shelf for early use. Avoid plate waste by preparing only the amount needed. Use leftovers in creative ways.

Cooking Food Well

Use cooking processes that retain maximum food value and maintain food safety. Prepare food with imagination and good sense. Give zest and appeal to dishes with a variety of seasonings, combinations, and serving arrangements. No matter how much they know about nutrition and health, people usually eat because they are hungry and the food looks and tastes good, not necessarily because it is healthy.

SUMMARY

Common public concerns about the safety of the community food supply center on the use of chemicals such as pesticides and food additives. These substances have produced an abundant food supply but also have brought dangers and require control. The FDA is the main government agency established to maintain this control and conducts activities related to areas such as food safety, food labeling, food standards, consumer education, and research.

Numerous organisms such as bacteria, viruses, and parasites that can contaminate food may cause food-borne disease. Rigorous public health measures control sanitation of food areas and personal hygiene of food handlers. The same standards should apply to home food preparation and storage.

Families under economic stress may benefit from counseling about financial assistance. Various U.S. food assistance programs help families in need, and referrals can be made to appropriate agencies. Families may also need assistance buying and handling food.

CRITICAL THINKING QUESTIONS

1. What is the basis of concern about food additives and pesticide residues?
2. What are some ways agriculture is changing to reduce the use of pesticides and their danger to workers, as well as to protect the land?
3. Describe ways that various organisms may contaminate food. What standards of food preparation and handling should be used to keep food safe?
4. Kaycee is a single mother with two children and is working part-time making minimum wage. During the school year, her children both receive free school breakfast and lunch. She is concerned for her kids' nutritional well-being during the summer months. For what assistance may Kaycee and her children qualify? What suggestions would you make to help establish a well-balanced diet for this family?
5. According to the wise food buying and handling practices described in this chapter, evaluate your own habits and describe potential hazardous points for food-borne illness contamination and ways to improve your food buying practices.

CHAPTER CHALLENGE QUESTIONS

True-False

Write the correct statement for each item you answer "false."

1. *True or False:* United States surveys reveal little or no real malnutrition.

2. *True or False:* The politics of a region or country is not involved in the nutritional status of the people.

3. *True or False:* The number of new processed food items using food additives has declined in recent years because of public pressure and concern.

4. *True or False:* The use of pesticides on farm crops and food additives in processed foods is controlled by the USDA and FDA.

5. *True or False:* Food poisoning is caused by viral contamination of food.

6. *True or False:* The WIC program buys agricultural food surpluses to support market prices of food and distributes these goods to needy persons.

7. *True or False:* The number of poor persons assisted by the Food Stamp Program has been increasing because of expanded federal support.

8. *True or False:* The Nutrition Services Incentive Program provides group meals for all persons over 60 years of age, regardless of their income.

Multiple Choice

1. Food additives are used in processed food items to do which of the following? *(Circle all that apply.)*

   a. Preserve food and lengthen its market life

   b. Enrich food with added nutrients

   c. Improve flavor, texture, and appearance

   d. Enhance or improve some physical property of the food

2. The use of food additives in food products is controlled by the

   a. U.S. Public Health Service.

   b. U.S. Department of Agriculture.

   c. Food and Drug Administration.

   d. Federal Trade Commission.

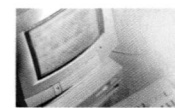

Please refer to the Students' Resource section of this text's Evolve web site for "Suggestions for Additional Study."

REFERENCES

1. The National Organic Program: *Organic food standards and labels: the facts*, Washington, DC, 2002 (accessed September 2003), NOP/U.S. Department of Agriculture [*www. ams.usda.gov/nop/Consumers/brochure.html*].

2. Falk MC and others: Food Biotechnology: benefits and concerns, *J Nutr* 132:1384, 2002.

3. Sevenier R and others: Increased production of nutriments by genetically engineered crops, *J Am Coll Nutr* 21:199S, 2002.

4. Division of Bacterial and Mycotic Diseases, National Center for Infectious Disease, Centers for Disease Control and Prevention: *Frequently asked questions about food irradiation*, Atlanta, 1999 (accessed September 2003), CDC [*www. cdc.gov/ncidod/dbmd/diseaseinfo/foodirradiation.htm*].

5. Neuhouser ML and others: Use of food nutrition labels is associated with lower fat intake, *J Am Diet Assoc* 99(1):45, 1999.

6. Staff: Practice points: translating research into practice: food labels benefit consumers and dietetic professionals, *J Am Diet Assoc* 99(1):53, 1999.

7. Center for Food Safety and Applied Nutrition, U.S. Food and Drug Administration: *Guidance on how to understand and use the nutrition facts panel on food labels*, Rockville, MD, 2003 (revised; accessed September 2003), CFSAN/ FDA [*http://vm.cfsan.fda.gov/~dms/foodlab.html*].

8. Center for Food Safety and Applied Nutrition, U.S. Food and Drug Administration: *A food labeling guide*. Appendix C, Rockville, MD, 2000 (revised; accessed September 2003), CFSAN/FDA [*www.cfsan.fda.gov/~dms/flg-6c. html*].

9. Dorner B: The four most serious causes of food-borne illness, *Today's Dietitian* 5(4):40, 2003.

10. Trevejo RT and others: Epidemiology of salmonellosis in California, 1990-1999: morbidity, mortality, and hospitalization costs, *Am J Epidemiol* 157:48, 2003.

11. Spake A: Death came with the water: *E. coli* breaks out at county fair, *U.S. News & World Report* 127(11):56, September 20, 1999.

12. Mahon BE and others: Consequences in Georgia of a nationwide outbreak of salmonella infections: what you don't

know might hurt you, *Am J Public Health* 89(1):31, 1999.

13. Henneman A: Don't mess with food safety myths, *Nutr Today* 34(1):23, 1999.

14. Food Safety Inspection Service, U.S. Department of Agriculture: *Basics for handling food safely*, Washington, DC, 2003 (revised; accessed September 2003), FSIS/USDA [*www.fsis.usda.gov/OA/pubs/facts_basics.htm*].

15. FDA Center for Food Safety and Applied Nutrition, Food Safety and Inspection Service, U.S. Department of Agriculture: *Foodborne illness: what consumers need to know*, Washington, DC, 2003 (updated; accessed September 2003), USDA [*www.fsis.usda.gov/OA/pubs/fact_fbi.htm*].

16. Division of Bacterial and Mycotic Disease, National Center for Infectious Diseases, Centers for Disease Control and Prevention: *Disease information: salmonellosis*, Atlanta, (accessed September 2003), CDC [*www.cdc.gov/ncidod/dbmd/diseaseinfo/salmonellosis_g.htm*].

17. Division of Bacterial and Mycotic Disease, National Center for Infectious Diseases, Centers for Disease Control and Prevention: *Disease information: shigellosis*, Atlanta, (accessed September 2003), CDC [*www.cdc.gov/ncidod/dbmd/diseaseinfo/shigellosis_g.htm*].

18. Division of Bacterial and Mycotic Disease, National Center for Infectious Diseases, Centers for Disease Control and Prevention: *Disease information: listeriosis*, Atlanta, (accessed September 2003), CDC [*www.cdc.gov/ncidod/dbmd/diseaseinfo/listeriosis_g.htm*].

19. Lanphear BP and others: Prevention of lead toxicity in U.S. children, *Ambul Pediatr* 3(1):27, 2003.

20. Jacobs DE and others: The prevalence of lead-based paint hazards in U.S. housing, *Environ Health Perspect* 110(10):A599, 2002.

21. Piomelli S: Childhood lead poisoning, *Pediatr Clin North Am* 49(6):1285, 2002.

22. Wright RO and others: Association between iron deficiency and blood lead level in a longitudinal analysis of children followed in an urban primary care clinic, *J Pediatr* 142(1):9, 2003.

23. Olson CM, Holben DH: Position of the American Dietetic Association: domestic food and nutrition security, *J Am Diet Assoc* 102(12):1840, 2003.

24. Food and Nutrition Service, Office of Analysis, Nutrition and Evaluation, U.S. Department of Agriculture: *Characteristics of food stamp households: fiscal year 2001*, Washington, DC, 2003 (accessed September 2003), OANE/USDA [*www.fns.usda.gov/oane/MENU/Published/FSP/FILES/Participation/Char01.htm*].

25. Food and Nutrition Service, Office of Analysis, Nutrition and Evaluation, U.S. Department of Agriculture: *WIC Participation and program characteristics 2000*, WIC-02-PC, Alexandria, VA, 2002, USDA.

26. Center for Nutrition Policy and Promotion, U.S. Department of Agriculture: *Official USDA food plans: cost of food at home at four levels, U.S. average, December 2002*, Alexandria, VA, (accessed March 2003), CNPP/USDA [*www.cnpp.usda.gov/FoodPlans/Updates/fooddec02.pdf*].

FURTHER READING AND RESOURCES

- U.S. Food and Drug Administration, Center for Food Safety and Applied Nutrition, *Food Labeling and Nutrition: www.cfsan.fda.gov/~dms/lab-gen.html*

- U.S. Department of Agriculture, Food Safety and Inspection Service, *Food Safety Publications: www.fsis.usda.gov/OA/pubs/consumerpubs.htm*

- U.S. Department of Agriculture, Agricultural Marketing Service, The National Organic Program, *Organic Food Standards and Labels: The Facts: www.ams.usda.gov/nop/Consumers/brochure.html*

- U.S. Department of Agriculture and Food and Drug Administration, Foodborne Illness Education Information Center: *www.nalusda.gov/fnic/foodborne/fbindex/033.htm*

- Centers for Disease Control and Prevention: *Health Topic: Foodborne Illnesses: www.cdc.gov/health/foodill.htm*

- Food Safety Training and Education Alliance: *www.fstea.org*

- International Food Safety Council, National Restaurant Association Educational Foundation: *www.foodsafetycouncil.org*

- U.S. Department of Agriculture, Cooperative State Research, Education, and Extension Service: *www.reeusda.gov*

- U.S. Food and Drug Administration, Center for Food Safety and Applied Nutrition: *www.cfsan.fda.gov*

 Explore the preceding web sites for current information and regulations on food safety, food-borne illness, and food labeling standards.

- Hamilton WL, Rossi PH: *Effects of food assistance and nutrition programs on nutrition and health*, ERS Food Assistance and Nutrition Research Report No. FANRR19-1, Washington, DC, 2002, Economic Research Service, U.S. Department of Agriculture.

 The USDA's food assistance and nutrition programs are under evaluation. This is the first of four reports to be released about the effectiveness of current programs on nutrition and health outcomes in the United States. This report, and reports to follow, can be viewed at www.ers.usda.gov/publications/fanrr19-1/.

CHAPTER 14

Food Habits and Cultural Patterns

KEY CONCEPTS

■ Personal food habits develop as part of one's social and cultural heritage, as well as individual lifestyle and environment.

■ Social and economic change usually results in alterations in food patterns.

■ Short-term food patterns, or fads, often stem from food misinformation that appeals to some human need.

Why do people eat what they eat? Food is necessary to sustain life and health, but people eat certain foods for many other reasons, least of all perhaps for good health and nutrition, although these are increasing concerns. As stated in Chapter 13, the broader food environment from which persons have to choose is often influenced by factors such as politics and poverty, which limit personal control and choice.

Many meanings are attached to food. All food habits are intimately related to one's whole way of life: one's values, beliefs, and situation. However, sometimes these food beliefs come from food misinformation and fads rather than sound nutrition knowledge. Some of these influences are examined here.

CULTURAL DEVELOPMENT OF FOOD HABITS

Food habits, like any other form of human behavior, do not develop in a vacuum. They grow from many personal, cultural, social, economic, and psychological influences. For each person, these factors are interwoven.

Strength of Personal Culture

Culture involves much more than the major and historic aspects of a person's communal life (e.g., language, religion, politics, and technology) but also develops from all the habits of everyday living and family relationships, such as preparing and serving food, caring for children, feeding them, and lulling them to sleep. People learn these things as they grow up. In a gradual process of conscious and unconscious learning, cultural values, attitudes, habits, and practices become a deep part of individual lives. Although parts of this heritage may be revised or rejected as adults, it remains within people to influence their lives and pass on to following generations. Americans have a broad heritage of food habits; influenced by a world of cultural diversity.

Food in a Culture

Food habits are among the oldest and most deeply rooted aspects of many cultures. Cultural background largely determines what is eaten, as well as when and how it is eaten, but much variation exists, of course. All types of customs, whether rational or irrational, beneficial or injurious, are found in every part of the world. However, whatever the situation, food habits are primarily based on food availability, economics, and personal food meanings and beliefs. Many foods in any culture take on symbolic meanings related to major life experiences (e.g., birth, death, religion, politics, and general social organization). From ancient times, ceremonies and religious rites involving food have surrounded certain events and seasons. Food gathering, preparing, and serving have followed specific customs, many of which remain today.

Traditional Cultural Food Patterns

The United States has been called a "melting pot" of ethnic and racial groups. In more recent years, however, this image is no longer appropriate. America's diversity has come to be recognized and even celebrated as a basis for national strength. This recognition is especially strong in the diversity of America's cultural food patterns.

Many different cultural food patterns are part of American family and community life. These patterns have contributed special dishes or modes of cooking to American eating habits. In turn, many of these cultural food habits have been Americanized. Older members of the family use traditional foods more regularly, with younger members of the family using them mainly on special occasions or holidays. Nevertheless, traditional foods have strong meanings and bind families and cultural communities in close fellowship. A few representative cultural food patterns are briefly reviewed here. Individual tastes and geographic patterns may vary somewhat, but food patterns are connected with culture and have a strong influence on how people eat.[1]

Religious Dietary Laws

The dietary practices within Christianity (Catholic, Protestant, and Eastern Orthodox churches), Judaism, Hinduism, Buddhism, and Islam vary according to their independent understanding and interpretation of what constitutes a healthy and proper diet. Such dietary laws may apply to what, how, and when specific foods are allowed or avoided. Some dietary laws are applicable at all times (no pork at any time for Islamic followers), whereas other laws apply only during religious ceremonies (e.g., Lent for Roman Catholics). The following are examples of two such religions and their dietary laws.

Jewish

Basic Food Pattern. All Jewish festivals are religious in nature and have historical significance,[2] but the observance of Jewish food laws differs among the three basic groups within Judaism: (1) Orthodox, strict observance; (2) Conservative, less strict; and (3) Reform, less ceremonial emphasis and minimum general use. The basic body of dietary laws is called the *Rules of Kashruth*. Foods selected and prepared according to these rules are called *kosher*, from the Hebrew word meaning "fit, proper." These laws originally had special ritual significance. Current Jewish dietary laws apply this significance to laws governing the slaughter, preparation, and serving of meat; the combining of meat and milk; and the use of fish and eggs. Various food restrictions exist, as follows:

- *Meat.* Appropriate meats should come from animals that chew their cud and have cloven hooves. Pork and birds of prey are avoided at all times. All forms of meat are rigidly cleansed of blood.
- *Meat and milk.* Meat and milk products are both part of the kosher Jewish diet; however, they are not to be eaten at the same meal or prepared using the

same dishes. Orthodox homes maintain two sets of regular dishes, one for serving meat and the other for meals using dairy products. An additional two sets of dishes are maintained especially for use during Passover.

- *Fish*. Only fish with fins and scales are allowed. These may be eaten with either meat or dairy meals. Shellfish and crustaceans are avoided.
- *Eggs*. No egg with a blood spot may be eaten. Eggs may be used with either meat or dairy meals.

Influence of Festivals. Many traditional Jewish foods relate to festivals of the Jewish calendar that commemorate significant events in Jewish history. Often, special Sabbath foods are used. A few representative foods, mostly of Eastern European influence, include the following:

- *Bagels*. Doughnut-shaped, hard yeast rolls
- *Blintzes*. Thin, filled, rolled pancakes
- *Borscht (borsch)*. Soup of meat stock, beaten egg or sour cream, beets, cabbage, or spinach; served hot or cold
- *Challah*. Sabbath loaf of white bread, shaped as a twist or coil, used at the beginning of the meal after the kiddush, the blessing over wine
- *Gefullte (gefilte) fish*. From a German word meaning "stuffed fish"; usually the first course of Sabbath evening meal; made of chopped and seasoned fish filet, stuffed back into the skin or rolled into balls
- *Kasha*. Buckwheat groats (hulled kernels), used as a cooked cereal or as a potato substitute with gravy
- *Knishes*. Pastry filled with ground meat or cheese
- *Lox*. Smoked, salted salmon
- *Matzo*. Flat, unleavened bread
- *Strudel*. Thin pastry filled with fruit and nuts, rolled, and baked

Muslim

Basic Food Pattern. Muslim dietary laws are based on the restriction or prohibition of some foods and the promotion of others, derived from Islamic teachings in the Koran. The laws are binding and must be followed at all times, even during pregnancy, hospitalization, or travel. These laws also are binding to visitors in the host Muslim country. Most all foods are permitted unless specifically conditioned or prohibited. The following listing outlines the permitted foods:

- *Milk products*. Permitted at all times
- *Fruits and vegetables*. Permitted except if fermented or poisonous
- *Breads and cereals*. Permitted unless contaminated or harmful

- *Meats*. Seafood (including fish, shellfish, eels, and sea animals) and land animals (except swine) are permitted; pork is strictly prohibited. Muslims typically eat kosher meats because the blood of the animal is not to be eaten. Halal meat is the equivalent of kosher meat.
- *Alcohol*. Strictly prohibited

Any food combinations are used as long as no prohibited items are included. Milk and meat may be eaten together, in contrast to Jewish kosher laws. The Koran mentions certain foods as being of special value, such as figs, olives, dates, honey, milk, and buttermilk. Prohibited foods by the Muslim dietary laws may be eaten when no other sources of food are available.

Representative Foods. A number of favorite foods and dishes are used as appetizers, main dishes, snacks, or salads. The following are some of these foods:

- *Bulgur (or burghel)*. Partially cooked and dried cracked wheat, available in coarse grind as a base for pilaf or fine grind for use in tabouli and kibbeh
- *Falafel*. A "fast food" made from a seasoned paste of ground soaked beans formed into shapes and fried
- *Fatayeh*. Snack or appetizer similar to a small pizza with toppings of cheese, meat, or spinach
- *Kibbeh*. Meat dish made of cracked wheat shell filled with small pieces of lamb and fried in oil
- *Pilaf*. Sautéed, seasoned bulgur or rice steamed in a bouillon, sometimes with poultry, meat, or shellfish
- *Pita*. Flat circular bread, torn or cut into pieces, stuffed with sandwich fillings or used as scoops for a dip such as *hummus* made from garbanzo beans
- *Tabouli*. Salad made from soaked bulgur combined with chopped tomatoes, parsley, mint, green onion, mixed with olive oil and lemon juice

Influence of Festivals. The fourth pillar of Islam commanded by the Koran is fasting. Among the Muslim people, a 30-day period of daylight fasting is required during **Ramadan,** the ninth month of the Islamic lunar calendar. Ramadan was chosen for the sacred fast because it was when Mohammed received the first of the revelations that were subsequently compiled to form the Koran, and it is also the month when his followers first drove their enemies from Mecca in 624 AD. During the month of Ramadan, Muslims all over the world observe daily fasting, taking no food or drink from dawn to sunset. However, nights are often spent in special feasts. First, an appetizer is taken, such as dates or a fruit drink, followed by the family's "evening breakfast," the *iftar*. At the end of Ramadan, a traditional feast lasting up to

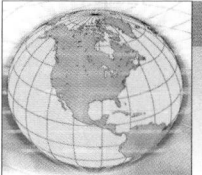

CULTURAL CONSIDERATIONS

ID AL-FITR: THE POST-RAMADAN FESTIVAL

In Muslim countries at the conclusion of Ramadan, Islam's holy month of prayer and fasting, wealthy merchants and princes traditionally hold public feasts for the needy. This is the festival of Id al-Fitr.

Over the years, many delicacies have been served to symbolize the joy of returning from fasting and the heightened sense of unity, brotherhood, and charity that the fasting experience has brought to the people. Among the foods served are chicken or veal sautéed with eggplant and onions, then simmered slowly in pomegranate juice and spiced with turmeric and cardamom seeds. The highlight

of the meal is usually kharuf mahshi, which is a whole lamb (symbol of sacrifice) stuffed with a rich dressing made of dried fruits, cracked wheat, pine nuts, almonds, and onions and seasoned with ginger and coriander. The stuffed lamb is baked in hot ashes for many hours, so that it is tender enough to be pulled apart and eaten with the fingers.

At the conclusion of the meal, rich pastries and candies are served. These may be flavored with spices or flower petals. Some of the sweets are taken home and savored as long as possible as a reminder of the festival.

---

3 days climaxes the observance. Special dishes, with delicacies such as thin pancakes dipped in powdered sugar, savory buns, and dried fruits, mark this occasion (see the Cultural Considerations box, "Id al-Fitr: The Post-Ramadan Festival").

All Muslims, regardless of medical condition, observe the fast of Ramadan. Individuals with diabetes, on medications, or who are pregnant or breastfeeding often experience complications during this time. Health care professionals must be sensitive to such religious practices when counseling with patients.[3]

Spanish and Native American Influences

Mexican

The food habits of the early Spanish settlers and Indian nations form the basis of the current food patterns of persons of Mexican heritage who now live in the United States, chiefly in the Southwest. The following three foods are basic to this pattern: dried beans, chili peppers, and corn. Variations and additions may be found in different places or among those of different income levels. Relatively small amounts of meat are used, and eggs are eaten occasionally. Fruit (e.g., mango and papaya) is consumed in varying amounts, depending on availability and price. For centuries, corn has been the basic grain used for bread in the form of tortillas, which are flat cakes baked on a hot surface or griddle. Wheat is also used in making tortillas; and rice and oats are added cereals. Coffee is a popular beverage. Major seasonings are chili peppers, onions, and garlic; the basic fat is lard.

Puerto Rican

The Puerto Rican people share a common heritage with the Mexicans, so much of their food pattern is similar (Figure 14-1).[4] Puerto Ricans, however, add tropical fruits and vegetables, many of which are available in their neighborhood markets in the United States. *Viandas*, which are starchy vegetables and fruits such as plantain and green bananas, are popular foods. Two other basic foods are rice and beans. Milk, meat, yellow and green vegetables, and other fruits are used in limited quantities; but dried codfish is a staple. Coffee is also a popular beverage for Puerto Ricans. The main cooking fat is usually lard.

Native American

The Native American population—Indian and Alaska Natives—is mainly composed of more than 500 federally recognized diverse groups living on reservations, in small rural communities, or in metropolitan cities.[1] Despite their individual diversity, the various groups share a spiritual attachment to the land and a determination to retain their culture. Food has great religious and social significance and is an integral part not only of celebrations and ceremonies but also of everyday hospitality, which includes a serious obligation for serving food.

Ramadan (Ar. *ramadān,* the host month) the ninth month of the Muslim year, a period of daily fasting from sunrise to sunset.

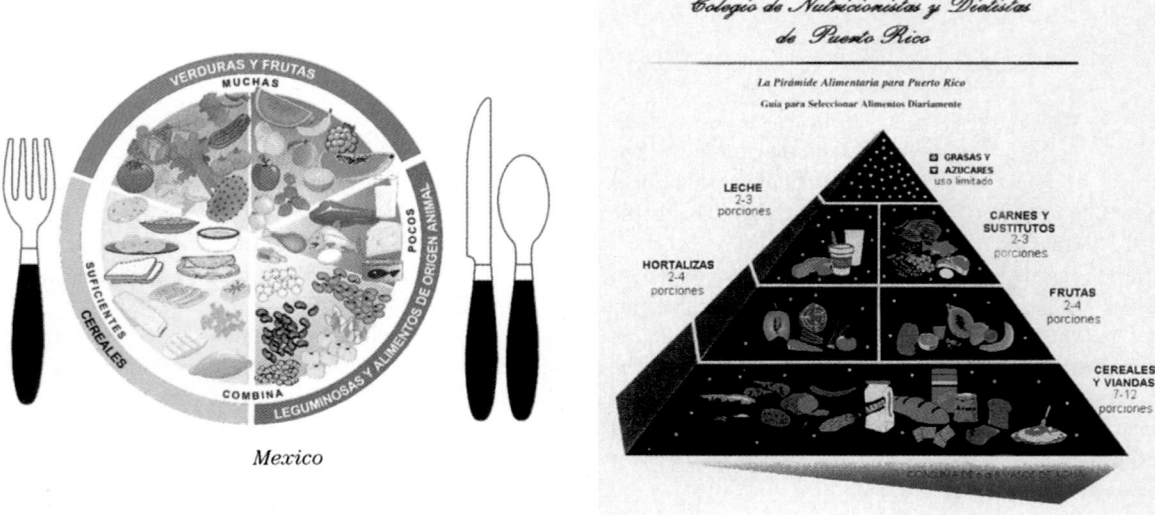

Figure 14-1 National food guides for Mexico and Puerto Rico. (From Painter J and others: Comparison of international food guide pictorial representations, *J Am Diet Assoc* 102(4):483, 2002, with permission from the American Dietetic Association.)

Foods may be prepared and used in different ways from region to region and vary according to what can be grown locally, harvested or hunted on the land or fished from its rivers, or is available in food markets.

Among the American Indian groups of the Southwest United States, the food pattern of the Navajo people, whose reservation extends over a 25,000-square mile area at the junction of three states, New Mexico, Arizona, and Utah, is one example.[1] The Navajos learned farming from the early Pueblo people, establishing corn and other crops as staples. They later learned herding from the Spaniards, making sheep and goats available for food and wool. Some families also raised chickens, pigs, and cattle. Today, Navajo food habits combine traditional dietary staples with modern food products from available supermarkets and fast-food restaurants (Figure 14-2). Meat (e.g., fresh mutton, beef, pork, chicken, or smoked or processed meat) is eaten daily. Other staples include bread (tortillas or fry bread, blue corn bread, and cornmeal mush); beverages (coffee, soft drinks, and other fruit-flavored sweet drinks); eggs; vegetables (corn, potatoes, green beans, and tomatoes); and some fresh or canned fruit. Frying is a common method of food preparation; lard and shortening are main cooking fats. Some health concerns are growing, however, about an increased use of modern convenience or snack foods that are high in fat, sugar, calories, and sodium, especially among children and teenagers (see the Cultural Considerations box, "Acculturation to an American Diet").

Other American Indian tribes in the United States have their own heritage and distinct dietary habits relative to custom and the region in which they live.

Influences of the Southern United States

African Americans

The African-American populations, especially in the Southern states, have contributed a rich heritage to American food patterns, particularly to Southern cooking as a whole. Similar to their moving music styles (e.g., spirituals, blues, gospel, and jazz), the food patterns of Southern African Americans were born of hard times and developed through a creative ability to turn any basic staples at hand into memorable food. Although regional differences occur, as with any basic food pattern, the representative use of foods from basic food groups is evident, as follows:

■ *Breads and cereals.* Traditional breads include hot breads such as biscuits, spoon bread (e.g., a souffle-like dish of cornmeal mush with beaten eggs), cornmeal muffins, and skillet cornbread. Cooked cereals such as cornmeal mush, hominy grits (ground corn), and oatmeal are commonly used.

■ *Eggs and dairy products.* Eggs and some cheese are used; but little milk is used, probably because of the

Native American Food Pyramid

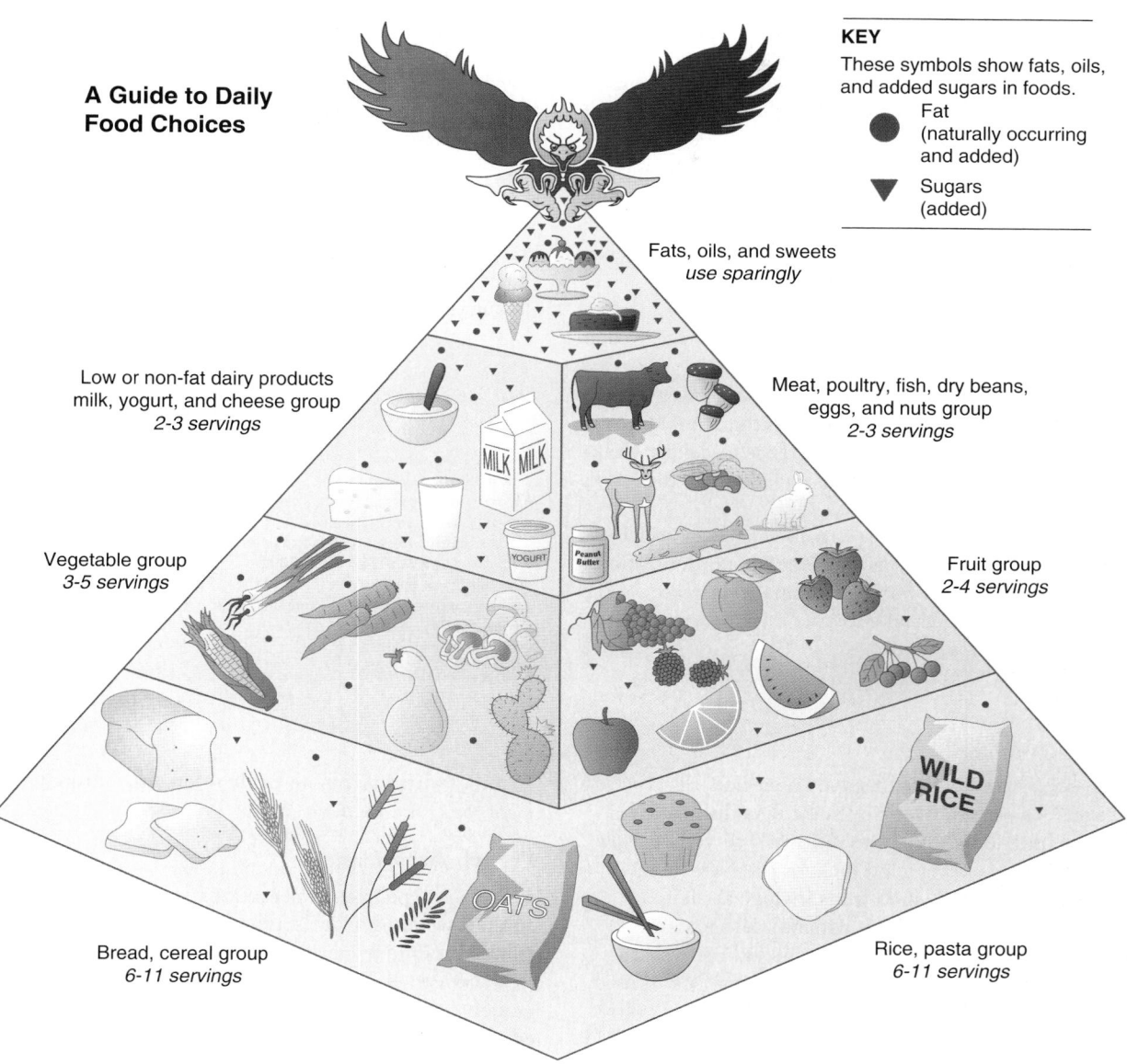

A Guide to Daily Food Choices

KEY

These symbols show fats, oils, and added sugars in foods.

● Fat (naturally occurring and added)

▼ Sugars (added)

Fats, oils, and sweets
use sparingly

Low or non-fat dairy products
milk, yogurt, and cheese group
2-3 servings

Meat, poultry, fish, dry beans, eggs, and nuts group
2-3 servings

Vegetable group
3-5 servings

Fruit group
2-4 servings

Bread, cereal group
6-11 servings

Rice, pasta group
6-11 servings

Note: These are only a few of the many Native American Foods that could fit within the Food Guide Pyramid

Figure 14-2   Native American Food Pyramid. (Designed by California Adolescent Nutrition and Fitness Program (CANFit) Youth Leadership Committee & Project Staff, Escondido Community Health Center, Funded by CANFit, Berkeley, Calif. [*www.canfit.org*]. Available online at the U.S. Department of Agriculture's web site: *www.nal.usda.gov/fnic/Fpyr/NAmFGP.html*).

greater prevalence of lactose intolerance among African Americans.

■ *Vegetables*. Leafy greens, such as turnip greens, collards, mustard greens, and spinach, are frequently used and usually cooked with bacon or salt pork. Cabbage is boiled or chopped raw with a salad dressing (e.g., coleslaw). Other vegetables used include okra (coated with cornmeal and fried), sweet potatoes (baked whole or sliced and "candied" with added sugar), green beans, tomatoes, potatoes, corn, butter beans (e.g., lima beans), and dried beans such as black-eyed peas or red or pinto beans cooked with

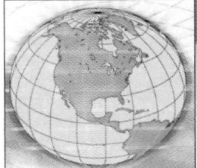

CULTURAL CONSIDERATIONS

ACCULTURATION TO AN AMERICAN DIET

A recent study looked at the major sources of energy intake among older Hispanic adults and evaluated the relationship with ethnicity, *acculturation*—the process of adopting the dietary practices of a new culture—and length of residency in the Unites States. When compared to non-Hispanic Caucasians in the United States, the Hispanic elderly consumed significantly less saturated fat and simple sugars and more complex carbohydrates. However, this healthy distinction is lost with those Hispanics who have lived in the United States for longer periods of time.* Hispanic adults are also noted to have significantly lower vitamin B$_{12}$ intake and plasma concentrations than non-Hispanic Caucasians, emphasizing the difference in dietary intake of such B$_{12}$ sources as meat and milk between the ethnic groups.†

One of the most notable negative effects of acculturation seems to be with the American Indian populations. Recent studies have noted a dramatic increase in the prevalence of diabetes, obesity, and cardiovascular disease among this population.‡ According to the CDC, the prevalence of death due to diabetes among American Indians is currently more than twice that of the total population.§ Researchers believe the increase in disease risk is directly associated with dietary and lifestyle adaptations to the typical American diet and a more sedentary lifestyle.

For more information on acculturation see the "Dietary acculturation: applications to nutrition research and dietetics" article referenced in the Further Reading and Resources section at the end of the chapter.

---

*Bermudez OI and others: Intake and food sources of macronutrients among older Hispanic adults: Association with ethnicity, acculturation, and length of residence in the United States, *J Am Diet Assoc* 100(6):665, 2000.
†Kwan LL and others: Low vitamin B-12 intake and status are more prevalent in Hispanic older adults of Caribbean origin than in neighborhood-matched non-Hispanic whites, *J Nutr* 132:2059, 2002.
‡Sewell JL and others: The increasing incidence of coronary artery disease and cardiovascular risk factors among a southwest Native American tribe, *Arch Intern Med* 162:1368, 2002.
§The burden of chronic diseases and their risk factors: national and state perspectives, U.S. Department of Health and Human Services, Centers for disease control and prevention, Feb. 2004, [*www.cdc.gov/ nccdphp/burdenbook2004/pdf/burden_book2004.pdf*]

smoked ham hocks and served over rice. Black-eyed peas served over rice make up a dish called "Hopping John" that is traditionally served on New Year's Day to bring good luck for the New Year.

■ *Fruits.* Commonly used fruits include apples, peaches, berries, oranges, bananas, and juices.
■ *Meat.* Pork is a common meat, including fresh cuts of ribs, sausage, and smoked ham. Some beef is used, mainly ground for meat loaf or hamburgers. Poultry is used frequently, mainly as fried chicken and baked holiday turkey. Organ meats, such as liver, heart, intestines (chitterlings), or poultry giblets (gizzard and heart), are used. Fish, including catfish, some flounder, and shellfish (e.g., crab and shrimp) are eaten when available. Frying is a common method of cooking; lard, shortening, or vegetable oils are fats used.
■ *Desserts.* Favorites include pies (e.g., pecan, sweet potato, and pumpkin) and deep-dish peach or berry cobblers; cakes (e.g., coconut and chocolate); and bread pudding to use up leftover bread.
■ *Beverages.* Coffee, apple cider, fruit juices, lemonade, iced sweet tea, carbonated soft drinks, and butter-

milk (which is a more easily tolerated, cultured form of milk) are used.

French Americans

The **Cajun** people, concentrated in the southwestern coastal waterways in southern Louisiana, have contributed a unique cuisine and food pattern to America's rich and varied fare. This pattern continues to provide a unique model for rapidly expanding forms of American ethnic food. The Cajuns are descendants of the early French colonists of Acadia, a peninsula on the eastern coast of Canada now known as Nova Scotia. In the pre-Revolutionary wars between France and Britain, both countries contended for the area of Acadia; but after Britain finally won control of all Canada, fear of an Acadian revolt led to a forcible deportation of the French colonists in 1755. After a long and difficult journey down the Atlantic coast, then westward along the Gulf of Mexico, a group of the impoverished Acadians finally settled along the bayou country of what is now Louisiana. To support themselves, they developed their unique food pattern from the seafood at hand and what they could grow and harvest. Over time, they blended their own French culinary background with the Creole cooking they found in their new homeland around New Orleans, which had combined classical French cuisine with other European, American Indian, and African styles of cooking.

Thus the unique Cajun food pattern of the Southern United States represents an ethnic blending of cultures using basic foods available in the area. Cajun foods are strong flavored and spicy, with the abundant seafood as a base, and usually cooked as a stew and served over rice. The well-known hot chili sauce, made of crushed and fermented red chili peppers blended with spices and vinegar and sold all over the world under the trade name Tabasco Sauce, is still made by generations of a Cajun family on Avery Island on the coastal waterway of southern Louisiana. The most popular shellfish native to the region is the crawfish, which is now grown commercially in the fertile rice paddies of the bayou areas. Catfish, red snapper, shrimp, blue crab, and oysters are some of the other popular seafoods used. Popular vegetables include onions, bell peppers, okra, parsley, shallots, and tomatoes; seasonings are Cayenne (red) pepper, hot pepper sauce (Tabasco), crushed black pepper, white pepper, bay leaves, thyme, and **filé powder.** Some typical Cajun dishes include seafood or chicken gumbo, **jambalaya,** red beans and rice, blackened catfish or red snapper, barbecued shrimp, breaded catfish with Creole sauce, and boiled crawfish. Breads and starches include French bread, hush puppies (fried cornbread-mixture balls, originally named because they were thrown to hungry hunting dogs around a hunting party's campfire to keep them from barking), cornbread muffins, cush-cush (cornmeal mush cooked with milk), grits (ground white corn), rice, and yams. Desserts include ambrosia (fresh peeled orange segments and juice with sliced bananas and freshly grated coconut), sweet potato pie, pecan pie, berry pie, bread pudding, or pecan pralines.

Asian Food Patterns

Chinese

Chinese cooks believe that refrigeration diminishes natural flavors, so they select the freshest foods possible, hold them the shortest time possible, and cook them quickly at a high temperature in a *wok* (e.g., a basic round-bottom pan) with small amounts of fat and liquid. The wok allows heat to be controlled in a quick stir-frying method that preserves natural flavor, color, and texture. Vegetables cooked just before serving are still crisp and flavorful when served. Meat is used more in small amounts in combined dishes than as a single main entree. Little milk is used, but eggs and soybean products (e.g., tofu) add other sources of protein. Foods that have been dried, salted, pickled, spiced, candied, or canned may be added as garnishes or relishes to

mask some flavors or textures or enhance others. Fruits usually are eaten fresh. Rice is the staple grain used at most meals. The traditional beverage is unsweetened green tea. Seasonings include soy sauce, ginger, almonds, and sesame seed. Peanut oil is the main cooking fat.[5] According to a recent study of nutrient intakes by ethnicity, the Chinese dietary patterns included significantly less total fat and saturated fat than the dietary patterns of African Americans, Caucasians, Hispanics, or Japanese.[6] Figure 14-3 illustrates the official food guides for China and Korea.

Japanese

In some ways, Japanese food patterns are similar to those of the Chinese. Rice is a basic grain at meals, soy sauce is used for seasoning, and tea is the main beverage. The Japanese diet contains more seafood, especially in the form of sushi. Many varieties of fish and shellfish are used. The term *sushi* does not necessarily mean raw fish. Some sushi is prepared with only vegetables or with cooked fish. Vegetables are usually steamed; pickled vegetables are also used. Fresh fruit is eaten in season; a tray of fruit is a regular course at main meals. The overall Japanese diet is high in sodium content and low in milk products (because of the high prevalence of lactose intolerance).

Southeast Asian

Since 1971, in the wake of the Vietnam War, more than 340,000 Southeast Asians have come to the United States as refugees. The largest groups of refugees are Vietnamese, but others have come from the adjacent war-torn countries of Laos and Cambodia. They have settled mainly in California, with other groups in Florida, Texas, Illinois, and Pennsylvania. As a whole, their food patterns are similar and are having an effect on American diet and

---

Cajun (derivative, *Acadian*) a group of people with an enduring tradition whose French-Catholic ancestors established permanent communities in the southern Louisiana coastal waterways after being expelled from Acadia (now Nova Scotia, Canada) by the reigning English in the late eighteenth century; developed unique food pattern from blend of native French influence and mix of Creole cooking found in the new land.

filé powder substance made from ground sassafras leaves; serves both to season and thicken the dish being made.

jambalaya a dish of Creole origin combining rice, chicken, ham, pork, sausage, broth, vegetables, and seasonings.

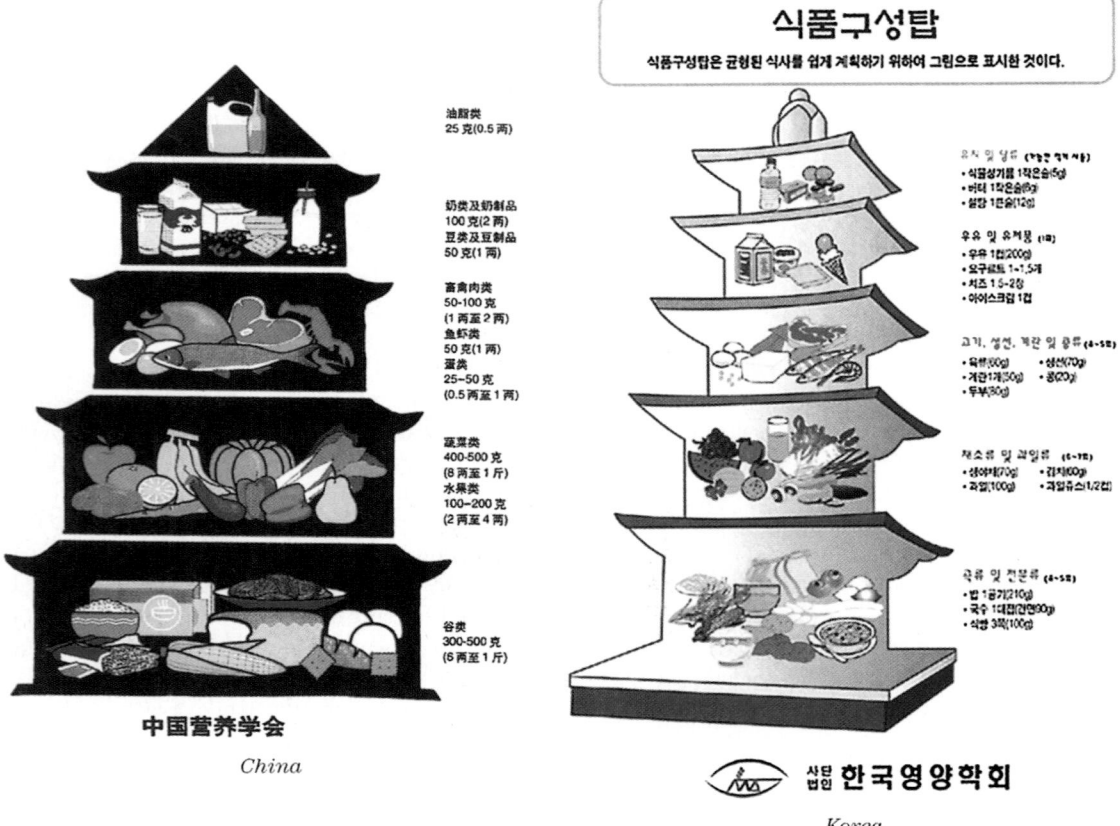

Figure 14–3   National food guides for China and Korea. (From Painter J and others: Comparison of international food guide pictorial representations, *J Am Diet Assoc* 102(4):483, 2002, with permission of the American Dietetic Association.)

agriculture. Asian grocery stores throughout the country stock many traditional Asian food items. Rice, both long grain and glutinous, forms the basis of the Indonesian food pattern and is eaten at most meals. The Vietnamese usually eat their rice plain in a separate rice bowl, not mixed with other foods, whereas other Southeast Asians may eat rice in mixed dishes.

Soups are also commonly used at meals. Many fresh fruits and vegetables are used along with fresh herbs and other seasonings such as chives, spring onions, chili peppers, ginger root, coriander, turmeric, and fish sauce. Many kinds of seafood (fish and shellfish) are used, as well as chicken, duck, and pork. Red meat usually is eaten only once or twice per month, and in small quantities. Stir-frying in a wok with a small amount of lard or peanut oil is a common method of cooking. A variety of vegetables and seasonings are used, with small amounts of seafood or meat added. In a traditional Asian diet, nuts and legumes are the primary sources of protein.

Since coming to the United States, Vietnamese have made some dietary changes that reflect American influence. These changes include the use of more eggs, beef, pork, candy and other sweet snacks, bread, fast foods, soft drinks, butter and margarine, and coffee.

Mediterranean Influences

Italian

The sharing of food is an important part of Italian life. Meals are associated with warmth and fellowship, and special occasions are shared with families and friends. Bread and pasta are the basic ingredients in most meals. Milk, seldom used alone, is typically mixed with coffee in equal portions. Cheese is a favorite food, with many popular varieties. Meats, poultry, and fish are used in many ways, and the varied Italian sausages and cold cuts are famous worldwide. Vegetables are used alone, in mixed main dishes or soups, in sauces, and in salads. Seasonings include herbs and spices, garlic, wine, olive oil, tomato

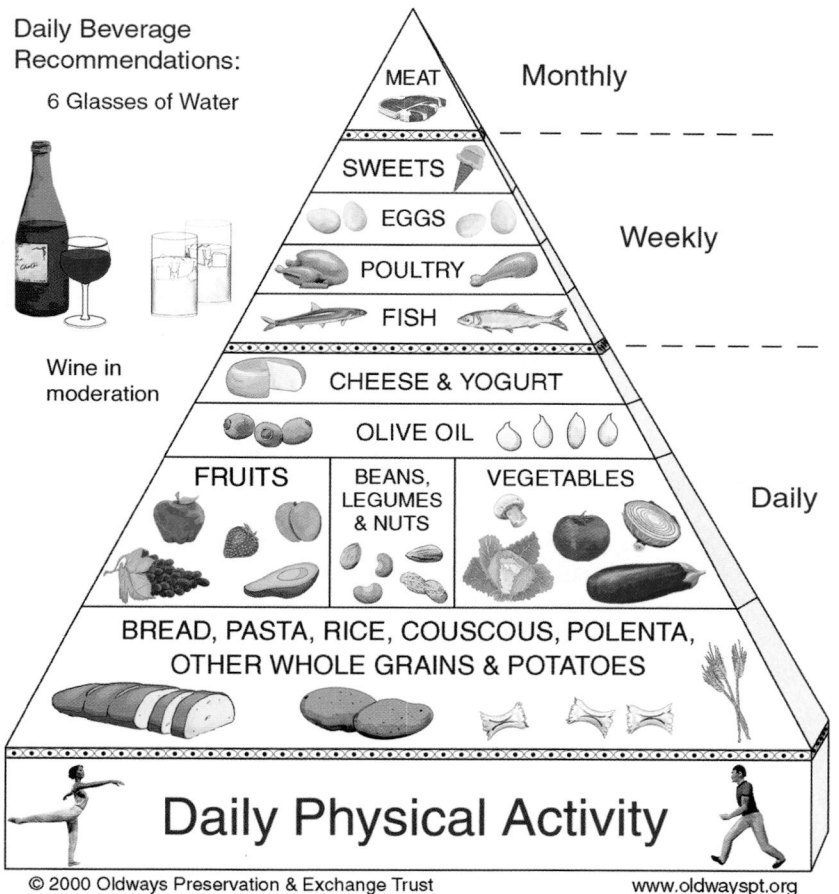

Figure 14–4   Mediterranean Diet Pyramid. (Copyright 2000, Oldways Preservation & Exchange Trust, Boston [*www.oldwayspt.org*].)

puree, and salted pork. Main dishes are prepared by initially browning vegetables and seasonings in olive oil; adding meat or fish for browning, as well; covering with such liquids as wine, broth, or tomato sauce; and simmering slowly on low heat for several hours. Fresh fruit is often eaten as dessert or a snack.

Greek

Everyday meals are simple, but Greek holiday meals are occasions for serving many delicacies. Bread is always the center of every meal, with other foods considered accompaniments. Milk is seldom used as a beverage but rather as the cultured form of yogurt. Cheese is a favorite food, especially *feta,* a special white cheese made from

sheep's milk and preserved in brine. Lamb is a favorite meat, but others, especially fish, also are used. Eggs are sometimes a main dish but never a breakfast food. Many vegetables are used, often as a main entree, cooked with broth, tomato sauce, onions, olive oil, and parsley. A typical salad of thinly sliced raw vegetables and feta cheese, dressed with olive oil and vinegar, is often served with meals. The traditional Greek salad is also a favorite at many American restaurants. Rice is a main grain in many dishes. Fruit is an everyday dessert, but rich pastries, such as *baklava,* are served on special occasions. Figure 14-4 illustrates the Mediterranean Diet Pyramid. See Appendix J for more information on traditional foods in various cultures.

SOCIAL, PSYCHOLOGICAL, AND ECONOMIC INFLUENCES ON FOOD HABITS

Social Influences

Social Structure

Human group behavior reveals many activities, processes, and structures that make up social life. In any society, social groups are formed largely by factors such as economic status, education, residence, occupation, and family. Values and habits vary in different groups. Subgroups also develop on the basis of region, religion, age, sex, social class, health concerns, special interests, ethnic backgrounds, politics, or other common concerns. All of our various group affiliations influence our habitual patterns, including our food attitudes and choices.

Food and Social Factors

Food is a symbol of acceptance, warmth, and friendliness in social relationships. People tend to accept food or food advice more readily from friends or acquaintances or from persons they view as trusted authorities. These influences are especially strong in family relationships. Food habits that are closely associated with family sentiments stay with people throughout life. During adulthood, certain foods may trigger a flood of childhood memories and are valued for reasons apart from any nutritional value.

Psychological Influences

Understanding Diet Patterns

Understanding dietary patterns better begins with recognition of the psychological influences involved. Food is a basic enjoyment of life and has many personal meanings and relationships. Social relationships, in turn, affect individual behavior. Many of these psychological factors are rooted in childhood experiences with food in the family. For example, when a child is hurt or disappointed, parents may offer a sweet food to help the child feel better. Then when adults feel hurt, they turn to those sweets to help them feel good again. Certain foods, especially sweets and other pleasurable tastes, stimulate "feel good" body chemicals in the brain called *endorphins* that give a mild "high" or help relieve pain.

Food and Psychosocial Development

Because food is so fundamental to physical survival, it also relates closely to psychosocial development as individuals. From infancy to old age, emotional maturity grows along with physical development. At each stage of human growth, food habits are part of both physical and psychosocial development. For example, when 2-year-old toddlers are struggling with their first steps toward eventual independence from their parents, they learn that they can control their parents through food and often become picky eaters, refusing to eat any new foods. Psychologists now believe that another normal developmental factor is involved, which they call *food neophobia,* or fear of unfamiliar foods. This universal trait may be an instinct from the evolutionary past that protected children from eating harmful foods when they were just becoming independent from their mothers.

Economic Influences

Family Income and Food Habits

Except perhaps for the relatively small group of very wealthy individuals, most American families live under socioeconomic pressures, especially in periods of recession and inflation. The problems of middle-income families differ in relative terms, but it is the low-income families—especially those in poverty situations—that suffer extreme needs. These families often lack adequate housing and may have little or no access to educational opportunities. As a result, they are poorly prepared for jobs and often only make a day-to-day living at low-paying work or are unemployed. Nearly one in every eight Americans lives in a family with an income below the federal poverty level, and about one in every four children younger than 6 years are members of such families.[7] It is no wonder that people with low incomes bear the greater burden of unnecessary illness and malnutrition.

Food habits are also manipulated by television, radio, magazines and other media messages. Influences from peers, convenience items, marketing at the local grocery store, and many other factors of persuasion may dictate the decision-making process for food choices throughout life. It is interesting to evaluate the food choices often made by those with the least available funds for food; oftentimes there is enough money for snack foods and soda, even when fresh fruits and vegetables are "too expensive."

Food Assistance Programs

Many low-income families can help improve their health by developing better food habits through community projects conducted by the U.S. Federal Extension Service working at the county level. These county Extension Educators, home economists, and their aides from the community, help families to use better food-buying practices, acquire skills in food preparation, and improve eating habits. Meals are more balanced, better use is made of government-donated commodity foods, and federal food stamps are spent more wisely. Some of the economical ways of handling food and available food-assistance programs are discussed in Chapter 13.

FOOD MISINFORMATION AND FADS

The word *fad* is a shortened form of an old word *faddle* (retained today in the phrase "fiddle-faddle"), meaning "to play with." A fad is something one "plays with" for a while. A fad is any popular fashion or pursuit, without substantial basis, that is embraced with fervor. Food fads are scientifically unsubstantiated beliefs about certain foods that may persist for a time in a given community or society. The word *fallacy* (L. *fallacia*, a trick to deceive) means "a deceptive, misleading, or false notion or belief." Therefore food fallacies are false or misleading beliefs that underlie food fads. The word *quack*, as used in this sense, is a shortened form of *quicksalver*, a term invented centuries ago by the Dutch to describe the pseudophysician or pseudoprofessor who sold worthless salves, "magic" elixirs, and cure-all tonics. He proclaimed his wares in a patter that skeptical people compared to the quacking of a duck. In medicine, nutrition, and allied health fields, a quack is a fraudulent pretender who claims to have skill, knowledge, or qualifications that he or she does not possess. The motive for such quackery is usually money, and the quack uses some cruel hoax to feed on the physical and emotional needs of his or her victims. The food quack exists because food faddists exist.

Unscientific statements about food often mislead consumers and contribute to poor food habits. False information may come from folklore or fraud. People should make wise food choices based on sound scientific knowledge from responsible authorities and recognize misinformation as such.

Food Fads

Types of Claims

Food faddists make exaggerated claims for certain types of food. These claims fall into four basic groups, as follows:

1. *Food cures.* Certain foods cure specific conditions.
2. *Harmful foods.* Certain foods are harmful and should be omitted from the diet.
3. *Food combinations.* Special food combinations restore health and are effective in reducing weight.
4. *"Natural" foods.* Only "natural" foods can meet body needs and prevent disease. The term *natural* may be used on unprocessed or minimally processed prod-

ucts that contain no artificial ingredients, coloring ingredients, or chemical preservatives. Some people consider all processed foods unhealthy, including those that are enriched or fortified. On the other hand, growing foods by organic farming is not a fad. It is an environmentally sound, positive practice now being developed by soil scientists that uses sustainable agriculture methods to avoid pesticides and restore the land (see Chapter 13).

Basic Error

These claims require a careful look. On the surface they seem to be simple statements about food and health. However, further observation reveals that each one focuses on foods per se, not on the specific chemical components in food, the *nutrients*, which are the actual physiologic agents of life and health. Certain individuals may be allergic to specific foods and obviously should avoid them. Also, certain foods may supply relatively large amounts of certain nutrients and therefore are good sources of those nutrients. However, the nutrients, not the whole foods, have specific functions in the body. Each nutrient is found in a wide variety of different foods. Remember, persons require specific nutrients, never specific foods.

Dangers

Why should health care workers be concerned about food fads and their effect on food habits? What harm do food fads cause? Food fads generally involve four possible dangers.

Dangers to Health. Responsibility for care of one's health is fundamental. Self-diagnosis and self-treatment can be dangerous, however, especially when such action follows questionable sources. By following such a course, persons with real illness may fail to seek appropriate medical care. Many ill and anxious people have been misled by fraudulent claims of cures and have postponed effective therapy.

Cost. Some foods and supplements used by faddists are harmless, but many are expensive. Money spent for useless items is wasted. When dollars are scarce, a family may neglect to buy foods that will fill its basic needs and instead purchase a "guaranteed cure."

Lack of Sound Knowledge. Misinformation hinders the development of individuals and society, while ignoring lines opened up by scientific progress. The perpetuation of certain superstitions can counteract sound teaching about health.

Distrust of the Food Market. America's food environment is changing. People should be watchful, but a blanket rejection of *all* modern food production is unwarranted. People must develop intelligent concerns and rational approaches to meet their nutritional needs. A wise course is to select a variety of primary foods "closer to the source" or those that have minimal processing and then add a few carefully selected processed items for specific uses. People can evaluate each food product on its own merits in terms of individual needs (e.g., nutrient contribution, personal values, safety, and cost).

Vulnerable Groups

Food fads appeal especially to certain groups of people with particular needs and concerns.

Elderly Persons

Fear of changes associated with aging may lead many middle-aged and older adults to grasp at exaggerated claims that some product restores vigor. Persons in pain living with chronic illness reach out for the "special supplement" that promises a sure cure. Desperately ill and lonely persons are easy prey for a cruel hoax.

Young Persons

Figure-conscious girls and muscle-minded boys may respond to crash programs and claims offering the "perfect body." Many who are lonely or have exaggerated ideas of glamour hope to achieve peer group acceptance by these means.

Obese Persons

Obesity is one of the most disturbing personal concerns and frustrating health problems in America today (see Chapter 15). Obese persons face a constant barrage of propaganda pushing diets, pills, candies, wafers, formulas, and devices. Many of these persons are likely to follow fads.

Athletes and Coaches

This group is a prime target for those who push miracle supplements. Always looking for the added something to give them the "competitive edge," athletes tend to fall prey to nutrition myths and hoaxes. Two such examples of substances being used by well-known athletes who influence many young players are the amino acid, creatine, and anabolic steroids.[8,9] Such misuse of drugs is harmful in the long run and dishonest behavior in young athletes in competition but also, at the dangerous rate taken by some aspiring young athletes, can be deadly.

Entertainers

Persons in the public eye are often taken in by false claims that certain foods, drugs, or dietary combinations will maintain the physical appearance and strength on which their careers depend.

Others

The vulnerability of the groups listed previously is obvious, but many other people in the general population follow the appeal of various food fads. Misinformation hinders the efforts of health professionals and concerned consumers to raise community nutrition standards.

What Is the Answer?

What can be done to counter food habits associated with food fads, misinformation, or even outright deception? What can, and *should*, health care workers do? An attitude of "do as I say, not as I do" achieves nothing. Health care workers cannot counsel or teach others until they have first examined their own habits. Helpful instruction is based on personal conviction, practice, and enthusiasm. Then the following approaches to positive teaching can be used.

Using Reliable Sources

Sound background knowledge is essential, as follows:

1. Know the product being pushed and the persons behind it.
2. Know how human physiology really works.
3. Know the scientific method of problem solving (e.g., collect the facts, identify the real problem, determine a reasonable solution or action, carry it out, and evaluate the results).

Sound community resources include the following:

■ Extension educators work in the community through state and county Extension Service offices and direct highly successful community nutrition activities, such as their Expanded Food and Nutrition Education Program (EFNEP). These specialists develop many food and nutrition guides, especially for those with limited education or little skill with English as a second language.
Information can be found at EFNEP: *www.reeusda.gov/f4hn/efnep/efnep.htm*.

■ The Food and Drug Administration (FDA) and U.S. Department of Agriculture (USDA) produce many educational materials related to food and nutrition (see Chapter 13). Requests for these mostly free materials can be directed to FDA and USDA agency offices.

Access to the *Cultural and Ethnic Food and Nutrition Education Materials* at *www.nal.usda.gov/fnic/pubs/bibs/gen/ethnic.html.*

■ Public Health nutritionists located in county and state public health offices and special programs, such as Women, Infants, and Children (WIC), can provide information.

WIC state agencies can be located on the Internet at *www.fns.usda.gov/wic/Contacts/statealpha.htm.*

■ Registered dietitians in local medical care centers and those serving hospitalized patients, outpatient clinics, and others in private practice also are valuable resources.

The American Dietetic Association's Nationwide Nutrition Network can be accessed at *www.eatright.org.*

In addition, state dietetic associations maintain lists of registered dietitians within the state.

Recognizing Human Needs

Consider the emotional needs that food and food rituals help fulfill. These needs are part of life. Use these needs in a positive way in nutrition teaching. Even if a person is using food as an emotional "crutch," the emotional need is very real. Never break crutches without offering a better and wiser way of support. Food, and all the associations with it, is a basic enjoyment of life. Maintaining a balance between "food as entertainment" and "food as fuel" is the challenge of identifying what human needs are being met by certain foods. Establishing a healthy diet must take all such human needs into consideration.

Remaining Alert to Teaching Opportunities

Use any opportunity that arises to present sound nutrition and health information, formally or informally. Learn about the available resources described previously (e.g., local or state university agricultural extension services, volunteer health agencies, clinic and hospital facilities, public health departments, and professional health organizations). Develop communication skills, avoid monotony, and use a well-disciplined imagination. Otherwise, the message will not convince consumers of the falsehoods behind the attractive skills of the food faddist or bogus "nutritionist" credentialed by a mail-order school or best-selling diet book.

Thinking Scientifically

Even very young children can be taught to use the problem-solving approach to everyday situations. Children are naturally curious. With their eternal "Why?" they often seek evidence to support statements they hear. They and others must be taught the value of three basic

---

> ### BOX 14–1 FANSA's 10 Red Flags of Junk Science
>
> 1. Recommendations that promise a quick fix
> 2. Dire warnings of danger from a single product or regimen
> 3. Claims that sound too good to be true
> 4. Simplistic conclusions drawn from a complex study
> 5. Recommendations based on a single study
> 6. Dramatic statements that are refuted by reputable scientific organizations
> 7. Lists of "good" and "bad" foods
> 8. Recommendations made to help sell a product
> 9. Recommendations based on studies published without peer review
> 10. Recommendations from studies that ignore differences among individuals or groups
>
> From Institute of Food Technologists, Food and Nutrition Science Alliance (FANSA): *Junk science: scientists issue 10 red flags for consumers* [news release], Chicago, 1995, FANSA [*www.faseb.org/ascn/fansa1.htm*]. Copyright American Society for Clinical Nutrition.

questions, as follows: (1) "What do you mean?" (2) "How do you know?" and (3) "What is your evidence?"

The Food and Nutrition Science Alliance (FANSA) is a partnership of four professional societies: American Dietetic Association, American Society for Nutritional Sciences, American Society for Clinical Nutrition, and Institute of Food Technologist. This organization issued a list of 10 red flags to help guide consumers in making educated decisions about nutrition and health issues. This list is an excellent guide when evaluating reports and claims about various diets, supplements, and other nutrition-related fads (Box 14-1).

Knowing Responsible Authorities

The FDA has the legal responsibility of controlling the quality and safety of the food and drug products marketed in the United States. However, this is a tremendous task and requires public help. Other government, professional, and private organizations can provide additional resources.

CHANGES IN AMERICAN FOOD HABITS

Personal Food Choices

Basic Determinants

As has been shown, universal factors determining personal food choices clearly arise from physical, social, and psychological needs. Box 14-2 summarizes some of these factors. Changing personal eating patterns is difficult enough; helping clients and patients to make needed

BOX 14-2 Factors Determining Food Choices

Physical Features

Food supply available
Food technology
Geography, agriculture, distribution
Personal economics, income
Sanitation, housing
Season, climate
Storage and cooking facilities

Social Factors

Advertising
Culture
General education and nutrition education
Political and economic policies
Religion and social class
Social problems, poverty, or alcoholism

Physiologic Factors

Allergy
Disability
Health-disease status
Heredity
Needs, energy, or nutrients
Therapeutic diets

Psychological Factors

Habit
Preference
Emotions
Cravings
Positive or negative experiences/associations
Personal food acceptance

---

changes for positive health reasons is even more difficult. Such teaching requires a sensitive and flexible understanding of the complex factors involved.

Factors Influencing Change

Ethnic patterns and regional cultural habits are strong influences. They establish early food habits and make changing those habits difficult. On the other hand, the changing society puts the old in conflict with the new. Some newer factors influence changes in food habits, as follows:[10]

■ *Income.* The generally improved economic situation of society provides sufficient income in most cases to give people more choice and time.

■ *Technology.* Expansion in the fields of science and technology increases the number and variety of food items available.

■ *Environment.* America's rapidly changing environment results in concerns about food and health.

■ *Vision.* America's expanding mass media, especially television, stimulates many options for new items and changes expectations and desires. The current market target for television advertisements is younger children, who then influence the family's buying habits.

Changing American Food Patterns

The stereotype of the all-American family of parents and two children eating three meals a day with no snacks in between is no longer the norm. There have been far-reaching changes in Americans' way of living and, subsequently, in their food habits.

Households

American households are increasing in number and changing in nature. Most new households are groups of unrelated persons or persons living together. The U.S. Census Bureau projections are that from 2000 to 2010 the number of nonfamily households will increase 17%, whereas family households will increase 9%.[11] The average size of American households is projected to decline from 2.59 persons in 2000 to 2.53 persons by 2010. Married couple households from 2000 to 2010 will decline from 54% to 52% of all households.[11] These changes reflect a rapidly changing society.

Working Women

The number of women in the work force continues to increase rapidly and is not likely to reverse. This trend is not restricted to any social, economic, or ethnic group. Women of all racial and ethnic groups will be the major entrants into the U.S. labor market. The U.S. Department of Labor reports that women were 46% of the total national work force in 1999.[11] This is a widespread change in society. Working parents increasingly rely on food items and cooking methods that save time, space, and labor.

Family Meals

Family meals, as they have been known, have changed. Breakfasts and lunches are seldom eaten in a family setting. Half of Americans between the ages of 22 and 40, as well as many children, skip breakfast regularly, and 25% skip lunch. One fourth of American households do not have a sit-down dinner as often as 5 nights a week. The Economic Research Service of the USDA recently

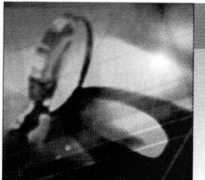

FOR FURTHER FOCUS

SNACKING: AN ALL-AMERICAN FOOD HABIT

The snack market in the United States continues to grow. Consumer spending for all foods has increased, with a greater portion of the increase being spent for snacks, mainly salty snacks, cookies, and crackers. Other popular snacks include soft drinks, candies, gum, fresh fruit, bakery items, milk, and chips.

Snacking is said to "ruin your appetite," and we certainly consume too many soft drinks, but is snacking all bad? Not necessarily. Surveys have shown a direct association between more complete nutrition and an in-

crease in snacking. Those who snack more show higher nutrient percentages in the "adequate" range of the DRI and RDA standards. Many people snack on foods that are not "empty extras" but essential contributions to total nutritional adequacy (e.g., fruit, cheese, eggs, bread, and crackers).

Snacking, or "grazing" as some persons do with more frequent nibbling, is clearly a significant component of food behavior. Rather than rule against the practice, we should promote snack foods that enhance nutritional well-being.

published a study comparing the food consumption patterns of individuals in 1977 to 1978 versus 1994 to 1996. Results show a dramatic decrease in the percent of food consumed from at-home meals over time. On average, 82% of all foods consumed in 1977 were at home, compared to 68% in 1996. From 1977 to 1996, the amount of food eaten at different locations, especially at fast-food restaurants, almost doubled.[12]

Meals and Snacks

Americans' habits have changed dramatically as to when they eat and whether they eat with their families. Mid-morning and midafternoon breaks at work usually involve food or beverages. Evening television snacks plus a midnight refrigerator raid are common. Nutrition hard liners of the old school may denounce this snacking behavior, but they are few and far between. Americans are moving toward a concept of *balanced days* instead of *balanced meals*. They are increasing the number of times a day they eat to as many as 11 "eating occasions," a pattern recently termed *grazing*. This shift is not necessarily bad, depending on the nature of the periodic snacking or more constant "grazing." In fact, studies indicate that frequent small meals are better for the body than three larger meals per day, especially when healthy snacking and grazing contribute to needed nutrient and energy intake (see For Further Focus box, "Snacking: An All-American Food Habit").

Health and Fitness

Americans' interest in health and fitness is increasing, which has affected food buying in several ways, with more nutrition awareness, weight concern, and inter-

est in gourmet or specialty foods. New lines of low-fat, fat-free, sugar-free, high-protein, and similar foods are popular.

Economical Buying

More Americans are making diet changes to save money. "No-frills" grocery stores, such as Food for Less, are becoming more and more popular across the country. With a warehouse-type store, the cost of overhead is significantly reduced and storeowners can pass that savings on to consumers. Many Americans are also members of bulk-food chains such as Costco and Sam's Club. Buying in bulk (economy size or family size) can save money, but only if one can efficiently use that much. There is no savings if food is not properly stored or used before it goes bad. Grocery stores also provide cost per unit pricing on the shelves to make it easier for consumers to compare the price of similar foods in different size containers or packages. Because the lowest cost per unit is the best buy, this is very beneficial for money-conscious shoppers!

Fast Foods

Most Americans have eaten in a fast-food restaurant at least once. From McDonald's modest beginning in 1955 in Des Plaines, IL, the fast-food business has grown into a multibillion-dollar enterprise that now captures almost half of the money spent on meals away from home. As family income rises, so does the consumption of fast foods, especially among the middle class. A recent article in the *Journal of the American Dietetic Association* compared portion sizes of selected foods from the year it was introduced to the sizes commonly found today. For example, a *regular* order of French fries from Burger King in 1954 was 2.6 oz. Today, a *medium* order of Burger King fries averages 4.1 oz. Similarly, in 1955 the only size fries McDonald's had to offer was a 2.4-oz portion. Today, the McDonald's portions range from small (2.4 oz) to supersize (7.1 oz). Such sizes dwarf the standard serving sizes on the USDA MyPyramid. A standard serving of soda according to MyPyramid is 12 fl oz. However, the average size soda served at a fast-food outlet is 23 fl oz.[13] Some researchers believe the expanding portion sizes in America's most popular restaurants are closely linked with America's expanding weight problem.

Tempting advertisements often lure consumers into ordering more food than they need. Deals like "two for one" or "value meals" could be a great bargain but often supply more food than is necessary for one person. In today's fast-food market, there are a variety of options outside of the customary hamburger and fries. Many fast-food chains offer grilled or baked chicken, turkey, or fish, deli fresh sandwiches with vegetables, side orders of salads or steamed vegetables, soup, and frozen yogurt. A well-balanced meal can be selected at most any restaurant, provided the consumer is astute in selecting the healthier choice. As with foods from any ethnic or cultural background, "all foods fit in moderation!"

SUMMARY

People all grow up and live in a social setting. Each inherits a culture and particular social structure, complete with its food habits and attitudes about eating. The effects on health that are associated with major social and economic shifts should be understood, as well as the current social forces (including cultural, religious, and psychological) to best help persons make dietary changes to benefit their health. Food fads and misinformation are increasingly popular within all facets of American society. Identifying harmful practices and providing accurate information are basic functions of the health care worker.

The food patterns of Americans are changing. They increasingly rely on new forms of food in fast, complex lives. More women are working; households are getting smaller; more people are living alone; and meal patterns are different. People search for less fancy, lower-cost food items, and also cook creatively. People are generally more nutrition and health conscious, and this consciousness is influencing the social patterns of eating from food choices at fast-food outlets to the number of times people eat per day.

CRITICAL THINKING QUESTIONS

1. What is the meaning of culture? How does it affect our food patterns?
2. This chapter outlines the dietary laws of two religious groups. What other dietary laws are you familiar with? Using the Internet for a reference, compare the dietary practices of another religious group to the ones given in the text. Are there any practices that could be problematic for children, elderly, or sick individuals?

3. What social and psychological factors influence our food habits? Give examples of personal meanings related to food.
4. Why does the public tend to accept nutrition misinformation and fads so easily? What groups of people are more susceptible? Select one such group and give some effective approaches you might use to educate them.
5. What are current trends in American food habits? Discuss their implications for nutrition and health.

CHAPTER CHALLENGE QUESTIONS

True-False

Write the correct statement for each item you answer "false."

1. *True or False:* Food habits result from instinctive behavioral responses throughout life.

2. *True or False:* The structure of American social classes is largely determined by occupation, income, education, and residence.
3. *True or False:* Lifestyles change as society's values change.

4. *True or False:* From the time of birth, eating is a social act that is built on social relationships.

5. *True or False:* Food fads are usually long lasting and seldom change.

6. *True or False:* Special food combinations are effective as weight-reducing diets and have special therapeutic effects.

Multiple Choice

1. A healthy body requires

   a. specific foods to control specific functions.

   b. certain food combinations to achieve specific physiologic effects.

   c. natural foods to prevent disease.

   d. specific nutrients in various foods to perform specific body functions.

2. Food habits in a given culture are largely based on which of the following? (*Circle all that apply.*)

   a. Food availability

   b. Genetic differences in food tastes

   c. Food economics, market practices, and food distribution

   d. Symbolic meanings attached to certain foods

3. In the Jewish food pattern, the word *kosher* refers to food prepared by which of the following? (*Circle all that apply.*)

   a. Ritual slaughter of allowed animals for maximum blood drainage

   b. Avoiding the combination of meat and milk in the same meal

   c. Special seasoning to avoid use of salt

   d. Special cooking of food combinations to ensure purity and digestibility

4. The basic grain used in the Mexican food pattern is

   a. rice.

   b. corn.

   c. wheat.

   d. oat.

5. Stir-frying is a basic cooking method used in the food pattern of

   a. Mexicans.

   b. Jews.

   c. Chinese.

   d. Greeks.

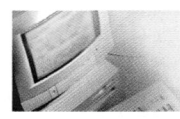

Please refer to the Students' Resource section of this text's Evolve web site for "Suggestions for Additional Study."

REFERENCES

1. Barer-Stein T: *You eat what you are: people, culture, and food traditions,* ed 2, New York, 1999, Culture Concepts.

2. Kittler PG, Sucher KP: *Cultural foods: traditions and trends,* New York, 1999, Wadsworth Publishing.

3. Burden M: Culturally sensitive care: managing diabetes during Ramadan, *Br J Commun Nurs* 6(11):581, 2001.

4. Painter J and others: Comparison of international food guide pictorial representations, *J Am Diet Assoc* 102(4): 483, 2002.

5. Davidson A: *The Oxford companion to food,* New York, 1999, Oxford University Press.

6. Huang M and others: Variation in nutrient intakes by ethnicity: results from the Study of Women's Health Across the Nation (SWAN), *Menopause* 9(5):309, 2002.

7. U.S. Department of Health and Human Services: *Healthy People 2010: understanding and improving health,* Washington, DC, 2000, USHHS/Government Printing Office.

8. Juhn MS, O'Kane JW, Vinci DM: Oral creatine supplement in male collegiate athletics: a survey of dosing habits and side effects, *J Am Diet Assoc* 99(5):593, 1999.

9. Pipe A, Ayotte C: Nutritional supplements and doping, *Clin J Sport Med* 12:245, 2002.

10. Southgate DAT: Dietary change: changing patterns of eating. In Meiselman HL, MacFie HJH, editors: *Food choices, acceptance, and consumption,* London, 1999, Chapman & Hall.

11. U.S. Census Bureau, U.S. Department of Commerce: *Statistical abstract of the United States 1999,* ed 119, Washington,

DC, 1999, U.S. Department of Commerce/Government Printing Office.

12. Economic Research Service, U.S. Department of Agriculture, *Briefing Room, Food consumption and nutrient intake tables, Table 6: sources of food energy intakes: individuals ages 2 and over*, Washington, DC, (accessed March 2003), USDA [*www.ers.usda.gov/Briefing/DietAndHealth/data/nutrients/table6.htm*].

13. Young LR, Nestle M: Expanding portion sizes in the U.S. marketplace: implications for nutrition counseling, *J Am Diet Assoc* 103:231, 2003.

FURTHER READING AND RESOURCES

• Satia-Abouta J and others: Dietary acculturation: applications to nutrition research and dietetics, *J Am Diet Assoc* 102(8):1105, 2002.

This article explores dietary acculturation by immigrants—the process of adopting the dietary practices of a new culture—in the United States and links specific practices with disease risk. The authors take an important look at the public health issues facing the U.S. immigrant population and how health care professionals can play a role in maintaining the healthiest combination of dietary practices.

• Juhn MS, O'Kane JW, Vinci DM: Oral creatine supplementation in male collegiate athletes: a survey of dosing habits and side effects, *J Am Diet Assoc* 99(5):593, 1999.

• Wagner DR: Hyperhydrating with glycerol: implications for athletic performance, *J Am Diet Assoc* 99(2):207, 1999.

These two articles provide sound scientific background to help athletes—especially younger, still growing athletes—who are straining to win, sometimes at whatever the cost to their bodies, and who thus are vulnerable to nutrition myths. In this effort, they may push to the limit, exceeding caution, and suffer harmful side effects. The potential misuse of two substances (creatine and glycerol) is clearly described, with the basis for caution presented in each case.

15

Weight Management

KEY CONCEPTS

- America's obsession with thinness carries social, physiologic, and biological costs.

- Underlying causes of obesity include a host of various genetic and environmental factors.

- Realistic weight management focuses on individual needs and health promotion.

A t least one out of every four Americans is on a weight-reduction diet. Use of these "diets" seems to increase daily, with a new diet book constantly appearing in the public press. Despite this obsession and the fact that weight loss is big business, Americans are actually getting heavier. The average American has gained about 2.25 kg (5 lbs) over the past decade or so. Why has this occurred?

Much of the answer lies in changing lifestyles. As technology advances, so do sedentary lifestyles, and none of these popular "diets" are working. Less than 5% of dieters maintain weight loss after such a diet. This chapter examines the problem of weight management and seeks a more positive and realistic health model that recognizes personal needs and sound weight goals.

OBESITY AND WEIGHT CONTROL

Body Weight and Body Fat

Definitions

An estimated 300,000 Americans die each year because of obesity-related diseases.[1] Obesity is not an "easy" problem. Obesity develops from many interwoven factors—including personal, physical, and genetic—and is difficult to define. As used in the traditional medical sense, *obesity* is a clinical term for excess body fat generally applied to persons who are at least 20% above a desired weight for height. The terms *overweight* and *obesity* often are used interchangeably, but they actually have different meanings. The word *overweight* simply means a body weight that is above a population weight-for-height standard. However, the word *obesity* is a more specific term that comes from a Latin root (*obedere*, to devour) and means "very fat." Thus it refers to the *degree of fatness* (e.g., the relative excess amount of fat in the total **body composition**), which is the real health problem. Over the past four decades the percentage of overweight (**body mass index [BMI]** ≥ 25) adults age 20 years or older has increased from 56% to 64%. The increase in persons meeting the criteria for clinical obesity (BMI ≥ 30) has increased even more dramatically from 13.4% of the population in 1960 to 31% in 2000.[2]

BMI can be tracked from childhood to adulthood with the new growth charts from the Centers for Disease Control and Prevention, and is a highly reliable method of predicting the relative risk of becoming an overweight adult based on the presence or absence of excess weight at various times during childhood. Studies show that 83% of children between the ages of 10 to 15 with a BMI greater than or equal to the 95th percentile become obese as adults.[3] However, one must always remember that every person is different, and *normal* values in healthy persons vary. Until recently, the important factor of *age* in setting a reasonable body weight for adults had been overlooked. With advancing age, body weight usually increases until about age 50 for men and age 70 for women, and then declines.

The exclusive use of BMI to define obesity has undergone some criticism because it does not actually measure body fat, per se, but total body weight. This method classifies some individuals as obese, when they do not actually have excessive body fatness.[4] For example, a football player in peak condition can be extremely "overweight" according to standard height-weight charts. That is, he can weigh considerably more than the average man of the same height, but much more of his weight is lean muscle mass, not excess fat (Figure 15-1).

Body Composition

Speaking in terms of body composition, instead of just absolute weight in pounds, provides a better evaluation of overall health relative to weight. Health professionals (e.g., usually the registered dietitian on the health care team) can measure body fatness with a variety of methods.

Body fat calipers measure the widths of skin folds at specific body sites, because most of the body fat is deposited in layers just under the skin. These measures are then used in specific formulas to calculate an estimated body fat composition. Calipers are an easy, portable, cheap, noninvasive way to measure body fat. However, reliability of the test is dependent on the skill of the technician and can vary greatly.

Hydrostatic weighing, a more precise method, is often used in athletic programs or research studies and ensures that obesity can be better defined in terms of body fat content. Hydrostatic weighing requires complete submersion of the patient or client in water. The person must exhale as much air as possible and stay underwater for a few seconds to get an accurate reading. Although this method is more accurate, it is not easy, portable, or cheap. Nor is it an option for many patients who cannot perform the test.

Bioelectrical impedance analysis is an easy, portable, inexpensive, and noninvasive body composition measurement tool. One type, a foot-to-foot analyzer, requires the person to stand on a modified scale with bare feet while a very light electrical current travels through the body. The analyzer determines body fat percentage based on gender, age, height, weight, total body water, and the rate at which the electrical current traveled. Fat impedes the current; therefore a lower total body fat composition will result in a faster travel time of the electrical current. Such

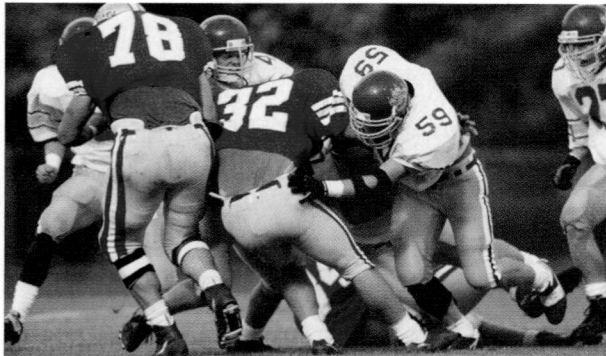

Figure 15–1   According to standard height-weight charts, some football players would be considered overweight. These charts should be used with discretion. (Credit: PhotoDisc.)

analyzers have both a standard adult and athletic setting. Although this method does not require any special skill on either the client or technician's part, discrepancies have been noted between total body fat percentages when measured via bioelectrical impedance versus hydrostatic weighing in some subsets of the population.[5]

Dual energy x-ray absorptiometry (DEXA), a much more accurate way of assessing body fat, is a relatively new method using radiation to distinguish bone, muscle, water, and fat density. Although this method is much less intimidating than hydrostatic weighing, it is very expensive.

Air displacement plethysmography, using the BOD POD Body Composition Tracking System (Life Measurement, Inc., Concord, CA), may prove to be a reliable method for assessing body composition that does not rely on technical expertise or radiation. However, it is also expensive and nonportable. The BOD POD calculates percent body fat using weight, body volume, thoracic lung volume, and body density. Current studies indicate that the BOD POD is a reliable measurement tool for most subgroups of the populations, but discrepancies may arise when measuring athletes.[6,7]

According to the American College of Sports Medicine, a body fat content within the range of 8% to 22% of total body weight is associated with the lowest risk of chronic disease for males ages 34 or less. For women it is somewhat larger: 20% to 35%.[8] Recommended body fat percentages do increase slightly with age, up to 25% and 38% for men and women, respectively. Health risks associated with obesity rise as the percentage of body fat exceeds these ranges.

Measures of Weight Maintenance Goals

Standard Height-Weight Tables

Height-weight tables are tools, or general population guides, and should be regarded only as such. Individual needs must be considered. One of the standard tables in use in the United States is the Metropolitan Life Insurance Company's "ideal" weight-for-height charts, which are based on life expectancy information gathered since the 1930s from its population of life insurance policy holders. Many people have questioned how well these tables represent the total current population because the data are based on such a select group of individuals (most of whom were Caucasian, middle- to upper-class men for the first couple of decades of gathering data) and may not take into consideration the wide variety of "norms" found within a diverse community.

More recent height-weight tables have been developed based on the National Research Council data on weight and health, the current *Dietary Guidelines for Americans*, and recent medical studies.[9] These more realistic guides, shown in Table 15-1, relate height and adult age ranges to good ranges of body weight.

Studies also show that health risks are as great, if not greater, for very thin low-weight persons as for extremely obese ones. Within each age group, both extremely thin and extremely fat persons have higher mortality rates.

Healthy Weight Range

A general calculation for determining healthy, or *ideal*, weight goals, are as follows:

- *Males:* 106 pounds for the first 5 feet, then add or subtract 6 pounds for each inch above or below 5 feet, respectively. A range is then taken by adding and subtracting 10% to account for small and large body frames.
- *Females:* 100 pounds for the first 5 feet, then add or subtract 5 pounds for each inch above or below 5 feet, respectively. A range is then taken by adding and subtracting 10% to account for small and large body frames.

Example: A 5 foot, 3-inch female would have an ideal body weight range of

$$100 \text{ lbs} + (3 \text{ in} \times 5 \text{ lbs}) = 115 \pm 10\%$$

Therefore her ideal body weight range is 103.5 to 126.5 lbs.

Similar to BMI, this calculation does not account for acceptable changes associated with age (loss of stature and slight increases in weight) or for individuals with very high lean body weight. A person's ideal weight may give him or her a "ballpark" figure for a healthy weight goal. However, there are two very important considerations to take into account when relying on ideal body weight calculations.

Individual Variation. The basic problem with "ideal weight" is that it varies with different people at different times under different circumstances. A person's ideal weight depends on many factors, including gender, age, body shape, metabolic rate, genetic make-up, and physical activity. Specific individual situations govern needs.

---

body composition   the relative sizes of the four basic body compartments that make up the total body: lean body mass (muscle mass), fat, water, and bone.

BMI (body mass index)   body weight in kilograms divided by the square of height in meters, kg/m^2.

TABLE 15–1	Good Body Weights-for-Height for Adults*								
	19-34 years		**35+ years**			**19-34 years**		**35+ years**	
Height (ft-in)†	Average weight (lbs)	Range (lbs)	Average weight (lbs)	Range (lbs)	Height (cm)	Average weight (kg)	Range (kg)	Average weight (kg)	Range (kg)
5'0"	112	97-128	123	108-138	152	51	44-58	55	49-62
5'1"	116	101-132	127	111-143	155	53	46-60	58	40-65
5'2"	120	104-137	131	115-148	157	54	47-62	59	52-67
5'3"	124	107-141	135	119-152	160	56	49-64	61	54-69
5'4"	128	111-146	140	122-157	163	58	51-66	64	56-72
5'5"	132	114-150	144	126-162	165	60	52-68	65	57-74
5'6"	136	118-155	148	130-167	168	62	54-71	68	59-76
5'7"	140	121-160	153	134-172	170	64	55-72	69	61-78
5'8"	144	125-164	158	138-178	173	66	57-75	72	63-81
5'9"	149	129-169	162	142-183	175	67	58-77	74	64-83
5'10"	153	132-174	167	146-188	178	70	60-79	76	67-86
5'11"	157	136-179	172	151-194	180	71	62-81	78	68-88
6'0"	162	140-184	177	155-199	183	74	64-84	80	70-90
6'1"	166	144-189	182	159-205	185	75	65-86	82	72-92
6'2"	171	148-195	187	164-210	188	78	67-88	85	74-95
6'3"	176	152-200	192	168-216	191	80	69-91	88	77-99
6'4"	180	156-205	197	173-222	193	82	71-93	89	78-101
6'5"	185	160-211	202	177-228	196	85	73-96	92	81-104
6'6"	190	164-216	208	182-234	198	86	75-98	94	82-106

Data from U.S. Department of Agriculture, U.S. Department of Health and Human Services: *Nutrition and your health: Dietary Guidelines for Americans,* ed 4, Washington, DC, 1995, Government Printing Office; and Bray GA: Pathophysiology of obesity, *Am J Clin Nutr* 55:448S, 1992.
*Expressed in pounds (for height, in feet-inches) and kilograms (for height, in centimeters)—without clothes.
†Without shoes.

Necessity of Body Fat. In the zeal to lose weight, people may forget that some body fat is essential to survival. Every cell membrane in the body has fat molecules within it. Fat is used for insulation and temperature regulation. Fat also protects the vital organs by providing cushioning. Victims of starvation die of fat loss, not protein depletion. For mere survival, males require 3% to 5% body fat, and females require 8% to 12%.[8] Menstruation begins when the female body reaches a certain size or, more precisely, when a young girl's body fat reaches a critical percent of body weight (e.g., ~20%). This is the amount needed for ovulation and to support a healthy pregnancy.[10]

Obesity and Health

Weight Extremes

Clearly massive, or *morbid*, obesity is a health hazard in itself and creates other medical problems by placing severe strain on all body systems. Both extremes of weight, fatness and thinness, pose health problems.

Overweight and Health Problems

The most recent National Health and Examination Survey (1999 to 2000) data indicated a marked increase in the prevalence of overweight persons in the United States.[2] Experts have estimated that more than 100 million American adults are overweight or obese, which increases their risk of related conditions such as hypertension; type 2 diabetes; heart disease; sleep apnea; gastroesophageal reflux disease; degenerative joint disease; and breast, prostate, and colon cancers.[1] The major problem affecting most Americans is the degree of excess weight that is a risk to positive health. Current studies indicate that direct relationships between excess weight and disease have been demonstrated in the following two conditions: type 2 diabetes mellitus and hypertension, which may contribute to cardiovascular disease. Health risks exist in *extreme* obesity, but unless a person is at least 30% over the normal weight-for-height ratio, the relation of weight to mortality is questionable. Weight loss can bring significant reductions in elevated blood glucose or blood pressure in

BOX 15–1   Kilocalorie Adjustment Necessary for Weight Loss

To lose 454 g (1 lb) a week = 500 fewer kcal daily

Basis of estimation:

1 lb body fat = 454 g
1 g pure fat = 9 kcal
1 g body fat = 7.7 kcal (some water in fat cells)
454 g × 9 kcal/g = 4086 kcals/454 g fat (pure fat)
454 g × 7.7 kcal/g = 3496 kcals/454 g body fat (or 3500 kcals)
500 kcal × 7 days = 3500 kcals = 454 g body fat

a role in determining a person's set-point for fat storage.[17] The researchers named the hormone *leptin,* from the Greek word *leptos,* meaning thin or slender. Leptin production, which varies greatly among people and situations, was first thought to control satiety in humans, but this theory has since been refuted. Women produce more leptin than men, and production increases after weight gain and during the luteal phase of the menstrual cycle.[17] Follow-up studies of leptin use in the treatment of obesity have reported disappointing results overall, although the hormone did prove effective in a small percentage of test participants.[18-20] Ongoing research seeks to learn what made the few who had a positive experience with leptin respond as they did.

Although there continue to be many unanswered questions about the exact mechanisms of leptin, the discovery of leptin receptors in the human brain has helped scientists in the search to understand how the hormone works in controlling body weight, and may enable them to develop antiobesity drugs.[21]

In other studies the focus is on population groups such as the Pima Indians, whose naturally low leptin concentration and low resting metabolic rate may be an expression of a "thrifty genotype."[22] Such researchers are exploring a possible genetic influence.

Genetic and Family Factors

Genetic inheritance probably influences a person's chance of becoming fat more than any other factor. Family food patterns then provide an environment allowing this genetic trait to present itself.

Genetic Control. Up to 80% of the predisposition to obesity is from genetic factors, thus making certain people highly susceptible to becoming obese in an environment that allows for such a genetic expression (see the Cultural Considerations box, "Genetics and the Predisposition for Obesity," for more information). In these types of obesity, genetic-metabolic controls regulate the amount of body fat an individual carries.[23] A person then eats to regain or lose whatever amount of fat the body is naturally set or programmed for, according to the weight below or above this internally regulated point (*set-point*). Thus persons who have unnaturally lost body fat below their programmed level, either by strenuous dieting or lack of food, eat to regain to their genetic set-point when food is available again. Similarly persons with lower programmed fat levels that have gained excess body fat above their genetic level by eating more, although their body metabolism remains unchanged by pushing food, lose this excess fat when they resume their regular food intake. This is not to say that a person has no control

obese persons with type 2 diabetes mellitus or hypertension.[11-14] In turn, these improvements reduce risks related to heart disease.

Causes of Obesity

Basic Energy Balance

How does a person become overweight? Although some persons suffer from congenital obesity, a major cause of obesity in sedentary Americans is *lack of physical activity.* In fact, a simple, well-defined walking program can help reduce the amount of body fat in overweight persons, even without any noticeable changes in dietary intake.[15] Thus regular exercise by itself has a significant effect on reducing fat and increasing lean body content.

The overall underlying energy imbalance (e.g., more energy intake as food than energy output as physical activity and basal metabolic needs) is the ultimate cause for excess weight. Excess intake is stored in the body as fat. About 3500 kcal is the equivalent of 1 lb (0.45 kg) of body fat (Box 15-1). A minor daily imbalance where energy intake exceeds output by a mere 5% can result in a weight gain of 5 kg in 1 year. This is part of the answer. However, it is also known that some overweight persons only eat moderate amounts of food and that some persons of average weight eat much more but never seem to gain unwanted pounds. Because many individual differences exist, more factors than just energy balance are involved in maintaining a healthy weight.

Obesity Gene

A research group at Rockefeller University first reported the obesity gene in test animals, an overweight strain of laboratory mice. Soon thereafter these researchers located the human equivalent of this gene.[16] The obesity gene encodes for a hormonelike protein thought to play

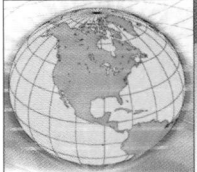

CULTURAL CONSIDERATIONS

GENETICS AND THE PREDISPOSITION FOR OBESITY

When comparing the prevalence of obesity in various racial and ethnic groups in the United States, researchers found a strong genetic influence, specifically in women.* Very few differences are seen between racial and ethnic groups among males. According to the National Health and Nutrition Examination Survey (NHANES): 1999 to 2000, the prevalence of obesity for racial/ethnic groups was as follows:

- Women: Non-Hispanic white: 30.1%
  Non-Hispanic black: 49.7%
  Mexican American: 39.7%
- Men: Non-Hispanic white: 27.3%
  Non-Hispanic black: 28.1%
  Mexican American: 28.9%

Thus non-Hispanic black women have a disproportionately high level of obesity when compared with other racial and ethnic groups. The exact cause for this differ-ence is not clearly defined; it is most likely a combination of genetics and environmental factors.

An even more dramatic trend noted throughout the NHANES data over the past few decades is the significant increase in obesity in both genders. The following summarizes the findings from these surveys. The percentages are the prevalence of obesity in both genders as a percent of the population:*

- 1960 to 1962: 13.4%
- 1971 to 1974: 14.5%
- 1976 to 1980: 15%
- 1988 to 1994: 23.3%
- 1999 to 2000: 30.9%

Although genetics do play a role in the prevalence and predisposition to obesity, such influences cannot explain such an increase in obesity for the entire population.

*Flegal KM and others: Prevalence and trends in obesity among U.S. adults: 1999-2000, *JAMA* 288(14):1723, 2002.

---

over his or her own body weight. A genetic influence is the *predisposing* factor, not the *determining* factor. The daily life, environment, and habits one chooses influence the expression of this genetic trait.

Family Reinforcement. However, in the long run excess body weight may have its start not so much in individual gene control as in the family food patterns learned in early years. An individual's genetic predisposition for in-creased body fat is reinforced by inappropriate family food patterns.[24] If one parent is obese, a child's chance of becoming obese is modest. This chance is greater if both parents are obese. Seldom does a child become obese if neither parent is overweight. In addition to genetic in-fluence, families also exert social pressure and teach chil-dren habits and attitudes toward food. Thus developing healthy eating habits, with fat-controlled cooking and the family enjoying meals together during childhood and teenage years is highly encouraged to establish balanced food patterns.

Physiologic Factors. The amount of body fat a person carries, whether through inheritance or eating habits, is related to the number and size of fat cells in the body.

Critical periods for developing obesity occur during early growth periods when cells are multiplying rapidly in childhood and adolescence. Once the body has added extra fat calls for more fuel storage, these cells remain and can store varying amounts of fat. Middle-aged and older adults may store more fat because of a decrease in basal metabolic rate, physical activity, and lean muscle mass.[9] Women also store more fat during pregnancy and after menopause in response to hormonal changes.

Other Environmental Factors. There are many environ-mental factors adding to the ever-increasing problem of obesity in the United States. The following are just a few: increase in food availability, fast and convenience foods, increase in portion sizes, decrease in food prepara-tion time and skills, decrease in physical activity, med-ications, and stressful lifestyles.[25] Many persons respond to emotional stress by eating, especially foods they regard as "comfort" foods. The primary stress hormone, cortisol, has been under the spotlight in recent years because of its relationship to weight gain. Cortisol levels rise in re-sponse to physical stressors and induce the fight-or-flight hormonal response. Under normal conditions, in which this type of stressor occurs only occasionally and normal cortisol levels return within a short period of time, no harm is done and the response to such stress is perfectly healthy. The problems with cortisol arise when continuous mental and emotional stressors such as deadlines at work, children, financial obligations, traffic, dieting, and so on induce a chronically high level of cortisol. Chronically elevated cortisol levels are associated with loss of muscle mass, increase in blood sugar levels, and increase in body fat, specifically abdominal fat.[26] Social pressures, especially on women, to maintain the cultural "ideal" thin body type contribute to the stress of constant dieting, which in turns creates a "catch-22" because this also increases cortisol levels, thus making weight loss even harder.

Individual Differences and Extreme Practices

Individual Energy-Balance Levels

Several factors influence a person's individual point of energy balance. Some persons have more genetic-based metabolic efficiency (e.g., the ability to "burn" food more readily than others do). Also, when calculating a person's energy intake, the figures indicate only an *estimated* value. Reported food values represent averages of many samples of that food tested. Many factors (e.g., including basal metabolic rate [BMR], body size, lean body mass, age, gender, and physical activity) also influence how much energy a person "burns." However, these calculations provide useful general information and indicate areas of individual needs and goals.

Extreme Practices

Individual differences in energy needs, along with social pressures, lead many overweight persons to use extreme measures to lose weight—often at the risk of their own health.

Fad Diets. A constant array of diet books and weight loss supplements promising to "melt the fat away" continue to flood the American market. These books and supplements usually sell briefly and then fade away, largely because their "quick fixes" do not work (Table 15-2). There are no magic, simple answers to such a complex problem. Most of the fad diets fail on the following two counts:

1. *Scientific inaccuracies and misinformation.* Fad diets or supplements are often nutritionally inadequate.
2. *Failure to address the necessity of changing long-term habits.* Persons often are set up for failure to main-

tain a healthy individual weight once it is achieved. The basic behavioral problem involved in changing food and exercise habits for life, actually a new lifestyle, is unrecognized.

For some persons the degree of energy restriction necessary places impossible demands, so they find themselves caught in a vicious cycle of **chronic dieting syndrome** and its harmful physical and psychological effects. These people often become caught up in the big business of the U.S. diet industry, where a large amount of money is spent each year on a wide range of weight loss diets, products, and services.

Fasting. This drastic approach takes many forms, from literal fasting to use of very-low-calorie diets of special formulas, possibly causing the effects of semistarvation (e.g., acidosis, low blood pressure, electrolyte loss, tissue protein loss, and decreased basal metabolic rate). Sometimes loss of sufficient heart muscle causes death. At best, some programs fail to help persons maintain the new weight after weight loss once refeeding begins.

Specific Macronutrient Restrictions. Avoiding any food group or macronutrient (e.g., carbohydrates, fats, and proteins) as the means for weight loss is unfounded. Such diets as that advocated by Dean Ornish (very, very low fat) or Robert Atkins (very low carbohydrate) are all together too restrictive to maintain for extended periods of time and carry their own health risk.

Clothing and Body Wraps. Special "sauna suits" or body wrapping has claimed to help weight loss in special spots of the body or clear up so-called *cellulite* tissue. The word *cellulite* was coined by a European beauty operator years ago and has no basis in scientific fact. Some persons endure such mummylike body wrapping in an attempt to reduce body size. The resulting small weight loss, how-

---

chronic dieting syndrome the cyclic pattern of weight loss by dieting to achieve an unnatural but culturally ideal body thinness, then regaining weight by compulsive food binges in response to stress, anxiety, and hunger. This abnormal psychophysiologic food pattern becomes chronic, changing a person's natural body metabolism and relative body composition to the abnormal state of a "metabolically obese" person of normal weight.

TABLE 15–2	Diet Summaries							
Diet	Philosophy	Foods to eat	Foods to avoid	Diet composition (average for 3 days)	Recommended supplements	Health claims scientifically proven?	Practicality	Lose and maintain weight?
Atkins*	Eating too many carbohydrates causes obesity and other health problems; ketosis leads to decreased hunger	Meat, fish, poultry, eggs, cheese, low-carbohydrate vegetables, butter, oil; no alcohol	Carbohydrates, specifically bread, pasta, most fruits and vegetables, milk	Protein: 27% Carbohydrates: 5% Fat: 68% (saturated: 26%)	Atkins supplement that includes chromium picolinate, carnitine, coenzyme Q10	No long-term validated studies published	Limited food choices; difficult to eat in restaurants because only plain protein sources and limited vegetables/salads allowed	Yes, but initial weight loss is mostly water; does not promote a positive attitude toward food groups; difficult to maintain long term because diet restricts food choices
Zone†	Eating right combination of foods leads to metabolic state at which body functions at peak performance, leading to decreased hunger, increased weight loss, and increased energy	Protein, fat, carbohydrates in exact portions only (40/30/30), low-glycemic-index foods, alcohol in moderation	Carbohydrates, specifically bread, pasta, fruit (some types), saturated fats	Protein: 34% Carbohydrates: 36% Fat: 29% (saturated: 9%) Alcohol: 1%	200 IU vitamin E	No; theories and long-term results not validated	Food must be eaten in required proportions of protein, fat, carbohydrates; menus plain and unappealing; vegetable portions very large; difficult to calculate portions	Yes, via caloric restriction; could result in weight maintenance if carefully followed; diet rigid and difficult to maintain

Diet	Theory	Foods Allowed	Foods Limited/Eliminated	Macronutrient Composition	Supplements	Long-Term Studies	Disadvantages	Weight Loss
Protein Power‡	Eating carbohydrates releases insulin in large quantities, which contributes to obesity and other health problems	Meat, fish, poultry, eggs, cheese, low-carbohydrate vegetables, butter, oil, salad dressings, alcohol in moderation	Carbohydrates	Protein: 26% Carbohydrates: 16% Fat: 54% (saturated: 18%) Alcohol: 4%	Multivitamin and mineral supplement	No long-term validated studies published	Not practical for long term; rigid rules	Yes, via caloric restriction; limited food choices not practical for long term
Sugar Busters§	Sugar is toxic to body and causes release of insulin, which promotes fat storage	Protein and fat; low-glycemic-index foods; olive oil, canola oil, and alcohol in moderation	Potatoes, white rice, corn, carrots, beets, white bread, all refined white flour products	Protein: 27% Carbohydrates: 52% Fat: 21% (saturated: 4%)	None	No long-term validated studies published	Eliminates many carbohydrate foods; discourages eating fruit with meals	Yes, via caloric restriction; limited food choices not practical for long term
Stillman¶	High-protein foods burn body fat; if carbohydrates are consumed, body stores fat instead of burning it	Lean meats, skinless poultry, lean fish and seafood, eggs, cottage cheese, skim-milk cheeses; no alcohol	All carbohydrates: bread, pasta, fruit, vegetables, fats, oils, dairy products	Protein: 64% Carbohydrates: 3% Fat: 33% (saturated: 13%)	Multivitamin and mineral supplement	No long-term validated studies published	Extreme limitations in food choices; very little variety	Yes, but loss is mostly water; maintenance based on strict calorie counting; very limited food choices not practical for long term

Modified from Jeor ST and others: Dietary protein and weight reduction: a statement for healthcare professionals from the Nutrition Committee of the Council on Nutrition, Physical Activity, and Metabolism of the American Heart Association, *Circulation* 104(15):1869, 2001 [http://circ.ahajournals.org/cgi/content/full/104/15/1869].

*Atkins C: *Dr. Atkins' new diet revolution*, New York, 1999, Avon Books.

†Sears B: *The zone*, New York, 1995, HarperCollins.

‡Eades MR, Eades MD: *Protein power*, New York, 1996, Bantam Books.

§Steward HL and others: *Sugar busters*, New York, 1998, Ballantine Books.

¶Stillman IM, Baker SS: *The doctor's quick weight loss diet*, New York, 1967, Dell.

ever, is only caused by temporary water loss. The only way to lose weight is to burn up more energy than consumed in the food eaten.

Drugs. Various amphetamine compounds, commonly called "speed," were once popular in the medical treatment of obesity but are no longer used because of their danger to health. Typical over-the-counter drugs have included phenylpropylamine (PPA; Dexatrim), which is a stimulant similar to amphetamine. Dexatrim has been linked to increased blood pressure and damage to blood vessels in the brain, which can lead to central nervous

system disorders such as confusion, stroke, hallucination, and psychotic behavior. No diuretics or hormones (e.g., thyroid hormone or steroids) should ever be used to alter body weight or leanness without strict medical indication and supervision.

A pair of related weight loss drugs, fenfluramine and phentermine, were produced and prescribed to be used together in the popular fen-phen combination for weight reduction. Shortly, however, physicians found that one in eight patients using these drugs developed valvular regurgitation, a sometimes fatal condition.[27] The U.S. Food and Drug Administration (FDA), with the support

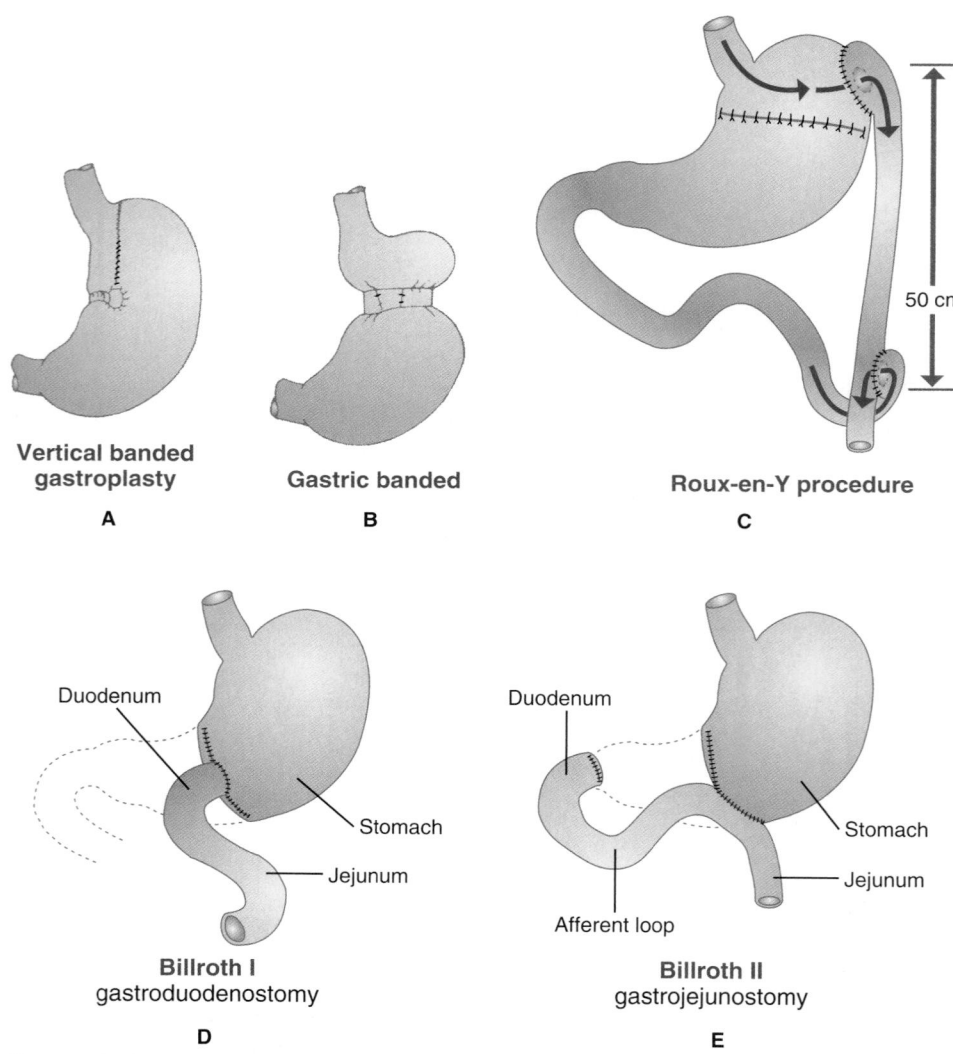

Figure 15-2 Surgical procedures for treatment of morbid obesity. (**A** and **B**, Modified from Grace DM: Gastric restriction procedures for treating severe obesity, *Am J Clin Nutr* 55:556S, 1992. **C-E**, From Mahan LK, Escott-Stump S: *Krause's food, nutrition, & diet therapy,* ed 11, Philadelphia, 2004, Saunders.)

of the medical community, quickly removed these drugs from the market. Although the pursuit of pharmacotherapy for the treatment of obesity is intense, there are few options currently available. Drugs used to treat obesity generally work in one of the following four ways:[28]

1. Reducing energy intake by suppressing the appetite
2. Increasing energy expenditure by stimulating the basal metabolic rate
3. Reducing the availability of nutrients to enter cells
4. Altering lipogenesis and lipolysis

The FDA has approved two medications, sibutramine and orlistat, for treatment of "clinically significant" obesity.[29] Sibutramine (Meridia) works by increasing the heart rate and thus increasing energy expenditure, whereas orlistat (Xenical) inhibits dietary fat absorption. Both medications have been successful with weight loss, but reports indicate that the weight returns when patients discontinue the medication.[25] As with many medications, there are also unpleasant side effects associated with these medications.

Surgery. Surgical techniques are usually reserved for the medical treatment of morbid obesity (BMI >40 or BMI 35 to 39 with at least one obesity-related disorder) in patients who have not had success with other methods of long-term weight loss. Although surgery historically has been the most successful method of permanent weight loss in morbid obesity, it is not without risk and complications. Greater than 90% of gastric bypass patients successfully lose 20% to 25% body weight and 50% to 80% maintain the weight loss for more than 5 years.[25] Current surgical procedures include vertical banded gastroplasty, Roux-en-Y gastric bypass, adjustable gastric banding, biliopancreatic diversion, and distal gastric bypass (Figure 15-2).[30-32] These types of surgical intervention are designed to reduce the space for food in the stomach, thus limiting appetite and eating, or by inducing malabsorption, thus decreasing nutrient availability to the body.[32] Weight loss surgeries require a skilled team of specialists, including nutritional care, careful patient selection, as well as continuous follow-ups in partnership with the patient and family.

A more limited type of cosmetic surgery that was developed in the 1980s and is still used is a form of local fat removal, **lipectomy,** which is commonly called liposuction. Lipectomy is used to remove fat deposits under the skin in places of cosmetic concern, such as the hips or thighs. A thin tube is inserted through a small incision in the skin, and the desired amount of fat is suctioned away. This procedure is quite painful, however, and carries risks such as infection, large disfiguring skin depressions, or blood clots that can lead to dangerous circulatory prob-

lems or even kidney failure. Any surgical procedure carries risk and may cause other problems and side effects.

SOUND WEIGHT-MANAGEMENT PROGRAM

Essential Characteristics

There are no shortcuts to successful weight control; it requires hard work and strong individual motivation. Weight management must be a personalized program that focuses on changed food and exercise behaviors and stress-relaxation habits. This program must build a healthy lifestyle and have support from the individual, family, or group with follow-ups.

Behavior Modification

Basic Principles

Food behavior is rooted in many human experiences and associations, as well as environmental situations. Addictive forms of eating responses and conditioning are common within many subgroups of the population. Behavior-oriented therapies are designed to help obese persons change patterns that contribute to excessive weight, such as excess food and eating, as well as lack of exercise. By understanding behaviors and changing associations with undesirable habits, reconditioning them into new desirable behavior patterns, overweight individuals can plan constructive actions to meet their personal health goals. This behavioral approach must begin with a detailed examination of each undesirable eating behavior with regard to the following three basic aspects:

1. *Cues or antecedents*. What stimulates the behavior?
2. *Response*. What happens during the eating or sedentary behavior after the cue?
3. *Consequences*. What happens after the response to the eating or sedentary behavior that serves to reinforce it?

Basic Strategies and Actions

A program of personal behavior modification for weight management is directed toward the following: (1) con-

---

lipectomy (Gr. *lipos,* fat; *ektomē,* excision) surgical removal of subcutaneous fat by suction through a tube inserted into a surface incision, or by removing larger amounts of subcutaneous fat by major surgical incision.

trol of eating behavior (e.g., the when, why, where, how, and how much); (2) promotion of physical activity to increase energy output; and (3) emotional, social, and psychological health. Three progressive actions follow in planning individual strategies.

Defining Problem Behavior. *Specifically* define the problem behavior and the desired behavior outcome. This process clearly establishes specific goals and contributing objectives.

Recording and Analyzing Baseline Behavior. Record eating and exercise behavior and analyze it carefully in terms of physical setting and persons involved. What types of

habit patterns emerge? How often do these patterns occur? What conditions seem to "trigger" the behavior? What consequent events seem to maintain the habits (e.g., time and pace, places, persons, social responses, hunger before and after, emotional mood, other factors)?

Planning Behavior-Management Strategy. Set up controls of the external environment involving the situational forces related to each of the three behavior areas involved: what goes before, the response, and the results. Then break these identified links to old undesirable behaviors and recondition them to the desired new eating and exercise behaviors. Think of as many creative ways as possible for reconditioning some personal food and ex-

CLINICAL APPLICATIONS

BREAKING OLD LINKS: STRATEGIES FOR CHANGING FOOD BEHAVIOR

Old habits die hard. They are never easy to change but, in the case of undesirable eating behaviors that contribute to excess body fat and are harmful to health, are worth the effort. Here are some behavioral suggestions.

1. Deal with Behavioral Cues

Eliminate as many cues for the problem behavior as possible. Avoid situations and contacts associated with problem foods, put temptation out of reach, and make the problem behavior as difficult as possible. Freeze leftovers, remove problem food items from the kitchen or store them in hard-to-get places, and take a route other than by the familiar bakery or candy shop home.

Suppress the cues that cannot be entirely eliminated. Control social situations that maintain the behavior, reward the alternate desired behavior, have a trusted person monitor eating patterns, reduce stress, minimize contact with excessive food, use smaller plates to make smaller food portions appear larger, control "poor me" moods with positive nonfood "treat" activities or physical activity.

Strengthen cues for desirable behaviors. Collect information and guides for a wide array of appropriate food choices and amounts. Use food behavior aids (e.g., records, a diary, or a journal). Distribute appropriate foods in desirable food meal/snack patterns. Make desirable food behavior as attractive and good-tasting as possible.

2. Deal with Actual Food Behavior in Response to Cues

Slow the pace of eating. Take one bite at a time and place utensil on the plate between bites. Chew each bite slowly. Sip a beverage. Consciously plan bits of conversation with meal companions for between bites. Visualize eating in slow motion. Enhance the social aspect of eating.

Savor the food. Eat slowly, sensing the taste, smell, and texture of the food. Develop and practice these sensory feelings to the extent that they can be described and brought to mind afterward. Look for food seasonings and combinations that will enhance this process and bring to mind positive feelings about the food experience.

3. Deal with the Follow-Up Behavior that Results

Decelerate the problem behavior. Slow down its frequency, and respond neutrally when it occurs rather than with negative talk or thoughts. Give social reinforcement to the decreasing number of times the problem behavior occurs. Focus on the ultimate consequences of the undesirable behavior in health problems.

Accelerate the desired behavior. Update the progress records or personal journal daily. Respond positively to all desired behavior; provide some sort of material reinforcement for positive behavior. Provide social reinforcement for all constructive efforts to modify behavior.

Such a program requires effort, motivation, and work. Continuously evaluate progress toward desired behavior while maintaining a realistic goal. Then plan individual or group maintenance and support activities during an extended follow-up period.

ercise behaviors that may need to change. The Clinical Applications box, "Breaking Old Links: Strategies for Changing Food Behavior," provides a few examples.

Dietary Principles

The central dietary approach in a weight-management program that could achieve a degree of *lasting* success must be based on five characteristics, as follows:

1. *Realistic goals.* Goals must be realistic in terms of overall weight loss and rate of loss, averaging $1/_2$ to 1 lb/week (no more than 1 to 2 lbs/week for morbidly obese patients).
2. *Energy (kcalories) reduced according to need.* The diet must have sufficient energy intake in relation to individual output of energy to produce a gradual weight loss.
3. *Nutritional adequacy.* The diet must be nutritionally adequate. Consuming less food may require vitamin/mineral supplements. In addition, the ratio of energy nutrients (e.g., carbohydrate, fat, and protein) should have an appropriate balance based on a wide variety of food sources.
4. *Cultural appeal.* The food plan must be similar enough to an individual's cultural eating pattern to form the basis for *permanent* alteration of eating habits. It must be a good, personal lifetime plan.
5. *Energy (kcalorie) readjustment to maintain weight.* When the desired weight level is reached, the energy level is adjusted according to maintenance needs. The changed basic habits of eating provide the continuing means of weight control.

Basic Energy-Balance Components

The two sides of energy balance are energy *intake* in the form of food and energy *output* in the form of metabolic work and physical activity. For successful weight reduction, both of these basic components must be addressed.

Energy Input: Food Behaviors

The energy value of the food intake must be reduced. To accomplish this, the usual amount of food served and eaten should be noted. Then smaller portions, attractively served, should be used. The food should be eaten *slowly*, and its taste and texture savored. Overall use of fat, sugar, and salt should be reduced; and the fiber content increased. A variety of foods should be chosen from a basic food guide, such as the food exchange lists (see Appendix F), in the amounts suggested in Table 15-3. These guides can serve as a focus for sound nutrition education.

Whole primary foods should be emphasized, and few processed foods used. Food intake should be fairly evenly distributed throughout the day. Some practical suggestions are provided in the Clinical Applications box, "Practical Suggestions for Changing Food Behaviors."

Energy Output: Exercise Behaviors

Energy output in physical activity must be increased relative to normal activity. For someone who has no planned physical activity, a regular daily exercise schedule, starting with simple walking for about a half hour each day and building to a brisk pace, is a great start. Some form of aerobic exercise (e.g., swimming or running) should be added, or a set of resistance exercises should be developed (see the For Further Focus box, "Benefits of Aerobic Exercise in Weight Management"). An exercise class may be helpful to maintain motivation (Figure 15-3).

Principles of a Sound Food Plan

On the basis of a careful diet history (see Chapter 17), a sound personalized food plan can be developed with the client and should involve each of the following principles of nutritional balance.

Energy Balance

As mentioned, there are no shortcuts to weight loss. Under normal circumstances, when energy expenditure is greater than energy intake, weight loss occurs. Because 1 pound of fat is equal to approximately 3500 kcal, an energy deficit of 500 kcal per day results in a weight loss of about 1 pound per week; a deficit of 250 kcal equals $1/_2$-pound weight loss per week (see Box 15-1). All persons pursuing weight loss should determine their current total energy needs as a basis for diet planning (Table 15-4). Then, adjustments to the diet (energy intake) and exercise program (energy output) can be balanced to produce a negative energy balance. As discussed throughout this text, individual energy needs and intake vary greatly. Therefore assuming all persons on a weight loss program should limit caloric intake to 1200 kcal per day (or any other prefabricated amount) is not appropriate. For a person who normally consumes 2000 kcal per day, the ideal scenario is a deficit of about 500 kcal per day. The total of those 500 kcal should not all come from diet. Reducing calorie intake by 25% (2000 × 25% = 500 kcal) would undoubtedly leave him or her hungry and constantly thinking about food. Instead, the weight loss program could include a 250-kcal reduction in energy intake and a 250 kcal increase in energy expenditure for a total deficit of 500 kcal.

TABLE 15–3	Weight-Reduction Food Plans Using the Exchange System of Dietary Control*†		
Food exchange groups	1200 kcal	1500 kcal	1800 kcal
TOTAL NUMBER OF EXCHANGES PER DAY			
Milk (nonfat)	2	2	2
Vegetable	3	4	4
Fruit	3	4	4
Starch/bread	5	7	9
Meat (lean or medium fat)	4	5	7
Fat	4	5	5
MEAL PATTERN OF FOOD EXCHANGES			
Breakfast			
Fruit	1	1	1
Meat	—	1	1
Starch/bread	1	2	2
Fat	1	1	1
Milk	½	½	½
Lunch/supper			
Meat	1	1	2
Vegetables	1	2	2
Starch/bread	2	2	3
Fat	1	2	2
Fruit	1	1	1
Milk	½	½	½
Dinner			
Meat	2	2	3
Vegetables	2	2	2
Starch/bread	1	2	3
Fat	2	2	2
Fruit	—	1	1
Milk	½	½	½
Snack (afternoon or evening)			
Milk	½	½	½
Meat	1	1	1
Starch/bread	1	1	1
Fruit	1	1	1

*Total kilocalorie distribution: 50% carbohydrate, 20% protein, 30% fat.
†See the food Exchange Lists in Appendix F.

Nutrient Balance

Basic energy nutrients are outlined in the diet to achieve the following nutrient balance:

- *Carbohydrate.* Approximately 45% to 65% of the total kcalories, with emphasis on complex forms such as starch with fiber, and a limit on simple sugars
- *Protein.* Approximately 10% to 35% of the total kcalories, with emphasis on lean food and small portions
- *Fat.* Less than or equal to 25% of the total kcalories, with emphasis on low animal fats, scant total use, and alternate nonfat seasonings

This nutrient balance meets the recommendations of the *Dietary Guidelines for Americans 2005* (see Figure 1-3). This can serve as a good general guide for long-term habits.

Distribution Balance

Spreading the food fairly evenly through the day helps meet energy needs. Hunger usually peaks every 4 to 5 hours. If an individual has certain "problem times" of the day, planning simple snacks for those periods helps maintain balance. Going for long periods of time with-

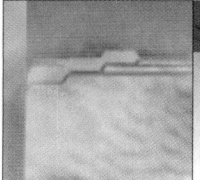

CLINICAL APPLICATIONS

PRACTICAL SUGGESTIONS FOR CHANGING FOOD BEHAVIORS

Goals

Be realistic. Do not set your goals too high. Adapt your rate of loss to $1/2$ to 1 lb per week. If visible tools are helpful motivation techniques, use them.

Kilocalories

Do not be an obsessive "calorie counter." Simply become familiar with food exchanges in your diet list and learn the general values of some of your home dishes, and then modify recipes or make occasional substitutes.

Plateaus

Anticipate plateaus; they happen to everyone. Plateaus are related to water accumulation as fat is lost. Increase exercises during these periods to help get started again.

Binges

Do not be discouraged when you break down and have a binge. This happens to most persons. Simply keep them infrequent and, when possible, plan ahead for special occasions. Adjust the following day's diet or the remainder of the same day accordingly.

Special Diet Foods

There is no need to purchase special "low-calorie" foods. Learn to read labels carefully. Most special diet foods are expensive foods that are not much lower in kilocalories than regular foods.

Home Meals

Try to avoid making a separate menu for yourself. Adapt your needs to the family meal, adjusting the seasoning or method of preparation to lower kilocalories, especially by reducing or omitting fat.

Eating away from Home

Watch portions. When you are a guest, limit extras such as sauces and dressings and trim meat well. In restaurants, select singly prepared items rather than combination dishes. Avoid items with heavy sauces or fat seasonings and fried foods. Select fruit or sherbet for dessert rather than pastries.

Appetite Control

Avoid dependence on appetite-depressant medications, which are usually only crutches. Try nibbling on food items from the free food list or save other meal items, such as fruit or bread exchanges, for use between meals.

Meal Pattern

Eat three or more meals a day. If you are used to three meals, then leave it at that. If snacks between meals help you, then plan part of your day's allowance to account for them. The main thing is that you do not consume your entire day's energy allowance at one time. Avoid the all-too-common pattern of no breakfast, little or no lunch, and a huge dinner.

---

out refueling can result in low blood sugar and subsequent periods of overeating, usually whatever can be found at the time. Everyone is probably guilty of skipping lunch on occasion and then raiding the vending machines for high-fat or -sugar foods later in the afternoon. Balanced meals require the foresight of planning and preparation.

Food Guide

The revised food exchange lists (Appendix F) follow the general *Dietary Guidelines for Americans*. Table 15-3 provides some examples of basic food plans for weight reduction. This basic food exchange system is a good general reference guide for comparative food values and portions, variety in food choices, and basic meal planning. A simple plan also can be outlined using the basic food groups of the MyPyramid guidelines (see Figure 1-2).

With either plan, food items can be combined into desired dishes. Alternate nonfat seasonings (e.g., herbs, spices, onion, garlic, lemon and lime juice, vinegar, wine, broth, mustard, and other condiments) can be used freely.

Preventive Approach

The most positive work with weight management is aimed at *prevention*. Current studies indicate that the U.S. population of children and adolescents are getting fatter, and these fatter individuals are becoming obese adults. A major culprit in this health epidemic is the lack of exercise, mainly from hours of television viewing. Support for young parents and children before an obese condition develops helps prevent many problems later in adulthood. This support and guidance should include early nutrition counseling and

FOR FURTHER FOCUS

BENEFITS OF AEROBIC EXERCISE IN WEIGHT MANAGEMENT

The goal of weight management is to reduce excess body fat and, in most cases, to build lean body mass (LBM). However, both tissues are lost when a person tries to reach a weight goal merely by reducing food intake.

Optimal body composition can be achieved by combining food restriction with aerobic exercise. Aerobic exercise consists of activities that are sustained long enough to draw on the body's fat reserve for fuel while oxygen intake is increased (thus the name aerobic). Lean body tissue burns fats in the presence of oxygen. Therefore aerobic activity is best suited for achieving the ideal balance of high LBM and low fatty tissue in the body.

The benefits of aerobic exercise to an overweight person in a weight-management program include the following:

● Lowered genetic setting for body fat
● Suppressed appetite
● Reduced total body fat

● Higher basal metabolic rate
● Increased circulatory and respiratory function
● Increased energy expenditure
● Retention of tissue protein and building of LBM levels

Sometimes persons complain about the slow rate of weight loss, difficulty in controlling appetite, and consistent "flabbiness" despite continuing diet management. These persons may welcome the suggestion of aerobic activity to help meet these needs. A brisk daily walk, jumping rope, swimming, bicycling, jogging, running, aerobic or spinning classes, or some other activity may be sustained long enough for it to have an aerobic effect. Carefully note the physical stress this activity may place on individuals who have not exercised for some time or who have medical problems related to exertion. These persons should have a medical checkup before beginning such a program on their own or joining a local gym or other community fitness center.

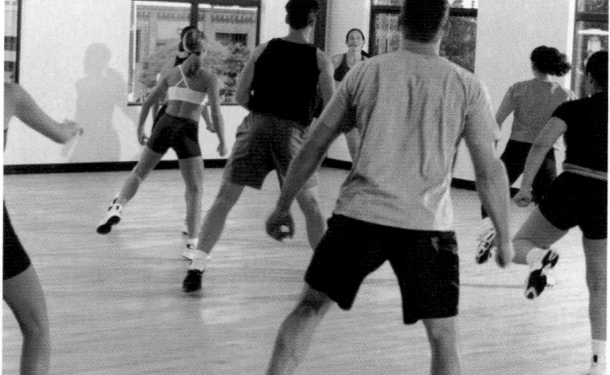

Figure 15–3 An exercise class provides regular support for an effective weight-management plan. (Credit: PhotoDisc.)

education, helping to build positive health habits, especially in positive eating behaviors and increased exercise through active play and physical activities for the entire family. Many programs for young children, such as Head Start, school lunch programs, the Women, Infants, and Children (WIC) program (see Chapter 13), and others are addressing obesity issues through education and prevention for both parents and children.

UNDERWEIGHT

General Causes and Treatment

Extremes in underweight, just as in overweight, can bring serious health problems. Although general underweight is a less common problem in the U.S. population than overweight, it does occur and usually is associated with poor living conditions or long-term disease. A person who is more than 10% below the average weight for height and age is considered underweight; and being at least 20% below the average is cause for concern. Serious results may occur in these persons, especially young children. Their resistance to infection is lowered, general health is poor, and strength is reduced.

Causes

Underweight is associated with conditions that cause general malnutrition, including the following:

■ *Wasting disease.* Long-term wasting disease with chronic infection and fever that raise the basal metabolic rate (BMR).
■ *Poor food intake.* Diminished food intake resulting from (1) psychological factors that cause a person to refuse to eat, (2) loss of appetite, or (3) personal poverty and limited available food supply.

TABLE 15–4 General Approximations for Daily Adult Basal and Activity Energy Needs

Daily energy needs (basis for calculations)	Activity energy needs above basal (%)	Male (70 kg) kcal	Female (58 kg) kcal
Basal energy needs			
1 kcal/kg per hour		70 kg × 24 hours = 1680	58 kg × 24 hours = 1392
Activity energy needs			
Sedentary	+20% basal	1680 + 336 = 2016	1392 + 278 = 1670
Very light	+30% basal	1680 + 504 = 2484	1392 + 418 = 1810
Moderate	+40% basal	1680 + 672 = 2352	1392 + 557 = 1949
Heavy	+50% basal	1680 + 840 = 2520	1392 + 696 = 2088

■ *Malabsorption.* Poor nutrient absorption resulting from (1) long-lasting diarrhea, (2) a diseased gastrointestinal tract, or (3) excessive use of laxatives.

■ *Hormonal imbalance.* Hyperthyroidism, or a variety of other hormonal imbalances, may increase the caloric needs of the body.

■ *Energy imbalance.* This can result from greatly increased physical activity without a corresponding increase in food.

■ *Poor living situation.* An unhealthy home environment can result in irregular and inadequate meals, where eating is considered unimportant and an indifferent attitude toward food exists.

Dietary Treatment

Underweight persons require special nutritional care to rebuild their body tissues and regain their health. Food plans should be adapted to each person's unique situation, whether it involves personal needs, living situation, economic needs, or any underlying disease. The dietary goal, according to each person's tolerance, is to increase both energy and nutrient intake, with adherence to the following needs:

■ *High-caloric diet:* significantly above the standard requirement for that individual
■ *High protein:* to rebuild tissues
■ *High carbohydrate:* to provide the primary energy source in an easily digested form
■ *Moderate fat:* to add energy without exceeding tolerance limits
■ *Good sources of vitamins and minerals:* including supplements when individual deficiencies require them

A variety of foods, attractively served, helps to revive the appetite and increase the desire to eat more. Nourishing meals and snacks should be spread through-

out the day and often include favorite foods. A basic aim is to help build good food habits, so that improved nutritional status and weight can be maintained once they are regained. Residents in long-term care facilities are especially vulnerable to weight-loss problems and have special needs (see the Clinical Applications box, "Problems of Weight Loss among Older Adults in Long-Term Care Facilities"). This rehabilitation process requires creative counseling of each individual and family, along with practical guides and support. In some cases, tube feeding or intravenous feeding (e.g., total parenteral nutrition [TPN]) may be necessary (see Chapter 22).

Ideal weight gain includes both lean and fat tissue. To gain lean tissue, or muscle, physical exercise also must be part of the equation for treatment. Resistance training increases lean tissue and, in turn, boosts appetite. A variety of weight lifting and strength training programs can be designed depending on the desires of the individual (e.g., where and when he or she can and will work out, etc.), and should be encouraged as an important part of healthy weight gaining.

Disordered Eating

Losing sight of what "normal" eating behavior is can be easy to do. Normal eating is when an individual: (1) eats when he or she is hungry and stops when full, (2) can demonstrate moderate constraint in food selection, (3) recognizes that it is okay to overeat sometimes and undereat sometimes and trust his or her body to establish a balance, and (4) can be flexible with his or her eating schedule.[33] Disordered eating can be defined as any eating pattern that is not normal, which can include a variety of subclinical problems. Disordered eating may be anything from an insurmountable fear of eating fat to an inability to eat in public. Sometimes family and personal tensions, as well as social pressures for

CLINICAL APPLICATIONS

PROBLEMS OF WEIGHT LOSS AMONG OLDER ADULTS IN LONG-TERM CARE FACILITIES

The American population of adults age 65 and older is rapidly increasing. The most rapid population increase over the next decade will be among those over 85 years of age. Many of these elderly persons will require long-term care in nursing homes.

One of the problems encountered with elderly residents is low body weight and rapid unintentional weight loss. These can become serious health problems and are a sensitive indicator of malnutrition, contributing to illness and death. Because weight loss is such a strong predictor of morbidity and mortality in clinical settings, early and continuing observation to assess needs is important, especially in relation to factors that contribute to weight loss.

In general, the weight loss can be caused by physical effects related to the metabolic changes of aging or disease or by factors that alter the amount and type of food eaten. Physical disease such as cancer can cause extreme weight loss from metabolic abnormalities, taste changes, loss of appetite, nausea, and vomiting. Other diseases underlying weight loss may be gastrointestinal problems, uncontrolled diabetes, and cardiovascular disorders such as congestive heart failure, pulmonary disease, infection, or alcoholism. Psychological factors or psychiatric disorders may also contribute to malnutrition and weight loss through depression, memory loss, disorientation, apathy, or appetite disturbance. Some altered mental states may be caused by nutritional deficiencies, such as low levels of folate and B-complex vitamins, as well as by protein-calorie malnutrition. These conditions can be corrected with specific nutritional support.

The following additional physiologic, psychological, and social factors may influence food intake and body weight and contribute to malnutrition in elderly persons:

● *Body composition changes*. Height and body weight gradually decline. Body weight usually peaks between the ages of 34 and 54 in men and 55 and 75 in women, decreasing thereafter. Body fat losses generally are not significant. The greatest cause of weight loss is a decline in body water, caused in part by weakening of the normal thirst mechanism. Therefore a feeling of thirst cannot be depended on to secure adequate water intake, so water must frequently be offered and encouraged. More constant attention to fluid intake also helps with the common problem of xerostomia (dry mouth) in older adults, which results from inadequate salivary secretions to help with eating, thus contributing to malnutrition. Lean body mass also declines with age, resulting in a lower basal metabolic rate, and decreased physical activity and energy requirements. Thus any possible increase in physical activity and use of nutrient-dense foods is encouraged.

thinness cause adolescent girls and boys (some even starting in grade school) and young adults to develop serious body image and eating problems that may become psychiatric disorders. No matter what they weigh, these individuals always see themselves as fat and develop a deep-seated fear of food and fatness. Historically, disordered eating behavior has been observed mostly in females. However, recent studies are finding that an increasing number of males are experiencing disordered eating as well.

Two forms of these extreme eating disorders are **anorexia nervosa** and **bulimia nervosa**. A third less extreme disorder, *compulsive overeating*, is fueled by the cultural drive for thinness and the resulting chronic dieting syndrome, and may sow the seeds of more dangerous extreme disorders. An estimated 5 million Americans are currently battling an eating disorder.

Anorexia Nervosa

This complex psychological problem results in self-imposed starvation. Anorexia nervosa patients generally are characterized as high achievers who constantly push themselves toward perfection. They see food and their body as things that can be controlled. Their distorted body image (seeing themselves as fat even when they are actually emaciated) (Figure 15-4), keeps them in a state of near panic. Anorexia nervosa patients may plan their days around ways of avoiding

- *Taste changes*. Regeneration of taste cells slows with age, but the extent and effect on food intake varies widely. The sense of smell also declines with age and may affect taste. Increased use of appropriate seasoning and flavoring in food preparation is needed.
- *Dentition*. About 50% of all Americans have lost their teeth by the age of 65. Many have dentures, but chewing problems often are present. About half of the nursing home populations report chewing, biting, and swallowing problems that interfere with eating and adequate food intake. Assessment of specific need and dental care solutions help correct eating problems.
- *Gastrointestinal problems*. Delayed gastric emptying may contribute to distention and lack of appetite. A decrease in gastric secretions, including hydrochloric acid, may hinder absorption of vitamin B_{12}, folate, and iron, thus contributing to anemia and loss of appetite. Constipation is a common complaint, often leading to laxative abuse and resulting in interference with nutrient absorption from chronic diarrhea. An increase in dietary fiber and liquids can help provide a more natural approach to establishing normal bowel movement.
- *Drug/nutrient interactions*. Elderly persons often take a number of prescribed and over-the-counter drugs, some of which are the direct cause of anorexia, nausea, and vomiting. Other drugs are indirect causes by inducing nutrient malabsorption, leading to deficiencies that in turn bring anorexia and weight loss. Drug

therapy for elderly patients should have constant medical, nutritional, and nursing attention to provide for appropriate use.
- *Functional disabilities*. Eating problems can prevent or alter the capacity of elderly persons to take in sufficient food. These problems may vary from more difficult functional disabilities that interfere with putting food into the mouth and swallowing (e.g., problems that often require a trained therapist) to dependence on feeding assistance that can be provided by sensitive nursing care.
- *Social problems*. Socioeconomic problems are often involved with care of the elderly. A specially trained geriatric social worker can help work out possible sources of financial assistance. A sense of social isolation can also lead to decreased food intake. Family support is necessary, as well as sensitive contacts with nursing home staff and residents and as much involvement as possible in group activities.

Health workers in geriatric settings need continuing education and sensitization to the potential dangers of low body weight and weight loss. Aged persons with acute and chronic illnesses and functional disabilities are at the greatest risk for nutrition-related problems. These persons need continuing nutrition assessment and monitoring of body weight. Some of the restrictions of "special diets" should be relaxed or discontinued when risk of malnutrition is evident, with the goal of increasing nutrient intake and making eating as enjoyable as possible.

food, which becomes a full-time obsession. Patients generally grow more depressed, irritable, and anxious as the disease progresses.

The American Psychiatric Association has established the following criteria as diagnostic for anorexia nervosa:

- Disturbed view of body size or shape
- Refusal to maintain or gain the minimal body weight for age and height
- Intense fear of weight gain or becoming fat
- Absence of at least three menstrual cycles for females

Individuals suffering from anorexia nervosa often are preoccupied with food, calories, and weight.

anorexia nervosa (Gr. *an-*, negative prefix; *orexis*, appetite) extreme psychophysiologic aversion to food resulting in life-threatening weight loss. A psychiatric eating disorder resulting from a morbid fear of fatness in which a person's distorted body image is reflected as fat when the body is actually malnourished and extremely thin from self-starvation.

bulimia nervosa (L. *bous*, ox; *limos*, hunger) a psychiatric eating disorder related to a person's fear of fatness, in which cycles of gorging on large quantities of food are followed by self-induced vomiting and use of diuretics and laxatives to maintain a "normal" body weight.

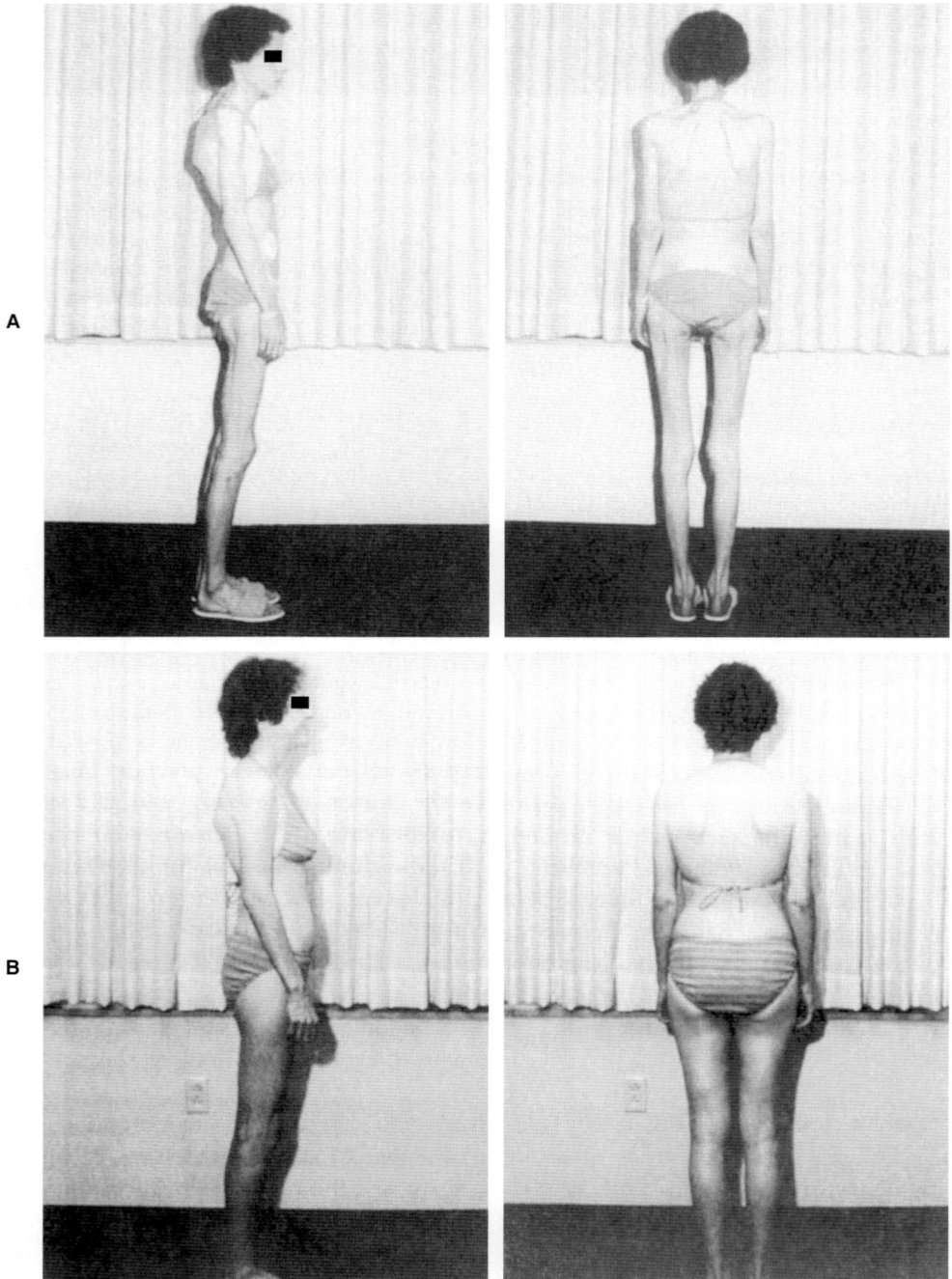

Figure 15–4 **A,** Anorectic woman before treatment. **B,** Same patient after gradual refeeding, nutrition management, and psychological therapy. (Courtesy Sycamore Hospital, a division of Kettering Medical Center, Dayton, OH.)

Warning signs include dramatic weight loss, avoiding food-related events, mood swings, excessive exercise, and other obsessive-compulsive behaviors.

Bulimia Nervosa

Individuals with bulimia nervosa also suffer from similar obsessions about body and food. Bulimia is an eating disorder involving repeated episodes of binge eating followed by a compensatory mechanism to rid the body of excess calories. Compensatory mechanisms include self-induced vomiting, laxative abuse, strict dieting/fasting, and excessive exercise. A "binge" varies among patients, but involves the consumption of very large quantities of food in a short period of time. Some individuals consume several thousand kcalories within 20 to 30 minutes. Oral and dental problems from the purging behavior may involve oral mucosal irritation, decreased salivary secretions and dry mouth (xerostomia), and irreversible enamel erosion.

The American Psychiatric Association has established the following criteria as diagnostic for bulimia nervosa:

■ Disturbed view of body size or shape with a feeling of lack of control over eating behavior during binge episodes
■ Recurrent episodes of binge eating (twice a week for at least 3 months)
■ Regular use of compensatory mechanisms (e.g., vomiting, laxatives or diuretic abuse, vigorous exercise, and strict dieting or fasting)

Individuals suffering from bulimia nervosa often go unnoticed and undiagnosed for much longer than anorexics. In general, body weight is within a normal weight range but may fluctuate regularly. Warning signs include excessive concern about weight, cycles of strict dieting and binge eating, self-criticism and low self-esteem, depression, and disappearance after meals.

Compulsive Overeating

This eating disorder includes binging episodes without the purging behavior of bulimics. This reactive type of eating often follows some stress or anxiety as an emotional eating pattern to soothe or relieve painful feelings. The binges may be triggered by psychological factors involving self and body image, with unrealistic weight goals. Dietary restriction and failure to achieve satiety or relieve hunger precede binges and relentlessly drive individuals toward a continuous, unsatisfying cycle. Persons who attempt to reach these unrealistic, and (for them) unnatural, weight goals are "forever dieting" (e.g., chronic dieting syndrome). After each weight loss, rebound eating occurs, followed by more attempts to lose weight. Thus the weight cycling, with its physiologic effects, continues.

Treatment

These psychological disorders require therapy from a team of skilled professionals, including physicians, psychologists, and nutritionists. Even with the best of care, recovery is slow, a day at a time, and the word *cure* is not used often. Approximately two thirds of eating disorder patients have persistent food and weight preoccupations throughout life. Patients with eating disorders often have neurologic disturbances. These chemical disturbances were first thought of as the cause for disordered eating behavior. However, researchers have found that once a normal weight and eating pattern is reestablished in the patient, the neurologic chemistry returns to normal. Therefore one of the first issues to address in treatment of an eating disorder is to establish a healthy weight in the patient. Psychological therapy is more successful once neurologic disturbances are reduced. Next, the team of professionals must work together to restore eating habits and attitudes toward food, optimize physical and mental health, and restore intrapersonal and interpersonal problems. Continuing support groups, including friends, family, and health care professionals, are critical for long-term treatment.

SUMMARY

In the traditional medical model, obesity has been viewed as an illness and a health hazard, which is true in cases of extreme or morbid obesity. Newer approaches view moderate overweight differently, however, in terms of the important aspect of fatness and leanness or body composition and propose a more person-centered positive health model (see the Clinical Applications box, "Case Study: John's Energy-Balance and Weight-Management Plan").

Planning a weight-management program, either for an overweight or underweight person, must involve the metabolic and energy needs of the individual. Personal food choices and habits, as well as fatty tissue needs during different stages of the life cycle, must be considered. Important aspects of such a weight-reduction program include changing food behaviors and increasing physical activity. A sound program is based on reduced energy intake for gradual weight loss and nutrient balance to meet

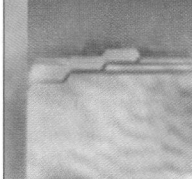

CLINICAL APPLICATIONS

CASE STUDY: JOHN'S ENERGY-BALANCE AND WEIGHT-MANAGEMENT PLAN

John is a college student leading a more or less sedentary life because of classes and study. He is interested in wrestling, however, and wants very much to make the team. To do so, he must lose some excess weight.

John begins to look carefully at his energy-balance picture. His weight is 180 pounds, and his average food intake each day is approximately 3000 kcal. He would like to plan a means of losing weight by reversing his energy balance.

Questions for Analysis

1. What is John's present daily total energy (kcalories) needs (based on weight and activity level)?
2. How does this total energy need compare with his food-energy intake?
3. To lose approximately 1 lb/week, how much should he reduce the caloric value of his daily diet?
4. Besides reducing his diet kcalories, what else could John do to help reverse his energy balance and improve his body condition?

the health standards of the U.S. dietary goals, with meals distributed throughout the day for energy needs. The ideal plan begins with prevention, stressing the formation of positive food habits in early childhood to prevent major problems later in life.

The American obsession with thinness has created extreme weight-management problems such as eating disorders that result in self-starvation. These psychological disorders require professional team therapy, including medical, psychological, and nutritional care.

CRITICAL THINKING QUESTIONS

1. Why is the term *ideal weight* difficult to define? Explain some of the problems in determining this measure. What role does it play in weight management?
2. What does *set-point* mean in relation to individual weight? How does it relate to diet and exercise in a personal weight-management program?

3. Describe the components of a positive health model for weight management. What are the basic principles of a sound food plan for such a program?
4. Describe the two major eating disorders associated with a growing obsession with thinness. What are the contributing social and psychological factors? What is the treatment? How does the chronic dieting syndrome relate and contribute to the prevalence of disordered eating?

CHAPTER CHALLENGE QUESTIONS

True-False

Write the correct statement for each item you answer "false."

1. *True or False:* Development of childhood obesity results exclusively from genetic inheritance.
2. *True or False:* Decreasing the energy expended in physical activity is a means of weight control.

3. *True or False:* A certain percentage of stored fat in the body is necessary for life.
4. *True or False:* A reasonable weight-reduction diet for an adult has an energy value of about 1200 to 1800 kcal, depending on individual size and need.
5. *True or False:* A weight-reduction diet should not use between-meal snacks.

Multiple Choice

1. Overweight is a direct risk factor in which of the following conditions? *(Circle all that apply.)*

   a. Surgery

   b. Type 2 diabetes mellitus

   c. Liver disease

   d. Hypertension

2. A 500-kcal deficit in the daily energy expenditure of an obese person enables him or her to lose weight at which of the following rates?

   a. 1 lb/week

   b. 2 lbs/week

   c. 3 lbs/week

   d. 4 lbs/week

3. An individual who has repeated binge-purge episodes, expresses severe self-criticism, and often is depressed may be suffering from which of the following?

   a. Anorexia nervosa

   b. Bulimia nervosa

   c. Compulsive overeating

   d. None of the above

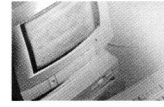

Please refer to the Students' Resource section of this text's Evolve web site for "Suggestions for Additional Study."

REFERENCES

1. O'Brien PE, Dixon JB: The extent of the problem of obesity, *Am J Surg* 184(6B):4S, 2002.

2. Flegal KM and others: Prevalence and trends in obesity among U.S. adults: 1999-2000, *JAMA* 288(14):1723, 2002.

3. Division of Nutrition and Physical Activity, National Center for Chronic Disease Prevention and Health Promotion, Centers for Disease Control and Prevention: *CDC growth charts PowerPoint presentation*, Atlanta, (accessed March 2003), DNPA/NCCDPHP/CDC [*www.cdc.gov/nccdphp/dnpa/growthcharts/training/powerpoint/slides/020.htm*].

4. Prentice AM, Jebb SA: Beyond body mass index, *Obesity* 2:141, 2001.

5. Swartz AM and others: Evaluation of a food-to-foot bioelectrical impedance analyzer in highly active, moderately active and less active young men, *Br J Nutr* 88(2):205, 2002.

6. Fields DA and others: Comparison of the BOD POD with the four-compartment model in adult females, *Med Sci Sports Exerc* 33(9):1605, 2001.

7. Vescovi JD, Miller W: Evaluation of the BOD POD for estimating percent fat in female college athletes, *J Strength Cond Res* 16(4):599, 2002.

8. American College of Sports Medicine: *ACSM's guidelines for exercise testing and prescription*, ed 6, Philadelphia, 2000, Lippincott Williams & Wilkins.

9. Food and Nutrition Board, Institute of Medicine: *Dietary reference intakes for energy, carbohydrate, fiber, fat, fatty acids, cholesterol, protein, and amino acids*, Washington, DC, 2002, National Academies Press.

10. Frisch RE: *Female fertility and the body fat connection*, Chicago, 2002, University of Chicago Press.

11. Vidal J: Updated review on the benefits of weight loss, *Int J Obes Relat Metab Disord* 26(4):S25, 2002.

12. Adler A: Obesity and target organ damage: diabetes, *Int J Obes Relat Metab Disord* 26(4):S11, 2002.

13. Schunkert H: Obesity and target organ damage: the heart, *Int J Obes Relat Metab Disord* 26(4):S15, 2002.

14. Miller ER and others: Results of the diet, exercise, and weight loss intervention trial (DEW-IT), *Hypertension* 40(5):612, 2002.

15. Asikainen T-M and others: Walking trials in postmenopausal women: effect of one vs two daily bouts on aerobic fitness, *Scand J Med Sci Sports* 12:99, 2002.

16. Zhang Y and others: Positional cloning of the mouse obese gene and the human homologue, *Nature* 372(6505):425, 1994.

17. Jequier E: Leptin signaling, adiposity, and energy balance, *Ann NY Acad Sci* 967:379, 2002.

18. Couzin J: Hormone research: leptin's uncertain promise, *U.S. News & World Report* 127(18):84, 8 November 1999.

19. Schultz S: Health: news you can use, why we're fat: gender and age matter more than you may realize, *U.S. News & World Report* 127(18):82, 8 November 1999.

20. Gura T: Obesity research: leptin not impressive in clinical trial, *Science* 286(5441):881, 29 October 1999.

21. Lee DW and others: Leptin and the treatment of obesity: its current status, *Eur J Pharmacol* 440(2-3):129, 2002.

22. Fox CS and others: Is a low leptin concentration, a low resting metabolic rate, or both the expression of the "thrifty genotype?" Results from the Pima Indians, *Am J Clin Nutr* 68(10):1053, 1998.

23. Dong C and others: Interacting genetic loci on chromosomes 20 and 10 influence extreme human obesity, *Am J Hum Genet* 72:115, 2003.

24. Birch LL, Davison KK: Family environmental factors influencing the developing behavioral controls of food in-

take and childhood overweight, *Pediatr Clin North Am* 48(4):893, 2001.

25. Cummings S: Position of the American Dietetic Association: weight management, *J Am Diet Assoc* 102(8):1145, 2002.

26. Talbott S: *The cortisol connection: Why stress makes you fat and ruins your health, and what you can do about it*, Alameda, CA, 2002, Hunter House.

27. Sachdev M and others: Effect of fenfluramine-derivative diet pills on cardiac valves: a meta-analysis of observational studies, *Am Heart J* 144(6):1065, 2002.

28. Fernandez-Lopez JA and others: Pharmacological approaches for the treatment of obesity, *Drugs* 62(6):915, 2002.

29. Fernstrom MH, Fernstrom JD: The new role of pharmacotherapy for weight reduction in obesity, *Int J Clin Pract* 56(9):683, 2002.

30. Barrow CJ: Roux-en-Y gastric bypass for morbid obesity, *AORN J* 76(4):590,593, 2002.

31. Ceelen W and others: Surgical treatment of severe obesity with a low-pressure adjustable gastric band: experimental data and clinical results in 625 patients, *Ann Surg* 237(1):10, 2003.

32. Fisher BL, Schauer P: Medical and surgical options in the treatment of severe obesity, *Am J Surg* 184(6B):9S, 2002.

33. Parker-Simmons S: *Eating disorders* [unpublished lecture hosted by University of Utah], Salt Lake City, 25 March 2003, University of Utah.

FURTHER READING AND RESOURCES

- Prentice AM, Jebb SA: Beyond body mass index, *Obesity* 2:141, 2001.

- Friedman JM: A war on obesity, not the obese, *Science* 299(5608):856, 2003.

  The preceding articles are excellent short reviews on the current status of obesity in the United States and the methods in which the obese are currently defined.

- Soliah L: The psychological appeal of fad diets, *Today's Dietitian* 5(4):22, 2003.

  The author takes a fascinating look into the psychological appeal and complications of fad diets.

16

Nutrition and Physical Fitness

KEY CONCEPTS

- Healthy muscle structure and function depend on appropriate energy fuels and tissue-building material, as well as oxygen and water.

- Different levels of physical activity and athletic performance draw on different body fuel sources.

- A sedentary lifestyle contributes to health problems.

- A healthy personal exercise program combines both strengthening and aerobic activities.

P ublic interest in physical fitness has continued to grow over the past few decades, sparked by the approach of preventive medicine and positive health promotion. This approach has been stimulated by an effort to prevent various chronic diseases in America's aging population and extend the number of healthy years.

This chapter demonstrates that nutrition and physical fitness are essential interrelated parts of positive health promotion. Both reduce risks associated with chronic diseases, and both are important therapies in dealing with already developed chronic conditions. Health care workers should provide their clients and patients with sound guidelines for physical fitness, while also practicing these sound guidelines themselves.

PHYSICAL ACTIVITY RECOMMENDATIONS AND BENEFITS

Guidelines and Recommendations

Americans are becoming less and less active on a daily basis. Technology is rapidly taking over the requirement for physical activity in everyday life. Of course, these are technologic advances, and society is proud of them—such things as moving sidewalks—yet some people are suffering the consequences of too much convenience in overall health. The reality is that fewer than 60% of American adults and 64% of adolescents engage in some form of leisure-time physical activity, and only 15% of adults participate in 30 minutes of moderate physical activity five or more times per week.[1]

Increased participation in regular physical activity is a national health goal. The U.S. Department of Health and Human Services has set nutrition and physical fitness goals for Americans, among many other health-related goals, in their *Healthy People 2010: Understanding and Improving Health* report. The 2010 target for participation in regular moderate-to-vigorous physical activity is set at 30% of adults and 85% of adolescents.[1] In addition to the goals of *Healthy People 2010*, the *Dietary Guidelines for Americans 2005*, the MyPyramid guidelines, and the Dietary Reference Intakes address the need to participate in physical activity on a daily basis. The most recent publication from the National Academy of Sciences increased its recommendations from 30 minutes of moderate exercise on most days of the week to 60 minutes of moderate exercise every day. The increased recommendations were made on the basis that the former was not enough to maintain a body weight within the recommended BMI range (18.5 to 25 kg/m^2).[2]

The National Academy of Sciences distinguishes between physical activity and exercise as such:

- *Physical activity.* Bodily movement that is produced by the contraction of muscle and that substantially increases energy expenditure.
- *Exercise.* Planned, structured, and repetitive bodily movement done to promote or maintain one or more components of physical fitness.[2]

Does walking the dog count toward 60 minutes of moderate exercise a day? Perhaps it does, if you are able to maintain a steady pace of 15 to 20 minutes per mile for the duration of the walk. The Food and Nutrition Board defines moderate activity as walking (3 to 4 mph), leisurely swimming/cycling, or playing golf. The recommendations state that to achieve health benefits from physical activity, the 60 minutes of moderate activity should be in addition to activities of daily living (house cleaning, walking to the bus stop, light gardening, etc.). Figure 16-1 suggests guidelines on how to incorporate the recommended activity into daily life.

Health Benefits

The health benefits of physical activity are not reserved just for athletes.[3] In a personally planned program to meet individual needs, any person can develop a healthy lifestyle. The longer people follow some form of regular exercise, the more committed they become.[4] Water aerobics, walking, and other "soft" workouts are becoming more and more popular in health clubs and have enabled more people to participate (e.g., those who cannot lift heavy weights or do "go-for-the-burn" aerobics). Several of these new gym members are older adults who have health problems that improve with moderate exercise.[5] Many elderly persons find that regular exercise not only helps manage their health but also assists them to feel more in control of their lives.

The sense of fitness exercise creates helps one to "feel good," physically, emotionally, and psychologically. However, in addition to this general sense of well-being, exercise (especially aerobic exercise) has special benefits for persons with certain health problems.

Coronary Heart Disease

Exercise reduces risks for heart disease in several ways, including improved heart function, blood cholesterol levels, and oxygen transport.

Heart Muscle Function. The heart is a four-chambered organ of muscle that is about the size of a fist in adults. Its ability to pump blood depends on its development. As with any muscle, this development depends on how much the heart is used. Exercise, especially aerobic conditioning, strengthens and enlarges this muscular organ, enabling it to pump more blood per beat, a capacity called *stroke volume*. The heart's ability to pump enough blood during exercise determines the degree of aerobic capacity in healthy persons.

Blood Cholesterol Levels. Exercise raises blood levels of high-density lipoprotein (HDL), known as the "good cholesterol," because it carries surplus cholesterol from the tissues to the liver for breakdown and removal from the body (see Chapter 19). Exercise also lowers blood levels of low-density lipoprotein (LDL), referred to as "bad cholesterol." LDL cholesterol carries at least two thirds of the total blood cholesterol to body tissues, raising the potential of cholesterol deposits in major arteries of the heart. Thus the beneficial effects of exercise on blood cholesterol profiles can lower the risks for diseased arteries.

Oxygen-Carrying Capacity. Exercise also enhances the circulatory system by increasing the oxygen-carrying capacity of the blood. The strengthened heart muscle can pump out more blood per beat, thus resulting in a healthy circulating blood volume without an increased heart rate (e.g., the number of beats per minute).

Hypertension

The risk for cardiovascular complications increases continuously with increasing levels of blood pressure.[6] When blood pressure is measured, persons with mild essential hypertension show a systolic blood pressure (e.g., the upper notation) of 140 to 159 mmHg or a diastolic blood pressure (e.g., the lower notation) of 90 to 104 mmHg (see Chapter 19) or both. According to the Centers for Disease Control and Prevention, approximately one in four adults in the United States has high blood pressure.[7] Persons with mild hypertension represent the overwhelming majority of hypertensive individuals in the general population. Exercise has become one of the most effective nondrug treatments for mild hypertension. Even for people with higher levels of blood pressure, exercise has proved to be an important adjunct to drug therapy, offsetting adverse drug effects and lowering drug needs.

Diabetes

Exercise helps control diabetes, especially type 2 diabetes (formerly called non–insulin-dependent diabetes mellitus) in obese adults.[8] Exercise improves the action of a person's naturally produced insulin by increasing the number of insulin receptor sites (e.g., areas where insulin

Figure 16–1   Physical Activity Pyramid. (Redrawn from Corbin RB, Lindsey R: *Fitness for life,* ed 4 (updated), Champaign, IL, 2002, Human Kinetics.)

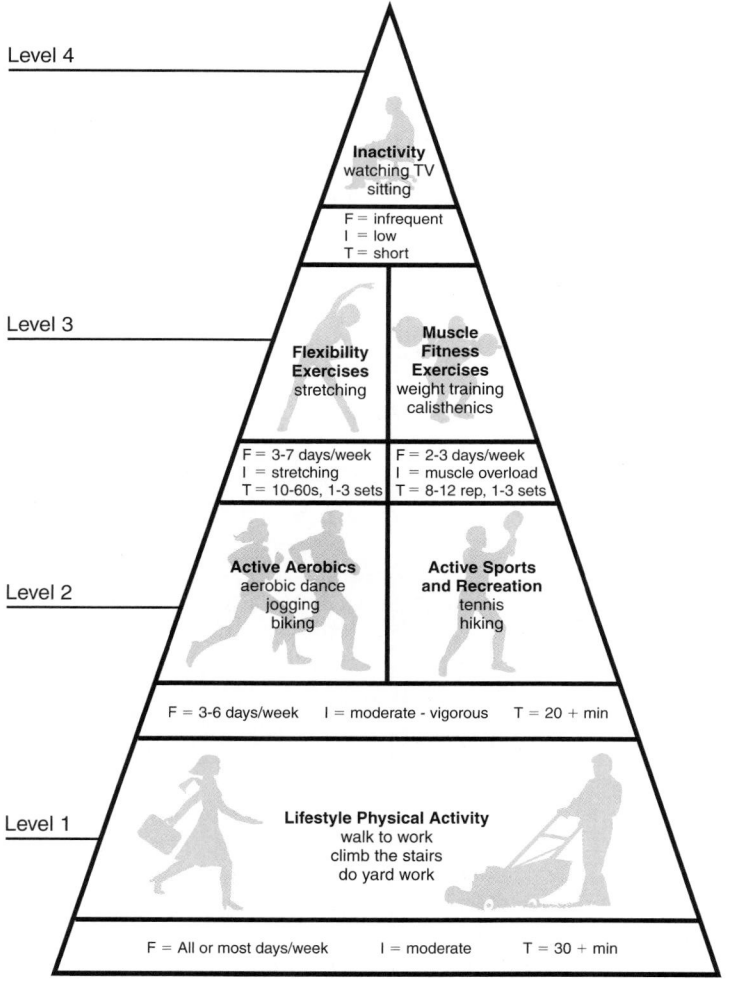

Level 4

Level 3

Level 2

Level 1

Inactivity
watching TV
sitting

F = infrequent
I = low
T = short

Flexibility Exercises
stretching

Muscle Fitness Exercises
weight training
calisthenics

F = 3-7 days/week
I = stretching
T = 10-60s, 1-3 sets

F = 2-3 days/week
I = muscle overload
T = 8-12 rep, 1-3 sets

Active Aerobics
aerobic dance
jogging
biking

Active Sports and Recreation
tennis
hiking

F = 3-6 days/week   I = moderate - vigorous   T = 20 + min

Lifestyle Physical Activity
walk to work
climb the stairs
do yard work

F = All or most days/week   I = moderate   T = 30 + min

may be carried into cells). In managing type 1 diabetes (formerly called *insulin-dependent diabetes mellitus*), the type of exercise and when it is done must be balanced with food and insulin injections to prevent reactions caused by drops in blood sugar.

Weight Management

Exercise is extremely beneficial to weight management in the following ways: (1) helps regulate appetite, (2) increases the basal metabolic rate, and (3) reduces the genetic fat deposit set-point level (see Chapter 15). Exercise also helps reduce stress-related eating and helps work off the hormonal effects of adrenaline produced by stress in the body.

Bone Disease

Weight-bearing exercises, such as walking and running, help strengthen bones. The weight-bearing load increases calcium deposits in bone, thus increasing bone density and reducing the risk for osteoporosis. The benefits of exercise on bone density are most notable during peak bone growth of the adolescent and young adult. However, excessive or extreme forms of training can have a rebound effect where bone density actually is lost because of overtraining or undernutrition.

Mental Health

Exercise stimulates the production of brain opiates, substances called *endorphins*. These natural chemicals decrease pain (this is how aspirin works, by stimulating production of endorphins) and improves mood, which may include an exhilarating kind of "high."

Types of Physical Activity

It is best to have a variety of exercises in one's fitness plan. A well-balanced exercise program incorporates resistance training, aerobic activities, flexibility and stretching exercises, along with a variety of activities of daily living. A good fitness plan is a combination of different enjoyable activities that most effectively reduce the risk of several chronic diseases.

Activities of Daily Living

Many activities of daily living do not reach aerobic levels (e.g., walking to work or the store, walking the dog, and playing catch with children) but are enjoyable and should be incorporated into daily life. If whatever one does is not fun, it will soon stop, reaping no benefit. Many people question whether exercise is most beneficial in the morning or at night. Again, the bottom line is it is best whenever one can commit to doing it *and* en-

joying it. There are no significant differences in the overall outcome as long as exercise is incorporated into a daily routine and consistently maintained.

Resistance Training

Resistance training creates and maintains muscle strength, a physical trait necessary for health and enhanced quality of life. Two position statements by the American College of Sports Medicine established guidelines for a beginning resistance training program and for progressive models of advanced training for healthy adults.[9,10] A beginning resistance program generally should include one set of 8 to 12 repetitions for 8 to 10 exercises, including one exercise for all major muscle groups performed 2 to 3 days per week.[9] A more progressive model incorporates gradual load increases to stimulate muscle overload, more muscle specificity and variation, and a training regimen of 4 to 5 days per week.[10]

Aerobic Exercise

Walking can be an aerobic exercise (Figure 16-2). It is convenient and requires no equipment except good walking shoes. Walking is also satisfying to many people for whom other forms may not be appropriate (e.g., running, biking, and aerobic dance). Start slowly and gradually increase the pace and distance. Table 16-1 lists examples of aerobic forms of exercise, whereas Table 16-2 provides information on energy expenditure per pound of body weight per hour for various activities.

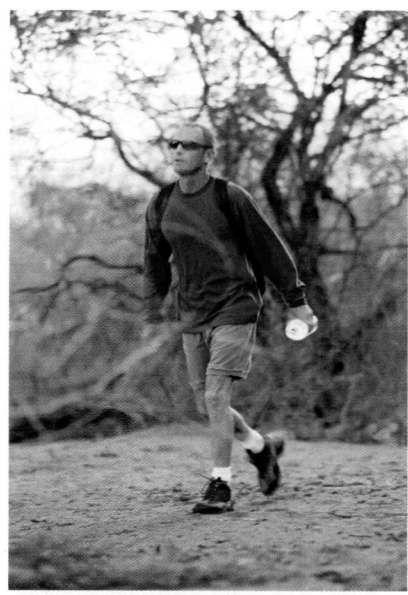

Figure 16–2   Aerobic walking is an enjoyable exercise that can fit into almost anyone's lifestyle.

Meeting Personal Needs

Health Status and Personal Gains

In planning a personal exercise program, check first on an individual's health status, present level of fitness, personal needs, and resources necessary for equipment or cost. The exercise chosen should be something that is both enjoyable and of aerobic value. Also, start slowly and build gradually to avoid discouragement and injury. Moderation and regularity are the chief guides.

Achieving Aerobic Benefits

To build aerobic capacity, the level of exercise needs to raise the pulse to within 60% to 90% of an individual's maximum heart rate. One's own *heart rate* can be calculated by subtracting one's age from 220, which gives the maximum heart rate. About 70% of this figure is the *target zone rate*, the level to which the pulse hopefully will be raised during exercise (Table 16-3). For aerobic benefits, this rate should be maintained for 30 to

TABLE 16–1 Aerobic Exercises for Physical Fitness*	
Type of exercise	**Aerobic forms**
Ball-playing	Handball
	Racquetball
	Squash
Bicycling	Stationary
	Touring
Dancing	Aerobic routines
	Ballet
	Disco
Jumping rope	Brisk pace
Running/jogging	Brisk pace
Skating	Ice skating
	Roller skating
Skiing	Cross-country
Swimming	Steady pace
Walking	Brisk pace

*Maintained at aerobic level for at least 30 minutes.

TABLE 16–2 Approximate Energy Expenditure per Hour during Various Activities	
Activity	**Kilocalories per hour**
Sleeping	63
Lying/sitting, awake	70
Standing, relaxed	84
Rapid typing, sitting	105
Dressing and undressing	140
Walking slowly (24 min/mile)	210
Water aerobics	280
High-impact aerobics	490
Football, flag/touch	560
Walking very fast (12 min/mile)	560
Stair, treadmill	630
Swimming, vigorous effort	700
Running (8 min/mile)	875

*For an adult weighing 70 kg (154 pounds).

TABLE 16–3 Target Zone Heart Rate According to Age to Achieve Aerobic Physical Effect of Exercise			
	Maximal attainable heart rate	Target zone	
Age	(pulse = 220 – age)	70% maximal rate	85% maximal rate
20	200	140	170
25	195	136	166
30	190	133	161
35	185	129	157
40	180	126	153
45	175	122	149
50	170	119	144
55	165	115	140
60	160	112	136
65	155	108	132
70	150	105	127
75	145	101	124

60 minutes about four to six times a week. Check the resting pulse before the exercise period, then again during and immediately after exercising.

Exercise Preparation and Care

Whatever the choice of exercise, preparation and continuing care are important. Before beginning, a person should stretch his or her muscles to prevent stress or injury, and take time to cool down afterward. A person should not go beyond his or her tolerance limits; but rather, listen to his or her own body. Rest when tired. Stop when hurting. When more challenge is desired, increase the exercise level, but only then; remember, it is an *individual* exercise plan.

DIETARY NEEDS DURING EXERCISE

Muscle Action and Fuel

Structure and Function

Millions of special cells and fibers make up skeletal muscle mass. These coordinated structures make all physical activity possible. They are stimulated by nerve endings to produce controlled muscle contraction and relaxation.

Fuel Sources

All of this action requires fuel to burn for energy. These fuel sources are the basic energy nutrients (e.g., primarily carbohydrate and some fat). Their metabolic products—glucose, glycogen, and fatty acids—provide ready fuels for immediate, short-, and long-term energy needs. A good diet to meet these needs is essential, whatever the level of physical activity.

Oxygen

The constant supply of oxygen necessary for life becomes all the more important during exercise. A person's ability to deliver this vital oxygen to the tissues for energy production determines how much exercise can be done. This **aerobic capacity** depends on two basic factors, as follows: (1) the fitness of the lungs, heart, and blood vessels; and (2) body composition.

Body Fitness. Physical fitness may be defined in terms of aerobic capacity, which is the body's ability to deliver and use oxygen in sufficient quantities to meet the demands of increasing levels of exercise, as measured in terms of maximal oxygen consumption (VO_2 max). The lungs, heart, and blood vessels deliver this necessary oxygen to the cells, so their health is essential to overall fitness. Aerobic capacity is measured by the amount of oxygen consumed per kilogram of body weight per minute. To measure VO_2 max, an individual must either run on a treadmill or ride a stationary bike to exhaustion while oxygen consumption is measured. As aerobic fitness improves, so does VO_2 max.

Body Composition. Body tissues that use more oxygen make up the *lean body mass*, which is mainly muscle mass. These tissues are the active metabolic tissues of the body. A person's aerobic capacity depends on the percentage of body fat and lean body mass. Body composition is determined by the relative amounts of these two components of body weight (see Chapter 15).

Fluid and Energy Needs

Fluid

More water is necessary, but often overlooked, for increased activity and exercise.[11] With continued exercise, the body temperature rises because of the release of heat as part of the energy produced. To control this temperature rise, the body sends as much heat as possible to the skin, where it is released in sweat. Over time, and especially in hot weather, this excessive sweating can lead to *dehydration*. To prevent dehydration, water must be replaced frequently. Athletes who are engaged in longer and more demanding endurance events, especially in a warm environment, however, may use one of the many mild saline and glucose (4% to 8% solution) sports drinks that have rapid gastric emptying and intestinal absorption times[11] (see the For Further Focus, "Sorting Out Sports Drinks," for more information).

Nutrient Stores

For athletes, as well as any active person, proper diet choices are essential for daily energy needs, nutrient reserves, and winning performances. When nutrient reserves become depleted during continuous exercise, the body burns its fuel stores to meet increasing energy demands and requires replenishing. With prolonged exercise, nutrient levels fall too low to sustain the body's continued demands. Fatigue follows, and exhaustion may result. Carbohydrate and fat are the fuels used to maintain these energy reserves; very little energy is drawn from protein.

Energy

Physical activity requires energy in the form of kcalories. Table 16-2 gives some examples of the amount of kcalories expended in general activities (see also Table 15-4 for a comparison of the energy expenditure for a very active person with that of an inactive person). Exercise raises the kcalorie need and helps regulate the appetite to meet this need. Exercise is the only way to adjust an individual's in-

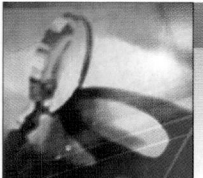

FOR FURTHER FOCUS

SORTING OUT SPORTS DRINKS

Sports drinks developed from the belief that water alone does not meet hydration needs during exercise. It is now known that the ideal fluid to prevent dehydration depends on how demanding the exercise is and how long it lasts.

For nonendurance exercise, physically fit athletes do perfectly well on plain water. However, long-term endurance athletes need both water and fuel (e.g., carbohydrate), especially in hot weather. For example, without carbohydrate replacement, a long-distance marathon runner would soon run out of muscle glycogen and the ability to utilize stored fat for energy and "hit the wall" or "bonk." Also, in such a demanding run when the body can sweat as much as 6% of its weight, it cannot keep cool enough and the overall system overheats, leading to heatstroke and collapse. Simply adding table sugar to water causes the water to remain in the stomach longer, where it does nothing for the immediate needs of the body tissues.

The first group of sports drinks began with a solution called *Gatorade*, named by its developers for their university's football team. They reasoned that if they analyzed their players' sweat they could appropriately replace lost minerals and water, thus better meeting the needs of athletes than plain water. (Of course, the manufacturers also added some flavoring, coloring, and sugars to make it more acceptable.) Although Gatorade was highly profitable for the university and the manufacturer, subsequent studies showed that regular nonendurance athletes did not need it. Plain water served their needs very well, and they obtained minerals in their diet.

A second category of sports drinks has been developed to meet both the water and energy needs of athletes in longer-lasting endurance events. More dilute 8% sugar solutions, using glucose or glucose polymers (e.g., short chains of about five glucose molecules) that are not sweet are being used. In the more dilute solutions, both energy-sustaining sugars quickly leave the stomach and provide a continuing fuel and water source for the endurance athlete.

Other products entering the sports drink market have been "Gatorade clones" that claim to add no sugar but supply ample amounts of fructose and glucose in their fruit juice base. Fructose does not leave the stomach rapidly and is absorbed more slowly from the intestine than glucose, often causing bloating or diarrhea. Still other products add multiple vitamins (e.g., yielding 137% of the RDA in a single 10-oz bottle) to their fruit juice base but contain no minerals. All of these vitamins do not help performance at all, and on a hot day a sweating athlete can easily down a megadose in four or five bottles.

Therefore sort out the claims of sports drinks; they are not for everyone. In the long run, special sports drinks meet the needs of athletes in endurance events. For nonendurance activities, however, most persons do not need them. After all, water is the best solution for regular needs, and costs far less.

---

ternal genetic *set-point*, which determines how much body fat the person will carry naturally (see Chapter 15). This body-fat point is raised (e.g., more body fat is stored) when the individual becomes more sedentary. Conversely, this point is lowered by regular exercise.

Macronutrient and Micronutrient Recommendations

Nutrient Ratios

Highly active persons and athletes have slightly increased protein requirements when compared with inactive persons, but recommendations for fat intake do not vary from standard guidelines. Carbohydrate is the preferred fuel and is the critical food for an active person, not only before an exercise period, but also during the

recovery period afterward. The complex carbohydrate forms (e.g., starches) not only sustain energy needs but also supply added fiber, vitamins, and minerals. Thus the recommended ratio of energy nutrients to support physical activity may be summarized as follows:

- *Carbohydrate:* 45% to 65% of total kcalories
- *Fat:* 25% to 30% of total kcalories
- *Protein:* 10% to 35% of total kcalories

aerobic capacity (Gr. *aer,* air or gas) requiring oxygen to proceed. Milliliters of oxygen consumed per kilogram of body weight per minute, as influenced by body composition.

Carbohydrate

The major nutrient used for energy support during exercise is the carbohydrate. The carbohydrate body-energy reserve comes from the following two sources: (1) circulating *blood glucose* and (2) *glycogen* stored in muscle cells and the liver. Thus for active persons, carbohydrates should contribute approximately 60% to 65% of the daily energy intake. Athletes competing in prolonged endurance events need more (e.g., 6 to 10 g/kg body weight) energy from carbohydrates.[11] Complex carbohydrates, or starches, are preferred more than simple sugars. On the whole, complex starches break down more slowly and help maintain blood sugar levels more evenly, avoiding high and low blood sugar spikes. Starches are also more readily converted to glycogen to maintain this store of constant primary fuel.

Simple sugars, on the other hand, are less efficient at maintaining the body's glycogen stores and are mainly converted to fat and stored as such. Simple sugars also trigger a sharper insulin response, contributing to the dangers of rebound **hypoglycemia.** Many studies have shown that low-carbohydrate diets hinder exercise performance. Athletes especially experience fatigue, dehydration, and hypoglycemia. Well-conditioned athletes sometimes use a glycogen-loading procedure (discussed later in this chapter) to build up glycogen stores for endurance events of 1 hour or more. In addition, complex carbohydrates supply needed fiber, vitamins, and minerals.

Fat

In the presence of oxygen, *fatty acids* serve as a fuel source from stored fat tissue. Note that fat as a fuel source is not drawn from the diet directly but from body fat stores. There is no evidence supporting improved physical performance with increased levels of fat in the diet. There is a need for some dietary fat, however, to supply *linoleic* and *linolenic acid*, the body's essential fatty acids. The total fat should not exceed approximately 25% to 30% of the total daily energy intake.

The relative use of stored fat for energy during exercise depends on the level of fitness of the person and the exercise intensity. Trained endurance athletes are more efficient at utilizing fat for energy than their untrained counterparts. However, the use of fat for energy declines as the exercise intensity increases above approximately 70% VO$_2$ max, at which point the body becomes more reliant on glucose utilization for immediate energy.[12] Mild or moderate intensity exercise, at 25% to 65% VO$_2$ max, increases fatty acid oxidation by fivefold to tenfold more than resting oxidation levels.

Protein

Some amino acid breakdown may occur during exercise, but protein is usually discounted as a fuel source because it makes an insignificant contribution to energy. No more than the usual adult requirement is needed to meet general needs of a healthy adult during exercise, which amount to about 10% to 35% of the total day's kcalories from protein. However, there is some evidence that endurance and strength-trained athletes may require as much as 1.2 to 1.7 g protein/kg body weight.[11] Protein recommendations, even for athletes, usually can be met through the diet alone because most Americans actually eat one and a half to two times the recommended amount of daily protein. Furthermore, excess protein from whole protein or amino acid supplements may put a taxing load on the kidneys, which can contribute to dehydration because the excess nitrogen must be excreted. High-protein diets also can lead to increased calcium loss in the urine.

Vitamins and Minerals

Vitamins and minerals cannot be used as fuel. They are not oxidized or used up in the energy production process. They are essential in this process but only as coenzyme partners (see Chapters 7 and 8). Increased exercise does not require increased vitamins or minerals. Exercise generally increases the body's efficient use of vitamins and minerals. Because athletes require more energy, their larger intake of nutrient-dense food also increases their dietary intake of vitamins and minerals. However, female and adolescent athletes should focus special attention on iron and may require dietary iron supplements if the levels of iron in their blood are consistently low.

ATHLETIC PERFORMANCE

General Training Diet

Anyone who exercises regularly (especially athletes in training) needs to apply the general principles of exercise and energy described in the previous discussion. Athletes involved in heavy training are more susceptible to immunosuppression because of the extreme demands placed on the body. A well-balanced diet with plenty of protein and carbohydrates from a variety of foods helps prevent exercise-induced malnutrition and risk for injury and infection.[13]

Carbohydrate

Moderate to high amounts, 5 to 7 g/kg body weight per day of carbohydrate, are needed to support general training. Endurance athletes have higher needs, 7 to 10 g/kg body weight per day. Female endurance athletes are the least likely group to achieve such dietary recommendations, despite evidence supporting enhanced performance from high carbohydrate intakes.[14]

Fat

Moderate amounts of fat, about 25% to 30% of the total kcalories, are needed to meet energy needs and maintain weight. Currently, 35% of the total kcalories in the typical American diet comes from fat.[15]

Protein

Protein should comprise the remainder of the diet, in moderate amounts (~10% to 30% total kcal or 1.2 to 1.7 g/kg body weight per day for highly active endurance or strength trainers).

Total Energy

Athletes need varying amounts of energy, depending on body size and the type of training or competition involved. A small person may need only about 1800 kcal/day to sustain body weight and normal daily activities, whereas a larger, muscular man may need about 3000 kcal/day.[11] Consider these different basic needs and add the additional energy needed for a given sport training. For example, endurance bicycle races in mountain areas may require an additional 2000 to 3000 kcal/day. Thus some athletes in training may require as many as 5000 to 7000 kcal/day just to maintain weight. A well-planned individual program is necessary.

Athletes should consume a variety of foods. The food groups of the MyPyramid guidelines (see Figure 1-2) may serve as a simple guide, with relative increases in servings as needed. Many choices and portions from the starch and fruit groups replace glycogen losses from the previous day's workouts and provide adequate glycogen stores in the muscles. Box 16-1 gives carbohydrate values for selected foods to use in planning an athlete's low-fat, moderate-protein, and high-carbohydrate diet, which should include 500 to 600 g carbohydrate each day.

Competition

Carbohydrate Loading

To prepare for an athletic event, especially an endurance event, athletes sometimes follow a dietary process called *carbohydrate* or *glycogen loading* (see the For Further Focus box, "Carbohydrate Loading for Endurance"). The current practice, which has been modified from earlier more stressful plans and takes place the week before the event, is a moderate, gradual tapering of exercise while total carbohydrate intake is increased in the diet (Table 16-4).

Pregame Meal

The ideal pregame meal depends on the tolerance of the athlete. It is usually a light meal eaten about 3 to 4 hours before the event. This meal should be high in complex carbohydrates (e.g., approximately 200 to 300 g carbohydrate) and relatively low in protein, with little fat or fiber.[11] This schedule gives the body time to digest, absorb, and transform the meal into stored glycogen. Good food choices include pasta, bread, bagels, muffins, and cereal with nonfat milk. Box 16-2 outlines a sample pregame meal.

Hydration

Dehydration can be a serious problem for athletes. Fluid needs depend on the following: (1) the intensity and duration of the exercise; (2) the surrounding temperature, altitude, and humidity; (3) the level of fitness; and (4) the pregame or pre-exercise state of hydration. The thirst mechanism cannot keep up with the loss of water during exercise; therefore to prevent dehydration athletes are advised to drink more water than they think they need (Figure 16-3). In addition to water loss (as much as 1.5 L/h), sweat also contains a relatively large amount of sodium and small amounts of other minerals (e.g., potassium, iron, and calcium).

Athletes are recommended to drink 6 to 12 oz of fluid every 15 to 20 minutes during athletic events. A number of sports drinks with added sugar, electrolytes, and flavorings have been marketed, but questions have been raised about their use or misuse (see the For Further Focus box, "Sorting Out Sports Drinks"). Adding electrolytes and sugar to water delays its emptying from the stomach. Except for endurance events lasting longer than 1 hour, plain water is usually the rehydration fluid of choice. Electrolytes will be replaced during the athlete's next meal. For events lasting longer than 1 hour, beverages containing 4% to 8% glucose concentrations and 0.5 to 0.7 g/L sodium are recommended.[11]

Ergogenic Aids

Since ancient times, athletes have been seeking and experimenting with "magic" substances or treatments to gain the competitive edge. Today these substances are known as **ergogenic** aids (Table 16-5). Most are worth-

---

hypoglycemia (Gr. *hypo*, under; *glykys*, sweet; *haima*, blood) an abnormally low blood sugar level that may lead to muscle tremors, cold sweat, headache, and confusion.

ergogenic (Gr. *ergon*, work; *gennan*, to produce) the tendency to increase work output; various substances that increase work or exercise capacity and output.

BOX 16–1 Grams of Carbohydrate in One Serving of Common Foods

Carbohydrate Group

Starches

Bread; Cereals and Grains; Starchy Vegetables; Crackers and Snacks; Beans, Peas, and Lentils; Starchy Foods Prepared with Fat

One serving contains 15 g carbohydrate; a serving is as follows:

½ cup bran cereal

¼ cup Grape-Nuts

1½ cups puffed cereal

½ cup grits

⅓ cup rice, white or brown

½ cup bulgur

½ cup pasta

⅓ cup baked beans

½ cup corn

½ cup beans and peas (garbanzo, pinto, kidney, white, split, black-eyed)

½ cup lentils

⅔ cup lima beans

½ cup green peas

1 cup winter squash (acorn, butternut, pumpkin)

½ cup yam, sweet potato, plain

1 small (3-oz) potato, baked or boiled

16 to 25 (3 oz) French-fried potatoes

½ (1 oz) bagel

1 (1½ oz) small muffin

½ English muffin

1 (1 oz) slice bread (white, whole wheat, pumpernickel, rye)

½ (1 oz) hot dog or hamburger bun

¾ oz pretzels

6 saltine-type crackers

1 waffle, 4½-inch square

2 pancakes, 4 inches across

2 taco shells, 6 inches across

1 tortilla, corn, 6 inches across

1 tortilla, flour, 6 inches across

1 biscuit, 2½ inches across

½ pita, 6 inches across

Fruits

One serving contains 15 g carbohydrate; a serving is as follows:

1 (4-oz) apple, unpeeled, small

4 whole (5½ oz) apricots, fresh

1 (4-oz) banana, small

½ (4 oz) pear, large, fresh

1¼ cup strawberries, whole

12 (3 oz) cherries, sweet, fresh

17 (3 oz) grapes, small

½ (11 oz) grapefruit, large

1 (5-oz) nectarine, small

1 (6½-oz) orange, small

1 (6-oz) peach, medium, fresh

1 slice (13½ oz) of 1¼ cup cubes of watermelon

2 (5 oz) plums, small

½ cup apple juice or cider

⅓ cup fruit juice blends, 100% juice

½ cup orange juice

½ cup grapefruit juice

Milk

One serving contains 12 g carbohydrate; a serving is as follows:

1 cup fat-free, 1%, or 2% milk

¾ cup plain low-fat yogurt

Other carbohydrates

One serving contains 15 g carbohydrate; a serving is as follows:

Cake, frosted, 2-inch square

Cake, unfrosted, 2-inch square

3 gingersnaps

5 Vanilla Wafers

2 small cookies or sandwich cookies with crème filling

½ cup ice cream

½ cup sherbet or sorbet

⅓ cup yogurt, frozen, low-fat or fat-free

1 granola bar

Vegetables

One serving is 5 g carbohydrate; a serving is as follows:

½ cup cooked vegetables

1 cup raw vegetables

½ cup vegetable juice

Examples: carrots, asparagus, beans (green, wax, Italian), beets, broccoli, cauliflower, onions, spinach, summer squash, greens (collard, kale, mustard, turnip), cucumbers, turnips.

Data from American Dietetic Association, American Diabetes Association: *Exchange lists for meal planning,* Chicago/Alexandria, VA, 2003, ADA/ADA.

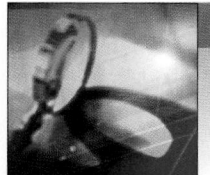

FOR FURTHER FOCUS

CARBOHYDRATE LOADING FOR ENDURANCE

Glycogen is the body storage form of carbohydrate, designed to provide an immediate source of backup fuel and protect blood glucose levels during the fasting hours of sleep. Glycogen is restored with each day's food intake, but during heavy exercise normal glycogen stores are quickly used up and the person reaches the point of exhaustion. This is a no-win situation in athletics.

During the 1960s trainers and coaches began to explore ways of avoiding this state of exhaustion in their players during endurance events. The trainers and coaches reasoned that if the athletes exercised heavily and ate a low-carbohydrate diet for 3 days to use up the stored glycogen,

and then only exercised lightly and ate a high-carbohydrate diet for the next 3 days, their glycogen stores would become supersaturated, enabling them to perform at a higher level. When this practice was tested, it was proved that the increase in glycogen stores in muscle and the athletes' performance was nearly twice their former workload.

This practice has become known as carbohydrate or glycogen loading and is specifically designed for endurance athletes. Today a less stressful, modified process of tapered depletion is used to prevent possible injury to muscle tissue. This method can be used more often than the previously used schedule and is more productive in the long run (see Table 16-4).

TABLE 16–4	Precompetition Program for Carbohydrate Loading	
Day	**Exercise**	**Diet**
1	90-minute period at 70%-75% VO$_2$ max	Mixed diet, 5 g carbohydrate/kg body weight
2-3	Gradual tapering of time and intensity: ~40-minute period	Same as Day 1
4-5	Continuation of tapering: ~20-minute period	Mixed diet, 10 g carbohydrate/kg body weight
6	Complete rest	Same as Days 4-5
7	Day of competition	High-carbohydrate pre-event meal

Modified from Coleman MA: Carbohydrate and exercise. In Rosenbloom CA, editor: *Sports nutrition: a guide for professionals working with active people*, ed 3, Chicago, 2000, The American Dietetic Association.

less fads, but one current practice, the use of **steroids**, is of great concern because it is dangerous and, in athletics, illegal. The use of steroids is widespread among athletes and body builders, sometimes starting as early as high school or even junior high school. These steroids are synthetic sex hormones that have two actions, as follows: (1) *anabolic* (tissue growth), and (2) *androgenic* (masculinization). Athletes often take these drugs in megadoses 10 to 30 times their normal body hormonal output to increase muscle size, strength, and performance. However, the physiologic side effects can be devastating, varying from premature closure of bone growth, thus stunting normal skeletal development, and liver injury to accelerated heart disease, high blood pressure, sterility, and many other physical effects.[16] Psychological effects vary from increased aggressiveness, drug dependence, and mood swings to depression, decreased sex drive, and violent rage. Many serious athletes confront

BOX 16–2 Sample Pregame Meal

1 cup spaghetti, tomato sauce
1 slice French bread
1 cup apple juice

This sample pregame meal includes approximately 300 kcal; high-complex carbohydrate; and low protein, fat, and fiber.

steroids (Gr. *stereos,* solid; L. *-ol, oleum,* oil) the group name for lipid-based sterols, including hormones, bile acids, and cholesterol.

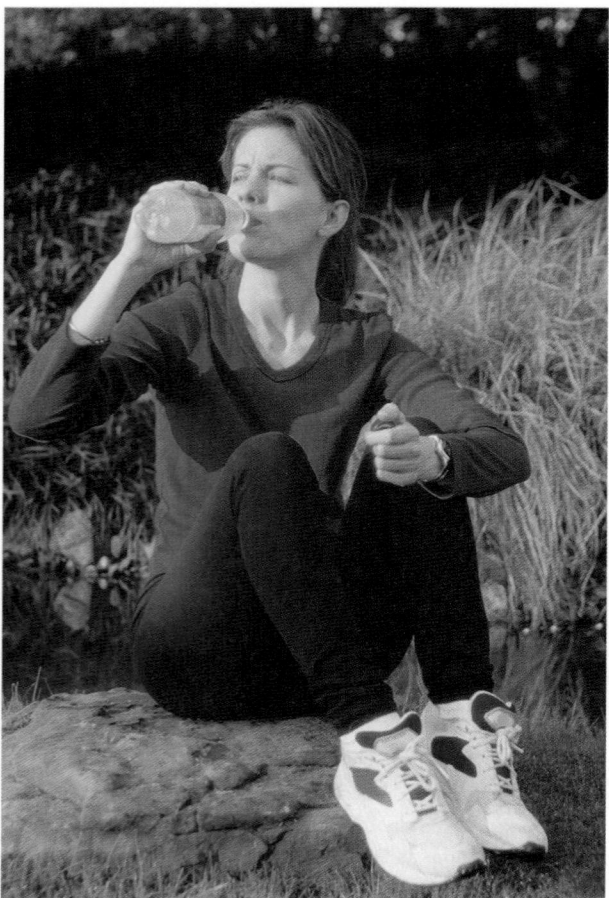

Figure 16–3 ■ Frequent small drinks of cold water during extended exercise prevent dehydration. (Credit: PhotoDisc.)

the hard choice of not using these dangerous drugs while facing a large field of opponents who are using them, or of using the drugs and risking the side effects and potential disqualification.

Misinformation

Athletes and their coaches are particularly susceptible to magic claims and myths about foods and dietary supplements. All athletes, particularly those involved in very competitive sports, constantly search for the competitive edge. Knowing this, manufacturers sometimes make distorted or false claims for products. In addition, the world of athletics holds numerous superstitions and myths about food and nutrients.

Myths and Superstitions

- Athletes need protein for extra energy.
- Extra protein builds bigger and stronger muscles.
- Muscle tissue breaks down during exercise, and protein supplements are needed to replace it.
- Mega doses of vitamin supplements enable athletes to use more energy.
- Vitamins and minerals are burned up in workouts and training sessions.
- Electrolyte solutions are important during daily exercise to replace sweat loss.
- A pregame meal of steak and eggs ensures maximum performance.
- Drinking water during exercise produces cramps.

Health care providers should be familiar with common fads and myths circulating in the community. Not only is knowing about these myths important, but also knowing how to approach them and what to recommend are necessary.

SUMMARY

Many fine muscle fibers and cells, triggered by nerve endings, work smoothly together to make physical activity possible. Carbohydrate, mainly in the form of complex carbohydrate foods or starches, is the primary fuel for energy to run this system. Carbohydrate metabolism yields circulating blood sugar and stored glycogen in muscles and liver for fuel. Stored body fat supplies additional fuel as fatty acids. However, protein provides insignificant energy for exercise. Vitamins and minerals cannot be burned for energy but are important coenzyme partners for the process of energy production.

Activities of daily living, aerobic exercises, and resistance training have many benefits, which increase with practice. Excellent aerobic exercises include sustained fast walking, swimming, jogging, running, and aerobic dancing or workouts. Resistance training increases muscle strength, a direct influence on metabolic rate and bone density.

Exercise does increase the need for energy and water. Water in small, frequent amounts is generally the best way to avoid dehydration. Electrolytes lost in sweat are replaced in the next meal. The optimal diet for athletes

TABLE 16–5	Ergogenic Aids Marketed to Athletes		
Substance	**Description**	**Claims**	**Actual effect**
Arginine, lysine, ornithine	Amino acids	Stimulate release of human growth hormone	No proven effect
Antioxidant vitamins C, E, beta-carotene	Compounds that may prevent free-radical damage	Prevent muscle damage from oxidation following high-intensity exercise	Some evidence of proven benefit
Caffeine*	Stimulant	Improves performance; increases fatty acid oxidation; spares glycogen	Some evidence of proven benefit
Carnitine	Facilitator of the transfer of long-chain fatty acids into the mitochondria	Enhances energy levels; decreases body fat	No proven effect
Creatine	Protein/amino acids	Increased intramuscular creatine; increases power output; promotes increase in lean body mass	Some evidence of proven benefit
DHEA	Hormone	Increases energy; increases muscle mass; decreases body fat	More research needed to confirm these observations
Ginseng	Extract of ginseng root	Reduces fatigue; improves endurance, strength, and recovery from exercise	No proven effect
HMB	Metabolite of the amino acid leucine	Increases in lean body mass; decreased body fat; increased strength	More research needed to confirm these observations

From Grodner M, Long S, DeYoung S: *Foundations and clinical applications of nutrition: a nursing approach*, ed 3, St Louis, 2004, Mosby.
*The use of caffeine is considered a form of doping by the International Olympic Committee (IOC). The IOC has set an upper limit of 12 μg per milliliter of caffeine in the urine.
DHEA = Dehydroepinandrosterone.
HMB = beta-hydroxy beta methybutyrate.

is approximately 60% of the kcalories from carbohydrate (mainly complex starches), 25% from fat, and 15% from protein. During the week before an athletic event, especially an endurance event, serious athletes may practice carbohydrate loading to meet the energy demands of competition. However, pregame meals should comprise small, mainly complex carbohydrates (starches), with little fat, protein, or fiber.

CRITICAL THINKING QUESTIONS

1. What is the primary role of each energy nutrient (carbohydrates, fats, protein) in terms of fuel for exercise?
2. Outline the nutrition and physical fitness principles you would discuss with a client who is an athlete. Plan a diet for this person that meets nutrient and energy needs.
3. Why is fluid balance vital during exercise periods? How are water and electrolyte balance achieved?
4. Describe the health benefits of exercise for a person with heart disease, as well as for a person with hypertension. Also describe the benefits of exercise for an overweight person with type 2 diabetes.
5. Describe several factors a person should consider when planning a personal exercise program. Define the term *aerobic exercise* and list its benefits.

CHAPTER CHALLENGE QUESTIONS

True-False

Write the correct statement for each item you answer "false."

1. *True or False:* Sports drinks containing electrolytes and sugar are the best way to replace fluids lost during short bouts of exercise, such as a 30-minute jog.

2. *True or False:* Drinking water immediately before and during an athletic event causes cramps.

3. *True or False:* Carbohydrate containing sports drinks are best absorbed from the stomach when in glucose concentrations of 4% to 8%.

4. *True or False:* Athletes need protein for extra energy.

5. *True or False:* Vitamins and minerals are burned for energy in workouts and training sessions.

6. *True or False:* Protein and fat do not contribute to glycogen stores.

7. *True or False:* Sweating is the main mechanism for dissipating body heat.

8. *True or False:* Aerobic exercise is of limited benefit in controlling heart disease and diabetes.

9. *True or False:* Walking can be an excellent form of aerobic exercise.

Multiple Choice

1. Which of the following activities is most likely to provide aerobic exercise?
   a. Golf
   b. Swimming
   c. Gardening
   d. Baseball

2. To develop aerobic capacity, an exercise should
   a. raise the pulse to 50% of the maximum heart rate.
   b. be maintained for alternating 10-minute periods.
   c. be practiced consistently every day.
   d. be practiced several times a week at an appropriate pulse rate for sustained periods of time.

3. Characteristics of a healthful exercise program should include which of the following? (*Circle all that apply.*)
   a. Enjoyable activities
   b. Moderation

   c. Regularity
   d. Going beyond tolerance limits

4. Exercise is beneficial in weight management because it serves which of the following purposes? (*Circle all that apply.*)
   a. Helps regulate appetite
   b. Decreases basal metabolic rate
   c. Reduces stress-related eating
   d. Increases the set-point for fat deposit

5. Which of the following meals is the best choice for an athlete's pregame meal?
   a. Large grilled steak, fried potatoes, ice cream
   b. Fried fish, vegetable salad with cream dressing, fresh fruit
   c. Spaghetti with tomato sauce, french bread, fruit
   d. Hamburger, french fries, cola

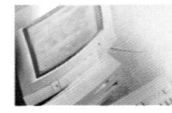

Please refer to the Students' Resource section of this text's Evolve web site for "Suggestions for Additional Study."

REFERENCES

1. U.S. Department of Health and Human Services: *Healthy people 2010: Understanding and improving health,* Washington, DC, 2000, Government Printing Office.
2. Food and Nutrition Board, Institute of Medicine: *Dietary reference intakes for energy, carbohydrate, fiber, fat, fatty acids, cholesterol, protein, and amino acids,* Washington, DC, 2002, National Academies Press.
3. Staff: Practice points: Translating research into practice: physical activity-it's not reserved for athletes, *J Am Diet Assoc* 99(2):212, 1999.

4. Simonen RL and others: Factors associated with exercise lifestyle-a study of monozygotic twins, *Int J Sports Med* 24(7):499, 2003.

5. Vidal J: Updated review on the benefits of weight loss, *Int J Obes Relat Metab Disord* 22(4):S25, 2002.

6. American Heart Association: *High blood pressure*, Dallas, 2002, (accessed April 2003), AHA [*www.americanheart. org*].

7. National Center for Health Statistics, Centers for Disease Control and Prevention: *Fast stats A to Z: hypertension*, Hyattsville, MD, (accessed April 2003), NCHS/CDC [*www. cdc.gov/nchs/fastats/hyprtens.htm*].

8. Adler A: Obesity and target organ damage: diabetes, *Int J Obes Relat Metab Disord* 26(4):S11, 2002.

9. American College of Sports Medicine: Position stand: The recommended quantity and quality of exercise for developing and maintaining cardiorespiratory and muscular fitness, and flexibility in healthy adults, *Med Sci Sports Exerc* 30:975, 1998.

10. American College of Sports Medicine: Position stand: Progressive models in resistance training for healthy adults, *Med Sci Sports Exerc* 34:364, 2002.

11. American College of Sports Medicine, American Dietetic Association, Dietitians of Canada: Joint position statement: Nutrition and athletic performance, *Med Sci Sports Exerc* 32(12):2130, 2000.

12. Horowitz JF, Klein S: Lipid metabolism during endurance exercise, *Am J Clin Nutr* 72(2):558S, 2000.

13. Gleeson M, Bishop NC: Elite athlete immunology: importance of nutrition, *Int J Sports Med* 21(1):S44, 2000.

14. Burke LM and others: Guidelines for daily carbohydrate intake: do athletes achieve them? *Sports Med* 31(4):267, 2001.

15. National Center for Health Statistics, Centers for Disease Control and Prevention: *Fast stats A to Z: diet (average daily intakes, 1988-1994)*, Hyattsville, MD, (accessed January 2003), NCHS/CDC [*www.cdc.gov/nchs/fastats/diet.htm*].

16. Ahrendt DM: Ergogenic aids: counseling the athlete, *Am Fam Physician* 63:913, 2001.

FURTHER READING AND RESOURCES

- Washington Coalition for Promoting Physical Activity: *www.beactive.org*

- *Physical activity and health: a report of the surgeon general*, National Center for Chronic Disease Prevention and Health Promotion, Centers for Disease Control and Prevention: *www.cdc.gov/nccdphp/sgr/sgr.htm*

- American College of Sports Medicine: *www.acsm.org*

- Office of Dietary Supplements, National Institutes of Health: *http://dietary-supplements.info.nih.gov*

- National Academies Press: *www.nap.edu*

  Review the above listed web sites for information, guidelines, research, and suggestions on exercise and physical fitness.

- Ahrendt DM: Ergogenic aids: counseling the athlete, *Am Fam Physician* 63:913, 2001.

  This review of the current ergogenic aids gives a useful summary report of the proposed action, possible side effects, and legality of many popular supplements.

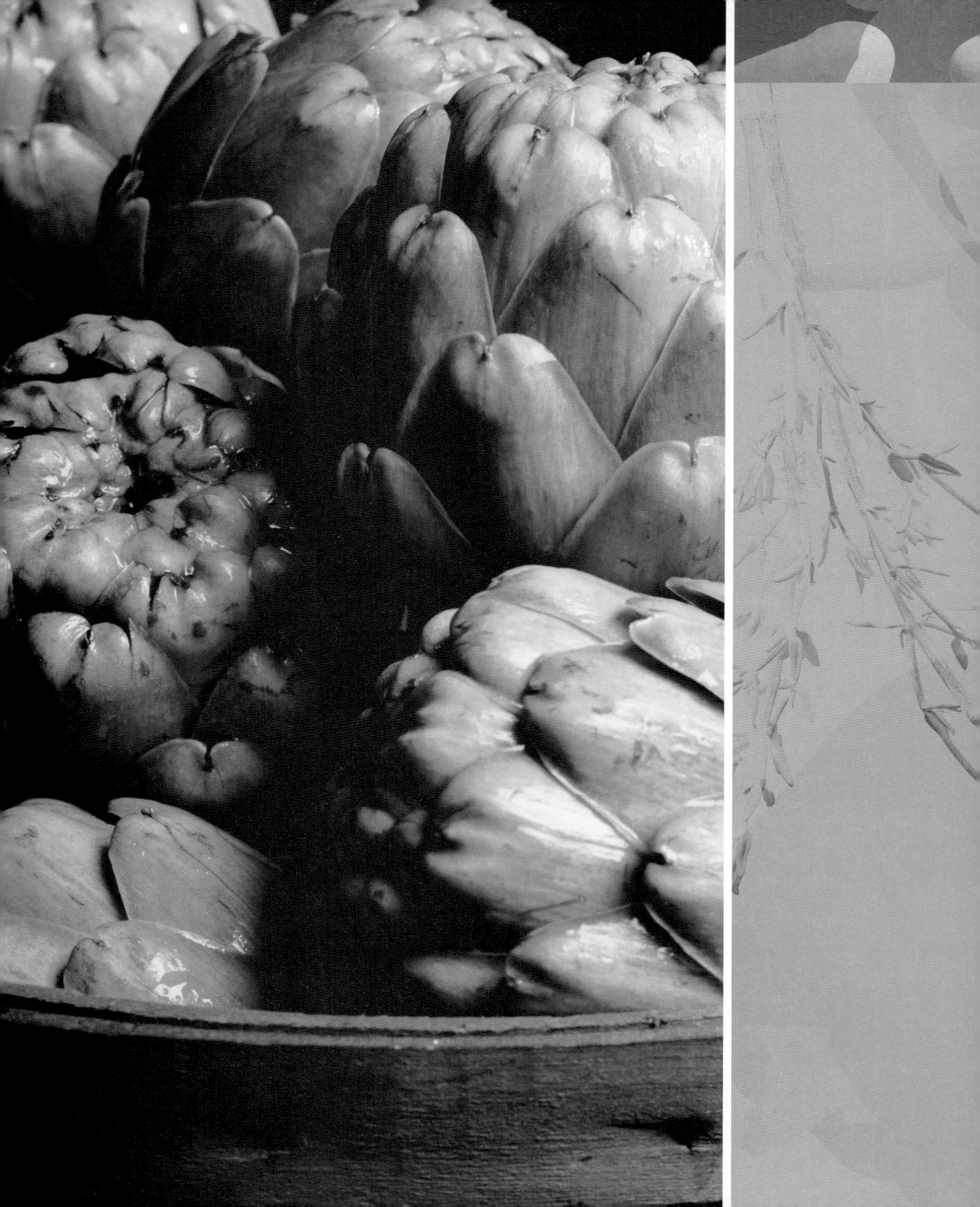

CHAPTER 17

Nutritional Care

P eople face acute illness or chronic disease and its treatment in a variety of settings: hospital, extended-care facility, clinic, or home. Nutritional support is fundamental in the successful treatment of disease, and is often the primary therapy. Sensitive care is always based on an individual's needs. To meet individual nutritional needs, a broad knowledge of nutritional state, requirements, and ways of meeting the identified needs is essential. The clinical dietitian, along with the physician, carries the major responsibility for this nutritional care. Each member of the health care team plays an important role in developing and maintaining a person-centered health care plan.

This chapter focuses on the comprehensive care of the patient's nutritional needs and explores the basic care process involved. The health care team, including the patient and family, must work together to support the healing process and promote health.

KEY CONCEPTS

■ Valid health care is based on individual care.

■ Comprehensive health care is best provided by a team of various health professionals and support staff persons.

■ A personalized health care plan, based on individual needs and goals, guides actions to promote healing and health.

THE THERAPEUTIC PROCESS

Setting and Focus of Care

Health Care Setting

Modern hospitals are a marvel of medical technology, but medical advances sometimes bring confusion to many patients, whose illnesses place them in the midst of a complex system of care. Various members of the medical staff come and go, and it is understandable when the day's scheduled course does not always run exactly as planned. Patients need personal advocates. Primary health care providers such as the nurse and dietitian can provide such essential support and personalized care.

Health Care Team

In the area of nutritional care, the registered dietitian (RD) carries the major responsibility. Working closely with the physician, the dietitian determines individual nutrition therapy needs and plan of care. Team support is essential throughout this process. Nurses are in a unique position to provide additional nutritional support, referring patients to the dietitian when necessary.

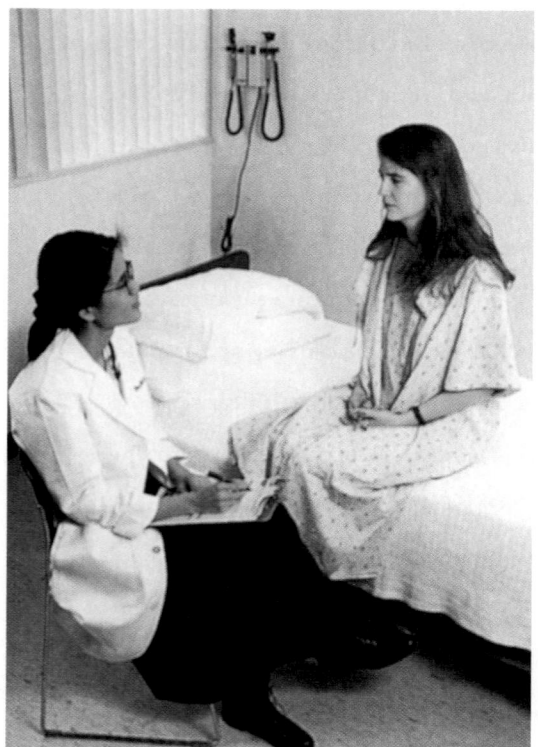

Figure 17–1 Interviewing patient to plan personal care. (From Seidel HM and others: *Mosby's guide to physical examination*, ed 3, St Louis, 1995, Mosby. Photographer: Patrick Watson.)

Of all the health care team members, nurses are in the closest continuous contact with patients and their families. A real partnership with patients and their families is essential to valid care. Patients and caretakers with emotional and social support have a much more positive experience with hospitalizations and overall medical care, regardless of clinical status.[1,2] Such a relationship is important to ensure the most beneficial health care approach. In developing this team relationship, all involved parties need each others' expertise and experience for a successful outcome.

Person-Centered Care

Nutritional care must be based on individual needs and must be *person-centered*. Needs must be constantly updated with the patient. Such personalized care demands a great commitment from health care workers. Despite all methods, tools, and technologies described here and elsewhere, remember this basic fact: *The most healing tool one will ever use is oneself.* This is a simple yet profound truth, because it is the *human* encounter to which health care workers bring themselves and their skills.

Phases of the Care Process

Collecting Information

To provide person-centered care, as much information about the patient's situation as possible must be collected. Family and medical history questionnaires are useful methods of gathering pertinent information upon admission or during the initial office visit of the patient. Appropriate care must take into consideration the nutritional status, food habits, and living situation, as well as the patient's needs, desires, and goals. The patient and family are the primary sources of this information (Figure 17-1). Other sources include the patient's medical chart, oral or written communication with hospital staff, and related research.

Identifying Problems

A careful study of all information gathered reveals basic patient needs. Other needs develop and guide the care plan as the hospitalization or consultation continues.

Planning Care

Objectives of the health care plan are designed to meet identified needs of the patient. This written care plan gives attention to personal needs and goals, as well as the identified requirements of medical care.

Implementing Care

Suitable and realistic actions then carry out the personal care plan. For example, nutritional care and teaching include an appropriate food plan with examples of food choices, food buying, or food preparation. Such activities ideally include family members as well.

Evaluating and Recording Results

Results of the implemented care plan must be checked to see if the patient's needs have been met so that the plan can be revised as necessary for continuing care. These actions and results must be carefully recorded in the patient's medical chart.

The remainder of this chapter briefly reviews each of the five phases of individual health care in terms of the nutritional aspects of overall patient care. Nutritional support is an essential component of all health care.

COLLECTING AND ANALYZING NUTRITION INFORMATION

Collection

Anthropometric Measurements

Practice taking anthropometric measurements correctly to avoid errors. Also maintain proper equipment and careful technique. Three types of measurements are common in clinical practice.

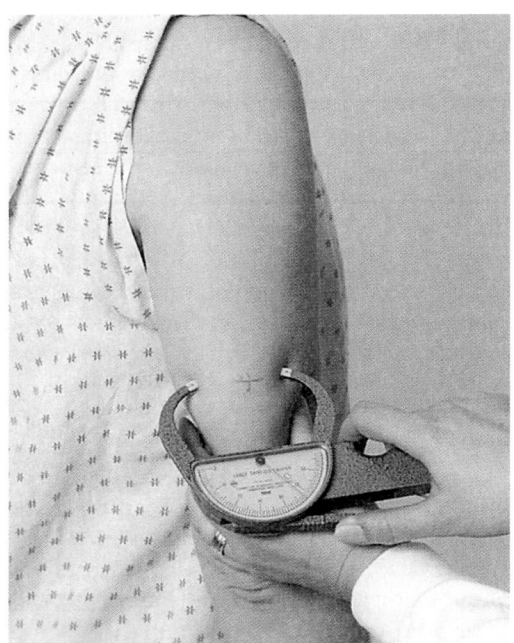

Figure 17–2   Assessment tools include skinfold calipers (shown in the figure), which measure the relative amount of subcutaneous fat tissues at various body sites. (From Seidel HM and others: *Mosby's guide to physical examination,* ed 4, St Louis, 1999, Mosby. Photographer: Patrick Watson.)

Weight. Weigh hospital patients at consistent times (e.g., in the early morning after the bladder is emptied and before breakfast). Weigh patients without shoes in light indoor clothing or an examination gown. Ask about their usual body weight and compare it with standard weight-height tables (see Chapter 15). Ask about any recent weight loss (e.g., how much over what time period). Rapid undesirable weight loss is significantly associated with increased health risks. Also ask if the cause is known, and ask about any recent weight gain, as well. Sometimes it is helpful to ask about general weight history over time (e.g., peaks and lows at what ages).

Height. Use a fixed measuring stick against the wall if possible. Otherwise, use the moveable measuring rod on the platform clinic scales. Have the person stand as straight as possible, without shoes or cap. Note the growth of children, as well as the diminishing height of older adults. Body mass index (BMI) is calculated using both weight and height measurements and is a helpful assessment tool throughout the life cycle.

Body Composition. The dietitian usually measures various aspects of body size and composition to determine relative levels of fat versus muscle. Various methods used to measure body composition were covered in Chapter 15. Some methods include: skinfold thickness measurement with calipers (Figure 17-2), hydrostatic weighing, bioelectrical impedance analysis (BIA), dual energy x-ray absorptiometry (DEXA), and the BOD POD body composition tracking system.

Medical Tests

Many laboratory and radiographic tests aid in nutritional status assessment. Such reports are generally available in the patient's chart for study. Several of the most frequently used tests are listed here.

Plasma Protein. Basic measures are hemoglobin, hematocrit, and serum albumin. Additional tests may include serum transferrin or total iron-binding capacity (TIBC) and ferritin. These tests help detect protein and iron deficiencies.

anthropometric measurements   physical measurements of the human body used for health assessment including height, weight, skinfold thickness, and circumference (head, hip, waist, wrist, mid-arm muscle).

Protein Metabolism. Basic 24-hour urine tests measure the products of protein metabolism (e.g., urinary creatinine and urea nitrogen). Elevated levels may indicate excess breakdown of body tissue.

Immune System Integrity. Basic tests determine the lymphocyte count, which is the ratio of these special white cells to the total white blood cell count. Skin testing also may be done to check for sensitivity to common antigens and, hence, the strength of the general immune system.

Skeletal System Integrity. Several tests may be used, especially with older patients, to determine the status of bone integrity and possible osteoporosis. Some tests commonly used are x-ray, DEXA, and a full body bone scan.

Gastrointestinal Function. X-rays are also useful to evaluate gastrointestinal function and problems, such as peptic ulcer disease or malfunctions along the gastrointestinal tract.

The medical tests used for nutrition assessment are generally reliable in persons of any age, but some conditions may interfere with test results and should be considered when evaluating laboratory values. For example, laboratory values are affected by hydration status, presence of chronic diseases, changes in organ function, and certain drugs.

Observations

Careful observation of various areas of the patient's body may reveal signs of poor nutrition. Table 17-1 lists some clinical signs of nutritional status that should be kept in mind when providing general patient care.

Diet History

Knowledge of the patient's basic eating habits may help identify possible nutritional deficiencies. The Clinical Applications box, "Nutrition History: Activity-Associated Food Pattern of a Typical Day," shows an example of a general guide for gathering a nutrition history. Sometimes a more specific food history is obtained using a 3-day food record; that is, recording everything consumed, food items used, and amounts and methods of preparation for 3 days. A more extended view of the diet may reveal additional information about food habits or problems.

Analysis

Nutritional Problems

A study of all the collected nutrition information helps to identify nutritional problems, which may include nutrient deficiencies (e.g., evidence of iron deficiency anemia) or underlying disease requiring a special modified diet.

Signs of general malnutrition requiring rebuilding of body tissue and nutrient stores may be evidenced. Special assistance in eating and swallowing may be necessary.

Drug Interactions

Information about all drugs—including over-the-counter self-medications and "street drugs," as well as alcohol and prescribed drugs—is essential. It is especially important for the nurse to be familiar with drug-food interactions because he or she is most commonly administering both drugs and food to patients. Research each drug to determine any possible problems from the interaction of drugs with foods or nutrients (Figure 17-3). Many such reactions exist and are encountered with multiple drug use, especially in elderly patients with chronic diseases. Patients may respond very differently from one another depending on their normal dietary habits, specific disease, compliance, and other medications or herbs currently taken.[3]

Drug-Food Interactions. Interactions in which food is unintentionally increasing or decreasing the effect of a drug can adversely influence the health of a patient. Certain foods may affect the absorption, distribution, metabolism, or elimination of a drug, thus altering the intended dose response. Timing, size, and composition of meals relative to medication administration are all common causes of drug-food interactions. For example, a high-fat meal increases the absorption of some drugs that are lipophilic ("fat loving"), whereas a high-fiber meal may bind other drugs and reduce their absorption.[3] The interaction of grapefruit juice and several drugs has been under critical evaluation in recent years. Researchers have found that grapefruit juice can dramatically increase the bioavailability of certain drugs to a toxic level.[3-5] The anticoagulation medication warfarin is a commonly prescribed drug for heart disease patients and is also one of the most highly interactive medications with certain foods, specifically those high in vitamin K.[6]

Drug-Nutrient Interactions. Drug-nutrient interactions refer primarily to those reactions occurring when prescription drugs are taken in combination with over-the-counter vitamin and mineral supplements. Unfortunately, the use of vitamin and mineral supplements are seldom reported to physicians or pharmacists by patients. It is imperative to ask patients what other medications they are taking and probe specifically into supplement use. Drug-nutrient interactions may result in a depletion of a nutrient (e.g., corticosteroids deplete vitamin C, antibiotics destroy the gut production of vitamin K) or the

TABLE 17-1 Clinical Signs of Nutritional Status

Body area	Signs of good nutrition	Signs of poor nutrition
General appearance	Alert, responsive	Listless, apathetic, cachectic
Weight	Normal for height, age, and body build	Overweight or underweight (special concern for underweight)
Posture	Erect, straight arms and legs	Sagging shoulders, sunken chest, humped back
Muscles	Well developed, firm, good tone; some fat under skin	Flaccid, poor tone; underdeveloped; tender, "wasted" appearance; inability to walk properly
Nervous control	Good attention span, not irritable or restless, normal reflexes, psychologic stability	Inattentive, irritable, confused; burning and tingling of hands and feet (paresthesia); loss of position and vibratory sense; weakness and tenderness of muscles (may result in inability to walk); decrease or loss of ankle and knee reflexes
Gastrointestinal function	Good appetite and digestion; normal, regular elimination; no palpable (perceptible to touch) organs or masses	Anorexia, indigestion, constipation or diarrhea, liver or spleen enlargement
Cardiovascular function	Normal heart rate and rhythm, no murmurs, normal blood pressure for age	Rapid heart rate (>100 beats/min tachycardia), enlarged heart, abnormal rhythm, elevated blood pressure
General vitality	Endurance, energetic, sleeps well, vigorous	Easily fatigued, no energy, falls asleep easily, looks tired or apathetic
Hair	Shiny, lustrous, firm, not easily plucked, healthy scalp	Stringy, dull, brittle, dry, thin, sparse; depigmented; can be plucked easily
Skin (general)	Smooth, slightly moist, good color	Rough, dry, scaly, pale, pigmented, irritated; bruises; petechiae
Face and neck	Skin color uniform; smooth, pink, healthy appearance; not swollen	Greasy, discolored, scaly, swollen; skin dark over cheeks and under eyes; lumpiness or flakiness of skin around nose and mouth
Lips	Smooth, good color; moist, not chapped or swollen	Dry, scaly, swollen; redness and swelling (cheilosis) or angular lesions at corners of the mouth or fissures or scars (stomatitis)
Mouth, oral membranes	Reddish-pink mucous membranes in oral cavity	Swollen, boggy oral mucous membranes
Gums	Good pink color, healthy, no swelling or bleeding	Spongy, bleed easily, marginal redness, inflamed, receding gums
Tongue	Good pink color or deep reddish in appearance, not swollen or smooth, surface papillae present, no lesions	Swelling, scarlet and raw, magenta color, beefy (glossitis), hyperemic and hypertrophic papillae, atrophic papillae
Teeth	No cavities, no pain, bright, straight, no crowding, well-shaped jaw, clean, no discoloration	Unfilled caries, absent teeth, worn surfaces, mottled (fluorosis), malpositioned
Eyes	Bright, clear, shiny; no sores at corner of eyelids; membranes moist and healthy pink color; no prominent blood vessels or amount of tissue or sclera; no fatigue circles beneath	Eye membranes pale (pale conjunctiva), redness of membrane (conjunctival infection), dryness, signs of infection, Bitot's spots, redness and fissuring of eyelid corners (angular palpebritis), dryness of eye membrane (conjunctival xerosis), dull appearance of cornea (corneal xerosis), soft cornea (keratomalacia)
Neck (glands)	No enlargement	Thyroid enlarged
Nails	Firm, pink	Spoon-shaped (koilonychia), brittle, ridged
Legs, feet	No tenderness, weakness, or swelling; good color	Edema, tender calf, tingling, weakness
Skeleton	No malformations	Bowlegs, knock-knees, deformity at diaphragm, beaded ribs, prominent scapulas

From Williams SR: Nutritional assessment and guidance in prenatal care. In Worthington-Roberts BS, Williams SR: *Nutrition in pregnancy and lactation*, ed 5, New York, 1993, McGraw-Hill.

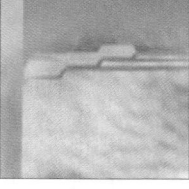

CLINICAL APPLICATIONS

NUTRITION HISTORY: ACTIVITY-ASSOCIATED FOOD PATTERN OF A TYPICAL DAY

Name _____ Date _____

Height _____ Weight (lb) _____ (kg) _____ Age_____ Ideal weight _____

Referral:

Diagnosis:

Diet order:

Occupation:

Recreation, physical activity:

Present food intake:

Time/location	Food (and method of preparation)	Serving size	Tolerance/comments
Breakfast			
Snack			
Lunch			
Snack			
Dinner			
Snack			

Summary: Total servings of foods in each category:

Breads/Grains: _____ Vegetables: _____ Fruits: _____ Dairy: _____ Meat: _____ Fat/Sugar: _____

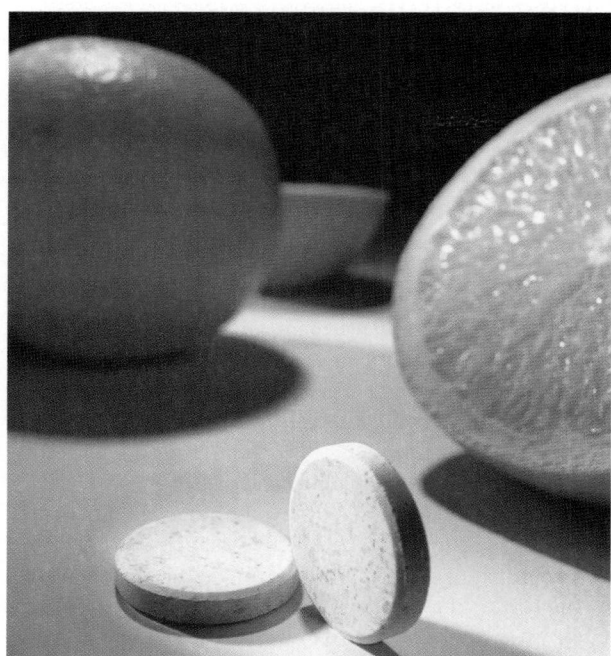

Figure 17–3   Many drugs, foods, and nutrients interact to cause nutritional problems. (Copyright 2004 JupiterImages Corporation.)

vitamin may induce metabolism of the drug (e.g. vitamin B_6 induces the anticonvulsant medication phenytoin by up to 50%).[7]

Drug-Herb Interactions. Interactions involving prescription drugs and herbs are the least well-defined of the drug interactions. St. John's Wort (*Hypericum perforatum*), one of the most commonly taken herbs for antidepression, has been studied extensively for drug interactions. It is unclear the exact mechanism in which St. John's Wort interacts with medications, because it is not the same with all drugs. Some researchers found the herb to decrease the activity of key enzymes involved in the metabolism of drugs, whereas others found the herb to increase the enzymatic activity.[7] Other common herbs involved in drug interactions include papaya extract (*Carica papaya*), devil's claw (*Harpagophytum procumbens*), *Ginkgo biloba*, evening primrose (*Oenothera biennis*), valerian (*Valeriana officinale*), kelp (*Fucus vesiculosus*), ginseng (*Panax ginseng*), ginger (*Zingiber officinale*), among many others.[7] Many herbs also have clinically documented medicinal properties and should be evaluated on an individual basis to determine appropriateness with the patient's current dietary habits and prescribed medications.

Personal Needs and Goals

Personal, cultural, and ethnic needs must be considered when helping a patient plan for meeting health needs (see the Cultural Considerations box, "Cultural Differences in Advanced Care Planning"). Psychological and emotional problems can weigh heavily on the overall outcome of a patient's prognosis and well-being. For example, geriatric patients in long-term health care facilities often suffer from depression and weight loss, confounding problems when individuals are already in poor health.

The most important link to this type of malnutrition is decreased food intake. Researchers have found everyday emotions to significantly influence food intake in this population.[8] Thus by addressing emotional tribulations, energy needs may be better met, and complications associated with malnutrition avoided. Unfortunately, such problems often are not discussed with the physician. In a study conducted in London, the two most common reasons given by patients for not discussing psychological problems with their physician was that the doctor did not have time and they feared there was nothing the doctor could do to help.[9] By probing patients with questions about their psychological well-being, perhaps some of the confounding factors can be alleviated. Likewise, economic needs are paramount for many persons in high-risk populations. In taking personal goals and needs into consideration, the health care team and patient can help establish priorities for immediate and long-term care.

PLANNING AND IMPLEMENTING NUTRITIONAL CARE

Basic Principles of Diet Therapy

Normal Nutrition Base

The primary principle of diet therapy is that it is based on a patient's normal nutritional requirements, which are important for patients to know. Any therapeutic diet is only a modification of normal nutritional needs and is only modified as an individual's specific condition requires.

Disease Modifications

Nutritional components of the normal diet may be modified in three basic ways, as follows:

1. *Energy.* The total energy value of the diet, expressed in kilocalories (kcal), may be increased or decreased.

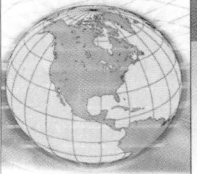

CULTURAL CONSIDERATIONS

CULTURAL DIFFERENCES IN ADVANCED CARE PLANNING

Advanced care planning is the process in which future treatment of a patient is determined before it is needed. Advanced directives and living wills are examples of documents recognized by law in the United States by all health care institutions. The Patient Self Determination Act of 1991 was intended to promote the use of advanced care procedures and strengthen the rights of patients during end-of-life medical procedures. Such documents are the only way in which treatment preferences of the patient can be ensured during times of unconsciousness or otherwise inability to communicate.

Medical nutrition therapy, such as enteral and parenteral nutrition, may be considered life-sustaining interventions by some individuals. There have been several recent studies comparing the cultural/racial discrepancy in attitudes about advanced care planning.*†‡§ Researchers suggest there are significant differences between various racial and ethnic patients and their caregivers about advanced care planning and end-of-life decisions. One study by Perkins and colleagues attempted to characterize those attitudes in three American ethnic cultures to enable health professionals to conduct culturally specific advanced care planning.* All three ethnic groups (European Americans, Mexican Americans, and African Americans) agreed that patients deserve a say in treatment and that advanced care planning can help

guide that decision. However, Mexican Americans and African Americans were much less likely to have advanced care planning documents than European Americans.

Other researchers have found African-American patients are more likely than Caucasians to request life-supportive treatments.†‡§ In recognizing such cultural differences in desired treatment and knowing the likelihood of patients having advanced care planning, health care professionals can assist the patient with greater awareness and sensitivity. Educate patients about advanced directives and living wills and explain all methods of life support that may be available. When such decisions are left in the hands of loved ones, even if the patient verbally expressed his or her wishes to the family, sometimes it is impossible for the family to then go through with the decision. Having advanced care planning can alleviate the burden on the family and ensure that the patient's wishes are granted.

*Perkins HS and others: Cross-cultural similarities and differences in attitudes about advance care planning, *J Gen Intern Med* 17:48, 2002.
†Phipps E and others: Approaching the end of life: attitudes, preferences, and behaviors of African-American and white patients and their family caregivers, *J Clin Oncol* 21(3):549, 2003.
‡Owen JE and others: End of life and reactions to death in African-American and white family caregivers of relatives with Alzheimer's disease, *Omega* 43(4):349, 2001.
§Hopp FP, Duffy SA: Racial variations in end-of-life care, *J Am Geriatr Soc* 48(6):658, 2000.

---

2. *Nutrients.* One or more of the basic nutrients (e.g., protein, carbohydrate, fat, mineral, or vitamin) may be modified in amount or form.
3. *Texture.* The texture or seasoning of the diet may be modified (e.g., liquid or low-residue diets).

Personal Adaptation

Successful nutrition therapy can occur only when the diet is *personalized* (e.g., adapted to meet individual needs). This can only be done by planning *with the patient or family.* Four areas must be explored together, as follows:

1. *Personal needs.* What personal desires, concerns, goals, or life situation needs must be met?

2. *Disease.* How does the patient's disease or condition affect the body and its normal metabolic functions?
3. *Nutrition therapy.* How and why must the diet be changed to meet needs created by the patient's particular disease or condition?
4. *Food plan.* How do these necessary nutritional modifications affect daily food choices? And how can these needs be met?

Routine House Diets

A schedule of routine "house" diets, based on some type of cycle menu, usually is followed in most hospitals. The basic modification is in texture, ranging from clear liquid (no milk) to full liquid (including milk) and soft food to

TABLE 17-2	Routine Hospital Diets			
Food	**Clear liquid**	**Full liquid**	**Soft**	**Regular**
Soup	Clear fat-free broth, bouillon	Same as clear, plus strained or blended cream soups	Same as clear and full, plus all cream soups	All
Cereal		Cooked refined cereal	Cooked cereal, corn flakes, rice, noodles, macaroni, spaghetti	All
Bread			White bread, crackers, melba toast, Zwieback	All
Protein foods		Milk, cream, milk drinks, yogurt	Same as full, plus eggs (not fried), mild cheese, cottage and cream cheeses, fowl, fish, tender beef, veal, lamb, liver, bacon	All
Vegetables			Potatoes: baked, mashed, creamed, steamed, scalloped; tender cooked whole, bland vegetables; fresh lettuce, tomatoes	All
Fruit and fruit juices	Fruit juices (as tolerated), flavored fruit drinks	All	Same as clear, plus cooked fruit: peaches, pears, applesauce, peeled apricots, white cherries; ripe peaches, pears, bananas, orange and grapefruit sections without membrane	All
Desserts and gelatin	Fruit-flavored gelatin, fruit ices and popsicles	Same as clear, plus sherbet, ice cream, puddings, custard, frozen yogurt	Same as clear and full, plus plain sponge cakes, plain cookies, plain cake, puddings, pie made with allowed foods	All
Miscellaneous	Soft drinks (as tolerated), coffee and tea, decaffeinated coffee and tea, cereal beverages such as Postum, sugar, honey, salt, hard candy, Polycose (Ross), residue-free supplements	Same as clear, plus margarine, pepper, all supplements	Same as clear and full, plus mild salad dressings	All

a full regular diet. Table 17-2 summarizes details of currently liberalized routine hospital diets.

Mode of Feeding

The method of feeding used in the nutritional care plan depends on the patient's condition. The dietitian and nurse work together to manage the diet by using oral, enteral, or parenteral feeding.

Oral Feeding

As long as possible, regular oral feedings are the preferred method of feeding. If needed, nutrient supplements may be added.

Assisted Oral Feeding

According to the patient's condition, the nurse may have to help the patient eat. Patients usually like to maintain independence as much as possible and should be encouraged to do so with whatever degree of assistance necessary. Making use of plate guards or special utensils to facilitate independence is usually welcomed by both patient and staff. Try to learn each patient's needs and limitations so that little things (e.g., having the meat cut up or the bread buttered before bringing the tray to the bedside) can be done without making a patient feel inadequate. When complete assistance is needed, have the tray securely placed within a patient's sight. Then relax; sit down beside the bed if this is more comfortable. Make simple conversation or remain silent as a patient's condition indicates. Offer small amounts and do not rush the feeding. Give ample time for a patient to chew and swallow or rest between mouthfuls. Offer liquids between the solids, using a drinking tube if necessary. Wipe the patient's mouth with a napkin during and after each meal. Let the patient hold the bread, if desired and able to do so. When feeding a patient who is blind or has eye dressings, describe the food on the tray so that a mental image helps create a desire to eat. Sometimes it is helpful to use the face of a clock to let a patient visualize the position of certain foods on the plate (e.g., indicating that the meat is at 12 o'clock, the potatoes are at 3 o'clock, etc.). Warn the patient that the soup feels particularly hot when taken through a straw, and identify each food being served beforehand.

Assisted feeding times can provide a special opportunity for nutrition counseling and support. Important observations can be made during this time. The nurse can closely observe the patient's physical appearance and responses to the foods served, appetite and tolerance for certain foods, as well as note the meaning of food to the person. These observations can help the nurse adapt the patient's diet to meet any particular individual needs. Helping patients learn more about their diets and nutritional needs is an important part of personal care. Persons who understand the role of good food in health (e.g., that it helps them regain strength and recover from illness) are more likely to accept the diet. They also feel more encouraged to maintain sound eating habits after discharge from the hospital, as well as improve their eating habits in general.

Enteral Feeding

When a patient cannot eat, but the remaining portions of the gastrointestinal tract can be used, an alternate form of **enteral** feeding by tube provides nutritional support. The saying, "if you don't use it, you lose it" also applies to gut function. Therefore any time the patient can tolerate feedings through the gut, it is the feeding method of choice. A small tube is placed through the patient's nasal cavity, running down the back of the throat into either the stomach or small intestine (nasogastric or nasojejunal, respectively) to administer an appropriate source of nutrients and energy. Various commercial formulas are available and usually are preferred over locally mixed ones. A blended formula, from table food, may be calculated and prepared but greater risk for contamination in preparation and storage exists. Enteral feedings, along with diagrams, are covered in much greater detail in Chapter 22.

Parenteral Nutrition

If a patient cannot tolerate food or formula through the gastrointestinal tract, intravenous (IV) feeding is necessary. Compared with tube feeding, **parenteral** feedings are more invasive, much more expensive, and introduce more risk. However, for patients in whom part or all of the gastrointestinal tract or accessory organs (liver, pancreas, etc.) are not functioning, it is necessary. There are two forms of parenteral nutrition: (1) peripheral vein feeding, and (2) central vein feeding. Again, both forms of parenteral nutrition are covered in greater detail, along with diagrams, in Chapter 22. A brief description follows.

Peripheral Vein Feeding. Various solutions of dextrose, amino acids, vitamins, minerals, and lipids can be fed directly into peripheral veins. The nutrient and energy intake is limited in this method of feeding, however, so peripheral vein feeding is only used when the need for nutritional support is not extensive or long term. It is helpful for patients to understand that this is still a method of "feeding."

Central Vein Feeding. When a patient's nutritional need is great (e.g., in massive injury or debilitating disease) and parenteral nutrition may be necessary for longer time, the use of a larger central vein is required. Total parenteral nutrition (TPN) through a central line involves a surgical procedure in which a catheter is inserted into the large subclavian vein for easy access. This mode of parenteral feeding allows for higher volumes of nutrients and can be used long term. A team of specialists (e.g., physicians, dietitians, pharmacists, and nurses) works closely together in the administration of parenteral nutrition. Throughout this procedure, the patient needs special care and support, including instruction for continued TPN use at home as needed (see Chapter 22 for more information about TPN).

EVALUATION OF NUTRITIONAL CARE

General Considerations

When the nutritional care plan is carried out, it is evaluated in terms of nutritional diagnosis and treatment objectives. This evaluation continues through the period of care and terminates at the point of discharge or the end of the care period. The various questions listed in the following sections are important.

Nutritional Goals

What is the effect of the diet or feeding method on the illness or the patient's situation? Is any change in the nutrients, energy, meal-snack patterns, or feeding methods necessary?

Accuracy of Care Plan Actions

Must any of the nutritional care plan components be changed? Is it necessary to change the type of food or feeding equipment, environment for meals, counseling procedures, or types of learning activities for nutrition education?

Ability to Follow Diet

Does any hindrance or disability prevent the patient from following the treatment plan? What is the effect of the diet on the patient, family, or staff? Was all the necessary nutrition information gathered correctly? Do the patient and family understand all the self-care instructions provided? Are needed community resources available and convenient? Has any necessary food-assistance program been sufficient for the patient's care?

Role of the Nurse and Clinical Dietitian

The nurse and dietitian form an important team for providing nutritional care. The dietitian determines nutritional needs, plans and manages nutrition therapy, evaluates plan of care, and records results. Throughout this entire process, the nurse helps to develop, support, and carry out the plan of care. Successful care depends on the close teamwork of the dietitian and nurse. When necessary, the nurse also may serve as an essential coordinator, advocate, interpreter, teacher, or counselor.

Coordinator and Advocate

Nurses work more closely with patients than any other practitioner. They are best able to coordinate the patient's special services and treatments and can consult and refer as needed. Unfortunately, malnutrition is common in hospital settings. There are many factors involved in malnutrition (lack of appetite because of pain, medicine-induced anorexia, surgery, emotional and psychological distress, etc.). However, sometimes patients have reduced food intake because of conflict with medical procedures or appointments during meal time. The nurse may be able to help resolve such conflicts by coordinating meal delivery times in consideration of the patient's scheduled procedures.

Interpreter

The nurse can help reduce a patient's anxiety by careful, brief, easily understood explanations about various treatments and plans of care. This help includes a basic reinforcement of special diet needs, resulting food choices from menus, and illustrations of needs from foods on the tray. These activities may be difficult with uninterested or unpleasant patients, but efforts to understand such patient behaviors are important. As mentioned, a patient's psychological and emotional status has a strong influence on his or her overall ability to deal with the medical problem at hand. Patients who are discharged without proper interpretation of their prognosis or plan of continued care may experience unnecessary stress and confusion. A group of researchers developed a useful questionnaire that may help identify gaps in patient understanding and may help direct the health care professional to address issues as yet resolved.[9] The questionnaire is short and focuses on communication, emotions, short-term outcome, barriers, and relations with auxiliary staff. Such tools may help the entire medical staff to identify and address the personal needs of each patient.

Teacher or Counselor

Basic teaching and counseling skills are essential in nursing. Many opportunities exist during daily care for planned conversations about sound nutrition principles, which will reinforce the dietitian's work with the patient. Learning about the patient's nutritional needs must begin with hospital admission or initial contact, must carry through the entire period of care, and must continue in the home environment, supported by community resources as needed.

---

enteral (Gr. *enteron,* intestine) a mode of feeding that uses the gastrointestinal tract through oral or tube feeding.

parenteral (Gr. *para,* alongside, accessory, beyond; *enteron,* intestine) a mode of feeding that does not use the gastrointestinal tract but instead provides nutritional support by intravenous delivery of nutrient solutions.

SUMMARY

The basis for effective nutritional care begins with the patient's nutritional needs and must involve the patient and family. Such person-centered care requires initial assessment and planning by the dietitian and continuous close teamwork among all team members providing primary care. Careful assessment of factors influencing nutritional status requires a broad foundation of pertinent information (e.g., physiologic, psychosocial, medical, and personal information). The patient's medical record is a basic means of communication among health care team members.

Nutrition therapy is based on the personal and physical needs of the patient. Successful therapy requires a close working relationship among dietetics, medical, and nursing staff in the health care facility. The nurse has a unique position to reinforce nutrition principles of the diet with the patient and family.

CRITICAL THINKING QUESTIONS

1. Identify and discuss the possible effects of various psychosocial factors on the outcome of nutrition therapy.
2. Describe commonly used measures for determining nutritional status in an outpatient setting and a long-term care facility. Include the following measurement tools: (1) anthropometric measures; (2) medical tests; (3) clinical observations; and (4) food habits.
3. Describe the roles of the dietitian and nurse in the nutritional care plan.

CHAPTER CHALLENGE QUESTIONS

True-False

Write the correct statement for each item you answer "false."

1. *True or False:* Nutritional care is based on the needs of individual patients.
2. *True or False:* Patients' housing situations have little relation to their illnesses or continuing care.
3. *True or False:* History-taking is an important skill in planning nutritional care.
4. *True or False:* A patient's social history has little value in planning his or her diet.
5. *True or False:* Once a diet treatment plan has been established, it should be followed continuously without change.
6. *True or False:* The involvement of the patient's family in the diet therapy and teaching usually creates problems and is best avoided.
7. *True or False:* Patients' personal goals do not relate to their diet therapy and instruction.

Multiple Choice

1. Which of the following personal details help(s) to determine a patient's nutritional needs? *(Circle all that apply.)*

   a. Gastrointestinal function

   b. Blood protein level

   c. Skinfold thickness

   d. Symptoms of illness

2. A nutrition history should include which of the following items of nutrition information? *(Circle all that apply.)*

   a. General food habits

   b. Food-buying practices

   c. Cooking methods

   d. Food likes and dislikes

3. Knowledge of which of the following items is necessary for carrying out valid diet therapy for a hospitalized patient? *(Circle all that apply.)*

   a. The specific diet and its relation to the patient's disease

   b. Foods affected by the diet modification

   c. The mode of the hospital's food service and the patient's need for any eating aids

   d. The patient's response to the diet

4. Which of the following actions would be helpful to a disabled patient who needs assistance in eating? *(Circle all that apply.)*

   a. Learning the extent of the disability and encouraging him or her to do as much of the feeding as he or she can himself

   b. Feeding the patient completely, regardless of the problem, because it saves him or her time and energy

   c. Hurrying the feeding to get in as much food as possible before the patient's appetite wanes

   d. Sitting comfortably by the patient's bed, offering mouthfuls of food, with ample time for chewing, swallowing, and rest as needed

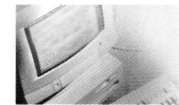

Please refer to the Students' Resource section of this text's Evolve web site for "Suggestions for Additional Study."

REFERENCES

1. Da Costa D and others: The relationship between health status, social support and satisfaction with medical care among patients with systemic lupus erythematosus, *Int J Qual Health Care* 11(3):201, 1999.
2. vom Eigen KA and others: Carepartner experiences with hospital care, *Med Care* 37(1):33, 1999.
3. Schmidt LE, Dalhoff K: Food-drug interactions, *Drugs* 62(10):1481, 2002.
4. Christensen H and others: Coadministration of grapefruit juice increases systemic exposure of diltiazem in healthy volunteers, *Eur J Clin Pharmacol* 58:515, 2002.
5. Charbit B and others: Pharmacokinetic and pharmacodynamic interaction between grapefruit juice and halofantrine, *Clin Pharmacol Ther* 72(5):514, 2002.
6. Heck AM and others: Potential interactions between alternative therapies and warfarin, *Health-Syst Pharm* 57:1221, 2000.
7. Sorensen JM: Herb-drug, food-drug, nutrient-drug, and drug-drug interactions: mechanisms involved and their medical implications, *J Altern Complement Med* 8(3):293, 2002.
8. Paquet C and others: Direct and indirect effects of everyday emotions on food intake of elderly patients in institutions, *J Gerontol A Biol Sci Med Sci* 58(2):153, 2003.
9. Steine S and others: A new, brief questionnaire (PEQ) developed in primary health care for measuring patients' experience of interaction, emotion and consultation outcome, *Fam Pract* 18(4):410, 2001.

FURTHER READING AND RESOURCES

- American Society for Parenteral and Enteral Nutrition (A.S.P.E.N.): *www.clinnutr.org*

   This association provides education, publications, conferences, and resources on clinical nutrition therapy for health care professionals. The association is made up of physicians, dietitians, nurses, pharmacist, scientists, and other allied health care professionals.

- American Dietetic Association, Practice Report Panel: Practice report of the American Dietetic Association: home care—an emerging practice area for dietetics, *J Am Diet Assoc* 99(11):1453, 1999.

   Home care, especially for the growing numbers of older persons in our population, is increasing and the accompanying need for nutritional and nursing care reflects this pressing situation. This excellent report identifies these needs and discusses possible ways of meeting them.

- Porter C and others: Dynamics of nutrition care among nursing home residents who are eating poorly, *J Am Diet Assoc* 99(11):1444, 1999.

   This article provides insight into the common problem of malnutrition among nursing home residents, and the apparently haphazard ways some staff members may respond, for example: (1) using liquid supplements for vitamins but not for minerals, (2) replacing regular meals with liquid supplement drinks, or (3) resorting to unpleasant and unethical measures such as force feeding.

18

Gastrointestinal and Accessory Organ Problems

KEY CONCEPTS

- Diseases of the gastrointestinal tract and its accessory organs interrupt the body's normal cycle of digestion, absorption, and metabolism.

- Allergic conditions produce sensitivity to certain food components.

- Underlying genetic diseases may cause metabolic defects that block the body's ability to handle specific food nutrients.

People often take for granted the body's highly organized and intricate system for handling food. However, when something goes wrong with the system it affects the whole being.

As the gastrointestinal tract and its handling of food are studied, the whole person, not just the physical system, actually is being looked at. The gastrointestinal tract is a sensitive mirror, both directly and indirectly, of the individual human condition.

This chapter looks at the sensitive system that handles food and its nutrients to provide energy and maintain body tissues. Nutrition therapy must be based not only on the functioning of this finely integrated network but also on the person whose life it affects.

THE UPPER GASTROINTESTINAL TRACT

Problems of the Mouth

Dental Problems

Although the incidence of dental caries has declined somewhat in the past few years, tooth decay still plagues children and adults.[1] Some of the decline is associated with increased use of fluoridated public water and toothpaste,[2] as well as better dental hygiene. In elderly persons, loss of teeth or ill-fitting dentures may cause problems with eating, swallowing, and overall nutrition. According to the Centers for Disease Control and Prevention, tooth decay is more common in lower socioeconomic individuals. More than one third of poor adults have at least one untreated decayed tooth.[1] Sometimes a *mechanical soft diet* is helpful for individuals lacking teeth. In such a diet, all foods are soft cooked and meats are ground and mixed with sauces or gravies, so that less chewing is necessary.

Surgical Procedures

A fractured jaw or other mouth or neck surgery poses obvious eating problems. Healing nutrients must be supplied, usually in the form of high-protein, high-caloric liquids. Table 18-1 provides an example of a simple milk shake. Other commercial formulas also are available. As healing progresses, soft foods requiring little chewing effort can be added, building to a full diet according to individual tolerance.

Oral Tissue Inflammation

The tissues of the mouth often reflect a person's general nutritional status. Malnutrition, especially severe states, causes deterioration of oral tissues, resulting in local infection or injury that brings pain and difficulty in eating. The following conditions of malnutrition in the oral cavity affect all its parts:

- *Gingivitis.* Inflammation of the gums, involving the mucous membrane and its supporting fibrous tissue circling the base of the teeth.
- *Stomatitis.* Inflammation of the oral mucous lining of the mouth.
- *Glossitis.* Inflammation of the tongue.
- *Cheilosis.* A cracking and dry scaling process at the corners of the mouth affecting the lips and corner angles, making opening the mouth to eat very painful.

Mouth ulcers may develop from three infectious sources: (1) herpes simplex virus, which causes mouth sores on the inside mucous lining of the cheeks and lips or on the external portion of lips, where they are commonly called cold sores or fever blisters; (2) *Candida albicans,* a fungus causing similar sores on the oral mucosa, which is a condition called candidiasis or thrush; or (3) *Hemolytic streptococcus,* a type of bacteria causing similar mucosal ulcers that are commonly called canker sores. These conditions are usually self-limiting and short-lived. Other causes may range from a simple toothbrush abrasion or allergies to a more serious underlying illness such as cancer, which lowers the body's immune system.

In any case, eating is painful and adequate nutrition becomes a major problem. Progressing from nutritionally dense liquids, high in protein and calories, to soft foods (e.g., usually nonacidic and nonspicy to avoid irritation) generally is well tolerated. Extremes in temperature are avoided if they cause pain. Room temperature soft or liquid foods usually are better accepted. In severe disease, as in cancer and its treatments, using a mouthwash containing a mild topical local anesthetic before meals helps to relieve the pain of eating.

TABLE 18–1	High-Protein, High-Kilocalorie Formula for Liquid Feedings		
Ingredients	**Amount**	**Approximate food value**	
Milk	1 cup	Protein:	40 g
Egg substitute	Equivalent of 2 eggs	Fat:	30 g
Skim milk powder or Casec	6-8 Tbsp	Carbohydrates:	70 g
	2 Tbsp	Kilocalories:	710
Sugar	2 Tbsp		
Ice cream	2.5-cm (1-inch) slice or 1 scoop		
Cocoa or other flavoring	2 Tbsp		
Vanilla	Few drops, as desired		

Salivary Gland Problems

Disorders of the salivary glands in the mouth also affect eating and related nutritional status. Problems may arise from infection, such as the mumps virus that attacks the **parotid gland.** Other problems arise from excess salivation, which occurs in numerous disorders affecting the nervous system (e.g., Parkinson's disease), from local mouth infections or injury, or from drug reactions. Conversely, a dry mouth from lack of salivation may be temporary, caused by fear, infection, or drug action. Permanent dry mouth, **xerostomia,** sometimes occurs in middle-aged and elderly adults, often associated with rheumatoid arthritis, radiation therapy, or as a side effect from many drugs necessary on a chronic basis. Xerostomia causes difficulty in swallowing and speaking, taste interference, and tooth decay. More liquid food items such as beverages, soups, stews, juicy fruits, and the use of gravies or sauces may facilitate the eating process. Extreme mouth dryness may be partially relieved by spraying an artificial saliva solution inside the mouth.

Swallowing Disorders

Swallowing is not as simple an act as it may seem. It actually involves highly integrated actions of the mouth, **pharynx,** and esophagus and, once started, is beyond voluntary control. Swallowing difficulty, **dysphagia,** is a fairly common problem with a variety of causes. It may be only temporary (e.g., a piece of food lodged in the back of the throat), for which the **Heimlich maneuver** is appropriate first aid. However, dysphagia is a more chronic problem in some patients and may be associated with insufficient production of saliva, dry mouth, abnormal peristaltic motility of the esophagus, complications of medication, or neurologic problems. To effectively treat dysphagia, the problem must be identified as either a mechanical obstruction or a neuromuscular disorder.[3] Such dysfunctional swallowing often causes persons to aspirate food particles, which may or may not be evident in coughing or choking episodes. Swallowing disorders are particularly common in cases of head trauma or brain tumor and stroke patients.[4,5]

It has been estimated that dysphagia affects 40% to 60% of nursing home residents.[6] Subtle symptoms include an unexplained drop in food intake or repeated episodes of pneumonia, possibly related to aspiration of food particles. Watch for warning signs of dysphagia and report them immediately. These signs may include a reluctance to eat certain food consistencies or any food at all, very slow chewing or eating, fatigue from eating, frequent throat clearing, complaints of food "sticking" in the throat, holding pockets of food in the cheeks, painful swallowing, regurgitation, or coughing or choking during attempts to eat.

The problem usually is referred to a team of specialists that includes a physician, nurse, dietitian, physical therapist, and an occupational therapist, who is especially important for evaluation and treatment of swallowing problems. Thin liquids are the most difficult food forms to swallow. Thus the diet is adapted to individual needs, in stages of added thickened liquids and pureed foods. Pureed foods are generally the consistency of mashed potatoes or pudding. Regular table food can be pureed in a food processor to achieve the desired consistency. There are also several manufacturers that produce pureed foods or food molds shaped like various meats or vegetables. Placing pureed foods in a food mold so that it takes the shape of the original food (e.g., corn on the cob or chicken breast) may enhance the appeal and appetite of patients faced with swallowing disorders.

Problems of the Esophagus

Central Tube Problems

The esophagus is a long muscular tube extending from the throat to the stomach. It is bound on both ends by circular muscles, or *sphincters,* that act as valves to con-

---

parotid glands (Gr. *para,* beyond, beside; *ous,* ear) the largest of three pairs of salivary glands situated near the ear. The parotid glands lie, one on each side, above the angle of the jaw, below and in front of the ear. They continually secrete saliva, which passes along the duct of the gland and into the mouth through an opening in the inner cheek, level with the second upper molar tooth. Normal saliva flow facilitates the chewing and swallowing of food and prevents dry mouth problems.

xerostomia (Gr. *xeros,* dry; *stoma,* mouth) dryness of the mouth from lack of normal secretions.

pharynx (Gr. *pharynx,* throat) the muscular membranous passage between the mouth and the posterior nasal passages and the larynx and esophagus.

dysphagia (Gr. *dys-,* painful; *phagein,* to eat) difficulty in swallowing.

Heimlich maneuver a first-aid maneuver to relieve a person who is choking from blockage of the breathing passageway by a swallowed foreign object or food particle. Standing behind the person, clasp the victim around the waist, placing one fist just under the sternum (breastbone) and grasping the fist with the other hand. Then make a quick, hard, thrusting movement inward and upward to dislodge the object.

trol food passage. The upper sphincter muscle remains closed except during swallowing, preventing airflow into the esophagus and stomach. Upon swallowing, the sphincter opens automatically and then closes immediately afterward. Various disorders along the tube may disrupt normal swallowing, including: (1) muscle spasms or uncoordinated contractions; and (2) stricture or narrowing of the tube caused by a scar from a previous injury, ingestion of caustic chemicals, a tumor, or *esophagitis* (an inflammation of the esophagus). These problems hinder eating and require medical attention through stretching procedures or surgery to widen the tube and drug therapy to heal the inflammation. The diet during such problems is liquid to soft in texture, depending on the extent of the closure problem and individual tolerance.

Lower Esophageal Sphincter Problems

Defects in the function of the lower esophageal sphincter (LES) may come from changes in the smooth muscle itself or from the nerve-muscle hormone control of *peristalsis* (see Chapter 5). Spasms occur when the LES muscles maintain an excessively high muscle tone, even while resting, thus failing to open normally when the person swallows. This condition is medically termed *achalasia*, from its tense muscle state, but is commonly called cardiospasm, from the proximity of the heart, although it does not relate to the heart at all. Symptoms include swallowing problems, frequent vomiting, a feeling of fullness in the chest, weight loss from eating difficulty, serious malnutrition, and pulmonary complications and infection caused by aspiration of food particles, especially during sleep. Surgical treatment involves dilating the LES or slitting the muscle, an *esophagomyotomy*. Both procedures can improve relaxation of the LES, but neither will affect the lack of peristalisis. The postoperative course starts with oral liquids and progresses to a regular diet within a few days, depending on tolerance. Patients should avoid very hot or cold foods, citrus juices, or highly spiced foods to prevent irritation. Patients should also eat frequent small meals as tolerated, and eat slowly in small bites and swallows.

Gastroesophageal Reflux Disease

Ongoing LES problems and esophageal motor impairment contribute to chronic gastroesophageal reflux disease (GERD).[7-9] Constant regurgitation of acid gastric contents into the lower part of the esophagus creates constant tissue irritation and inflammation, *esophagitis*. GERD is a serious and difficult problem that physicians graphically describe as "acid setting up shop in the esophagus." They further indicate that the problem is more widespread than the number of cases reported, because only the "tip of the iceberg" of chronic sufferers seeks medical help. Gastric acid and pepsin from the stomach cause tissue erosion, resulting in the most common symptom of frequent, severe heartburn that occurs 30 to 60 minutes after eating. The pain sometimes moves into the neck or jaw or down the arms. A hiatal hernia may or may not be present. In addition, the acid reflux may be caused by pregnancy, obesity, pernicious vomiting, or nasogastric tubes. The most common complications are *stenosis*, which is a narrowing or stricture of the esophagus, and esophageal ulcer.

Treatment for GERD and its relentless esophagitis includes weight management, because obesity is often a causative factor. Other conservative measures relate to acid control (e.g., during sleep, mealtime, and the use of antacids). Patients must avoid lying down after eating and must sleep with the head of the bed elevated. Frequent use of antacids helps control the symptoms. The goals and actions of dietary care are outlined in Table 18-2.

TABLE 18-2	**Dietary Care of Gastroesophageal Reflux Disease (GERD)**
Goal	**Action**
Decrease esophageal irritation	Avoid common irritants such as coffee, carbonated beverages, tomato and citrus juices, and spicy foods
Increase lower esophageal sphincter pressure	Increase protein foods
	Decrease fat to approximately 45 g/day or less; use nonfat milk
	Avoid strong tea, coffee, and chocolate if poorly tolerated
	Avoid peppermint and spearmint
Decrease reflux frequency and volume	Eat small, frequent meals
	Sip only a small amount of liquid with meal; drink mostly between meals
	Avoid constipation; straining increases abdominal pressure reflux
Clear food materials from the esophagus	Sit upright at the table or elevate the head of the bed
	Do not recline for 2 hours or more after eating

Hiatal Hernia

The lower end of the esophagus normally enters the chest cavity through an opening in the diaphragm membrane called the *hiatus*. A hiatal hernia occurs when a portion of the upper stomach also protrudes through this opening, as shown in Figure 18-1. Hiatal hernias are not uncommon problems, especially in obese adults, for whom weight reduction is essential. Hiatal hernia patients are advised to eat small amounts of food at a time, avoid lying down after meals, and sleep with the head of the bed elevated to prevent reflux of acidic stomach contents. Frequent use of antacids helps control the symptoms of heartburn, which is caused by the acid-enzyme-food mixture irritating the lower esophagus and the upper herni-

ated area of the stomach. Of persons with esophagitis and gastritis, 85% to 90% respond to weight reduction and other conservative measures. Large hiatal hernias or smaller sliding hernias may require surgical repair.

Problems of the Stomach and Duodenum: Peptic Ulcer Disease

Incidence

Throughout the United States, peptic ulcer disease (PUD) affects about 25 million people at some point in their life.[10] It can occur at any age but is seen mostly in middle adulthood, between the ages of 45 and 55. Gastric and duodenal ulcers, along with the complication of

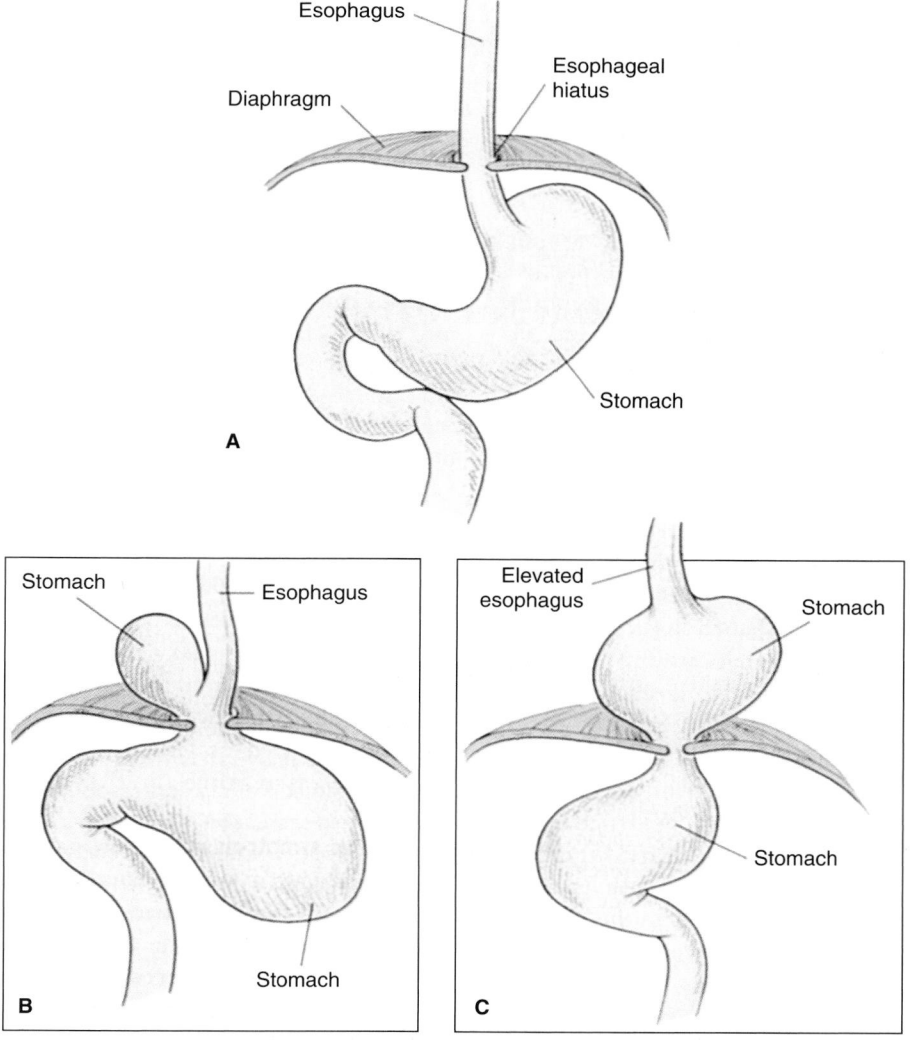

Figure 18–1   Hiatal hernia in comparison with normal stomach placement. **A,** Normal stomach. **B,** Paraesophageal hernia (esophagus in normal position). **C,** Esophageal hiatal hernia (elevated esophagus). (Credit: Bill Ober.)

perforation, occur more often in men. Other diseases and injuries, such as burns, may exacerbate the development of stress ulcers.

Causes

The underlying cause of PUD has been identified as *Helicobacter pylori* infection.[11,12] *H. pylori*, responsible for 80% to 90% of gastric and duodenal ulcers, are common spiraling, rod-shaped bacteria inhabiting the gastrointestinal area around the pyloric valve. This muscular valve connects the lower part of the stomach to the head of the small intestine, the duodenal bulb. Infection by *H. pylori* is a major determinant of chronic active gastritis and is also a necessary ingredient, along with gastric acid and pepsin, in the ulcerative process. Although approximately two thirds of the world's population is infected with *H. pylori*, not all persons develop ulcers (see the Cultural Considerations box, "The Risk for Gastric Ulcer Disease: Environmental or Genetic?"). However, those individuals who are infected have a twofold to sixfold higher risk of developing gastric cancer and lymphoma.[10] Tobacco smoking was also found highly correlated to incidence of PUD in a recent large-scale study in Denmark, thus confirming it as a major risk factor. The same study noted a negative association with physical activity and occurrence of PUD, suggesting a protective role against PUD in some individuals.[13]

Chronic use of *nonsteroidal antiinflammatory drugs* (NSAIDs) also may contribute to PUD development in susceptible persons.[14] These widely used drugs, including ibuprofen (Advil, Motrin) and aspirin (acetylsalicylic acid, ASA), irritate the gastric mucosa and cause bleeding, erosion, and ulceration, especially with prolonged or excessive use. The NSAIDs, including at least a dozen antiinflammatory drugs, are so-named to distinguish them from the steroid drugs, which are synthetic variants of the natural adrenal hormones. However, both physical and psychological factors are involved in the progression of PUD development.

Physical Factors. The general term *peptic ulcer* refers to an eroded mucosal lesion in the central portion of the gastrointestinal tract. This lesion can occur in the lower esophagus, stomach, or first portion of the duodenum,

---

CULTURAL CONSIDERATIONS

THE RISK FOR GASTRIC ULCER DISEASE: ENVIRONMENTAL OR GENETIC?

Before discovering the bacteria *Helicobacter pylori* in 1982, peptic ulcer disease was thought to be the exclusive result of excess stress, acid, and spicy food. Although these factors may still contribute to the disease, it is now known that infection with *H. pylori* causes 80% to 90% of duodenal and gastric ulcers, whereas chronic use of nonsteroidal antiinflammatory drugs is responsible for most of the rest.

Infection with *H. pylori*

H. pylori infection is more common in certain ethnic and age groups than others. In the United States, older adults, African Americans, and Hispanics have the highest prevalence of infection. Also, individuals of a lower socioeconomic status have a higher risk of *H. pylori* infection than individuals of a higher status. The mechanism by which *H. pylori* infection is transmitted is not yet known; however, it is believed to be spread through fecal-oral or oral-oral routes. This may be one of the reasons that *H. pylori* infection is higher in developing countries than in developed countries. Remember that not all carriers of the bacteria develop a peptic ulcer.

Active *H. pylori* Ulcers

These ulcers are more common in men than women in the United States. In other countries, such as Japan where peptic ulcer disease is very common, men are reported to have twice the prevalence of peptic ulcers as women. The risks for developing an ulcer are not easily defined by genetics, gender, ethnicity, or environment. It seems to be a combination of all the preceding that leads to ulceration. Researchers believe that genetics are less important than environment in determining risk of ulceration but both physiologic and psychological factors are involved in the overall environmental risk.

Physiologic trauma and emotional stress can lead to excess acid secretions in the stomach. For individuals already infected with *H. pylori* bacteria, that may be the missing link for creating a perfect environment for rapid growth and inflammation, and ultimately resulting in an ulcer. Therefore treatment for peptic ulcers must focus on eliminating the cause (bacteria, drugs, or other) and focus on the environmental cues involved in promoting excessive acidic secretions.

the *duodenal bulb*. Most ulcers occur in the duodenal bulb, because the gastric contents emptying there are most concentrated. The lesion results from an imbalance between the following two factors: (1) the amount of gastric acid and pepsin secretions (a powerful gastric enzyme for digestion of protein) and the extent of the *H. pylori* infection; and (2) the degree of tissue resistance to these secretions and the infection. The more acidic the environment, the more favorable the conditions for *H. pylori* colonization.

Psychological Factors. The influence of psychological factors in the development of peptic ulcer varies. No distinct personality type is free from the disease. However, stress during the young and middle adult years when personal and career strivings are at a peak, may contribute to peptic ulcer development in predisposed individuals (Figure 18-2). The stress of emergency trauma and injury, as well as the long-term rehabilitation processes, often exacerbate stress ulcers.

Clinical Symptoms

General symptoms include increased gastric muscle tone and painful contractions when the stomach is empty. With duodenal ulcers, the amount and concentration of hydrochloric acid secretions are increased; with gastric ulcers, the secretions may be normal. Low plasma protein levels, anemia, and weight loss reveal nutritional deficiencies. Hemorrhage may be one of the first signs. Diagnosis is confirmed by x-ray tests and visualization by **gastroscopy.**

Medical Management

In treating patients with PUD, physicians have four basic goals, as follows: (1) to alleviate the symptoms, (2) to promote healing, (3) to prevent recurrences by eliminating the cause, and (4) to prevent complications. In addition to general traditional measures, the recently expanded knowledge base about the cause of PUD and the development of a number of new drugs has increased the physician's available management tools.[14]

Rest. Adequate rest, relaxation, and sleep have long been the foundation of general care to enhance the body's natural healing process. Positive stress-coping and relaxation skills, which help patients deal with personal psychosocial stress factors, can be learned and practiced. Encouraging patients to talk about anxieties, anger, and frustrations may help them feel better. As soon as they are able, appropriate physical activity helps work out tensions. Habits that contribute to ulcer development, such as smoking and alcohol use, should be eliminated. Common drugs (e.g., aspirin) and NSAIDs (e.g., ibuprofen) should be avoided. Sometimes sedatives are prescribed to aid rest.

Drug Therapy. Advances in knowledge and therapy have currently provided physicians with four basic types of drugs for managing peptic ulcer disease, as follows:[15]

- *Blocking agents* (two types) that control acid secretion (e.g., cimetidine [Tagamet], ranitidine [Zantac]; and omeprazole [Prilosec])
- *Mucosal protectors* that inactivate pepsin and produce a gel-like substance to cover the ulcer and protect it from acid and pepsin while it heals itself (e.g., sucralfate [Carafate])
- *Antibiotics* that control the *H. pylori* bacterial infection (e.g., amoxicillin, proton pump inhibitor, tetracycline, and metronidazole)
- *Antacids* that counteract or neutralize the acid. Usually magnesium-aluminum compounds (e.g., Mylanta II or Maalox TC [therapeutic choice]) are the antacids of choice in treating peptic ulcer disease.

Maintenance drug therapy is imperative after large initial doses stabilize the growth rate of the bacteria. A continuous low-dose drug therapy follows initial treatment, with intermittent full-dose treatment or symptomatic self-care with the same agents used to heal the initial ulcer in-

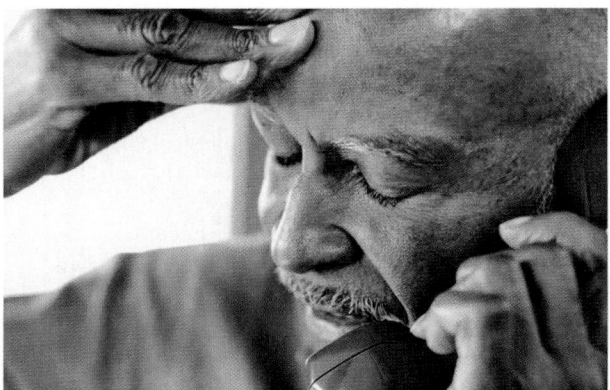

Figure 18–2 Stress may contribute to peptic ulcer disease in predisposed individuals. (Credit: PhotoDisc.)

gastroscopy (*gastro,* stomach; *scopy,* to view or see) examination of upper intestinal tract using a flexible tube with a small camera on the end. The tube is about 9 mm in diameter and takes color pictures as well as biopsy samples, if necessary.

fection.[15] Success rates depend on the relative strengths of the risk factors that influence recurrence (Box 18-1).

Dietary Management

In the past, a highly restrictive, bland diet was used in the care of patients with peptic ulcer disease. A bland diet has long since proved to be ineffective and lacking in adequate nutritional support for the healing process. Such a restrictive diet is unnecessary today because newer and better drugs are available to control acid secretions and assist healing. Thus current diet therapy is based on a liberal individual approach, guided by individual responses to any food. In this positive nutritional support for medical management, two basic goals guide food habits.

Eating a Well-Balanced Healthy Diet. Supply a well-balanced regular healthy diet to aid tissue healing and maintenance. Nutrient-energy needs are outlined in the current Recommended Dietary Allowances and Dietary Reference Intakes (see inside front book cover) and expressed in simple food choices in the Food Guide Pyramid (see Figure 1-2). Further focus is supplied by the goals of the *Dietary Guidelines for Americans* (see Chapter 1).

Avoiding Acid Stimulation. Avoid stimulating excess gastric acid secretion, which irritates gastric mucosa. Only a few food-related habits have been shown to affect acid secretion, as follows:

■ *Meal pattern.* Eat three regular meals a day without frequent snacks, especially at bedtime. Any food intake stimulates more acid output.
■ *Food quantity.* Do not eat large quantities at a meal to avoid stomach distention.
■ *Milk intake.* Avoid drinking milk frequently because it stimulates significant acid secretion, has only a transient buffering effect, and its animal fat content is undesirable. The milk sugar, lactose, also creates abdominal cramping, gas, and diarrhea for many persons with lactose intolerance caused by a deficiency of the enzyme lactase (see Chapter 2).
■ *Seasonings.* Individual tolerance is the rule, but the following agents have caused variable results and perhaps should be limited: hot chili peppers, black pepper, and chili powder.
■ *Dietary fiber.* There is no evidence for restricting dietary fiber. Some fibers, especially soluble forms, are beneficial.
■ *Coffee.* Avoid regular and decaffeinated coffee. Coffee stimulates acid secretion and may cause indigestion. The comparative effect of regular tea and colas may be milder to some persons, but these beverages also stimulate acid secretion.
■ *Citric acid juices.* These juices may cause gastric reflux and discomfort in some persons.
■ *Alcohol.* Avoid alcohol in concentrated forms, such as 40% (80 proof) alcohol. Other less concentrated forms of wine, taken with food in moderation, are tolerated well by some persons. Avoid beer; it has been shown to be a potent stimulant of gastric acid. For those who find it difficult to avoid alcohol and coffee completely, a small glass of dinner wine occasionally or a small cup (*demitasse*) of coffee at the close of a meal may minimize the acid secretion.
■ *Smoking.* Smoking is best eliminated completely at any time as it hinders ulcer healing. It not only affects gastric acid secretion but also hinders the effectiveness of drug therapy.
■ *Food environment.* Finally, consider the food environment. Eat slowly and savor the food in a calm environment. Respect individual responses or tolerances

---

BOX 18–1   Risk Factors for Recurring Peptic Ulcer

High-Risk

Medical/physical

Hypersecretion of gastric acid
Previous recurrences of peptic ulcer with complications
Helicobacter pylori infection

Emotional

Continuous, unrelieved emotional stress
Denial of emotional problems

Behavioral

Poor dietary habits
Failure to maintain prescribed diet and drug therapy
Cigarette smoking (10 or more/day)

Moderate-Risk

Medical/physical

Family history of peptic ulcer disease among close relatives
Recurring discomfort after eating

Emotional

Emotionally stressful environment
Recognition of emotional problems

Behavioral

Frequent use of aspirin and other NSAIDs
Distilled alcohol consumption
Irregular meals

NSAIDs= Nonsteroidal antiinflammatory drugs

to specific foods. Remember that the same food may bring different responses at different times depending on stress factors.

In the long run, a wide range of foods that are attractive to the eye and taste and regular, relaxed eating habits provide the best course of action.

THE LOWER GASTROINTESTINAL TRACT

Small Intestine Diseases

Diarrhea

In some cases, diarrhea may result from intolerance to specific foods or nutrients, as in lactose intolerance (see Chapter 2) or acute food poisoning from a specific foodborne organism or toxin (see Chapter 13). A variety of parasites (*Giardia lamblia, Cryptosporidium parvum, Cyclospora cayetanensis, Entamoeba histolytica*), bacteria (*Campylobacter, Clostridium difficile, Escherichia coli, Listeria monocytogenes, Salmonella enteritidis, Shigella*), and viral infections (HIV, rotavirus, Norwalk agent) are known causes of diarrhea.[16] So-called traveler's diarrhea, from irregular meals, unfamiliar foods, and travel tensions, is also a well-known gastrointestinal disturbance.[17]

Chronic diarrhea (diarrhea lasting more than 2 weeks) could be a life-threatening illness for young children or individuals with a weak immune system. Diarrhea in infants is a more serious problem, especially if prolonged, that can quickly lead to dehydration and nutrient losses and is associated with infection. Intravenous fluid and electrolyte replacement may be necessary, or an oral solution of water, glucose, and electrolytes (e.g., Polycose [Ross]) may be used. As soon as it is tolerated, a regular refeeding schedule is needed to avoid malnutrition.

Malabsorption

There are multiple causes of malabsorption, including the following:[18]

- *Maldigestion problems*. Pancreatic disorders, biliary disease, bacterial overgrowth, ileal disease (inflammatory bowel disease)

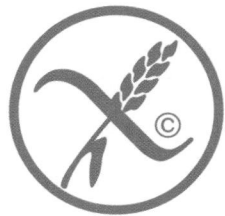

Figure 18–3   Gluten-free symbol. (Copyright Coeliac UK, Bucks, United Kingdom, 2004.)

- *Intestinal mucosal changes*. Mucosal surface alterations, intestinal surgery (e.g., as resections that shorten the bowel and absorbing surface area)
- *Genetic disease*. Cystic fibrosis with its complications of pancreatic insufficiency and lack of pancreatic enzymes
- *Intestinal enzyme deficiency*. Lactose intolerance caused by lactase deficiency (see Chapter 2)
- *Cancer and its treatment*. Absorbing surface effect of radiation and chemotherapy (see Chapter 23)
- *Metabolic defects*. Absorbing surface effects of pernicious anemia or gluten-induced mucosal disease (e.g., celiac sprue)

Three of these malabsorption conditions—celiac sprue, cystic fibrosis, and inflammatory bowel disease—are reviewed in this chapter.

Celiac Sprue

Disease Process. The childhood disorder *celiac disease* and the adult disease *nontropical sprue* are now known to be a single disease, called *celiac sprue*. In all cases, the cause is hypersensitivity to the protein gluten in certain grains. The eroded mucosal surface shows villi that are malformed and deficient in number with few microvilli. This damaged mucosa effectively reduces the absorbing surface by as much as 95%. The underlying cause is as yet unknown but probably involves an enzyme deficiency and a genetic base. The major symptom of **steatorrhea** (e.g., approximately 80% of ingested fat appears in the stools) and the progressive malnutrition are secondary effects to the gluten reaction.

Nutrition Management. The goal of nutrition management is to control the dietary gluten intake and prevent malnutrition. Wheat and rye are the main sources of gluten, but it is also present to some extent in oats and barley. Thus these grains are eliminated from the diet, and corn and rice are used as substitutes. Careful label reading is important for parents and children, because many commercial products use gluten-containing grains as thickeners or fillers. Some commercial products are using a gluten-free symbol on their food labels to assist in identification of acceptable foods (Figure 18-3). With an increasing number of processed foods and ethnic dishes, it is difficult to detect all food sources of gluten. Home test kits for gluten are available and may be beneficial for

steatorrhea   (Gr. *steatos*, fat; *rhoia*, flow) fatty diarrhea; excessive amounts of fat in the feces often caused by malabsorption diseases.

individuals consuming foods for which they do not have access to the ingredient list. Adhering to a low-gluten or gluten-free diet (Box 18-2) is the only effective treatment in maintaining a healthy mucosa and must be followed for life. Because of the nature of the malabsorption disorder, it is also important for patients with celiac sprue to be monitored for potential vitamin and mineral deficiency and partake in supplementation as necessary.

Cystic Fibrosis

Disease Process. Cystic fibrosis (CF) is the most common fatal genetic disease in North America and is currently affecting 30,000 people in the United States alone.[19] It is a generalized genetic disease of childhood, occurring mainly in Caucasian populations, in which 1 in 28 persons is a carrier. In past years, children with CF generally lived to about age 10, dying from complications such as damaged airways and lung infections, as well as a fibrous pancreas and lack of essential pancreatic enzymes to digest nutrients. However, recent discovery of the CF gene and the underlying metabolic defect has improved management of the disease and helped push the life expectancy up into adulthood. Nonetheless, mortality rates from CF have a strong correlation with poverty status. A recent study reported individuals in the lowest socioeconomic category having a 44% in-

---

BOX 18–2 Low-Gluten Diet for Children with Celiac Sprue Disease

Dietary Principles

- Kilocalories—high, usually approximately 20% above normal requirement to compensate for fecal loss
- Protein—high, as tolerated to promote growth in children and maintenance in adults
- Fat—low, but not fat-free, because of impaired absorption
- Carbohydrates—simple, easily digested sugars (fruits, vegetables) should provide approximately one half of the kilocalories
- Feedings—small, frequent feedings during ill periods; afternoon snack for older children
- Texture—smooth, soft, avoiding irritating roughage initially, using strained foods longer than usual for age, adding whole foods as tolerated and according to age of child
- Vitamins—supplements of B vitamins, vitamins A and E in water-miscible forms, and vitamin C
- Minerals—iron supplements if anemia is present

Selection of Foods

Food groups	Foods included	Foods excluded
Milk	Milk (plain or flavored with chocolate or cocoa) Buttermilk	Malted milk; preparations such as Cocomalt, Hemo, Postum, Nestle's chocolate
Meat or substitute	Lean meat, trimmed well of fat Eggs, cheese Poultry, fish Creamy peanut butter (if tolerated)	Fat meats (sausage, pork) Luncheon meats, corned beef, frankfurters, all common prepared meat products with any possible wheat filler Duck, goose Smoked salmon Meat prepared with bread, crackers, or flour
Fruits and juices	All cooked and canned fruits and juices Frozen or fresh fruits as tolerated, with no skins and seeds	Prunes, plums (unless tolerated)
Vegetables	All cooked, frozen, canned as tolerated (prepared *without* wheat, rye, oat, or barley products); raw as tolerated	Any causing individual discomfort All prepared with wheat, rye, oat, or barley products
Cereals	Corn or rice	Wheat, rye, oat, barley; any product containing these cereals
Breads, flours, cereal products	Breads, pancakes, or waffles made with suggested flours (cornmeal, cornstarch; rice, soybean, lima bean, potato, buckwheat)	All bread or cereal products made with gluten; wheat, rye, oat, barley, macaroni, noodles, spaghetti; any sauces, soups, or gravies prepared with gluten flour, wheat, rye, oat, or barley
Soups	Broth, bouillon (no fat or cream; no thickening with wheat, rye, oat, or barley products); soups and sauces may be thickened with cornstarch	All soups containing wheat, rye, oat, or barley products

creased risk of death compared with patients of the highest income category.[20] Identifying and addressing differences between socioeconomic classes in terms of treatment factors, environment, and overall care is important to improve the life of all patients with CF.

The metabolic defect coupled with CF inhibits the normal movement of chloride (Cl) and sodium (Na) ions in body tissue fluids (see Chapter 9). These ions become trapped in cells, causing thick mucus to form that clogs ducts and passageways. Involved organ tissues are damaged so that they no longer function normally. The classic CF symptoms include the following:

- *Thick mucus in the lungs*, which leads to damaged airways, more difficult breathing, and lung infections
- *Pancreatic insufficiency*, which leads to lack of normal pancreatic enzymes (see Chapter 5) to digest the macronutrients and progressive loss of insulin-producing beta cells and eventual diabetes mellitus (see Chapter 20)
- *Malabsorption* of undigested food nutrients, with consequential malnutrition and stunted growth
- *Liver disease* from progressive degeneration of functional liver tissue, initiated by clogged bile ducts
- *Salt (NaCl) concentration* increased in body perspiration, resulting in salt depletion

Nutrition Management. Current nutrition management of CF follows the guidelines developed by the U.S. Cystic Fibrosis Foundation. Nutritional support is a critical component of the treatment regime and can have a significant impact on normal growth.[21] Treatment is based on the following three factors: (1) increased knowledge of the disease process, (2) early newborn screening and diagnosis, and (3) improved pancreatic-enzyme replacement products. These products, such as Pancrease (McNeil), contain the normal pancreatic enzymes for each energy nutrient (e.g., lipase for fat digestion, amylase for starch digestion, and the protein enzymes trypsin, chymotrypsin, and carboxypeptidase [see Chapter 5]). These enzymes are processed into very small enteric-coated beads encased in capsules that are designed not to open or dissolve until they reach the alkaline medium of the intestine. Generous doses of these special enzyme-replacement capsules, varying with a child's age (e.g., an average of about 25 to 30 capsules per day), are divided between the three meals and usually are taken just before eating. Adequate enzyme replacement is the foundation that makes aggressive diet therapy a possibility for meeting growth needs.

Children with CF require 105% to 150% of the recommended nutrients for their age, depending on the severity of the disease. The former low-fat diet is no longer used. Instead, a nutritionally adequate high protein, normal-to-high-fat diet is recommended and provides about 20% of the kcalories as protein, 40% as carbohydrate, and 40% as fat. Routine care is based on regular nutrition assessment, diet counseling, food plans, enzyme replacement, vitamin supplements (especially fat-soluble vitamins A, D, E, and K), nutrition education, and exploration of individual problems, as outlined in Table 18-3. Try applying these principles of care in the Clinical Applications box, "Case Study:

TABLE 18–3	**Levels of Nutritional Care for Management of Cystic Fibrosis**	
Level of care	**Patient groups**	**Nutrition actions**
Level I—Routine care	All	Diet counseling, food plans, enzyme replacement, vitamin supplements, nutrition education, exploration of problems
Level II—Anticipatory guidance	Above 90% ideal weight-height index but at risk for energy imbalance, severe pancreatic insufficiency, frequent pulmonary infections, normal periods of rapid growth	Increased monitoring of dietary intake, complete energy-nutrient analysis, increased kcalorie density as needed, assessment of behavioral needs, counseling and nutrition education
Level III—Supportive intervention	85%-90% ideal weight-height index, decreased weight-growth velocity	Reinforcement of all the above actions, addition of energy-nutrient–dense oral supplements
Level IV—Rehabilitative care	Consistently below 85% ideal weight-height index, nutritional and growth failure	All the above plus enteral nutritional support by nasoenteric or enterostomy tube feeding (see Chapter 22)
Level V—Resuscitative or palliative care	Below 75% ideal weight-height index, progressive nutritional failure	All the above plus continuous enteral tube feedings or TPN (see Chapter 22)

Modified from CFF Consensus Report, Ramsey B and others: Nutrition assessment and management in cystic fibrosis: a consensus report, *Am J Clin Nutr* 55:108, 1992. Copyright the American Society for Clinical Nutrition.

TPN = Total parenteral nutrition.

CLINICAL APPLICATIONS

CASE STUDY: PAUL'S ADAPTATION TO CYSTIC FIBROSIS

Paul is a 12-year-old boy with cystic fibrosis. He is hospitalized with pneumonia and has difficulty breathing. Paul is a thin child with little muscle development who tires easily, although he has a large appetite. His stools are large and frequent and contain undigested food material.

Questions for Analysis

1. What is cystic fibrosis? Account for the clinical effects of the disease as evidenced by Paul's appearance and symptoms.

2. What are the basic goals of treatment in cystic fibrosis? Why is vigorous nutrition therapy a main part of treatment? Describe the current role of enzyme replacement therapy in this aggressive nutritional support.

3. Outline a day's food plan for Paul. Check the amount of protein and kcalories by calculating the total food values in your food plan to ensure the extra amount he needs is provided.

4. Why does Paul require therapeutic doses of multivitamins, including B-complex vitamins? Why does he need to have these in water-soluble form?

Paul's Adaptation to Cystic Fibrosis." This specialized care is administered by the medical genetics division of hospitals, with a team of CF specialists and their staff assistants, using guidelines provided by the U.S. Cystic Fibrosis Foundation.

Inflammatory Bowel Disease

The term *inflammatory bowel disease* applies to both *ulcerative colitis* and *Crohn's disease*. The related condition *short-bowel syndrome* results from repeated surgical removal of parts of the small intestine as the disease progresses. It was recently estimated by the Centers for Disease Control and Prevention that more than a half-million persons in the United States suffer from Crohn's disease alone.[22] All of these conditions can have severe, often devastating, nutritional results as more and more of the absorbing surface area becomes involved. Restoring positive nutrition is a basic requirement for tissue healing and health. **Elemental formulas** of amino acids, glucose, fat, minerals, and vitamins are more easily absorbed and support initial healing in response to antibacterial and antiinflammatory medications. The diet is gradually advanced to restore optimal nutrient intake. The principles of continuing dietary management include the following: (1) high-protein, about 100 g/day, omitting milk at first because it causes difficulty in many patients; (2) high-energy, approximately 2500 to 3000 kcal/day; (3) increased vitamins and minerals, usually with supplements.[23,24]

The former practice of reducing fiber or residue in the diet has been questioned. The bland, low-residue diets of the past mainly have been based on tradition or anecdotal belief rather than scientific studies on humans. These diets tended to be less appetizing and nourishing than regular diets. Current study and clinical practice indicate the benefit of a regular nourishing diet, respecting individual tolerances and disease status. A close working relationship among the physician, dietitian, and nurse is essential. Appetite is often poor, but adequate nutrition intake is imperative. A range of feeding modes, including enteral and parenteral nutritional support as needed, are explored in individual cases to achieve the vigorous nutritional care necessary. However, whatever the mode of feeding, it always must be provided with personal support, warmth, and encouragement.

Large Intestine Diseases

Diverticular Disease

Diverticulosis is a lower intestinal condition characterized by the formation of many small pouches, or pockets, along the muscular mucosal lining, usually in the colon (Figure 18-4). These little pouches are called *diverticula*. Most often they occur in older persons and develop at points of weakened muscles in the bowel wall, along the track of blood vessels entering the bowel from without. The direct cause is a progressive increase in pressure within the bowel from segmental circular muscle contractions that normally move the remaining food mass along and form the feces for elimination. When pressures become sufficiently high in one of these segments and there is insufficient fiber to maintain the necessary bulk for preventing these high internal pressures within the colon, small diverticula develop. As the pockets become infected, a condition called **diverticulitis,** the affected area is painful.

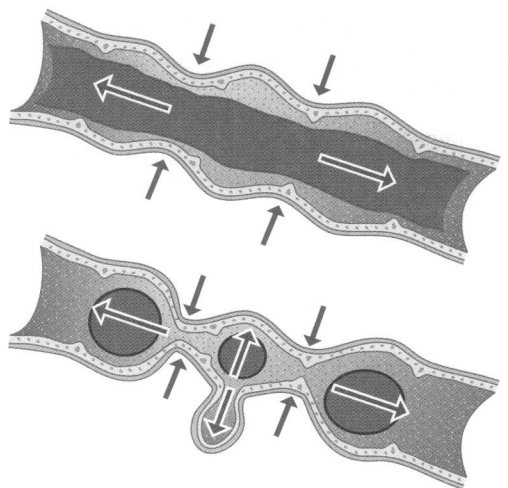

Figure 18-4 Mechanism by which low-fiber, low-bulk diets might generate diverticula. Where the colon contents are bulky *(top),* muscular contractions exert pressure longitudinally. If the lumen is small in diameter *(bottom),* contractions can produce occlusions and exert pressure against the colon wall, which may produce a diverticular "blowout." (From Mahan LK, Escott-Stump S: *Krause's food, nutrition, & diet therapy,* ed 11, Philadelphia, 2004, Saunders.)

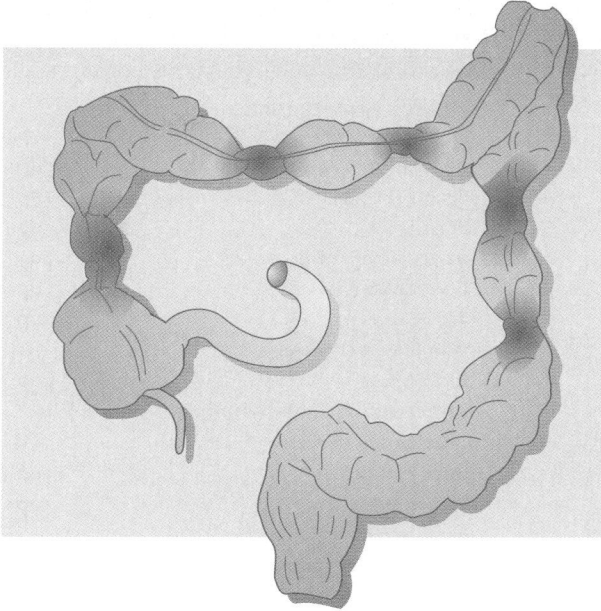

Figure 18-5 Irritable bowel syndrome. (From Mahan LK, Escott-Stump S: *Krause's food, nutrition, & diet therapy,* ed 10, Philadelphia, 2000, Saunders.)

The commonly used collective term covering diverticulosis and diverticulitis is *diverticular disease.* As the inflammatory process advances, increased pain and tenderness are localized in the lower left side of the abdomen and are accompanied by nausea, vomiting, distention, diarrhea, intestinal spasm, and fever. Sometimes perforation occurs, and surgery is indicated. There also may be underlying malnutrition. Aggressive nutrition therapy hastens recovery from an attack, shortens the hospital stay, and reduces costs. Current studies and clinical practice have demonstrated better management of chronic diverticular disease with an increased amount of dietary fiber rather than with the older practice of restricting fiber.[25] Certain foods, such as nuts and seeds, can act as irritants by accumulating in the small diverticula pouches and thus are restricted as a preventative measure against inflammation.

Irritable Bowel Syndrome

Gastroenterologists currently estimate that 15% to 20% of the general U.S. population has problems consistent with the condition now called *irritable bowel syndrome* (IBS), yet a large majority of victims do not seek medical attention. Although IBS (Figure 18-5) is one of the most common gastrointestinal disorders, its precise nature and cause continue to puzzle practitioners.

Accumulating evidence indicates, however, that IBS is a multicomponent disorder of physiologic, emotional, environmental, and psychologic function.[26,27] Medical guidelines define IBS as a benign functional (e.g., medical), nonorganic disorder displaying three major types of symptoms, as follows: (1) chronic and recurrent pain in any area of the abdomen; (2) small-volume bowel dysfunction, varying from constipation or diarrhea to a combination of both; and (3) excess gas formation with increased distention and bloating, accompanied by rumbling abdominal sounds, belching, and passing of gas. Patients appear tense and anxious, and stress is a major triggering factor. A highly individual and personal approach to nutritional care is essential, based on careful nutrition

elemental formula a nutritional support formula composed of simple elemental nutrient components that require no further digestive breakdown and are thus readily absorbed; formulas with the protein as free amino acids and the carbohydrate as the simple sugar glucose.

diverticulitis (L. *divertere,* to turn aside) inflammation of pockets of tissue (diverticula) in the lining of the mucous membrane of the colon.

TABLE 18–4 Dietary Fiber and Kilocalorie Values for Selected Foods

Foods	Serving size	Kilocalories	Dietary fiber (g)
BREADS AND CEREALS			
Fiber One	½ cup	59	14.4
All Bran	⅓ cup	70	8.5
Bran (100%)	½ cup	75	8.4
Bran Buds	⅓ cup	75	7.9
Barley whole grain	½ cup	135	6.8
Corn Bran	⅔ cup	100	5.4
40% Bran	¾ cup	119	5.2
Whole wheat bagel	1 small	145	5.1
Bran Chex	⅔ cup	90	4.6
Whole wheat English muffin	1	134	4.4
Cracklin' Oat Bran	⅓ cup	110	4.3
Bran Flakes	¾ cup	90	4.0
Wheat germ	¼ cup	108	3.6
Bran muffin	1	172	3.5
Whole wheat matzo	2	100	3.4
Wheaties	1 cup	107	3.0
Shredded Wheat	1 oz	101	2.8
Bulgur	⅓ cup	50	2.7
Air-popped popcorn	1 cup	25	2.5
Oatmeal	1 cup	144	2.2
Wheat Chex	⅔ cup	69	2.2
Whole wheat roll	1	75	2.1
Whole wheat pita	1 small	75	2.1
Brown rice	½ cup	109	1.8
Grape nuts	¼ cup	100	1.4
Whole wheat bread	1 slice	60	1.4
Corn tortilla	1 medium	58	1.4
Triscuits	3	53	1.3
Rye Krisp	3	22	1
Wild rice	¼ cup	41	0.7
Total	1 cup	84	0.6
Graham cracker	2 squares	59	0.4
LEGUMES, COOKED			
Cooked dried peas	½ cup	116	8.1
Cooked lentils	½ cup	115	7.8
Cooked dry black beans	½ cup	114	7.5
Cooked dry pinto beans	½ cup	117	7.4
Kidney beans	½ cup	110	7.3
Cooked dry northern beans	½ cup	104	6.2
Cooked dry navy beans	½ cup	129	5.8
Lima beans	½ cup	130	4.5
VEGETABLES, COOKED			
Green peas	½ cup	55	3.6
Corn	½ cup	70	2.9
Parsnip	½ cup	50	2.7
Potato, with skin	1 medium	95	2.5
Brussels sprouts	½ cup	30	2.3

TABLE 18–4	Dietary Fiber and Kilocalorie Values for Selected Foods—*cont'd*		
Foods	Serving size	Kilocalories	Dietary fiber (g)
VEGETABLES, COOKED—*cont'd*			
Carrots	½ cup	25	2.3
Broccoli	½ cup	20	2.2
Spinach	½ cup	21	2.2
Beans, green	½ cup	15	1.6
Tomato, chopped	½ cup	17	1.5
Cabbage, red and white	½ cup	15	1.4
Kale	½ cup	20	1.4
Cauliflower	½ cup	15	1.1
Lettuce (fresh)	1 cup	7	0.8
FRUITS			
Raspberries	½ cup	30	4.2
Apple	1 medium	80	3.5
Raisins	¼ cup	110	3.1
Prunes, dried	3	60	3.0
Strawberries	1 cup	45	3.0
Orange	1 medium	60	2.6
Pear	½ large	62	2.5
Banana	1 medium	105	2.4
Blueberries	½ cup	40	2.0
Dates, dried	3	70	1.9
Peach	1 medium	35	1.9
Apricot, fresh	3 medium	50	1.8
Grapefruit	½ cup	40	1.6
Apricot, dried	5 halves	40	1.4
Cherries	10	50	1.2
Pineapple	½ cup	40	1.1

assessment (see Chapter 17). Guided by this personal food and symptoms pattern, a reasonable food plan can be devised with the patient. In general, the food plan should give attention to the following basic principles:

■ *Increase dietary fiber.* A regular diet with optimal energy-nutrient composition and dietary fiber food sources (e.g., whole grains, legumes, fruits, and vegetables) provides basic therapy (Table 18-4).
■ *Recognize gas formers.* Some foods are recognized gas formers because of known constituents (e.g., indigestible short chains of glucose [oligosaccharides] in the case of legumes). Others may cause gaseous discomfort on an individual basis.
■ *Respect food intolerances.* Lactose intolerance, for example, in people who lack the digestive enzyme lactase is well known (see Chapter 2).
■ *Reduce total fat content.* Excess fat delays gastric emptying and contributes to malabsorption problems.

■ *Avoid large meals.* Large amounts of food in one meal create discomfort from gastric distention and gas. Smaller, more frequent meals usually reduce these symptoms.
■ *Decrease air-swallowing habits.* These habits include eating rapidly and in large amounts, excessive fluid intake, especially of carbonated beverages, and gum-chewing.

Patients are very individualized in the symptoms they suffer most. For example, the predominant symptom may be diarrhea, constipation, abdominal pain, gas, or bloating, but not necessarily all of these. Therefore the dietary recommendations are equally as individualized. Experienced practitioners have learned that in helping patients manage IBS, an honest and creative relationship is essential. Lifestyle and diet are highly personal, and wise nutrition management involves realistic counseling toward a healthier life.

Constipation

This general complaint, real or imagined, is common. Americans spend a quarter of a billion dollars each year on laxatives to treat their so-called regularity problem. "Normal" intestinal elimination is ill defined and can vary greatly. However, a daily bowel movement is not necessary for good health. This common short-term problem usually results from various sources of nervous tension and worry, changes in routines, constant laxative use, low-fiber diets, or lack of exercise. Improved diet, exercise, and bowel habits usually remedy the situation. Any regular laxative or enema routine should be avoided. The diet should include increased fiber, naturally laxative fruits (e.g., dried prunes and figs), and adequate fluid intake, based on the assessment of current fiber and fluid intake, as well as any diuretic drug use. Constipation occurs at all ages but is almost epidemic among elderly persons. In all cases, a personalized approach to management is fundamental.

FOOD ALLERGIES AND INTOLERANCES

Food Allergies

The Problem

Several conditions may cause certain food allergies or intolerances. Intolerances, unlike true allergies, are not life threatening and are nonimmunologic in etiology. The underlying problem of an allergic reaction is the body's immune system reacting to a protein as if it was a threatening foreign object and launching a powerful attack against it. The word **allergy** comes from two Greek words meaning "altered reactivity" and refers to the abnormal reactions of the immune system to a number of substances in the environment. A particular allergic condition results from a disorder of the immune system.

Common Food Allergens

The most common food allergens are peanuts, tree nuts, shellfish, fish, milk, soy, egg, and wheat.[28] Early foods of infancy and childhood are often offenders in sensitive individuals, especially if introduced to the child before the gastrointestinal tract is fully capable of sophisticated digestion. In a child's diet, solid foods should be added one at a time, with common offenders excluded in early feedings. If a child is showing signs of allergic reaction, a process of *food elimination* is sometimes used to identify disagreeable foods. A core of less-often offending foods is used at first, and then other single foods gradually are added to test the response. If a given food causes an allergic reaction, the food is identified as an allergen and eliminated from use. The food may be tried again later to see if it still causes the same reaction, validating the initial response. It is not uncommon for in-

dividuals to outgrow allergies to milk, soy, and eggs. However, peanuts, tree nuts, and shellfish tend to elicit an allergic response, sometimes fatally, throughout life. In the case of peanuts, however, a research team at Johns Hopkins University, noting the allergic reaction encountered from the small packet of peanuts on commercial airlines, is currently developing an oral vaccine to induce tolerance in persons with severe peanut allergies.

Recognizing signs and symptoms of allergic reactions may save a life. *Anaphylactic shock* is the most severe form of allergic reaction and can result in death in a relatively short period of time. The victim's throat, lips, and tongue swell to the point of blocking the airway, ultimately suffocating the individual. The most common symptoms of food allergies are: hives, nausea, diarrhea, and abdominal pain. Individuals suffering from anaphylactic shock experience swelling of the face and throat, difficulty breathing, anxiety, increased heart rate, and if not treated, decreased blood pressure and loss of consciousness.

It is helpful to refer any person with food allergies to a dietitian to provide family support, education, and counseling. Guidance on food substitutions or special food products and modified recipes to maintain nutritional needs for growth are necessary. Children tend to become less allergic as they grow older, but family education about the label reading of all food products and cooking guides is essential from the beginning.

Genetic Disease and Food Intolerances

The Genetic Defect

Certain food intolerances stem from underlying genetic disease. In each genetic disease, the specific cell enzyme (all enzymes are proteins) controlling the cell's metabolism of a specific nutrient is missing, thus blocking the normal handling of the nutrient at that point. Three examples of genetic defects are phenylketonuria, galactosemia, and lactose intolerance.

Phenylketonuria. Phenylketonuria (PKU) is an autosomal recessive genetic disorder. PKU results when phenylalanine hydroxylase, the enzyme responsible for breaking down the essential amino acid phenylalanine to tyrosine (another amino acid) is not produced by the body. If left untreated, this condition causes profound mental retardation and central nervous system damage, with irritability, hyperactivity, convulsive seizures, and bizarre behavior. PKU affects approximately 1 in every 10,000 babies born in the United States. Today mandatory newborn-screening programs in all areas of the United States can identify affected babies, so treatment is started immediately. With treatment, these babies grow normally and have healthy lives. The treatment is a low-phenylalanine diet, using special formulas and low-protein food products for life. Much family counseling by the metabolic team at each care center is also needed.

Galactosemia. This genetic disease affects carbohydrate metabolism. The missing cell enzyme (known as GALT) is one that converts galactose to glucose. Because galactose comes from the breakdown of lactose (milk sugar), all sources of lactose in an infant's diet must be eliminated. When not treated, this condition causes brain and liver damage. Newborn-screening programs also identify affected babies, so treatment can begin immediately to avoid such damage and enable the child to grow normally. Treatment is a galactose-free diet, with special formulas for infants and lactose-free food guides. Similar to PKU, galactosemia is also an autosomal recessive disorder and the treatment diet must be followed for life.

Lactose Intolerance. A deficiency of any one of the disaccharidases (e.g., lactase, sucrase, or maltase) in the small intestine may produce a wide range of GI problems and abdominal pain because the specific sugar involved cannot be digested. Lactose intolerance is the most com-

mon. In this condition, there is insufficient lactase to break down the milk sugar lactose; thus lactose accumulates in the intestine, causing abdominal cramping and diarrhea. Milk and all products containing lactose are carefully avoided. Milk treated with a commercial lactase product or soy milk products are safe substitutes.

PROBLEMS OF THE GASTROINTESTINAL ACCESSORY ORGANS

Three major accessory organs—the liver, gallbladder, and pancreas—produce important digestive agents that enter the intestine and aid in the handling of food substances (Figure 18-6). Diseases of these organs easily affect normal GI function and cause problems with the

> **allergy**   (Gr. *allos,* other; *ergon,* work) a state of hypersensitivity to particular substances in the environment that works on body tissues to produce problems in functions of affected tissues; the agent involved (allergen) may be a certain food eaten or a substance (e.g., pollen) inhaled.

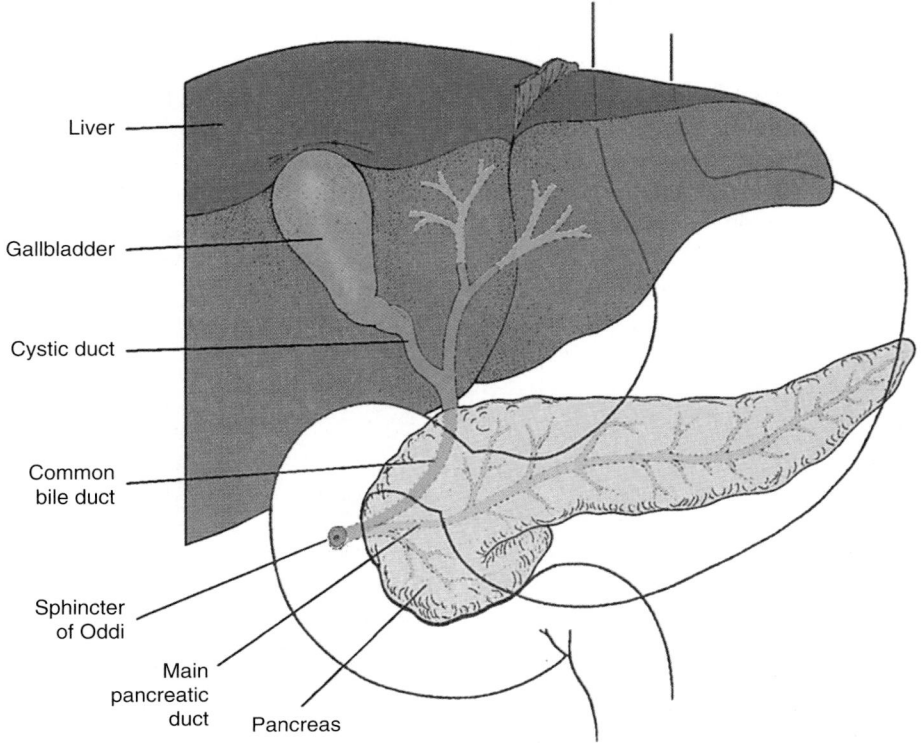

Liver

Gallbladder

Cystic duct

Common bile duct

Sphincter of Oddi

Main pancreatic duct

Pancreas

Figure 18–6   Biliary system organs.

handling of specific types of food. The normal structure of the liver's functional units, the *lobule* and its cells, is shown in Figure 18-7.

Liver Disease

The liver has several critical roles in basic metabolism and regulation of body functions. Some essential functions include: bile production (for fat digestion), synthesis of proteins and blood clotting factors, metabolism of hormones, medications, macronutrients and micronutrients, the regulation of blood glucose levels, and urea production (to remove waste products of normal metabolism). Diseases of the liver are the twelfth leading cause of death in the United States.[29]

Hepatitis

Acute hepatitis is an inflammatory condition caused by viruses, alcohol, drugs, or toxins. The viral agent causing infection is often transmitted by the oral-fecal route, which is common in many epidemic diseases. The carrier is usually contaminated food or water. In other cases, the virus may be transmitted by transfusions of infected blood or contaminated syringes or needles. Symptoms include anorexia and jaundice, with underlying malnutrition. Treatment is based on bed rest and nutrition therapy to support healing of the involved liver tissue. The following requirements govern the principles of the diet therapy and relate to the liver's function in metabolizing each nutrient:

■ *High-protein.* Protein is essential for building new liver cells and tissues. It also combines with fats (lipoproteins) to remove them, preventing damage from fatty infiltration in liver tissue. The diet should supply 0.8 to 1 g/kg of high-quality protein daily if there are no complications. If the individual is suffering from complications and a positive nitrogen balance is desirable, 1.2 to 1.3 g/kg of protein is warranted (Box 18-3).

■ *High-carbohydrate.* Available glucose restores protective glycogen reserves in the liver. It also helps meet the energy demands of the disease process, as well as preventing the breakdown of protein for energy, thus ensuring its use for the vital tissue-building necessary for healing. Glucose intolerance and hypoglycemia are sometimes problematic with liver disease. Therefore the amount of carbohydrates in the diet depends on individual needs and condition.

■ *Moderate-fat.* Some fat helps season food to encourage eating despite a poor appetite. A moderate amount of easily used fat, from milk products and vegetable oil, is beneficial. The diet should incorporate 25% to 40% of total calories from fat. Energy supply is more dependent on fat as the disease progresses.

■ *High-energy.* From 2500 to 3000 kcal (approximately 120% of basal energy expenditure) is needed daily to meet energy demands. This increased amount is necessary to support the healing process, to make up losses from fever and general debilitation, and to renew strength for recuperating from the disease.

■ *Meals and feedings.* At first, liquid feedings (e.g., milk shakes high in protein and kcalories [see Table 18-1] or special formula products) may be necessary. As a patient's appetite and food tolerance improve, a full diet is needed, while observing likes and dislikes and

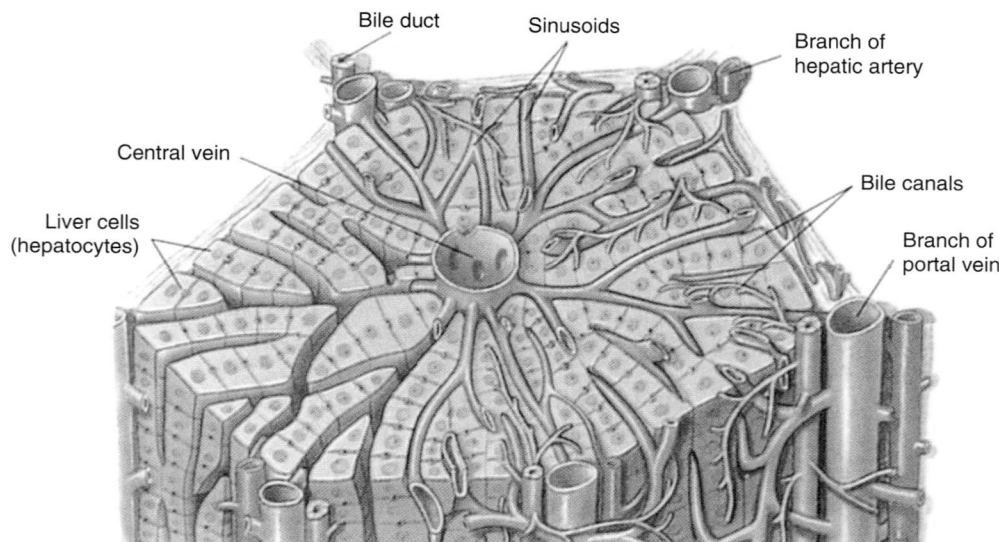

Figure 18–7 Liver structure showing hepatic lobule and hepatic cell. (Credit: Medical and Scientific Illustration.)

planning ways to encourage an optimal food intake. Nutrition is the basic therapy during acute hepatitis (see the Clinical Applications box, "Case Study: Bill's Bout with Infectious Hepatitis").

Cirrhosis

Liver disease may advance to a chronic state of cirrhosis (Figure 18-8). The most common problem is fatty cirrhosis associated with malnutrition and alcoholism. This relentless malnutrition leads to multiple nutritional deficiencies as alcohol increasingly replaces balanced meals. Alcohol and its metabolic by-products also can cause direct damage to liver cells. The accompanying fatty infiltration kills liver cells, and only nonfunctioning fibrous scar tissue remains. Low plasma protein levels eventually lead to *ascites*, abdominal fluid accumulation. Scar tissue impairs blood circulation, resulting in elevated venous blood pressure and esophageal **varices**. The rupture of these enlarged veins with massive hemorrhage is often the cause of death. Treatment is difficult when alcoholism is the underlying problem. Nutrition therapy focuses on as much healing support as possible, as follows:

■ *Protein according to tolerance.* In the absence of impending hepatic coma, the diet should supply 80 to 100 g of protein per day to correct severe malnutrition, heal liver tissue, and restore plasma proteins. If signs of coma begin, the protein has to be reduced according to individual tolerance.

BOX 18–3 High-Protein, High-Carbohydrate, Moderate-Fat Daily Diet

1 L (1 qt) milk
¼ cup egg substitute (e.g., Egg Beaters)
224 g (8 oz) lean meat, fish, poultry
4 servings vegetables:
    2 servings potato or substitute
    1 serving green leafy or yellow vegetable
    1 to 2 servings other vegetables, including 1 raw
3 to 4 servings fruit (including juices often):
    1 to 2 citrus fruits (or other good source of ascorbic acid)
    2 servings other fruit
6 to 8 servings bread and cereal (whole grain or enriched):
    1 serving cereal
    5 to 6 slices bread, crackers
2 to 4 Tbsp butter or fortified margarine
Additional jam, jelly, honey, and other carbohydrate foods as patient desires and is able to eat them
Sweetened fruit juices to increase both carbohydrates and fluid

---

varices dilated blood vessels within the wall of the esophagus used to redirect blood flow from the liver. During cirrhosis, blood flow is significantly reduced in the liver. As a result, alternative pathways form, expand, and crowd the esophagus. These vessels can continue to expand to the point of rupturing and can lead to death.

CLINICAL APPLICATIONS

CASE STUDY: BILL'S BOUT WITH INFECTIOUS HEPATITIS

Bill is a college student who spent part of his summer vacation in Mexico. Shortly after he returned home, he began to feel ill. He had little energy, no appetite, and severe headaches. Nothing he ate seemed to agree with him. He felt nauseated, began to have diarrhea, and soon developed a fever. He began to show evidence of jaundice.

Bill was hospitalized for diagnosis and treatment, and his tests indicated impaired liver function. His liver and spleen were enlarged and tender. The physician's diagnosis was infectious hepatitis. Bill's hospital diet was high in proteins, carbohydrates, and kcalories and moderately low in fats, but Bill had difficulty eating. He had no appetite, and food seemed to nauseate him even more.

Questions for Analysis

1. What are the normal functions of the liver in relation to the metabolism of carbohydrates, proteins, and fats? What other metabolic functions does the liver have?
2. What is the relationship of the normal liver functions to the effects or clinical symptoms that Bill experienced during his illness?
3. Why does vigorous nutrition therapy in liver disease (e.g., hepatitis) present a problem in planning a diet?
4. Outline a day's food plan for Bill. Calculate the amount of kilocalories and protein to ensure that he is getting the necessary amount.
5. What vitamins and minerals would be significant aspects of Bill's nutrition therapy? Why?

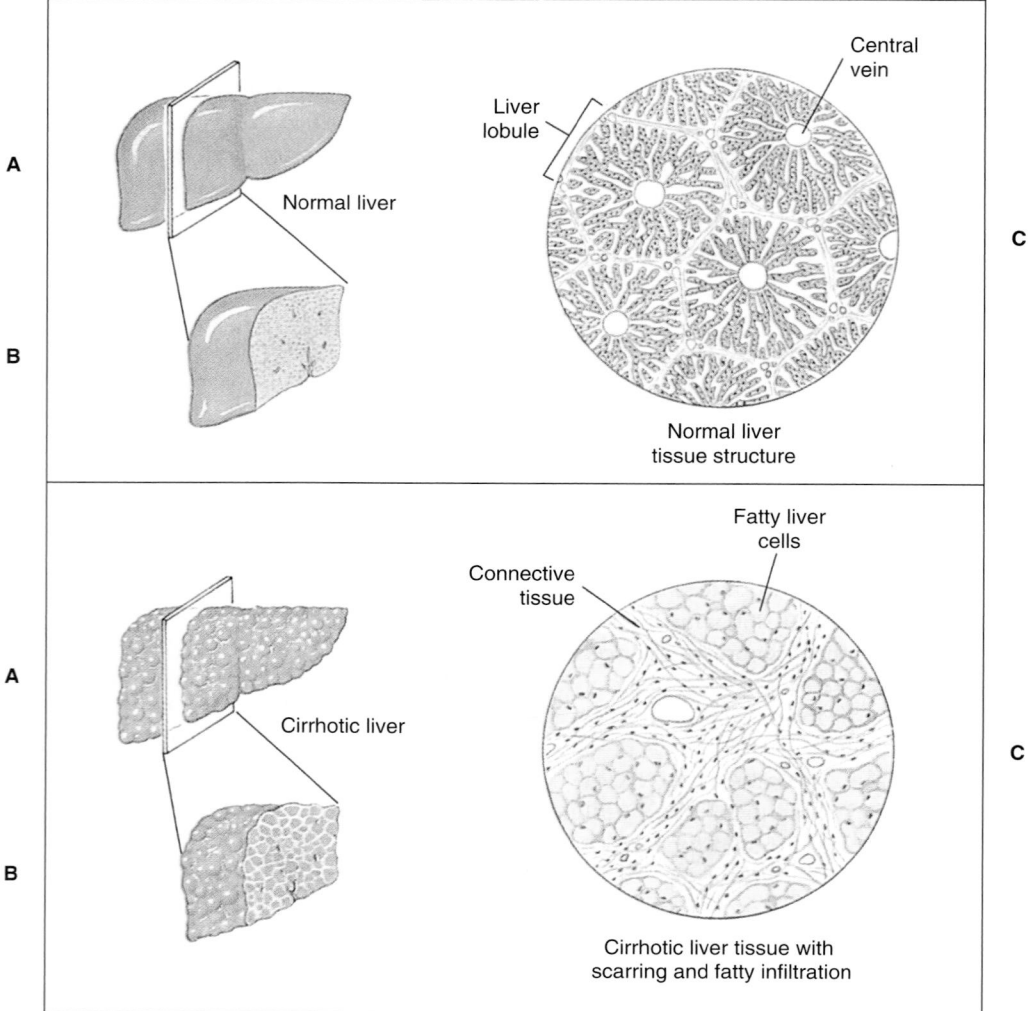

Figure 18–8 Comparison of normal liver and liver with cirrhotic tissue changes. **A,** Anterior view of organ. **B,** Cross-section. **C,** Tissue structure. (Credit: Medical and Scientific Illustration.)

- *Low sodium.* Sodium is restricted to 500 to 1000 mg per day to help reduce the fluid retention (ascites).
- *Soft texture.* If esophageal varices develop, soft foods help prevent the danger of rupture and hemorrhage.
- *Optimal general nutrition.* The remaining diet principles outlined for hepatitis are continued for cirrhosis for the same reasons. Kcalories, carbohydrates, and vitamins, especially B-complex vitamins including thiamin and folate, are important. Moderate fat is used. Alcohol is prohibited.

Hepatic Coma

One of the main functions of the liver is to remove ammonia, and hence nitrogen (see Chapter 4), from the

blood by converting it to urea for urinary excretion. When cirrhosis continues and fibrous scar tissue replaces more and more functional liver tissue, the blood can no longer circulate normally through the liver. Therefore other vessels develop around this scar tissue, bypassing the liver. The blood, carrying its ammonia load, cannot get to the liver for its normal removal of the ammonia and nitrogen. Instead, it must follow the bypass and proceed to the brain, producing ammonia intoxication and coma. The resulting *hepatic encephalopathy* brings about apathy, confusion, inappropriate behavior, drowsiness, and eventually progresses to coma. Treatment focuses on removing the sources of excess ammonia. Because ammonia is a nitrogen compound and its main source is pro-

---

BOX 18–4   Low-Protein Diets: 15 g, 30 g, 40 g, and 50 g Protein

General Directions

■ The following diets are used when dietary protein is to be restricted.

■ The patterns limit foods containing large percentages of protein (e.g., milk, eggs, cheese, meat, fish, fowl, and legumes).

■ Meat extractives, soups, broth, bouillon, gravies, and gelatin desserts also should be avoided.

Basic Meal Patterns (contain approximately 15 g protein)

Breakfast

½ cup fruit or fruit juice
½ cup cereal
1 slice toast
Butter
Jelly
Sugar
2 Tbsp cream
Coffee

Lunch

1 small potato
½ cup vegetable
Salad (vegetable or fruit)
1 slice bread
Butter
1 serving fruit
Sugar
Coffee or tea

Dinner

1 small potato
½ cup vegetable
Salad (vegetable or fruit)
1 slice bread
Butter
1 serving fruit
Sugar
Coffee or tea

For 30 g Protein

Add: 1 cup milk
     28 g (1 oz) meat, 1 egg, or equivalent

Examples of meat portions:

■ 28 g (1 oz) meat = 1 thin slice roast,
   4 × 5 cm (1½ × 2 inches)
■ 1 rounded Tbsp cottage cheese
■ 1 slice American cheese

For 40 g Protein

Add: 1 cup milk
     70 g (2½ oz) meat, or 1 egg and 42 g (1½ oz) meat

Examples of meat portions:

■ 70 g (2½ oz) meat = Ground beef patty
   (5 from 448 g [1 lb])
■ 1 slice roast

For 50 g Protein

Add: 1 cup milk
     112 g (4 oz) meat, or 2 eggs and 56 g (2 oz) meat

Examples of meat portions:

■ 112 g (4 oz) meat = 2 lamb chops
■ 1 small steak

---

tein, the chief dietary goal is to reduce protein intake. Box 18-4 provides a guide for reducing the diet's protein to 15 g/day, with additional increases according to individual tolerance.

Gallbladder Disease

The basic function of the gallbladder is to concentrate and store bile and then release the concentrated bile into the small intestine when fat is present there. In the intestine, the bile emulsifies the fat, preparing it for initial digestion, and then carries it into the cells of the intestinal wall for its continued metabolism.

Cholecystitis and Cholelithiasis

Inflammation of the gallbladder, *cholecystitis*, usually results from a low-grade chronic infection. Cholesterol in bile, which is not soluble in water, is normally kept in solution. When continued infection alters the solubility of bile ingredients, however, cholesterol separates out and forms gallstones. This condition is called *cholelithiasis*. When infection, stones, or both are present, the normal contraction of the gallbladder, triggered by fat entering the intestine, causes pain. Thus fatty foods usually are avoided. The treatment is surgical removal of the gallbladder, a *cholecystectomy*. If a patient is obese, some weight loss before surgery may be indicated. In any case,

BOX 18–5 Low-Fat and Fat-Free Diets

Low-Fat Diet

General description

- This diet contains foods that are low in fat.
- Foods are prepared without the addition of fat.
- Fatty meats, gravies, oils, cream, lard, avocados, and desserts containing eggs, butter, cream, and nuts are avoided.
- Foods should be used in the specified amounts and only as tolerated.
- The sample pattern contains approximately 85 g protein, 50 g fat, 220 g carbohydrates, and 1670 kcal.

Selection of Foods

Foods	*Foods allowed*	*Foods not allowed*
Beverages	Skim milk, coffee, tea, carbonated beverages, fruit juices	Whole milk, cream, evaporated and condensed milk
Bread and cereals	All kinds	Rich rolls or breads, waffles, pancakes
Desserts	Gelatin, sherbet, water ices, fruit whips made without cream, angel food cake, rice and tapioca puddings made with skim milk	Pastries, pies, rich cakes and cookies, ice cream
Fruits	All fruits, as tolerated	Avocado
Eggs	3 allowed per week, cooked any way except fried	Fried eggs
Fats	3 tsp butter or margarine daily	Salad and cooking oils, mayonnaise
Meats	Lean meat such as beef, veal, lamb, liver, lean fish and fowl—all baked, broiled, or roasted without added fat	Fried meats, bacon, ham, pork, goose, duck, fatty fish, fish canned in oil, cold cuts
Cheese	Dry or fat-free cottage cheese	All other cheese
Potato or substitute	Potatoes, rice, macaroni, noodles, spaghetti—all prepared without added fat	Fried potatoes, potato chips
Soups	Bouillon or broth, without fat; soups made with skim milk	Cream soups
Sweets	Jam, jelly, sugar candies without nuts or chocolate	Chocolate, nuts, peanut butter
Vegetables	All vegetables, as tolerated	The following should be omitted if they cause distress: broccoli, cauliflower, corn, cucumber, green pepper, radishes, turnips, onions, dried peas, and beans
Miscellaneous	Salt in moderation	Pepper, spices, highly spiced food, olives, pickles, cream sauces, gravies

Suggested Menu Pattern

Breakfast	*Lunch and dinner*
Fruit	Meat, broiled or baked
Cereal	Potato
Toast, jelly	Vegetable
1 tsp butter or margarine	Salad with fat-free dressing
	Bread, jelly
Egg 3 times/week	1 tsp butter or margarine
Skim milk, 1 cup	Fruit or dessert, as allowed
Coffee, sugar	Skim milk, 1 cup
	Coffee, sugar

Fat-Free Diet

General description

The following additional restrictions are made to the low-fat diet to make it relatively fat-free:

1. Meat, eggs, and butter or margarine are omitted.
2. A substitute for meat at the noon and evening meals is 84 g (3 oz) fat-free cottage cheese.

diet therapy centers on controlling fat intake. Box 18-5 outlines a general low-fat diet guide, but the degree of its application depends upon individual need.

Pancreatic Disease

The pancreas is a key organ in normal digestion and metabolism, acting as both an exocrine and endocrine gland. Digestive enzymes and bicarbonate, necessary for the breakdown of carbohydrates, proteins, and fats, are excreted by the pancreas under hormonal control during digestion. The endocrine functions of the pancreas are primarily related to blood glucose regulation by the hormones glucagon and insulin.

Pancreatitis

Acute inflammation of the pancreas, *pancreatitis*, results when the very enzymes the organ produces (e.g., principally trypsin [see Chapter 4]) digest the organ tissue. Obstruction of the common duct through which the inactive enzymes normally enter the intestine causes the enzymes and bile to back up into the pancreas. This mixing of digestive materials activates the powerful enzymes within the gland. In this active form, they begin to "digest" the pancreatic tissue itself, causing severe pain. Mild or moderate episodes may subside completely, but the condition tends to recur, leading to chronic pancreatitis. Excessive alcohol consumption and gallstones are the major culprits leading to pancreatitis in the United States. Initial care includes the following measures for acute disease involving shock: intravenous feeding, replacement of fluid and electrolytes, blood transfusion, antibiotics, pain medications, and gastric suction. As healing progresses, oral feedings are resumed. A light diet is used to reduce stimulation of pancreatic secretions. Alcohol and excess coffee also should be avoided to decrease pancreatic stimulation.

SUMMARY

Nutrition management of gastrointestinal disease is based on the degree of interference in the normal process of ingestion, digestion, absorption, and metabolism that the disease causes. Problems in the upper GI tract relate to conditions that hinder chewing, swallowing, or transporting the food mass down the esophagus into the stomach. Esophageal problems such as muscle constriction, acid reflux causing esophagitis, or a hiatal hernia at the entry of the esophagus into the chest cavity, interfere with passage of the food into the stomach. These problems cause general acid tissue irritation and discomfort after eating. Peptic ulcer disease, a common GI problem, is an acidic erosion of the mucosal lining of the stomach or the duodenal bulb, which is where the concentrated acidic food mass enters the duodenum, the first section of the small intestine. The ulcerated tissue brings about nutritional problems such as anemia and weight loss. Medical management consists of drug therapy and rest. Diet therapy is liberal and individual, with a goal of correcting malnutrition and supporting the healing process.

Problems of the lower GI tract include common functional disorders such as malabsorption and diarrhea, for which symptomatic and personalized treatment is indicated. Diseases such as celiac sprue, which is caused by sensitivity to gluten in certain grains and results in malabsorption problems, and the genetic disease, cystic fibrosis, require individualized nutritional support. The inflammatory bowel diseases (e.g., Crohn's disease and ulcerative colitis) involve extensive tissue damage that often requires surgical resection, as well as the resulting short bowel syndrome from the decreased absorbing surface area. Large intestine problems (e.g., diverticular disease, irritable bowel disease, and constipation) often involve anxiety and stress, and thus are more difficult to resolve. Nutrition therapy requires modification of the diet's protein and energy content and food texture, increased vitamins and minerals, and replacement of fluids and electrolytes. Continuous adjustment of the diet is made according to individual need.

Other food intolerances may be caused by allergies or underlying genetic disease. Genetic diseases of metabolism result from missing cell enzymes that control the metabolism of specific nutrients. The special diet in each case limits or eliminates the particular nutrient involved.

Diseases of the GI accessory organs also contribute to nutritional problems. Common liver disorders include hepatitis and cirrhosis. Uncontrolled cirrhosis leads to hepatic coma and eventual liver failure and death. Nutrient and energy levels of the necessary diet therapy vary with the progression of the disease process. Gallbladder disease, infection, and stones involve some limit to fat tolerance, which is modified according to individual need. The treatment for gallstones is surgical removal of the organ, followed by moderate use of dietary fat. Pancreatic disease (pancreatitis) is a serious condition requiring immediate measures to counter the shock symptoms, followed by restorative nutritional support.

CRITICAL THINKING QUESTIONS

1. What general nutritional guidance would you give to a person with a hiatal hernia? What would be the basic goal of your suggestions?
2. What are the basic principles of diet planning for patients with peptic ulcer disease? How do these principles differ from the traditional therapy formerly used?
3. Describe the causes, clinical signs, and treatment of each of the following diseases: diverticular disease, celiac sprue, and inflammatory bowel disease.
4. What is the rationale for treatment in the progressive course of liver disease (e.g., hepatitis, cirrhosis, and hepatic coma)?

CHAPTER CHALLENGE QUESTIONS

True-False

Write the correct statement for each item you answer "false."

1. *True or False:* A high-fiber diet, rich in raw vegetables, is indicated for a person with dental problems.
2. *True or False:* Lying down after eating helps a person with hiatal hernia relieve discomfort.
3. *True or False:* The fundamental cause of peptic ulcer disease is unknown.
4. *True or False:* Peptic ulcer pain is reduced when consuming decaffeinated coffee and colas versus the full caffeinated forms of these beverages.
5. *True or False:* A low-fiber diet is encouraged for treatment of diverticulosis.
6. *True or False:* All food sources of wheat must be eliminated in the gluten-free diet for treatment of celiac disease.
7. *True or False:* Phenylketonuria is a genetic disease requiring dietary control of the essential amino acid phenylalanine.
8. *True or False:* Soy products are often used for individuals allergic to milk.
9. *True or False:* The nutritional objective in cystic fibrosis is to meet growth needs and help compensate for nutrient losses, along with enzyme replacement therapy.

Multiple Choice

1. In a gluten-free diet for celiac disease, which of the following foods is eliminated?
   a. Eggs
   b. Milk
   c. Rice
   d. Whole wheat crackers
2. The symptoms of anemia in malabsorption diseases are caused by poor absorption of which of the following nutrients?
   a. Vitamins B_2 and C
   b. Iron and folic acid
   c. Calcium and phosphorus
   d. Fats and protein
3. Lactose intolerance in certain population groups is caused by a genetic deficiency of which of the following enzymes?
   a. Sucrase
   b. Pepsin
   c. Lactase
   d. Maltase
4. Treatment for hepatic coma includes
   a. increased protein to aid healing of liver cells.
   b. decreased protein to reduce ammonia levels in blood.
   c. increased kcalories to reduce the metabolic load.
   d. increased fluid intake to stimulate output.

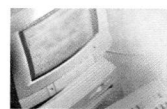
Please refer to the Students' Resource section of this text's Evolve web site for "Suggestions for Additional Study."

REFERENCES

1. Centers for Disease Control and Prevention, National Center for Chronic Disease Prevention and Health Promotion, Oral Health Resources: *Fact Sheet: Oral health for adults*, Atlanta, 2002 (accessed April 2003), CDC/NCCDPHP [*www.cdc.gov/OralHealth/factsheets/adult.htm*].

2. Centers for Disease Control and Prevention, National Center for Chronic Disease Prevention and Health Promotion, Oral Health Resources: *Fact Sheet: Using fluoride to prevent and control dental caries in the United States*, Atlanta, 2002 (accessed April 2003), CDC/NCCDPHP [*www.cdc.gov/OralHealth/factsheets/fl-caries.htm*].

3. Spieker MR: Evaluating dysphagia, *Am Fam Physician* 61:3639, 2000.

4. Mukand JA and others: Incidence of neurologic deficits and rehabilitation of patients with brain tumors, *Am J Phys Med Rehabil* 80(5):346, 2001.

5. Kumlien S, Axelsson K: Stroke patients in nursing homes: eating, feeding, nutrition and related care, *J Clin Nurs* 11:498, 2002.

6. Shanley C, O'Loughlin G: Dysphagia among nursing home residents: an assessment and management protocol, *J Gerontol Nurs* 26(8):35, 2000.

7. Birnbaum A: Gastroesophageal reflux in children, *Food Allergy News* 8(4):1, 1999.

8. Cohen S, Parkman HP: Diseases of the esophagus. In Goldman L, Bennett JC, editors: *Cecil's textbook of medicine*, ed 21, vol 1, Philadelphia, 2000, Saunders.

9. Chrysos E and others: Factors affecting esophageal motility in gastroesophageal reflux disease, *Arch Surg* 138:241, 2003.

10. Centers for Disease Control and Prevention, National Center for Infectious Diseases, Division of Bacterial and Mycotic Diseases: *Helicobacter pylori and peptic ulcer disease: fact sheet for health care providers*, Atlanta, 2001 (accessed April 2003), CDC/NCID/DBMD [*www.cdc.gov/ulcer/md.htm*].

11. Ganga-Zandzou PS and others: Natural outcome of *Helicobacter pylori* infection in asymptomatic children: a two-year follow-up study, *Pediatrics* 104(2):216, 1999.

12. Covacci A and others: *Helicobacter pylori* virulence and genetic geography, *Science* 284(5418):1328, 1999.

13. Rosenstock S and others: Risk factors for peptic ulcer disease: a population based prospective cohort study comprising 2416 Danish adults, *Gut* 52:186, 2003.

14. Shiotani A and Graham DY: Pathogenesis and therapy of gastric and duodenal ulcer disease, *Med Clin North Am* 86(6):1447, 2002.

15. Weissman G: NSAIDS: aspirin and aspirin-like drugs. In Goldman L, Bennett JC, editors: *Cecil's textbook of medicine*, ed 21, vol 1, Philadelphia, 2000, Saunders.

16. Centers for Disease Control and Prevention, National Center for Infectious Diseases, Division of Parasitic Diseases, *Fact sheet: chronic diarrhea*, Atlanta, 1999 (accessed April 2003), CDC/NCID/DPD [*www.cdc.gov/ncidod/dpd/parasites/diarrhea/factsht_chronic_diarrhea.htm*].

17. Juckett G: Prevention and treatment of traveler's diarrhea, *Am Fam Physician* 60(1):119, 1999.

18. Semrad CE, Chang EB: Malabsorption syndromes. In Goldman L, Bennett JC, editors: *Cecil's textbook of medicine*, ed 21, vol 1, Philadelphia, 2000, WB Saunders.

19. Cystic Fibrosis Foundation: *What is CF*, Bethesda, MD, 2003 (accessed April 2003), CFF [*www.cff.org/about_cf/what_is_cf.cfm?CFID-907515&CFTOKEN-19214244*].

20. O'Connor GT and others: Median household income and mortality rate in cystic fibrosis, *Pediatrics* 111(4):333, 2003.

21. Hankard R and others: Nutrition and growth in cystic fibrosis, *Horm Res* 58(1):16, 2002.

22. Ashford D, Imhoff B, Angulo F, and the FoodNet working group, CDC: *Over a half-million persons may have Crohn's disease in the United States*, San Francisco, October 2001, Infectious Diseases Society of America.

23. Stenson WF: Chronic inflammatory bowel disease. In Goldman L, Bennett JC, editors: *Cecil's textbook of medicine*, ed 21, vol 1, Philadelphia, 2000, Saunders.

24. Wilcox CM: Miscellaneous inflammatory diseases of the intestine. In Goldman L, Bennett JC, editors: *Cecil's textbook of medicine*, ed 21, vol 1, Philadelphia, 2000, Saunders.

25. Snape WJ Jr: Disorders of gastrointestinal motility. In Goldman L, Bennett JC, editors: *Cecil's textbook of medicine*, ed 21, vol 1, Philadelphia, 2000, WB Saunders.

26. Tally NJ: Functional gastrointestinal disorders: irritable bowel syndrome, non-ulcer dyspepsia, and non-cardiac chest pain. In Goldman L, Bennett JC, editors: *Cecil's textbook of medicine*, ed 21, vol 1, Philadelphia, 2000, Saunders.

27. Viera AJ and others: Management of irritable bowel syndrome, *Am Fam Physician* 66(10):1867, 2002.

28. Allergic Reaction Central: *Causes of anaphylaxis: food*, Napa, CA, 2003 (accessed April 2003), DEY, an affiliate of EMD, Inc. [*www.allergic-reactions.com/consumer/2_1.cfm*].

29. U.S. Department of Health and Human Services, Centers for Disease Control and Prevention, National Center for Health Statistics: *Fast stats A to Z: chronic liver disease/cirrhosis*, Hyattsville, MD, 2003 (accessed April 2003), USDHHS/CDC/NCHS [*www.cdc.gov/nchs/fastats/liverdis.htm*].

FURTHER READING AND RESOURCES

- Cystic Fibrosis Foundation: *www.cff.org*
- Cystic Fibrosis.com: *www.cysticfibrosis.com*
- Celiac Sprue Association: *www.csaceliacs.org*
- Crohn's and Colitis Foundation of America: *www.ccfa.org*
- International Foundation for Functional Gastrointestinal Disorders: *www.iffgd.org*
- National PKU News: *www.pkunews.org*
- Parents of Galactosemic Children, Inc.: *www.galactosemia.org*

   The preceding organizations provide support for individuals affected by a disorder of the gastrointestinal tract. As a health care provider, it is advisable to be familiar with these organizations, as well as their web sites, to refer patients to organizations that can continue to give them support, understanding, and up-to-date information about their disease.

- Aldrich JK, Massey LK: A liberalized geriatric diet fits most dietary prescriptions for long-term-care residents, *J Am Diet Assoc* 99(4):4, 478, 1999.

   This brief article describes an excellent program for care of elderly persons in a long-term care facility that focuses on quality care with an emphasis on good food that is well presented. Therapeutic diets are liberalized to encourage eating and balancing good tasting "normal food" with the necessity for diet therapy.

- Spanier JA and others: A systematic review of alternative therapies in the irritable bowel syndrome, *Arch Intern Med* 163:265, 2003.

   Irritable bowel syndrome (IBS) is a frustrating disorder of the gastrointestinal tract. A variety of medical and psychological factors contribute to the disorder, which is more prevalent in women than men, and a variety of treatment modalities have been explored. This article reviews the wide array of alternative and complementary treatment methods proposed for IBS.

CHAPTER 19

Coronary Heart Disease and Hypertension

KEY CONCEPTS

■ Several risk factors contribute to the development of heart disease, most of which are preventable factors associated with lifestyle.

■ Essential hypertension, believed to be predominantly a genetic risk factor for heart disease, has very few symptoms but can be identified and controlled.

■ Most cardiovascular risk factors are associated with nutrition and can be reduced by changing food habits and lifestyles.

Cardiovascular disease is the number one cause of death in the United States, accounting for more than 700,000 deaths each year.[1] A similar situation exists in most other developed Western societies. Every day, thousands of people suffer heart attacks and strokes and more than a million others continue to suffer from various forms of rheumatic and congestive heart disease.

During the past 20 years, the cardiovascular death rate has declined somewhat, mostly because of improved emergency care for heart attacks, but cardiovascular disease remains the top "killer disease." This chapter's discussion looks at the primary underlying disease process, atherosclerosis, and the various risk factors involved; and explores ways to use nutritional approaches to reduce these risk factors and help prevent disease.

CORONARY HEART DISEASE

Atherosclerosis

Disease Process

The major cardiovascular disease and the underlying pathologic process in coronary heart disease is **athero-sclerosis**. Ongoing studies have strengthened the earlier association of key risk factors (including diet) to the progressive development of the atherosclerotic process.[2] This process is characterized by fatty fibrous plaques that may begin in childhood and develop into fatty streaks, largely composed of cholesterol, on the inside lining of major blood vessels. When tissue is examined, crystals of cholesterol can be seen with the unaided eye in the softened cheesy debris of advanced disease. This fatty debris sug-

gested its name to early investigators, from the Greek words *athera*, meaning "gruel," and *skleros*, meaning "hardening." This fatty fibrous process gradually thickens over time, narrowing the interior part of the blood vessel and often forming blood clots from irritation of the vessel tissue. The thickening of the vessel or a blood clot may eventually cut off blood flow, as shown in Figure 19-1.

Cells die when deprived of their normal blood supply. The local area of dying or dead tissue is called an *infarct*. If the affected blood vessel is a major artery supplying vital blood nutrients and oxygen to the heart muscle, the *myocardium*, the event is called an acute **myocardial infarction (MI)** or a *heart attack*. If the affected vessel is a major artery supplying the brain, the event is called a **cerebrovascular accident (CVA)** or *stroke*. The major arteries and their many branches serving the heart are

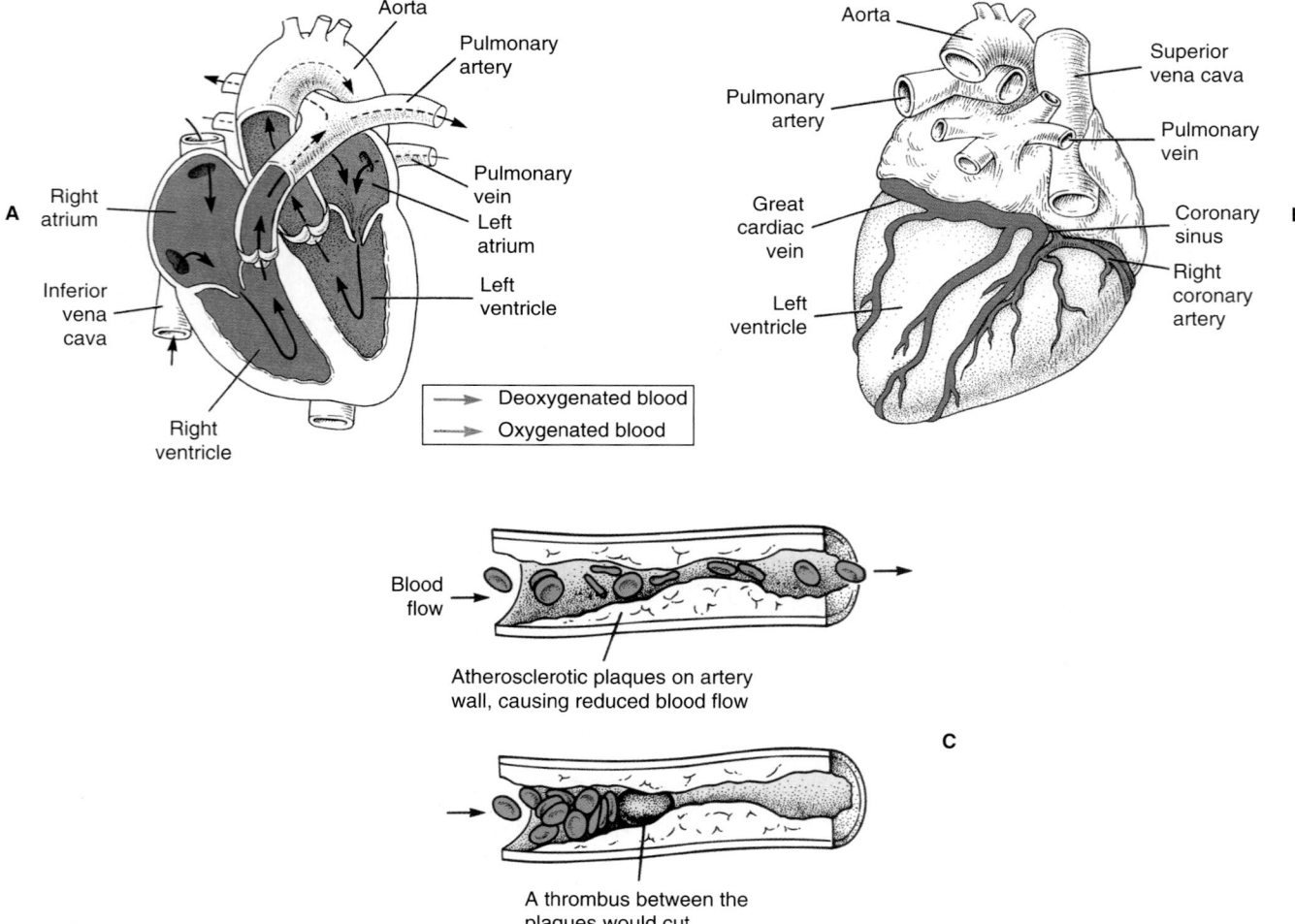

Figure 19–1 **A** and **B,** The normal human heart. **A,** Anterior view showing cardiac circulation. **B,** Posterior external view showing coronary arteries. **C,** Atherosclerotic plaque in artery.

called *coronary* arteries because they lie across the brow of the heart muscle and resemble a crown. Thus the overall disease process is identified as **coronary heart disease.**[3] A common symptom of its presence is **angina pectoris**, or chest pain, usually radiating down the arm and sometimes brought on by excitement or physical effort.

Relation to Fat Metabolism

Major research studies have found elevated blood **lipids** associated with coronary heart disease and related heart attacks. *Lipid* is the class name for all fats and fat-related compounds. Lipid substances involved in the disease process are described in more detail in Chapter 3. Three of these substances are emphasized in this chapter.

Triglycerides. The chemical name for fat, describing its basic structure, is *triglyceride*. All simple fats, whether in the body or in food, are triglycerides. The blood test for total triglycerides measures the level circulating in blood. Major research studies of heart disease have shown a definite association between high consumption of saturated fat and an elevated blood lipid level. Studies of body fat distribution, especially using waist measurements in children, help to identify persons more likely to have adverse lipid levels.[2]

Cholesterol. Cholesterol is the fat-related compound produced in the body and is an important part of normal cell functioning. Cholesterol is also found in foods of animal origin (e.g., meat, dairy, and butter); it is not found in any plant foods. Although it is an essential compound in the body, an excess amount of cholesterol is clearly associated with heart disease. When blood cholesterol levels rise above that needed by the body, the excess is deposited in arteries throughout the body, which is the beginning of atherosclerosis. Estimates indicate that 19% of American adults (20 to 74 years of age) have high blood cholesterol,[4] many of whom have the related problems of obesity and hypertension, requiring medical advice and intervention using diet as the primary treatment. A reduction in dietary cholesterol has been shown to lower total blood cholesterol levels and reduce the risk of heart disease in predisposed individuals.[5] A total blood cholesterol level of less than 200 mg/dl is considered desirable. However, the average cholesterol level in American adults is 203 mg/dl.[4]

Lipoproteins. Because fat is not soluble in water, it is carried in the blood stream in small packages wrapped with protein, which are called *lipoproteins*. These compounds are produced in the intestinal wall after a meal containing fat and in the liver as part of the regular ongoing process of fat metabolism. Lipoproteins carry fat and cholesterol to tissues for cell metabolism and back to the liver for breakdown and excretion as needed. Lipoproteins are grouped and named according to their protein, fat, and cholesterol content (e.g., their density). Those with the highest protein content have the highest density and vice versa. Three of these types of lipoproteins that are formed in the liver are significant in relation to heart disease risk, as follows:

- *Very low-density lipoproteins* (VLDL) carry a relatively large load of fat to cells but also include approximately 15% cholesterol.
- *Low-density lipoproteins* (LDL) carry, in addition to other lipids, at least two thirds of the total plasma cholesterol to body tissues. They are formed in the liver and in serum from catabolism of VLDL. Because

atherosclerosis (Gr. *athere*, gruel; *skleros*, hard) the underlying pathology of coronary heart disease; a common form of arteriosclerosis that is characterized by the formation of yellow cheeselike fatty streaks containing cholesterol that develop into hardened plaques in the inner lining of major blood vessels such as the coronary arteries.

myocardial infarction (MI) (Gr. *mys*, muscle; *kardia*, heart; L. *infarcire*, to stuff in) a heart attack; caused by failure of the heart muscle to maintain normal blood circulation, because of blockage of coronary arteries with fatty cholesterol plaques that cut off delivery of oxygen to the affected part of the heart muscle.

cerebrovascular accident (CVA) (L. *cerebrum*, brain, *vas*, vessel) a stroke, caused by arteriosclerosis within blood vessels of the brain that cuts off oxygen supply to the affected portion of brain tissue, thus paralyzing body muscle actions controlled by the affected brain area.

coronary heart disease term designating the overall medical problem resulting from the underlying disease of atherosclerosis in the coronary arteries, which serve the heart muscle with blood oxygen and nutrients.

angina pectoris (L. *angina*, severe pain; *pectus*, breast) spasmodic, choking chest pain caused by lack of oxygen to the heart muscle, symptom of a heart attack; also may be caused by severe effort or excitement.

lipids (Gr. *lipos*, fat) the chemical group name for fats and fat-related compounds such as cholesterol and lipoproteins.

LDLs constantly send cholesterol to tissues, they have been called the source of "bad cholesterol." In blood lipid tests, the total LDL is the major cholesterol of concern. A blood LDL level of up to 129 mg/dl is considered healthy, and the person is without risk. Borderline risk occurs in the range of 130 to 159 mg/dl; any level above 160 mg/dl carries high risk.

■ *High-density lipoproteins* (HDL) carry less total fat and more protein. They transport cholesterol from the tissues to the liver for catabolism and elimination from the body. HDL cholesterol is not found in food; rather, it is produced in the body. When compared with LDL cholesterol, HDL cholesterol is often called "good cholesterol," and higher serum levels are considered protective against cardiovascular disease. The desirable HDL range is 40 mg/dl or higher. Values below 40 mg/dl imply increased risk for cardiovascular disease and a value of 60 mg/dl or greater contributes protection and decreased risk. HDL cholesterol is more closely associated with regular exercise than diet.

Table 19-1 outlines the recommended blood levels of each lipid component.

Risk Factors

Several important facts have been learned from major studies of heart disease, as follows:

1. The underlying disease process of atherosclerosis is caused by multiple risk factors, as shown in Box 19-1. Note the personal risk factors over which people do have control versus those they cannot control, such as the following:
   ■ *Sex.* Occurs more in men than women; after menopause women catch up with men in cholesterol level and potential heart disease risk.
   ■ *Age.* Occurs at an earlier age in families carrying a positive family history for heart disease; general risk increases with the aging process.
   ■ *Family history.* A positive family history is defined as a history of premature (before age 55 years) cardiovascular disease in a parent or grandparent or parental high blood cholesterol above 240 mg/dl.

TABLE 19–1	Cholesterol and Lipoprotein Profile Classification	
Cholesterol reading	**Classification**
TOTAL CHOLESTEROL (mg/dl)	
<200	Desirable
200-239	Borderline high risk
≥240	High risk
LDL CHOLESTEROL (mg/dl)	
<100	Optimal
100-129	Near optimal
130-159	Borderline high risk
160-189	High risk
≥190	Very high risk
HDL CHOLESTEROL (mg/dl)	
≥60	Optimal
40-59	Desirable
<40	High risk
TRIGLYCERIDES (mg/dl)	
<150	Optimal
150-199	Borderline high risk
≥200	High risk

BOX 19–1 Multiple Risk Factors in Cardiovascular Disease

**Personal Characteristics
(no control)**

Sex
Age
Family history

**Learned Behaviors
(intervention and change)**

Stress/coping
Cigarette smoking
Sedentary lifestyle
Obesity, especially in the abdominal region

**Learned Behaviors
(intervention and change)—*cont'd***

Food habits
    Excess fat
    Excess sugar
    Excess salt

Background Conditions (screening and treatment)

Hypertension
Diabetes mellitus
Hyperlipidemia (especially hypercholesterolemia)

Early screening for children and adolescents with a high risk resulting from family history is important so that appropriate therapy (e.g., diet [low fat and weight control] with cholesterol-lowering drugs as needed) may be started when the fatty streaks in coronary arteries are just beginning.

2. Elevated serum cholesterol is one of the *major* risk factors for the disease process, which is worsened by obesity, lack of exercise, excess food intake, stress, and smoking. The National Cholesterol Education Program recommends cholesterol screening every 5 years for adults without existing risk factors and more often for those with higher risk.

3. Compounding diseases such as diabetes, hypertension, and metabolic syndrome (as defined in Table 19-2) increase the risk for developing cardiovascular disease.[6,7]

4. Dietary fat *can* affect serum cholesterol. Thus diets aimed at lowering saturated fat and cholesterol intake are an important part of the treatment for cardiovascular disease.

Dietary Recommendations for Reduced Risk

Dietary Guidelines for Americans. Because control of dietary fat and cholesterol is important in reducing risks for heart disease, the *Dietary Guidelines for Americans* (see Chapter 1) issued by the U.S. Departments of Agriculture and of Health and Human Services, as well as other national health agencies for heart disease, cancer, and diabetes, recommend dietary restriction in both nutrients. The following are three primary factors in a heart-healthy diet for the general public:

1. Reduce the total amount of fat. No more than 30% of total energy (kilocalories) intake should come from fat.

2. Reduce the use of animal fat. No more than approximately one third of the total fat kilocalories should

come from saturated animal fat, with the remainder coming from unsaturated plant fat (see Chapter 3).

3. Reduce the intake of cholesterol. Dietary cholesterol should be limited to about 300 mg/day.

National Cholesterol Education Program (NCEP) Adult Treatment Panel III Guidelines. The National Heart, Lung, and Blood Association's NCEP began a campaign against high blood cholesterol in 1988 with the release of its Report of the Expert Panel on Detection, Evaluation, and Treatment of High Blood Cholesterol in Adults (ATP). The NCEP designed the Step I and Step II diets, also endorsed by the American Heart Association, to lessen the risk of cardiovascular disease by reducing high blood cholesterol levels. Since the inception of the Step I and II diets, the NCEP has released two follow-up reports. In the most recent, the Third Report of the Expert Panel on Detection, Evaluation, and Treatment of High Blood Cholesterol in Adults (ATP III), the organization moved toward an intensive life-habit intervention that is focused on appropriate weight, diet, physical activity, and other controllable risk factors.[8] Table 19-3 gives a comparison of the recommendations for each of the three diets. This approach is referred to as the Therapeutic Lifestyle Changes (TLC) diet and includes the following recommendations:

■ Total energy intake should reflect energy expenditure to maintain desirable body weight and prevent weight gain.

■ Total fat intake should not exceed 25% to 35% of total kcalories with saturated fat contributing no more than 7%, polyunsaturated fat up to 10%, and monounsaturated fats up to 20%. Individuals with metabolic syndrome or diabetes can increase intake of unsaturated fats in place of carbohydrates.

■ Carbohydrates, mainly from complex carbohydrates such as whole grains, fruits, and vegetables should make up 50% to 60% of the total energy intake per day. The diet should allow for 10 to 25 g of soluble fiber and 2 g of plant-derived sterols or stanols per day (see the For Further Focus box, "Soy Protein and Heart Disease").

■ Total protein intake should account for approximately 15% of the total energy intake. Soy protein is encouraged as a low-fat alternative to other animal products.

■ Total intake should be less than 200 mg dietary cholesterol per day.

A diet rich in vegetables, fruits, whole grains, low in saturated and trans fatty acids, with moderate use of polyunsaturated and monounsaturated food fats (e.g., mostly from olive oil or corn oil and other vegetable oils

TABLE 19–2	Diagnosing Metabolic Syndrome	
Risk factor	**Defining level**
Abdominal obesity	Waist circumference
Men	>40 inches
Women	>35 inches
Triglycerides	≥150 mg/dl
HDL cholesterol	
Men	<40 mg/dl
Women	<50 mg/dl
Blood pressure	≥130/≥85 mmHg
Fasting blood glucose	≥110 mg/dl

TABLE 19-3 | **American Heart Association and National Cholesterol Education Program Recommendations for Lowering Cholesterol**

Nutrient*	Recommended intake as percent of total calories		
	Step I diet	Step II diet	TLC diet in ATP III
Total fat	30% or less	30% or less	25%-35%
Saturated	7%-10%	Less than 7%	Less than 7%
Polyunsaturated	Up to 10%	Up to 10%	Up to 10%
Monounsaturated	Up to 15%	Up to 15%	Up to 20%
Carbohydrate	55% or more	55% or more	50%-60%
Protein	~15%	~15%	~15%
Cholesterol	<300 mg/day	<200 mg/day	<200 mg/day
Total calories	To achieve and maintain desired weight	To achieve and maintain desired weight	Balance energy intake and expenditure to maintain desirable body weight and prevent weight gain

Modified from Krauss RM and others: AHA dietary guidelines (revision 2000): a statement for healthcare professionals from the Nutrition Committee of the American Heart Association, *Circulation* 102(18):2284, 2000; and National Cholesterol Education Program (NCEP) Expert Panel on Detection, Evaluation, and Treatment of High Blood Cholesterol in Adults (Adult Treatment Panel III): Third Report of the NCEP Expert Panel on Detection, Evaluation, and Treatment of High Blood Pressure in Adults (Adult Treatment Panel III), *Circulation* 106:3143, 2002.
*Calories from alcohol not included.
ATP = Adult Treatment Panel; TLC = Therapeutic Lifestyle Changes.

and products) is the basic guideline.[8,9] Low-fat and fat-free dairy products, and lean meat, fish, and poultry are used instead of their high-fat alternatives.

When the risk factor of obesity is present, the overall excess energy value of the diet (kcalories) is also reduced accordingly, and increased exercise is encouraged (see Chapter 15). A treadmill exercise tolerance test is used to determine the exercise limit for a person with a cardiac history (Figure 19-2). The American Heart Association still recommends the Step I diet as a heart-healthy diet for the general public as a means to prevent heart disease, but the TLC diet has been adopted as the preferred diet for individuals with known cardiovascular disease or multiple existing risk factors.[10]

Acute Cardiovascular Disease

When cardiovascular disease progresses to the point of cutting off the blood supply to major coronary arteries, a critical vascular event—a heart attack or MI—may occur (see the Clinical Applications box, "Case Study: The Patient with a Myocardial Infarction [Heart Attack]"). In the initial, acute phase of the attack, additional diet modifications are necessary to allow for healing.

Objective: Cardiac Rest

All care, including diet, is directed toward ensuring cardiac rest so that the damaged heart may be restored to normal functioning.

Principles of Diet Therapy

The diet is modified in energy value and texture, as well as in fat and sodium content.

Energy. A brief period of reduced energy intake during the first day or so after the heart attack reduces the metabolic workload on the damaged heart. The metabolic demands for digestion, absorption, and metabolism of food require a generous cardiac output volume. Thus to decrease the level of metabolic activity that the weakened heart can accommodate, small feedings are spread over the day when an oral diet is started. The patient progresses to eating more as healing occurs. During the initial recovery period, the diet may be limited to about 1200 to 1500 kcal to continue cardiac rest from metabolic workloads. Afterward, if the patient is overweight, this kcalorie level may be continued to help the patient begin gradually losing excess weight.

Texture. Early feedings generally include foods that are relatively soft in texture or easily digested to avoid excess effort in eating or the discomfort of gas formation. Some patients benefit from assistance in the feeding process for a short period, especially those patients with poor appetite or weakness, or those who become short of breath from the exertion of feeding themselves. Smaller, more frequent meals may give needed nourishment without undue strain or pressure. Depending on the patient's condition, gas-forming foods, caffeine-containing beverages, and hot or cold temperature extremes in foods (both solids and liquids) also generally should be avoided.

FOR FURTHER FOCUS

SOY PROTEIN AND HEART DISEASE

The health benefits of soy protein seem to be boundless! In recent years, this humble protein has been linked to a reduced risk for cancer, osteoporosis, menopausal symptoms, and coronary heart disease. In regard to coronary heart disease, ingestion of soy protein has specifically been linked to a reduction in LDL cholesterol, the bad cholesterol; an increase in HDL cholesterol, the good cholesterol; and a reduction in triglycerides. The findings are so significant that the FDA has approved an official health claim linking soy protein consumption and a reduced risk of coronary heart disease.*

One of the main focuses of research in this area is to narrow the recommendations for the amount and type of phytosterols and phytostanols needed on a daily basis to receive the most beneficial results. Phytosterols and phytostanols are the molecules found in plant foods that have the cholesterol lowering effect. One way in which they work is by preventing the absorption of cholesterol in the digestive tract. Previous research had found a huge range (18 to 124 g/day) in the amount of soy protein needed to achieve the desired results. One reason for this large difference results from the low water solubility of the compounds. Because the compound requires fat as a carrier, consuming that amount of soy protein could drastically increase total fat consumption. (Even if it is the "heart-healthy fat," it still carries the potential for increasing weight gain.) The FDA recommends consuming four servings per day of soy protein with each serving containing a minimum of 6.25 g, for a total of 25 g/day. Researchers are exploring alternative methods for introducing the protein without drastically changing the diet or fat intake. One study found that a low-dose soy protein supplement in b-sitosterol produced a modest reduction in LDL cholesterol and may be an effective alternative, or addition, to soy protein foods.† A similar study combined soy protein with small amounts of lecithin, dried it, and added it to otherwise fat-free foods as an alternative source of phytosterols and phytostanols.‡ Both b-sitosterol and lecithin increase the water solubility of the compound and allowed for better absorption without the fat. In both cases, the beneficial effects of soy protein were seen in the form of lowered cholesterol and improved lipid profiles.

Incorporating soy protein into a low-fat, high-fiber diet with plenty of fruits and vegetables is a sound start to reducing the risk for coronary heart disease. Soy protein can be found in the following foods:

- Meat alternatives
- Miso
- Nondairy frozen desserts
- Okara
- Soy beverages
- Soy cheese
- Soy nut butter
- Soy yogurt
- Soybeans
- Soybean oil
- Soy milk
- Soy nuts
- Tempeh
- Textured vegetable protein
- Tofu

*U.S. Food and Drug Administration: *Health claim: soy protein and coronary heart disease (CHD)*, Code of Federal Regulations, Title 21, Vol 2, Sec 101.82, Rockville, MD, revised 2002, (accessed May 2003), FDA [*www.cfsan.fda.gov/~lrd/cf101-82.html*].
†Cicero AF and others: Effects of a new soy/b-sitosterol supplement on plasma lipids in moderately hypercholesterolemic subjects, *J Am Diet Assoc* 102(12):1807, 2002.
‡Spilburg CA and others: Fat-free foods supplement with soy stanol-lecithin powder reduce cholesterol absorption and LDL cholesterol, *J Am Diet Assoc* 103(5):577, 2003.

Fat. The general Step I diet controls the amount and types of fat, as well as cholesterol (see Table 19-3). Table 19-4 outlines the maximum amount of fat allowed in Step I, Step II, and TLC diets.

Sodium. General attention to reduced sodium content in food selection is important as well. Usually a mild sodium restriction to about 2 to 3 g/day is sufficient (Box 19-2).

This restriction can be achieved by only using salt lightly in cooking, adding none when eating, and avoiding salty processed foods. Appendixes D and E provide the sodium values of foods and a salt-free seasoning guide. Food labels on canned and other processed foods, as mandated by the U.S. Congress and administered by the Food and Drug Administration (FDA), provide specific information about the sodium content of such foods (see Chapter 13).

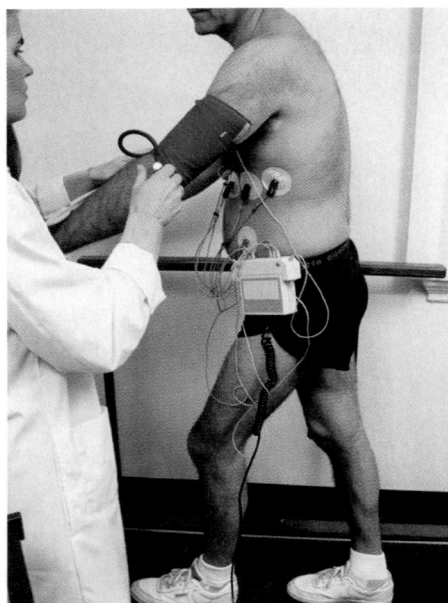

Figure 19–2 Patient with history of cardiac disease is evaluated for exercise tolerance with treadmill test. (Credit: PhotoDisc.)

Chronic Heart Disease

In chronic heart disease, congestive heart failure may develop over time. The progressively weakened heart muscle is unable to maintain an adequate cardiac output to sustain normal blood circulation. The resulting fluid imbalances cause edema, especially pulmonary edema. This condition makes breathing difficult and places more stress on the laboring heart.

Objective: Control of Cardiac Edema

The basic objective of diet therapy in this condition is to control the fluid imbalance that results in cardiac edema.

Principles of Diet Therapy

Because of sodium's role in tissue fluid balance (see Chapter 9), the diet used to treat cardiac edema restricts sodium intake. The main source of dietary sodium is common table salt, sodium chloride. The taste for salt is acquired. Some people salt food heavily by habit without even tasting it first, thus habituating their taste to high salt levels. Others acquire a taste for less salt by gradually using smaller and smaller amounts. Therefore in American diets common daily adult intakes of sodium range widely, from 3 to 4 g up to 10 to 12 g with heavy use. Besides the salt used in cooking or added at the table, a large amount is used in food processing. Remaining

sources of sodium include that found as a naturally occurring mineral in certain foods. The American Heart Association has outlined the following three main levels of sodium restriction, which can be achieved by progressively deleting the main dietary sodium sources:

1. **Mild sodium restriction (2 to 3 g).** Salt may be used *lightly* in cooking, assuming that fresh foods are used, but *no added salt* is allowed. In addition, no salty processed foods (e.g., pickles, olives, bacon, ham, corn chips, or potato chips) are used. Some processed foods with less salt added are available in food markets.
2. **Moderate sodium restriction (1000 mg).** No salt is used in cooking, and no added salt or salty foods are used. Beginning at this level, some control of foods with natural sodium is started. Vegetables higher in natural sodium are limited. Fresh foods are used, rather than those processed with salt. Salt-free baked products generally are used. Foods higher in natural sodium (e.g., meat and milk) are only used in moderate portions.
3. **Strict sodium restriction (500 mg).** In addition to the mild and moderate deletions, the natural sodium food sources of meat, milk, and eggs are used in smaller portions. Per day milk is limited to 2 cups in any form, meat to 5 oz, and eggs to 1 oz. Higher-sodium vegetables are deleted. Box 19-2 provides a general deletion list for all three levels of sodium restriction.

ESSENTIAL HYPERTENSION

The Problem of Hypertension

Incidence and Nature

Hypertension, or high blood pressure, is a health problem for 50 million Americans. About 23% of American adults (20 to 74 years) have high blood pressure, with the numbers increasing with age.[11] The incidence is highest among older African-American women. When speaking of the chronic disease of elevated blood pressure, the term *hypertension* is actually more appropriate than *high blood pressure* because blood pressure occasionally may be elevated in situations such as overexertion or stress. In general, the disease hypertension means essential (or primary) hypertension, and 90% of cases fall in this category. The specific cause is unknown, although injury to the inner lining of the blood vessel wall appears to be an underlying link. *Secondary hypertension* is the result of a known cause and is a symptom or side effect of

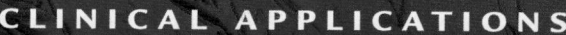

CLINICAL APPLICATIONS

CASE STUDY: THE PATIENT WITH A MYOCARDIAL INFARCTION (HEART ATTACK)

Charles Carter is a successful young businessman who works long hours and carries the major responsibility of his struggling small business. At his last physical checkup, the physician cautioned him about his pace because he was already showing some mild hypertension. His blood cholesterol was elevated, and he was overweight. In his desk job he got little exercise and found himself smoking more and eating irregularly under the stress of his increasing financial pressures.

One day while commuting in the heavy freeway traffic, he felt a pain in his chest and became increasingly apprehensive. When he arrived home, the pain persisted and increased. He broke out into a cold sweat and felt nauseated. When he became more ill after trying to eat dinner, his wife called their physician and Mr. Carter was admitted to the hospital.

After emergency care and tests, the physician placed Mr. Carter in the coronary care unit at the hospital. His test results showed elevated total cholesterol, triglycerides, and lipoproteins, especially LDL, but low HDL. The electrocardiogram revealed an infarction of the posterior myocardium wall.

When Mr. Carter was first able to take oral nourishment, he had only a liquid diet. As his condition stabilized, his diet was increased to 800 kcal (soft diet) with low cholesterol and low fat. By the end of the first week, his diet was increased again to 1200 kcal (full diet) with low cholesterol and only 25% of the total kcalories from fat and a polyunsaturated/saturated ratio of 1:1.

Mr. Carter gradually improved over the next few days and was able to go home. The physician, nurse, and dietitian discussed with Mr. Carter and his wife the need for care at home during a period of convalescence. They explained that he had an underlying lipid disorder and was to continue his weight loss and follow a TLC diet.

Questions for Analysis

1. Identify factors in Mr. Carter's personal and medical history that place him at high risk for coronary heart disease. Give reasons why each factor contributes to heart disease.
2. Identify as many of the laboratory tests the physician ordered as you can. Relate these tests to Mr. Carter's condition.
3. Why did Mr. Carter receive only a liquid diet at first? What is the reason for each modification in his first diet of solid food?
4. What occurs in the underlying disease process that causes a heart attack? What relation do fat and cholesterol have to this underlying process?
5. Outline a day's menu for Mr. Carter on his 1200 kcal TLC diet.
6. What needs might Mr. Carter have when he goes home? How would you help him prepare to go home? Name some community resources you might use to help him understand his illness and plan self-care.

---

another primary condition. For example, individuals with kidney disease often suffer from secondary hypertension.

Hypertension has been called the "silent disease" because no signs indicate its presence. It can have serious effects if not detected, treated, and controlled. Hypertension is usually an inherited disorder; children of hypertensive parents may develop the condition at early ages, often in their adolescent years. Obesity worsens the condition because it forces the heart to work harder, thus maintaining higher pressure, to circulate blood through the excess tissue. Smoking also increases blood pressure because nicotine constricts the small blood ves-

congestive heart failure chronic condition of gradually weakening heart muscle unable to pump normal blood flow through the heart-lung circulation, resulting in congestion of fluids in the lungs.

pulmonary edema (L. *pulmonis*, lung; Gr. *oidema*, swelling) accumulation of fluid in lung tissues.

essential hypertension an inherent form of high blood pressure with no specific discoverable cause, considered to be familial; also called *primary hypertension*.

TABLE 19-4	Maximum Amount of Fat Allowed per Day on a Step I, Step II, and TLC Diet at Various Calorie Levels			
	Total fat (g)		Saturated fat (g)	
Total calories	Step I and II	TLC	Step I	Step II and TLC
1200	40	33-47	9-13	9
1400	47	39-54	11-16	11
1600	53	44-62	12-18	12
1800	60	50-70	14-20	14
2000	67	56-78	16-22	16
2200	73	61-86	17-24	17
2400	80	67-93	19-27	19
2600	87	72-101	20-29	20
2800	93	78-109	22-31	22
3000	100	83-117	23-33	23

Based on recommendations from Krauss RM and others: AHA Dietary Guidelines: revision 2000: A statement for healthcare professionals from the Nutrition Committee of the American Heart Association, *Circulation* 102:(18):2284, 2000; and National Cholesterol Education Program (NCEP) Expert Panel on Detection, Evaluation, and Treatment of High Blood Cholesterol in Adults (Adult Treatment Panel III): Third Report of the NCEP Expert Panel on Detection, Evaluation, and Treatment of High Blood Pressure in Adults (Adult Treatment Panel III), *Circulation* 106:3143, 2002.

sels. Other risk factors include lack of exercise, chronic stress, certain drugs (e.g., birth control pills), and—for some sensitive persons—caffeine.

Types of Hypertensive Blood Pressure Levels

Common blood pressure measurements indicate the pressure of the blood surge in the arteries of the upper arm with each heartbeat. The power of each surge is measured in units called *millimeters of mercury* (mmHg). Two forces are counted and represented by two numbers. The number on the top of the fraction measures the force of the blood surge when the heart contracts, the *systolic* pressure. The number on the bottom measures the pressure remaining in the arteries when the heart relaxes between beats, the *diastolic* pressure. Adult blood pressure usually is considered normal if recorded as <140/<90 mmHg. Current hypertension screening and treatment programs identify persons with hypertension according to degree of severity of these pressures (Table 19-5). Specific care is then outlined depending on the severity, limiting drugs as much as possible.

Stage 1 Hypertension. The initial focus is on approaches of diet therapy (without drugs) to reduce excess weight and restrict sodium.

Stage 2 Hypertension. In addition to the diet therapy for Stage 1, drugs are used according to need and usually include a diuretic agent. Continuous use of some, although not all, diuretic drugs cause loss of potassium along with the increased loss of water from the body. Because potassium is necessary for maintaining normal heart muscle

action, depletion could become dangerous. Potassium replacement is necessary. Dietary replacement by increased use of potassium-rich foods (e.g., fruits, especially bananas and orange juice, vegetables, legumes, nuts, and whole grains) is an important part of therapy. Appendix D provides the sodium and potassium values of foods.

Stage 3 Hypertension. In addition to the diet for Stage 2 hypertension, vigorous drug therapy is necessary. Nutritional support is important for all types of hypertension, along with other nondrug therapies of physical exercise and stress reduction.[12]

Principles of Nutrition Therapy

Weight Management

According to individual need, weight management requires losing excess weight and maintaining an appropriate weight for height. A sound approach to managing weight loss is given in Chapter 15, and guidance for increasing physical exercise is given in Chapter 16. Because the overweight state has been closely associated with hypertension risk factors, a wisely planned personal program of weight reduction and physical activity is a cornerstone of therapy.

Sodium Control

In sodium-sensitive persons, additional attention is given to restricting sodium in the diet. The mild 2-g sodium level generally is sufficient (see Box 19-2). The equivalent of 2.4 g of sodium is approximately 6 g sodium chlo-

BOX 19–2   Sodium-Restricted Diet Recommendations

**Restrictions for Mild Low-Sodium Diet
(2 to 3 g sodium/day)**

The following should not be used:

- Salt at the table (to be used lightly in cooking)
- Salt-preserved foods such as salted or smoked meat (bacon and bacon fat, bologna, dried or chipped beef, corned beef, frankfurters, ham, kosher meats, luncheon meats, salt pork, sausage, smoked tongue), salted or smoked fish (anchovies, caviar, salted and dried cod, herring, sardines), sauerkraut, olives
- Highly salted foods such as crackers, pretzels, potato chips, corn chips, salted nuts, salted popcorn
- Spices and condiments such as bouillon cubes,* catsup,* chili sauce,* celery salt, garlic salt, onion salt, monosodium glutamate, meat sauces, meat tenderizers,* pickles, prepared mustard, relishes, Worcestershire sauce, soy sauce
- Cheese,* peanut butter*

**Restrictions for Moderate Low-Sodium Diet
(1000 mg sodium/day)**

The same measures as for the mild low-sodium diet should be taken, plus the following items should be avoided:

- Salt in cooking
- Buttermilk (unsalted buttermilk may be used) instead of skim milk
- Frozen peas, frozen lima beans, frozen mixed vegetables, any frozen vegetables to which salt has been added

*Low-sodium brands may be used.

**Restrictions for Moderate Low-Sodium Diet
(1000 mg sodium/day)—cont'd**

- More than one serving of any of these vegetables per day: artichokes, beet greens, beets, carrots, celery, dandelion greens, kale, mustard greens, spinach, Swiss chard, turnips (white)
- Regular bread, rolls,* crackers*
- Dry cereals,* except puffed rice, puffed wheat, and shredded wheat
- Quick-cooking Cream of Wheat
- Shellfish: clams, crab, lobster, shrimp (oysters may be used)
- Salted butter, salted margarine, commercial French dressings,* mayonnaise,* other salad dressings*
- Regular baking powder,* baking soda, or anything containing them; self-rising flour
- Prepared mixes: pudding,* gelatin,* cake, biscuit
- Commercial candies

**Restrictions for Strict Low-Sodium Diet
(500 mg sodium/day)**

The same measures as for the mild and moderate low-sodium diets should be taken, plus the following items should be avoided:

- More than 2 cups of skim milk per day, including that used on cereal
- Any commercial foods made of milk (ice cream, ice milk, milk shakes)
- The following vegetables: artichokes, beet greens, beets, carrots, celery, dandelion greens, kale, mustard greens, spinach, Swiss chard, turnips (white)

---

ride or table salt. However, in more severe cases of hypertension the moderate 1-g sodium level may be indicated.

Other Minerals

In addition to sodium control, especially for sodium-sensitive persons, other minerals have been discussed in relation to hypertension. Some evidence suggests that increased calcium and magnesium intake is beneficial for some persons with hypertension. As indicated, increased potassium to replace loss with diuretic use and supply normal dietary needs is also an important part of diet therapy.

The DASH Diet

The DASH diet is the result of a successful landmark study called "Dietary Approaches to Stop Hypertension" that was able to significantly lower blood pressure by diet alone within a short period of time (14 days).[13] The diet

recommends eating four to six servings of fruits, four to six servings of vegetables, and two to three servings of low-fat dairy foods per day, in addition to lean meats and high fiber grains. Studies have found that individuals following the diet have an average decrease in systolic blood pressure of 6 to 11 mmHg.[13] When combining the DASH diet with a low sodium diet, the blood pressure–lowering effects are even greater.[14] More recent studies have found that the DASH diet also can produce a slight reduction in LDL cholesterol, an added benefit for preventing heart disease[15] (although findings indicate the diet may cause a slight decrease in HDL cholesterol as well.)

The DASH diet is recommended for individuals with high blood pressure, blood pressure in the "high-normal" range, a family history of high blood pressure, or for those who are trying to get off blood pressure medications. The first step in following the DASH diet is to determine the

TABLE 19–5	Classification of Blood Pressure for Adults* (Ages 18 Years and Older)				
				Initial drug therapy	
BP classification	**SBP* (mmHg)**	**DBP* (mmHg)**	**Lifestyle modification**	**Without compelling indication**	**With compelling indication**
Normal	<120	and <80	Encourage		
Prehypertension	120-139	or 80-89	Yes	No antihypertensive drug indicated	Drug(s) for compelling indications†
Stage 1 hypertension	140-159	or 90-99	Yes	Thiazide-type diuretics for most; may consider ACEI, ARB, BB, CCB, or combination	Drug(s) for the compelling indications;† other antihypertensive drugs (diuretics, ACEI, ARB, BB, CCB) as needed
Stage 2 hypertension	≥160	or ≥100	Yes	Two-drug combination for most‡ (usually thiazide-type diuretic and ACEI or ARB or BB or CCB)	

National Heart, Lung, and Blood Institute, National Institutes of Health: *Seventh Report of the Joint National Committee on Prevention, Detection, Evaluation, and Treatment of High Blood Pressure (JNC 7) express,* NIH publication #03-5233, Bethesda, MD, 2003, NHLBI/NIH. [*www.nhlbi.nih.gov/guidelines/hypertension/jncintro.htm*].

*Treatment determined by highest blood pressure category.
†Patients with chronic kidney disease or diabetes should be treated to blood pressure goal of <130/80 mmHg.
‡Initial combined therapy should be used cautiously in those individuals at risk for orthostatic hypotension.
ACEI = Angiotensin-converting enzyme inhibitor; *ARB* = angiotensin receptor blocker; *BB* = beta blocker; *CCB* = calcium channel blocker; *DBP* = diastolic blood pressure; *SBP* = systolic blood pressure.

appropriate energy (kcalorie) level based on desired weight and activity level (Chapter 6). Then, the appropriate number of servings per day of each food group should be based on the total energy need. Table 19-6 outlines the DASH diet and serving sizes, whereas Box 19-3 provides a 1-day sample menu based on a 2000-calorie diet.

Additional Lifestyle Factors

The National High Blood Pressure Education Program recommends limiting alcohol intake to 1 oz ethanol per day for men and 0.5 oz per day for most women and lightweight persons. One ounce ethanol is equal to 24 oz regular beer, 10 oz wine, or 2-oz 100-proof whiskey. Additional recommendations to prevent or treat hypertension include: stop smoking, limit saturated fat and cholesterol intake, and increase aerobic type physical activity to a minimum of 30 to 45 minutes per day on most days of the week.[13]

EDUCATION AND PREVENTION

Practical Food Guides

Food Planning and Purchasing

The *Dietary Guidelines for Americans* (see Chapter 1) provide a basic outline to guide sound food habits. The food exchange lists described in Chapter 20 and listed in Appendix F for reference list the food groups with the fat and sodium modifications discussed in this chapter.

These lists also provide a guide for controlling energy intake to help plan for any needed weight management. An important part of purchasing food is reading labels carefully. The Nutrition Facts labels provide basic nutrition information in a standard format so that it is easily recognized and clearly expressed (see Chapter 13).

All processed food products that make any health claims must follow the strict guidelines provided by the FDA. A good general guide is to use primarily fresh foods with informed selection of processed foods as necessary. Refer to Chapter 13 for background material about food supply and health.

Food Preparation

The public is more aware of the need to prepare foods with less fat and salt than ever before. Consequently, the cookbook industry has responded by providing an abundance of guides and recipes for various age groups and customs. Many seasonings (e.g., herbs, spices, lemon, wine, onion, garlic, nonfat milk and yogurt, and fresh fat-free meat broth) can help train the taste for less salt and fat (see Appendix E). Less meat in leaner and smaller portions can be combined with more complex carbohydrate foods (e.g., starches such as potato, pasta, rice, bulgur, and beans) to make more healthful main dishes. Whole grain breads and cereals can provide needed fiber, and more use of fish can add healthier forms of fat in smaller quantities. A variety of vegetables may

TABLE 19-6   Servings per Day for Each Food Group According to the DASH Diet

Calorie-intake range	Grains	Vegetables	Fruits	Dairy foods	Meats, poultry, and fish	Nuts, seeds, and legumes	Added fats and oils	Sweets
1400-1800	6	4	4	2	1½	¼	1	½
1800-2200	7	4	4	2½	1½	½	2	½
2200-2600	9	5	5	3	2	½	3	1
2600-3000	11	6	6	3½	2½	½	4	2
Example of serving sizes	1 slice bread ½ cup dry cereal or cooked rice	1 cup raw leafy vegetable ½ cup cooked vegetable 6 oz vegetable juice	6 oz fruit juice 1 medium fruit ¼ cup dried fruit ½ cup fresh, frozen, or canned fruit	8 oz milk 1 cup yogurt 1½ oz cheese	3 oz cooked meats, poultry, or fish	1½ oz or ⅓ cup nuts 2 tablespoons seeds ½ cup cooked legumes	1 tsp regular soft margarine, butter, or regular mayonnaise 1 Tbsp low-fat mayonnaise or regular salad dressing 2 Tbsp light salad dressing	1 Tbsp jelly, jam, sugar, or maple syrup ½ oz jelly beans or 3 pieces hard candy ½ cup low-fat or nonfat frozen yogurt or sherbet

From Moore T and others: *The DASH diet for hypertension: lower your blood pressure in 14 days—without drugs*, New York, 2001, The Free Press, a Division of Simon & Schuster Adult Publishing Group. Copyright © 2001 by Thomas Moore, Laura Scetkey, Lawrence Appel, George Bray, and William Vollmer.

BOX 19-3 Sample 1-Day Menu on DASH Diet (2000 kcal)

Breakfast

1 cup apple juice
⅔ cup shredded wheat
3 Tbsp raisins
1 slice whole wheat toast
1 tsp unsalted margarine
1 tsp jelly
1 cup skim milk

Lunch

1 cup apple juice
1 serving tomato soup
1 cup steamed green beans
2 whole wheat rolls
1 tsp unsalted margarine

Lunch—cont'd

2 medium plums
½ cup skim milk

Dinner

1 serving sweet-and-sour pork with vegetables
1 cup cooked brown rice
1 serving salad
2 tsp fresh lemon juice
1 serving vanilla pudding with banana
½ cup skim milk

From Moore T and others: *The DASH diet for hypertension: lower your blood pressure in 14 days—without drugs,* New York, 2001, The Free Press, a Division of Simon & Schuster Adult Publishing Group. Copyright © 2001 by Thomas Moore, Laura Scetkey, Lawrence Appel, George Bray, and William Vollmer.

---

be used (e.g., in salads or steamed and lightly seasoned), and fruits add interest, taste appeal, and nourishment to meals. *The American Heart Association* publishes several cookbooks that are excellent guides to newer, lighter, tasteful, and healthier food preparation.

Special Needs

Individual adaptation of diet principles is important in all nutrition teaching and counseling. Special attention must be given to personal desires, ethnic diets, individual situations, and food habits as discussed in Chapter 14. Any diet must meet both personal and health needs.

Education Principles

Starting Early

Prevention of hypertension and heart disease begins in childhood, especially with children in high-risk families. With close attention to normal growth needs, some preventive measures in family food habits relate to weight control and avoidance of foods high in salt and fat. For adults with heart disease and hypertension, learning should be an integral part of all therapy. If a heart attack does occur, education should begin early in convalescence, not at hospital discharge, to give patients and their families clear and practical knowledge of positive needs.

Focusing on High-Risk Groups

Education on the risks of heart disease and hypertension should be directed particularly to persons and families with these risks (see Box 19-1). For example, hyperten-sion has been closely associated with certain high-risk groups, including African Americans, persons with strong family histories, and obese individuals (see the Cultural Considerations box, "Influence of Ancestors on a Person's Risk for Heart Disease").

Using a Variety of Resources

As researchers learn more about heart disease and hypertension, the American Heart Association and other health agencies are providing many excellent resources. The American Dietetic Association provides a series of pamphlets that are helpful in client education, several of which are useful here: "Weight Expectations," "Fiber Facts," "Cholesterol Countdown," and "The Sodium Story" (P.O. Box 10960, Chicago, IL 60610, *www. eatright.org*). As the public and professionals have become more aware of health needs and disease prevention, an increasing number of resources and programs also can be found in most communities. These include various weight-management programs, registered dietitians in private practice or in health care centers who provide nutrition counseling, and practical food-preparation materials found in a number of recent "light cuisine" cooking classes and cookbooks. Bookstores and public libraries, as well as health education libraries in health centers and clinics, provide an abundance of materials on health promotion and self-care. For example, local health care centers teach persons with hypertension and their families how to take their own blood pressure, so they can assume more control in managing their health needs, as well as provide resources for such self-care.

CULTURAL CONSIDERATIONS

INFLUENCE OF ANCESTORS ON A PERSON'S RISK FOR HEART DISEASE

Although the mortality rate from heart disease has declined since the 1960s, it is still the number one cause of death in the United States. The United States ranks 16th in the incidence of cardiovascular disease among the industrialized nations. According to the 1999 heart and stroke statistical update, the countries of Russian Federation, Bulgaria, Hungary, Romania, Czech Republic, and Poland have much higher incidences of cardiovascular disease—specifically among men. Unlike weight and dietary habits, family history is an unmodifiable risk factor for cardiovascular disease. Therefore distinguishing between environmental factors and the genetics associated with a culture is important for identifying the specifics with regard to cause of disease. Only when those factors have been recognized can prevention and treatment programs be directed on an individual basis.

Interestingly, the major conditions of heart disease (hypertension and high blood cholesterol) are more prevalent in certain ethnic and age groups within the United States than others. The prevalence of both hypertension and high blood cholesterol increases with age. However, hypertension is most prevalent in the African-American population, whereas hypercholesterolemia (high blood cholesterol) is most common in Caucasian, and non-Hispanic females, and least common in African-American males. As a health care provider, be aware of the risk associated with cardiovascular disease among various ethnic groups. By acknowledging the risk associated with ethnicity, warning signs may be detected earlier than they would otherwise.

SUMMARY

Coronary heart disease is the leading cause of death in the United States. Its underlying blood vessel disease is *atherosclerosis*, which involves build-up of the fatty substance containing cholesterol on the interior surfaces of blood vessels, interfering with blood flow and damaging blood vessels. If this fatty build-up becomes severe, it cuts off the supply of oxygen and nutrients to tissue cells, which in turn die. When this occurs in a major coronary artery, the result is a *myocardial infarction* or heart attack.

The risk for atherosclerosis increases with the amount and type of blood lipids (fats), or *lipoproteins*, available. Elevated *serum cholesterol* is a primary risk factor for development of atherosclerosis.

Current recommendations to help prevent coronary heart disease involve a low-fat balanced diet, weight management, and increased exercise. Such a diet limits fats to 25% to 30% of total energy intake, sodium intake to 2 to 3 g per day, and cholesterol intake to 300 mg/day. Dietary recommendations for acute cardiovascular disease (e.g., heart attack) include measures to ensure cardiac rest (e.g., energy restriction, soft foods, and small meals, modified in fat, cholesterol, and sodium). Persons with chronic heart disease involving congestive heart failure benefit from a low-sodium diet to control cardiac edema. Persons with hypertension can improve their condition with weight control, exercise, sodium restriction, and adequate calcium and potassium intake.

CRITICAL THINKING QUESTIONS

1. Why are fat and cholesterol primary factors in heart disease? How are they carried in the blood stream? Which of these "fat packages" carry so-called "good cholesterol" and which carry "bad cholesterol," the cholesterol of concern? How can people influence the relative amounts of these fat and cholesterol carriers in the blood? Describe the food changes involved.

2. Identify the risk factors for heart disease. What control do people have over these risk factors?

3. Identify four dietary recommendations for a patient who has had a heart attack. Describe how each recommendation facilitates recovery.

4. Discuss the three main levels of sodium restriction, describing general food choices and preparation methods.

5. What does the term *essential hypertension* mean? Why would weight control and sodium restriction contribute to its control? What other nutrient factors may be involved in hypertension?

CHAPTER CHALLENGE QUESTIONS

True-False

Write the correct statement for each item you answer "false."

1. *True or False:* In the disease process underlying heart disease (atherosclerosis), the fatty deposits in blood vessel linings are composed mainly of cholesterol.

2. *True or False:* Hypertension occurs more frequently in Caucasian than African-American persons.

3. *True or False:* The problem of cardiovascular disease could be solved if cholesterol could be removed entirely from the body.

4. *True or False:* Cholesterol is a dietary essential because humans depend entirely on food sources for their supply.

5. *True or False:* Lipoproteins are the major transport form of lipids in the blood.

6. *True or False:* The basic clinical objective in treating acute cardiovascular disease (e.g., a heart attack) is cardiac rest.

7. *True or False:* In chronic congestive heart disease, the heart eventually may fail because its weakened muscle must work at a faster rate to pump out the body's necessary blood supply.

8. *True or False:* The taste for salt is instinctive in humans to ensure a sufficient supply.

9. *True or False:* High sodium intake is an effective therapy for congestive heart failure and hypertension.

10. *True or False:* Essential hypertension can be cured by drugs and diet.

Multiple Choice

1. A low-cholesterol diet restricts which of the following foods? *(Circle all that apply.)*
   a. Fish
   b. Liver
   c. Butter
   d. Nonfat milk

2. Helpful seasonings to use in a sodium-restricted diet include which of the following? *(Circle all that apply.)*
   a. Lemon juice
   b. Soy sauce
   c. Herbs and spices
   d. Seasoned salt

3. Which of the following foods may be used freely on a low-sodium diet?
   a. Fruits
   b. Milk
   c. Meat
   d. Spinach and carrots

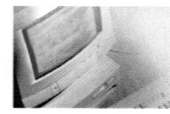

Please refer to the Students' Resource section of this text's Evolve web site for "Suggestions for Additional Study."

REFERENCES

1. Minino AM and others: *National Vital Statistics Report,* vol 50, no 15, Atlanta, 2002, Centers for Disease Control and Prevention.

2. Freedman DS and others: Relation of circumferences and skinfold thicknesses to lipid and insulin concentrations in children and adolescents: the Bogalusa Heart Study, *Am J Clin Nutr* 69(2):308, 1999.

3. National Heart, Lung, and Blood Institute, National Institutes of Health: *Coronary heart disease explained,* Bethesda, MD, (accessed October 2003), NHLBI/NIH [*www.nhlbisupport.com/chd1/chdexp.htm*].

4. National Center for Health Statistics, Centers for Disease Control and Prevention: *Cholesterol,* Hyattsville, MD, 2003 (accessed April 2003), NCHS/CDC [*www.cdc.gov/nchs/fastats/cholest.htm*].

5. National Center for Chronic Disease Prevention and Health Promotion, Centers for Disease Control and Prevention: *Cholesterol fact sheet,* Atlanta, 2003 (accessed April 2003), NCCDPHP/CDC [*www.cdc.gov/cvh/library/fs-cholesterol.htm*].

6. Blumenthal RS: Overview of the adult treatment panel (ATP) III guidelines, *JHASIM* 2(5):148, 2002.

7. Liu S, Manson JE: Dietary carbohydrates, physical inactivity, obesity, and the "metabolic syndrome" as predictors of coronary heart disease, *Curr Opin Lipidol* 12(4):395, 2001.

8. National Cholesterol Education Program (NCEP) Expert Panel on Detection, Evaluation, and Treatment of High Blood Cholesterol in Adults (Adult Treatment Panel III): Third Report of the NCEP Expert Panel on Detection, Evaluation, and Treatment of High Blood Pressure in Adults (Adult Treatment Panel III), *Circulation* 106:3143, 2002.

9. Krauss RM and others: AHA Dietary Guidelines: revision 2000: A statement for healthcare professionals from the Nutrition Committee of the American Heart Association, *Circulation* 102(18):2284, 2000.

10. American Heart Association: *Step I, step II and TLC diets*, Dallas (accessed April 2003), AHA [*www.americanheart. org/presenter.jhtml?identifier=4764*].

11. National Center for Health Statistics, Centers for Disease Control and Prevention: *Hypertension*, Hyattsville, MD, 2003 (accessed May 2003), NCHS/CDC [*www.cdc.gov/ nchs/fastats/hyprtens.htm*].

12. Appel LJ and others: A clinical trial of the effects of dietary patterns on blood pressure. DASH Collaborative Research Group, *N Engl J Med* 336(16):1117, 1997.

13. National Heart, Lung, and Blood Institute, National Institutes of Health: *Seventh Report of the Joint National Committee on Prevention, Detection, Evaluation, and Treatment of High Blood Pressure* (JNC 7) express, NIH publication #03-5233, Bethesda, MD, 2003, NHLBI/NIH (accessed June 2003), [*www.nhlbi.nih.gov/guidelines/hypertension/jncintro.htm*].

14. Sacks FM and others: Effects on blood pressure of reduced dietary sodium and the Dietary Approaches to Stop Hypertension (DASH) diet, *N Engl J Med* 344:3, 2001.

15. Obarzanek E and others: Effects on blood lipids of a blood pressure-lowering diet: the Dietary Approaches to Stop Hypertension (DASH) trial, *Am J Clin Nutr* 74:80, 2001.

FURTHER READING AND RESOURCES

- American Heart Association: *www.americanheart.org*

- National Cholesterol Education Program: *www.nhlbi.nih. gov/chd/*

- National Center for Chronic Disease Prevention and Health Promotion, Cardiovascular health: *www.cdc.gov/cvh/index.htm*

   The organizations listed above are valuable sources of information on the most current recommendations for healthy lifestyles to prevent and treat heart disease. The web sites also provide educational materials for health care professionals.

- National Cholesterol Education Program (NCEP) Expert Panel on Detection, Evaluation, and Treatment of High Blood Cholesterol in Adults (Adult Treatment Panel III): Third Report of the NCEP Expert Panel on Detection, Evaluation, and Treatment of High Blood Pressure in Adults (Adult Treatment Panel III), *Circulation* 106:3143, 2002.

   As large-scale research studies continue to uncover the underlying factors associated with heart disease, the national recommendations for preventative measures are continually updated. This report outlines the most recent recommendations for preventing and treating high blood pressure.

20

Diabetes Mellitus

The Centers for Disease Control and Prevention estimates that 17 million Americans have diabetes, which accounts for 6.2% of the total population.[1] Diabetes is currently the sixth-ranking cause of death from disease in the United States.

Diabetes mellitus is an ancient disease. Historically, it claimed the lives of its victims at a young age. Greater knowledge of the disease and proper self-care practices have enabled persons with diabetes to live long and fruitful lives. For the most part, with professional guidance and support, persons with diabetes can remain healthy and reduce the risk of health problems by consistently practicing good self-care skills.

This chapter looks at diabetes to learn its nature and understand why daily self-care is essential for health.

KEY CONCEPTS

- Diabetes mellitus is a metabolic disorder of glucose metabolism with many causes and forms.

- A consistent, sound diet is the keystone of diabetes care and control.

- Good self-care skills practiced daily enable a person with diabetes to remain healthy and reduce risks for complications.

- A personalized care plan, balancing food intake, exercise, and insulin regulation, is essential to successful diabetes management.

THE NATURE OF DIABETES

Etiology of the Disease

Glucose is the primary, and preferred, source of energy for the body. As discussed in Chapter 2, carbohydrate foods break down during digestion and are absorbed into the blood stream mainly as glucose. That glucose is then transported throughout the body to be used as energy. However, for glucose to be used by the cells in the body, it first has to be taken out of the blood and into the cell. For this process to happen, the hormone insulin must be present. Insulin is produced by the β cells of the pancreas (see the For Further Focus box, "The History and Dis-covery of Insulin"). Individuals with diabetes either do not produce insulin or cannot effectively use the insulin produced. Without insulin, glucose accumulates in the blood stream. The Expert Committee on the Diagnosis and Classification of Diabetes Mellitus defines diabetes as "a group of metabolic diseases characterized by **hyper-glycemia** (elevated blood glucose) resulting from defects in insulin secretion, insulin action, or both."[2]

hyperglycemia (Gr. *hyper,* above; *glykys,* sweet) blood sugar elevated above normal limits.

FOR FURTHER FOCUS

THE HISTORY AND DISCOVERY OF INSULIN

Early History and Name

The symptoms of diabetes were described on an Egyptian papyrus, the Ebers Papyrus, which dates to about 1500 BC. In the first century, the Greek physician Areatus wrote of a malady in which the body "ate its own flesh" and gave off large quantities of urine. He named it *diabetes,* from the Greek word meaning "siphon" or "to pass through." In the seventeenth century, the word *mellitus,* from the Latin word meaning "honey," was added because of the sweet nature of the urine. The addition of *mellitus* distinguished the disorder from an-other disorder, *diabetes insipidus,* in which large urine out-put was also observed. However, diabetes insipidus is a much rarer and quite different disease that is caused by lack of the pituitary antidiuretic hormone (ADH). Today, the simple term *diabetes* refers to diabetes mellitus.

Diabetic Dark Ages

Throughout the Middle Ages and the dawning of our sci-entific era, many early scientists and physicians contin-ued to puzzle over the mystery of diabetes, but the cause remained obscure. For physicians and their patients these years could be called the "Diabetic Dark Ages." Pa-tients had short life spans and were maintained on a va-riety of semistarvation and high-fat diets.

Discovery of Insulin

The first breakthrough came from a clue pointing to the pancreas's involvement in the disease process. This clue was provided by a young German medical student, Paul Langerhans (1847 to 1888), who found special clusters of cells scattered about the pancreas forming little "islands" of cells. Although he did not yet understand their function, Langerhans could see that these cells were different from the rest of the tissue and assumed that they must be im-portant. When his suspicions later proved true, these little clusters of cells were named for their young discoverer, the *islands of Langerhans.* In 1922, using this important clue, two Canadian scientists, Frederick Banting and his assis-tant, Charles Best, together with two other research team members, physiologists J.B. Collip and J.J.R. Macleod, ex-tracted the first insulin from animals. It proved to be a hormone that regulates the oxidation of blood glucose and helps to convert it to heat and energy. They called the hor-mone *insulin,* from the Latin word *insula* meaning "island." Insulin did prove to be the effective agent for treating diabetes. The first child treated in January, 1922, Leonard Thompson, lived to adulthood but died at age 27, not from his diabetes but from coronary heart disease caused by the "diabetic diet" of the day, which was based on 70% of its total kcalories from fat! It is not surprising that his autopsy showed marked atherosclerosis.

Successful Use of Diet and Insulin

The insulin discovery team was more successful on their third try with a young girl diagnosed as having diabetes at age 11. She had initially been put on a starvation diet, and her weight fell from 75 to 45 pounds (34 to 21 kg) over a 3-year period. However, fortunately the medical research team had learned the importance of a well-balanced diet for normal growth and health. Thus with good diet and the new insulin therapy, this child, Elizabeth Hughes, gained weight and vigor and lived a normal life. She married, had three children, took insulin for 58 years, and died at age 73 of heart failure. No dia-betes has appeared among her immediate descendants.

BOX 20–1 Risk Factors for Type 2 Diabetes Mellitus

- A family history of diabetes
- Age 45 years or older
- Overweight (BMI ≥25 kg/m²)
- Not physically active on a regular basis
- Race/ethnicity (African American, Hispanic American, Native American, Asian American, and Pacific Islander)
- History of gestational diabetes
- Woman who has delivered an infant weighing more than 9 pounds
- Previously identified as *impaired glucose tolerance*

Classification of Diabetes Mellitus and Glucose Intolerance

There are various types of diabetes mellitus, which are dependent on the pathogenic process of the disease.

Type 1 Diabetes Mellitus

Type 1 diabetes mellitus accounts for 5% to 10% of all cases of diabetes. Previously called insulin-dependent diabetes or juvenile-onset diabetes, type 1 diabetes develops rapidly and tends to be more severe and unstable than other types of diabetes. This form of diabetes is caused by an autoimmune destruction of the β cells in

---

CULTURAL CONSIDERATIONS

RISK FACTORS FOR DIABETES: GENETIC VS. ENVIRONMENTAL

Type 2 diabetes has been known for years as "adult onset diabetes" because it rarely affected anyone under the age of 40. However, this form of diabetes is rapidly becoming a health care concern in children and adolescents. As with the occurrence of type 2 diabetes in adults, it has been reported mostly among minority populations. Pima Indian children have been diagnosed with type 2 diabetes as young as 3½ years of age. In an effort to define the contributing factors to increased prevalence of type 2 diabetes, researchers are considering in utero exposure to diabetes from mother to fetus and shared maternal-child environmental factors.

It is well accepted that there is a positive association between family history of type 2 diabetes and insulin resistance in adults. However, this association has not been fully researched in children with a family history. A recent study evaluated parental history and early-onset type 2 diabetes in African-American and Latino children in Chicago.* The average onset of type 2 diabetes in this study was 13.28 years, less than 5 years older than the average onset for type 1 diabetes in this same population. The authors concluded that children and adolescents with type 2 diabetes were more likely to have a positive parental history of diabetes in either or both parents than their type 1 diabetes counterparts. Yet, it is unclear if this association is caused by genetic or environmental factors.

A separate study by Goran and colleagues evaluated the influence of family history on insulin sensitivity in children.† The researchers in this study controlled for other factors known to increase the risk for type 2 diabetes (increased body fat, ethnicity, and onset of puberty). African-American, Hispanic, and Native American children have a higher risk for developing type 2 diabetes than Caucasian children. Although this was a small study (21 paired children), the results indicate that family history may not influence insulin resistance during childhood. Such findings indicate that the environmental factor associated within family settings could be more influential at this point of development in children than genetic factors.

Diabetes, impaired glucose tolerance, obesity and even cardiovascular disease are beginning to plague the children of American in a similar fashion as our adults. As research continues to uncover the pathophysiology, risk factors, and methods of prevention and treatment, hopefully this trend in disease progression will come to a halt. For a review on the current research about obesity and risk of type 2 diabetes and cardiovascular disease in children, Goran and colleagues recently published an excellent review (see references below).‡

*Onyemere KU, Lipton RB: Parental history and early-onset type 2 diabetes in African Americans and Latinos in Chicago, *J Pediatr* 141(6): 825, 2002.
†Goran MI and others: Influence of family history of type 2 diabetes on insulin sensitivity in prepubertal children, *J Clin Endocrinol Metab* 88(1):192, 2003.
‡Goran MI and others: Obesity and risk of type 2 diabetes and cardiovascular disease in children and adolescents, *J Clin Endocrinol Metab* 88(4):1417, 2003.

the pancreas. At least four different autoantibodies have been identified as the cause for destruction (islet cell autoantibodies, autoantibodies to insulin, autoantibodies to glutamic acid decarboxylase, and autoantibodies to the tyrosine phosphatases IA-2 and IA-2β). The rate of destruction determines the onset of diabetes. The initial onset of type 1 diabetes occurs rapidly in children and adolescences; hence, the old terminology of "juvenile-onset diabetes," but it can occur at any age. For some individuals, the rate of destruction is slower and may not present symptoms of diabetes until adulthood. Individuals with this type of diabetes rely on exogenous insulin for survival, which is where the old terminology of "insulin-dependent diabetes" came from. Persons with type 1 diabetes are usually underweight and at higher risk for acidosis.

Type 2 Diabetes Mellitus

Approximately 90% to 95% of the individuals with diabetes have type 2 diabetes. This form has a strong genetic link and is more prevalent in older, obese, inactive individuals.[3] Box 20-1 lists additional risk factors for the development of type 2 diabetes. Unlike type 1 diabetes, type 2 is not caused from an autoimmune response. This form of diabetes results from an insulin resistance or insulin defect—the body is either not pro-

ducing enough insulin or the insulin it is producing cannot be used. These individuals usually do not need exogenous insulin for survival, but rather rely on diet, exercise, and (usually) oral medications for disease management. This form of diabetes, previously called adult-onset or non–insulin-dependent diabetes, has an initial onset primarily in adults above age 40, but is now also being diagnosed in children.[4] As American children get heavier, the occurrence of type 2 diabetes in young people is on the rise (see the Cultural Considerations box, "Risk Factors for Diabetes: Genetic vs. Environmental"). Many adults and children with type 2 diabetes can improve or reduce their symptoms with weight loss and are maintained on diet therapy and balanced exercise programs alone. Table 20-1 summarizes the differences between type 1 and type 2 diabetes mellitus.

Gestational Diabetes

Gestational diabetes mellitus (GDM) is a temporary form of diabetes occurring during pregnancy, with normal blood glucose control usually regained after delivery. Women who have diabetes before conception (type 1 or 2) are considered to have pregestational diabetes and do not fall into this category during pregnancy. GDM can present complications for both mother and infant if not carefully monitored and controlled. Persistent hyper-

TABLE 20–1	**Differentiating Type 1 and Type 2 Diabetes Mellitus**	
Factor	**Type 1**	**Type 2**
Gender	Males and females	Increased rate among females
Ethnicity	Increased rates among persons with Northern European heritage	Increased rate among persons with heritage from equatorial countries; highest rates found with Native American, Hispanic, African-American, Asian, Pacific Islander, and Mediterranean heritage
Age of onset	Generally under 30 years of age, with peak onset before puberty	Generally over 40 years of age, although genetic predisposition is inherited and onset may be seen at younger ages
Weight	Usually normal or underweight; unintentional weight loss often precedes diagnosis	Usually overweight but may be of normal weight
Treatment	Insulin injections are necessary to prevent death; food and exercise have to be balanced with insulin injections	Weight loss is usually the first goal; reduction of sugar and fat and increase of fiber (soluble) are helpful. Oral hypoglycemic agents or insulin or both may be necessary for good blood glucose management but are not necessary to prevent imminent death. Exercise is important.
β cell* functioning	Totally absent (no insulin produced) after the "honeymoon period;" residual insulin produced for approximately 1 year after diagnosis	Excess insulin production is usually evident (hyperinsulinemia), but because of insulin resistance at the cell level, relative insulin insufficiency is present. Insulin production may also be normal or below normal.

From Peckenpaugh NJ: *Nutrition essentials and diet therapy,* ed 9, Philadelphia, 2003, Saunders.
*β cells are found in the pancreas.

glycemia is associated with an increased risk of intrauterine fetal death and **macrosomia.**

Approximately 7% of all pregnant women develop GDM.[5] Risk factors for GDM are the same as risk factors for type 2 diabetes (see Box 20-1). Women at high risk for developing GDM should be screened with a glucose tolerance test as soon as possible. Women who do not present multiple risk factors, but are at moderate risk, undergo screening at 24 to 28 weeks of gestation. The only women who are exempt from GMD screening are those who meet the following criteria:[5]

■ Less than 25 years of age
■ Healthy prepregnancy weight
■ Member of an ethnic group with a low prevalence of GDM (see Box 20-1 for high-risk ethnic groups)
■ No known diabetes in first-degree relatives
■ No history of abnormal glucose tolerance
■ No history of poor obstetric outcome

Screening for GDM should follow one of two approaches:

1. *One-step approach:* 100-g oral glucose tolerance test (OGTT). In this test, the patient is given a 100-g solution of glucose and then the venous blood glucose is measured at 1, 2, and 3 hours after administration of the glucose to monitor response. The test must be given in the morning after an overnight fast (8 to 14 hours of nothing to eat) and after at least 3 days of unrestricted diet and physical activity. If two or more of the following criteria are met, the individual is diagnosed with GDM:

   ■ Fasting glucose: ≥95 mg/dl
   ■ Glucose after 1 hour: ≥180 mg/dl
   ■ Glucose after 2 hours: ≥155 mg/dl
   ■ Glucose after 3 hours: ≥140 mg/dl

2. *Two-step approach:* 50 g oral glucose challenge test (GCT) and OGTT. The patient is first screened for glucose intolerance with the 50-g oral glucose challenge test (using the same protocol as for the 100-g OGTT) and if his or her blood glucose levels do not fall below 140 mg/dl within 1 hour after administration, an OGTT is then performed. The American Diabetes Association states that the threshold value of 140 mg/dl cutoff point identifies 80% of women with GDM.[5]

If a fasting plasma glucose test meets the general diagnostic criteria for diabetes (discussed further in this chapter under the section on general management of diabetes), a glucose tolerance test may not be necessary for diagnosis of GDM.

For women who develop gestational diabetes, their blood glucose levels are monitored carefully and they are taught to follow a tightly managed program of diet and self-testing of blood glucose levels, blood pressure, and urinary protein. For those women who are unable to maintain blood glucose levels within an acceptable range (≤95 mg/dl fasting, ≤140 mg/dl 1 hour postprandial, or ≤120 mg/dl 2 hours postprandial), insulin therapy is recommended. Complications of GDM for mother and child are greatly reduced, if not eliminated, by tight control of blood glucose levels.

Other Specific Types of Diabetes

Secondary diabetes may be caused by a number of conditions or agents affecting the pancreas. Examples include the following:

■ *Genetic defects.* Defects in the β cells or insulin action may result in several forms of diabetes.[2] These forms of diabetes are not characteristic of the autoimmune destruction found in type 1 diabetes. Mutations on at least three genetic loci have been identified, resulting in impaired insulin secretion (although not the action of the insulin). Other less common defects in the action of the insulin (but not the amount secreted) also result in hyperglycemia and diabetes. Two such syndromes identified in the pediatric population are Leprechaunism and Rabson-Mendenhall syndrome.[2]
■ *Pancreatic conditions or disease.* Any condition causing damage to the pancreatic cells can result in diabetes. Such conditions are: tumors affecting the islet cells, acute viral infection by a number of agents such as the mumps virus, acute pancreatitis from biliary disease and gallstones, chronic pancreatic insufficiency such as that which occurs in cystic fibrosis, pancreatic surgery as may occur in cancer of the pancreas, or severe traumatic abdominal injury. One of the most common causes of chronic pancreatitis is alcohol abuse.
■ *Endocrinopathies.* Insulin works in conjunction with several other hormones in the body. Hormones such as growth hormone, cortisol, glucagon, and epinephrine are all antagonistic to the functions of insulin. Therefore in disorders where excessive amounts of these antagonistic hormones are produced, the action of insulin is hindered and hyperglycemia ensues. **Cushing's syndrome,** hyperthyroidism, and **aldosteronoma** are examples of endocrinopathies that ultimately cause symptoms of diabetes. Usually, when the primary disorder (excessive antagonistic hormone secretion) is removed, the resulting hyperglycemia is resolved.

■ *Drug- or chemical-induced diabetes.* Certain drugs and toxins can impair insulin secretion or insulin action. The following drugs/toxins have been linked to impaired glucose tolerance and diabetes: pentamidine, nicotinic acid, glucocorticoids, thyroid hormone, diazoxide, thiazides, diazoxide, Dilantin, β-adrenergic agonist, and α-interferon.[2]

Impaired Glucose Tolerance

Individuals whose fasting blood glucose is above normal ($\geq$110 mg/dl), but not high enough for diagnosis of diabetes (<126 mg/dl), fall into the impaired glucose tolerance classification, also referred to as prediabetes. Impaired glucose tolerance (IGT) is a risk factor for developing type 2 diabetes. Treatment guidelines follow those designed for type 2 diabetes (later in this chapter) and can help prevent or prolong the progression into full-blown type 2 diabetes. Individuals with IGT often have a complicated assortment of underlying conditions (e.g., hypercholesterolemia, obesity, or hypertension) that build on one another to create the condition known as syndrome X, or metabolic syndrome, which is a significant risk factor for cardiovascular disease. See Table 19-2 for diagnostic criteria of metabolic syndrome.

Symptoms of Diabetes

Initial Signs

Early signs of diabetes include three primary symptoms: (1) increased thirst (*polydipsia*), (2) increased urination (*polyuria*), and (3) increased hunger (*polyphagia*). Unintentional weight loss may occur with type 1, or weight gain with type 2.

Laboratory Test Results

Various laboratory tests show the following results: *glycosuria* (sugar in the urine), *hyperglycemia* (elevated blood sugar), and abnormal glucose tolerance tests.

Other Possible Symptoms

Additional signs may include blurred vision, skin irritation or infection, and general weakness and loss of strength. In elderly persons with diabetes, the skin irritation may be perineal itching and the weakness may be general drowsiness.

Progressive Results

Continued symptoms may occur if the disease is left uncontrolled. These symptoms may include water and electrolyte imbalance, **ketoacidosis,** and coma.

THE METABOLIC PATTERN OF DIABETES

Energy Balance and Normal Blood Glucose Controls

Energy Balance

Diabetes has been called a disease of carbohydrate metabolism, but it is a general metabolic disorder involving all three of the energy nutrients—carbohydrate, fat, and protein. Diabetes is especially related to the metabolism of the two main fuels, carbohydrate and fat, in the body's overall energy system. The following three basic stages of normal glucose metabolism are illustrated in Figure 20-1:

1. Initial interchange with glycogen and reduction to a smaller central compound (*glycolysis pathway*)
2. Joining with the other two energy nutrients fat and protein (*pyruvate link*)
3. Final common energy production (*citric acid cycle*)

Normal Blood Glucose Balance

Control of blood glucose within its normal range of 70 to 110 mg/dl is important for general health. Normal control mechanisms ensure that people always have sufficient circulating blood sugar, glucose, to meet the constant energy needs—even the basal metabolic energy needs during sleep—because glucose is the body's preferred fuel. Note the balanced sources and uses of blood glucose as shown in Figure 20-2.

---

macrosomia   (Gr. *macro,* large; *sōma,* body) excessive fetal growth resulting in an abnormally large infant carrying high risk for perinatal mortality.

Cushing's syndrome   excess secretion of glucocorticoids from the adrenal cortex. Symptoms and complications include protein loss, obesity, fatigue, osteoporosis, edema, excess hair growth, diabetes, and skin discoloration.

aldosteronoma   excess secretion of aldosterone from the adrenal cortex. Symptoms and complications include sodium retention, potassium wasting (loss in the urine), alkalosis, weakness, paralysis, polyuria, polydipsia, hypertension, and cardiac arrhythmias.

ketoacidosis   excess production of ketones; a form of metabolic acidosis as occurs in uncontrolled diabetes or starvation from burning body fat for energy fuel; a continuing, uncontrolled state can result in coma and death.

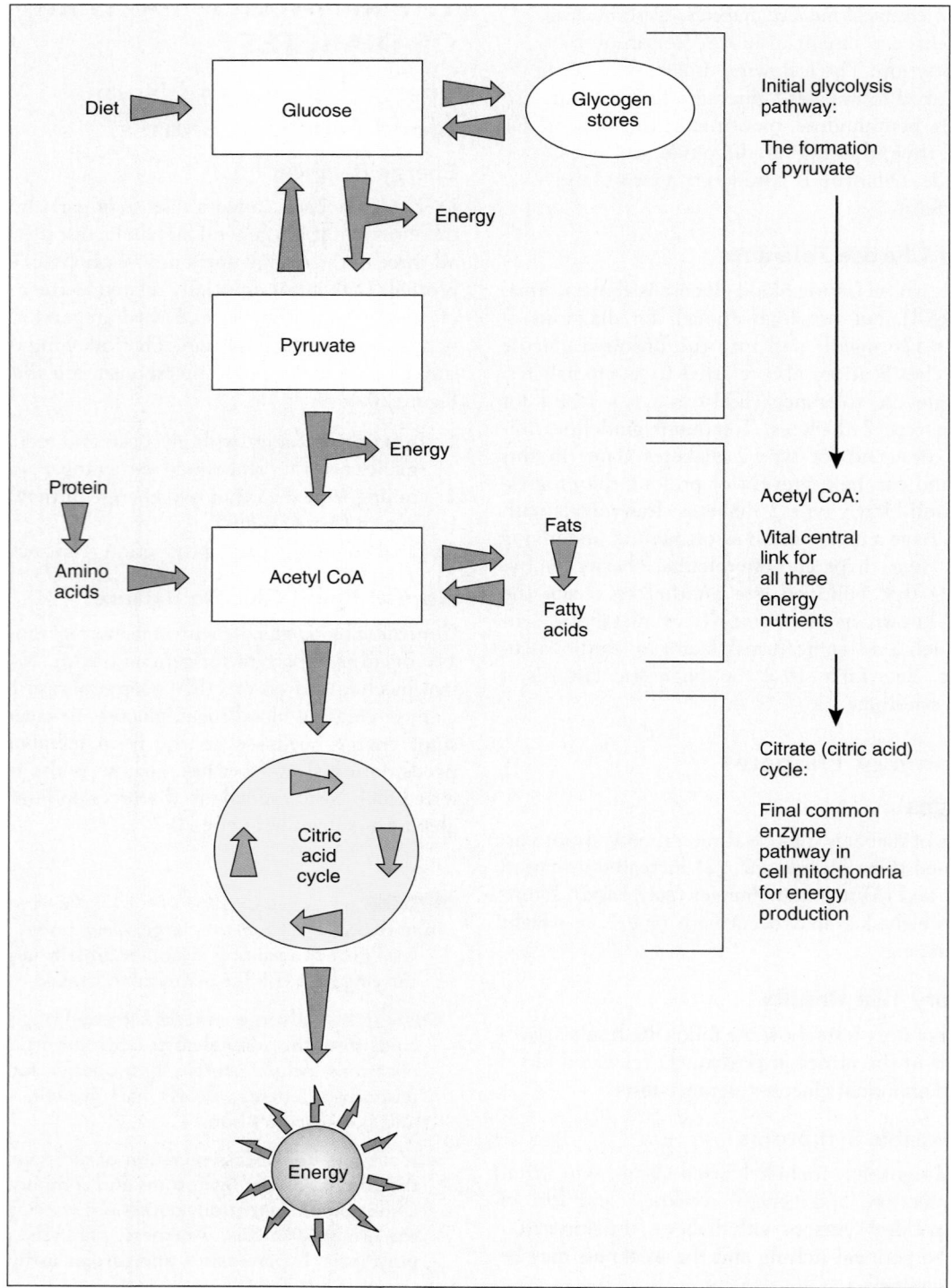

Figure 20–1   Basic glucose metabolism and interaction with fat and protein to yield energy.

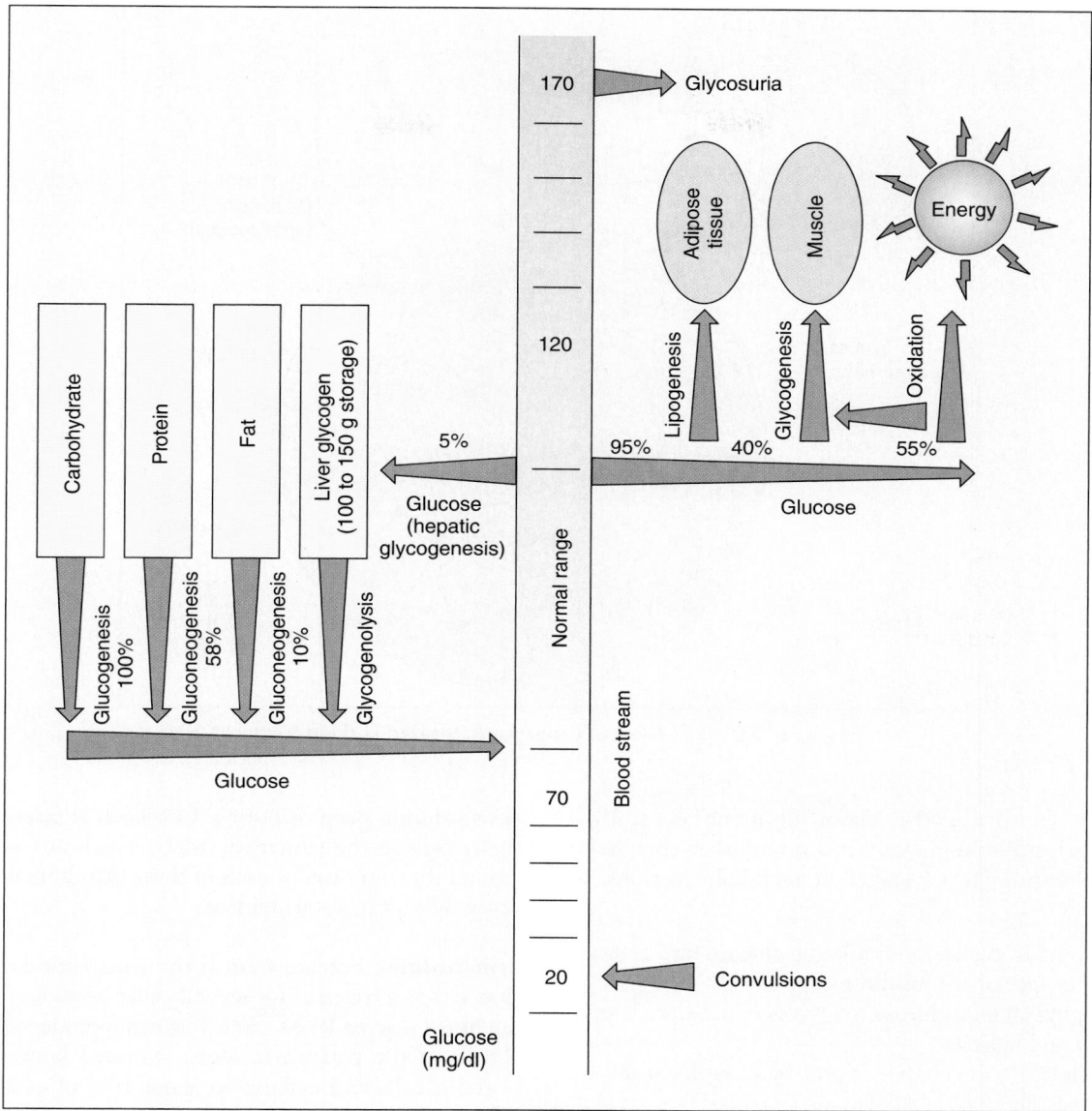

Figure 20–2   Sources of blood glucose (e.g., food and stored glycogen) and normal routes of control.

Sources of Blood Glucose. To ensure a constant supply of the body's main fuel, the following two sources of blood glucose exist:

1. *Diet.* The energy nutrients in food (e.g., dietary carbohydrate, fat, and, as needed, protein)
2. *Glycogen.* The back-up source from constant turnover of stored glycogen in liver and muscles

Uses of Blood Glucose. To prevent blood glucose from continually rising above a normal range, the body uses glucose as needed by (1) burning it by cell oxidation for

immediate energy needs; (2) changing it to glycogen, which is briefly stored in muscles and liver, then withdrawn and changed back into glucose for short-term energy needs; and (3) changing it to fat, which is stored for longer periods as body fat.

Pancreatic Hormonal Control

The specialized cells of the islets (islands) of Langerhans in the pancreas provide three hormones that work together to regulate blood glucose levels: (1) insulin, (2) glucagon, and (3) somatostatin. The specific arrangement of human islet cells is illustrated in Figure 20-3.

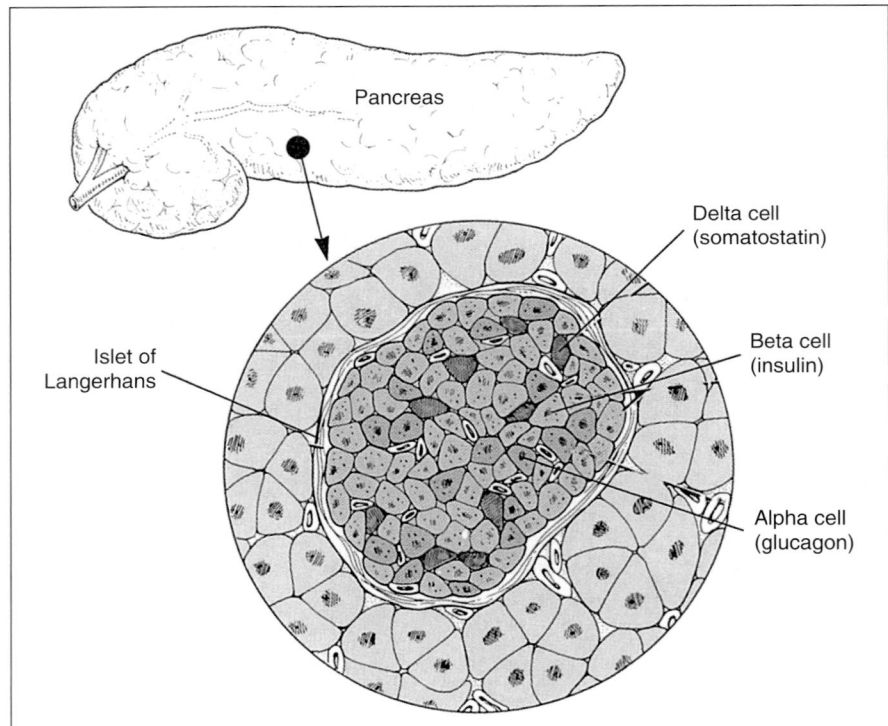

Figure 20–3   Islets of Langerhans, located in the pancreas.

Insulin. Insulin is the major hormone controlling the level of blood glucose. It accomplishes this major function through a number of metabolic actions, as follows:

■ Helping to transport circulating glucose into cells by way of specialized insulin receptors
■ Helping change glucose to glycogen and store it in liver and muscles
■ Stimulating the change of glucose to fat for storage as body fat
■ Inhibiting breakdown of tissue fat and protein
■ Promoting uptake of amino acids by skeletal muscles, increasing tissue protein synthesis
■ Influencing the burning of glucose for constant energy as needed

Insulin is produced in the β cells of the islets, which fill its central zone and make up about 60% of each islet gland.

Glucagon. Glucagon is a hormone that acts in an opposite manner of insulin to balance the overall blood glucose control. It can rapidly break down stored glycogen and, to a lesser extent, fat. This action raises blood glucose concentrations as needed to protect brain and other tissues during sleep or fasting. Glucagon is produced in the α cells of the pancreatic islets, which are arranged around the outer rim of each of these glands, making up about 30% of its total cell mass.

Somatostatin. Somatostatin is the pancreatic hormone that acts as a "referee" for several other hormones affecting blood glucose levels. Somatostatin is produced in the δ cells of the pancreatic islets, scattered between the α and β cells and making up about 10% of each islet's cells. Somatostatin inhibits the secretion of insulin, glucagon, and other gastrointestinal hormones such as gastrin and cholecystokinin. Because it has more generalized functions in the regulation of circulating blood glucose, somatostatin is also produced in other parts of the body (e.g., the hypothalamus).

Abnormal Metabolism in Uncontrolled Diabetes

When normal insulin activity is lacking, such as in uncontrolled diabetes, the normal controls for blood glucose levels do not function properly. As a result, abnormal metabolic changes and imbalances occur among the three energy nutrients.

Glucose

Glucose cannot enter cells for oxidation through its normal cell pathways to produce energy without the action of insulin. Thus it builds up in the blood, creating hyperglycemia.

Fat

In the absence of functioning insulin, fat tissue formation (*lipogenesis*) decreases, and fat tissue breakdown (*lipolysis*) increases. However, normal lipolysis requires an adequate supply of glucose, which in turn relies on the help of insulin to accept glucose into the cell. Therefore intermediate products of fat breakdown, called **ketones,** accumulate in the body. Increased fat breakdown leads to excess formation of ketones, causing ketoacidosis. The appearance of one of these ketones, **acetone,** in the urine indicates the adverse development of ketoacidosis.

Protein

Protein tissues are also broken down in the body's effort to secure energy sources, causing weight loss and urinary nitrogen loss.

Long-Term Complications

The long-term complications associated with diabetes are results of continuous hyperglycemia. These health problems mainly relate to tissue changes affecting blood vessels in vital organs. Individuals with good blood glucose control can avoid many such complications.

Retinopathy

Retinopathy involves small hemorrhages from broken arteries in the retina, with yellow, waxy discharge or retinal detachment. Diabetic retinopathy is the leading cause of new cases of blindness in adults.[1] The risk for retinopathy significantly increases with incessant hyperglycemia (fasting blood glucose ≥120 mg/dl). There are few warning signs of retinopathy; however, nearly all type 1 diabetic patients develop some degree of retinopathy and up to 21% of patients with type 2 diabetes have retinopathy at the time of diagnosis.[6] There are treatment modalities (laser photocoagulation therapy) that can prevent, or at least delay the onset, and thus ongoing eye evaluations are an important part of the care plan. The American Diabetes Association position statement on diabetic retinopathy recommends individuals with type 1 diabetes go for a first-time examination within 3 to 5 years after diagnosis and those with type 2 diabetes have their first examination at the time of diagnosis. Examinations should continue on a yearly basis from that point forward.[6] Retinopathy is not to be confused with the blurry vision that sometimes occurs as one of the first signs of diabetes. Blurry vision is caused by the increased glucose concentration in the fluids of the eye, bringing brief changes in the curved, light-refracting surface of the eye.

Nephropathy

Diabetes is the number one cause of end-stage renal disease in the United States.[1] Approximately 20% to 30% of diabetic patients develop some form of nephropathy, with a much higher prevalence in Native Americans, Hispanics, and African Americans than in non-Hispanic Caucasians.[7] As with retinopathy, nephropathy is exacerbated by poor blood glucose control. The primary symptom is microalbuminuria (low but abnormal levels of albumin in the urine). Nephropathy and end-stage renal disease cannot be cured, but with better blood glucose control and antihypertensive therapy, the disease progression can be slowed. Recommendations for screening are the same as for retinopathy, within 5 years of diagnosis for type 1 and at diagnosis for type 2 with annual follow-ups.

Neuropathy

Current statistics indicate that 60% to 70% of people with diabetes suffer mild to severe forms of nervous system damage.[1] These changes in the nerves involve injury and disease in the peripheral nervous system, especially in the legs and feet, causing prickly sensations, increasing pain, and eventual loss of sensation resulting from damaged nerves. The loss of nerve reaction can lead to further tissue damage and infection from unfelt foot injuries such

---

glucagon (Gr. *glykys,* sweet; *gonē,* seed) a hormone secreted by the a cells of the pancreatic islets of Langerhans in response to hypoglycemia; it has an opposite balancing effect to that of insulin, raising the blood glucose, and thus is used as a quick-acting antidote for a low blood glucose reaction of insulin. It also counteracts the overnight fast during sleep by breaking down liver glycogen to keep blood glucose levels normal and maintain an adequate energy supply for normal nerve and brain function.

ketones chemical name for a class of organic compounds, including three ketoacid bases that occur as intermediate products of fat metabolism, one of which is acetone.

acetone a major ketone compound that results from fat breakdown for energy in uncontrolled diabetes; persons with diabetes periodically do urinary acetone tests to monitor the status of their diabetes control.

as bruises, burns, and deeper cellulitis. Amputations and foot ulcerations are the most common results of severe neuropathy. The risk for such complications are increased for those individuals who have had diabetes for greater than 10 years, are male, have poor glucose control, or have cardiovascular, retinal, or renal complications.[8]

Heart Disease

Cardiovascular disease (CVD) is the major cause of death for persons with diabetes and occurs two to four times as often in persons with diabetes than in the general population.[1] The standards of medical care for individuals with diabetes include recommendations for the prevention and management of CVD, specifically aimed at blood lipid levels and blood pressure.[9] Glycemic control is not as strongly related to dyslipidemia and hypertension as it is to other long-term complications of diabetes (e.g., retinopathy, nephropathy, and neuropathy). However, the comorbid conditions greatly increase the risk of CVD and evaluation and treatment must be part of the overall health care plan for individuals with diabetes.

Dyslipidemia. Elevated triglyceride levels and decreased HDL cholesterol are characteristic of dyslipidemia in type 2 diabetic patients. Management of dyslipidemia is prioritized as: (1) lower low-density lipoprotein (LDL) cholesterol, (2) raise high-density lipoprotein (HDL) cholesterol, and (3) lower triglycerides. Recommendations for lipid profiles for adults with diabetes are as follows:[10]

■ LDL cholesterol: <100 mg/dl
■ HDL cholesterol: >40 mg/dl for men and >50 mg/dl for women
■ Triglycerides: <150 mg/dl

Hypertension. Depending on other risk factors, such as obesity, ethnicity, and age, hypertension affects between 20% and 60% of individuals with diabetes and is a major comorbid complication.[11] The risk for CVD is doubled for people with both diabetes and hypertension, making blood pressure evaluation and treatment an important part of the health care plan. The recommendation for blood pressure in adults with diabetes is a blood pressure of less than 130/80 mmHg.

GENERAL MANAGEMENT OF DIABETES

Early Detection and Monitoring

The guiding principles for the treatment of diabetes are early detection and prevention of complications. Community screening programs and testing of family members help

to identify persons with elevated blood glucose levels who may benefit from a *glucose tolerance test* (e.g., fasting and 2-hour tests with a measured glucose dose) and medical evaluation. An additional monitoring aid is the glycosylated *hemoglobin* A_{1c} assay (normal range 4% to 6%), which provides an effective tool for evaluating long-term management of diabetes and degree of control. This test reflects the level of blood glucose over the preceding 3-month period of time because the glucose attaches itself to the hemoglobin molecule over the life of the red blood cell. Other tests such as *fructosamine* (an amino sugar formed from glucosamine) or *C-peptide* (an antibody radioimmunoassay after a special test meal to determine the type of diabetes) sometimes may be used for diagnostic purposes. However, the glycosylated hemoglobin assay, HbA_{1c}, is currently the most accurate assessment for monitoring ongoing blood glucose control. Box 20-2 outlines the criteria for diagnosis of diabetes mellitus, and Table 20-2 gives the correlation between HbA_{1c} values and plasma glucose.

Basic Goals of Care

General Overall Objectives

The health care team is guided by three basic objectives when working with a person with diabetes.

Maintaining Optimal Nutrition. The first objective is to sustain a high level of nutrition for general health promotion, adequate growth and development, and maintenance of an appropriate lean weight.

Avoiding Symptoms. This objective seeks to keep a person relatively free from symptoms of *hyperglycemia* and *glycosuria*, which indicate poor control.

Preventing Complications. This third objective recognizes the increased risk a person with diabetes carries for developing the significant tissue changes already described. Consistent control of blood glucose levels helps to reduce these risks.

Special Objectives in Pregnancy

When a woman with diabetes becomes pregnant or the pregnancy induces gestational diabetes, her body metabolism changes to meet the increased physiologic needs of the pregnancy while battling the manifestations of diabetes (see Chapter 10). A team of specialists usually works closely with the mother. Careful team monitoring of the mother's diabetes management is essential to ensure her health and the health of her baby. Potential problems of fetal damage, perinatal mortality, stillbirth, prematurity, or delivery of a very large baby (*macrosomia*) are serious concerns during this time.

BOX 20-2 Criteria for the Diagnosis of Diabetes Mellitus

1. Symptoms of diabetes plus casual plasma glucose concentration ≥200 mg/dl
   Casual is defined as any time of day without regard to time since last meal. The classic symptoms of diabetes include polyuria, polydipsia, and unexplained weight loss.
2. *Fasting* plasma glucose ≥126 mg/dl
   Fasting is defined as no caloric intake for at least 8 hours.
3. Two-hour plasma glucose ≥200 mg/dl during an oral glucose tolerance test (OGTT)
   The OGTT should be performed using a glucose load equivalent of 75 g anhydrous glucose dissolved in water.

Note: In the absence of unequivocal hyperglycemia with acute metabolic decompensation, these criteria should be confirmed by repeat testing on a different day. The third measure (OGTT) is not recommended for routine clinical use.
From The Expert Committee on the Diagnosis and Classification of Diabetes Mellitus: Report of the Expert Committee on the Diagnosis and Classification of Diabetes Mellitus, *Diabetes Care* 26 (1 suppl):55, 2003. Copyright American Diabetes Association.

TABLE 20-2 Correlation between HbA$_{1c}$ and Plasma Glucose Levels

HbA$_{1c}$	Mean plasma glucose	
	mg/dl	mmol/l
6	135	7.5
7	170	9.5
8	205	11.5
9	240	13.5
10	275	15.5
11	310	17.5
12	345	19.5

Basic Elements of Diabetes Management

Balancing three basic elements is essential in good control of diabetes. First, the healthy *diet* described here forms the foundation for good management. Second, physical *exercise* provides the important balance to maintain good blood glucose control. Third, to ensure adequate insulin activity, some persons need *drugs* (e.g., insulin injections or oral hypoglycemic agents). However, a fourth element, *stress-coping skills*, may well be added in today's stressful world.

Importance of Good Self-Care Skills

To accomplish these objectives, a person with diabetes must learn and regularly practice good self-care. Daily self-discipline and informed self-care are necessary for sound diabetes management because all persons with diabetes must ultimately treat themselves, with the support of a good health care team. More emphasis is now being given to comprehensive diabetes education programs that encourage self-monitoring of blood glucose levels and more self-care responsibility.

DIET THERAPY FOR INDIVIDUALS WITH DIABETES

The Diabetes Control and Complications Trial

Based on the need for a more comprehensive program of care for diabetes, a large-scale United States clinical research study supported by the National Institutes of Health was conducted. This project (the Diabetes Control and Complications Trial [DCCT]), compared the effects of intensive insulin therapy aimed at achieving blood glucose levels as close as possible to the normal nondiabetic range with the effects of conventional therapy on early microvascular complications of type 1 diabetes mellitus. The positive results of this important study, supported by both the American Dietetic Association and the American Diabetic Association, remain highly significant. There was a decrease of approximately 60% in risk of retinopathy, nephropathy, and neuropathy with the individuals who underwent intensive treatment and rigorous control of blood glucose levels.[12] Results from DCCT confirmed the association between long-term complications of diabetes and blood glucose control and provided support for the development of the current standards of medical care.

Application in Clinical Practice

Revised Recommendations

Based on the remarkable positive research results, the American Diabetes Association issued a revised position paper in January 2003 on nutrition recommendations and principles of care for persons with diabetes mellitus.[9] These guidelines defined the goal of medical nutrition therapy as: to assist patients with diabetes in making changes in nutrition and exercise habits in balance with insulin from both internal or external sources.

cellulitis diffuse inflammation of soft or connective tissues (e.g., in the foot) from injury, bruises, or pressure sores that lead to infection; poor care may result in ulceration and abscess or gangrene.

Core Problem

The primary focus in diabetes care is glycemic control, the regulation of the body's primary fuel, blood glucose. Based on the concept of balance, three main principles of nutrition therapy are as follows:

1. Total energy balance
2. Nutrient balance
3. Food distribution balance

Personal diet is then expressed in terms of the following:

1. Total kcalories necessary for energy balance
2. Ratio of these kcalories in relative amounts of the three energy nutrients: carbohydrate, fat, and protein
3. A food distribution pattern for the day

A fundamental personal principle underlies the whole plan. The diet for any person with diabetes is always based on the normal nutritional needs of that person for positive health.

Total Energy Balance

Normal Growth and Weight Management

Because type 1 diabetes usually begins in childhood (typically before puberty), the normal height-weight charts for children provide a standard for adequate growth. During adulthood, maintaining a lean weight continues to be a basic goal. Because type 2 diabetes usually occurs in overweight adults, the major goal is weight reduction and control.

Energy Intake

The total energy value of the diet for a person with diabetes should be sufficient to meet individual needs for normal growth and development, physical activity and exercise, and maintenance of a desirable lean weight. Exercise is always an important factor in diabetes control because it improves the body's ability to use glucose by increasing insulin-receptor sites in the tissues. Energy intake in the diet is constantly balanced with energy output in work and exercise and metabolic body work. The Recommended Dietary Allowance (RDA) and Dietary Reference Intakes (DRI) standards for children and adults (see front of book) can serve as guides for total energy needs, with appropriate reductions in kilocalories for overweight adults, as described in Chapter 15.

Nutrient Balance

The ratio of carbohydrate, fat, and protein in the diet is based on current recommendations for ideal glucose reg-

ulation and lower fat intake to reduce risks of cardiovascular complications. Carbohydrate and monounsaturated fat intake should provide 60% to 70% of the total energy intake with protein and other sources of fat providing the rest.

Carbohydrate

Starch and Sugar. In years past it was thought that ingestion of simple sugars resulted in a more profound increase in blood glucose levels than ingestion of complex carbohydrates. However, recent research evaluating the *glycemic index* (GI) of carbohydrate foods indicates that starchy foods greatly differ from one another in their ability to raise plasma glucose levels, thus contradicting the notion that all complex carbohydrates are created equal.[13] A food's glycemic index is determined by measuring the increase in blood glucose after ingestion of a 50-g carbohydrate sample of the food compared with a 50-g sample from a known source, usually white bread or pure glucose. The rate of digestion and absorption determine the GI value. Although it is clear that carbohydrates differ in their ability to raise blood glucose, there is no clear trend separating simple sugars from complex carbohydrates. For example, potatoes and white bread—both complex carbohydrates—have a similar GI to pure glucose. Current recommendations for carbohydrate intake are based on studies in which the glycemic response of individuals with diabetes was not significantly different when consuming either complex carbohydrates or simple sugars, as long as the total amount of carbohydrate was the same.[14]

Fiber. As with all people, consumption of dietary fiber is encouraged for a healthy diet. There are no reasons for individuals with diabetes to consume greater amounts than the general public.

Sugar Substitute Sweeteners. Nutritive and nonnutritive sweeteners may be used in the diet in moderation. Various sugar substitutes are available. Approved noncaloric sweeteners include products such as saccharin, aspartame, acesulfame-K, and sucralose. Aspartame is made from two amino acids, phenylalanine and aspartic acid, and is metabolized as such. Small amounts of caloric sweeteners, such as the very small amounts of sucrose, fructose, and sorbitol must be accounted for in a meal. However, many persons cannot tolerate sorbitol and have significant diarrhea when it is used. In summary, nutritive and nonnutritive sweeteners are safe to consume in moderation and as part of a nutritious and well-balanced diet.

Guidelines for carbohydrate intake are based on the following recommendations from the American Diabetes Association position statement:[14]

■ Foods containing carbohydrate from whole grains, fruits, vegetables, and low-fat milk should be included in a healthy diet.
■ With regard to the glycemic effects of carbohydrates, the total amount of carbohydrate in meals or snacks is more important than the source or type.
■ Because sucrose does not increase glycemia to a greater extent than isocaloric amounts of starch, sucrose and sucrose-containing foods should not be restricted in people with diabetes; however, they should be substituted for other carbohydrate sources or, if added, covered with insulin or other glucose-lowering medication.
■ Nonnutritive sweeteners are safe when consumed within the acceptable daily intake levels established by the Food and Drug Administration.

Protein

Most Americans eat much more protein than they need. Normal age requirements as outlined in the DRI standards can be a guide for protein intake. In general, approximately 15% to 20% of the total energy as protein is sufficient to meet growth needs in children and maintain tissue integrity in adults. High protein intakes generally are not recommended because of their saturated fat content and unnecessary stress on the kidneys to excrete excess nitrogen.

Fat

No more than 25% to 30% of the diet's total kcalories should come from fat, with saturated fat (animal fat) composing less than 10%. Lower cholesterol intake—no more than 300 mg/day—also is recommended. Control of fat-related foods, which contribute to the development of atherosclerosis and coronary heart disease, helps reduce the increased risk for CVD. Individuals with elevated LDL cholesterol are recommended to limit saturated fat intake to less than 7% of total energy intake and cholesterol to less than 200 mg/day.[14]

Food Distribution Balance

As a general rule, fairly even amounts of food should be eaten at regular intervals throughout the day, adjusted to blood glucose self-monitoring. This basic pattern helps provide a more even blood glucose supply and prevent swings between low and high levels. Snacks between meals may be needed.

Daily Activity Schedule

Food distribution must be planned ahead, especially by persons using insulin, and adjusted according to each day's scheduled activities and blood glucose monitoring to prevent episodes of hypoglycemia from insulin reactions. Careful distribution of food and snacks is especially important for children and adolescents with diabetes to balance with insulin during growth spurts and changing hormone patterns of puberty. Practical consideration should be given to school and work schedules and demands, athletics, social events, and stress periods. A stressful event caused by any source (e.g., injury, anxiety, fear, or pain) brings an adrenaline (epinephrine) rush, which is the common "fight-or-flight" effect that counteracts insulin activity and can contribute to a glycemic response.

Exercise

For persons using insulin, it is especially important that any exercise or additional physical activity is covered in the food distribution plan (Table 20-3). The energy demands of exercise are discussed in Chapter 16.

The American Diabetes Association position statement on physical activity/exercise and diabetes recommends the following guidelines for regulating the glycemic response to exercise:[15]

1. Achieve metabolic control before physical activity.
   a. Avoid physical activity if fasting glucose levels are higher than 250 mg/dl and ketosis is present, and use caution if glucose levels are higher than 300 mg/dl and no ketosis is present.
   b. Ingest added carbohydrate if glucose levels are less than 100 mg/dl.
2. Monitor blood glucose before and after physical activity.
   a. Identify when changes in insulin or food intake are necessary.
   b. Learn the glycemic response to different physical activity conditions.
3. Monitor food intake.
   a. Consume added carbohydrate as needed to avoid hypoglycemia.
   b. Carbohydrate-based foods should be readily available during and after physical activity.

For adults with type 2 diabetes, regular exercise is an essential part of successful weight-management and glucose control programs. Long-term studies have found regular, moderate-intensity exercise programs help individuals with type 2 diabetes control blood glucose and reduce the risk of cardiovascular disease, hyperlipidemia, hypertension, and obesity.

TABLE 20-3	Meal-Planning Guide for Active People with Type 1 Diabetes	
Activity level	**Exchange needs**	**Sample menus**
MODERATE		
30 minutes	1 bread	1 bran muffin
	or	*or*
	1 fruit	1 small orange
1 hour	2 bread + 1 meat	Tuna sandwich
	or	*or*
	2 fruit + 1 milk	½ cup fruit salad + 1 cup milk
STRENUOUS		
30 minutes	2 fruit	1 small banana
	or	*or*
	1 bread + 1 fat	½ bagel + 1 tsp cream cheese
1 hour	2 bread + 1 meat + 1 milk	Meat and cheese sandwich + 1 cup milk
	or	*or*
	2 bread + 2 meat + 2 fruit	Hamburger + 1 cup orange juice

Drug Therapy

The food distribution pattern also is influenced by any form of drug therapy (type, amount, and dose schedule of insulin or oral hypoglycemic agent) that is necessary for control of the diabetes.

Diet Management

General Planning according to Type of Diabetes

Because forms of diabetes vary widely, the nature of an individual's diabetes and its treatment regime largely determine the necessary personal diet management. Table 20-4 provides guidelines for diet strategies necessary for each of the two main types of diabetes, types 1 and 2.

Individual Needs

Every person with diabetes is unique, having not only a particular form and degree of diabetes but also a different living situation, background, and food habits. All of these personal needs must be considered, as discussed in Chapters 14 and 17, if appropriate and realistic care is to be planned. The nutrition counselor, who is usually the clinical dietitian, always seeks to discover these various individual needs in a careful initial nutrition assessment that includes medical and psychosocial needs, as well as personal lifestyle characteristics. This information provides the basis for determining the diet prescription and calculating nutritional requirements. A personal diet plan using the balance principles described here then can be outlined.

A major principle of diabetes management is the variety of methods and dietary guidelines that the clinical dietitian, assisted by the nutrition team, can use in planning and supporting patients. Among these various dietary guides, the familiar food exchange method, tailored to meet individual needs, remains a commonly used approach. Materials used in the variable research methods are available from the American Dietetic Association and the American Diabetes Association.

Food Exchange System

The dietitian uses this familiar tool to calculate the patient's energy and nutrient needs, as well as to distribute foods in a balanced meal/snack pattern. The food exchange system is so called because persons with diabetes use the system to select a variety of foods from the various food groups according to their personal food plan.

In this system, commonly used foods are grouped into three basic *exchange lists* according to roughly equal food values in the portions indicated. Thus a variety of foods may be chosen from these lists to fulfill the basic food plan, while the basic diet prescription of total energy and balanced ratio of nutrients is maintained. The designated food values for each of the food exchange groups are shown in Table 20-5. The booklet "Exchange Lists for Meal Planning" is available from both the American Diabetes Association and the American Dietetic Association. Its colorful illustrations, clear content, and style provide a helpful tool for patient and client education. These exchange lists are included in Appendix F. Table 20-6 illustrates a calculated 2200-kcal diet and

TABLE 20–4 Dietary Strategies for Type 1 and Type 2 Diabetes Mellitus

Dietary strategy	Type 1	Type 2
Decrease energy intake (kcalories)	No	Yes, if weight loss is recommended
Increase frequency and number of feedings	Yes	Usually no
Have regular daily intake of kcalories from carbohydrate, protein, and fat	Very important	Yes
Plan consistent daily ratio of protein, carbohydrate, and fat for each feeding	Desirable	Yes, but not as tightly controlled
Use extra or planned food to treat or prevent hypoglycemia	Very important	Usually not necessary
Plan regular times for meals and snacks	Very important	Yes
Use extra food for unusual exercise	Yes	Usually not necessary
During illness, use small, frequent feedings of carbohydrates to prevent starvation ketoacidosis	Important	Usually not necessary because of resistance to ketoacidosis

TABLE 20–5 Amount of Nutrients in One Serving from Each Exchange List

Groups/lists	Carbohydrate (g)	Protein (g)	Fat (g)	Kilocalories
CARBOHYDRATE GROUP				
Starch	15	3	0-1	80
Fruit	15	—	—	60
Milk				
Fat-free	12	8	0-3	90
Reduced-fat	12	8	5	120
Whole	12	8	8	150
Other carbohydrates	15	Varies	Varies	Varies
Vegetables	5	2	—	25
MEAT AND MEAT SUBSTITUTE GROUP				
Very lean	—	7	0-1	35
Lean	—	7	3	55
Medium-fat	—	7	5	75
High-fat	—	7	8	100
FAT GROUP	—	—	5	45

Data from American Diabetes Association, American Dietetic Association: *Exchange lists for meal planning,* Alexandria, VA; Chicago, 2003, ADA/ADA.

resulting food pattern using the exchange system, whereas Box 20-3 outlines a sample menu based on this food pattern.

Special Concerns

Special concerns come up in daily living and become an important part of ongoing dietary counseling. Some suggestions for these concerns are given here.

Special Diet Food Items. Little need exists for special "dietetic" or "diabetic" foods. Persons with diabetes should eat the regular, well-balanced diet (e.g., modified in the same areas of fat, cholesterol, sugar, fiber, and salt) that is recommended for the general population to promote health and prevent disease. This kind of a healthful diet primarily uses regular fresh foods from all the basic food groups, with limited use of processed foods (noting the grams of carbohydrate per serving on the label) and more use of nonfat seasonings. The simple principles of moderation and variety guide food choices and amounts.

Alcohol. Occasional use of alcohol in an adult diabetic diet can be planned, but caution must be the guide. Individuals with type 1 diabetes who consume alcohol must be reminded of the following: (1) to eat when they drink, because food slows alcohol absorption; and (2) to not in-

TABLE 20–6   Calculation of Diabetic Diet Using Exchange System (2200 kcal)

Food group	Total day's exchanges	Carbohydrates: 275 g (50% kcal)	Protein: 110 g (20% kcal)	Fat: 75 g (30% kcal)	Breakfast	Lunch	Dinner	Snacks Afternoon	Snacks Bedtime
CARBOHYDRATES									
Fruit	3	45	—	—	1	1	1	1	—
Vegetable	4	20	8	—	—	2	2	—	—
Other carbohydrates	1	15	Varies	Varies	—	—	1	—	—
Milk									
Fat-free	2	24	16	—	1	—	—	—	1
Reduced fat	—	—	—	—	—	—	—	—	—
Whole	—	—	—	—	—	—	—	—	—
Starch	11.5	172	34.5	—	3	3	3	1	1.5
MEAT AND MEAT SUBSTITUTES									
Very lean	2	—	14	0-1	—	—	—	1	1
Lean	3	—	21	9	—	—	3	—	—
Medium-fat	2	—	14	10	1	1	—	—	—
High-fat	—	—	—	—	—	—	—	—	—
FAT	11	—	—	55	3	3	3	1	1
TOTAL GRAMS		276	107.5	75					

BOX 20–3 Sample Menu Prescription: 2200 kcal

275 g carbohydrate (50% kcal)
110 g protein (20% kcal)
75 g fat (30% kcal)

Breakfast

1 medium, sliced fresh peach
Shredded wheat cereal
1 poached egg on whole-grain toast
1 bran muffin
1 tsp margarine
1 cup low-fat milk
Coffee or tea

Lunch

Vegetable soup with wheat crackers
Tuna sandwich on whole wheat bread
    Filling: Tuna (½ cup, drained)
          Mayonnaise (2 tsp)
          Chopped dill pickle
          Chopped celery
Fresh pear

Afternoon Snack

10 crackers with 2 Tbsp peanut butter
Orange

Dinner

Pan-broiled pork chop (well-trimmed)
1 cup brown rice
½ to 1 cup green beans
Tossed green salad
   Italian dressing (1 to 2 Tbsp)
½ cup applesauce
1 bran muffin

Evening Snack

3 cups popped, plain popcorn
1 oz cheese
1 cup low-fat milk

---

crease insulin dose because the overall effect of alcohol is to lower the blood glucose level. Occasional use is defined as moderate intake (e.g., less than 6% of the total energy on a given day) and not more than 1 or 2 equivalent portions once or twice a week. An equivalent portion is 1 oz of liquor, 4 oz of wine, or 12 oz of beer. The same precautions for the use of alcohol that apply to the general public apply to people with diabetes. When a person with type 1 diabetes uses a small amount of alcohol, it should *not* be substituted for food exchanges in the diet, but only used in addition, to avoid the possibility of hypoglycemic reactions. Alcohol may be used in cooking as desired because it vaporizes in the cooking process and only contributes its flavor to the finished product.

Hypoglycemia. Persons with diabetes must learn how to avoid **hypoglycemia,** low blood glucose levels. The body's vital "brain food" is glucose. The brain depends on a constant supply of glucose for metabolism and proper func-

tion; a prolonged lack of glucose can lead to permanent brain damage. Hypoglycemia can occur from too high a dose of insulin, or from hypoglycemic oral drugs that act by stimulating the islet cells in the pancreas to secrete more insulin. Hypoglycemia also can occur if a person with diabetes delays a meal or snack, does not eat enough carbohydrate, or exercises too much without sufficient food. Table 20-7 lists symptoms of both hyperglycemia and hypoglycemia. Because behavior is often irrational

---

hypoglycemia (Gr. *hypo-*, below; *glykys,* sweet) low blood glucose; a serious condition in insulin-dependent diabetes management that requires immediate sugar intake to counteract, followed by a snack of complex carbohydrate food (e.g., bread or crackers) and a protein (e.g., lean meat, peanut butter, or cheese) to maintain the normal blood glucose.

TABLE 20-7	Symptoms of Hyperglycemia and Hypoglycemia	
Factor	Hyperglycemia (high blood glucose)	Hypoglycemia (low blood glucose)
Cause	Too much food, not enough insulin, illness, or stress	Not enough food, too much insulin, or too much exercise
Onset	Gradual	
Symptoms	Polydipsia*	Sudden shaking
	Polyuria†	Rapid heartbeat
	Polyphagia‡	Sweating
	Dry skin	Anxiety and irritability
	Blurred vision	Dizziness
	Drowsiness	Polyphagia
	Nausea	Impaired vision
		Weakness
		Headache

*Polydipsia = extreme thirst.
†Polyuria = frequent urination.
‡Polyphagia = excessive hunger.

and movements are uncoordinated, this state may be mistaken for drunkenness, and the person may lapse into coma. Thus an identification bracelet or pendant is an important means of informing others of the true condition so that proper treatment—a glucose replacement in food or beverage or an injection of glucagon—can be given. Note the 15-g carbohydrate-replacement portions listed in the Bread/Cereal (starch) and Fruit exchange groups (see Table 20-5 and Appendix F). Persons with type 1 diabetes should always carry a convenient form of sugar (e.g., sugar lumps or glucose tablets) with them to take at the first sign of a hypoglycemic attack, and then follow this sugar as soon as possible with a snack of complex carbohydrate and protein.

Illness. When general illness occurs, food and insulin should be adjusted accordingly. The texture of the food can be modified to use easily digested and absorbed liquid foods (Table 20-8). This type of liquid substitution can be used for meals not eaten. In general, persons with diabetes who are ill should do the following:

- Maintain food intake every day, not skipping meals.
- Do not omit insulin but follow an adjusted dosage if needed.
- Replace carbohydrate solid foods with equal liquid or soft foods.

- Monitor blood glucose level frequently.
- Contact physician if the illness lasts more than a couple of days.

Travel. When a trip is planned, the diet counselor and the client should confer to decide on food choices, depending on what will be available to the traveler. In general, preparation activities can include the following:

- Review meal planning skills, the number and type of exchanges at each meal, basic portion sizes, and tips on eating out.
- Learn about foods that will be available (e.g., ordering a diabetic diet ahead from airlines).
- Select appropriate snacks to carry and plan time intervals for their use.
- Plan for any time-zone changes.
- Carry some quick-acting form of carbohydrate at all times and tell companions about signs, symptoms, and treatment of hypoglycemia.
- Wear an identification bracelet or pendant.
- Secure a physician's cover letter concerning syringes and insulin prescription.

Eating Out. In general, persons with diabetes should plan ahead so that food eaten at home before and after a meal out can be accommodated to maintain the continuing day's balance. Choosing restaurants that have the appropriate food available also makes menu selection easier.

Stress. Any form of physiologic or psychosocial stress affects diabetes control because of the hormonal responses that are antagonistic to insulin action. Persons with diabetes, especially those using insulin, should learn useful stress-reduction exercises and activities as part of their self-care skills and practices.

DIABETES EDUCATION PROGRAM

Goal: Person-Centered Self-Care

In the past few years, the traditional roles of health care professionals and their patients and clients have been changing. Patients and clients are taking a much more active and informed role in their own health care. This action is especially true in the case of persons with diabetes. By the nature of the disease process and the necessity of daily "survival" skills, persons with diabetes must practice regular, daily self-care (see the Clinical Applications box, "Case Study: Richard

TABLE 20–8	Modifying a Diabetic Meal Plan for Illness	
Food intake	**Exchange**	**Carbohydrate (g)**
USUAL INTAKE		
½ chicken breast, roasted	3 meat	0
1 tsp margarine	1 fat	0
½ cup rice	1 bread	15
Tossed green salad, lemon wedge	Free food	0
¾ cup strawberries	1 fruit	10
1 cup skim milk	1 milk	12
TOTAL		37
SICK-DAY INTAKE*		
2 cups broth	Free food	0
1 cup gelatin	1 other carbohydrate	15
1 cup ginger ale (regular)	1 other carbohydrate	15
2 cups herbal tea	Free food	0
TOTAL		30

*Objective: To provide adequate amounts of carbohydrate for times when the person with diabetes has a poor appetite.

CLINICAL APPLICATIONS

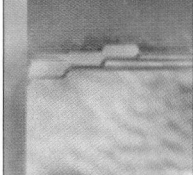

CASE STUDY: RICHARD MANAGES HIS DIABETES

Richard Smith, age 21, has type 1 diabetes mellitus. He gives himself two injections a day, each a combination of medium-acting insulin and regular short-acting insulin. He does one injection before breakfast and one before dinner and usually tests his blood glucose level before each meal and at bedtime. Richard is a college student, who is usually active in athletics.

However, this is final exam week and Richard's schedule is irregular. He is putting in long hours of study and is under considerable stress. On the day before a particularly difficult examination, he is reviewing his study materials at home and forgets to do his blood test or eat lunch. About mid-afternoon, he begins to feel faint and realizes that his blood glucose is low and an insulin reaction is imminent if he does not get a quick source of energy. He looks in the kitchen, and all he can find is orange juice, milk, butter, a loaf of bread, and a jar of peanut butter.

Questions for Analysis

1. Which of the foods should Richard eat immediately? Why?

2. Later, when he is feeling better, Richard makes a peanut butter and butter sandwich, pours a glass of milk, and eats his snack while he continues studying. What carbohydrate food sources of energy are in his snack?

3. Are these carbohydrate sources in a form that the cells can burn for energy? What changes must Richard's body make in these sources to get them into the basic carbohydrate fuel form? What is the complex form of carbohydrate in his snack? Why is this a valuable form of carbohydrate in his diet? What is the basic form of carbohydrate fuel circulating in the blood for use by the cells?

4. What is the relationship of carbohydrate and fat in the final production of energy in the body? If Richard did not take his insulin to provide the necessary control agent for metabolizing the carbohydrate, what would happen to him as the result of improper handling of fat and accumulation of ketones?

Manages His Diabetes"). Thus any effective and successful diabetes education program must focus on personal needs and informed self-care skills. Professional communication must reflect this personal focus and supportive concern.

Content: Tools for Self-Care

Necessary Skills

Diabetes educators and the American Diabetes Association have developed guidelines for diabetes education based on the learning needs and necessary skills and con-

TABLE 20–9	Types of Insulin			
Type of insulin	**Examples**	**Onset of action**	**Peak action**	**Duration of action**
Rapid-acting	Humalog (Lispro)	5-15 minutes	30-90 minutes	3-5 hours
	NovoLog (Aspart)	15 minutes	40-50 minutes	
Short-acting (regular)	Humulin R	30-60 minutes	60-120 minutes	5-8 hours
	Novolin R			
Intermediate-acting (NPH)*	Humulin N	1-3 hours	8 hours	20 hours
	Novolin N			
	Humulin L	1-2.5 hours	7-14 hours	18-24 hours
	Novolin L			
Long-acting	Ultralente	4-8 hours	8-12 hours	36 hours
	Lantus (Glargine)	1 hour	None	24 hours

*Intermediate and short-acting mixtures also are available.

FOR FURTHER FOCUS

COMPARATIVE TYPES OF INSULIN

A common method of insulin use is a mixture of short-acting and longer-acting types injected twice a day (see Table 20-9). Persons with unstable diabetes or irregular mealtimes may inject short-acting insulin before each meal or snack, as well as use a longer-acting type of insulin once or twice a day. Many experienced persons often self-test their blood glucose levels with finger pricks to secure a blood sample and use a glucose monitor to read the result. These persons have learned to adjust their insulin dosage to their test results, food pattern, work-school-social activities, and exercise schedule. In difficult cases, a device that continuously delivers insulin into the bloodstream, an insulin pump, may be used to maintain a finer control over the body's varying insulin needs.

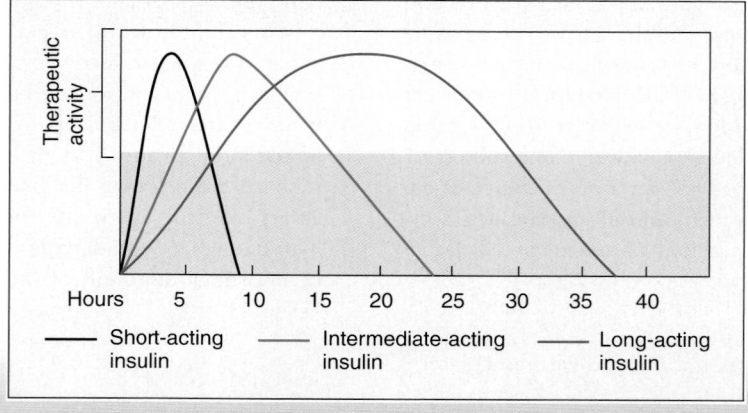

tent areas necessary for self-care of diabetes. Persons with diabetes must have essential skills for the best possible control, as well as favorable surrounding factors related to life situations and psychosocial needs. The tools for self-care involve seven basic content areas.

Nature of Diabetes. Persons should have a basic general knowledge of the nature of diabetes and how their individual form and degree of diabetes relates to this process. This means comparing the general "big picture" with their particular "personal picture." Such a comparison includes evaluating initial basic survival needs, as well as fulfillment of their own fundamental needs, especially support for personal concerns and feelings, in dealing with their diabetes.

Nutrition. Together with their nutrition counselor (e.g., usually the clinical dietitian), persons with diabetes should develop a sound food plan based on individual nutritional needs, living and working situations, and food habits. Such planning includes understanding how the food plan relates to maintaining good diabetes control and promoting positive health.

Insulin. According to their treatment plan, persons with diabetes should understand the following about their insulin activity medications:

■ *Insulin* types and duration of action (Table 20-9), as well as combinations of insulin use (see the For Further Focus box, "Comparative Types of Insulin"), which include learning how insulin works in the body, and how its action relates to the food plan. Learning good insulin-injection technique is also an important part of the treatment plan. In addition to the standard insulin injections (Figure 20-4), there are also alternative methods for insulin administration using an insulin pump (Figure 20-5).

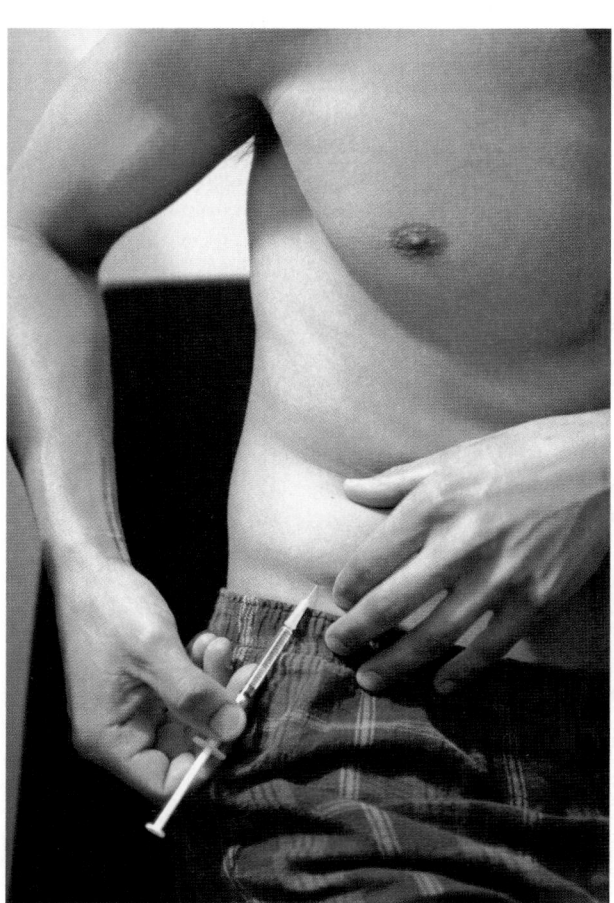

Figure 20–4   Man with diabetes injecting himself with insulin. (Credit: PhotoDisc.)

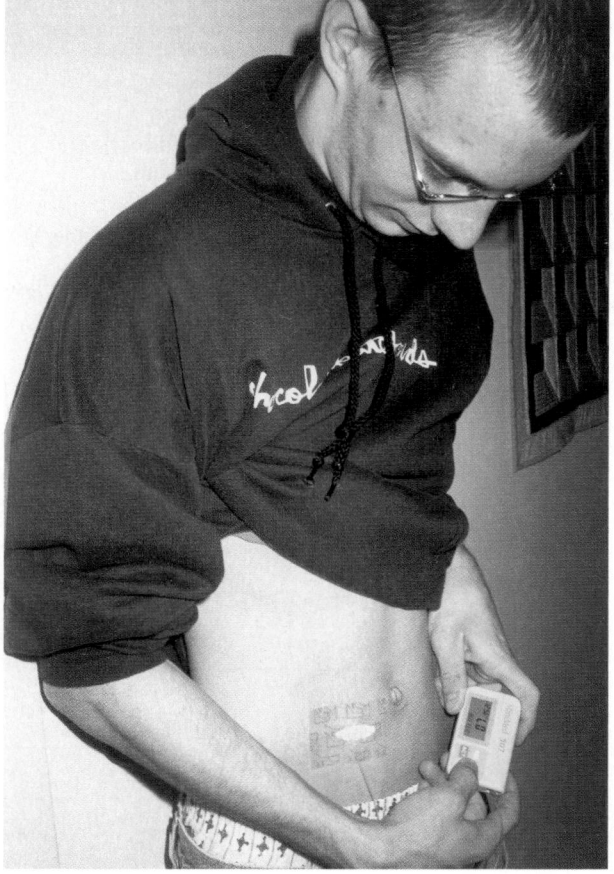

Figure 20–5   Insulin injection using an insulin pump (From Peckenpaugh NJ: *Nutrition essentials and diet therapy*, ed 9, Philadelphia, 2003, Saunders.)

■ *Oral hypoglycemic agents* that stimulate insulin activity, their comparative types and effects (Table 20-10), and how to regulate them are key points that should be well understood by the patient or caretaker.

Monitoring Glucose Levels. Monitoring of blood glucose levels, as well as urinary acetone to note possible ketoacidosis, is important. This monitoring includes learning accurate self-testing procedures, as well as understanding the meaning of the results and knowing what action to take accordingly in relation to food, insulin, or exercise. A variety of self-tests are now available for quick blood glucose monitoring. Small glucose testing kits can fit into purses, backpacks, or glove compartments for easy access and convenience. Techniques now exist using very small amounts of blood from the finger or arm, and more advanced methods using oil secretions on the skin are currently under evaluation for accuracy of use.

Controlling Emergencies. Persons should recognize the early signs of hypoglycemia and its causes and treatment. This recognition includes knowledge of hypoglycemia's relation to the interactive balances among insulin, food, and exercise as the basis of the diabetes care plan (Figure 20-6); daily diabetic care and how to prevent such episodes; the immediate emergency treatment with some form of quick-acting simple carbohydrate to counteract it; and the need to follow the emergency sugar with a snack of complex carbohydrate and protein as soon as possible to sustain a normal blood glucose.

Illness and Special Needs. Persons with diabetes should learn how to deal with illness and other special needs, several of which have been discussed. This knowledge should include how to adjust diet and insulin, as well as planning ahead for events of daily living such as travel, eating out, exercise, or stress.

TABLE 20–10	Oral Hypoglycemic Medications	
Category of medication	**Examples**	**Action**
Alpha-glucose inhibitor	Acarbose (Precose) Miglitol (Glyset)	Slows breakdown of starches, delaying the rise in blood glucose following a meal
Biguanide	Metformin (Glucophage)	Increases sensitivity of endogenous insulin
Meglitinide	Repaglinide (Prandin)	Stimulates release of insulin from beta cells
Nateglinide	Nateglinide (Starlix)	Stimulates release of insulin from beta cells
Sulfonylurea	Chlorpropamide (Diabinese) Glipizide (Glucotrol) Glyburide (DiaBeta/Micronase/Glynase) Glimepiride (Amaryl)	Stimulates release of insulin from beta cells
Thiazolidinedione	Rosiglitazone (Avandia) Pioglitazone (Actos)	Increases insulin sensitivity in muscle and fat

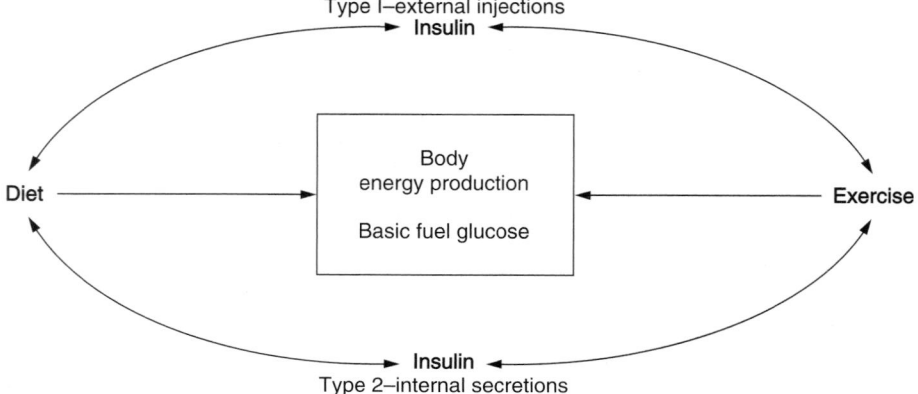

Figure 20–6 Basis of diabetes management: body energy balance. Interacting relations among diet (energy source), insulin (hormone controlling body use of basic fuel glucose), and exercise (physical activity using blood glucose).

Personal Identification. Persons also should obtain a personal identification bracelet or pendant. Obtaining such identification should entail an understanding of why having it at all times is important, especially for persons using insulin.

Levels of Educational Needs

These educational needs can be organized in a diabetes education program on the following three levels as a learning aid: (1) survival level, (2) home-management level, and (3) lifestyle level.

Resources

A number of useful resources are available from health agencies such as the American Diabetes Association and the American Heart Association, including informational materials and a useful cookbook with nutritional values of recipes. More cookbooks for consumers on "light" cooking that reduces fat, sugar, and salt and suggests many alternative seasonings and methods of preparation are also being offered. In addition, resource persons include hospital and clinic dietitians, dietitians in private practice, public health nutritionists, and local chapters of the American Diabetes Association. Any resource materials used must be evaluated in terms of individual needs.

Staff Education

In the final analysis, the success of the diabetes education program in any health care facility depends on the sensitivity and training of the staff conducting the program. Continuing education is essential for all professionals and their assistants. Educational games are often useful tools as part of the staff education program, which the staff can then use in teaching their patients and clients. Many such resources can be developed.

SUMMARY

Diabetes mellitus is a syndrome of varying forms and degrees that have the common characteristic of hyperglycemia. Its underlying metabolic disorder involves all three of the energy nutrients—carbohydrate, fat, and protein—and influences energy balance. The major controlling hormone involved is insulin from the pancreas, and persons with diabetes have either a lack of insulin or a resistance to its action.

Type 1 diabetes affects approximately 5% to 10% of all persons with diabetes; it usually presents itself first during childhood and is more severe and unstable. Treatment of type 1 diabetes involves regular meals and snacks balanced with insulin and exercise. Self-monitoring of blood glucose levels is an important part of disease management.

Type 2 diabetes occurs mostly in adults, especially those who are overweight. Acidosis is rare. Treatment involves weight reduction and maintenance along with regular exercise.

The keystone of care for all forms of diabetes is sound diet therapy. The basic food plan should be rich in complex carbohydrates and dietary fiber; low in simple sugars, fats (especially saturated fats), and cholesterol; and moderate in protein. Food should be distributed throughout the day in fairly regular amounts and at regular times and tailored to meet individual needs.

CRITICAL THINKING QUESTIONS

1. Define *diabetes mellitus*. Describe the nature of the underlying metabolic disorder. What is the one common characteristic of all forms of diabetes mellitus?
2. Describe the major characteristics of the two main types of diabetes mellitus. Explain how these characteristics influence differences in nutrition therapy. List and describe medications used to control these conditions.
3. Identify and explain symptoms of uncontrolled diabetes mellitus. How would you explain to a patient the differences between hyperglycemia and hypoglycemia and how to treat these symptoms?
4. Describe the possible long-term complications of poorly controlled diabetes mellitus. Can these complications be avoided? Is so, how?
5. In terms of the balance concept, describe the principles of a sound diet for a person with diabetes mellitus.

CHAPTER CHALLENGE QUESTIONS

True-False

Write the correct statement for each item you answer "false."

1. *True or False:* Most persons with type 2 diabetes are underweight when the disease is discovered.

2. *True or False:* The two nutrients whose metabolism is most closely affected in diabetes are fat and protein.

3. *True or False:* Insulin is a hormone produced by the pituitary gland.

4. *True or False:* Insulin action is influenced by both glucagon and somatostatin.

5. *True or False:* Acetone in the urine of a person with diabetes usually indicates that the diabetes is in poor control.

6. *True or False:* Persons with diabetes usually are taught to test their own blood glucose daily and regulate their insulin, food, and exercise accordingly.

7. *True or False:* Coronary artery disease occurs in persons with diabetes at 2 to 4 times the rate of the general population.

8. *True or False:* Diabetic complications occur in a relatively small number of persons with long-term diabetes.

9. *True or False:* A diabetic diet is a combination of specific foods that should remain constant.

10. *True or False:* Persons with unstable type 1 diabetes should follow a low-carbohydrate diet for better control.

Multiple Choice

1. The caloric value of the diet for a person with diabetes should be

   a. increased above normal requirements to meet the increased metabolic demand.

   b. decreased below normal requirements to prevent glucose formation.

   c. sufficient to maintain the person's appropriate lean weight.

   d. contributed mainly by fat to spare the carbohydrate for energy needs.

2. The exchange system of diet control is based on which of the following principles? (*Circle all that apply.*)

   a. Equivalent food values

   b. Variety of food choices

   c. Nutritional balance

   d. Reeducation of eating habits

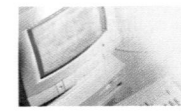 Please refer to the Students' Resource section of this text's Evolve web site for "Suggestions for Additional Study."

REFERENCES

1. Diabetes Public Health Resource, National Center for Chronic Disease Prevention and Health Promotion, Centers for Disease Control and Prevention: *National diabetes fact sheet: national estimates on diabetes,* Atlanta, 2003 (accessed May 2003), DPHR/NCCDPHP/CDC [*www.cdc.gov/diabetes/pubs/estimates.htm*].

2. The Expert Committee on the Diagnosis and Classification of Diabetes Mellitus: Report of the Expert Committee on the Diagnosis and Classification of Diabetes Mellitus, *Diabetes Care* 26(1 suppl):5, 2003.

3. Ferber D: New clues found to diabetes and obesity, *Science* 283(5407):1423, 1999.

4. Goran MI, Ball GD, Cruz ML: Obesity and risk of type 2 diabetes and cardiovascular disease in children and adolescents, *J Clin Endocrinol Metab* 88(4):1417, 2003.

5. American Diabetes Association: Gestational diabetes mellitus, *Diabetes Care* 26(1 suppl):103, 2003.

6. Fong DS and others: Diabetic retinopathy, *Diabetes Care* 26(1 suppl):99, 2003.

7. American Diabetes Association: Diabetic nephropathy, *Diabetes Care* 26(1 suppl):94, 2003.

8. American Diabetes Association: Preventive food care in people with diabetes, *Diabetes Care* 26(1 suppl):78, 2003.

9. American Diabetes Association: Standards of medical care for patients with diabetes mellitus, *Diabetes Care* 26(1 suppl):33, 2003.

10. American Diabetes Association: Management of dyslipidemia in adults with diabetes, *Diabetes Care* 26(1 suppl):83, 2003.

11. American Diabetes Association: Treatment of hypertension in adults with diabetes, *Diabetes Care* 26(1 suppl):80, 2003.

12. American Diabetes Association: Implications of the diabetes control and complications trial, *Diabetes Care* 26(1 suppl):25, 2003.

13. Liu S, Manson JE: Dietary carbohydrates, physical inactivity, obesity, and the "metabolic syndrome" as predictors of coronary heart disease, *Curr Opin Lipidol* 12(4):395, 2001.

14. American Diabetes Association: Evidence-based nutrition principles and recommendations for the treatment and prevention of diabetes and related complications, *Diabetes Care* 26(1 suppl):51, 2003.

15. American Diabetes Association: Physical activity/exercise and diabetes mellitus, *Diabetes Care* 26(1 suppl):73, 2003.

FURTHER READING AND RESOURCES

- American Diabetes Association: *www.diabetes.org*
- National Institute of Diabetes & Digestive & Kidney Diseases: *www.niddk.nih.gov*

  The preceding organizations are dedicated to providing the most current information on evaluation, treatment, and prevention of diabetes. The web sites provided are excellent resources for health care professionals and patients.

- For men only, fatherhood: will your kids get diabetes? *The Diabetes Advisor* 1(1 [Jan/Feb]):21, 1999.
- Treatment topics: type 2 diabetes now threatens kids, *The Diabetes Advisor* 6(6 [Nov/Dec]):30, 1999.

  These two articles give you a taste of the helpful information in this little journal published every two months by The American Diabetes Association. For example, these articles indicate that type 2 diabetes, which was once considered a disease of older adults, is now becoming more common in children and teenagers. The writers indicate that the whole family will be healthier if they make eating healthful meals a family affair. Everyone benefits by being active and eating healthful meals together.

CHAPTER 21

Renal Disease

More than 2.8 million Americans have been diagnosed with some form of kidney disease, and 37,000 persons die from such diseases each year.[1] Data from the Third National Health and Nutrition Examination Survey (NHANES III) indicates that decreased kidney function goes largely undiagnosed; 8.3 million individuals (4.7% of the U.S. population) have abnormal kidney function.[2] These kidney problems are costly in lost work, time, and pay, as well as in personal quality of life. In all, they are now the ninth leading cause of death in America.[3]

This chapter looks at the nutritional care of persons with kidney disease, mainly the extensive problem of chronic renal failure. Although dialysis extends the lives of persons with this irreversible disease, it does so at tremendous personal cost emotionally, physically, and financially. Renal disease is a serious national and personal health problem.

KEY CONCEPTS

- Renal disease interferes with the normal capacity of nephrons to filter waste products of body metabolism.

- Short-term renal disease requires basic nutritional support for healing rather than dietary restriction.

- The progressive degeneration of chronic renal failure requires nutrient modification according to individual disease status and dialysis treatment.

- Current therapy for renal stones depends more on the basic nutrition and health support for medical treatment than on major food and nutrient restrictions.

BASIC PHYSIOLOGY OF THE KIDNEY

Fundamental Role of the Kidneys

The kidneys perform the following two major functions:

1. Make urine, through which they excrete most of the waste products of metabolism
2. Control the concentrations of most constituents of body fluids, especially blood

Tremendous quantities of fluid (~180 L) are filtered through the kidneys each day. All but 1 to 1.5 L of this fluid is reabsorbed back into circulation to maintain necessary balance, particularly with circulating blood volume and all its essential components. Thus as the blood continuously circulates through the kidneys, these marvelous twin organs repeatedly "launder" the blood to monitor and maintain its precious quantity and quality. Indeed the composition of various body fluids are determined not so much by what the mouth takes in as by what the kidneys keep; they are the "master chemists" of the internal environment.

Renal Nephrons

Basic Functional Unit

The basic functional unit of the kidney is the **nephron.** Each human kidney is made up of approximately 1 million nephrons, all of which are capable of forming urine independently. Many of today's advances in treating kidney disease are based on providing maximal support for the nephron's vital functions. Nephron structure is adapted in fine detail to its vital function of maintaining the balanced internal fluid environment necessary for life. At birth, each person has far more nephrons than actually needed, but they are gradually lost after approximately age 30. Many researchers have related this loss to the excessive protein in a typical Western diet.

Major Nephron Functions

The following life-supporting tasks are performed while the body fluid flows through the finely built nephron units:

- *Filtration.* Most materials of the entering blood are filtered out except for the larger components of red blood cells and proteins.
- *Reabsorption.* As the filtrate continues through the winding tubules, substances the body needs are selectively reabsorbed and returned to the blood.
- *Secretion.* Along the tubules, additional hydrogen ions (H^+) are secreted as needed to maintain acid-base balance.

- *Excretion.* Unneeded waste materials are excreted in the now-concentrated urine.

Special Additional Functions

In addition to major functions in regulating blood constituents and making and excreting concentrated urine, the kidneys perform the following other special functions related to maintaining body fluid pressures, producing red blood cells, and activating vitamin D:

- *Renin secretion.* When arteriole pressures fall, the kidneys activate and secrete renin, an enzyme that initiates the renin-angiotensin-aldosterone mechanism operating on the kidneys' nephrons to reabsorb sodium and maintain hormonal control of body water balance (see Chapter 9).
- *Erythropoietin secretion.* The kidneys are responsible for producing the body's major supply (e.g., 80% to 90%) of *erythropoietin,* a circulating hormone that is the principal factor in stimulating red blood cell production in response to decreased tissue oxygen.
- *Vitamin D activation.* The kidneys convert an intermediate inactive form of vitamin D to the final active vitamin D hormone in the proximal tubules of the nephrons (see Chapter 7). This action is stimulated by the parathyroid hormone.

Nephron Structures

The unique metabolic tasks of the kidney are performed by specific nephron structures. Key parts of the nephron include the **glomerulus** and the different tubules, as shown in Figure 21-1.

Glomerulus

At the head of each nephron, a cup-shaped membrane holds the entering blood capillary and its branching tuft of smaller vessels. This cup-shaped capsule is named

---

nephron   (Gr. *nephros,* kidney) microscopic anatomical and functional unit of the kidney that selectively filters and reabsorbs essential blood factors, secretes hydrogen ions as needed to maintain acid-base balance, reabsorbs water to protect body fluids, and forms and excretes a concentrated urine for elimination of wastes. There are approximately 1 million nephrons in each kidney.

glomerulus   (L. *glomus,* ball, cluster) the first section of the nephron, a cluster of capillary loops cupped in the nephron head that serves as an initial filter.

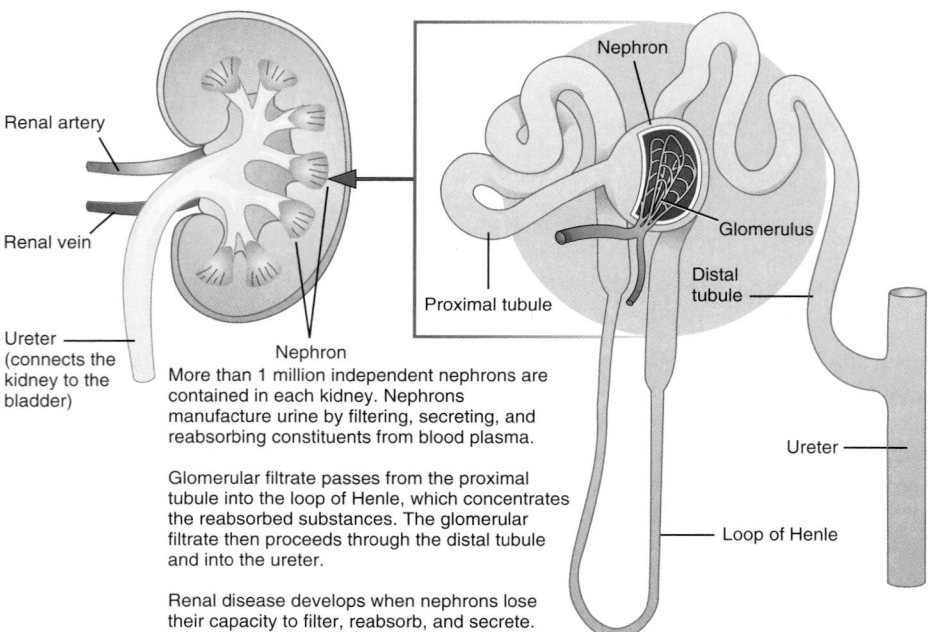

Renal artery

Renal vein

Ureter
(connects the
kidney to the
bladder)

Nephron

More than 1 million independent nephrons are
contained in each kidney. Nephrons
manufacture urine by filtering, secreting, and
reabsorbing constituents from blood plasma.

Glomerular filtrate passes from the proximal
tubule into the loop of Henle, which concentrates
the reabsorbed substances. The glomerular
filtrate then proceeds through the distal tubule
and into the ureter.

Renal disease develops when nephrons lose
their capacity to filter, reabsorb, and secrete.

Nephron

Glomerulus

Distal
tubule

Proximal tubule

Ureter

Loop of Henle

Figure 21–1   Anatomy of the kidney. (From Peckenpaugh NJ: *Nutrition essentials and diet therapy*, ed 9, Philadelphia, 2003, Saunders.)

Bowman's capsule, for the young English physician, Sir William Bowman, who in 1843 first clearly established the basis of plasma filtration and consequent urine secretion based on the intimate relationship of the blood-filled glomeruli and the filtration across the enveloping membrane. This cupped membrane and its tuft or cluster of branching capillaries is called the glomerulus, from the Latin word *glomus* meaning "ball." Only the larger blood proteins and cells remain behind in the circulating blood as it leaves the glomerulus. The rate at which blood is filtered through the glomerulus, the glomerular filtration rate (GFR), is the preferred method for monitoring kidney function.[4] Chronic kidney disease is defined as GFR less than 60 ml/min per 1.73 m² for 3 or more months. Often, diet therapy is based on a patient's GFR.

Tubules

From the cupped head of each nephron, a small tubule carries the filtered fluid through its winding pathway and empties into the central area of the kidney. Specific materials are reabsorbed along the way in each of the four parts of these tubules.

Proximal Tubule. Most of the needed nutrients are reabsorbed in this first part of the tubule and returned to the blood. Glucose and amino acids, as well as about 80% of

the water and other substances, usually are reabsorbed here. Only approximately 20% of the filtered fluid remains to enter the next section of the tube.

Loop of Henle. This midsection of the tubule narrows and dips down into the central part of the kidney. Here, the important exchange of sodium and water occurs. This fluid environment maintains the necessary *osmotic pressure* to concentrate the urine as it passes through the central area later, on its way out.

Distal Tubule. The latter part of the tubule winds back up into the outer area of the kidney. Here, secretion of H⁺ occurs as needed to provide acid-base balance. Sodium also is reabsorbed as needed under the influence of the adrenal hormone **aldosterone.**

Collecting Tubule. In this final section of the tubule, a normal concentrated urine is produced by the following important water-reabsorbing actions: (1) influence of the pituitary hormone **antidiuretic hormone (ADH),** also called *vasopressin;* and (2) the osmotic pressure from the more dense surrounding fluid in the central area of the kidney. The urine, which is now concentrated and ready for excretion, only amounts to 0.5% to 1% of the original fluid and materials filtered through the glomerulus at the head of the nephron.

DISEASE PROCESS AND DIETARY CONSIDERATIONS

General Causes of Kidney Disease

Several disease conditions may interfere with the normal functioning of the nephrons, resulting in kidney disease. These conditions are discussed in greater detail in the following sections.

Inflammatory and Degenerative Disease

The small blood vessels and membranes in the nephrons may become inflamed for a short time (e.g., in acute *glomerulonephritis*). In other cases, entire nephrons or sections of nephrons may be involved, stopping normal function and producing *nephrotic syndrome*. These nephrotic lesions may continue to affect more and more nephrons, leading to progressive *chronic renal failure*. As a result, the impaired metabolism of protein, electrolytes, and water creates nutritional disturbances.

Damage from Other Diseases

Circulatory disorders such as prolonged, poorly controlled hypertension can cause degeneration of the small renal arteries and interfere with normal nephron function. The increased demand on other nephrons in turn can cause more hypertension and still more damage to nephrons. Diabetes mellitus is the number one cause of end-stage renal disease (ESRD) in the United States, accounting for approximately 40% of all new cases. Hyperglycemia and hypertension associated with uncontrolled diabetes can damage small renal arteries leading to *glomerulosclerosis* (e.g., loss of functioning nephrons) and eventual chronic renal failure.[5,6] Kidney abnormalities present from birth also may lead to poor function, infection, or obstruction within the kidneys.

Infection and Obstruction

Symptoms of bacterial urinary tract infection may range from the occasional mild discomfort of bladder infections to more involved chronic recurrent disease and obstruction from kidney stones. Obstruction anywhere in the urinary tract blocks drainage and causes further infection and general tissue damage.

Damage from Other Agents

Various environmental agents (e.g., chemical pesticides, solvents, and similar materials), animal venom, certain plants, and some drugs are nephrotoxic (poisonous to the kidney) that can cause kidney damage.[7,8] Malnutrition, often a consequence of renal failure, also can exacerbate the rate of renal tissue destruction by (1) increasing the rate of cell deterioration, and (2) impairing the immune system thus increasing susceptibility to infection.[9,10]

Genetic Defect

Congenital abnormalities of both kidneys can contribute to predisposing renal disease with extensive distortion of renal structure. Cystic diseases (e.g., polycystic kidney disease, medullary cystic disease) are genetically linked kidney diseases accounting for 6% of the total patient population with ESRD in the United States.[9] Being born with only one kidney does not necessarily constitute kidney disease or even impaired function. Many people are born with one kidney, some of whom are never even aware of the fact, and never have any problems. Box 21-1 lists risk factors and common causes of kidney disease. (See also the Cultural Considerations box, "Prevalence of Kidney Disease among Ethnic Groups in the United States and Potential Causes for Differences," for more information.)

Nutrition Therapy in Renal Disease

In the treatment of renal disease, nutrition therapy in each case is based on the nature of the disease process and individual responses.

Length of Disease

In short-term acute disease, medical therapy with antibiotics usually controls the disease, and nutrition therapy is aimed toward optimal nutritional support for healing and normal growth. Long-term chronic disease involves more specific nutrient modifications.

Degree of Impaired Renal Function

In milder acute disease with few nephrons involved, less interference occurs with general renal function because

---

aldosterone   a potent hormone of the outside layer of the adrenal glands that acts on the distal nephron tubule to cause reabsorption of sodium in an ion exchange with potassium. The aldosterone mechanism is essentially a sodium-conserving mechanism but also indirectly conserves water because water absorption follows the sodium resorption.

antidiuretic hormone (ADH)   a hormone of the pituitary gland that acts on the distal nephron tubule to conserve water by causing its reabsorption; also called *vasopressin*.

BOX 21-1 Risk Factors and Common Causes of Kidney Disease

Sociodemographic Factors

Older age
U.S. ethnic minority status: African American, American Indian, Hispanic, Asian, or Pacific Islander
Exposure to certain chemical and environmental conditions
Low income/education

Clinical Factors

Poor glycemic control in diabetes
Hypertension
Autoimmune disease
Systemic infections
Urinary tract infections
Urinary stones
Lower urinary tract obstruction
Neoplasia
Family history of chronic kidney disease
Recovery from acute kidney failure
Reduction in kidney mass
Exposure to certain nephrotoxic drugs
Low birth weight

From Eknoyan G, Levin NW: K/DOQI clinical practice guidelines for chronic kidney disease: evaluation, classification, and stratification, *Am J Kidney Dis* 39(2 suppl):1, 2002. Copyright National Kidney Foundation.

---

hematuria (Gr. *haima*, blood; *ouron*, urine) the abnormal presence of blood in the urine.

proteinuria (Gr. *protos*, first, protein; *ouron*, urine) an abnormal excess of serum proteins (e.g., albumin) in the urine.

edema (Gr. *oidema*, swelling) excess accumulation of fluid in the body tissues.

hypertension high blood pressure.

oliguria (Gr. *oligos*, little; *ouron*, urine) the secretion of small amounts of urine in relation to fluid intake ($\leq$0.5 mg/kg per hour).

anuria (Gr. *an-*, negative prefix; *ouron*, urine) an absence of urine production, indicating kidney shutdown or failure.

blood urea nitrogen (BUN) a basic test of nephron function by measuring its ability to normally filter urea nitrogen, a product of protein metabolism, from the blood.

---

the large number of back-up nephrons can meet basic needs. However, in progressive chronic disease more and more nephrons become involved and renal failure finally results. In such cases, extensive nutrition therapy is required to help maintain renal function as long as possible.

Individual Clinical Symptoms

In continuing disease, nutrient modifications are designed to meet individual needs according to specific clinical symptoms. This personalized nutrition therapy is especially important when advanced renal disease is treated with dialysis.

This chapter's discussion focuses primarily on the more serious degenerative process of chronic renal failure and dialysis that requires much nutrition therapy. Brief reviews of nutritional support for short-term conditions provide reference for general nutritional care.

NEPHRON DISEASE PROBLEMS

Glomerulonephritis

Disease Process

This inflammatory process affects the *glomeruli*, the small blood vessels in the cupped membrane at the head of the nephron. Glomerulonephritis occurs mostly in young children and usually follows a brief course in its acute form.

Clinical Symptoms

Classic symptoms include **hematuria** and **proteinuria,** although **edema** and mild **hypertension** also may occur. These patients usually have little appetite, which contributes to feeding problems. If the disease progresses to more renal involvement, signs of **oliguria** or **anuria** may develop.

Nutrition Therapy

General care in uncomplicated disease focuses mainly on bed rest and antibiotic drug therapy. Pediatricians and dietitians favor overall optimum nutritional support for growth with adequate protein. Salt usually is not restricted. Diet modifications are not crucial in most patients with acute short-term disease, especially children with poststreptococcal disease. Fluid intake is adjusted to output as a rule.

However, if the disease process advances more specific nutrition therapy may be indicated according to individual needs, as follows:

■ *Protein.* If the **blood urea nitrogen (BUN)** is elevated and urine output is decreased, dietary protein may be restricted. The diet usually is modified to a

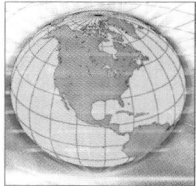

CULTURAL CONSIDERATIONS

Prevalence of Kidney Disease among Ethnic Groups in the United States and Potential Causes for Differences

According to the U.S. Renal Data System Annual Report, the incidence of kidney disease continues to rise at an alarming rate. The National Institutes of Health estimates that more than 651,000 patients in the year 2010 will experience kidney failure requiring dialysis therapy or kidney transplant.* Part of this escalating occurrence results from the average increase in age and the high prevalence of diabetes in the elderly population (diabetes is the number one cause of kidney disease). What is even more alarming is that those estimates are only considering patients who meet the clinical definition of chronic kidney disease: structural or functional abnormalities of the kidney for at least 3 months, most often defined as decreased GFR less than 60 ml/min per 1.73 m^2. When researchers evaluated GFR in 15,625 adults participating in the Third National Health and Nutrition Examination Survey (NHANES III), an additional 31.2% of the population had a mild reduction in GFR (60 to 89 ml/min per 1.73 m^2).† Underlying decline in kidney function goes largely unnoticed and untreated, yet the number of individuals suffering from it are potentially very large.

Many factors increase one's risk for chronic kidney disease (CKD) such as diabetes, hypertension, age, and ethnicity. Historically, African Americans have had a significantly higher incidence of CKD than Caucasians (2.7 times higher). Recent studies have evaluated causes of CKD in these two ethnic groups in an attempt to identify and explain this racial disparity. One such study found that almost one half of the excess risk of CKD in African-American adults could be explained on the basis of modifiable risk factors.‡ The author defines modifiable risk factors as socioeconomic factors, lifestyle factors, and clinical factors (glycemic control in diabetes mellitus and blood pressure). In comparing individuals with CKD, this study found African Americans more likely to have less education; live below the poverty level; be unmarried, less physically active, and more obese; smoke cigarettes, and have a higher prevalence of diabetes and hypertension than their Caucasian counterparts.‡ Such findings lend important information to health care providers in regard to prevention and treatment of CKD. Although these factors do not account for all causes of racial disparity, they are modifiable, and therefore achievable in terms of goals for reducing the risk of CKD.

Another recent study evaluated the health-related quality of life (HRQOL) and associated outcomes among hemodialysis patients of different ethnicities in the United States.§ The HRQOL questionnaire assesses each patient on a mental, physical, and disease process level and is associated with mortality. Questions about symptoms, effects of disease on daily life, burden of disease, work status, cognitive function, quality of social interaction, sexual function, sleep, social support, staff encouragement, and patient satisfaction also were taken into consideration. Mortality risk in CKD is significantly higher in Caucasians than African Americans. An interesting find in this study was that African Americans treated by dialysis scored higher than Caucasians in several components of the questionnaire. In combining the results of these two studies, we find that African Americans are at greater risk for developing CKD; however, their health-related quality of life remains higher than those Caucasians who suffer CKD, even though African Americans have a lower level of socioeconomic status. The risk for mortality is higher among Caucasians with low HRQOL.

In a nutshell, African Americans are at a higher risk for CKD, but a large portion of these risk factors are modifiable and potentially can be prevented. Caucasian Americans, on the other hand, suffer CKD much less frequently than African Americans; however, their mortality rate or outcome is much worse. Basically, Caucasians on dialysis do not cope as well in terms of quality of life as African Americans. As research continues to advance, hopefully the disparities between ethnicity and disease outcome will become clearer, making a prevention or treatment mechanism available.

---

*U.S. Renal Data System: *USRDS 2001 annual data report,* Bethesda, MD, 2001, National Institute of Diabetes and Digestive and Kidney Disease, National Institutes of Health.
†Coresh J and others: Prevalence of chronic kidney disease and decreased kidney function in the adult U.S. population: Third National Health and Nutrition Examination Survey, *Am J Kidney Dis* 41:1, 2003.
‡Tarver-Carr ME and others: Excess risk of chronic kidney disease among African-American versus white subjects in the United States: a population-based study of potential explanatory factors, *J Am Soc Nephrol* 13(9):2363, 2002.
§Lopes AA and others: Health-related quality of life and associated outcomes among hemodialysis patients of different ethnicities in the United States: the Dialysis Outcomes and Practice Patterns Study (DOPPS), *Am J Kidney Dis* 41(3):605, 2003.

lowered protein intake of 0.6 g/kg ideal body weight. As long as renal function is adequate to maintain a normal BUN level, dietary protein intake may be held at 0.75 to 1 g/kg body weight.

■ *Carbohydrate.* To provide sufficient energy in dietary kcalories, carbohydrates should be given liberally, which also helps combat catabolism of tissue protein and prevent starvation **ketosis.**

■ *Sodium.* If low urine output indicates impaired renal function, sodium may be restricted to 500 to 1000 mg/day (see Chapter 19). As recovery occurs, the normal sodium intake of 2 to 3 g/day may be resumed.

■ *Potassium.* If oliguria becomes severe, renal clearance of potassium is impaired. Thus potassium intake must be monitored carefully according to individual needs.

■ *Water.* Fluid intake is restricted according to urine output. If restriction is not indicated, fluids can be consumed as desired.

Nephrotic Syndrome

Disease Process

Nephrotic syndrome, or **nephrosis,** results from nephron tissue damage to both the glomerulus and tubule. The primary damage is to the major filtering membrane of the glomerulus, allowing large amounts of protein to pass into the tubule. This high-protein concentration then causes further damage to the tubule. Both filtration and reabsorption functions of the nephron are disrupted. Nephrosis may be caused by progressive glomerulonephritis, by other diseases such as diabetes or connective tissue disorders (**collagen disease**), or by other agents such as drugs, heavy metals, or toxic venom from stinging insects.

Clinical Symptoms

Nephrotic syndrome is characterized by a group of symptoms resulting from the nephron tissue damage and impaired function. The large protein loss leads to massive edema and **ascites,** as well as proteinuria. The abdomen becomes distended as fluid accumulates, and plasma protein level is greatly reduced, especially in the albumin fraction, because of large losses in the urine. As protein loss continues, tissue proteins are broken down and general malnutrition follows. Severe edema and ascites often mask the extent of body tissue wasting.

Nutrition Therapy

The former standard recommendation for patients with nephrotic syndrome was a high-protein diet, sometimes as high as 3 to 4 g/kg body weight per day. However, current evidence indicates that high-protein diets may accelerate loss of renal function and moderately low-protein diets reduce albuminuria and albumin catabolism, with no change in the GFR. Nutrition therapy is now directed toward controlling major symptoms (e.g., edema and malnutrition), resulting from the massive protein losses. Therefore physicians and dietitians are now managing these patients with diets containing less protein, as follows:

■ *Protein.* Protein intake should meet nutritional and growth needs, without excess (e.g., 0.6 to 0.75 g/kg of body weight/day).

■ *Energy.* Sufficient energy always must be provided to free protein for tissue rebuilding. High daily intakes of 30 to 40 kcal/kg per ideal body weight may be required. Because appetite is usually poor, food must be as appetizing as possible and in a form most easily tolerated.

■ *Sodium.* Dietary sodium may be moderately reduced (e.g., to approximately 1 to 3 g/day) if necessary to help prevent edema.

■ *Other minerals and vitamins.* There is no need for potassium restriction. Iron and vitamin supplements may be helpful.

RENAL FAILURE

The two types of renal failure, acute and chronic, have a number of symptoms that reflect interference with normal nephron functions in nutrient metabolism. Both forms have similar nutrition therapy, depending on the extent of renal tissue damage.

Acute Renal Failure

Disease Process

Renal function in healthy kidneys may shut down suddenly after some metabolic insult or traumatic injury, causing a life-threatening situation. This is a medical emergency in which the dietitian and nurse play important supportive roles. Varying causes may be to blame, as follows:

■ *Severe injury,* such as extensive burns or a crushing injury involving extensive tissue damage

■ *Infectious disease,* such as peritonitis

■ *Toxic agents* in the environment, such as carbon tetrachloride or poisonous mushrooms, insect stings, or animal bites

■ *Drug reactions* in allergic or sensitive persons, such as a penicillin or cyclosporine reaction

Acute renal failure can last from days to weeks, with normal function returning when the condition causing the kidney failure is treated. Depending on the extent of renal tissue damage, it may take months to regain full function. However, some individuals do not regain normal kidney function, and the disease progresses to chronic renal failure.

Clinical Symptoms

The major sign of acute renal failure is oliguria, which is caused when cellular debris from the tissue damage blocks the tubules. This diminished urine output often is accompanied by proteinuria or hematuria. Other symptoms may include nausea and vomiting, fatigue and muscle weakness, swelling in the lower extremities, itchy skin, and confusion. Water balance becomes a crucial factor. Short-term dialysis may be needed to support renal function.

Nutrition Therapy

The major challenge during acute renal failure is to improve or maintain nutritional status while the patient is faced with marked catabolism. Loss of appetite is common, and parenteral nutrition therapy may be required. Recommendations for protein intake during acute renal failure have been debated over the years. Current standards indicate the need for very individualized therapy based on the patient's renal function, as indicated by the GFR.

Chronic Renal Failure

Disease Process

Chronic renal failure, or chronic renal insufficiency, is caused by the progressive breakdown of renal tissue, which impairs all renal functions. Few functioning nephrons remain and then gradually deteriorate. Chronic renal failure develops slowly and there is no true cure, with exception of a kidney transplant.

Chronic renal insufficiency may result from a variety of diseases involving the nephrons, as follows: (1) primary glomerular disease; (2) metabolic disease with renal involvement, such as diabetes; (3) renal vascular disease; (4) renal tubular disease; (5) congenital abnormality of both kidneys; (6) hypertension; and (7) heart or lung disease.

Clinical Symptoms

Depending on the nature of the underlying renal disease, chronic renal changes may involve extensive scarring of renal tissue, which distorts the kidney structure and brings vascular changes from prolonged hypertension. As the nephrons are lost one by one, the remaining nephrons gradually lose their ability to sustain vital metabolic balances.

- *Water balance.* In the beginning stages of chronic renal failure the kidneys are unable to reabsorb water and properly concentrate urine. Therefore large amounts of dilute urine are produced (polyuria). Dehydration is a risk factor at this point and may become critical. As the disease progresses, urine production declines to a point of oliguria and finally

anuria. Without urinary excretion of waste products, dangerous levels of urea accumulate in the blood.
- *Electrolyte balances.* Several imbalances among electrolytes result from decreasing nephron function. The failing kidney cannot appropriately maintain the vital sodium-potassium balance that guards body water (see Chapter 9). A concentration of materials (e.g., phosphate, sulfate, and organic acids) is produced by metabolism of food. Without appropriate filtering, these materials accumulate in the blood, causing metabolic acidosis. The disturbed metabolism of calcium and phosphate from lack of activated vitamin D, a process that occurs in the kidneys, leads to bone pain from a disease called **osteodystrophy**.
- *Nitrogen retention.* Increasing loss of nephron function results in elevated amounts of nitrogenous metabolites, such as **urea** and **creatinine**.
- *Anemia.* The damaged kidney cannot accomplish its normal participation in the production of red blood cells—production of erythropoietin. There-

---

ketosis the accumulation of ketones, intermediate products of fat metabolism, in the blood.

nephrosis (Gr. *nephros*, kidney) a nephrotic syndrome caused by degenerative lesions of the renal tubules of the nephrons, especially the thin basement membrane of the glomerulus that helps support the capillary loops; marked by edema, albuminuria, and decreased serum albumin.

collagen disease (Gr. *kolla*, glue; *gennan*, to produce) a disease attacking collagen tissues, the protein substance of the white fibers (collagenous fibers) of skin, tendon, bone, cartilage, and other connective tissues; any of a group of diseases that cause widespread changes in the connective tissue (e.g., rheumatoid arthritis, lupus erythematosus, scleroderma, and rheumatic fever).

ascites (Gr. *askites*, from; *askos*, bag) outflow and accumulation of serous (blood and lymph serum) fluid in the abdominal cavity; also known as *abdominal* or *peritoneal dropsy*.

osteodystrophy (Gr. *osteon*, bone; *dys*, painful, disordered, abnormal; *trephein*, to nourish) bone disease resulting from defective bone formation. The general term *dystrophy* applies to any disorder arising from faulty nutrition.

urea chief nitrogen-carrying product of dietary protein metabolism; appears in blood, lymph, and urine.

creatinine nitrogen-carrying product of tissue protein breakdown, excreted in the urine.

fore fewer red cells are produced, and those that are produced survive a shorter time.

▪ *Hypertension.* When blood flow to renal tissue is increasingly impaired, renal hypertension develops. In turn, hypertension causes cardiovascular damage and further deterioration of the kidneys.

▪ *Azotemia.* Elevated BUN, serum creatinine, and serum uric acid levels are reflected in the characteristic laboratory finding of **azotemia.**

In its clinical practice guidelines, the National Kidney Foundation categorizes chronic kidney disease into five stages, depending on GFR (Table 21-1).[9]

General Signs and Symptoms

Increasing loss of renal function causes progressive weakness, shortness of breath, general lethargy, and fatigue. Thirst, appetite loss, weight loss, diarrhea, and vomiting may occur. Increasing capillary fragility causes skin, nose, oral, and gastrointestinal bleeding. Nervous system involvement brings muscular twitching, burning sensations in the extremities, or convulsions. Irregular cyclic breathing (e.g., Cheyne-Stokes respiration) indicates acidosis, and ulceration of the mouth, a bad taste, and fetid breath also occur. Malnutrition lowers resistance to infection. Bone and joint pain continue.

Nutrition Therapy

Basic Objectives. Treatment always must be individual and must be adjusted according to progression of the illness, the type of treatment being used, and the patient's response. However, the general basic therapy objectives in care of chronic renal failure are the following:

▪ Reduce protein breakdown.
▪ Avoid dehydration or excess hydration.
▪ Correct acidosis.
▪ Correct electrolyte imbalances.
▪ Control fluid and electrolyte losses from vomiting and diarrhea.
▪ Maintain optimal nutritional status.
▪ Maintain appetite, general morale, and sense of well-being.
▪ Control complications of hypertension, bone pain, and nervous system involvement.
▪ Retard rate of renal failure, postponing the ultimate need for dialysis.

Principles. Nutrition for chronic renal failure involves variable nutrient adjustments according to individual need, as follows:

▪ *Protein.* The critical problem is to provide just enough protein to maintain tissue integrity while

TABLE 21–1	Stages of Chronic Kidney Disease*	
Stage	**Description**	**GFR (ml/min/1.73m²)**
1	Kidney damage, with normal or elevated GFR	≥90
2	Kidney damage, with mild decrease in GFR	60-89
3	Moderate decrease in GFR	30-59
4	Severely decreased GFR	15-29
5	Kidney failure	<15 (or dialysis)

GFR, glomerular filtration rate.
From Eknoyan G and Levin NW: K/DOQI clinical practice guidelines for chronic kidney disease: evaluation, classification, and stratification, *Am J Kidney Dis* 39(2 suppl):1, 2002. Copyright National Kidney Foundation.
*Chronic kidney disease is defined as either kidney damage or GFR <60 ml/min/1.73m² for 3 or more months. Kidney damage is defined as pathologic abnormalities or markers of damage, including abnormalities in blood or urine tests or imaging studies.

avoiding a damaging excess. Protein is generally limited to 0.6 to 0.75 g/kg body weight per day for individuals with a GFR less than 25 ml/min, of which at least 50% should come from high-biological value protein (see Chapter 4) to ensure an adequate intake of essential amino acids.

▪ *Amino acid supplements.* Mixtures of essential amino acids or amino acid precursors provide necessary protein supplementation for low-protein diets. Commercial formulas are available for nondialysis patients. Other supplements are made up of nitrogen-free "copies" of essential amino acids called *analogs.*

▪ *Energy.* Carbohydrate and fat must supply sufficient nonprotein kilocalories to spare protein for tissue synthesis, as well as to supply energy. For individuals younger than 60 years of age with chronic renal failure and GFR less than 25 ml/min, the recommended dietary energy intake is 35 kcal/kg body weight per day. Energy needs are less for individuals more than age 60 (30 to 35 kcal/kg per day).

▪ *Water.* With nondialyzed patients, fluid intake should be sufficient to maintain adequate urine volume. Intake usually is balanced with output.

▪ *Sodium.* The need for sodium varies. If hypertension and edema are present, sodium intake must be restricted. Sodium intake usually ranges from 500 to 2000 mg/day (see Chapter 19).

▪ *Potassium.* The damaged kidney cannot clear potassium adequately, so the dietary intake is kept at approximately 1500 to 2000 mg/day.

▪ *Phosphate and calcium.* Moderate dietary phosphorus restriction (e.g., to approximately 500 to 600 mg/day), along with the protein restriction, is an effective

CLINICAL APPLICATIONS

CASE STUDY: THE PATIENT WITH CHRONIC RENAL FAILURE

Charles Brown, age 49, is an active man working at a large company who has begun to tire more easily. He has little appetite and feels generally ill most of the time. He recently noticed some ankle swelling and some blood in his urine. At his wife's insistence, he finally decided to see his physician.

After a complete work-up, his physician's findings included the following:

1. No prior illness except a case of the flu with a throat infection during Charles' overseas service in the Army
2. Laboratory tests: albumin, red and white cells in the urine; abnormal blood urea nitrogen and glomerular filtration rate
3. Other symptoms: hypertension, edema, headache, occasional vision blurring, and low-grade fever

The physician discussed the findings and the serious prognosis of advanced renal disease with Charles and his wife, and together they explored the immediate medical and nutritional needs for treatment. They also discussed the ultimate need for medical management with dialysis. The physician prescribed medications to control Charles' growing symptoms and discomfort.

As time went by, Charles' symptoms increased. He lost more weight, was anemic, and experienced increased bone and joint pain. Gastrointestinal bleeding and nausea also increased, and he had occasional muscle twitching or spasms. Small mouth ulcers made eating a painful effort. Charles and his wife made visits to the clinic dietitian to learn how to manage his present predialysis diet at home.

Questions for Analysis

1. What metabolic imbalances in chronic renal failure do you think accounted for the symptoms Charles was having?
2. What are the objectives of treatment in chronic renal failure?
3. What are the basic principles of Charles' predialysis diet? Describe this type of diet. What foods would be included? Plan a 1-day menu for Charles.
4. What nutrient-related medications and supplements would Charles' physician and clinical dietitian probably use in his treatment plan? Why?

---

means of delaying progressive renal failure. A calcium supplement is used to correct for hypocalcemia.

■ *Vitamins.* A multivitamin supplement is usually added to the diet of renal patients on protein restriction. A diet of up to 40 g of protein does not contribute the full daily need of all the vitamins (see the Clinical Applications box, "Case Study: The Patient with Chronic Renal Failure").

End-Stage Renal Disease

Disease Process

When chronic renal failure advances to an end stage, life-support decisions face the patient, family, and physician. ESRD occurs when the patient's GFR decreases to 15 ml/min. This decrease is caused by irreversible damage to a majority of the kidneys' nephrons. At this point, the patient has two options, chronic kidney **dialysis** or kidney transplant. The lives of an estimated 50,000 persons in the United States who develop kidney disease each year have been prolonged by dialysis and kidney transplants. Kidney transplantation has several advan-

tages. Current advances in surgical techniques, immunosuppressive drugs to prevent rejection, and antibiotics to control infection have helped ensure successful outcomes. In addition, the organ donor system has improved. A successful renal transplant can provide an improved quality of life and is more cost-effective than dialysis. Long-term effects of dialysis include bone disorders, nutritional depletion, anemia, and hormonal im-

azotemia (Gr. *a-*, negative prefix; *zoe*, life; *azote*, nitrogen; *haima*, blood) an excess of urea and other nitrogenous substances in the blood.

dialysis (Gr. *dia*, through; *lysis*, dissolution) the process of separating crystalloids (crystal-forming substances) and colloids (gluelike substances) in solution by the difference in their rates of diffusion through a semipermeable membrane; crystalloids (e.g., blood sugar and other simple metabolites) pass through readily; and colloids (e.g., plasma proteins) pass through slowly or not at all.

balances, as well as psychological depression and diminished quality of life from constant dependence on treatments. However, dialysis has become the major treatment for advanced renal disease, at a considerable cost; some $1.4 billion each year is covered by Medicare. Two forms of dialysis are used: hemodialysis and ambulatory peritoneal dialysis.

Therapy

Hemodialysis. Hemodialysis using an artificial kidney machine (Figure 21-2) removes toxic substances from the blood and helps restore nutrients and metabolites to normal blood levels. To prepare a patient for hemodialysis therapy, a surgical fistula is made by joining an artery and a vein on the forearm just beneath the skin. After this attachment has healed, a needle is inserted through the healed tissue and connected by tubes to the dialysis machine.

A patient with chronic renal failure usually requires two to three treatments per week, each of which lasts 4 to 8 hours. During each treatment, the patient's blood makes several round trips through the dialysis solution in the machine, which removes excess waste material to maintain normal blood levels of life-sustaining substances that the patient's own kidneys can no longer accomplish. Two compartments in the machine are separated by a filter. One compartment contains blood from the patient that contains all the excess fluids and waste materials; the other contains the *dialysate*, a solution that may be thought of as a "cleaning fluid." As in normal capillary filtration, the blood cells are too large to pass through the pores in the filter. However, the remaining smaller molecules in the blood pass through the filter and are carried away by the dialysate. If the patient's blood is deficient in certain materials, these may be added to the dialysate.

The diet of a hemodialysis patient is an important aspect of maintaining biochemical control. Several basic objectives govern an individual's diet and are designed to perform the following four tasks:

1. Maintain protein and energy balance
2. Prevent dehydration or fluid overload
3. Maintain normal serum potassium and sodium levels
4. Maintain acceptable phosphate and calcium levels

Controlling infection is always an underlying goal. In most cases nutrition therapy can be planned with more liberal nutrient allowances, as follows:

■ *Protein.* Protein-energy malnutrition (PEM) is a major concern in patients on dialysis and is considered one of the most significant predictors of adverse outcomes. Fifty to seventy percent of patients on dialysis suffer from PEM resulting from metabolic and hormonal disturbances, anorexia, nausea, and vomiting.[9] For most adult dialysis patients, a protein allowance of 1.2 g/kg lean body weight is carefully calculated by the dialysis center's clinical dietitians. This amount provides for nutritional needs, maintains positive nitrogen balance, does not produce ex-

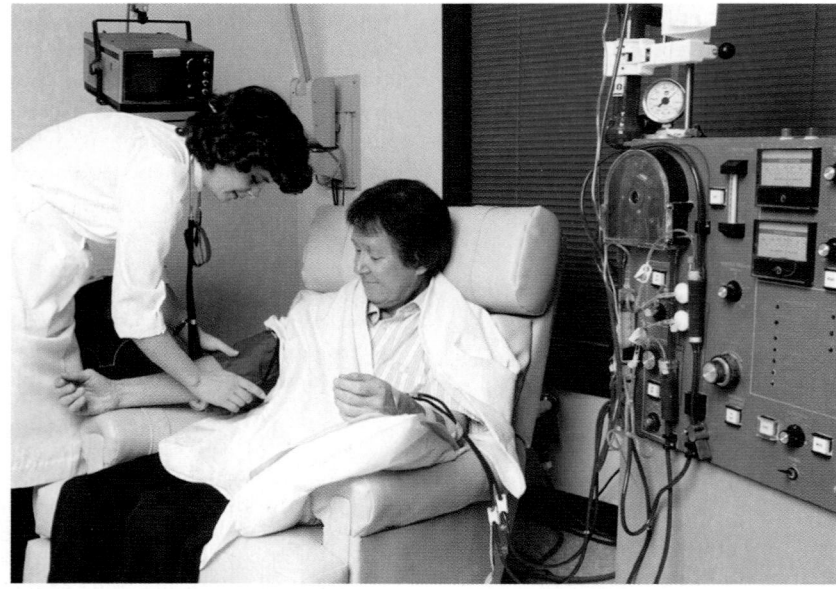

Figure 21–2   Patient with end-stage chronic renal disease undergoing hemodialysis treatment. (Credit: PhotoDisc.)

cessive nitrogenous waste, and replaces the amino acids lost during each dialysis treatment. At least 75% of this daily allowance should consist of protein foods of high biological value (e.g., eggs, meat, fish, and poultry) but little if any milk. Milk is restricted because it adds more fluid and has a high content of sodium, phosphate, and potassium.

- *Energy.* It is recommended that dialysis patients maintain a body mass index (BMI) within the upper 50th percentile (23.6 to 24 kg/m^2) because of the association between malnutrition and clinical outcomes. The unfortunate combination is that kidney failure is closely related to a decrease in appetite when GFR falls below 60 ml/min per 1.73 m^2.[9] A generous amount of carbohydrates with some fat continue to supply needed kilocalories for energy and protein sparing. An intake of 35 kcal/kg of lean body weight helps avoid catabolism, which would further complicate kidney function. The Kidney Disease Outcomes Quality Initiative (K/DOQI) dietary guidelines recommend monitoring nutritional status of patients with chronic kidney disease at regular intervals: every 1 to 3 months for patients with GFR <30 ml/min per 1.73 m^2 and every 6 to 12 months for patients with GFR 30 to 59 ml/min per 1.73 m^2 to identify anorexia and help prevent malnutrition.[9]
- *Water balance.* Fluid is usually limited to 1000 ml/day, plus an amount equal to any urine output.
- *Sodium.* To control body fluid retention and hypertension, sodium is limited to 1000 to 3000 mg/day. Sodium intake is not as stringently regulated for patients on dialysis as it is for those with kidney failure and not yet on dialysis because the dialysis process will rid the body of excess sodium.
- *Potassium.* To prevent potassium accumulation, which can cause cardiac problems, potassium intake is restricted to 1500 to 3000 mg/day.
- *Vitamins.* A supplement of the water-soluble vitamins (e.g., B complex and C) is given to replace their loss during the dialysis treatment.

Peritoneal Dialysis. An alternative form of treatment some patients can use is *peritoneal dialysis,* which has the convenience of home use. In this process, the patient introduces the dialysate solution directly into the peritoneal cavity four or five times a day, where it can be exchanged for fluids that contain the metabolic waste products. Because this form of dialysis is continuous within the body, the process is called *continuous ambulatory peritoneal dialysis* (CAPD). First, the patient is prepared by surgical insertion of a permanent catheter. Treatments are carried out by attaching a disposable bag containing the dialysate solution to the abdominal catheter leading into the peritoneal cavity, waiting 20 to 30 minutes for the solution exchange, and then lowering the bag to allow the force of gravity to cause the waste-containing fluid to drain into it. When the bag is empty, it can be folded around the waist or tucked into a pocket, providing the patient mobility. Intermittent use of peritoneal dialysis, self-administered at home, gives the patient more mobility and a sense of control. An automated device sometimes is used to provide several solution exchanges during night sleep hours and one continuous exchange during the day, a technique called *continuous cyclic peritoneal dialysis* (CCPD). A more liberal diet may be used with peritoneal dialysis and good self-care. The patient can do the following:

- Increase protein intake to 1.2 to 1.5 g/kg body weight.
- Limit phosphorus to 1200 to 1500 mg/day by restricting phosphorus-rich foods (e.g., nuts and legumes) to 1 serving per week and dairy or egg products to a half-cup portion or one egg or its equivalent each day.
- Increase potassium by eating a wide variety of fruits and vegetables each day (2000 to 4000 mg/day).
- Encourage liberal fluid intake to prevent dehydration.
- Avoid sweets and fats to control triglyceride and low-density lipoprotein levels.
- Maintain lean body weight by accounting for the energy provided by the dialysate solution into the total meal plan.

Moderate-protein commercial formulas are also available for use by dialysis patients.

Comorbid Complications

Osteodystrophy. Bone disease or disorders are found in about 40% of patients suffering from decreased kidney function and almost 100% of patients with kidney failure. A combination of factors contributes to osteodystrophy during kidney disease. Decreased activation of vitamin D has a cascade effect resulting in: (1) elevated parathyroid hormone (PTH), and (2) reduced serum calcium levels. Patients also suffer from elevated serum

---

peritoneal cavity (Gr. *per*, around; *teinein*, to stretch) a strong, smooth surface; a serous membrane lining the abdominal and pelvic walls and undersurface of the diaphragm, forming a sac enclosing the body's vital visceral organs within the peritoneal cavity. Peritoneal dialysis is a form of dialysis through the peritoneum into and out of the peritoneal cavity.

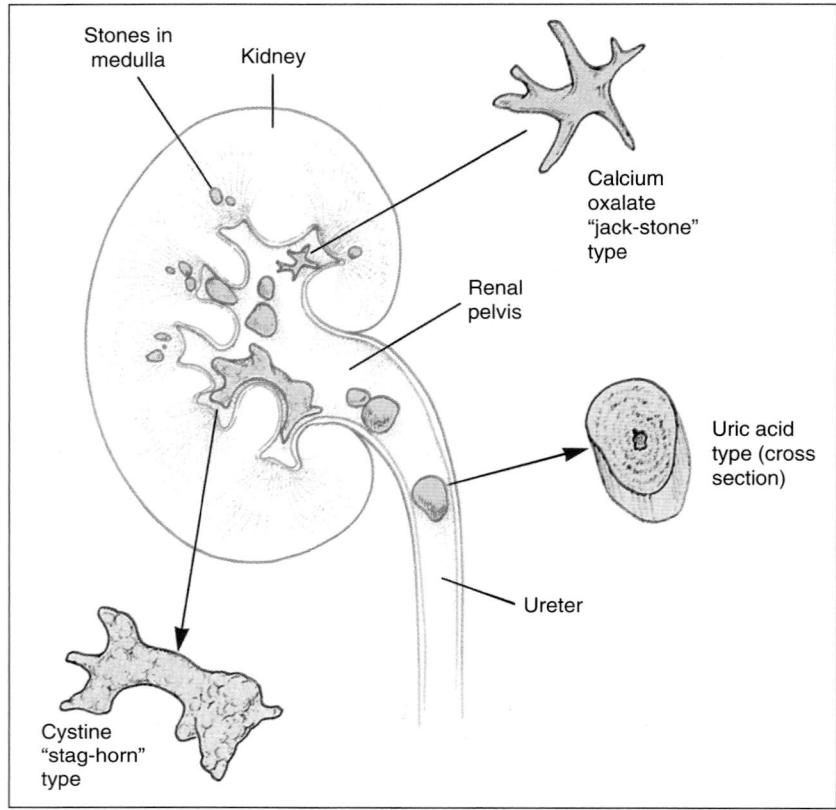

Figure 21–3 Renal calculi: stones in kidney, pelvis, and ureter.

BOX 21–2 Risk Factors for the Development of Kidney Stones

Male gender—2.5 times more likely to develop stones than women

Age—most common in individuals ages 20 to 40

Family history—accounts for 45% of all cases

Diet—high animal protein and low in fiber and fluids, or other dietary patterns causing prolonged imbalances in acidity of urine

Weight—overweight or severely underweight increases risk

Lifestyle—high stress

Medical conditions—hypertension, gout, bedridden status

Medications—for AIDS, thyroid hormones, chemotherapy, long-term antacid use

---

AIDS = acquired immunodeficiency syndrome.

---

phosphorus levels combined with the inability to excrete this phosphorus by the kidney. This combination causes abnormal changes in bone structure and function. The use of aluminum-based phosphate binders to reduce phosphorus absorption may introduce toxic amounts of aluminum in the body, further disrupting bone mineral-

ization.[11] It is recommended to evaluate patients with any level of kidney dysfunction for bone disease and disorders of calcium and phosphorus metabolism.[9]

Neuropathy. Central and peripheral neurologic disturbances are present in up to 65% of patients at the initiation of dialysis and are even more common in patients with diabetes. Symptoms of neuropathy may not be present until GFR falls below 12 to 20 ml/min per 1.73 m²; however, patients should be assessed periodically for implications of uremia or disease progression.[9]

KIDNEY STONE PROBLEMS

Disease Process

The basic cause of kidney stones is unknown, but many factors relating to the nature of the urine itself or conditions of the urinary tract environment contribute to their formation. The major stones are formed from calcium, struvite, and uric acid. Figure 21-3 illustrates the formation of these various stones. In addition, Box 21-2 lists risk factors associated with kidney stone development.

BOX 21-3 Food Sources of Oxalates

Fruits

Berries, all
Concord grapes
Currants
Figs
Fruit cocktail
Plums
Rhubarb
Tangerines

Vegetables

Baked beans
Beans, green and wax
Beet greens
Beets
Celery
Chard, Swiss
Chives
Collards
Eggplant
Endive
Kale
Leeks
Mustard greens
Okra
Peppers, green

Vegetables—*cont'd*

Rutabagas
Spinach
Squash, summer
Sweet potatoes
Tomatoes
Tomato soup
Vegetable soup

Nuts

Almonds
Cashews
Peanut butter
Peanuts

Beverages

Cocoa
Draft beer
Tea

Other

Grits
Tofu, soy products
Wheat germ

Calcium Stones

In North America, 5% of women and 12% of men suffer from kidney stones, 70% to 80% of which are composed of calcium oxalate.[12] Almost half of all calcium-stone cases likely result from genetic predisposition. However, other cases may be initiated by imbalances of compounds in the urine or blood, such as the following:

- Excess calcium in the blood (hypercalcemia)
- Excess calcium in the urine (hypercalciuria)
- Excess oxalate in the urine (hyperoxaluria; Box 21-3 shows food sources of oxalates)
- Low levels of citrate in the urine (hypocitraturia)
- Infection

Uric Acid Stones

Excess excretion of uric acid may be caused by some impairment with the metabolism of **purine,** a nitrogen end product of dietary protein from which uric acid is formed. This impairment occurs in diseases such as gout and also can occur in rapid tissue breakdown during wasting disease.

Struvite Stones

Struvite stones are composed of a single compound, magnesium ammonium phosphate ($MgNH_4PO_4$), and are often called *infection stones* because they mainly are caused by urinary tract infections, not an association with any specific nutrient. Thus no specific diet therapy is involved. Struvite stones usually are large "staghorn" stones that are removed surgically.

Other Stones

Cystine and xanthine stones are the rarest kidney stones. Cystine stones are caused by a genetic metabolic defect in the renal reabsorption of the amino acids cystine, ornithine, lysine, and arginine, causing an accumulation in the urine. Because this disorder is of genetic origin, it occurs rarely and only in individuals with this

---

purines (L. *purum,* pure; Gr. *ouron,* urine) nitrogen-containing compounds that yield uric acid as a metabolic end product eliminated in the urine.

genetic history. Xanthine stones are associated with treatment for gout and a family history of gout.

General Symptoms and Treatment

Clinical Symptoms

The main symptom of kidney stones is severe pain. Many other urinary symptoms may result from the presence of the stones. Usually general weakness and sometimes fever are present. Laboratory examination of the urine and any passed stones help determine treatment.

Treatment

General treatment may include several considerations, as discussed in the following sections.

Fluid Intake. A large fluid intake is a primary therapy that helps to produce more dilute urine and prevent accumulation of materials that form stones.

Stone Composition. In some cases, dietary control of the stone constituents may help reduce the recurrence of such stone formation, thus helping to pre-

---

BOX 21–4 Acid, Alkaline, and Neutral Food Groups

Meat/Dairy Group

Acid Ash
Beef
Cheese
Eggs
Fish
Peanuts
Poultry

Alkaline Ash
Milk and milk products

Neutral
—

Starch Group

Acid Ash
Pasta
Rice
Whole grain bread and crackers

Alkaline Ash
—

Neutral
Corn-based products (e.g., corn tortillas)

Vegetables

Acid Ash
Corn
Lentils

Alkaline Ash
All vegetables other than corn and lentils

Neutral
—

Fruits

Acid Ash
Cranberries
Plums
Prunes

Alkaline Ash
All fruits other than cranberries, plums, and prunes

Neutral
—

Beverages

Acid Ash
—

Alkaline Ash
—

Neutral
Coffee, tea

Fats/Sweets

Acid Ash
Bacon
Cake
Cookies

Alkaline Ash
—

Neutral
Butter
Hard candy
Honey
Margarine
Syrup
Vegetable oil

vent the accumulation of these metabolic substances in the urine available for stone formation.

Urinary pH. In the past, urinary pH was given much emphasis in relation to diet therapy for renal stones, but for some years now has been questioned. Research has indicated that acidification of the urine by traditional acid/alkaline ash diets may have little effect on urinary tract infections or the formation of stones in the urinary tract because calculation methods for determining the effect of specific foods on urinary pH have not proved to be valid. It is only in general, not precise, terms that vegetables, fruits, and milk are called alkaline ash foods or that meat, cheese, eggs, and whole grains are called acid ash foods. A desired pH of the urine is better achieved by medical means than by traditional acid/alkaline ash diets (Box 21-4).

Binding Agents. Materials that bind potential stone elements in the intestine can prevent their absorption and eliminate them from the body. For example, phytate is used to bind calcium. Phytates are found in high-fiber plant foods such as whole wheat, bran, and soybeans. Glycine has a similar effect on oxalates.

Drug Therapy. A variety of drugs is useful in the treatment of kidney stones, in combination with diet therapy.

For medications to be most effective, the specific type of stone should be identified. This is not always possible, thus limiting drug therapy in some individuals. Common drugs for kidney stones include the following:[12]

- *For calcium stones:* diuretics, citrates, phosphates, and cholestyramine
- *For uric acid stones:* sodium bicarbonate, potassium citrate, and allopurinol
- *For struvite stones:* medications to eliminate the infection, organic acids, and aluminum hydroxide gels

Nutrition Therapy

The nutritional care plan mainly relates to the nature of the stone. The diet is designed to reduce intake of nutrients that lead to the formation of a particular type of stone.

Calcium Stones

Dietary calcium intake is protective against kidney stones in most people. However, a low-calcium diet of approximately 400 mg/day is sometimes recommended for individuals who have supersaturation of calcium in the urine and are not at risk for bone loss (Table 21-2).

TABLE 21–2	**Low-Calcium Diet***	
Group	**Foods allowed**	**Foods not allowed**
Beverage†	Carbonated beverage, coffee, tea	Chocolate-flavored drinks, milk, milk drinks
Bread	White and light rye bread or crackers	
Cereals	Refined cereals	Oatmeal, whole grain cereals
Desserts	Cake, cookies, gelatin desserts, pastries, pudding, sherbets—all made without chocolate, milk, or nuts; if egg yolk is used, it must be from one-egg allowance	
Fat	Butter, cream (2 Tbsp daily), French dressing, margarine, salad oil, shortening	Cream (except in amount allowed), mayonnaise
Fruit	Canned, cooked, or fresh fruit or juice except rhubarb	Dried fruit, rhubarb
Meat, eggs	224 g (8 oz) daily of any meat, fowl, or fish except clams, oysters, or shrimp; not more than one egg daily, including those used in cooking	Clams, oysters, shrimp, cheese
Potato or substitute	Potato, hominy, macaroni, noodles, refined rice, spaghetti	Whole grain rice
Soup	Broth, vegetable soup made from vegetables allowed	Bean or pea soup, cream or milk soup
Sweets	Honey, jam, jelly, sugar	
Vegetables	Any canned, cooked, or fresh vegetables or juices except those listed	Dried beans, broccoli, green cabbage, celery, chard, collards, endive, greens, lettuce, lentils, okra, parsley, parsnips, dried peas, rutabagas
Miscellaneous	Herbs, pickles, popcorn, relishes, salt, spices, vinegar	Chocolate, cocoa, milk gravy, nuts, olives, white sauce

*Approximately 400 mg calcium.
†Depends on the calcium content of the local water supply. In instances of high calcium content, distilled water may be indicated.

This lower level mainly is achieved by removal of milk and dairy products, the main dietary sources of calcium. Other secondary calcium sources are whole grains and leafy vegetables. If a stone is calcium phosphate, additional sources of phosphorus (e.g., meats, legumes, and nuts) should be controlled. If a stone is calcium oxalate, foods high in oxalate (see Box 21-3) should be avoided.

Other dietary factors to consider in the case of calcium stones are sodium, fluid, and fiber intake. High intake of salt increases the amount of calcium excretion in the urine, thus precipitating hypercalciuria. Drinking plenty of fluids is beneficial in preventing all types of kidney stones by diluting the urine. Fiber foods high in phytates help prevent crystallization of oxalate calcium salts.

Uric Acid Stones

Approximately 7% of the total incidence of renal calculi is uric acid stones. Because uric acid is a metabolic product of purines, a low-purine diet sometimes is recommended. If dietary control of purines is desired, the following foods should be avoided: organ meats, alcoholic beverages, anchovies, sardines, yeast, legumes, mushrooms, spinach, asparagus, cauliflower, and poultry.

Cystine Stones

Cystine is derived from the essential amino acid methionine, so a low-methionine diet sometimes is used. Because this diet is essentially a low-protein diet and the rare genetic cystinuria condition occurs mainly in children, the treatment of choice is usually a regular diet to support growth. Medical drug therapy is used to control infection or produce more alkaline urine. General dietary principles in regard to renal stone disease are summarized in Table 21-3.

TABLE 21–3	Summary of Dietary Principles in Renal Stone Disease	
Stone chemistry	Nutrient modification	Dietary ash (urinary pH)
Calcium	Low calcium (400 mg)	Acid ash
Phosphate	Low phosphorus (1000-1200 mg)	
Oxalate	Low oxalate	
Struvite ($MgNH_4PO_4$)	Low phosphorus (1000-1200 mg; associated with urinary infections)	Acid ash
Uric acid	Low purine	Alkaline ash
Cystine	Low methionine	Alkaline ash

SUMMARY

The nephrons are the functional units of the kidneys. Through these unique structures, the kidney maintains life-sustaining blood levels of materials required for life and health. The nephrons accomplish their tremendous task by constantly "laundering" the blood over and over many times each day, returning necessary elements to the blood and eliminating the remainder in concentrated urine. Various diseases that interfere with the vital function of nephrons can cause serious renal disease if damage is extensive.

At its end stage, chronic renal failure is treated by dialysis or kidney transplant. Dialysis patients require close monitoring for protein, water, and electrolyte balance. Renal diseases have predisposing factors (e.g., recurrent urinary tract infections may lead to renal calculi, and progressive glomerulonephritis may lead to chronic nephrotic syndrome and renal failure). The Western diet is suspect as a predisposing factor in the development of chronic renal failure. The modern diet of excess protein may overtax human nephrons, which were not originally designed to handle a steady diet of protein-rich foods.

CRITICAL THINKING QUESTIONS

1. For each of the following conditions, outline the nutritional components of therapy, explaining the effect of each on kidney function: glomerulonephritis, nephrotic syndrome, and chronic renal failure.
2. Consider the nutritional factors that must be monitored in persons undergoing renal dialysis. How would

you suggest a client self-monitor fluid intake to both meet hydration needs while not exceeding restrictions? Make a general list of all dietary sources of fluid.
3. Outline the medical and nutrition therapy for various types of renal stones. Why are acid/alkaline diet modifications no longer valid therapies?

CHAPTER CHALLENGE QUESTIONS

True-False

Write the correct statement for each item you answer "false."

1. *True or False:* The basic functional unit of the kidney is the nephron.

2. *True or False:* There are only a few nephrons in each kidney, so metabolic stress can easily cause problems.

3. *True or False:* The operation of the nephrons relates little to the rest of the body.

4. *True or False:* The glomerulus' main function is filtration.

5. *True or False:* The tasks of the various parts of the nephron tubules are reabsorption, secretion, and excretion.

6. *True or False:* Dietary modifications in acute glomerulonephritis usually involve crucial restrictions of protein and sodium.

7. *True or False:* The primary symptom in nephrotic syndrome is massive albuminuria.

8. *True or False:* The nephrotic syndrome is best treated by a very low protein diet.

9. *True or False:* The multiple symptoms of advanced chronic renal failure basically result from metabolic imbalances in the body's inability to handle protein, electrolytes, and water.

10. *True or False:* Prolonged immobilization (e.g., with full body casts or disability) may lead to withdrawal of bone calcium and the formation of calcium renal stones.

Multiple Choice

1. Acute glomerulonephritis is best treated by which of the following methods? *(Circle all that apply.)*

   a. Reducing protein because filtration is impaired

   b. Using a normal amount of protein for optimum tissue nutrition and growth

   c. Restricting sodium to help control edema

   d. Allowing moderate salt use in uncomplicated cases

2. Diet therapy in nephrotic syndrome is designed to perform which of the following functions? *(Circle all that apply.)*

   a. Increase protein to replace the massive losses.

   b. Decrease protein moderately to reduce albumin losses.

   c. Increase kilocalories to provide energy and spare protein for tissue need.

   d. Restrict sodium moderately to help prevent edema.

3. The general diet needs in chronic renal failure include which of the following? *(Circle all that apply.)*

   a. Reduced protein intake

   b. Increased carbohydrate and moderate fat for needed energy

   c. Careful control of sodium and potassium according to need

   d. Increased fluids to stimulate kidney function

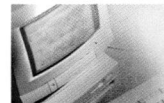

Please refer to the Students' Resource section of this text's Evolve web site for "Suggestions for Additional Study."

REFERENCES

1. U.S. Department of Health and Human Services, Centers for Disease Control and Prevention, National Center for Health Statistics, *Kidney disease*, Hyattsville, MD, 2003 (accessed May 2003), USHHS/CDC/NCHS [*www.cdc. gov/nchs/fastats/kidbladd.htm*].

2. Coresh J and others: Prevalence of chronic kidney disease and decreased kidney function in the adult U.S. pop-

ulation: Third National Health and Nutrition Examination Survey, *Am J Kidney Dis* 41:1, 2003.

3. Minino AM, Smith BL: Deaths: preliminary data for 2000, *Natl Vital Stat Rep* (12): 2001.

4. Churchill DN and others: Clinical practice guidelines for initiation of dialysis, *J Am Soc Nephrol* 10(13 suppl):289, 1999.

5. American Diabetes Association: Diabetic nephropathy, *Diabetes Care* 26(1 suppl):94, 2003.
6. Kikkawa R, Koya D, Haneda M: Progression of diabetic nephropathy, *Am J Kidney Dis* 41(1 suppl):19, 2003.
7. Satarug S and others: A global perspective on cadmium pollution and toxicity in non-occupationally exposed population, *Toxicol Lett* 137(1-2):65, 2003.
8. Karras A and others: Tenofovir-related nephrotoxicity in human immunodeficiency virus infected patients: three cases of renal failure, Fanconi syndrome, and nephrogenic diabetes insipidus, *Clin Infect Dis* 36(8):1070, 2003.
9. Eknoyan G, Levin NW: K/DOQI clinical practice guidelines for chronic kidney disease: evaluation, classification, and stratification, *Am J Kidney Dis* 39(2 suppl):1, 2002.
10. Vanhoulder R, Glorieux G, and Lameire N: The other side of the coin: impact of toxin generation and nutrition on the uremic syndrome, *Semin Dialysis* 15(5):311, 2002.
11. Malluche HH: Aluminum and bone disease in chronic renal failure, *Nephrol Dial Transplant* 17(2):21, 2002.
12. MD Consult: *Kidney stones* [patient handout], St Louis, 2002 (accessed May 2003), MD Consult/Elsevier [http://home.mdconsult.com/das/patient/view/36547852-2.

FURTHER READING AND RESOURCES

- National Institute of Diabetes & Digestive & Kidney Disease: *www.niddk.nih.gov*
- National Kidney Foundation: *www.kidney.org*
- American Foundation for Urologic Disease: *www.afud.org*
- Nephrology Forum, on Nephrology Channel: *www.nephrologychannel.com*

    Review the preceding web sites for additional information on various forms of kidney disease. There are several national organizations that provide free education and support for health care providers, patients, and family. Dietary restrictions for patients with kidney disease can sometimes be overwhelming for patients and loved ones. To fully understand such diets, continuous follow-up and feedback are needed. Such sites as these can help provide much needed information.

- Hebert CJ: Preventing kidney failure: primary care physicians must intervene earlier, *Cleve Clin J Med* 70(4):337, 2003.
- Szromba C, Thies MA, Ossman SS: Advancing chronic kidney disease care: new imperatives for recognition and intervention, *Nephrol Nurs J* 29(6):547, 2002.

    The preceding articles highlight the risk factors and early signs of decreased kidney function and address the important roles of physicians and nurses in identifying such factors.

22

Surgery and Nutritional Support

KEY CONCEPTS

■ Surgical treatment requires added nutritional support for tissue healing and rapid recovery.

■ The special nutritional problems of gastrointestinal surgery require diet modifications because of the surgery's effect on normal food passage.

■ Diet management for surgery patients to ensure optimal nutritional support involves both oral and intravenous feeding methods.

Malnutrition continues to occur among hospitalized patients, many of whom are surgical patients. Surveys in developed countries show that 20% to 50% of hospital patients have clinical signs of protein-energy malnutrition, which hinders healing.[1] Effective nutritional support must reverse malnutrition, improve prognosis, and speed recovery in a cost-effective manner.[2] The surgical process also places physiologic and psychological stress on patients, bringing added nutritional demands and risks for clinical problems.

This chapter looks at the nutritional needs of surgery patients and the enteral and parenteral feeding methods of providing nutritional support. Careful attention to both preoperative and postoperative nutritional support can reduce complications and provide essential resources for healing and health.

NUTRITIONAL NEEDS OF GENERAL SURGERY PATIENTS

A patient undergoing surgery faces large physiologic and psychological stress. Subsequently, nutritional demands are greatly increased during this period and deficiencies can easily develop, leading to serious malnutrition and clinical complications. Therefore careful attention *must* be given to a patient's nutritional status in preparation for surgery, as well as to the individual nutrition therapy needs that follow for wound healing and a more rapid recovery. A significant amount of research has been dedicated to understanding the association between protein-energy malnutrition and clinical outcomes. Although the defining factors for diagnosing protein-energy malnutrition have varied, poor nutritional status and the following associations are well accepted:[3]

- Impaired wound healing
- Increased risk of postoperative infection
- Reduced quality of life
- Impaired function of gastrointestinal tract
- Impaired immune system
- Impaired functioning of the cardiovascular and respiratory systems
- Increased hospital stay
- Increased cost
- Increased rate of mortality

Preoperative Nutritional Care: Nutrient Reserves

When the surgery is elective (i.e., not necessary or emergency), body nutrient stores can be built up to fortify a patient for the demands of the surgery and the period immediately following, when food intake may be limited. Commercial formulas provide needed nutrition supplementation. Particular needs center on protein, energy, vitamins, and minerals.

Protein

Protein deficiencies among surgical patients upon admission are common (see the For Further Focus box, "Protein-Energy Malnutrion during Surgery and Illness"). Every patient facing surgery needs to be fortified with adequate body protein in tissue and plasma to counteract blood losses during surgery and prevent tissue breakdown in the immediate postoperative period. For example, extensive bone healing is involved in orthopedic surgery. Protein is essential for forming the sound foundation that anchors mineral matter in bone tissue and is espe-

cially important with the occurrence of bone fractures in the growing U.S. population of elderly persons, particularly older women.[4]

Energy

Sufficient energy always must be provided when increased protein is necessary for tissue building. The increased source of kilocalories support the added energy demands and spare protein for its tissue-building work. For example, increased carbohydrate intake is needed to maintain optimal glycogen stores in the liver as a necessary resource for immediate energy fuel, thus directing protein to its tissue synthesis task. If a person is underweight, extra energy may be required to increase the weight to an ideal maintenance level before surgery. If a person is overweight and the surgery is not immediately necessary, some weight reduction may help reduce surgical complications.

Vitamins and Minerals

When increased protein and energy are necessary for any purpose, the appropriate intake of vitamins and minerals involved in protein and energy metabolism also must be supplied. Any deficiency state (e.g., anemia) should be corrected. Water balance should be assessed because both electrolytes and fluids are necessary to prevent dehydration.

Immediate Preoperative Period

Usual preparation for surgery calls for nothing to be taken orally for at least 8 hours before the surgery. This preparation is necessary to ensure that the stomach retains no food at surgery, which may cause complications such as vomiting or aspiration of food particles during anesthesia or recovery from anesthesia. In addition, any food present in the stomach may interfere with the surgical procedure or increase the risk for postoperative gastric retention and expansion. Especially before gastrointestinal surgery, a nonresidue diet (Box 22-1) may be followed for several days to clear the operative site of any food residue. Commercial nonresidue elemental formulas can provide a complete diet in liquid form. These formulas can be administered by tube or made more palatable for oral use with various flavorings.

Emergency Surgery

If the surgery is an emergency, no time is available for building up ideal nutritional reserves. Thus it is more important for persons to maintain a good nutritional status through a healthy diet as a regular habit so that optimum nutrient reserves are available to supply needs at times of stress.

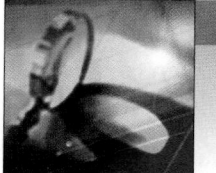

FOR FURTHER FOCUS

PROTEIN-ENERGY MALNUTRITION DURING SURGERY AND ILLNESS

Protein-energy malnutrition (PEM) compromises quality of life and ability to recover from surgery and injury. As general health declines with age, and the risk for unplanned surgery increases, so does the prevalence of PEM.* Actively evaluating the nutritional status of older people in either home, hospital or nursing home settings may provide valuable information about the preoperative needs of these individuals.†‡ Providing oral supplements or enteral feeding tubes for malnourished elderly patients before surgery may be a cost effective way to improve outcome, reduce hospital stay, and reduce the risk of complications associated with surgery.§

Even without a formal nutrition assessment, PEM can be identified by monitoring unplanned weight loss. The following table provides a quick guide to evaluate weight loss:

| Initial weight (lbs) | Weight loss (%) and resulting weight (lbs) | |
	5%	10%
80	76	72
85	81	77
90	86	81
95	90	86
100	95	90
110	105	99
120	114	108
130	124	117
140	133	126
150	143	135
160	152	144
170	162	153
180	171	162

Unplanned weight loss is indicative of PEM and compromised ability to deal with physiologic stress. An unplanned weight loss of 5% over a 1-month period, or 10% over a 6-month period, is considered a significant loss. A loss of greater than 5% in 1 month or greater than 10% in 6 months is classified as severe. Identifying and treating those individuals at risk for PEM also may prevent poor outcome in the event of surgery or injury.

*Crogan NL, Pasvogel A: The influence of protein-calorie malnutrition on quality of life in nursing homes, *J Gerontol A Biol Sci Med Sci* 58(2): 159, 2003.
†Van Nes MC and others: Does the Mini Nutritional Assessment predict hospitalization outcomes in older people? *Age Ageing* 30:221, 2001.
‡Beck AM, Ovensen L, Schroll M: A six months' prospective follow-up of 65+y-old patients from general practice classified according to nutritional risk by the Mini Nutritional Assessment, *Eur J Clin Nutr* 55(11): 1028, 2001.
§Nourhashemi F and others: Nutritional support and aging in preoperative nutrition, *Curr Opin Clin Nutr Metab Care* 2(1):87, 1999.

Postoperative Nutritional Care: Nutrient Needs for Healing

Adequate nutritional support is necessary to aid recovery from surgery when nutrient losses are great. At the same time, food intake is greatly diminished or even absent for

elemental formula a nutritional support formula composed of simple elemental nutrient components that require no further digestive breakdown and are thus readily absorbed.

BOX 22–1 Nonresidue Diet and Postsurgical Nonresidue Diet

Nonresidue Diet

General Description

1. This diet includes only those foods free from fiber, seeds, and skins and with the minimum amount of residue.
2. Fruits and vegetables are omitted except for strained fruit juices.
3. Milk is omitted.
4. The diet is adequate in protein and energy, containing approximately 75 g protein, 100 g fat, 250 g carbohydrate, and 2260 kcal. It is likely to be inadequate in vitamin A, calcium, and riboflavin.
5. If patients are to remain a long time on this diet, supplementary vitamins and minerals should be administered.

Selection of Foods

Foods	Foods Allowed	Foods Not Allowed
Beverages	Carbonated beverages, coffee, tea	Milk, milk drinks
Bread	Crackers, melba or rusks	Whole grain bread
Cereals	Refined as Cream of Wheat, Farina, fine cornmeal, Malt-o-Meal, pablum, rice, strained oatmeal, cornflakes, puffed rice, Rice Krispies	Whole grain and other cereals
Cheese		None allowed
Desserts	Plain cakes and cookies, gelatin desserts, water ices, angel food cake, arrowroot cookies, tapioca puddings made with fruit juice only	Pastries, all others
Eggs	As desired, preferably hard-cooked	Fried eggs
Fats	Butter or substitute, small amount of cream	None
Fruits	Strained fruit juices	All others
Meat, fish, poultry	Tender beef, chicken, fish, lamb, liver, veal; crisp bacon	Fried or tough meat, pork
Potatoes or substitute	Only macaroni, noodles, spaghetti, refined rice	Potatoes, corn, hominy, unrefined rice
Soup	Bouillon and broth only	All others
Sweets	Hard candy, fondant, gumdrops, jelly, marshmallows, sugar, syrup, honey	Other candy, jam, marmalade
Vegetables	Tomato juice	All others
Miscellaneous	Salt	Pepper

Postsurgical Nonresidue Diet

General Description

1. This diet is slightly higher in residue but has greater variety, including potatoes, white bread products, processed cheese, sauces, desserts made with milk, and cream for coffee and cereal.
2. The average daily menu contains 85 g protein, 2300 kcal, and slightly more vitamins and minerals.

Selection of Foods

To the selections listed for the nonresidue diet outlined previously, add the following:

● *Cheese:* Processed cheese, mild cream cheeses
● *Potatoes:* Prepared any way, skin removed
● *Bread:* Any kind without bran, white bread, rolls, pancakes, waffles
● *Fats:* 2 oz cream or half-and-half per meal, cream sauce, cream gravy
● *Desserts:* All desserts except those containing fruit and nuts
● *Condiments:* As desired

Note: Fruit juice and hard candies may be taken between meals to increase caloric intake.

a period. To supply this additional nutritional support, several nutrients require particular attention.

Protein

Optimal protein intake in the postoperative recovery period is of primary concern for all patients. Protein is needed to replace losses during surgery and supply the increased demands of the healing process. During the period immediately after surgery, the body tissues usually undergo considerable **catabolism,** which means that the process of tissue breakdown and loss exceeds the process of tissue buildup (see Chapter 4). A negative nitrogen balance of as much as 20 g/day also may occur during this time. This negative balance represents an actual loss of more than 0.5 kg (1 lb) of tissue protein per day. In addition to the protein losses from tissue breakdown caused by metabolic imbalances, other losses of protein from the body also occur, including plasma protein loss from hemorrhage, wound bleeding, and various body fluid losses or **exudates.** Increased loss of plasma protein also may occur from extensive tissue destruction, inflammation, infection, and trauma. If any degree of prior malnutrition or chronic infection existed, a patient's protein deficiency could easily become severe and cause serious complications. There are several reasons for this increased protein demand.

Building Tissue. The process of wound healing requires building a great deal of new body tissue, which can only be done when enough of the essential amino acids (see Box 4-1) from dietary protein intake or body stores can be brought to the tissue by the circulating blood. These necessary amino acids must come from dietary protein or from intravenous feeding if a patient cannot eat normally for an extended period of time. Such protein needs usually can be met through oral feedings, so patients are encouraged to eat as soon as possible after surgery. Dietary protein intake sometimes must be increased to 100 to 150 g/day to restore lost protein and build new tissues at the wound site.

Controlling Shock. A sufficient supply of plasma protein, mainly albumin, is necessary to maintain blood volume (see Chapter 9). If the plasma protein level drops, pressure to keep tissue fluid circulating between the capillaries and cells is insufficient. Without adequate pressure, water leaves the blood capillaries and cannot be drawn back into circulation. Shock symptoms result from a shrinking blood volume and the body's effort to restore it.

Controlling Edema. When serum protein levels are low, a loss of osmotic pressure (necessary to maintain normal movement of fluid between the capillaries and surrounding tissue) is lost and **edema** develops. Edema is char-

acterized by puffiness or swelling of the tissue from the excess fluid being held there instead of returning to circulation. Generalized edema may adversely affect heart and lung function. Local edema at the wound site also interferes with closure of the wound and hinders the normal healing process.

Healing Bone. Protein, as well as mineral matter, is essential to the foundation of bone tissue for proper formation and healing. Protein provides a matrix for calcium and phosphorus to be laid down to form proper bone **callus** and strong bones.

Resisting Infection. Protein tissues are the major components of the body's immune system, providing its defense against infection. These defense agents include special white cells called *lymphocytes,* as well as antibodies and various other blood cells, hormones, and enzymes. Tissue strength is a major defense barrier against infection at all times.

Transporting Lipids. Fat is also an important component of tissue structure, forming the center of cell walls and participating in many other necessary metabolic activities. Protein is necessary to carry fat in the blood stream to all tissues (see Chapter 19) for maintaining tissue

---

catabolism (Gr. *katabole,* a throwing down) the process by which body tissues are broken down, the opposite of anabolism. Catabolism includes all the processes in which complex substances are progressively broken down into simpler ones, usually with the release of energy. Together, anabolism and catabolism constitute metabolism, which is the coordinated operation of anabolic (building up) and catabolic (breaking down) processes into a dynamic balance of energy and substance.

exudate (L. *exsudare,* to sweat out) various materials such as cells, cellular debris, and fluids, usually resulting from inflammation, that have escaped from the blood vessels and are deposited in or on the surface tissues; protein content is high.

edema (Gr. *oidema,* swelling) an unusual accumulation of fluid in the interstitial (e.g., small structural spaces between tissue parts) spaces of the body.

callus (L. *callositis,* callus, bone) unorganized meshwork of newly grown, woven bone developed on a pattern of the original clot of fibrin, formed after fracture or surgery, and normally replaced in the healing process by hard adult bone.

structures and activities. Protein is also necessary to carry fat to the liver for necessary work in fat metabolism. Protein in the liver combines with and removes fat, thus avoiding the danger of fatty infiltration, which could lead to liver disease.

Because protein has many important functions during recovery from surgery, protein deficiency at this time obviously can lead to many clinical problems. Such problems include poor wound healing, rupture of the suture lines **(dehiscence),** delayed healing of fractures, depressed heart and lung function, anemia, failure of gastrointestinal **stomas** (discussed later in this chapter) to function, reduced resistance to infection, liver damage, extensive weight loss, and increased mortality risk.

Water

Water balance after surgery is a constant concern. Sufficient fluid intake is necessary to prevent dehydration, especially in elderly persons whose thirst mechanism may be depressed and cannot be depended on to ensure adequate fluid intake. In patients who have complications or are seriously ill and have extensive drainage, as much as 7 L of fluid may be necessary daily. During the postoperative period, large water losses also may occur from vomiting, hemorrhage, fever, or excessive urination. The usual intravenous fluids after surgery will supply some initial needs, but oral intake should begin as soon as possible and be sufficiently maintained.

Energy

As always, when increased protein is demanded for tissue building, enough nonprotein kcalories must be supplied for energy to spare protein for its vital tissue-building function. The fuel sources, carbohydrate and fat, therefore must be sufficiently supplied in the total diet. Because excess fat presents general health problems, carbohydrates become the major source of needed fuel. A minimum of 100 g carbohydrates must be supplied by the diet on a daily basis to spare protein from catabolism and use as energy. In situations of acute metabolic stress (e.g., in extensive surgery or burns), energy needs may increase to as much as 1.2 to 2 kcal/kg body weight per day over basal energy requirements. Energy requirements can be estimated by first calculating basal energy needs using the Harris-Benedict equations (see Chapter 6) and then multiplying by an injury factor (1.2 to 2) to meet added energy needs for stress and sepsis. Energy needs for burn patients are directly dependent on percent of body surface area (BSA) burned and are calculated as follows:[5]

$$20 \text{ kcal/kg} + [40 \times \% \text{ of BSA burned}]$$

Carbohydrates not only spare protein for tissue building but also help avoid liver damage by maintaining glycogen reserves in the liver tissue. However, excessive fuel storage as body fat should be avoided because fatty tissue heals poorly and is more susceptible to infection.

Vitamins

Several vitamins require particular attention in wound healing. Vitamin C helps to build connective tissue, new capillary walls, and general tissue ground substance. *In vitro* studies demonstrate that addition of vitamin C to cell culture media improves the cells epidermal barrier, metabolic viability, DNA synthesis, and ability to heal.[6] If extensive tissue building is necessary, as much as 3000 mg vitamin C per day for 3 or more days may be beneficial in the immediate period after injury.[7] (It is not recommended to continue supplementing at this level long-term.) As energy and protein intake are increased, the B vitamins that have important coenzyme roles in protein and energy metabolism (e.g., especially thiamin, riboflavin, and niacin) also must be increased. Other B-complex vitamins—folate, B_{12}, pyridoxine, and pantothenic acid—also play important roles in building hemoglobin and thus must meet the demands of an increased blood supply and general metabolic stress. Vitamin K, which is essential for blood clotting, is usually present in a sufficient amount because it is synthesized by intestinal bacteria.

Minerals

Attention to any mineral deficiencies is essential. When tissue is broken down (as occurs after surgery), cell potassium and phosphorus are lost. Electrolyte imbalances of sodium and chloride also result from fluid losses. Iron deficiency anemia may develop from blood loss or faulty iron absorption. Another mineral important in wound healing is zinc. An adequate amount of protein usually meets this need because most dietary zinc is found in protein foods of animal origin. Sometimes zinc supplements may be recommended for extensive surgery and poor zinc stores.

GENERAL DIETARY MANAGEMENT

Initial Intravenous Fluid and Electrolytes

Most general surgical patients can and should progress to oral feedings as soon as possible to provide adequate nutrition. Remember that routine postoperative intravenous (IV) fluids are used to supply hydration needs and electrolytes, not to sustain energy and nutrients. Ordinary postsurgery IVs are not designed to supply complete nutrient needs or compete with oral feedings. For example, a 5% dextrose solution (D_5W) with normal saline (0.9% NaCl solution) contains only 5 g dextrose/dl (e.g., about 20 kcal or 200 kcal/L), although the total energy need is more than 10 times that amount. A rapid return to regular eating should be encouraged and maintained.

Methods of Feeding

Two basic methods for dietary management are available, as follows:

1. **Enteral.** Taking in nourishment through the regular gastrointestinal route as long as it can be used, either by regular oral feedings or by tube feedings
2. **Parenteral.** Taking in nourishment through veins, either small peripheral veins or a large central vein

Enteral Feedings

When the gastrointestinal tract can be used, it is the preferred route of feeding, orally if possible and if not, by feeding tube.[8]

Oral Feeding. Most general surgical patients can and should receive oral feedings as soon as possible. Oral feedings allow more needed nutrients to be added and help stimulate normal action of the gastrointestinal tract. Food usually can be taken orally as soon as regular bowel sounds return. When oral feedings begin, the patient usually progresses from clear to full liquids and then to a soft or regular diet. Examples of these progressive "routine house diets" used in hospitals are given in Chapter 17. Individual tolerance and needs are always the guide, but encouragement and help should be supplied in general care of postsurgery patients to enable them to eat as soon as possible. Depending on a patient's condition, a general energy-nutrient food supplement formula may be added orally, with or between meals.[8] The energy value of foods in the regular diet also may be increased as tolerated with added sauces, seasonings, and dressings. More frequent, less bulky, concentrated small meals may be helpful, making every bite count.

Tube Feeding. When regular oral feedings are not tolerated, as with patients who are comatose or severely debilitated or have undergone radical neck or face surgery, nutrient formulas may be fed by tube. The most common route is the nasogastric (NG) tube, which is inserted through the nose and into the stomach (Figure 22-1, *A*). For patients at risk for aspiration, reflux, or continuous vomiting, a nasoduodenal (ND) or nasojejunal (NJ) tube may be more appropriate. In both cases, a tube is first inserted through the nose into the stomach. Then

it is passed through the stomach and into the appropriate portion of the small intestines via peristaltic activity or endoscopic or fluoroscopic guidance. Modern small-bore nasoenteric feeding tubes made of softer, more flexible polyurethane and silicone materials have replaced large-bore stiff tubing. These modern feeding tubes are more comfortable for the patient and easily carry the variety of nutrient materials now available in enteral nutrition-support formulas. With the development of improved formulas and feeding equipment, the question of using blender-mixed formulas of regular foods seldom arises. Using blenderized table food for tube feedings may present the following problems:

■ *Physical form.* Foods broken down and mixed in a blender yield a sticky, larger-particle mixture that does not go through the small feeding tubes easily and thus requires the more uncomfortable large-bore tubing.
■ *Safety.* Such blender-mixed formulas carry problems of bacterial growth and infection, as well as inconsistent nutrient composition because the solid components settle out.
■ *Digestion and absorption.* Blenderized food requires a fully functioning digestive and absorptive system to digest the food and absorb its released nutrients. Many patients have gastrointestinal deficits that require nutrients with varying degrees of predigestion (hydrolysis) or smaller molecular structure.

In overall comparison, commercial formulas provide a sterile, homogenized solution suitable for the more comfortable, modern, small-bore feeding tubes and ensure a fixed profile of nutrients in intact or predigested form. No matter what type of feeding tube or formula used to

dehiscence (L. *dehiscere*, to gape) a splitting open; the separation of layers of a surgical wound—partial or superficial or complete—with total disruption requiring resuturing.

stoma (Gr. *stoma*, mouth, opening) the opening established in the abdominal wall, connecting with the ileum or colon, for elimination of intestinal wastes after surgical removal of diseased portions of the intestines.

enteral (Gr. *enteron*, intestine) a mode of feeding that uses the gastrointestinal tract through oral or tube feeding.

parenteral (Gr. *para-*, beyond, beside; *enteron*, intestine) a mode of feeding that does not use the gastrointestinal tract but provides nutritional support by intravenous delivery of nutrient solutions.

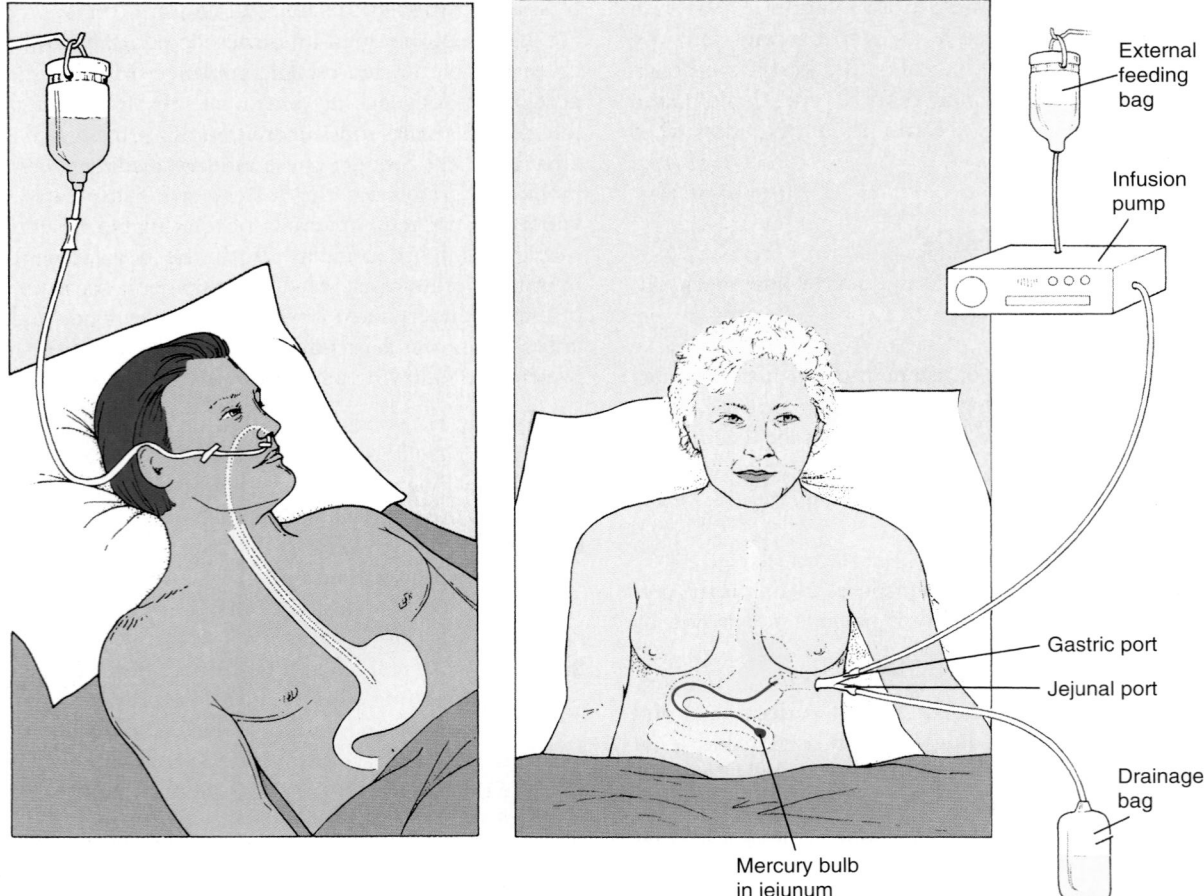

External
feeding
bag

Infusion
pump

Gastric port

Jejunal port

Drainage
bag

Mercury bulb
in jejunum

Figure 22–1 Types of tube feeding. Common nasogastric feeding tube *(left)*. Gastrostomy-jejunal enteral feeding tube *(right)*.

meet a patient's physiologic needs, such a method of feeding may contribute to a patient's psychological stress. Much support for a patient's quality of life is an important part of patient care planning.

Alternative Routes for Enteral Tube Feeding. The nasoenteric route described is usually indicated for short-term therapy (e.g., 3 to 4 weeks) in many clinical situations. For long-term feedings, however, *enterostomies*—surgical placement of the tube at progressive points along the gastrointestinal tract—provide a more comfortable route, as follows:

■ *Esophagostomy.* A cervical esophagostomy is placed at the level of the cervical spine to the side of the neck after head and neck surgeries for cancer or traumatic injury. This placement removes the discomfort of the nasal route and enables the entry point to be easily concealed under clothing.

■ *Percutaneous endoscopic gastrostomy (PEG).* A gastrostomy tube may be surgically placed through the abdominal wall into the stomach if a patient is not at risk for aspiration (see Figure 22-1, *B*).
■ *Percutaneous endoscopic jejunostomy (PEJ).* A jejunostomy tube is surgically placed through the abdominal wall and passed through the duodenum into the jejunum, the middle section of the small intestine, if the patient is at risk for aspiration. This procedure is indicated for patients who lack a competent gag reflex or have gastric cancer or gastric ulcerative disease.

The tube-feeding formula generally is prescribed by the physician and clinical dietitian according to the patient's nutritional need and tolerance. In any form of tube feeding, it is important to regulate the amount of formula and the rate at which it is given. Highly concentrated formulas should be started at one-quarter to one-half the goal rate of final delivery and advanced every 8 to 12 hours as tolerated. Patients who have not been fed in 5 days will not be able to tolerate large feedings and should start with 25 to 50 ml/hour, with gradual increases to goal rate.[9] In most tube-feeding cases, diarrhea is the most frequently reported gastrointestinal complication. Formulas supplemented with the soluble fiber pectin in a 1% solution (1 ml pectin/100 ml formula) may improve bowel function and reduce the incidence of diarrhea in some patients. However, fiber supplemented formulas are contraindicated for patients with impaired gastric emptying.[10] Medications and *Clostridium difficile* enterocolitis are common culprits in causing diarrhea and should be ruled out before farther investigation or changes are made.

A wide variety of commercial formulas are available and designed to meet particular needs. These products may be made from *intact nutrients* for use with a fully functioning gastrointestinal system able to digest and absorb them. Others may be made from predigested *elemental or semielemental nutrients*, which are readily absorbed with only minimal residue.[10] Still others may be formulated for special problems or single-nutrient products (modules) of protein, carbohydrate, and fat mixed together as calculated by the clinical dietitian or clinical pharmacist to meet a patient's specific needs. Commercial enteral formulas have the advantage of being standard in composition and immediately available for use. These formulas are also sterile and may be stored. Some examples are given in Table 22-1.

Parenteral Feedings

Parenteral nutrition refers to any feeding method other than the normal gastrointestinal route. In current medical and nutritional usage, *parenteral* specifically refers to the special feeding of basic predigested nutrient elements directly into the blood circulation through certain veins when the gastrointestinal tract cannot be used. Depending on the nutritional support necessary, the following two routes are available:

1. *Peripheral parenteral nutrition (PPN)*. PPN is used when a solution of no more than 800 to 900 mOsm/kl is sufficient to provide needs and when feeding is necessary for only a brief period (10 days). The osmolality, or mOsm/L, of a solution depends on the concentration of its total particles, including dextrose, protein, and electrolytes. Small peripheral veins, usually in the arm, are used to deliver the less concentrated solutions (Figure 22-2). There are catheters in use now that will allow an extended feeding period in a peripheral vein for individuals with large veins and can tolerate the *extended dwell catheter.*

2. *Total parenteral nutrition (TPN)*. TPN is used when the energy and nutrient requirement is large or when needed to supply full nutritional support for longer periods of time. A large central vein, usually the subclavian vein leading directly into the rapid flow of the superior vena cava to the heart, is used for surgical placement of the feeding catheter (Figure 22-3). Nutritional support solutions of much higher osmolality are tolerated in this vein.

TPN is used in cases of major surgery or complications, especially those involving the gastrointestinal tract, or when the patient is unable to obtain sufficient nourishment orally. TPN provides crucial nutritional support from solutions containing large amounts of glucose, amino acids, electrolytes, minerals, and vitamins. Fat in the form of lipid emulsions is also used to supply needed energy and the essential fatty acids. A basic TPN solution may contain between 3.5% and 15% crystalline amino acids and 2.5% to 70% dextrose with added electrolytes, vitamins, and trace elements (Table 22-2). The physician and clinical dietitian on the nutritional support team determine the individual formula needed based on detailed individual nutrition assessment. The pharmacist on the nutritional support team carefully mixes the solutions according to the prescription. Then the administration of the solution is an important nursing responsibility (Box 22-2). Long-term home use of TPN has been a lifesaving measure for many persons but is expensive and requires thorough training.

SPECIAL NUTRITIONAL NEEDS AFTER GASTROINTESTINAL SURGERY

Because the gastrointestinal system is uniquely designed to handle food, a surgical procedure on any part of this system requires special dietary attention or modification.

Mouth, Throat, and Neck Surgery

Surgery involving the mouth, jaw, throat, or neck requires modification in the mode of eating. A patient usually cannot chew or swallow normally, so accommodations must be made according to individual limitations.

TABLE 22–1	Examples of Enteral Formulas and Macronutrient Components*			
		Sources		
Brand name	**Manufacturer**	**Carbohydrate**	**Protein**	**Fat**
STANDARD COMPLETE DIETS: INTACT MACRONUTRIENTS				
Sustacal HC	Mead Johnson (Evansville, IN)	Corn syrup, sucrose	Casein	Soy oil
Isocal HN	Mead Johnson	Corn syrup	Casein	Soy and MCT oils
Magnacal	Mead Johnson	Maltodextrins	Casein	Soy oil
Ensure	Ross Products (Columbus, OH)	Corn syrup, sucrose	Casein	Corn oil
Osmolite	Ross Products	Corn syrup	Casein, soy protein isolate	Soy, corn, and MCT oils
Jevity (Plus)	Ross Products	Maltodextrins, corn syrup	Casein	Safflower, canola, and MCT oils
Travasorb	Nestle (Glendale, CA)	Corn syrup, sucrose	Soy protein isolate	Soy oil
STANDARD COMPLETE DIETS: SEMIELEMENTAL AND ELEMENTAL				
Vital HN	Ross Products	Glucose oligosaccharides	Small peptides	Safflower oil
Reabilan HN	Nestle	Maltodextrin	Small peptides	MCT oil, EFA
Critacare HN	Mead Johnson	Maltodextrin	Free amino acids and small peptides	Safflower oil, fatty acids
Optimenal	Ross Products	Maltodextrin, sucrose	Small peptides	MCT
SPECIALTY DIETS: TRAUMA				
Vivonex TEN	Novartis (Basil, Switzerland)	Glucose oligosaccharides	Crystalline amino acids	Safflower oil
Traumacal	Mead Johnson	Corn syrup	Casein	Soybean oil, MCT
IntensiCal	Mead Johnson	Maltodextrin, corn starch	Casein	Canola oil, MCT
Advera for HIV	Ross Products	Maltodextrin, sucrose	Soy protein hydrolysate	Canola oil, MCT
SPECIALTY DIETS: RENAL				
Travasorb HN	Nestle	Glucose oligosaccharides	Crystalline amino acids	Sunflower oil, MCT
Suplena	Ross Products	Maltodextrin, sucrose	Casein	Safflower oil, soy oil
SPECIALTY DIETS: HEPATIC				
Travasorb MCT	Nestle	Glucose oligosaccharides, sucrose	Crystalline amino acids	Sunflower oil, MCT
SPECIALTY DIETS: CHILDREN AGES 1 TO 10				
PediaSure	Ross Products	Corn syrup, sucrose	Casein-whey	Safflower-soy oils, MCT
Kindercal	Mead Johnson	Maltodextrin, sucrose	Milk protein	Canola, sunflower, corn, and MCT oils

EFA = Essential fatty acids; *HC* = high-calorie; *HIV* = human immunodeficiency virus; *HN* = high-nitrogen; *MCT* = medium-chain triglycerides; *TEN* = total enteral nutrition.
*All formulas are enriched with essential micronutrients—vitamins and minerals—as needed.

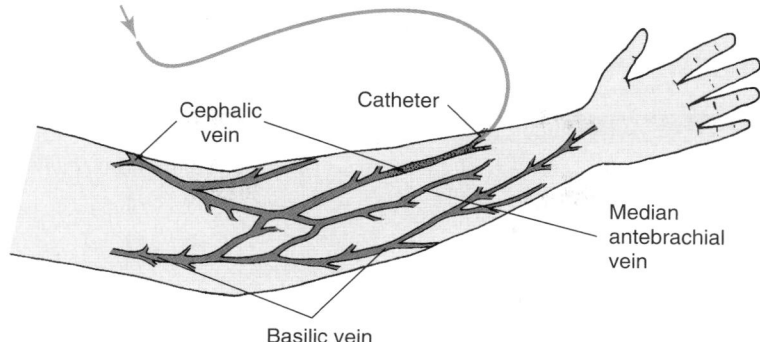

Figure 22–2   Peripheral parenteral nutrition feeding into small veins in the arm.

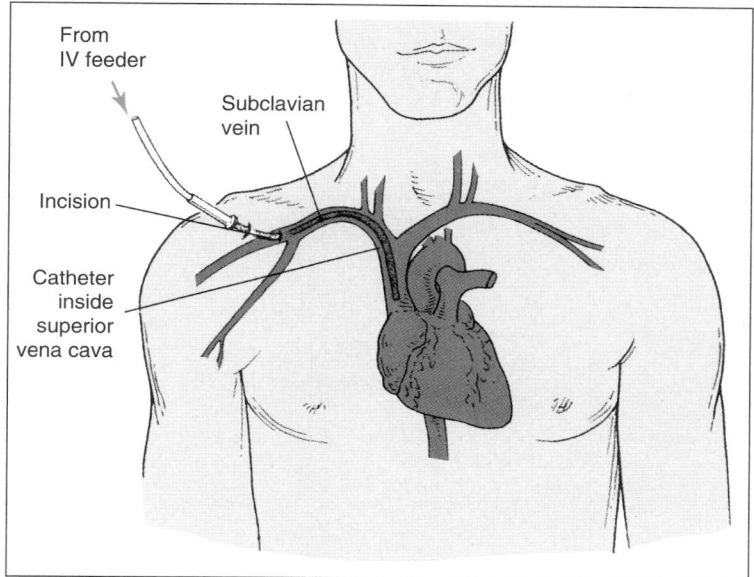

Figure 22–3   Catheter placement for total parenteral nutrition (TPN) made for feeding via subclavian vein to superior vena cava.

Oral Liquid Feedings

Concentrated liquid feedings should be planned to ensure adequate nutrition in a smaller amount of food. An enriched commercial formula can be used several times a day to supply needed nourishment.

Tube Feedings

In cases of radical neck or facial surgery, or when a patient is comatose or severely debilitated, tube feedings may be indicated. For long-term needs, improved equipment and standardized commercial formulas have made continued home tube feeding possible for many patients. A nasogastric tube usually is used, but if there is obstruction in the esophagus, or other complications, the tube is

inserted into an opening in the abdominal wall, a gastrostomy, which the surgeon makes at the time of surgery.

Stomach Surgery

Nutritional Problems

Because the stomach is the first major food reservoir in the gastrointestinal tract, stomach surgery poses special problems in maintaining adequate nutrition. Some of these problems may develop immediately after the surgery, depending on the type of surgical procedure (Figure 22-4) and the individual patient's response. Other complications may occur later when the person begins to eat a regular diet.

TABLE 22–2	Example of Basic Total Parenteral Nutrition Formula Components
Component	**Amount**
BASIC SOLUTION	
Crystalline amino acids	4%
Dextrose	25%
ADDITIVES	
Electrolytes	
Na	50 mEq/L
Cl	50 mEq/L
K	40 mEq/L
HPO_4	25 mEq/L
Ca	5 mEq/L
Mg	8 mEq/L
Vitamins	
Multiple (MV)	1.7 ml conc/L
Vitamin C (per day)	500 mg
Trace elements solution (per day)	
Zn	3 mg
Cu	1.6 mg
Cr	2 μg
Se	120 μg
Mn	2 μg
I	120 μg
Fe	1.5 μg
Other additives (as needed)	
Regular insulin	0-25 U/L
Heparin	1000 U/L

TPN = Total parenteral nutrition.

BOX 22–2 Administration of Total Parenteral Nutrition Formula

Careful administration of total parenteral nutrition (TPN) formulas is essential. Specific protocols vary somewhat but usually include the following points:

- *Start slowly.* Allow time to adapt to the increased glucose concentration and osmolality of the solution.
- *Schedule carefully.* During the first 24 hours, 1 to 2 L is administered by continuous drip, with the slow rate usually regulated by an infusion pump.
- *Monitor closely.* Note the metabolic effects of glucose (not to exceed 200 mg/dl) and electrolytes.
- *Increase volume gradually.* After the first day, increase by 1 L/day to reach the desired daily volume.
- *Make changes cautiously.* Watch the effect of all changes and proceed slowly.
- *Maintain a constant rate.* Keep the correct hourly infusion rate, with no "catch-up" or "slow-down" effort to meet the original volume order.
- *Discontinue slowly.* Take the patient off the TPN feeding gradually, reducing the rate and daily volume approximately 1 L/day.

Immediate Postoperative Period

Serious nutritional deficits may occur immediately after surgery, especially after a total gastrectomy. Increased gastric fullness and distention may result if the gastric resection also involved a *vagotomy* (i.e., cutting of the vagus nerve, which supplies a major stimulus for gastric secretions). Lacking the normal nerve stimulus, the stomach becomes *atonic* (i.e., without normal muscle tone) and empties poorly. Food fermentation occurs, producing *flatus*, or gas, and diarrhea. Weight loss is common after extensive gastric surgery; at least half of patients fail to reach their optimal weight level.

To cover this immediate postoperative nutritional need after the gastrectomy procedure, surgeons usually leave a temporary catheter in place with a *jejunostomy* (e.g., an opening to the jejunum) through which the patient can be fed an elemental formula to ensure optimal nutritional support during this important recovery

period. Frequent small oral feedings are generally resumed according to a patient's tolerance. A typical pattern of simple dietary progression may cover about a 2-week period. The basic principles of such general diet therapy for the immediate postgastrectomy period involve the following: (1) size of meals: small and frequent; and (2) nature of meals: simple, easily digested, nonspicy, and low in bulk.

'Dumping Syndrome'

Dumping syndrome is a frequently encountered complication after extensive gastric resection. After the initial recovery from surgery, when the patient begins to feel better and eats a regular diet in greater volume and variety, discomfort may occur 30 to 60 minutes after meals. A cramping, full feeling develops, the pulse becomes rapid, and a wave of weakness, cold sweating, and dizziness may follow. Nausea, vomiting, or diarrhea typically conclude the event. These distressing reactions to food intake only increase anxiety. As a result, less and less food is eaten. Weight loss and general malnutrition follow (see the Clinical Applications Box, "Case Study: John Has a Gastrectomy").

This complex of symptoms constitutes a shock syndrome that results when a meal containing a large proportion of readily soluble carbohydrates rapidly enters, or "dumps," into the small intestine. When the stomach

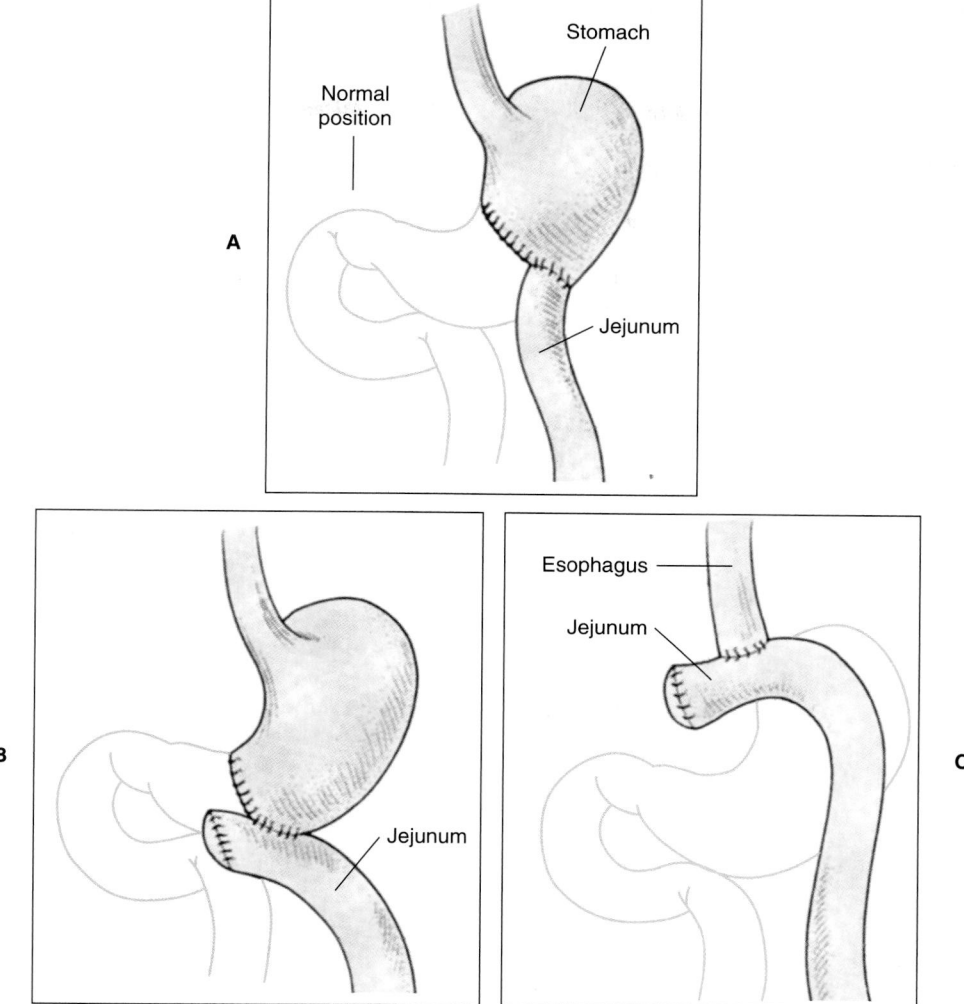

Figure 22-4 Gastric surgery. A, Partial gastrectomy, Billroth I. B, Partial gastrectomy, Billroth II. C, Total gastrectomy.

has been removed, food passes directly from the esophagus into the small intestine (see Figure 22-4). This rapidly entering food mass is a concentrated solution (higher osmolality) in relation to the surrounding circulation of blood. To achieve an osmotic balance (i.e., a state of equal concentrations of fluids within the small intestine and surrounding blood circulation), water is drawn from the blood into the intestine. This water shift rapidly shrinks the vascular fluid volume. As a result, blood pressure drops and signs of rapid heart action to rebuild the blood volume appear: rapid pulse, sweating, weakness, and tremors. In about 2 hours, a second sequence of events usually follows. The initial concentrated solution of carbohydrate has been rapidly digested and absorbed, so the blood glucose rises rapidly and stimulates an overproduction of insulin. Blood sugar eventu-

ally drops below normal levels with symptoms of mild *hypoglycemia* (low blood sugar). Dramatic relief from these distressing symptoms, as well as gradual stabilization of weight, follows careful control of the diet (Box 22-3). Careful reintroduction of milk in small amounts may later be used to test tolerance. Patients also may find that eating slowly and lying down for 15 to 30 minutes after eating helps decrease the rate of gastric emptying.

Gallbladder Surgery

For patients suffering from acute gallbladder disease, *cholecystitis*, or from gallstones, *cholelithiasis* (Figure 22-5), the treatment is usually removal of the gallbladder, *cholecystectomy*. The modern procedure for this removal requires only minimal surgery involving small skin punc-

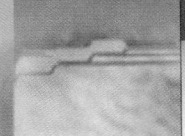

CLINICAL APPLICATIONS

CASE STUDY: JOHN HAS A GASTRECTOMY

After long experience with persistent peptic ulcer disease involving more and more gastric tissue, John and his physician decided that surgery was needed. John then entered the hospital for a total gastrectomy. John withstood the surgery well and received some initial nutritional support from an elemental formula fed through a tube the surgeon had placed into his jejunum. After a few days, the tube was removed and, over the next 2-week period, John was gradually able to take a soft diet in small oral feedings. He soon recovered enough to go home and gradually felt his strength returning. He was relieved to be free of his former ulcer pain and began to resume more and more of his usual activities, eating a regular diet of increasing volume and variety of foods.

However, as time went by John began having more discomfort after meals. He felt a cramping sensation and increased heartbeat, and then a wave of weakness with sweating and dizziness. John would often become nauseated and vomit. As his anxiety increased, he began to eat less and less and his weight began to drop. He was soon in a state of general malnutrition.

John finally returned to seek medical help. The physician and clinical dietitian outlined a change in his eating habits, and a special food plan was worked out for him. Although the diet seemed strange to him, John followed it faithfully because he had felt so ill. To his surprise, he

soon found that his previous symptoms after eating had almost completely disappeared. Because he felt so much better on the new diet plan, he formed new eating habits around it. His weight gradually returned to normal, and his state of nutrition markedly improved. John found that he would always fare better if he would "nibble" on food items throughout the day rather than consume large meals as he used to do.

Questions for Analysis

1. What were John's nutritional needs immediately after surgery and over the next 2 weeks? Why was it necessary for his feedings to be resumed cautiously?
2. Why is emphasis given to postsurgical protein sources? How should this nutrient be provided?
3. Why must sufficient energy be consumed after surgery?
4. Why is fluid therapy paramount after surgery?
5. What minerals and vitamins need special attention after surgery? Why?
6. When John began to feel better and resumed regular eating, why did he become ill? Describe his symptoms and why they developed.
7. Outline the principles of the special diet the dietitian provided to relieve John's symptoms. Plan a day's meal/snack pattern for John with basic instructions and suggestions you would discuss with him.

tures, called *minilaparoscopic cholecystectomy (MLC)*, rather than the previous surgery with a long abdominal incision.[11] Through these small openings, the surgeon can insert needed instruments and a laparoscope fitted with a miniature camera and bright fiberoptic lighting. With only a single stitch and a small bandage closing each opening, the patient can go home almost immediately and be fully recovered, and have a videotape of the whole procedure!

Because the function of the gallbladder is to concentrate and store bile, aiding in the digestion and absorption of fat, some moderation in dietary fat usually is indicated. After surgery, control of fat in the diet facilitates wound healing and comfort because the hormonal stimulus for bile secretion still functions in the surgical area, causing pain with intake of fatty foods. The body also needs a period of time to readjust to the more dilute supply of liver bile available to assist fat digestion and absorption. Depending on individual tolerance and re-

sponse, a relatively low-fat diet may be needed, such as the guide given previously for gallbladder disease (see Chapter 18).

Intestinal Surgery

In cases of intestinal disease involving tumors, lesions, or obstructions, the affected intestinal area should be resectioned. In complicated cases involving large sections of the bowel and requiring surgical removal of most of the small intestine, nutritional support is difficult. In such cases, TPN is used to supply major support with a small allowance of oral feeding for personal food desires. After general resection for less severe cases, a diet relatively low in dietary fiber may be briefly used to allow for healing and comfort. The surgery sometimes requires making an opening in the abdominal wall to the outside from the intestine, a *stoma* (Figure 22-6), for the elimination of fecal waste. If the opening is in the area of the *ileum*, the

BOX 22–3 Diet for Postoperative Gastric Dumping Syndrome

General Description

1. Five or six small meals should be administered daily.
2. A relatively high fat content helps retard the passage of food and maintain weight.
3. A high protein content (meat, eggs, cheese) helps rebuild tissue and maintain weight.
4. A relatively low simple carbohydrate content helps prevent rapid passage of quickly used foods.
5. No milk, sugar, sweets, desserts, alcohol, or sweet carbonated beverages are allowed.
6. Fluids should be avoided for at least 1 hour before and after meals and limited to 4 oz during meals.
7. Relatively low-roughage foods are allowed; raw foods are allowed as tolerated.
8. Very hot or very cold foods or liquids should be avoided.

Meal Pattern

Breakfast	2 scambled eggs with 1-2 Tbsp butter or margarine
	½-1 slice bread or small serving cereal with butter or margarine
	1 tsp low-calorie jelly
	1 serving solid fruit*
Midmorning snack	*Sandwich*
	1 slice bread with butter or margarine
	2 oz (56 g) lean meat
Lunch	4 oz (112 g) lean meat with 1-2 Tbsp butter or margarine
	Green or colored vegetable† with butter or margarine
	½-1 slice bread with butter or margarine
	½ banana or other solid fruit*
Midafternoon snack	Same as midmorning snack
Dinner	4 oz (112 g) lean meat with 1-2 Tbsp butter or margarine
	Green or colored vegetable† with butter or margarine
	½-1 slice bread with butter or margarine (or small serving starchy vegetable substitute)
	1 serving solid fruit*
Bedtime snack	2 oz (56 g) meat or 2 eggs or 2 oz (56 g) cheese or cottage cheese
	1 slice bread or 5 crackers with butter or margarine

*Fruit choice: applesauce, baked apple, canned fruit (drained), banana, orange, or grapefruit sections.
†Vegetable choice: spinach, green beans, squash, beets, carrots, green peas.

first section of the large intestine, it is called an *ileostomy*. In this area, the food mass is still fairly liquid and more problems are encountered in management. If the opening is farther along the colon in the last part of the large intestine, it is called a *colostomy*. In this area, the water is largely reabsorbed by the large intestine and the remaining feces are more formed, making management much easier. More radical surgery involving a *proctocolectomy* (e.g., removal of rectal tissue and lower colon) and construction of an *ileoanal reservoir* may be necessary. For many patients, this procedure is a desirable alternative to stoma formation and care.

Coping with any ostomy is difficult at best, and patients need much support and practical help in learning about self-care. A relatively low-fiber diet may be helpful at first, but the aim is to advance as soon as possible to a regular diet. Progression to a regular diet is important both for nutritional value and emotional support. Regular food provides much psychological comfort to a patient, and dietary adjustments to individual tolerances for specific foods can be made easily. Patients can revert to a low-fiber intake occasionally when diarrhea occurs.

Rectal Surgery

For a brief period after rectal surgery, or *hemorrhoidectomy*, a clear fluid or nonresidue diet (see Box 22-1) may be indicated to reduce painful elimination and allow healing. In some cases, a nonresidue commercial elemental formula such as Vivonex (Novartis) may be used to delay bowel movements until the surgical area has healed. Return to a regular diet usually is rapid.

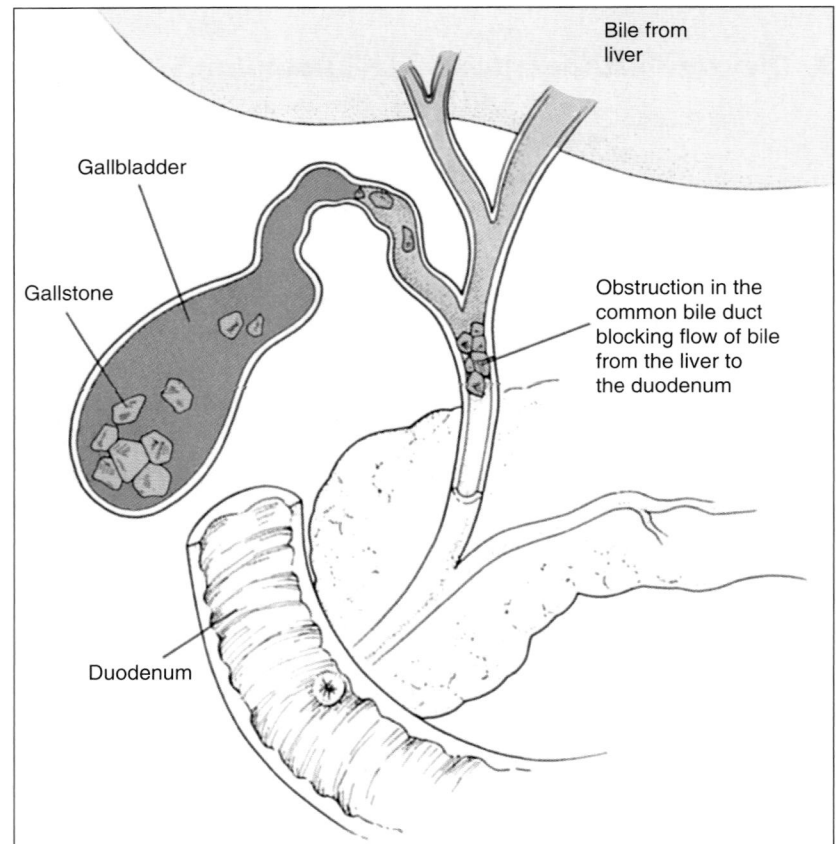

Figure 22–5 Gallbladder with stone (cholelithiasis).

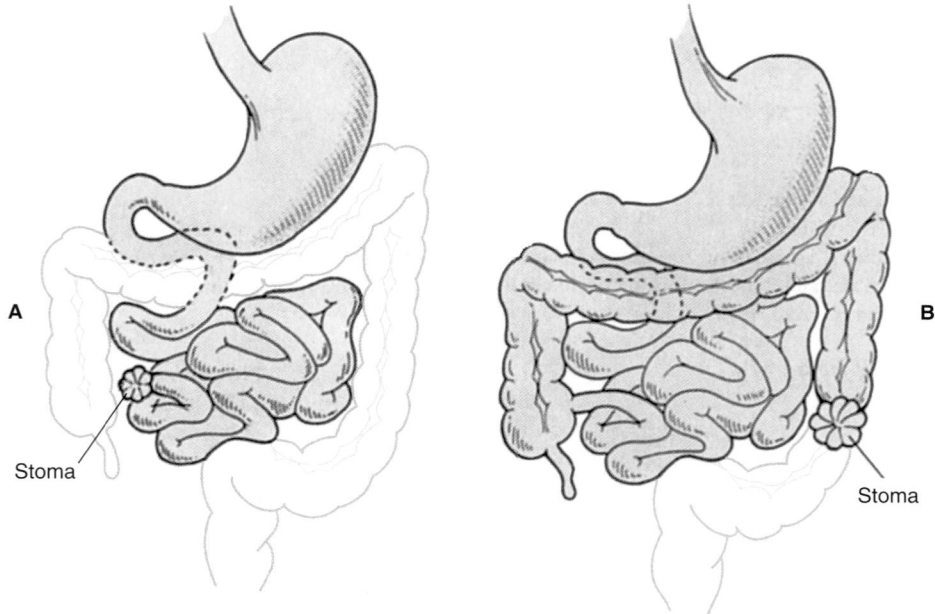

Figure 22–6 A, Ileostomy. B, Colostomy.

SPECIAL NUTRITIONAL NEEDS FOR PATIENTS WITH BURNS

Nutritional Support Base

Treatment and Prognosis

Each year, more than 100,000 persons are burned severely enough to require special hospitalization and care. Treatment of these extensive burns presents a tremendous nutritional challenge. The following factors influence the plan of care and its outcome:

- *Age.* Elderly persons and very young children are more vulnerable to poor outcome.
- *Health condition.* Any preexisting health problems or other injuries complicate care.
- *Burn severity.* The location and severity of the burns and the time elapsed before treatment are significant.

Degree and Extent of Burns

The depth of the burn affects its treatment and healing process (Figure 22-7). *First-degree burns* only involve cell damage in the top layer of skin, the *epidermis*. *Second-degree burns* involve cell damage in both the top and second layers of skin, the *dermis*. *Third-degree burns* result

in full-thickness skin loss, including the underlying fat layer. Second- and third-degree burns covering at least 15% to 20% of the total body surface—or even 10% loss in children and elderly persons—are serious and require extensive care. Burns of severe depth covering more than 50% of the body surface are often fatal. Patients with major burn injuries usually are transferred to a regional burn unit facility for specialized burn team care.

Stages of Nutritional Care

The nutritional care of adults and children with massive burns presents a great challenge and must be constantly adjusted to individual needs and responses. At each stage, critical attention is given to amino acid needs for tissue rebuilding, fluid-electrolyte balance, and energy (kcalorie) support. Three periods of care generally occur during the immediate shock, recovery, and secondary feeding periods.

Stage 1

Part 1: Immediate Shock Period. From the first hours until about the second day after a burn, massive flooding edema occurs at the burn site. Loss of protective skin leads to immediate losses of water, electrolytes (e.g., mainly sodium), and protein. As water is drawn from sur-

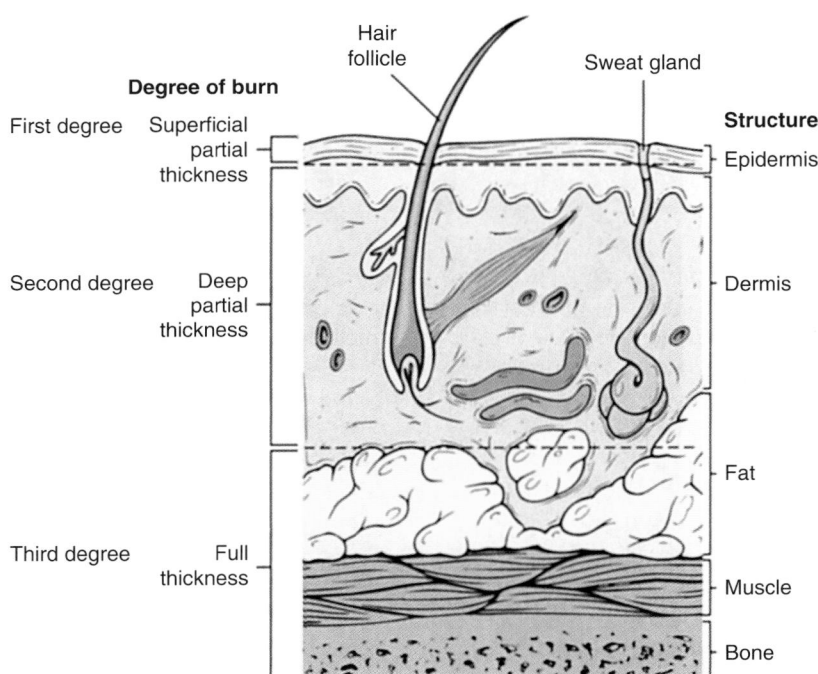

Figure 22–7 Depth of skin area involved in burns. (From Lewis SM, Heitkemper MM, Dirksen SR: *Medical-surgical nursing: assessment and management of clinical problems,* ed 5, St Louis, 2000, Mosby.)

rounding blood to replace the losses, general loss continues, blood volume and pressure drop, and urine output decreases. *Cell dehydration* (critical loss of cell water) follows as cell water is drawn out to balance the loss of tissue fluid. Cell potassium is also withdrawn and circulating serum potassium levels rise.

Immediate intravenous fluid therapy with a salt solution such as 6% hetastarch in saline or balanced salt solution or **lactated Ringer's solution** replaces water and electrolytes and helps to prevent shock.[12,13] After approximately 12 hours, when vascular permeability returns to normal and losses begin to decrease at the burn site, albumin solutions or plasma can be used to help restore blood volume. During this initial period, little attempt is made to meet protein and energy requirements because of the following: (1) infusion of glucose at this time may cause *hyperglycemia* (high blood sugar); (2) amino acids would be lost at the burn site; and (3) *adynamic ileus* (e.g., obstruction of the intestines caused by loss of normal bowel muscle action) may develop after the injury.

Part 2: Recovery Period. After approximately 48 to 72 hours, tissue fluids and electrolytes are gradually reabsorbed, balance is re-established, and the pattern of massive tissue loss is reversed. A sudden *diuresis* (e.g., increased excretion of urine) occurs, indicating successful initial therapy. Constant attention to fluid intake and output, with checks for any signs of dehydration or overhydration, are essential. Studies evaluating early (within 24 hours) versus delayed (after 48 hours) enteral nutritional support indicate that initiating nutritional support shortly (within 24 hours) after the burn injury may stimulate protein retention but this has not been associated with an improved recovery rate and thus remains inconclusive.[14]

Stage 2

Part 1: Secondary Feeding Period. Toward the end of the first week after the burn, adequate bowel function returns and a vigorous feeding program must begin. Despite a patient's depression and lack of appetite, at this point life may depend on rigorous nutrition therapy. Three major reasons exist for these increased nutrient and energy demands, as follows:

1. *Tissue destruction* has brought large losses of protein and electrolytes that must be replaced.
2. *Tissue catabolism* has followed the injury with further loss of lean body mass and nitrogen.
3. *Increased metabolism* brings added nutritional needs to cover the additional energy costs of infection or fever and the increased protein metabolism of tissue replacement and skin grafting.

Part 2: Nutrition Therapy. Successful nutrition therapy during this critical feeding period is based on vigorous protein and energy intake, as follows:

■ *High protein.* Aggressive supplementation of protein is crucial to promote early wound healing and support immune function. Depending on the extent of the burn injury and catabolic losses, individual protein needs vary from 1.8 to 2.5 g/kg body weight per day.[5] Children may require 2.5 to 3 g/kg body weight per day to meet increased metabolic needs of stress and injury, tissue regeneration, and normal needs of growth.
■ *High energy.* Caloric needs are calculated based on the total body surface area (BSA) burned as follows: 20 kcal/kg body weight + [40 × % BSA burned], with a maximum of 50% BSA used.[5] Beyond 50% BSA burned, little increases in total energy needs occur. There is a possibility for overfeeding, however, which would further increase metabolic stress and should be avoided. Such high energy needs are necessary to spare the protein essential for tissue rebuilding and supply the greatly increased metabolic demands for healing. A liberal portion of the total kcalories should come from carbohydrate, with a moderate amount of fat supplying the remaining need.
■ *High vitamin, high mineral.* Increased vitamin C, as much as 1 to 2 g/day, may be needed as a partner with amino acids for tissue rebuilding. Vitamin A and zinc are specifically important for optimal immune function and often are supplemented. Increased thiamin, riboflavin, and niacin are necessary for increased energy and protein metabolism. Special attention to electrolyte imbalances and calcium:phosphorus ratios in the blood are warranted during this period.

Part 3: Dietary Management. Either enteral or parenteral methods of feeding may be used to meet these crucial nutrient demands. With any method, a careful intake record must be maintained to measure progress toward the increased nutritional goals.

Enteral Feeding. Oral feedings are desired if tolerated. Concentrated liquids are given using added protein or amino acids. Commercial formulas such as Ensure (Ross) may be used as added interval nourishment. Solid foods based on individual preferences usually are tolerated by about the second week. Some patients may require calculated tube feedings to ensure adequate intake in correct nutrient proportions. In such cases, low-bulk defined formula solutions are given through small-bore feeding tubes. Continuous support and encouragement always are necessary, with food presented as attractively and appetizingly as possible.

Parenteral Feeding. For some patients, oral intake and tube feedings may be inadequate to meet the increased nutritional demands, or enteral feeding may be impossible because of associated injuries or complications. In such cases, parenteral feeding can provide essential nutritional support.

Stage 3

Follow-Up Reconstruction. Continued nutritional support is essential to maintain tissue strength for successful skin grafting or reconstructive plastic surgery. Patients need not only the physical rebuilding of body resources any

surgery requires but also much personal support to rebuild their will and spirit, because disfigurement or disability is possible. Health team members can do much to help instill courage and confidence to face the future again. Optimal physical stamina gained through persistent supportive medical, nutritional, and nursing care helps patients rebuild the personal resources needed to cope.

Lactated Ringer's solution sterile solution of calcium chloride, potassium chloride, sodium chloride, and sodium lactate in water given to replenish fluid and electrolytes; developed by English physiologist Sidney Ringer (1835-1910).

SUMMARY

The nutritional demands of surgery begin before a patient reaches the operating table. Before surgery, the task is to correct any existing deficiencies and build nutritional reserves to meet surgical demands. After surgery, the task is to replace losses and support recovery. The additional task of encouraging eating is often necessary during this period of healing.

Postsurgical feedings are given in a variety of ways. The oral route is always preferred. However, inability to eat or

damage to the intestinal tract may require feeding through a tube or into veins. Special formulas are used for such alternate means of nourishment and are designed to meet specific individual needs. For patients undergoing surgery on the gastrointestinal tract, special diets are modified according to the surgical procedure performed. For patients with massive burns, increased nutritional support is necessary in successive stages in response to the burn injury and to the continuing tissue rebuilding requirements.

CRITICAL THINKING QUESTIONS

1. Describe the general effect of imbalances on the following nutritional factors through the preoperative, immediate postoperative, and long-term postoperative periods: protein, energy, vitamins and minerals, and fluids.
2. Describe the major surgical effects for which nutrition therapy must be planned after these procedures: mouth, throat, or neck surgery; gastric resection; cholecystectomy; and rectal surgery.

3. Write a 1-day meal plan for a person experiencing postgastrectomy "dumping syndrome." What general dietary guidelines are used?
4. How do an ileostomy and a colostomy differ? What are the dietary needs for each one?
5. Outline the nutritional care of a burn patient from treatment for immediate shock through recovery and tissue reconstruction.

CHAPTER CHALLENGE QUESTIONS

True-False

Write the correct statement for each item you answer "false."

1. *True or False:* Nothing is usually given by mouth for at least 8 hours before surgery to avoid food aspiration during anesthesia.

2. *True or False:* The most common nutrient deficiency related to surgery is that of protein.
3. *True or False:* Negative nitrogen balance is a rare finding after surgery.

4. *True or False:* Extensive drainage in complicated surgery cases increase water loss to dangerous levels if constant replacement is not provided.

5. *True or False:* Vitamin C is essential to wound healing because it is involved in building strong connective tissue.

6. *True or False:* Regardless of the type, oral liquid feedings usually provide little nourishment.

7. *True or False:* Tube feedings can only be successfully prepared from complete commercial preparations.

8. *True or False:* A postgastrectomy patient can usually return to regular eating habits within a few days.

9. *True or False:* After a diseased gallbladder is surgically removed, a patient can freely tolerate any foods containing fats.

10. *True or False:* A careful diet record of the total food and liquid intake is important for a burn patient to ensure that increased nutrient and energy demands are met.

Multiple Choice

1. Postsurgical edema develops at the wound site as a result of
   a. decreased plasma protein levels.
   b. excess water intake.
   c. excess sodium intake.
   d. lack of early ambulation and physical exercise.

2. In a postoperative orthopedic patient's diet, protein is essential to
   a. provide extra energy needed to regain strength.
   b. provide a matrix to anchor mineral matter and form bone.
   c. control the basal metabolic rate.
   d. give more taste to the diet, thus increasing appetite.

3. Complete high-quality protein is essential to wound healing because it
   a. supplies the essential amino acids needed for tissue synthesis.
   b. is used to meet the bodies increased energy demands.

   c. is not a source of nitrogen to the body.
   d. provides the most concentrated source of kilocalories.

4. A diet for postgastrectomy "dumping syndrome" should include which of the following? (*Circle all that apply.*)
   a. Small frequent meals
   b. No liquid with meals
   c. No milk, sugar, sweets, or desserts
   d. High protein content

5. For a burn patient, a diet high in protein and energy is essential to do which of the following? (*Circle all that apply.*)
   a. Replace the extensive loss of tissue protein at the burn sites
   b. Provide essential amino acids for extensive tissue healing
   c. Counteract the negative nitrogen balance from loss of lean body mass
   d. Meet added metabolic demands of infection or fever

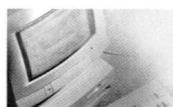

Please refer to the Students' Resource section of this text's Evolve web site for "Suggestions for Additional Study."

REFERENCES

1. Corish CA, Kennedy NP: Protein-energy undernutrition in hospital in-patients, *Br J Nutr* 83:575, 2000.
2. Wilmore DW: Postoperative protein sparing, *World J Surg* 23:545, 1999.
3. Corish CA: Pre-operative nutritional assessment, *Nutr Soc* 58:821, 1999.
4. Lane JM, Russell L, Khan SN: Osteoporosis, *Clin Orthop* 372:139, 2000.
5. Orr PA, Case KO, Stevenson JJ: Metabolic response and parenteral nutrition in trauma, sepsis, and burns, *J Infus Nurs* 25(1):45, 2002.
6. Boyce ST and others: Vitamin C regulates keratinocyte viability, epidermal barrier, and basement membrane *in vitro*, and reduces wound contraction after grafting of cultured skin substitutes, *J Invest Dermatol* 118:565, 2002.

7. Long CL and others: Ascorbic acid dynamics in the seriously ill and injured, *J Surg Res* 109(2):144, 2003.

8. Hall JC: Choosing nutrition support: how and when to initiate, *Nurs Case Manag* 4(5):212, 1999.

9. Haddad RY, Thomas DR: Enteral nutrition and enteral tube feeding: review of the evidence, *Clin Geriatr Med* 18(4):867, 2002.

10. Mechanick JI, Brett EM: Nutrition support of the chronically critically ill patient, *Crit Care Clin* 18(3):597, 2002.

11. Hsieh CH: Early minilaparoscopic cholecystectomy in patients with acute cholecystitis, *Am J Surg* 185(4):344, 2003.

12. Moretti EW and others: Intraoperative colloid administration reduces postoperative nausea and vomiting and improves postoperative outcomes compared with crystalloid administration, *Anesth Analg* 96(2):611, 2003.

13. Martin G and others: A prospective, randomized comparison of thromboelastographic coagulation profile in patients receiving lactated Ringer's solution, 6% hetastarch in a balanced-saline vehicle, or 6% hetastarch in saline during major surgery, *J Cardiothorac Vasc Anesth* 16(4):441, 2002.

14. Gottschlich MM and others: An evaluation of the safety of early vs delayed enteral support and effects on clinical, nutritional, and endocrine outcomes after severe burns, *J Burn Care Rehabil* 23(6):401, 2002.

FURTHER READING AND RESOURCES

- Corish CA, Kennedy NP: Protein-energy undernutrition in hospital in-patients, *Br J Nut* 83:575, 2000.

  This article highlights the adverse effects of protein-energy malnutrition in hospitalized patients. It also gives a thorough review of the literature over the past few decades about clinical outcomes and methods of nutrition assessment.

- Baxter JP: Problems of nutritional assessment in the acute setting, *Nutr Soc* 58:39, 1999.

  This article complements Corish and Kennedy's article by summarizing the appropriate methods of nutrition assessment for the hospitalized patient and expressing the importance of recognizing and treating macronutrient deficiencies as soon as possible.

23

Nutritional Support in Cancer and AIDS

KEY CONCEPTS

■ Environmental agents, genetic factors, and any weaknesses in the body's immune system can contribute to the development of cancer.

■ The strength of the body's immune system relates to its overall nutritional status.

■ Nutritional problems affect the nature of the disease process and the medical treatment methods in patients with cancer or AIDS.

■ The progressive effect of the human immunodeficiency virus (HIV) through its three stages of white T-cell destruction requires aggressive nutrition therapy.

With the accumulating environmental problems and changing lifestyles of the past few years, cancer has become a more prevalent health problem. Because cancer generally is associated with aging, the increasing life expectancy has somewhat contributed to this increasing incidence. Although AIDS and cancer share a direct relation to the body's immune system and basic nutritional needs, their courses and fatal outcomes are distinct.

This chapter looks at nutritional support in relation to both cancer and AIDS. Both conditions threaten life and have important nutritional connections in prevention and therapy.

PROCESS OF CANCER DEVELOPMENT

The Nature of Cancer

Multiple Forms

One of the problems in the study and treatment of cancer is that it is not a single problem; it has a highly varying nature and expresses itself in multiple forms. In these multiple genetic forms, cancer has become one of our major health problems—second only to heart disease—and accounts for about 22% of the total deaths in the United States each year.[1,2] The general term *cancer* is used to designate a malignant tumor or **neoplasm,** a term that refers to new growth. However, there are many forms of cancer that vary worldwide and change as populations migrate to different environments.

Nutrition Relationships

No one specific treatment or special diet for cancer exists, despite various fad diets and claims. Instead, relationships of nutrition and cancer care focus on the following two fundamental areas:

1. *Prevention* in relation to the environment and the body's natural defense system
2. *Therapy* in relation to nutritional support for medical treatment and rehabilitation

The Normal Cell

Human life results from the process of individual cell growth and reproduction. This process goes on over and over again, almost without error, guided by a cell's *genes*. In adults approximately 3 to 4 million cells complete the life-sustaining process of cell division every second, largely without mistake, guided by the "genetic code" contained in the specific cell nucleus material in each gene, *deoxyribonucleic acid* (DNA). Each gene carries unique genetic information that controls the synthesis of proteins and transmits genetic inheritance. Thus cells only arise from cell division of preexisting cells and carry their genetic patterns. Normal cell structure and function operates in an orderly manner under this constant gene control, with regulatory genes switching on and off as needed to control cell activities.

The Cancer Cell

However, this orderly cell operation can be lost with **mutation** or changes in the genes, especially in the regulatory genes. Cell growths may become malignant tumors when normal gene control is lost. Thus the misguided cell and its tumor tissue represent normal cell growth that has "gone wild." Cancer tumors are identified by their primary site of origin and stage of growth. *Sarcomas* arise from connective tissue; *carcinomas* arise from epithelial tissue. Stages of tumor development depend on its rate of growth, degree of functional self-control, and amount of penetration or spread into surrounding tissue. Also the incidence of cancer increases with age because a relationship exists between cancer cell development and the aging process of cells, tissues, and organ systems.

Causes of Cancer Cell Development

The underlying cause of cancer is thus the fundamental loss of cell control over normal cell reproduction. Several factors may contribute to this loss and change a normal cell into a cancer cell.

Mutations

As indicated, mutations, or changes in a cell's genes, are caused by loss of one or more of the regulatory genes in the cell nucleus or damage to a specific gene. Such a mutant gene may be inherited or arise from an environmental stimulus. Some cancers have strong genetic causes and tend to run in families (e.g., colon cancer).

Chemical Carcinogens

Agents that cause cancer are called *carcinogens*. Several chemical substances can interfere with the structure or function of regulatory genes. Exposure to such agents may

---

neoplasm (Gr. *neos*, new; *plasma*, formation) any new or abnormal cellular growth, specifically one that is uncontrolled and aggressive.

mutation (L. *mutare*, to change) a permanent transmissible change in a gene.

be by individual choice (e.g., cigarette smoking)[3] or may result from general exposure to environmental contaminants (e.g., pesticides, fungicides, and industrial chemicals such as dichlorodiphenyltrichloroethane (DDT), tetradifon, and dicofol).[4-8] The actions of such substances may result in gene mutation, damage to gene regulation, or activation of a dormant virus.

Radiation

Radiation damage to genes may come from x-rays, radioactive materials, sunlight, or atomic wastes. An estimated 1 million Americans develop skin cancer every year and overexposure to the ultraviolet radiation of the sun is the most important environmental factor contributing to this form of cancer.[9,10] The three major types of skin cancer are associated with specific gene mutations as follows:[11]

1. Basal cell carcinoma—*patched* (PTC) gene mutations
2. Squamous cell carcinoma—p53 gene mutations
3. Melanoma—p16 gene mutations.

Common forms of cancer on the head and neck are usually basal cell carcinoma and are relatively easy to cure by surgical removal.

The most lethal form of skin cancer, *malignant melanoma*, occurs in the skin cells that produce the pigment melanin and accounts for 75% of all skin cancer deaths. About 54,000 cases occur in the United States each year, with approximately 7400 deaths annually.[9] In the United States the incidence varies with latitude, with the greater number occurring in the southern states.

Viruses

Oncogenic, tumor-inducing, viruses that interfere with the function of regulatory genes have been identified in animals and are the focus of much ongoing research. Although oncogenes were first found in viruses, their history indicates that they also function in normal vertebrate cells. A virus is little more than a packet of a few genes, usually fewer than five, whereas cells of complex organisms such as humans have thousands. Disease viruses act as parasites, taking over the cell machinery to reproduce themselves.

Epidemiologic Factors

Epidemiology is the study of disease incidence in populations. Studies of cancer distribution involve factors such as race, region, age, heredity, occupation, and diet (see the Cultural Considerations box, "Types and Incidence of Cancer and AIDS in American Populations"). Racial incidence changes as population groups migrate to new environments and then acquire the cancer characteristics of the new population. The American incidence of

breast cancer, for example, has been used as a model for the diet-cancer connection in relation to obesity and the American high-fat diet, thus initiating studies such as the Women's Healthy Eating and Living (WHEL) Study. The WHEL study was designed as a comprehensive intervention trial promoting a diet high in vegetables, fruit, fiber, and low in fat in women with early-stage breast cancer.[12]

Stress Factors

Health care professionals recognize psychological stress as a disease risk factor in our complex society, especially in high-risk populations that lack social and economic supports. Psychic trauma, especially the loss of central personal relationships, takes its toll. Studies of people under stress have shown increased incidence of cancer and measured reduction of immune response to disease, especially in the response of the "natural killer cells" of the immune system.[13,14] Through their influence on the integrity of the immune system, poor food behaviors, nutritional status, and overall level of oxidative stress make a person more vulnerable to cancer-producing factors.[15]

Dietary Factors

The relationship between diet and cancer is complex. Although it has been the subject of much research, there are many unanswered questions. Foods contain both carcinogenic and *anti*carcinogenic compounds. Although studies have found conflicting results about the dietary intake of specific nutrients (individual vitamins or minerals), there is a general agreement in the research community about the preventative role of fruit and vegetable consumption and several types of cancer. There is also a convincing amount of research linking dietary *deficiencies* of specific nutrients (iron, zinc, folate, vitamins B_{12}, B_6, and C) with an increased risk of DNA damage and cancer.[16]

The Body's Defense System

The body's defense system is remarkably efficient and complex. Special cells protect not only against external invaders such as bacteria and viruses but also against internal "aliens" such as cancer cells.

Defensive Cells of the Immune System

Two major cell populations provide the immune system's primary "search and destroy" defense for detecting and killing alien, non-self substances that carry potential disease. These two populations of *lymphocytes*, a special type of white blood cell, develop early in life from a common stem cell in the bone marrow. The two types are called *T cells*, derived from thymus cells, and *B cells*, derived from bursal intestinal cells (Figure 23-1). A major func-

CULTURAL CONSIDERATIONS

TYPES AND INCIDENCE OF CANCER AND AIDS IN AMERICAN POPULATIONS

Cancer

It is interesting to see the changes over time in incidences of various forms of cancer. According to the Centers for Disease Control Vital Statistics, there have been significant changes between 1990 and 1998, specifically with regard to prostate, stomach, lung, and bronchus cancer. However, these changes are not equal across all gender and racial groups. For instance, the incidence of lung and bronchus cancer in men has decreased for all racial groups (Caucasian, African American, Asian or Pacific Islander, and Hispanic). However, the same type of cancer is on a slight rise for both African-American and Caucasian women. Cancers of the oral cavity and pharynx, stomach, pancreas, and bladder are on a decline in almost all gender and racial groups represented by the Vital Statistics report in the United States, whereas breast cancer continues to claim more and more lives. Melanoma cancer deaths affect disproportionately more men than women (4.1 vs. 1.8 per 100,000 deaths) and more Caucasians than any other racial group. The confounding factors associated with cancer risk are slowly being uncovered and explored. Hopefully, the trend toward prevention will become stronger with advanced research.

AIDS

The incidence of AIDS cases and death has been on a slight decline in the past few decades. However, there are cur-

rently more than 325,000 people living with AIDS in the United States. Seventy percent of new HIV infections each year occur in men. According to risk, 25% of new cases are injection drug users, with heterosexual men and women accounting for 33%, and men who have sex with men (MSM) representing the largest portion of new cases, 42%.

The percentage of new HIV infections according to race is disproportionate to the total U.S. population. For example, African Americans only make up 13% of the total U.S. population, but 54% of new HIV infection cases are African Americans. Although Hispanics represent 12% of the total U.S. population, 19% of new cases are of Hispanic origin. In addition, 26% of new cases are in Caucasians and 1% is in all other racial groups combined.

The method of transmission is very different for men and women. Seventy-five percent of the new cases in women are transmitted via heterosexual activity, whereas 60% of new cases in men are transmitted via homosexual activity. Injection drug use is the method of HIV infection for 25% of both male and female populations. As of December 2000, 448,060 deaths have been reported resulting from AIDS in the United States. Because there are currently no cures and no vaccines for HIV, prevention is the only means of protection regardless of race or gender.

Data from Centers for Disease Control and Prevention: *A glance at the HIV epidemic:* [HIV/AIDS Update], Atlanta, (accessed June 2003), CDC [*www.cdc.gov/nchstp/od/news/At-a-Glance.pdf*].

---

tion of T cells is to activate the *phagocytes,* special cells that destroy invaders, as well as to act as "killer cells" that attack and kill disease-carrying **antigens.** A major function of B cells is to produce proteins known as **antibodies,** which also kill antigens. Specially tailored proteins called *monoclonal antibodies* have been grown in laboratory mice from specific, single-cell "clones" of original antibodies, giving medical researchers a tool to diagnose and treat several diseases, including cancer.

Relation of Nutrition to Immunity

Nutritional support is necessary to maintain the integrity of the human immune system. Severely malnourished persons show changes in the structure and function of their immune system. These changes result from **atrophy** or losses in the basic tissues involved (e.g., liver, bowel wall, bone marrow, spleen, and lymphoid tissue). Nutrition is fundamental in maintaining normal immunity and com-

bating sustained attacks of disease such as cancer. The very core of the immune system, antibodies, are proteins in structure. A direct and simple example of the important role of nutrition in immunity is the link between protein-energy malnutrition and suppressed immune function.

---

antigen   (antibody + Gr. *gennan,* to produce) any foreign or "nonself" substances (e.g., toxins, viruses, bacteria, and foreign proteins) that stimulate the production of antibodies specifically designed to counteract their activity.

antibody   any of numerous protein molecules produced by B cells as a primary immune defense for attaching to specific related antigens.

atrophy   (L. *a-,* negative prefix; *trophē,* nourishment) a wasting away.

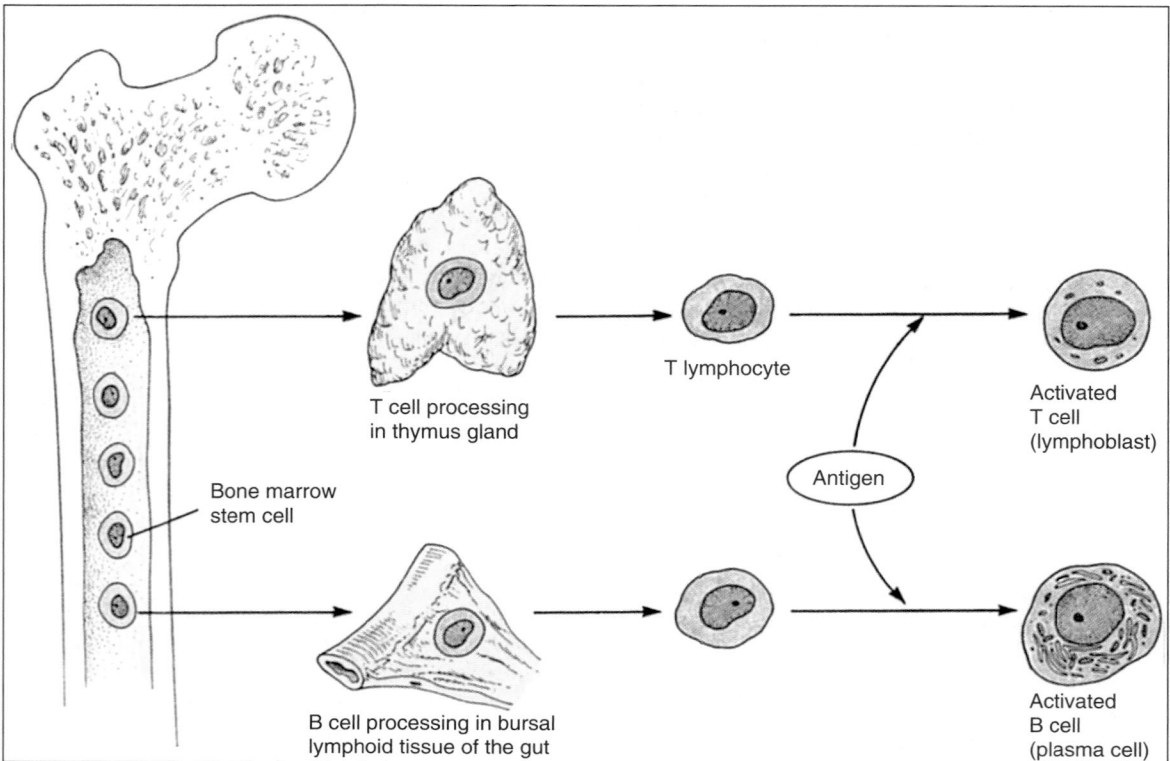

Figure 23-1 Development of the T and B cells, lymphocyte components of the body's immune system. (Credit [color]: Eileen Draper.)

In the figure: Bone marrow stem cell; T cell processing in thymus gland; T lymphocyte; Antigen; Activated T cell (lymphoblast); B cell processing in bursal lymphoid tissue of the gut; Activated B cell (plasma cell)

The Healing Process and Nutrition

The strength of any body tissue is maintained through constant synthesis—building and rebuilding—of tissue protein. Such strong tissue is a front line of the body's defense. This process of tissue building and healing requires optimal nutrition intake. Specific nutrients—protein and key vitamins and minerals, as well as nonprotein energy sources—must be constantly supplied in the diet. Wise and early use of vigorous nutritional support for cancer patients has been shown to provide recovery of normal nutritional status, including **immunocompetence,** thus improving their response to therapy and prognosis.[17]

NUTRITIONAL SUPPORT FOR CANCER TREATMENT

Three major forms of therapy are used today as medical treatment for cancer, as follows:

1. Surgery
2. Radiation
3. Chemotherapy

Each one requires nutritional support.

Surgery

Any surgery, as discussed in Chapter 22, requires nutritional support for the healing process. This requirement is particularly true for patients with cancer because their general condition is often weakened by the disease process and its drain on the body's resources. With early diagnosis and sound nutritional support before and after surgery, many tumors can be removed successfully and recovery is often ensured. Nutrition therapy also includes any needed modifications in food texture or specific nutrients, depending on the site of the surgery or the function of the organ involved. Various methods of feeding patients after surgery are reviewed in Chapter 22.

Radiation

Radiation therapy is often used by itself or in conjunction with surgery. This type of therapy involves treatment with high-energy x-rays targeted on the cancer site to kill or shrink cancerous cells. Radiation may be administered to the body by an external machine (Figure 23-2) or by implanted radioactive materials at the cancer site. Although the goal is for only the cancer cells to die, other cells within close range of the target site and rapidly growing cells often die as well. The site and intensity of the radiation treatment determine the nature of the nutritional problems the patient may experience. For example, radiation to the head, neck, or esophagus affects the oral mucosa and salivary secretions, thus affecting taste sensations and sensitivity to food texture and temperature, with increasing anorexia and nausea. Means of enhancing the appetite through food appearance and aroma as well as texture must be explored. Similarly radiation to the abdominal area affects the intestinal mucosa, causing loss of villi and absorbing surface; therefore malabsorption problems may follow. Ulcers or inflammation and obstruction or *fistulas* also may develop from tissue breakdown. A fistula, from the Latin word for "pipe," is an abnormal opening or passageway within the body or to the outside. As such, it interferes with normal functioning of the involved tissue. General malabsorption within the gastrointestinal (GI) tract may be further compounded by lack of food intake resulting from loss of appetite and nausea.

Chemotherapy

Chemotherapy drugs kill rapidly growing cancer cells. Unlike radiation therapy, chemotherapy is administered via the blood stream, coursing through the entire body. However, because these drugs are highly toxic they also affect normal healthy cells. This accounts for their side effects on rapidly growing tissues such as those of the bone marrow, GI tract, and hair, as well as for problems in nutrition management. General complications include the following:

- *GI effects.* Numerous problems may develop that interfere with food tolerance: nausea and vomiting, loss of normal taste sensations and lack of appetite, diarrhea, ulcers, malabsorption, or *stomatitis*, an inflammation of the tissues around the mouth or other orifices of the body.
- *Bone marrow effects.* Interference with the production of specific blood factors causes related problems: reduced red blood cells causing anemia, reduced white blood cells causing lowered resistance to infections, and reduced blood platelets causing bleeding.
- *Hair follicle effects.* Interference with normal hair growth results in general hair loss.

Other problems may relate to the use of pretreatment antidepressant drugs that have special blood pressure effects when used with certain tyramine-rich foods. These drugs are the *monoamine oxidase* (MAO) inhibitors, and their use requires a tyramine-restricted diet (Box 23-1).

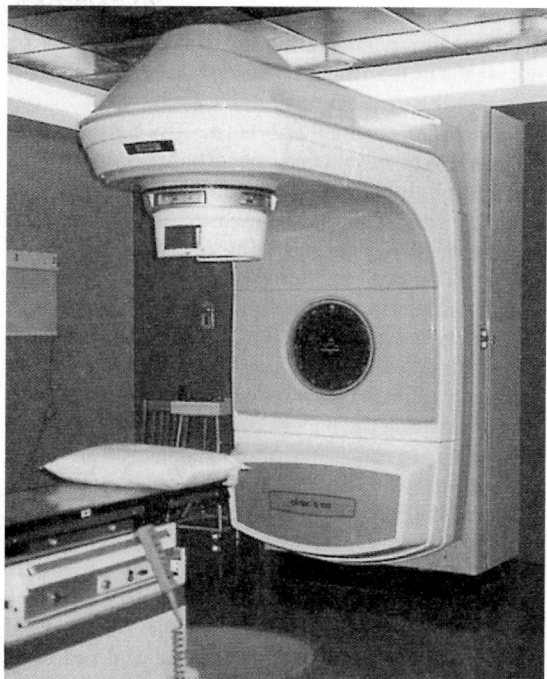

Figure 23–2   Radiation treatment machine. (From Lewis SM, Heitkemper MM, Dirksen SR: *Medical-surgical nursing: assessment and management of clinical problems,* ed 5, St Louis, 2000, Mosby.)

NUTRITION THERAPY IN THE CANCER PATIENT

Problems Related to the Disease Process

General feeding problems pose a great challenge to the clinical dietitian planning care and the nurse providing important supportive assistance. These problems relate to the overall systemic effects of cancer, as well as to the specific individual responses to the type of cancer involved.

General Systemic Effects

Cancer generally causes the following three basic systemic effects:

1. Anorexia, or loss of appetite, resulting in poor food intake

---

immunocompetence (L. *immunis,* free, exempt) the ability or capacity to develop an immune response (i.e., antibody production or cell-mediated immunity) after exposure to an antigen.

BOX 23–1   Tyramine-Restricted Diet

General Directions

- The diet was designed for patients on monoamine oxidase (MAO) inhibitors, drugs that have been reported to cause hypertensive crises when used with tyramine-rich foods, in which aging, protein breakdown, and putrefaction are used to increase flavor. Studies indicate that as little as 5 to 6 mg tyramine can produce a response and that 25 mg is a dangerous dose.
- Food sources of other pressor amines, such as histamine, dihydroxyphenylalanine, and hydroxytyramine, are also avoided.
- All foods listed should be avoided. Limited amounts of foods with a lower tyramine amount, such as yeast bread, may be included in a specific diet.
- Over-the-counter drugs such as decongestants, cold remedies, and antihistamines should be avoided.

Restricted Foods

Foods to Avoid	Representative Tyramine Values (μg/g or ml)
Cheeses	
N.Y. state cheddar	1416
Gruyére	516
Stilton	466
Emmenthaler	225
Brie	180
Camembert	86
Processed American	50
Wines	
Chianti	25.4
Sherry	3.6
Riesling	0.6
Sauternes	0.4
Beer, ale (varies with brand)	
Highest	4.4
Average	2.3
Least	1.8

Additional Foods to Avoid

Other aged cheeses
  Blue
  Boursault
  Brick
  Cheddars (other)
  Gouda
  Mozzarella
  Parmesan
  Provolone
  Romano
  Roquefort
Yeast and products made with yeast
  Homemade bread
  Yeast extracts such as soup cubes, canned meats, and Marmite
Italian broad beans with pod (fava beans)
Meat
  Aged game
  Liver
  Canned meats with yeast extracts
Fish (salted, dried)
  Herring, cod, capeline
  Pickled herring
Other
  Cream, especially sour
  Yogurt
  Soy sauce, vanilla, chocolate
  Salad dressings

---

2. Increased metabolism, resulting in increased nutrient and energy needs
3. Negative nitrogen balance, resulting in more *catabolism*, or breaking down of body tissues

Continuing weight loss ensues. The extent of these effects may vary widely, from a mild response to an extreme form of debilitating **cachexia** seen in advanced disease. This extreme weight loss and weakness are caused by an inability to ingest or use nutrients causing a patient's body to feed off its own tissue protein.[18] About half of all cancer patients suffer from this debilitating syndrome. An involuntary weight loss of greater than 5% of premorbid weight within a 6-month period is indicative of cachexia. The best way to cure cachexia is to alleviate the cancer. However, because this is not always an immediate possibility, aggressive nutrition therapy is the next best thing. There are a variety of drugs currently in use to increase appetite, decrease nausea, spare protein degradation, and improve caloric intake such as: glucocorticoids, progestational drugs (megestrol), cyprohepta-dine, prokinetic agents (metoclopramide), branched-chain amino acids, eicosapentaenoic acid, cannabinoids (THC), and 5'-deoxyfluorouridine.[18]

Specific Effects Related to the Type of Cancer

In addition to the primary nutritional problems caused by the disease process itself, secondary problems in eating or use of nutrients results from specific tumors causing obstructions or lesions in the GI tract or adjacent tissue. Such conditions limit food intake and digestion, as well as absorption of nutrients. Depending on the nature and location of the tumor, as well as its medical treatment, a variety of individual nutritional problems may occur and require personal attention.

Basic Objectives of Nutrition Therapy

Prevention of Catabolism

Every effort is made to meet the increased metabolic demands of the disease process, thus preventing extensive catabolic effects in tissue breakdown. It is far easier to maintain nutrition from the beginning than to rebuild the body from extensive malnutrition. The medical treatment may increase this catabolic effect.

Relief of Symptoms

The symptoms of the disease or side effects of the treatment can be devastating for a patient. Relief requires much individual and family counseling to devise ways of meeting needs and helping the patient to eat. The types of foods used, their preparation and service, or the process of feeding should be individualized according to situation, response, and need.

Although the clinical dietitian and the physician have the primary responsibility for planning and managing the nutrition therapy program, a tremendous contribution is made by the nursing staff and other health care personnel in the day-to-day support and counsel in helping the patient to eat. It is often this kind of constant care and support that differentiates combating the course of the disease and ensuring the comfort and well-being of the patient.

Principles of Nutritional Care

The following basic principles underlie all sound patient care, as discussed in Chapter 17:

1. Identifying needs
2. Planning care based on these needs

Only by acting upon these principles can one determine if real needs are being met. Thus nutrition assessment and care planning are primary concerns.

Nutrition Assessment

Determining and monitoring the nutritional status of each patient is the primary responsibility of the clinical dietitian, but other nursing support staff often assists. Various members of the health care team may take part in body measurements and calculations of body composition, laboratory tests and interpretation of results, physical examination and clinical observations, and dietary analysis.

Personal Care Plan

Based on the detailed information gathered about each patient, including living situation and other personal and social needs, the clinical dietitian, in consultation with the physician, develops a personal plan of nutrition therapy for each patient. This outline then can be incorporated into the nursing care plan because the dietitian works with the nursing staff to carry it out. The day-to-day plan is constantly checked with the patient and family and changed as needed to meet the nutritional demands of the patient's condition and individual desires and tolerances.

Nutritional Needs

Although individual needs vary, guidelines for nutrition therapy must meet specific nutrient needs and goals related to the accelerated metabolism, which demands increased protein-tissue synthesis and energy production.

Energy

The hypermetabolic nature of the disease and its healing requirements place great energy demands on a cancer patient. Sufficient fuel from carbohydrate and, to a lesser extent, fat must be available to spare protein for vital tissue building. An adult patient with good nutritional status needs about 2000 kcal, or 25 to 30 kcal/kg body weight, for maintenance requirements. More kilocalories may be needed according to the degree of individual stress or amount of tissue synthesis needed. A malnourished patient requires 2500 to 3500 kcal, or 35 to 40 kcal/kg, depending on the degree of malnutrition or extent of tissue injury.

---

cachexia (Gr. *kakos*, bad; *hexis*, habit) a specific profound syndrome caused by malnutrition and a disturbance in glucose and fat metabolism usually seen in patients with terminal cancer or AIDS; general poor health indicated by an emaciated appearance.

Protein

Necessary tissue building for healing, and to offset tissue breakdown by the disease, requires essential amino acids and nitrogen. Efficient protein use depends on an optimal protein: energy ratio to promote tissue building and prevent tissue catabolism. An adult patient with good nutritional status needs approximately 80 to 100 g of high-quality protein to meet maintenance requirements. A malnourished patient needs between 100 and 150 g to replenish deficits and restore positive nitrogen balance.

Vitamins and Minerals

Key vitamins and minerals control protein and energy metabolism through their coenzyme roles in specific cell enzyme pathways (see Chapters 7 and 8) and also play important roles in building and maintaining strong tissue. Therefore an optimal intake of vitamins and minerals, at least to the Dietary Reference Intakes/Recommended Dietary Allowance standards but more often to higher therapeutic levels, is needed. Vitamin and mineral supplements usually are indicated to ensure dietary intake.

Fluid

Adequate fluid intake must be ensured for the following two reasons:

1. To replace GI losses from fever, infection, vomiting, or diarrhea
2. To help the kidneys dispose of metabolic breakdown products from destroyed cancer cells and from the toxic drugs used in chemotherapy

Some chemotherapeutic drugs (e.g., cyclophosphamide [Cytoxan]) require as much as 2 to 3 L of forced fluids daily to prevent hemorrhagic cystitis.

Nutrition Management

Achieving these nutritional objectives and needs in the face of frequent poor food tolerance or inability to eat presents a great challenge to the nutritional support team and patient. The specific method of feeding depends on the patient's condition. The dietitian and physician may manage a patient's nutritional care using either enteral or parenteral modes of feeding (see Chapter 22).

Enteral: Oral Diet with Nutrient Supplementation

An oral diet with supplementation is the most desired form of feeding when tolerated. A personal food plan, based on the nutrition assessment information gathered, must be worked out with the patient and family. This food plan must include adjustments in food texture and temperature, food choices, and tolerances and should provide as much energy and nutrient density as possible in smaller volumes of food (see the Clinical Applications box, "Strategies for Improving Food Intake in Cancer or AIDS Patients"). The plan also must give special attention to eating problems with loss of appetite, mouth problems, and GI problems.

Loss of Appetite. Anorexia is a major problem in cancer patients and curtails food intake when it is needed most. Anorexia often sets up a vicious cycle that can lead to the gross malnutrition of cancer cachexia. A vigorous program of eating, *not dependent on appetite for stimulus,* must be planned with the patient and family. The overall goal is to provide food with as much *nutrient* density as possible so that "every bite counts."

Mouth Problems. Various problems contributing to eating difficulties may stem from sore mouth, stomatitis, or taste and smell changes. Decreased saliva and sore mouth often result from radiation to the head and neck area or from chemotherapy. Spraying the mouth with artificial saliva is helpful. Frequent small snacks, soft and bland and cool or cold, are often better accepted. The treatment may alter the tongue's taste buds, causing taste distortion, "taste blindness," and the inability to distinguish sweet, sour, salt, or bitter, bringing more food aversions. Strong food seasonings (for those who can tolerate them) and high-protein liquid drinks may be helpful. Because the treatment also may alter salivary secretions, foods with a high liquid content should be favored. Solid foods may be swallowed more easily with the use of sauces, gravies, broth, yogurt, or salad dressings. A food processor or blender can render foods in semisolid or liquid forms for easier swallowing. Any dental problems should be corrected to help with chewing.

GI Problems. Chemotherapy often causes nausea and vomiting, which need special individual attention (see the Clinical Applications box, "Strategies for Improving Food Intake in Cancer or AIDS Patients"). Food that is hot, sweet, fatty, or spicy sometimes exacerbates nausea and should be avoided according to individual tolerances. Small, frequent feedings of soft to liquid cold foods, eaten slowly with rests in between, may be helpful. The physician's use of antinausea drugs such as prochlorperazine (Compazine) may help with food tolerances. Special surgical treatment involving the GI tract requires related dietary modifications, as discussed in Chapter 22. Chemotherapy or radiation treatment can affect the mu-

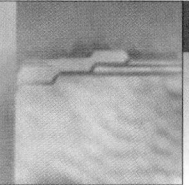

CLINICAL APPLICATIONS

STRATEGIES FOR IMPROVING FOOD INTAKE IN CANCER OR AIDS PATIENTS

Suggestions for Controlling

Nausea and Vomiting

- Try small, frequent meals.
- Eat more when feeling better.
- Eat drier foods with fluids in between.
- Try cold foods and saltier foods.
- Avoid fatty or overly sweet foods.
- Do not recline right after eating.
- If vomiting, replace fluids and electrolytes with juices, broths, ginger ale, and sports drinks.
- Experiment with spices and flavoring.
- Use foods and special dishes with pleasant-smelling aromas.

Tips for Increasing Energy and Protein Intake

- Fortify foods with high caloric condiments, sauces, and dressings.
- Add extra ingredients such as dry milk and cream during food preparation.

- Use interval drinks of commercial food supplements.
- Use regular calorie-containing foods and beverages, not low-calorie substitutes.
- Prepare favorite foods in small quantities and freeze extra in small serving sizes for snacks.
- Eat by the clock: have a meal or snack every 1 or 2 hours.
- Eat more when appetite is good.
- Enjoy meals with pleasant surroundings, company, and music.
- Keep a supply of easy-to-prepare and convenient foods on hand.
- Try mild exercise, according to physical status.
- If mouth is sore, use soft foods, avoid hot or cold temperature extremes, and check with physician or nurse for topical anesthetic mouth rinses to use before eating.

---

cosal cells secreting lactase and thus create lactose intolerance. In such cases, a non–milk-based nutrient supplement (e.g., Ensure [Ross Products, Columbus, OH], which is a soy-based product) may be used.

Pain and Discomfort. Patients are more able to eat if any severe pain is controlled and they are positioned as comfortably as possible. Physicians previously tended to withhold pain medications for fear of addictions, but the current medical consensus is to administer pain control medication as needed, in close consultation with the patient and family, and monitor responses carefully. This is especially true for children with cancer undergoing painful treatments.

Enteral: Tube Feeding

When the GI tract can still be used but the patient is unable to eat and requires more assistance to achieve essential intake goals, tube feeding may be indicated (see Chapter 22). However, many patients have negative feelings about tube feeding, especially about the use of a nasogastric tube. Table 23-1 lists some helpful procedures to use with such patients. On the other hand, some highly motivated patients have even learned to pass their small-caliber tubes themselves. In some in-

stances, patients can be fed by pump-monitored slow drip during the night and be free from the tube during the day. The use of special formulas and delivery system equipment also has made home enteral nutrition possible and practical.

Parenteral: Peripheral Vein Feeding

When the GI tract cannot be used and nutritional support is vital, intravenous feeding must be initiated. For brief periods—in cases requiring less concentrated intakes of energy and nutrients—solutions of dextrose, amino acids, vitamins, and minerals, with concurrent use of lipid emulsions may be fed into smaller peripheral veins. Use of smaller peripheral veins carries less risk than use of a larger central vein and can supply necessary support when nutrient needs are not excessive. Peripheral vein feeding is combined with tube feeding to supply additional needs in some cases, avoiding the use of a central vein.

Parenteral: Central Vein Feeding

When nutritional needs are greater and must continue over an extended period of time, central vein feeding has often provided a life-saving alternative. This total parenteral nutrition (TPN) process requires surgical place-

TABLE 23–1	Problem-Solving Tips for Patients Receiving Enteral Nutrition
Problem	**Suggested solutions**
Thirst, oral dryness	Lubricate lips
	Chew sugarless gum
	Brush teeth
	Rinse mouth frequently
	Caution: Use lemon drops sparingly because of cariogenic effects; other hard candies are appropriate alternatives.
Tube discomfort	Gargle with a mixture of warm water and mouthwash
	Gently blow nose
	Clean tube regularly with water or water-soluble lubricant
	If persistent, pull out tube gently, clean it, and reinsert
	Request smaller tube
Tension, fullness	Relax, breathe deeply after each feeding
Loud stomach noises	Take feedings in private
Limited mobility	Change positions in bed or chair
	Walk around the house or hospital corridor
Gustatory Distress	
General dissatisfaction with feeding	Warm or chill feedings
	Caution: Feedings that are too cold may cause diarrhea.
	Serve favorite foods that have been liquefied
Persistent hunger	Chew a favorite food; then spit it out
	Chew gum
	Suck hard candy
Inability to drink	Rinse mouth frequently with water and other liquids

ment of the feeding catheter, along with careful assessment, monitoring, and administration. Although TPN carries risks, thus requiring skilled team management, this hyperalimentation process has provided a significant means of turning the metabolic status of cancer patients from catabolism to anabolism, often avoiding the serious development of cancer cachexia. Details of these alternate enteral and parenteral methods of feeding are discussed in Chapter 22.

CONCLUSIONS: CANCER THERAPY AND PREVENTION

Therapy

Ample evidence at this point indicates that vigorous nutritional support increases the chances for successful medical treatments in the care of cancer. The fundamental reasons for this improved possible outcome are briefly reviewed here. It is also evident that much effort on the part of the health care team, the patient, and the family, all working together, is absolutely necessary for vigorous nutritional support to become a reality.

Prevention

On the basis of studies concerning possible associations of nutritional factors and food forms with cancer, the American Cancer Society has issued guidelines for the public to help persons make generally healthy food choices to reduce the risk of cancer.[19] These guidelines are established by a national panel of experts and are updated every 5 years. The statements are intended to serve as guiding principles based on the most current information in cancer research and prevention. In addition, the U.S. Food and Drug Administration has defined specific food labeling guidelines linking foods, or nutrients, to decreased cancer risk.[20] A variety of other government and privately funded research studies are ongoing in the hopes of identifying a more specific cause and cure for cancer.

American Cancer Society Guidelines

■ *Eat a variety of healthful foods, with an emphasis on plant sources.* Specifically, the American Cancer Society recommends that individuals: (1) eat five or more vegetables and fruits every day; (2) choose whole grains instead of processed (refined) grains and sugars; (3) limit consumption of red meats, especially processed and high-fat meats; and (4) choose foods that help maintain a healthful weight. Based on research reviewed and accepted by the American Cancer Society, there is enough evidence to indicate that following these guidelines can reduce the risk for the following types of cancer: colorectal, breast, prostate, lung, esophageal, oral, stomach, pancreatic, bladder, and endometrial.[19]

■ *Adopt a physically active lifestyle.* Children and adolescents are encouraged to participate in at least 60 minutes per day of moderate-to-vigorous physical activity at least 5 days per week. Adults should engage in at least moderate activity for a minimum of 30 minutes on 5 or more days per week. Examples of moderate activity are: walking, skating, yoga, softball or baseball, downhill skiing, garden maintenance, or lawn care. Vigorous activities include: running, aerobics, fast bicycling, circuit weight training, soccer, singles tennis, basketball, cross-country skiing, and heavy manual labor. There is convincing evidence that increasing physical activity can produce protective benefits against colorectal and breast cancer.[19]

■ *Maintain a healthful weight throughout life.* By balancing energy intake with physical activity and losing weight if currently overweight, the risk for colorectal cancer, breast cancer, esophageal and oral cancer, and pancreatic cancer are reduced.[19] The American Cancer Society recommends maintaining a body mass index (BMI) between 18.5 and 25.0 kg/m^2.

■ *If you drink alcoholic beverages, limit consumption.* The U.S. Department of Health and Human Services and American Cancer Society recommend men and women who drink alcohol limiting their alcohol intake to two drinks per day for men and one drink per day for women.[19,21] One drink is defined as 12 oz of beer, 5 oz of wine, or 1.5 oz of 80-proof distilled spirits. Limiting alcohol intake is associated with beneficial affects against colorectal, breast, esophageal, oral, and pancreatic cancers.[19]

Dietary choices and physical activity are the most modifiable risk factors for cancer development. It is estimated that 35% of all cancer deaths in the United States are attributed to diet, be it either too much or too little of specific nutrients. Thus following the preceding guidelines could make a significant difference in the lives of many.

U.S. Food and Drug Administration Health Claims

Health claims approved for use on food labels are regulated by the U.S. Food and Drug Administration (see Chapter 13). The following food/nutrient-cancer associations have been approved for use on food labels in the United States:[20]

■ A diet low in total fat may reduce the risk of some cancers.
■ Low-fat diets rich in fiber-containing grain products, fruits, and vegetables may reduce the risk of some types of cancer.
■ Low-fat diets rich in fruits and vegetables (foods that are low in fat and may contain dietary fiber, vitamin A, or vitamin C) may reduce the risk of some types of cancer.

On the basis of this consistent and strong association, the U.S. National Cancer Institute has developed a program to encourage Americans to eat five or more servings of fruits and vegetables every day, which is one of the nation's health-promotion and disease-prevention objectives.[22] The 5-A-Day for Better Health program is now underway with many associated projects through participating state public health agencies and public-private partnerships with the food industry and food service operations. The program is serving as a model for such partnerships in community nutrition.

Ongoing Cancer Research

Many studies have shown that diets high in fat and low in fiber, fruits, and vegetables—major sources of micronutrients and phytochemicals—are associated with increased incidence and mortality from various cancers.[23] The exact mechanism by which such diets promote cancer are not yet clearly defined for each association and thus are still under investigation. The protective roles of several food components such as fish oils, garlic, soy products, various teas and dietary supplements (e.g., folic acid, vitamin A, vitamin C, vitamin E, and selenium) are currently under analysis for definitive correlations and mechanisms associated with decreased cancer risk.[19,24,25] In addition to preventative cancer research, there also are emerging reports on dietary guidelines for cancer survivors and alternative or complementary diet therapies.[26]

The Centers for Disease Control and Prevention (CDC) hosts many programs aimed at preventing and controlling cancers, as well as researching cause and effect relationships. The following programs and initiatives are examples of such programs ongoing through the CDC: National Comprehensive Cancer Control Program, National Breast and Cervical Cancer Early Detection Program, National Program of Cancer Registries, Tobacco Control Program, and initiatives such as the colorectal cancer prevention and control initiative, prostate cancer control initiative, skin cancer primary prevention education initiative, and the ovarian cancer control initiative.[27]

2

Acquired Immunodeficiency Syndrome

PROCESS OF AIDS DEVELOPMENT

This portion of the chapter looks at acquired immunodeficiency syndrome (AIDS) and compares its relation to the body's immune system and course of development with that of cancer. Similarly, a brief review is presented on the process of AIDS development, its medical treatment, nutritional support, and conclusions about AIDS therapy and prevention.

In the late 1970s physicians in New York City and San Francisco first puzzled over an uncommon medical problem appearing among their patients. No known cause of immune suppression could be found, but persons were nonetheless suffering and dying from complications of common infections, largely pneumonia, that were ordinarily easily handled by the human immune system and the usual antibiotics or other antibacterial drugs. Its **virus** source and **pandemic** effects were soon to become alarmingly evident worldwide. According to the National Institutes of Health, 14,000 people worldwide are infected with HIV *every day*, and six people under the age of 25 are infected *per minute*[28] (see the Cultural Considerations box, "Types and Incidence of Cancer and AIDS in American Populations").

Evolution of Human Immunodeficiency Virus

Early Pandemic Spread

The earliest known case of AIDS was identified in a blood sample collected in 1959 from a Bantu man living in what is currently called the *Democratic Republic of Congo*, an area from which the current world epidemic is believed to have originated.[29] Early in the 1960s, first in the African country of Uganda, strange deaths began to occur from simple common infections such as pneumonia that did not respond to the usual antibiotic drugs. By the late 1970s and early 1980s the same strange deaths were occurring in Europe and America. Similar reports of unexplained immune system failure increased rapidly in various parts of the world, and the pandemic spread alarmingly. These early cases came from people with diverse social and medical backgrounds, including heterosexual and homosexual men, intravenous drug users exchanging needles, and recipients of transfused blood and blood products (e.g., children with hemophilia and medical/surgical patients). After feverish research, the underlying infectious agent was finally discovered in May 1983. The French scientist Luc Montagnier, a leading pioneer of AIDS research, reported that he and his team at the Pasteur Institute in Paris had isolated the viral cause, now known as *human immunodeficiency virus (HIV)*.

Evolution and Spread of the Virus

Where did this deadly virus come from, and how did it gain such strength so rapidly? From studies thus far, scientists are beginning to find some answers. Apparently HIV is not a new virus but an old one that only recently grew deadly in humans while gaining strength during the social upheavals of the 1960s and 1970s. The uprooting effect of rapid social change, urbanization, and world travel allowed the virus to spread rapidly through world populations and reproduce aggressively in its human host.

Parasitic Nature of the Virus

No virus can have a life of its own. By their structure and reproductive nature, viruses are the ultimate **parasites.** They are mere shreds of genetic material, a small packet of genetic information encased in a protein coat. Viruses only contain a small chromosome of nucleic acids (RNA or DNA), usually with fewer than five genes. They can only live through a host, whom they invade and infect, hijacking the host's cell machinery to run off a multitude of copies of themselves. Scientists agree that HIV, which is genetically similar to viruses found in African primates (e.g., simian immunodeficiency virus [SIV]), was probably transmitted to humans in an earlier age as ancient hunters cut themselves while butchering their kills for food.[30] The current deadly strength of HIV results from its aggressive growth within an increasing number of hosts. Today, more than 800,000 people throughout the United States and more than 30 million worldwide, are infected with HIV.

Stages of Disease Progression

The individual clinical course of HIV infection varies substantially, but the following three distinct stages mark the progression of the disease:

1. Primary HIV infection and extended well period of viral incubation
2. AIDS-related complex (ARC) of illnesses
3. Terminal AIDS

Stage 1: Primary HIV infection

HIV is transmitted from an infected person to another person through sexual contact, sharing needles or syringes, or blood transfusions. Blood donations are now very closely screened for HIV antibodies in most countries, thus reducing this form of transmission. Pregnant women with HIV also may infect their babies during delivery. About 2 to 4 weeks after initial exposure and infection, a mild flulike episode lasting about 1 week may occur. This brief mild response reflects the initial development of antibodies to the viral infection. Any subsequent HIV testing is positive. Then for the next 8 to 10 years, the person typically feels well, not knowing the infection is present unless an HIV test is done. This long well period is deceptive, however, because it is actually a critical stage of viral incubation. The virus is actually "hiding away" in lymphoid tissues (e.g., lymph nodes, spleen, adenoid glands, and tonsils), where it is rapidly multiplying in its parasite life cycle within the host, taking over more and more of its special T-helper white blood cells (CD4) and gaining strength.[31] Researchers emphasize the crucial nature of this incubation period and the importance of earlier medical treatment intervention after an HIV-positive test to slow this viral-strengthening time while drugs and vaccines are being developed to combat its steady progression.

Stage 2: AIDS-Related Complex

After the extended "well" HIV-positive stage, a period of associated infectious illnesses begins to invade the body. This ARC period of opportunistic illnesses is so named because by this period the HIV infection has killed enough host-protective white T cells (e.g., T helper lymphocytes) to severely damage the immune system and lower the body's normal disease resistance so that even the most common everyday infections have an opportunity to take root and grow (Box 23-2). Common symptoms during this pre-AIDS period include persistent fatigue, mouth sores of thrush (e.g., oral *Candida albicans*), night sweats, diarrhea, fever greater than 100° F, unintentional weight loss, remarkable headache, new skin rash, new or unusual cough, sore throat or mouth, unusual bruises or skin discoloration, and shortness of breath.[32]

Stage 3: Final Stage of AIDS

The terminal stage of full-blown HIV infection, designated as AIDS, is marked by rapidly declining T-helper lymphocyte counts from the normal healthy level of about 1000 per cubic millimeter of blood ($1000/mm^3$). Persons infected with HIV usually lose about 40 to $80/mm^3$ of T-helper lymphocytes every year. When falling T-helper lymphocyte counts are roughly between 200 and 500 mm^3, various diseases (e.g., tuberculosis or Kaposi's sarcoma) generally occur. Kaposi's sarcoma is the most common AIDS-associated cancer, characterized by malignant, rapidly growing tumors of the skin and mucous linings of the GI and respiratory tracts, where they may cause severe internal bleeding. Low-dose radiation therapy or anticancer drugs may be used to slow the spread of tumors. At T-helper lymphocyte counts below $200/mm^3$, *protozoan parasites* (i.e., primitive single-cell organisms) appear and infect a number of body organs. At counts under $50/mm^3$, *cytomegalovirus* (CMV), a herpes virus causing lesions on mucous linings of body organs) or *lymphoma* (any cancer of the lymphoid tissue) can flourish. This series of HIV effects on the body brings marked changes in body weight in both men and women, with women losing disproportionately more body fat. When the AIDS virus finally kills enough white cells to overwhelm the immune system's weakened resistance to the disease complications, death follows.

---

virus (L. *virus*, poison; *virion*, individual virus particle) a minute microscopic infectious organism characterized by lack of independent metabolism and the ability to reproduce with genetic continuity only within a living host. Each particle (virion) basically consists of nucleic acids (genetic material) and a protein shell that protects and contains the genetic material and any enzymes present.

pandemic (Gr. *pan*, all; *dēmos*, people) a widespread epidemic, distributed through a region, a continent, or the world.

parasite (Gr. *para*, along side; *sitos*, food, grain; *parasitos*, one who eats at another's table in ancient Greece, a term for a person who received free meals in return for amusing or flattering conversation) an organism that lives in or on an organism of another species known as the host, from whom all life cycle nourishment is obtained.

BOX 23–2 Common Types of Microorganisms Causing Clinical Complications in AIDS

Parasites

Pneumonia
Focal encephalitis
Malabsorption, diarrhea
Meningitis

Bacteria

Bacteremia
Diarrhea
Pneumonia
Meningitis
Tuberculosis
Encephalitis

Fungi

Fungemia
Pneumonia
Thrush, stomatitis, esophagitis
Skin lesions

Viruses

Multiple mucosal lesions, herpes simplex
Pneumonia
Non-Hodgkin's lymphomas
Multiple skin lesions, herpes zoster
Nausea, vomiting, diarrhea, fever

AIDS = Acquired immunodeficiency syndrome.

NUTRITION MANAGEMENT IN THE HIV/AIDS PATIENT

Support for Medical Management

Basic Current Goals

Medical management of HIV infection during all of its stages is constantly evolving. Intensive medical research for drugs and vaccines to halt this devastating virus continues. Current studies are aimed at preventing progressive immunodeficiency, stopping HIV transmission to uninfected individuals, and restoring depressed immune function to normal to prevent AIDS-associated complications. Thus basic current medical goals are to do the following:

1. Delay progression of the infection and improve the immune system
2. Prevent opportunistic illnesses
3. Recognize the infection early and provide rapid treatment for complications, including infections and cancers

Initial Evaluation: AIDS Team

The initial medical evaluation of a person newly diagnosed with HIV is critical in providing guidelines for ongoing comprehensive care by the AIDS team. This professional team includes medical, nutritional, nursing, and psychosocial health care specialists. Box 23-3 outlines an initial evaluation guide that emphasizes special coordinated medical care and the importance of nutritional, nursing, and psychosocial support.

Drug Therapy

Developing effective drugs is difficult because of the highly evolved nature of the virus. One of the earliest findings in the drug research for HIV has been a group of compounds called *nucleoside/nucleotide reverse transcriptase inhibitors* (NRTIs) that inhibit the virus's necessary enzyme for copying itself, thus effectively preventing viral increase. There have been multiple toxic side effects (Box 23-4), however, some of which (e.g., nausea) may be helped by dietary modifications. Other types of antiretroviral drugs approved by the U.S. Food and Drug Administration (FDA), and currently in use in the United States, are *non-nucleoside reverse transcriptase inhibitors* (NNRTIs), *protease inhibitors* (PIs), and most recently, *fusion inhibitors* (Box 23-5).[33] Protease inhibitors help stop HIV by inhibiting the basic enzyme, protease, which is essential to its development. Unfortunately, the HIV virus is capable of mutation in response to some drugs, specifically protease inhibitors, thus becoming resistant to treatment.[34] In addition to these antiretroviral drugs, there are many other drugs approved by the FDA to prevent or treat AIDS-related illnesses.

Vaccine Development

A successful HIV vaccine would train the body's immune system to identify and destroy the HIV virus. The development and testing of vaccines takes several years. Once a potential vaccine is identified, it must go through the following three phases of testing and be determined effective before the FDA can approve it for public use:

1. *Phase I.* The vaccine is tested in small groups of healthy, low-risk participants. This phase lasts 12 to 18 months.

BOX 23-3 Initial Evaluation of Newly Diagnosed HIV-Infected Patients

Routine history and physical examination, to include:
  History of exposure to infectious complications of AIDS
  Assessment of baseline mental status
Baseline laboratory studies
  CBC, differential, platelets
  Biochemistry screening profile
  Urinalysis
  Chest x-ray
  Tuberculin test with energy panel
  Serologic test for syphilis
  Toxoplasma serology
  T-lymphocyte subsets
  Hepatitis B serology (optional)

Nutrition assessment and counseling; nutritional support, and follow-up
Psychosocial and financial status assessment
Referral to and involvement in psychosocial support, including:
  Social worker, nurse, psychologist or psychiatrist, patient support group, community support group, and agencies
Rehabilitation program for substance abusers
Planning for family members and children, including issues of testing and providing for their care

Modified from Gold JWM: HIV-1 infection: diagnosis and management, *Med Clin North Am* 76(1):1, 1992.
AIDS = Acquired immunodeficiency syndrome; *CBC* = complete blood count; *HIV* = human immunodeficiency virus.

BOX 23-4 Toxic Effects of AIDS Drugs

AZT (azidothymidine, zidovudine)

Bone marrow suppression, decreased red and white blood cell counts
Anemia, muscle pain
Nausea and vomiting
Headache, malaise, fatigue, fever
Confusion, tremulousness, disordered brain function
Bluish color of fingernails and toenails

ddl (dideoxyinosine)

Painful peripheral nerves
Occasional pancreatitis

ddl (dideoxyinosine)—cont'd

Headache, insomnia, restlessness
Occasional hepatitis

ddC (dideoxycytidine)

Painful peripheral nerves
Stomatitis, fevers
Bone pain, edema

d4T (dideoxythymidine)

Painful peripheral nerves
Anemia

AIDS = Acquired immunodeficiency syndrome.

2. *Phase II.* The vaccine is tested in hundreds of high- and low-risk participants. This phase can last up to 2 years.
3. *Phase III.* Thousands of high-risk participants are tested for both safety and effectiveness of the vaccine. This phase usually lasts an additional 3 to 4 years.

In February 1999, Thailand became the first country to begin a Phase III HIV vaccine trial. Thailand has one the fastest growing HIV-infected populations in the world. The CDC and the National Institutes of Health are the two agencies involved in coordinating vaccine research in the United States and are working in conjunction with other agencies worldwide to expedite the development of an effective vaccine.

Wasting Effects of HIV Infection on Nutritional Status

Severe Malnutrition and Weight Loss

Patients with HIV typically suffer from decreased appetite and insufficient energy intake coupled with elevated resting energy expenditure. Major weight loss follows and eventually leads to extreme cachexia, similar to that seen in cancer patients. Malnutrition suppresses cellular immune function, thus perpetuating the onset of opportunistic infections, the primary cause of death in AIDS patients. The chronic, relentless body wasting of AIDS is so striking that in Africa it is called "slim disease." This wasting process plays

---

BOX 23–5 FDA-Approved Antiretroviral Drugs

Nucleoside/Nucleotide Reverse Transcriptase Inhibitors (NRTIs)

abacavir (Ziagen)
didanosine (Videx, ddI)
lamivudine (Epivir, 3T3)
stavudine (Zerit, d4T)
tenofovir DF (Viread)
zalcitabine (HIVID, ddC)
zidovudine (Retrovir, AZT, ZDV)

Nonnucleoside Reverse Transcriptase Inhibitors (NNRTIs)

delavirdine (Rescriptor)
efavirenz (Sustiva)
nevirapine (Viramune)

Protease Inhibitors (PIs)

amprenavir (Agenerase)
indinavir (Crixivan)
lopinavir + ritonavir (Kaletra)
nelfinavir (Viracept)
ritonavir (Norvir)
saquinavir (Fortovase, Invirase)

Fusion Inhibitor

enfuvirtide (Fuzeon, T-20)

---

a major role in the decreased quality of life, debilitating weakness, and fatigue of AIDS patients.

Causes of Body Wasting

The characteristic body wasting of HIV infection may result from any of the following processes, alone or combined:

- *Inadequate food intake.* An important factor in the profound weight loss is severe *anorexia*, loss of appetite. This state is probably related to the patient's life-changing situation, as well as to the body's physiologic changes from the disease.
- *Malabsorption of nutrients.* Diarrhea and malabsorption are common in AIDS patients. These symptoms have been related to drug-diet interactions and the progressive effects of HIV infection. The viral infection causes blunting of the intestinal villi and secretion of abnormal intestinal enzymes. In later stages of AIDS, the damaged intestinal tissues are open to opportunistic organisms, resulting in severe diarrhea and malabsorption.
- *Disordered metabolism.* In the final stage of weight loss in AIDS patients, changes in metabolism (e.g., hypermetabolism and altered energy metabolism) occur. Progressive depletion of lean body mass and increased resting energy expenditure also result.

Lipodystrophy

Encouraging results initially came with use of the drug megestrol (Megace) in treating cachexia and wasting

syndrome in patients with AIDS or cancer. This drug is a synthetic hormone similar to the natural hormone progesterone, which improves appetite and food intake, leading to weight gain. However, the majority of the weight gained is fat mass as opposed to lean tissue. Disproportionate gaining of fat mass, lipodystrophy, and continued wasting of lean tissue contribute to the abnormal body composition changes seen in AIDS patients. The use of human growth hormone, cytokine inhibitors, and resistance training appears to be more effective in preventing lean tissue losses.[35-37]

Nutrition Assessment

A comprehensive nutrition assessment provides the baseline information necessary for starting and continuing nutritional care. The clinical dietitian on the AIDS team conducts this assessment and calculates daily energy and protein needs, assessing and monitoring weight changes and evaluating laboratory tests. These tests and evaluations are especially necessary for certain patients on special nutritional support, enteral or parenteral. Further person-centered nutritional care necessary for all HIV-infected patients is evident in the ABCDs of nutrition assessment outlined (see the Clinical Applications box, "The ABCDs of Nutrition Assessment of AIDS Patients.") On first contact with a health professional, all patients should be referred to the AIDS team clinical dietitian for screening to detect the degree of any nutritional problems. Together with the patient, the dietitian can then plan for ongoing nutritional care and support.

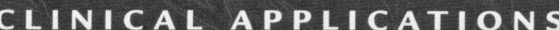

CLINICAL APPLICATIONS

THE ABCDs OF NUTRITION ASSESSMENT OF AIDS PATIENTS

The initial nutrition-assessment visit with a patient infected with HIV is important because it sets the pattern and direction for all of the continuing nutritional care that is to follow.

This vital encounter serves both informational and relational functions. It provides the necessary baseline information for planning practical, individual nutritional support. More importantly, however, the initial visit establishes the essential provider–patient relationship, which is the very human context in which continuing nutritional care and support are provided. The basic ABCDs of nutrition assessment provide a practical guide, with special EFs added for HIV-infection patients.

Anthropometry

● Age, sex, height
● Weight: current, usual, percent of usual, ideal, percent of ideal, weight loss over a defined period
● Body composition: bioelectrical impedance test, dual-energy x-ray absorptiometry (DEXA)
● Mid-upper arm measures: circumference, triceps skinfold thickness; calculated mid-arm muscle circumference

Biochemical Tests

● Serum proteins: albumin, prealbumin, transferrin
● Liver function test (evaluate liver function)
● Blood urea nitrogen, serum electrolytes (evaluate renal function)
● Urinary urea nitrogen excretion

● Creatinine height index (evaluate protein tissue breakdown)
● Complete blood count (evaluate for anemia)
● Fasting glucose (evaluate for high or low blood glucose levels)

Clinical Observations

● General signs of nutritional status (see Table 17-1)
● Drug effects

Diet Evaluations

● Usual intake, current intake, restrictions, modifications (use 24-hour recall and food diaries)
● Nutrition supplements, vitamin or mineral supplements
● Food allergies, intolerances
● Activity level (average energy expended per day)
● Support system (caregivers to help with nutritional care plan)

Environmental, Behavioral, and Psychological Assessment

● Living situation, personal support
● Food environment, types of meals, eating assistance needed

Financial Assessment

● Medical insurance
● Income, financial support through caregivers
● Ability to afford food, enteral supplements, additional vitamins or minerals

---

Suggested guidelines for developing such patient-centered care plans are outlined in Table 23-2.

Nutrition Counseling, Education, and Supportive Care

Counseling Principles

An adolescent client once defined a counselor as "someone to talk to while I make up my mind," and client-centered counseling in the care of persons with HIV infection must be just that. The basic goal of nutrition counseling is to make the least amount of changes necessary in a person's lifestyle and food patterns to promote optimal nutritional status while providing maximum comfort and quality of life.

In this person-centered care process, the following counseling principles are particularly important:

■ *Motivation.* Changed behavior in any area requires the motivation, desire, and ability to achieve one's goals. AIDS is no exception. Until a patient perceives food patterns and behaviors as appropriate goals, it is best to wait for a better time and simply start with establishing a general supportive climate in which to continue working together. Any specific obstacle raised by the patient (e.g., time, physical

TABLE 23–2	Planning Nutrition Care for Patients with AIDS	
Type of problem	**Possible causes**	**Patient care plan considerations**
Food intake	Anorexia	Patient, caregiver roles
	Drug-food interaction	Motivation, patient decision making
	HIV, other infection	Education, counseling
	Taste alteration	Resource materials
	Food intolerances, allergies	Nutrition supplements
	Lack of access or ability to prepare food	Vitamin, mineral supplements
	Depression	Drug-food reactions
		Special enteral-parenteral nutrition support
		Monitoring, adjustments as needed
Nutrient absorption	HIV-related infections or cancers	Treatment of underlying disease or disorder
	Diminished gastric HCl secretion	Pancreatic enzymes supplement
	Altered mucosal absorbing surface	Drug-nutrient reactions
	Organ involvement: liver, pancreas, gall-bladder, kidney	Special enteral-parenteral nutrition support, appropriate formula design
	Drug-nutrient interaction	Monitoring, adjustments as needed
Altered metabolism, excretion	HIV infection	Review of drug dosage, schedule
	Associated infections, diseases	Modification of diet, meal plan
	Drug-nutrient interactions	Treatment of infection, symptoms
	Altered hormonal function	Review of diet nutrients, increase or decrease
	Organ dysfunction	Special enteral-parenteral nutrition support, appropriate formula design
		Monitoring, adjustments as needed

Data from Newman CF: *Practical guidelines for improving nutritional status in HIV-related disease,* University of California, Davis Medical School Fifth Annual Conference on Clinical Nutrition, Nutrition in the Treatment of Serious Medical Problems, Feb 28-29, 1992.
AIDS = Acquired immunodeficiency syndrome; *HIV* = human immunodeficiency virus; *HCL* = hydrochloric acid.

limitations, money, or increased anxiety) can be met with related suggestions to think about.

■ *Rationale.* Any diet or food behavior change, with possible benefits or risks, must be clearly explained to the patient. The question "Why?" is always important. As with cancer patients at such points of stress, AIDS patients are more vulnerable to the lure of unproven therapies.

■ *Provider–patient agreement.* When the patient is ready, any change must be an agreement and must fit daily routines and include any caregivers as needed. Throughout the process, the nutrition counselor should provide necessary information and encouragement.

■ *Manageable steps.* All information or actions should proceed in manageable steps, as small as necessary, in order of complexity and difficulty. Do simple, easy things first. Information overload can discourage anyone. Clinicians should also keep in mind any brain or central nervous system decline in the patient. Such decline may contribute to memory loss and inability to follow nutrition advice.

Personal Food Management Skills

The patient's living situation and general practical skills in planning, purchasing, and preparing food must be considered. Any need for information and guidance in developing these skills or providing sources of help should be provided.

Community Programs

Information about available community food programs (e.g., Meals-on-Wheels, for delivery of prepared meals when the patient is too ill to shop for food or prepare it) may be needed. Information about food assistance programs (e.g., food stamps or food commodities [see Chapter 13]), for which lower-income persons may qualify, also may be needed.

Psychosocial Support

In the final analysis, every aspect of care provided should be given in a form and manner that provide genuine psychosocial support. All health care providers working with HIV-infected patients must be particularly sensitive to the special psychological and social issues that confront them. Major stress areas may include issues relating to autonomy and dependency, a sense of uncertainty and fear of the unknown, grief, change and loss, fear of symptoms and abandonment, and spiritual questions that arise when someone confronts a life-threatening disease. Common emotions are hostility, denial, withdrawal, depression, anxiety, guilt, and confusion. Health care providers always must be aware of how the patient and caregivers are relating to the disease, using assistance of social workers or clinical psychologists as needed. Stress-reduction groups, including exercise training, are help-ful, as they have proved to be in other life-threatening situations (e.g., cancer and coronary heart disease).

However, most of all health care workers must examine their own stresses, values, and fears about sexual orientation and behavior, intravenous drug use, and fear of AIDS transmission. Preconceived judgments are easily picked up by patients and threaten the provider-patient relationship. Before they can be effective with patients, all health care workers must first deal with their own fears and prejudices and learn to let go of judgmental behavior.

SUMMARY

The general term *cancer* is given to various abnormal, malignant tumors in different tissue sites. The cancer cell is derived from a normal cell that loses control over its growth and reproduction. Cancer cell development occurs via mutation of regulatory genes and is influenced by environmental chemical carcinogens, radiation, and special viruses. Other lifestyle factors associated with an increased risk for cancer include diet, excessive alcohol use, and smoking, as well as physical and psychological stress. Cell integrity is mediated by the body's immune system, primarily through its two types of special white blood cells: T cells that can kill invading agents that cause disease, and B cells that can make specific antibodies to attack these agents.

Cancer therapy primarily consists of surgery, radiation, and chemotherapy with specific drugs. Supportive nutritional care must be highly individualized according to body responses to the disease and its treatment. This care is based on nutrition assessment and provided by the following routes: oral, tube feeding, peripheral vein, and TPN through a large central vein. In any case, nutrition management must meet the physical and psychological needs of individual patients.

Likewise, nutritional care of patients with AIDS must be built on knowledge and compassion, with a sensitiv-ity and concern for individual patient needs. The current worldwide spread of HIV and its fatal consequences have reached epidemic proportions and are still growing. The overall disease progression follows the three distinct stages: (1) HIV infection, (2) ARC with associated opportunistic illnesses, and (3) full-blown AIDS with complicating diseases leading to death.

Medical management of HIV infection, which is still without a cure or vaccine, involves supportive treatment of associated illnesses and diseases. In the terminal AIDS stage, the virus eventually gains enough strength to destroy the host's immune system (e.g., T-helper white cells), and death follows. New drugs are being used to slow the disease process, while intensive ongoing research seeks a vaccine and cure.

Nutrition management centers on providing individual nutrition support to counteract the severe body wasting and malnutrition characteristic of the disease. The process of nutritional care involves comprehensive nutrition assessment and evaluation of personal needs, planning care with patient and caregivers, and meeting practical food needs. Throughout the care process, nutrition counseling, education, and strategic services also help provide psychosocial support for each patient, according to individual needs.

CRITICAL THINKING QUESTIONS

1. What is cancer? Describe several major causes of cancer cell formation. Why is cancer an increasing health problem?
2. In what two main ways does nutrition relate to cancer? Give examples of each.
3. Describe the major types of defense cells that are the major components of the body's immune system. How does nutrition relate to immunity?
4. Describe nutritional problems associated with each of the three medical treatments of cancer.
5. Outline the general procedure for nutrition management of a cancer patient.
6. List and describe the American Cancer Society's dietary guidelines for reducing the risk for cancer.
7. Describe the evolutionary history of HIV and its current worldwide epidemic spread. How is it

transmitted, and why do you think it has spread so rapidly? Identify major population groups at risk.

8. Describe the nature of the AIDS virus and its action in the human body.

9. Describe the three stages of HIV infection from initial infection to death.

10. Outline basic parts of a comprehensive initial nutrition assessment of a patient with HIV infection, and describe the reasons for each type of information and its evaluation.

11. Describe the general process of planning nutritional care on the basis of the patient assessment information and the main types of nutritional problems in patients with HIV. Devise a related plan of action for each type of problem. Give an example of how you might follow up to see what worked or did not work and make adjustments.

CHAPTER CHALLENGE QUESTIONS

True-False

Write the correct statement for each item you answer "false."

1. *True or False:* A cancer cell is unrelated to a normal cell.

2. *True or False:* Genes consist of cell nucleus material that controls protein synthesis and transmits hereditary information.

3. *True or False:* Chemical carcinogens are substances that can cause cancer to develop.

4. *True or False:* The incidence of cancer is not related to age.

5. *True or False:* Cancer-causing mutant genes may be inherited, making a person more susceptible to the influence of some added environmental agent.

6. *True or False:* Antigens are specialized protein components of our immune systems that protect us against disease.

7. *True or False:* Cachexia is a muscle wasting syndrome occurring only in AIDS patients.

8. *True or False:* Unlike patients with cancer, individuals with AIDS do not require nutritional support.

9. *True or False:* Lipodystrophy is the abnormal fat redistribution syndrome characteristic in some AIDS patients suffering from protein wasting and body fat gaining, often in abnormal places.

10. *True or False:* Individuals with AIDS have severely weakened immune systems, such that parasites and bacteria that are not normally lethal to a healthy individual could result in death.

Multiple Choice

1. Special blood cells that are major components of the immune system are

   a. erythrocytes.

   b. lymphocytes.

   c. neurotransmitters.

   d. platelets.

2. A serious primary problem resulting from prolonged vomiting from cancer chemotherapy relates to

   a. nitrogen balance.

   b. calcium balance.

   c. fluid and electrolyte balance.

   d. vitamin E balance.

3. Side effects of cancer chemotherapy that reflect the toxic effect of the drugs on rapidly reproducing cells include

   a. severe headaches.

   b. GI symptoms.

   c. increased urination.

   d. increased appetite.

4. An adequate amount of high-quality protein is essential in a cancer patient's diet to

   a. prevent catabolism.

   b. meet increased energy demands.

   c. prevent anabolism.

   d. stimulate hypermetabolism.

5. Small amounts of which of the following types of food would most likely help treat the nausea caused by cancer chemotherapy?

   a. Hot liquids

   b. Dry, spicy foods

   c. Warm, fat-seasoned foods

   d. Soft, cold foods

6. Which of the following is not a method by which HIV can be transmitted?

   a. Sexual contact

   b. Social kissing

   c. Sharing needles

   d. Blood transfusions

7. An individual with HIV infection is said to have AIDS when

   a. he or she loses 10 lbs.

   b. he or she has a rapid increase in T-helper lymphocytes.

   c. he or she starts taking medications such as protease inhibitors.

   d. he or she has a rapid decrease in T-helper lymphocytes.

8. Body wasting in the AIDS patient is usually a result of which of the following?

   a. Inadequate food intake

   b. Malabsorption of nutrients

   c. Disordered metabolism

   d. All of the above

9. Which of the following medications has shown promising results in maintaining lean tissue in AIDS patients?

   a. Human growth hormone

   b. Protease inhibitors

   c. Megace

   d. Fusion inhibitors

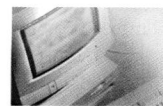

Please refer to the Students' Resource section of this text's Evolve web site for "Suggestions for Additional Study."

REFERENCES

1. U.S. Department of Health and Human Services, Centers for Disease Control and Prevention, National Center for Health Statistics, *Cancer*, Hyattsville, MD, 2003 (accessed June 2003), USDHHS/CDC/NCHS [*www.cdc.gov/nchs/fastats/cancer.htm*].

2. Centers for Disease Control and Prevention: *National vital statistics report*, vol 50, no 16, Atlanta, September 16, 2002, CDC.

3. Miller DP and others: Association between self-reported environmental tobacco smoke exposure and lung cancer: modification by GSTP1 polymorphism, *Int J Cancer* 104(6):758, 2003.

4. Settimi L and others: Prostate cancer and exposure to pesticides in agricultural settings, *Int J Cancer* 104:458, 2003.

5. Settimi L and others: Cancer risk among male farmers: a multi-site case-control study, *Int J Occup Med Environ Health* 14(4):339, 2001.

6. Sharpe CR, Siemiatycki J, Parent ME: Activities and exposures during leisure and prostate cancer risk, *Cancer Epidemiol Biomarkers* 10(8):855, 2001.

7. Meinert R and others: Leukemia and non-Hodgkin's lymphoma in childhood and exposure to pesticides: results of a register-based case-control study in Germany, *Am J Epidemiol* 151(7):639, 2000.

8. Ji BT and others: Occupational exposure to pesticides and pancreatic cancer, *Am J Ind Med* 39(1):92, 2001.

9. Centers for Disease Control and Prevention, Division of Cancer Prevention and Control: *Skin cancer: preventing America's most common cancer* [2003 program fact sheet], Atlanta, 2003 (accessed June 2003), CDC/DCPC [*www.cdc.gov/cancer/nscpep/skin.htm*].

10. de Gruijl FR, van Kranen HJ, Mullenders LH: UV-induced DNA damage, repair, mutations and oncogenic pathways in skin cancer, *J Photochem Photobiol B* 63(1-3):19, 2001.

11. Cleaver JE, Crowley E: UV damage, DNA repair and skin carcinogenesis, *Front Biosci* 7:1024, 2002.

12. Pierce JP and others: A randomized trial of the effect of a plant-based dietary pattern on additional breast cancer events and survival: the Women's Healthy Eating and Living (WHEL) study, *Control Clin Trials* 23(6):728, 2002.

13. Perera FP: Uncovering new clues to cancer risk, *Sci Am* 274(5):54, 1996.

14. Lillberg K and others: Stressful life events and risk of breast cancer in 10,808 women: a cohort study, *Am J Epidemiol* 157(5):415, 2003.

15. Kang DH: Oxidative stress, DNA damage, and breast cancer, *AACN Clin Issues* 13(4):540, 2002.

16. Ames BN, Wakimoto P: Are vitamin and mineral deficiencies a major cancer risk? *Natl Rev Cancer* 2:694, 2002.

17. Aiko S and others: Beneficial effects of immediate enteral nutrition after esophageal cancer surgery, *Surg Today* 31(11):971, 2001.

18. Inui A: Cancer anorexia-cachexia syndrome: current issues in research and management, *CA Cancer J Clin* 52:72, 2002.

19. Byers T and others: American Cancer Society guidelines on nutrition and physical activity for cancer prevention: reducing the risk of cancer with healthy food choices and physical activity, *CA Cancer J Clin* 52:92, 2002.

20. U.S. Food and Drug Administration, Center for Food Safety and Applied Nutrition: *A food labeling guide, appendix C*, College Park, MD, 2000 [rev] (accessed June 2003), FDA/CFSAN [*www.cfsan.fda.gov/~dms/flg-6c.html*].

21. U.S. Department of Health and Human Services: *USDA dietary guidelines for Americans*, ed 5, Washington, DC, 2000 (accessed June 2003), USDHHS [*http://198.102.218.57/dietaryguidelines/dga2000/10guidelines.pdf*].

22. U.S. Department of Health and Human Services: *Healthy people 2010: understanding and improving health*, Washington, DC, 2000, Government Printing Office.

23. Ames BN: DNA damage from micronutrient deficiencies is likely to be a major cause of cancer, *Mutat Res* 475 (1-2):7, 2001.

24. Weisburger JH: Lifestyle, health and disease prevention: the underlying mechanisms, *Eur J Cancer Prev* 11(2 suppl): 1, 2002.

25. Abdulla M, Gruber P: Role of diet modification in cancer prevention, *Biofactors* 12(1-4):45, 2000.

26. Brown J and others: Nutrition during and after cancer treatment: a guide for informed choices by cancer survivors, *CA Cancer J Clin* 51:153, 2001.

27. Centers for Disease Control and Prevention, National Center for Chronic Disease Prevention and Health Promotion, *Chronic disease prevention-preventing and controlling cancer: the nation's second leading cause of death*, Atlanta, 2003 (accessed June 2003), CDC/NCCDPHP [*www.cdc.gov/nccdphp/aag/aag_dcpc.htm*].

28. National Institute of Allergy and Infectious Disease, National Institutes of Health: *HIV vaccines explained*, Bethesda, MD, (accessed June 2003), NIAID/NIH [*www.niaid.nih.gov/publications/pdf/HIVvaccinebrochure.pdf*].

29. Tuofu Z and others: An African HIV-1 sequence from 1959 and implications for the origin of the epidemic, *Nature* 391(6667):594, 1998.

30. Christensen D: AIDS virus jumped from chimps, *Sci News* 155(6):84, 1999.

31. Christensen D: Why AIDS? The mystery of how HIV attacks the immune system, *Sci News* 155(13):204, 1999.

32. Kotler DP and others: Relative influences of sex, race, environment, and HIV infection on body composition in adults, *Am J Clin Nutr* 69(3):432, 1999.

33. AIDSinfo: *Overview of drugs*, Rockville, MD, (accessed June 2003), National Institutes of Health, U.S. Department of Health and Human Services [*www.aidsinfo.nih.gov/drugs*].

34. Wu TD and others: Mutation patterns and structural correlates in human immunodeficiency virus type 1 protease following different protease inhibitor treatment, *J Virol* 77(8):4836, 2003.

35. Kotler DP: Cachexia, *Ann Intern Med* 133:622, 2000.

36. Kotler DP: Nutritional alterations associated with HIV infection, *J Acquir Immune Defic Syndr* 25(1 suppl):8, 2000.

37. Engelson ES: HIV lipodystrophy diagnosis and management. Body composition and metabolic alterations: diagnosis and management, *AIDS Read* 13(4 suppl):10, 2003.

FURTHER READING AND RESOURCES

- National Cancer Institute: *www.nci.nih.gov*

- American Cancer Society: *www.cancer.org*

- Centers for Disease Control and Prevention: *www.cdc.gov*

- AIDS: *Official Journal of the International AIDS Society: www.aidsonline.com*

- AIDS Treatment News, part of AIDS.ORG: *www.aids.org/index.html*

- Johns Hopkins AIDS Service: *www.hopkins-aids.edu*

- National Center for HIV, STD, and TB Prevention, a division of the Centers for Disease Control and Prevention: *www.cdc.gov/nchstp/od/nchstp.html*

- The NIAID Division of AIDS: *www.niaid.nih.gov/daids/vaccine/news.htm*

  The preceding organizations and societies provide current information and updates on research, education, treatment, incidence, and mechanism of prevention for cancer or AIDS.

- Kang DH: Oxidative stress, DNA damage, and breast cancer, *AACN Clin Issues* 13(4):540, 2002.

  This article explains the role of oxidative stress and the development of breast cancer, the second leading cause of cancer deaths in women. The author believes nurses have a fundamental role in cancer research.

- Nerad J and others: General nutrition management in patients infected with Human Immunodeficiency Virus, *CID* 36(2 suppl):52, 2003.

  The authors give an overview of the nutrition management, levels of care, and appropriate screening tools involved in the care of HIV infected patients. This article also includes a table of HIV medications and common food interactions.

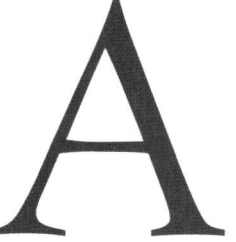

Food Composition Table

The following food composition table was developed by SureQuest Systems, Inc., and includes all of the foods listed in *Mosby's NutriTrac Nutrition Analysis CD-ROM, Version III,* which accompanies every copy of this text. Please note, however, that you can find some nutrient information in *Mosby's NutriTrac Nutrition Analysis CD-ROM* that is not listed here in the food composition table.

The easiest way to look for a food is to use the "Search For" feature in *Mosby's NutriTrac Nutrition Analysis CD-ROM.* However, if you do not have access to a computer or your computer time is limited, you can easily look for a food using this food composition table. The foods in the table are arranged alphabetically, within groups.

The code number before each food listing corresponds to the food data bank in *Mosby's NutriTrac Nutrition Analysis CD-ROM.* When you input your dietary intake into the CD-ROM program, you may choose to use these code numbers. Alternatively, you may choose to enter your dietary intake into *Mosby's NutriTrac Nutrition Analysis CD-ROM* by typing a food's name or partial name and using the "Search For" option.

Column heading key: *g,* grams; *mg,* milligrams; *mcg,* micrograms; *re,* retinol equivalent.

*NOTE: The "Weight in Grams" column provides the weight in grams of the serving or of one unit of measure (e.g., if a serving is 3 oz, the "Weight in Grams" column may indicate the weight of 1 oz).

USDA ID Code	Food Name	Weight in Grams*	Quantity of Units	Unit of Measure	Protein (g)	Fat (g)	Carbohydrate (g)	Kilocalories	Caffeine (g)	Fiber (g)	Cholesterol (mg)	Saturated Fat (g)
Baby Food												
	Babyfood, Applesauce	170.0000	3.000	Ounce	0.00	0.00	17.51	62.90	0.00	2.89	0.00	0.00
	Babyfood, Bananas w/ Tapioca	170.0000	3.000	Ounce	0.68	0.34	30.26	113.90	0.00	2.72	0.00	0.14
	Babyfood, Barley, Ppd w/ Whole Milk	28.3500	3.000	Ounce	1.30	0.94	4.62	31.47	0.00	0.00	0.00	0.00
	Babyfood, Beef	71.0000	3.000	Ounce	10.30	3.48	0.00	75.26	0.00	0.00	19.53	1.84
	Babyfood, Beef and Rice	170.0000	3.000	Ounce	8.50	4.93	14.96	139.40	0.00	0.00	0.00	0.00
	Babyfood, Beef Lasagna	170.0000	3.000	Ounce	7.14	3.57	17.00	130.90	0.00	0.00	0.00	0.00
	Babyfood, Beef Noodle	170.0000	3.000	Ounce	4.25	3.23	12.58	96.90	0.00	1.87	13.60	1.31
	Babyfood, Beef Stew	170.0000	3.000	Ounce	8.67	2.04	9.35	86.70	0.00	1.87	21.30	0.99
	Babyfood, Beets	224.0000	1.000	Cup	2.91	0.22	17.25	76.16	0.00	4.26	0.00	0.04
	Babyfood, Carrots	224.0000	1.000	Cup	1.79	0.45	16.13	71.68	0.00	3.81	0.00	0.09
	Babyfood, Chicken	71.0000	3.000	Ounce	10.44	6.82	0.00	105.79	0.00	0.00	41.68	1.75
	Babyfood, Chicken Noodle	170.0000	3.000	Ounce	4.03	2.01	14.94	93.50	0.00	1.53	15.30	0.58
	Babyfood, Chicken Soup	229.0000	1.000	Cup	3.66	3.89	16.49	114.50	0.00	2.52	9.16	0.64
	Babyfood, Chicken Sticks	71.0000	3.000	Ounce	10.37	10.22	0.99	133.48	0.00	0.14	55.38	2.90
	Babyfood, Cookies, Arrowroot	28.3500	1.000	Ounce	2.15	4.05	20.19	125.31	0.00	0.06	0.30	0.94
	Babyfood, Corn, Creamed	240.0000	1.000	Cup	3.36	0.96	39.12	156.00	0.00	5.04	2.40	0.17
	Babyfood, Cottage Cheese w/ Fruit	28.3500	3.000	Ounce	0.85	0.20	4.51	22.11	0.00	0.00	0.00	0.00
	Babyfood, Egg Yolks	28.3500	3.000	Ounce	2.84	4.90	0.28	57.55	0.00	0.00	208.37	1.47
	Babyfood, Egg Yolks and Bacon	170.0000	3.000	Ounce	4.25	8.50	10.54	134.30	0.00	1.53	159.80	2.79
	Babyfood, Fruit Dessert	170.0000	3.000	Ounce	0.51	0.00	29.24	107.10	0.00	1.02	0.00	0.00
	Babyfood, Green Beans	240.0000	1.000	Cup	2.88	0.24	13.68	60.00	0.00	4.56	0.00	0.05
	Babyfood, Ham	71.0000	3.000	Ounce	10.72	4.76	0.00	88.75	0.00	0.00	20.66	1.59
	Babyfood, Juice, Apple	131.0000	4.200	Fl Oz	0.00	0.13	15.33	61.57	0.00	0.13	0.00	0.03
	Babyfood, Juice, Mixed Fruit	127.0000	3.000	Ounce	0.13	0.13	14.73	59.69	0.00	0.13	0.00	0.03
	Babyfood, Juice, Orange	127.0000	3.000	Ounce	0.76	0.38	12.95	55.88	0.00	0.13	0.00	0.03
	Babyfood, Macaroni and Cheese	170.0000	3.000	Ounce	4.42	3.40	13.94	103.70	0.00	0.51	10.20	2.01
	Babyfood, Macaroni and Tomato and Beef	170.0000	3.000	Ounce	4.25	1.87	15.98	100.30	0.00	1.87	6.80	0.70
	Babyfood, Meat Sticks	71.0000	3.000	Ounce	9.51	10.37	0.78	130.64	0.00	0.14	49.70	4.13
	Babyfood, Mixed Vegetable	170.0000	3.000	Ounce	1.70	0.00	13.43	56.10	0.00	0.00	0.00	0.00
	Babyfood, Noodles and Chicken	170.0000	3.000	Ounce	2.89	3.74	15.47	108.80	0.00	1.87	0.00	0.00
	Babyfood, Peach Cobbler	220.0000	3.000	Ounce	0.66	0.00	40.26	147.40	0.00	1.54	0.00	0.00
	Babyfood, Peach Melba	28.3500	3.000	Ounce	0.09	0.00	4.65	17.01	0.00	0.00	0.00	0.00
	Babyfood, Peaches w/ Sugar	170.0000	3.000	Ounce	0.85	0.34	32.13	120.70	0.00	2.55	0.00	0.03
	Babyfood, Pears	170.0000	3.000	Ounce	0.51	0.17	19.72	73.10	0.00	6.12	0.00	0.02
	Babyfood, Peas, Buttered	28.3500	3.000	Ounce	0.99	0.37	3.20	17.01	0.00	0.00	0.00	0.00
	Babyfood, Plums w/ Tapioca	170.0000	3.000	Ounce	0.17	0.00	34.68	125.80	0.00	2.04	0.00	0.00
	Babyfood, Rice, Ppd w/ Whole Milk	28.3500	1.000	Ounce	1.11	1.02	4.73	32.60	0.00	0.02	3.21	0.66
	Babyfood, Rice, w/ Mixed Fruit	170.0000	3.000	Ounce	1.53	0.34	31.11	134.30	0.00	1.02	0.00	0.10
	Babyfood, Spaghetti and Tomato and Meat	170.0000	3.000	Ounce	4.37	2.33	19.41	115.60	0.00	1.87	8.50	0.92
	Babyfood, Spinach, Creamed	28.3500	3.000	Ounce	0.85	0.40	1.81	11.91	0.00	0.51	0.00	0.00
	Babyfood, Split Pea and Ham	28.3500	3.000	Ounce	0.94	0.37	3.20	20.13	0.00	0.31	0.00	0.00
	Babyfood, Squash	224.0000	1.000	Cup	1.79	0.45	12.54	53.76	0.00	4.70	0.00	0.09
	Babyfood, Sweet Potatoes	224.0000	1.000	Cup	2.46	0.22	31.14	134.40	0.00	3.36	0.00	0.04
	Babyfood, Teething Biscuits	28.3500	1.000	Ounce	3.03	1.19	21.66	111.13	0.00	0.40	0.00	0.43
	Babyfood, Tropical Fruit	113.0000	3.000	Ounce	0.23	0.00	18.53	67.80	0.00	0.00	0.00	0.00
	Babyfood, Turkey	71.0000	3.000	Ounce	10.93	5.04	0.00	91.59	0.00	0.00	37.70	1.64
	Babyfood, Turkey and Rice	170.0000	3.000	Ounce	4.03	1.56	16.27	95.20	0.00	1.70	6.80	0.41
	Babyfood, Turkey Sticks	71.0000	3.000	Ounce	9.73	10.08	0.99	129.22	0.00	0.36	46.15	2.94
Baked Goods												
	Bagels, Blueberry	56.7000	1.000	Each	5.96	0.90	30.28	155.92	0.00	1.30	0.00	0.12
	Bagels, Cinnamon-raisin	56.7000	1.000	Each	5.56	0.96	31.30	155.36	0.00	1.30	0.00	0.16
	Bagels, Cinnamon-raisin, Toasted	56.7000	1.000	Each	6.02	1.02	33.62	166.70	0.00	1.42	0.00	0.18

Page Key: A2 = Baby Food   A2 = Baked Goods   A8 = Beverages   A14 = Breads/Grains and Pasta   A18 = Breakfast Foods/Cereals   A26 = Dairy and Eggs   A40 = Fats and Oils   A42 = Fruits and Vegetables   A52 = Meats and Beans   A60 = Nuts and Seeds   A62 = Frozen Entrees and Packaged Foods   A76 = Restaurant Chains–Fast Foods   A92 = Restaurant Chains–Other   A106 = Seafood and Fish   A110 = Snacks and Sweets   A120 = Soups   A122 = Supplements   A126 = Toppings and Sauces

Monounsaturated Fat (g)	Polyunsaturated Fat (g)	Vitamin D (mg)	Vitamin K (mg)	Vitamin E (mg)	Vitamin A (re)	Vitamin C (mg)	Thiamin (mg)	Riboflavin (mg)	Niacin (mg)	Vitamin B₆ (mg)	Folate (mcg)	Vitamin B₁₂ (mcg)	Calcium (mg)	Iron (mg)	Magnesium (mg)	Phosphorus (mg)	Potassium (mg)	Sodium (mg)	Zinc (mg)
0.00	0.00	0.00	0.00	1.02	1.70	64.26	0.02	0.05	0.10	0.05	2.89	0.00	8.50	0.37	5.10	10.20	130.90	3.40	0.07
0.03	0.07	0.00	0.00	1.02	6.80	43.69	0.03	0.03	0.37	0.24	10.88	0.00	13.60	0.51	20.40	15.30	183.60	15.30	0.12
0.00	0.00	0.00	0.00	0.00	0.00	0.00	0.14	0.16	1.70	0.03	2.52	0.09	65.21	3.50	8.51	42.53	54.43	13.89	0.24
1.31	0.11	0.00	0.00	0.28	22.01	1.35	0.01	0.11	2.33	0.09	4.05	1.04	5.68	1.17	6.39	51.12	134.90	46.86	1.42
0.00	0.00	0.00	0.00	0.00	134.30	6.63	0.03	0.12	2.28	0.24	10.20	0.87	18.70	1.17	13.60	59.50	204.00	606.90	1.56
0.00	0.00	0.00	0.00	0.00	265.20	3.23	0.12	0.15	2.30	0.12	10.20	0.87	30.60	1.48	18.70	68.00	207.40	771.80	1.19
1.43	0.15	0.00	0.00	0.68	149.60	2.38	0.05	0.07	0.99	0.05	20.40	0.17	13.60	0.73	11.90	51.00	78.20	28.90	0.68
0.75	0.17	0.00	0.00	0.41	425.00	5.10	0.02	0.12	2.23	0.12	10.20	0.87	15.30	1.22	18.70	74.80	241.40	586.50	1.48
0.04	0.09	0.00	0.00	1.16	6.72	5.38	0.02	0.09	0.29	0.04	68.99	0.00	31.36	0.72	31.36	31.36	407.68	185.92	0.27
0.02	0.20	0.00	0.00	1.16	2645.44	12.32	0.04	0.09	1.12	0.18	38.75	0.00	51.52	0.87	24.64	44.80	452.48	109.76	0.40
3.07	1.65	0.00	0.00	0.28	8.52	1.07	0.01	0.11	2.43	0.13	7.88	0.28	39.05	0.70	7.81	63.90	86.62	36.21	0.72
0.80	0.46	0.00	0.00	0.31	294.10	0.17	0.05	0.07	1.19	0.09	11.90	0.00	35.70	0.65	11.90	134.30	66.30	132.60	0.68
0.98	2.06	0.00	0.00	0.55	393.88	2.29	0.05	0.07	0.66	0.09	11.91	0.27	84.73	0.62	11.45	54.96	151.14	36.64	0.50
4.45	2.12	0.00	0.00	0.28	2.13	1.21	0.01	0.14	1.43	0.07	7.88	0.28	51.83	1.11	9.94	85.91	75.26	340.09	0.72
2.55	0.24	0.00	0.00	0.00	0.00	1.56	0.14	0.12	1.63	0.01	9.92	0.02	9.07	0.85	6.24	32.89	44.23	104.90	0.15
0.29	0.43	0.00	0.00	1.25	19.20	5.28	0.02	0.12	1.20	0.10	30.48	0.05	43.20	0.65	19.20	79.20	194.40	124.80	0.55
0.00	0.00	0.00	0.00	0.17	0.57	6.75	0.00	0.01	0.01	0.00	1.45	0.02	8.79	0.04	1.13	11.06	11.91	14.46	0.05
1.96	0.64	0.00	0.00	0.22	106.60	0.40	0.02	0.08	0.01	0.05	26.11	0.44	21.55	0.78	1.98	81.36	21.83	11.06	0.54
3.76	1.09	0.00	0.00	0.46	47.60	1.53	0.09	0.14	0.46	0.05	6.97	0.15	47.60	0.80	8.50	85.00	59.50	81.60	0.46
0.00	0.00	0.00	0.00	0.39	40.80	5.10	0.03	0.02	0.24	0.05	5.95	0.00	15.30	0.36	8.50	13.60	161.50	22.10	0.09
0.00	0.12	0.00	0.00	1.25	103.20	20.16	0.05	0.24	0.77	0.10	78.48	0.00	156.00	2.59	52.80	45.60	307.20	4.80	0.46
2.26	0.65	0.00	0.00	0.28	7.10	1.49	0.10	0.13	2.02	0.14	1.49	0.07	3.55	0.72	7.81	63.19	149.10	47.57	1.21
0.00	0.04	0.00	0.00	0.79	2.62	75.85	0.01	0.03	0.10	0.04	0.13	0.00	5.24	0.75	3.93	6.55	119.21	3.93	0.04
0.01	0.05	0.00	0.00	0.25	5.08	80.77	0.03	0.01	0.15	0.05	8.51	0.00	10.16	0.43	6.35	6.35	128.27	5.08	0.04
0.06	0.08	0.00	0.00	0.76	7.62	79.38	0.06	0.04	0.30	0.06	33.53	0.00	15.24	0.22	11.43	13.97	233.68	1.27	0.08
0.90	0.22	0.00	0.00	0.41	5.10	2.21	0.10	0.10	0.94	0.03	18.70	0.05	86.70	0.51	11.90	100.30	74.80	129.20	0.54
0.77	0.14	0.00	0.00	0.41	185.30	2.55	0.09	0.10	1.28	0.09	15.30	0.41	23.80	0.61	11.90	74.80	122.40	28.90	0.61
4.60	1.13	0.00	0.00	0.28	14.91	1.70	0.04	0.12	1.05	0.06	6.32	0.21	24.14	0.98	7.81	73.13	80.94	388.37	1.35
0.00	0.00	0.00	0.00	0.00	414.80	5.61	0.02	0.03	0.70	0.14	11.39	0.00	28.90	0.53	17.00	37.40	190.40	15.30	0.41
0.00	0.00	0.00	0.00	0.00	221.00	1.36	0.07	0.07	1.16	0.03	5.78	0.15	44.20	0.83	18.70	56.10	100.30	44.20	0.54
0.00	0.00	0.00	0.00	0.51	30.80	45.10	0.02	0.04	0.57	0.02	2.42	0.00	8.80	0.22	4.40	13.20	123.20	19.80	0.07
0.00	0.00	0.00	0.00	0.00	5.67	7.37	0.00	0.01	0.08	0.00	0.54	0.00	3.12	0.09	0.57	1.42	26.37	2.55	0.08
0.12	0.15	0.00	0.00	1.02	30.60	32.13	0.02	0.05	1.11	0.03	6.63	0.00	8.50	0.46	8.50	18.70	263.50	8.50	0.10
0.03	0.03	0.00	0.00	1.02	5.10	37.40	0.02	0.05	0.32	0.02	6.46	0.00	13.60	0.43	15.30	20.40	195.50	3.40	0.14
0.00	0.00	0.00	0.00	0.00	11.62	3.60	0.02	0.02	0.39	0.04	10.26	0.00	12.76	0.29	0.00	33.17	1.42	0.08
0.00	0.00	0.00	0.00	1.02	15.30	1.36	0.02	0.05	0.36	0.05	1.53	0.00	10.20	0.37	6.80	10.20	141.10	13.60	0.14
0.00	0.00	0.00	0.00	0.00	7.35	0.34	0.13	0.14	1.48	0.03	2.32	0.09	67.76	3.46	12.76	49.61	53.87	13.04	0.18
0.07	0.09	0.00	0.00	0.12	3.40	15.81	0.22	0.27	3.60	0.19	1.70	0.03	27.20	4.42	8.50	35.70	85.00	17.00	0.24
0.85	0.32	0.00	0.00	0.12	214.20	0.34	0.09	0.12	1.65	0.10	45.90	0.05	25.50	0.90	18.70	59.50	207.40	127.50	0.90
0.00	0.00	0.00	0.00	0.15	104.33	1.02	0.01	0.02	0.07	0.02	19.50	0.02	32.04	0.40	17.86	13.89	62.65	15.59	0.10
0.00	0.00	0.00	0.00	0.07	22.68	0.54	0.01	0.01	0.14	0.01	3.69	0.01	6.52	0.14	0.00	13.89	38.56	3.97	0.18
0.04	0.18	0.00	0.00	1.16	450.24	17.47	0.02	0.16	0.85	0.16	34.50	0.00	53.76	0.78	26.88	35.84	414.40	2.24	0.18
0.00	0.09	0.00	0.00	1.16	1487.36	21.50	0.07	0.07	0.85	0.25	23.07	0.00	35.84	0.87	26.88	53.76	544.32	49.28	0.25
0.41	0.24	0.00	0.00	0.12	3.40	2.58	0.07	0.15	1.23	0.03	13.89	0.02	74.56	1.01	9.92	46.49	91.57	102.63	0.26
0.00	0.00	0.00	0.00	0.00	2.26	21.24	0.01	0.03	0.09	0.03	3.73	0.00	11.30	0.29	5.65	9.04	65.54	7.91	0.06
1.87	1.25	0.00	0.00	0.28	7.10	1.70	0.01	0.18	2.47	0.12	8.59	0.76	19.88	0.96	8.52	67.45	127.80	51.12	1.28
0.51	0.39	0.00	0.00	0.27	319.60	0.51	0.05	0.07	1.17	0.09	13.60	0.03	40.80	0.70	15.30	62.90	146.20	136.00	0.80
3.32	2.57	0.00	0.00	0.28	4.26	1.07	0.01	0.11	1.24	0.06	8.02	0.71	51.12	0.88	11.36	73.13	64.61	342.93	1.30
0.08	0.40	0.00	0.00	0.02	0.00	0.00	0.30	0.18	2.58	0.02	49.90	0.00	41.96	2.02	16.44	54.44	57.26	302.78	0.50
0.10	0.38	0.00	0.00	0.08	0.00	0.40	0.22	0.16	1.74	0.04	51.04	0.00	10.78	2.16	15.88	56.70	83.92	182.58	0.64
0.10	0.40	0.00	0.00	0.10	3.96	0.34	0.18	0.16	1.68	0.04	43.66	0.00	11.34	2.32	13.04	47.06	92.42	196.18	0.46

USDA ID Code	Food Name	Weight in Grams*	Quantity of Units	Unit of Measure	Protein (g)	Fat (g)	Carbohydrate (g)	Kilocalories	Caffeine (g)	Fiber (g)	Cholesterol (mg)	Saturated Fat (g)
	Bagels, Egg	56.7000	1.000	Each	6.02	1.20	30.06	157.62	0.00	1.30	13.60	0.24
	Bagels, Egg, Toasted	66.0000	1.000	Each	7.52	1.45	37.62	197.34	0.00	0.00	17.16	0.30
	Bagels, Oat Bran	56.7000	1.000	Each	6.06	0.68	30.22	144.58	0.00	2.04	0.00	0.10
	Bagels, Oat Bran, Toasted	66.0000	1.000	Each	7.59	0.86	37.82	180.84	0.00	0.00	0.00	0.14
	Bagels, Plain	56.7000	1.000	Each	5.96	0.90	30.28	155.92	0.00	1.30	0.00	0.12
	Bagels, Plain, Toasted	66.0000	1.000	Each	7.46	1.12	37.95	194.70	0.00	0.00	0.00	0.16
	Biscuits, Plain or Buttermilk	56.7000	1.000	Each	7.04	9.36	27.50	206.38	0.00	0.74	0.56	1.42
	Cake, Angelfood	28.3500	1.000	Slice	1.67	0.23	16.39	73.14	0.00	0.43	0.00	0.03
	Cake, Boston Cream Pie	28.3500	1.000	Slice	0.68	2.41	12.16	71.44	0.00	0.40	10.49	0.69
	Cake, Carrot, w/ Cream Cheese Frosting	111.0000	1.000	Slice	5.11	29.30	52.39	483.96	0.00	0.00	59.94	5.43
	Cake, Chocolate w/ Chocolate Frosting	28.3500	1.000	Slice	1.16	4.65	15.48	104.04	0.00	0.79	11.91	1.35
124	Cake, Chocolate, Double, Layer-Sara Lee	79.0000	1.000	Piece	3.00	13.00	33.00	260.00	0.00	2.00	25.00	11.00
125	Cake, Chocolate, German, Layer-Sara Lee	83.0000	1.000	Piece	4.00	15.00	34.00	280.00	0.00	2.00	30.00	11.00
126	Cake, Coconut Layer-Sara Lee	81.0000	1.000	Piece	3.00	14.00	34.00	280.00	0.00	2.00	30.00	12.00
	Cake, Fruitcake	28.3500	1.000	Slice	0.82	2.58	17.46	91.85	0.00	1.05	1.42	0.30
127	Cake, Fudge Golden Layer-Sara Lee	80.0000	1.000	Piece	3.00	13.00	34.00	270.00	0.00	1.00	25.00	11.00
	Cake, German Chocolate, w/ Frosting	111.0000	1.000	Slice	3.89	20.65	55.17	404.04	0.00	0.00	53.28	5.26
	Cake, Gingerbread	67.0000	1.000	Slice	2.68	6.83	33.97	207.03	0.00	2.14	23.45	1.74
	Cake, Pineapple Upside-down	28.3500	1.000	Slice	0.99	3.43	14.32	90.44	0.00	0.23	6.24	0.83
	Cake, Pound	30.0000	1.000	Slice	1.65	5.97	14.64	116.40	0.00	0.15	66.30	3.47
128	Cake, Pound, All Butter, Family	76.0000	1.000	Piece	4.00	17.00	36.00	310.00	0.00	0.50	75.00	9.00
129	Cake, Pound, All Butter-Sara Lee	76.0000	1.000	Piece	4.00	16.00	38.00	320.00	0.00	0.50	85.00	9.00
130	Cake, Pound, Chocolate Swirl-Sara Lee	83.0000	1.000	Piece	5.00	16.00	42.00	330.00	0.00	0.50	75.00	8.00
131	Cake, Pound, Reduced, Fat-Sara Lee	76.0000	1.000	Piece	4.00	11.00	42.00	280.00	0.00	1.00	65.00	3.00
132	Cake, Pound, Strawberry Swirl-Sara Lee	83.0000	1.000	Piece	4.00	11.00	44.00	290.00	0.00	0.50	60.00	3.00
	Cake, Sponge	28.3500	1.000	Slice	1.53	0.77	17.32	81.93	0.00	0.16	28.92	0.23
133	Cake, Vanilla Layer-Sara Lee	80.0000	1.000	Piece	2.00	13.00	31.00	250.00	0.00	0.00	35.00	10.00
	Cake, White, w/ Coconut Frosting	28.3500	1.000	Slice	1.25	2.92	17.92	100.93	0.00	0.28	0.28	1.11
134	Cake, White, w/o Frosting	74.0000	1.000	Slice	4.00	9.18	42.33	264.18	0.00	0.00	1.48	2.42
	Cake, Yellow, w/ Chocolate Frost	28.3500	1.000	Slice	1.08	4.93	15.71	107.45	0.00	0.51	15.59	1.32
	Cake, Yellow, w/ Vanilla Frosting	28.3500	1.000	Slice	0.99	4.11	16.67	105.75	0.00	0.09	15.59	0.67
169	Cheesecake, 25% Reduced Fat, Crm	120.0000	1.000	Piece	9.00	13.00	40.00	310.00	0.00	2.00	70.00	8.00
170	Cheesecake, Cherry Cream-Sara Lee	135.0000	1.000	Piece	6.00	12.00	55.00	350.00	0.00	2.00	35.00	5.00
171	Cheesecake, Chocolate Chip-Sara	120.0000	1.000	Piece	8.00	21.00	47.00	410.00	0.00	2.00	65.00	14.00
	Cheesecake, Commercially Prepared	28.3500	1.000	Slice	1.56	6.38	7.23	91.00	0.00	0.12	15.59	2.81
172	Cheesecake, French-Sara Lee	111.0000	1.000	Piece	5.00	21.00	24.00	350.00	0.00	1.00	20.00	13.00
	Cheesecake, Homemade	85.0000	1.000	Slice	0.50	22.10	21.42	303.45	0.00	0.00	102.85	12.21
	Cheesecake, No-bake Type	28.3500	1.000	Slice	1.56	3.60	10.06	77.68	0.00	0.54	8.22	1.90
173	Cheesecake, Original Cream-Sara Lee	121.0000	1.000	Piece	7.00	18.00	39.00	350.00	0.00	1.00	50.00	9.00
	Cheesecake, Plain, w/ Cherry Top	90.0000	1.000	Slice	4.50	16.65	23.85	258.30	0.00	0.00	76.50	9.11
174	Cheesecake, Strawberry Cream-Sara Lee	135.0000	1.000	Piece	6.00	12.00	49.00	330.00	0.00	2.00	40.00	5.00
175	Cheesecake, Strawberry French-Sara Lee	123.0000	1.000	Piece	4.00	14.00	43.00	320.00	0.00	1.00	20.00	9.00
	Coffeecake	28.3500	1.000	Slice	1.93	6.61	13.24	118.50	0.00	0.57	9.07	1.64
198	Coffeecake, Butter Streusel-Sara Lee	54.0000	1.000	Piece	4.00	12.00	25.00	220.00	0.00	0.50	35.00	6.00
	Coffeecake, Cheese	28.3500	1.000	Slice	1.98	4.31	12.56	96.11	0.00	0.28	24.10	1.53
199	Coffeecake, Cheese, Reduced Fat,	54.0000	1.000	Piece	3.00	6.00	28.00	180.00	0.00	0.00	20.00	1.50
200	Coffeecake, Crumb-Sara Lee	57.0000	1.000	Piece	3.00	9.00	32.00	220.00	0.00	0.50	15.00	1.50
	Coffeecake, Fruit	28.3500	1.000	Slice	1.47	2.89	14.60	88.17	0.00	0.71	1.98	0.71
201	Coffeecake, Pecan-Sara Lee	54.0000	1.000	Piece	4.00	12.00	24.00	230.00	0.00	0.50	25.00	4.50
202	Coffeecake, Raspberry-Sara Lee	54.0000	1.000	Piece	3.00	8.00	27.00	220.00	0.00	0.50	15.00	2.50
	Cream Puffs, Shell, w/ Custard Filling	28.3500	1.000	Each	1.90	4.39	6.49	73.14	0.00	0.11	37.99	1.04
	Crisp, Apple	282.0000	1.000	Cup	5.08	10.15	91.09	459.66	0.00	0.00	0.00	2.03
	Croissant, Apple	28.3500	1.000	Ounce	2.10	2.47	10.52	72.01	0.00	0.71	8.79	1.41

Page Key: A2 = Baby Food   A2 = Baked Goods   A8 = Beverages   A14 = Breads/Grains and Pasta   A18 = Breakfast Foods/Cereals   A26 = Dairy and Eggs   A40 = Fats and Oils   A42 = Fruits and Vegetables   A52 = Meats and Beans   A60 = Nuts and Seeds   A62 5 Frozen Entrees and Packaged Foods   A76 = Restaurant Chains–Fast Foods   A92 = Restaurant Chains–Other   A106 = Seafood and Fish   A110 = Snacks and Sweets   A120 = Soups   A122 = Supplements   A126 = Toppings and Sauces

Monounsaturated Fat (g)	Polyunsaturated Fat (g)	Vitamin D (mg)	Vitamin K (mg)	Vitamin E (mg)	Vitamin A (re)	Vitamin C (mg)	Thiamin (mg)	Riboflavin (mg)	Niacin (mg)	Vitamin B₆ (mg)	Folate (mcg)	Vitamin B₁₂ (mcg)	Calcium (mg)	Iron (mg)	Magnesium (mg)	Phosphorus (mg)	Potassium (mg)	Sodium (mg)	Zinc (mg)
0.24	0.36	0.00	0.00	0.00	18.72	0.34	0.30	0.14	1.96	0.06	49.90	0.10	7.38	2.26	14.18	47.62	38.56	286.34	0.44
0.30	0.46	0.00	0.00	0.00	21.12	0.33	0.30	0.15	2.20	0.06	11.22	0.11	9.24	2.82	17.82	59.40	48.18	358.38	0.55
0.14	0.28	0.00	0.00	0.08	0.00	0.12	0.18	0.20	1.68	0.02	45.92	0.00	6.80	1.74	17.58	62.38	65.20	287.46	0.52
0.18	0.35	0.00	0.00	0.00	0.00	0.07	0.19	0.22	1.89	0.13	23.10	0.00	8.58	2.18	40.92	116.82	144.54	359.70	1.48
0.08	0.40	0.00	0.00	0.02	0.00	0.00	0.30	0.18	2.58	0.02	49.90	0.00	41.96	2.02	16.44	54.44	57.26	302.78	0.50
0.09	0.49	0.00	0.00	0.00	0.00	0.00	0.31	0.20	2.91	0.03	11.22	0.00	12.54	2.52	20.46	67.98	71.94	378.84	0.62
3.92	3.52	0.00	0.00	1.66	0.56	0.00	0.24	0.16	1.90	0.02	33.46	0.08	27.78	1.88	9.64	243.82	127.00	596.48	0.28
0.02	0.10	0.00	0.00	0.00	0.00	0.00	0.03	0.14	0.25	0.01	9.92	0.02	39.69	0.15	3.40	9.07	26.37	212.34	0.02
1.29	0.29	0.00	0.00	0.30	6.52	0.06	0.12	0.08	0.05	0.01	4.25	0.05	6.52	0.11	1.70	13.89	11.06	40.82	0.05
7.24	15.10	0.00	0.00	0.00	426.24	1.22	0.15	0.17	1.13	0.08	13.32	0.11	27.75	1.39	19.98	78.81	124.32	273.06	0.54
2.48	0.52	0.00	0.00	0.00	7.09	0.03	0.01	0.04	0.16	0.01	4.82	0.04	12.19	0.62	9.64	34.59	56.70	94.69	0.20
0.00	0.00	0.00	0.00	0.00	20.00	0.00	0.00	0.00	0.00	0.00	0.00	0.00	40.00	1.00	0.00	0.00	0.00	180.00	0.00
0.00	0.00	0.00	0.00	0.00	20.00	0.00	0.00	0.00	0.00	0.00	0.00	0.00	40.00	0.70	0.00	0.00	0.00	160.00	0.00
0.00	0.00	0.00	0.00	0.00	0.00	0.00	0.00	0.00	0.00	0.00	0.00	0.00	40.00	1.00	0.00	0.00	0.00	170.00	0.00
1.19	0.94	0.00	0.00	0.47	1.13	0.14	0.01	0.03	0.22	0.01	5.39	0.00	9.36	0.59	4.54	14.74	43.38	76.55	0.08
0.00	0.00	0.00	0.00	0.00	20.00	0.00	0.00	0.00	0.00	0.00	0.00	0.00	40.00	0.50	0.00	0.00	0.00	130.00	0.00
8.71	5.46	0.00	0.00	0.00	23.31	0.00	0.11	0.14	1.10	0.02	4.44	0.10	53.28	1.22	18.87	173.16	150.96	368.52	0.49
3.75	0.90	0.00	0.00	0.00	10.72	0.07	0.13	0.12	1.05	0.03	6.70	0.05	46.23	2.22	10.72	112.56	161.47	306.86	0.27
1.47	0.93	0.00	0.00	0.38	18.43	0.34	0.04	0.05	0.34	0.01	7.37	0.02	34.02	0.42	3.69	23.25	31.75	90.44	0.09
1.77	0.32	0.00	0.00	0.00	46.80	0.00	0.04	0.07	0.39	0.01	12.30	0.08	10.50	0.41	3.30	41.10	35.70	119.40	0.14
0.00	0.00	0.00	0.00	0.00	80.00	0.00	0.00	0.00	0.00	0.00	0.00	0.00	20.00	1.20	0.00	0.00	0.00	310.00	0.00
0.00	0.00	0.00	0.00	0.00	80.00	0.00	0.00	0.00	0.00	0.00	0.00	0.00	20.00	0.70	0.00	0.00	0.00	280.00	0.00
0.00	0.00	0.00	0.00	0.00	40.00	0.00	0.00	0.00	0.00	0.00	0.00	0.00	60.00	1.20	0.00	0.00	0.00	350.00	0.00
0.00	0.00	0.00	0.00	0.00	60.00	0.00	0.00	0.00	0.00	0.00	0.00	0.00	20.00	1.00	0.00	0.00	0.00	350.00	0.00
0.00	0.00	0.00	0.00	0.00	20.00	0.00	0.00	0.00	0.00	0.00	0.00	0.00	40.00	0.70	0.00	0.00	0.00	140.00	0.00
0.27	0.13	0.00	0.00	0.08	13.04	0.00	0.07	0.08	0.55	0.01	11.06	0.07	19.85	0.77	3.12	38.84	28.07	69.17	0.14
0.00	0.00	0.00	0.00	0.00	0.00	0.00	0.00	0.00	0.00	0.00	0.00	0.00	20.00	0.50	0.00	0.00	0.00	140.00	0.00
1.05	0.61	0.00	0.00	0.20	3.12	0.03	0.04	0.05	0.30	0.01	6.24	0.02	25.52	0.33	3.40	19.85	28.07	80.51	0.09
3.93	2.33	0.00	0.00	0.00	11.84	0.15	0.14	0.18	1.13	0.02	5.18	0.06	96.20	1.12	8.88	68.82	70.30	241.98	0.24
2.72	0.60	0.00	0.00	0.64	9.36	0.00	0.03	0.05	0.35	0.01	6.24	0.05	10.49	0.59	8.51	45.64	50.46	95.54	0.18
1.73	1.46	0.00	0.00	0.00	5.39	0.00	0.03	0.02	0.14	0.01	7.65	0.04	17.58	0.30	1.70	40.54	15.03	97.52	0.07
0.00	0.00	0.00	0.00	0.00	60.00	0.00	0.00	0.00	0.00	0.00	0.00	0.00	100.00	1.00	0.00	0.00	0.00	310.00	0.00
0.00	0.00	0.00	0.00	0.00	20.00	15.00	0.00	0.00	0.00	0.00	0.00	0.00	40.00	0.70	0.00	0.00	0.00	320.00	0.00
0.00	0.00	0.00	0.00	0.00	60.00	1.20	0.00	0.00	0.00	0.00	0.00	0.00	60.00	1.20	0.00	0.00	0.00	300.00	0.00
2.45	0.45	0.00	0.00	0.45	41.39	0.11	0.01	0.05	0.06	0.01	5.10	0.05	14.46	0.18	3.12	26.37	25.52	58.68	0.14
0.00	0.00	0.00	0.00	0.00	20.00	1.20	0.00	0.00	0.00	0.00	0.00	0.00	40.00	0.50	0.00	0.00	0.00	280.00	0.00
6.87	1.75	0.00	0.00	0.00	272.85	0.34	0.03	0.18	0.34	0.04	10.20	0.21	49.30	1.06	6.80	81.60	86.70	240.55	0.47
1.28	0.23	0.00	0.00	0.00	28.07	0.14	0.03	0.07	0.14	0.01	8.51	0.09	48.76	0.13	5.39	66.34	59.82	107.73	0.13
0.00	0.00	0.00	0.00	0.00	20.00	0.00	0.00	0.00	0.00	0.00	0.00	0.00	80.00	0.50	0.00	0.00	0.00	320.00	0.00
5.21	1.38	0.00	0.00	0.00	216.90	0.63	0.03	0.14	0.32	0.04	9.00	0.15	38.70	1.11	6.30	63.90	83.70	182.70	0.36
0.00	0.00	0.00	0.00	0.00	0.00	18.00	0.00	0.00	0.00	0.00	0.00	0.00	40.00	0.70	0.00	0.00	0.00	320.00	0.00
0.00	0.00	0.00	0.00	0.00	0.00	12.00	0.00	0.00	0.00	0.00	0.00	0.00	40.00	0.50	0.00	0.00	0.00	230.00	0.00
3.68	0.88	0.00	0.00	0.97	9.36	0.09	0.06	0.07	0.48	0.01	17.29	0.05	15.31	0.54	6.24	30.62	34.87	99.51	0.23
0.00	0.00	0.00	0.00	0.00	60.00	0.00	0.00	0.00	0.00	0.00	0.00	0.00	20.00	0.50	0.00	0.00	0.00	240.00	0.00
2.02	0.47	0.00	0.00	0.44	24.66	0.03	0.03	0.04	0.19	0.02	11.06	0.10	16.73	0.18	4.25	28.63	81.93	96.11	0.17
0.00	0.00	0.00	0.00	0.00	0.00	0.00	0.00	0.00	0.00	0.00	0.00	0.00	40.00	0.50	0.00	0.00	0.00	230.00	0.00
0.00	0.00	0.00	0.00	0.00	0.00	0.00	0.00	0.00	0.00	0.00	0.00	0.00	20.00	0.50	0.00	0.00	0.00	210.00	0.00
1.58	0.42	0.00	0.00	0.24	5.67	0.23	0.01	0.05	0.73	0.01	13.32	0.01	12.76	0.69	4.82	33.45	25.52	109.15	0.18
0.00	0.00	0.00	0.00	0.00	20.00	0.00	0.00	0.00	0.00	0.00	0.00	0.00	20.00	0.70	0.00	0.00	0.00	170.00	0.00
0.00	0.00	0.00	0.00	0.00	0.00	0.00	0.00	0.00	0.00	0.00	0.00	0.00	0.00	0.50	0.00	0.00	0.00	220.00	0.00
1.85	1.18	0.00	0.00	0.63	56.42	0.09	0.03	0.08	0.24	0.02	7.94	0.10	18.71	0.33	3.40	30.90	32.60	96.67	0.17
4.31	2.99	0.00	0.00	0.00	87.42	6.49	0.24	0.20	2.19	0.12	14.10	0.00	78.96	2.12	19.74	70.50	273.54	513.24	0.45
0.68	0.18	0.00	0.00	0.00	27.78	0.14	0.07	0.05	0.45	0.01	16.16	0.06	8.51	0.31	3.69	16.44	25.52	77.68	0.29

USDA ID Code	Food Name	Weight in Grams*	Quantity of Units	Unit of Measure	Protein (g)	Fat (g)	Carbohydrate (g)	Kilocalories	Caffeine (g)	Fiber (g)	Cholesterol (mg)	Saturated Fat (g)
	Croissant, Butter	28.3500	1.000	Ounce	2.32	5.95	12.98	115.10	0.00	0.74	18.99	3.31
	Croissant, Cheese	28.3500	1.000	Ounce	2.61	5.93	13.32	117.37	0.00	0.74	16.16	3.01
	Croissant, Chocolate	56.0000	1.000	Medium	5.21	14.07	25.15	234.61	0.00	2.20	38.00	8.07
218	Croissants, Petite-Sara Lee	57.0000	2.000	Each	6.00	11.00	26.00	230.00	0.00	1.00	3.00	4.00
219	Croissants, Sara Lee	43.0000	1.000	Each	4.00	8.00	20.00	170.00	0.00	1.00	4.00	3.00
	Danish Pastry, Cheese	28.3500	1.000	Small	2.27	6.21	10.55	106.03	0.00	0.27	4.54	1.92
	Danish Pastry, Cinnamon	28.3500	1.000	Small	1.98	6.35	12.64	114.25	0.00	0.37	5.95	1.61
	Danish Pastry, Fruit	28.3500	1.000	Small	1.53	5.24	13.55	105.18	0.00	0.54	32.32	1.38
	Danish Pastry, Lemon	28.3500	1.000	Small	1.53	5.24	13.55	105.18	0.00	0.54	11.34	0.80
	Danish Pastry, Nut	28.3500	1.000	Small	2.01	7.14	12.96	121.91	0.00	0.57	13.04	1.65
	Danish Pastry, Raspberry	28.3500	1.000	Small	1.53	5.24	13.55	105.18	0.00	0.54	11.34	0.80
	Doughnuts, Chocolate, Sugared or Glazed	28.3500	1.000	Each	1.28	5.64	16.27	118.22	0.28	0.62	16.16	1.45
	Doughnuts, French Crullers, Glazed	28.3500	1.000	Each	0.88	5.19	16.87	116.80	0.00	0.34	3.12	1.32
	Doughnuts, Glazed	28.3500	1.000	Each	1.81	6.46	12.56	114.25	0.00	0.34	1.70	1.65
	Doughnuts, Plain	28.3500	1.000	Each	1.42	6.49	14.09	119.35	0.00	0.43	10.49	1.03
	Doughnuts, Plain, Chocolate-coated	28.3500	1.000	Each	1.42	8.79	13.61	134.38	0.57	0.57	17.29	2.30
	Doughnuts, Plain, Sugared or Glazed	28.3500	1.000	Each	1.47	6.49	14.40	120.77	0.57	0.43	9.07	1.68
	Doughnuts, w/ Creme Filling	28.3500	1.000	Each	1.81	6.95	8.51	102.34	0.00	0.22	6.80	1.54
	Doughnuts, w/ Jelly Filling	28.3500	1.000	Each	1.67	5.30	11.06	96.39	0.00	0.24	7.37	1.37
	Doughnuts, Whole Wheat, Sugared	28.3500	1.000	Each	1.79	5.47	12.08	102.06	0.00	0.63	5.67	0.86
	Eclairs, Custard-filled w/ Chocolate	28.3500	1.000	Small	1.81	4.45	6.86	74.28	0.57	0.17	36.00	1.17
612	Mousse, Chocolate-Sara Lee	122.0000	1.000	Piece	5.00	25.00	37.00	400.00	0.00	2.00	30.00	20.00
	Muffins, Banana Nut	95.0000	1.000	Each	6.00	12.00	53.00	340.00	0.00	2.00	35.00	0.90
	Muffins, Blueberry	28.3500	1.000	Small	1.56	1.84	13.61	78.53	0.00	0.74	8.51	0.40
	Muffins, Corn	28.3500	1.000	Small	1.67	2.38	14.43	86.47	0.00	0.96	7.37	0.38
	Muffins, Oat Bran	28.3500	1.000	Small	1.98	2.10	13.69	76.55	0.00	1.30	0.00	0.31
	Muffins, Plain	28.3500	1.000	Small	1.96	3.23	11.74	83.92	0.00	0.77	11.06	0.61
	Muffins, Wheat Bran	28.3500	1.000	Small Sl	0.68	3.54	10.52	75.13	0.00	0.00	0.00	0.86
641	Pie, Apple, 45% Reduced Fat-Sara Lee	128.0000	1.000	Slice	4.00	8.00	51.00	290.00	0.00	2.00	4.00	1.50
642	Pie, Apple, Dutch, Homestyle-Sara Lee	131.0000	1.000	Slice	3.00	15.00	53.00	350.00	0.00	2.00	0.00	3.00
643	Pie, Apple, Homestyle-Sara Lee	131.0000	1.000	Slice	3.00	16.00	46.00	340.00	0.00	1.00	0.00	3.50
	Pie, Banana Cream	65.0000	1.000	Large	4.62	7.93	27.24	183.95	0.00	0.00	21.45	1.47
	Pie, Apple	28.3500	1.000	Small Sl	1.25	3.86	9.33	76.26	0.00	0.20	14.46	1.07
	Pie, Blueberry	28.3500	1.000	Small Sl	0.51	2.84	9.89	65.77	0.00	0.29	0.00	0.48
644	Pie, Blueberry, Homestyle-Sara Lee	131.0000	1.000	Slice	3.50	15.00	54.00	360.00	0.00	2.00	0.00	3.50
	Pie, Butterscotch Pudding	127.0000	1.000	Slice	5.97	18.16	42.29	354.33	0.00	0.00	77.47	5.09
	Pie, Cherry	28.3500	1.000	Small Sl	0.57	3.12	11.28	73.71	0.00	0.23	0.00	0.73
	Pie, Cherry, Fast Food	28.3500	1.000	Small	0.85	4.56	12.08	89.59	0.00	0.74	0.00	0.70
645	Pie, Cherry, Homestyle-Sara Lee	131.0000	1.000	Slice	3.00	16.00	42.00	320.00	0.00	2.00	0.00	3.50
	Pie, Chocolate Creme	28.3500	1.000	Small Sl	0.74	5.50	9.53	86.18	0.00	0.57	1.42	1.41
	Pie, Chocolate Mousse	28.3500	1.000	Small Sl	0.99	4.37	8.39	73.71	0.28	0.00	9.92	2.32
646	Pie, Chocolate Silk Supreme-Sara Lee	136.0000	1.000	Slice	4.00	32.00	49.00	500.00	0.00	2.00	4.00	16.00
647	Pie, Coconut Cream-Sara Lee	136.0000	1.000	Slice	4.00	31.00	47.00	480.00	0.00	2.00	0.00	14.00
	Pie, Coconut Creme	28.3500	1.000	Small Sl	0.60	4.71	10.55	84.48	0.00	0.37	0.00	1.98
	Pie, Coconut Custard	28.3500	1.000	Small Sl	1.67	3.74	8.56	73.71	0.00	0.51	9.92	1.66
	Pie, Egg Custard	28.3500	1.000	Small Sl	1.56	3.29	5.90	59.54	0.00	0.45	9.36	0.67
	Pie, Fruit, Fried	28.3500	1.000	Small Sl	0.85	4.56	12.08	89.59	0.00	0.74	0.00	0.70
	Pie, Lemon Meringue	28.3500	1.000	Small Sl	0.43	2.47	13.38	75.98	0.00	0.34	12.76	0.50
648	Pie, Lemon Meringue-Sara Lee	142.0000	1.000	Slice	2.00	11.00	59.00	350.00	0.00	5.00	0.00	2.50
	Pie, Lemon, Fried	28.3500	1.000	Small	0.85	4.56	12.08	89.59	0.00	0.74	0.00	0.70
	Pie, Mince Meat	28.3500	1.000	Small Sl	0.74	3.06	13.61	81.93	0.00	0.74	0.00	0.76
649	Pie, Mince, Homestyle-Sara Lee	131.0000	1.000	Slice	3.00	17.00	56.00	390.00	0.00	3.00	0.00	4.00
650	Pie, Peach, Homestyle-Sara Lee	131.0000	1.000	Slice	3.00	14.00	46.00	320.00	0.00	2.00	0.00	3.00

Monounsaturated Fat (g)	Polyunsaturated Fat (g)	Vitamin D (mg)	Vitamin K (mg)	Vitamin E (mg)	Vitamin A (re)	Vitamin C (mg)	Thiamin (mg)	Riboflavin (mg)	Niacin (mg)	Vitamin B6 (mg)	Folate (mcg)	Vitamin B12 (mcg)	Calcium (mg)	Iron (mg)	Magnesium (mg)	Phosphorus (mg)	Potassium (mg)	Sodium (mg)	Zinc (mg)
1.57	0.31	0.00	0.00	0.12	52.73	0.06	0.11	0.07	0.62	0.02	17.58	0.05	10.49	0.58	4.54	29.77	33.45	210.92	0.21
1.85	0.67	0.00	0.00	0.29	55.85	0.06	0.15	0.09	0.61	0.02	20.98	0.09	15.03	0.61	6.80	36.86	37.42	157.34	0.27
3.31	0.89	0.00	0.00	0.00	76.41	0.11	0.22	0.15	1.22	0.02	16.11	0.16	23.89	1.18	10.89	63.20	69.69	376.34	0.43
0.00	0.00	0.00	0.00	0.00	40.00	0.00	0.00	0.00	0.00	0.00	0.00	0.00	40.00	1.00	0.00	0.00	0.00	200.00	0.00
0.00	0.00	0.00	0.00	0.00	40.00	0.00	0.00	0.00	0.00	0.00	0.00	0.00	20.00	0.70	0.00	0.00	0.00	200.00	0.00
3.21	0.73	0.00	0.00	0.72	12.76	0.03	0.05	0.07	0.57	0.01	17.01	0.05	9.92	0.45	4.25	30.62	27.78	127.58	0.20
3.55	0.83	0.00	0.00	0.84	0.85	0.03	0.09	0.07	0.81	0.01	17.58	0.03	20.13	0.56	5.39	30.33	35.44	105.18	0.20
2.84	0.67	0.00	0.00	0.70	6.24	1.11	0.07	0.06	0.56	0.01	9.36	0.03	13.04	0.50	4.25	25.23	23.53	100.36	0.15
1.68	0.43	0.00	0.00	0.42	15.03	1.11	0.02	0.03	0.22	0.01	4.54	0.03	13.04	0.21	4.25	25.23	23.53	100.36	0.15
3.88	1.21	0.00	0.00	1.03	3.97	0.48	0.06	0.07	0.65	0.03	23.53	0.06	26.65	0.51	9.07	31.19	26.93	102.91	0.25
1.68	0.43	0.00	0.00	0.42	17.01	1.11	0.02	0.03	0.22	0.01	4.54	0.03	13.04	0.21	4.25	25.23	23.53	100.36	0.15
3.20	0.70	0.00	0.00	0.76	3.12	0.03	0.01	0.02	0.13	0.01	10.77	0.01	60.39	0.64	9.64	45.93	30.05	96.39	0.16
2.96	0.65	0.00	0.00	0.70	0.85	0.00	0.05	0.07	0.60	0.01	9.92	0.01	7.37	0.69	3.40	34.87	22.11	97.81	0.07
3.65	0.82	0.00	0.00	0.87	1.13	0.03	0.10	0.06	0.81	0.02	12.19	0.03	12.19	0.58	6.24	26.37	30.62	96.96	0.22
2.64	2.23	0.00	0.00	1.09	4.82	0.06	0.06	0.07	0.52	0.02	13.32	0.08	12.47	0.55	5.67	76.26	36.00	154.79	0.16
4.96	1.07	0.00	0.00	1.18	3.12	0.06	0.04	0.03	0.37	0.01	8.22	0.07	9.92	0.70	11.34	57.27	55.57	121.62	0.17
3.60	0.82	0.00	0.00	0.00	0.85	0.03	0.07	0.06	0.43	0.01	13.04	0.07	17.01	0.30	4.82	33.17	28.92	113.97	0.12
3.42	0.87	0.00	0.00	0.78	5.39	0.00	0.10	0.04	0.64	0.02	18.14	0.04	7.09	0.52	5.67	21.55	22.68	87.60	0.23
2.90	0.67	0.00	0.00	0.70	4.54	0.00	0.09	0.04	0.61	0.03	17.58	0.06	7.09	0.50	5.67	24.10	22.40	83.07	0.21
2.30	2.01	0.00	0.00	1.02	4.25	0.06	0.06	0.07	0.52	0.03	5.67	0.05	13.89	0.31	6.24	29.48	41.96	100.64	0.19
1.84	1.12	0.00	0.00	0.60	54.15	0.09	0.03	0.08	0.23	0.02	7.94	0.10	17.86	0.33	4.25	30.33	33.17	95.54	0.17
0.00	0.00	0.00	0.00	0.00	40.00	0.00	0.00	0.00	0.00	0.00	0.00	0.00	60.00	1.20	0.00	0.00	0.00	190.00	0.00
1.50	2.40	0.00	0.00	0.00	21.00	0.03	0.18	0.12	0.04	0.01	13.20	0.00	44.00	1.01	16.10	108.20	371.00	210.00	0.20
0.56	0.71	0.00	0.00	0.30	2.55	0.31	0.04	0.03	0.31	0.01	12.76	0.16	16.16	0.46	4.54	55.85	34.87	126.72	0.14
0.60	0.91	0.00	0.00	0.52	10.21	0.00	0.08	0.09	0.58	0.02	17.58	0.03	20.98	0.80	9.07	80.51	19.56	147.70	0.15
0.48	1.17	0.00	0.00	0.37	0.00	0.00	0.07	0.03	0.12	0.05	14.74	0.00	17.86	1.19	44.51	106.60	143.73	111.42	0.52
0.78	1.62	0.00	0.00	0.00	11.34	0.09	0.08	0.09	0.65	0.01	14.46	0.04	56.70	0.68	4.82	43.38	34.30	132.39	0.16
1.91	4.09	0.00	0.00	0.00	162.50	5.07	0.22	0.29	2.62	0.21	33.80	0.09	121.55	2.72	50.70	185.25	206.70	382.20	1.79
1.53	0.95	0.00	0.00	0.00	3.40	0.48	0.04	0.03	0.35	0.01	6.80	0.00	1.98	0.32	1.98	7.94	22.40	59.82	0.05
0.00	0.00	0.00	0.00	0.00	0.00	0.00	0.00	0.00	0.00	0.00	0.00	0.00	20.00	1.20	0.00	0.00	0.00	400.00	0.00
0.00	0.00	0.00	0.00	0.00	0.00	1.20	0.00	0.00	0.00	0.00	0.00	0.00	0.00	1.00	0.00	0.00	0.00	350.00	0.00
0.00	0.00	0.00	0.00	0.00	0.00	1.20	0.00	0.00	0.00	0.00	0.00	0.00	0.00	0.70	0.00	0.00	0.00	310.00	0.00
1.62	0.93	0.00	0.00	0.42	19.85	0.45	0.04	0.06	0.30	0.04	7.65	0.07	21.26	0.29	4.54	26.08	46.78	68.04	0.14
1.20	1.00	0.00	0.00	0.57	9.64	0.77	0.00	0.01	0.09	0.01	6.24	0.00	2.27	0.09	1.42	6.52	14.18	92.14	0.05
0.00	0.00	0.00	0.00	0.00	0.00	2.40	0.00	0.00	0.00	0.00	0.00	0.00	0.00	0.70	0.00	0.00	0.00	340.00	0.00
7.64	4.35	0.00	0.00	0.00	106.68	0.64	0.18	0.27	1.26	0.07	13.97	0.38	128.27	1.64	21.59	134.62	220.98	335.28	0.69
1.66	0.58	0.00	0.00	0.43	15.31	0.26	0.01	0.01	0.06	0.01	6.24	0.00	3.40	0.14	2.27	8.22	22.96	69.74	0.05
2.11	1.53	0.00	0.00	0.00	4.82	0.37	0.04	0.03	0.41	0.01	5.10	0.02	6.24	0.35	2.84	12.19	18.43	106.03	0.07
0.00	0.00	0.00	0.00	0.00	80.00	0.00	0.00	0.00	0.00	0.00	0.00	0.00	0.00	0.00	0.00	0.00	0.00	290.00	0.00
3.15	0.68	0.00	0.00	0.77	0.00	0.00	0.01	0.03	0.19	0.01	3.69	0.00	10.21	0.30	5.95	19.28	36.00	38.56	0.07
1.44	0.23	0.00	0.00	0.00	28.63	0.14	0.01	0.04	0.17	0.01	7.37	0.06	21.83	0.31	9.07	65.49	80.80	130.41	0.17
0.00	0.00	0.00	0.00	0.00	0.00	0.00	0.00	0.00	0.00	0.00	0.00	0.00	40.00	1.20	0.00	0.00	0.00	440.00	0.00
0.00	0.00	0.00	0.00	0.00	0.00	0.00	0.00	0.00	0.00	0.00	0.00	0.00	40.00	0.70	0.00	0.00	0.00	430.00	0.00
2.06	0.44	0.00	0.00	0.53	0.00	0.00	0.01	0.02	0.06	0.02	1.98	0.03	8.22	0.23	5.67	24.10	18.43	72.29	0.13
1.56	0.33	0.00	0.00	0.00	7.65	0.17	0.03	0.04	0.11	0.00	3.69	0.03	22.96	0.23	5.10	34.59	49.61	94.97	0.19
1.36	1.05	0.00	0.00	0.53	18.99	0.17	0.01	0.06	0.08	0.01	5.67	0.12	22.68	0.16	3.12	31.75	30.05	68.04	0.15
2.11	1.53	0.00	0.00	0.84	0.85	0.37	0.04	0.03	0.41	0.01	5.10	0.02	6.24	0.35	2.84	12.19	18.43	106.03	0.07
0.76	1.03	0.00	0.00	0.62	14.74	0.91	0.02	0.06	0.18	0.01	3.69	0.05	15.88	0.17	4.25	29.77	25.23	41.39	0.14
0.00	0.00	0.00	0.00	0.00	0.00	0.00	0.00	0.00	0.00	0.00	0.00	0.00	0.00	1.00	0.00	0.00	0.00	460.00	0.00
2.11	1.53	0.00	0.00	0.00	0.85	0.00	0.04	0.03	0.41	0.01	5.10	0.02	6.24	0.35	2.84	12.19	18.43	106.03	0.07
1.32	0.81	0.00	0.00	0.53	0.57	1.67	0.04	0.03	0.34	0.02	6.52	0.00	6.24	0.42	3.97	11.91	57.55	72.01	0.06
0.00	0.00	0.00	0.00	0.00	0.00	2.40	0.00	0.00	0.00	0.00	0.00	0.00	20.00	1.00	0.00	0.00	0.00	450.00	0.00
0.00	0.00	0.00	0.00	0.00	40.00	21.00	0.00	0.00	0.00	0.00	0.00	0.00	0.00	1.00	0.00	0.00	0.00	250.00	0.00

USDA ID Code	Food Name	Weight in Grams*	Quantity of Units	Unit of Measure	Protein (g)	Fat (g)	Carbohydrate (g)	Kilocalories	Caffeine (g)	Fiber (g)	Cholesterol (mg)	Saturated Fat (g)
	Pie, Pecan	28.3500	1.000	Small Sl	1.13	5.24	16.22	113.40	0.00	0.99	9.07	1.01
651	Pie, Pecan, Homestyle-Sara Lee	121.0000	1.000	Slice	5.00	24.00	70.00	520.00	0.00	3.00	45.00	4.50
	Pie, Pumpkin	28.3500	1.000	Small Sl	1.11	2.69	7.74	59.54	0.00	0.77	5.67	0.51
652	Pie, Pumpkin, Homestyle-Sara Lee	131.0000	1.000	Slice	4.00	11.00	37.00	260.00	0.00	2.00	30.00	2.50
653	Pie, Raspberry, Homestyle-Sara Lee	131.0000	1.000	Slice	3.00	19.00	48.00	380.00	0.00	2.00	4.00	4.50
	Pie, Vanilla Creme	28.3500	1.000	Small Sl	1.36	4.08	9.24	78.81	0.00	0.17	17.58	1.14
696	Shortcake, Strawberry-Sara Lee	71.0000	1.000	Piece	2.00	7.00	27.00	180.00	0.00	0.50	15.00	5.00
	Strudel, Apple	28.3500	1.000	Small	0.94	3.18	11.65	77.68	0.00	0.62	1.70	0.58
	Sweet Rolls w/ Raisins and Nuts	57.0000	1.000	Each	3.76	7.30	29.58	196.08	0.00	0.00	13.11	1.35
	Sweet Rolls, Cheese	28.3500	1.000	Small	2.01	5.19	12.39	102.06	0.00	0.34	21.55	1.72
	Sweet Rolls, Cinnamon w/ Raisins	28.3500	1.000	Small	1.76	4.65	14.43	105.46	0.00	0.68	18.71	0.87
729	Sweet Rolls, Cinnamon, Deluxe-Sara Lee	76.0000	1.000	Roll	5.00	15.00	41.00	370.00	0.00	1.00	40.00	9.00

Beverages

USDA ID Code	Food Name	Weight in Grams*	Quantity of Units	Unit of Measure	Protein (g)	Fat (g)	Carbohydrate (g)	Kilocalories	Caffeine (g)	Fiber (g)	Cholesterol (mg)	Saturated Fat (g)
	Beef Broth and Tomato Juice, Cnd	168.0000	5.500	Fl Oz	1.01	0.17	14.28	62.16	0.00	0.17	0.00	0.05
	Beer, Dark	356.000	12.000	Fl Oz	0.09	0.00	1.10	12.18	0.00	0.06	0.00	0.00
	Beer, Killians	356.000	12.000	Fl Oz	0.09	0.00	1.10	12.18	0.00	0.06	0.00	0.00
	Beer, Light	354.0000	12.000	Fl Oz	0.71	0.00	4.60	99.12	0.00	0.00	0.00	0.00
	Beer, Regular	356.000	12.000	Fl Oz	1.07	0.00	13.17	145.96	0.00	0.71	0.00	0.00
	Beverage, Strawberry Flavor	266.000	1.000	Cup	7.98	8.25	32.72	234.08	0.00	0.00	31.92	5.08
	Bloody Mary	29.7000	1.000	Fl Oz	0.15	0.03	0.98	23.17	0.00	0.00	0.00	0.00
	Choc Mix, Hot, No Sugar-Swiss M	20.0000	1.000	Packet	3.00	1.50	13.00	70.00	4.00	0.00	0.00	0.00
	Choc Mix, Hot, No Sugar, Fat Free	15.0000	1.000	Packet	4.00	0.00	9.00	50.00	4.00	0.00	0.00	0.00
	Coffee, Brewed	237.0000	1.000	Cup	0.24	0.00	0.95	4.74	137.46	0.00	0.00	0.00
	Coffee, Brewed, Decaf.	29.6000	6.000	Fl Oz	0.03	0.00	0.12	0.59	0.18	0.00	0.00	0.00
	Coffee, Instant, Cappuccino Flav	29.3000	6.000	Fl Oz	0.06	0.32	1.64	9.38	12.16	0.00	0.00	0.28
	Coffee, Instant, Decaffeinated	179.0000	6.000	Fl Oz	0.18	0.00	0.72	3.58	1.79	0.00	0.00	0.00
	Coffee, Instant, Mocha Flavor	29.3000	6.000	Fl Oz	0.09	0.29	1.32	7.91	6.83	0.00	0.00	0.25
	Coffee, Instant, Regular	179.0000	6.000	Fl Oz	0.18	0.00	0.72	3.58	57.28	0.00	0.00	0.00
203	Cola	369.0000	12.000	Fl Oz	0.10	0.10	38.50	151.00	7.60	0.00	0.00	0.00
	Cola, Diet	369.0000	12.000	Fl Oz	0.20	0.00	0.30	2.00	7.60	0.00	0.00	0.00
	Crystal Lite	29.5750	8.000	Fl Oz	0.00	0.00	0.00	0.63	0.00	0.00	0.00	0.00
	Gatorade Thirst Quencher	244.0000	8.000	Fl Oz	0.00	0.00	14.00	50.00	0.00	0.00	0.00	0.00
	Gatorlode High Carb, Loading Rec	354.0000	11.600	Fl Oz	0.00	0.00	71.00	280.00	0.00	0.00	0.00	0.00
	Gatorpro Sports Nutrition Sup.	336.0000	11.000	Fl Oz	17.00	6.00	59.00	360.00	0.00	0.00	0.00	0.50
	Juice Drink, Cranberry-apple, Bo	245.0000	1.000	Cup	0.25	0.00	41.90	164.15	0.00	0.25	0.00	0.00
	Juice Drink, Cranberry-apricot,	245.0000	1.000	Cup	0.49	0.00	39.69	156.80	0.00	0.25	0.00	0.00
	Juice Drink, Cranberry-grape, Bo	245.0000	1.000	Cup	0.49	0.25	34.30	137.20	0.00	0.25	0.00	0.07
	Juice Drink, Grape, Cnd	250.0000	1.000	Cup	0.25	0.00	32.25	125.00	0.00	0.25	0.00	0.00
	Juice Drink, Orange and Apricot,	250.0000	1.000	Cup	0.75	0.25	31.75	127.50	0.00	0.25	0.00	0.03
	Juice Drink, Pineapple and Grape	250.0000	1.000	Cup	0.50	0.25	29.00	117.50	0.00	0.25	0.00	0.03
	Juice Drink, Pineapple and Orang	250.0000	1.000	Cup	3.25	0.00	29.50	125.00	0.00	0.25	0.00	0.00
	Juice, Apple, Unsweetened	248.0000	1.000	Cup	0.15	0.27	28.97	116.56	0.00	0.25	0.00	0.05
	Juice, Carrot, Cnd	236.0000	1.000	Cup	2.24	0.35	21.92	94.40	0.00	1.89	0.00	0.07
	Juice, Clam and Tomato, Cnd	166.0000	5.500	Fl Oz	1.00	0.33	18.18	79.68	0.00	0.33	0.00	0.08
	Juice, Cranberry, Bottled	252.5860	0.750	Cup	0.00	0.25	36.37	143.97	0.00	0.00	0.00	0.00
	Juice, Grape, Cnd Or Bottle, Uns	253.0000	1.000	Cup	1.42	0.20	37.85	154.33	0.00	0.25	0.00	0.08
	Juice, Grapefruit, Cnd. Sweetened	250.0000	1.000	Cup	1.45	0.23	27.83	115.00	0.00	0.25	0.00	0.03
	Juice, Grapefruit, Cnd. Unsweetened	247.0000	1.000	Cup	1.28	0.25	22.13	93.86	0.00	0.25	0.00	0.02
	Juice, Grapefruit, Pink, Fresh	247.0000	1.000	Cup	1.24	0.25	22.72	96.33	0.00	0.25	0.00	0.02
	Juice, Grapefruit, White, Fresh	247.0000	1.000	Cup	1.24	0.25	22.72	96.33	0.00	0.25	0.00	0.02
	Juice, Guava	239.9120	0.750	Cup	0.00	0.00	21.63	87.86	0.00	0.00	0.00	0.00
	Juice, Mango	239.9120	0.750	Cup	0.00	0.00	21.63	87.86	0.00	0.00	0.00	0.00
	Juice, Orange, Fresh	248.0000	1.000	Cup	1.74	0.50	25.79	111.60	0.00	0.50	0.00	0.05

Monounsaturated Fat (g)	Polyunsaturated Fat (g)	Vitamin D (mg)	Vitamin K (mg)	Vitamin E (mg)	Vitamin A (re)	Vitamin C (mg)	Thiamin (mg)	Riboflavin (mg)	Niacin (mg)	Vitamin B6 (mg)	Folate (mcg)	Vitamin B12 (mcg)	Calcium (mg)	Iron (mg)	Magnesium (mg)	Phosphorus (mg)	Potassium (mg)	Sodium (mg)	Zinc (mg)
3.04	0.90	0.00	0.00	0.52	13.32	0.31	0.03	0.03	0.07	0.01	7.65	0.03	4.82	0.29	5.10	21.83	20.98	120.20	0.16
0.00	0.00	0.00	0.00	0.00	0.00	0.00	0.00	0.00	0.00	0.00	0.00	0.00	20.00	0.70	0.00	0.00	0.00	480.00	0.00
1.14	0.89	0.00	0.00	0.48	105.46	0.28	0.02	0.04	0.05	0.02	5.67	0.07	17.01	0.22	4.25	20.13	43.66	79.95	0.13
0.00	0.00	0.00	0.00	0.00	150.00	0.00	0.00	0.00	0.00	0.00	0.00	0.00	60.00	1.00	0.00	0.00	0.00	460.00	0.00
0.00	0.00	0.00	0.00	0.00	0.00	4.80	0.00	0.00	0.00	0.00	0.00	0.00	0.00	1.00	0.00	0.00	0.00	330.00	0.00
1.71	0.98	0.00	0.00	0.38	24.10	0.14	0.04	0.06	0.28	0.01	7.37	0.09	25.52	0.29	3.69	29.48	35.72	73.71	0.15
0.00	0.00	0.00	0.00	0.00	0.00	9.00	0.00	0.00	0.00	0.00	0.00	0.00	20.00	0.20	0.00	0.00	0.00	140.00	0.00
0.93	1.51	0.00	0.00	0.87	2.55	0.48	0.01	0.01	0.09	0.01	3.97	0.06	4.25	0.12	2.55	9.36	42.24	76.26	0.05
2.66	2.85	0.00	0.00	0.00	60.42	0.34	0.16	0.16	1.33	0.05	17.67	0.06	36.48	1.46	15.96	62.70	123.12	185.25	0.38
2.57	0.58	0.00	0.00	0.00	21.83	0.06	0.04	0.04	0.24	0.02	12.19	0.09	33.45	0.22	5.39	27.78	38.84	101.21	0.18
1.36	2.12	0.00	0.00	1.22	18.14	0.57	0.09	0.08	0.67	0.03	14.74	0.04	20.41	0.45	4.82	21.55	31.47	108.58	0.17
0.00	0.00	0.00	0.00	0.00	60.00	0.00	0.00	0.00	0.00	0.00	0.00	0.00	20.00	0.70	0.00	0.00	0.00	300.00	0.00
0.05	0.03	0.00	0.00	0.00	21.84	1.51	0.00	0.05	0.27	0.03	7.22	0.08	18.48	0.97	5.04	21.84	161.28	220.08	0.03
0.00	0.00	0.00	0.00	0.00	0.00	0.00	0.00	0.01	0.14	0.02	1.78	0.01	1.49	0.01	1.78	3.56	7.43	1.49	0.01
0.00	0.00	0.00	0.00	0.00	0.00	0.00	0.00	0.01	0.14	0.02	1.78	0.01	1.49	0.01	1.78	3.56	7.43	1.49	0.01
0.00	0.00	0.00	0.00	0.00	0.00	0.00	0.04	0.11	1.38	0.11	14.51	0.04	17.70	0.14	17.70	42.48	63.72	10.62	0.11
0.00	0.00	0.00	0.00	0.00	0.00	0.00	0.04	0.11	1.60	0.18	21.36	0.07	17.80	0.11	21.36	42.72	89.00	17.80	0.07
2.37	0.29	0.00	0.00	0.00	74.48	2.39	0.11	0.43	0.21	0.11	12.24	0.88	292.60	0.21	31.92	228.76	369.74	127.68	0.93
0.00	0.01	0.00	0.00	0.00	10.10	4.10	0.01	0.01	0.13	0.02	3.95	0.00	2.08	0.11	2.38	4.16	43.36	66.53	0.03
0.00	0.00	0.00	0.00	0.00	0.00	0.00	0.00	0.00	0.00	0.00	0.00	0.00	80.00	0.40	0.00	0.00	0.00	220.00	0.00
0.00	0.00	0.00	0.00	0.00	0.00	0.00	0.00	0.00	0.00	0.00	0.00	0.00	80.00	0.20	0.00	0.00	0.00	180.00	0.00
0.00	0.00	0.00	0.00	0.00	0.00	0.00	0.00	0.00	0.52	0.00	0.24	0.00	4.74	0.12	11.85	2.37	127.98	4.74	0.05
0.00	0.00	0.00	0.00	0.00	0.00	0.00	0.00	0.00	0.07	0.00	0.03	0.00	0.59	0.01	1.48	0.30	15.98	0.59	0.01
0.02	0.01	0.00	0.00	0.00	0.00	0.00	0.00	0.00	0.05	0.00	0.00	0.00	1.17	0.02	1.47	4.10	18.17	15.82	0.01
0.00	0.00	0.00	0.00	0.00	0.00	0.00	0.00	0.02	0.50	0.00	0.00	0.00	5.37	0.07	7.16	5.37	62.65	5.37	0.05
0.02	0.01	0.00	0.00	0.00	0.00	0.00	0.00	0.00	0.04	0.00	0.00	0.00	1.17	0.04	1.47	4.40	18.46	5.57	0.02
0.00	0.00	0.00	0.00	0.00	0.00	0.00	0.00	0.00	0.50	0.00	0.00	0.00	5.37	0.09	7.16	5.37	64.44	5.37	0.05
0.00	0.00	0.00	0.00	0.00	0.00	0.00	0.00	0.00	0.00	0.00	0.00	0.00	0.00	0.13	3.00	46.00	4.00	14.00	0.05
0.00	0.00	0.00	0.00	0.00	0.00	0.00	0.00	0.00	0.00	0.00	0.00	0.00	0.00	0.11	4.00	30.00	0.00	21.00	0.28
0.00	0.00	0.00	0.00	0.00	0.00	0.75	0.00	0.00	0.00	0.00	0.00	0.00	0.00	0.00	0.00	0.00	0.00	0.00	0.00
0.00	0.00	0.00	0.00	0.00	0.00	0.00	0.00	0.00	0.00	0.00	0.00	0.00	0.00	0.00	0.00	0.00	30.00	110.00	0.00
0.00	0.00	0.00	0.00	0.00	0.00	18.00	0.11	0.39	4.50	0.45	0.00	0.00	0.00	0.00	0.00	0.00	0.00	0.00	0.00
0.00	0.00	0.05	0.00	3.50	160.00	50.00	1.10	0.50	6.00	0.64	63.00	0.80	280.00	3.00	70.00	400.00	1310.00	300.00	3.60
0.00	0.00	0.00	0.00	0.00	0.00	78.40	0.02	0.05	0.15	0.05	0.49	0.00	17.15	0.15	4.90	7.35	66.15	4.90	0.10
0.00	0.00	0.00	0.00	0.00	112.70	0.00	0.02	0.02	0.29	0.05	1.47	0.00	22.05	0.37	7.35	12.25	149.45	4.90	0.10
0.00	0.05	0.00	0.00	0.00	0.00	78.40	0.02	0.05	0.29	0.07	1.72	0.00	19.60	0.02	7.35	9.80	58.80	7.35	0.10
0.00	0.00	0.00	0.00	0.00	0.00	40.00	0.03	0.03	0.25	0.05	2.00	0.00	7.50	0.25	10.00	10.00	87.50	2.50	0.08
0.08	0.05	0.00	0.00	0.00	145.00	50.00	0.05	0.03	0.50	0.08	14.50	0.00	12.50	0.25	10.00	20.00	200.00	5.00	0.13
0.03	0.08	0.00	0.00	0.00	10.00	115.00	0.08	0.05	0.68	0.10	26.25	0.00	17.50	0.78	15.00	15.00	152.50	35.00	0.15
0.00	0.00	0.00	0.00	0.00	132.50	56.25	0.08	0.05	0.53	0.13	27.25	0.00	12.50	0.68	15.00	10.00	115.00	7.50	0.15
0.02	0.07	0.00	0.00	0.02	0.00	103.17	0.05	0.05	0.00	0.07	0.25	0.00	17.36	0.92	7.44	17.36	295.12	7.44	0.07
0.02	0.17	0.00	0.00	0.02	2584.20	20.06	0.21	0.14	0.92	0.52	8.97	0.00	56.64	1.09	33.04	99.12	689.12	68.44	0.42
0.02	0.03	0.00	0.00	0.00	36.52	6.81	0.07	0.05	0.32	0.13	26.39	50.80	19.92	1.00	36.52	129.48	149.40	600.92	1.79
0.00	0.00	0.00	0.00	0.00	0.00	89.42	0.02	0.02	0.09	0.05	0.51	0.00	7.58	0.38	5.05	5.05	45.47	5.05	0.18
0.00	0.05	0.00	0.00	0.00	2.53	0.25	0.08	0.10	0.66	0.18	6.58	0.00	22.77	0.61	25.30	27.83	333.96	7.59	0.13
0.03	0.05	0.00	0.00	0.13	0.00	67.25	0.10	0.05	0.80	0.05	26.00	0.00	20.00	0.90	25.00	27.50	405.00	5.00	0.15
0.02	0.05	0.00	0.00	0.12	2.47	72.12	0.10	0.05	0.57	0.05	25.69	0.00	17.29	0.49	24.70	27.17	377.91	2.47	0.22
0.02	0.05	0.00	0.00	0.00	108.68	93.86	0.10	0.05	0.49	0.10	25.19	0.00	22.23	0.49	29.64	37.05	400.14	2.47	0.12
0.02	0.05	0.00	0.05	0.12	2.47	93.86	0.10	0.05	0.49	0.10	25.19	0.00	22.23	0.49	29.64	37.05	400.14	2.47	0.12
0.00	0.00	0.00	0.00	0.00	0.00	40.55	0.00	0.00	0.00	0.00	0.00	0.00	0.00	0.00	0.00	0.00	0.00	23.65	0.00
0.00	0.00	0.00	0.00	0.00	0.00	40.55	0.00	0.00	0.00	0.00	0.00	0.00	0.00	0.00	0.00	0.00	0.00	23.65	0.00
0.10	0.10	0.00	0.10	0.22	49.60	124.00	0.22	0.07	0.99	0.10	75.14	0.00	27.28	0.50	27.28	42.16	496.00	2.48	0.12

USDA ID Code	Food Name	Weight in Grams*	Quantity of Units	Unit of Measure	Protein (g)	Fat (g)	Carbohydrate (g)	Kilocalories	Caffeine (g)	Fiber (g)	Cholesterol (mg)	Saturated Fat (g)
	Juice, Orange, From Concentrate	249.0000	1.000	Cup	1.69	0.15	26.84	112.05	0.00	0.50	0.00	0.02
	Juice, Orange, w/ Added Calcium	248.5900	0.750	Cup	1.69	0.15	26.80	111.87	0.00	0.50	0.00	0.02
	Juice, Passion-fruit, Purple, Fr	247.0000	1.000	Cup	0.96	0.12	33.59	125.97	0.00	0.49	0.00	0.00
	Juice, Passion-fruit, Yellow, Fr	247.0000	1.000	Cup	1.65	0.44	35.69	148.20	0.00	0.49	0.00	0.05
	Juice, Pineapple, Cnd	250.0000	1.000	Cup	0.80	0.20	34.45	140.00	0.00	0.50	0.00	0.03
	Juice, Prune, Cnd	256.0000	1.000	Cup	1.56	0.08	44.67	181.76	0.00	2.56	0.00	0.00
	Juice, Tangerine, Cnd Sweetened	249.0000	1.000	Cup	1.25	0.50	29.88	124.50	0.00	0.50	0.00	0.02
	Juice, Tangerine, Fresh	247.0000	1.000	Cup	1.24	0.49	24.95	106.21	0.00	0.49	0.00	0.05
	Juice, Tomato, Cnd w/ Added Salt	243.0000	1.000	Cup	1.85	0.15	10.28	41.31	0.00	0.97	0.00	0.02
	Juice, Tomato, Cnd w/o Salt	243.0000	1.000	Cup	1.85	0.15	10.28	41.31	0.00	1.94	0.00	0.02
	Juice, Tropical Fruit, Blend	247.0000	1.000	Cup	0.00	0.00	28.90	113.62	0.00	0.25	0.00	0.00
558	Juice, V-8 Splash, Berry Blend	240.0000	8.000	Fl Oz	0.00	0.00	28.00	110.00	0.00	0.00	0.00	0.00
559	Juice, V-8 Splash, Strawberry Kiwi	240.0000	8.000	Fl Oz	0.00	0.00	28.00	110.00	0.00	0.00	0.00	0.00
560	Juice, V-8 Splash, Tropical Blend	240.0000	8.000	Fl Oz	0.00	0.00	30.00	120.00	0.00	0.00	0.00	0.00
	Juice, V-8, Low Salt	243.0000	8.000	Fl Oz	1.60	0.00	8.20	40.00	0.00	0.25	0.00	0.00
	Juice, Vegetable, Cnd.	242.0000	1.000	Cup	1.52	0.22	11.01	45.98	0.00	1.94	0.00	0.02
	Kool-Aid	236.0000	8.000	Fl Oz	0.00	0.00	25.10	98.00	0.00	0.00	0.00	0.00
	Lemonade Flavor Drink	266.0000	1.000	Cup	0.00	0.00	28.73	111.72	0.00	0.00	0.00	0.05
	Lemonade, Low Calorie	237.0000	1.000	Cup	0.00	0.00	1.19	4.74	0.00	0.00	0.00	0.00
	Lemonade, Pink	247.0000	1.000	Cup	0.25	0.00	25.94	98.80	0.00	0.00	0.00	0.02
	Lemonade, White	248.0000	1.000	Cup	0.25	0.00	26.04	99.20	0.00	0.25	0.00	0.02
	Liqueur, Coffee w/ Cream, 34 Proof	47.0000	1.500	Fl Oz	1.32	7.38	9.82	153.69	7.05	0.00	7.05	4.54
	Liqueur, Coffee, 53 Proof	52.0000	1.500	Fl Oz	0.05	0.16	24.34	174.72	13.52	0.00	0.00	0.06
	Liqueur, Coffee, 63 Proof	52.0000	1.500	Fl Oz	0.05	0.16	16.74	160.16	13.52	0.00	0.00	0.06
	Liqueur, Creme De Menthe, 72 Proof	50.0000	1.500	Fl Oz	0.00	0.15	20.80	185.50	0.00	0.00	0.00	0.01
	Liquor Drink, Bourbon and Soda	29.0000	1.000	Fl Oz	0.00	0.00	0.00	26.10	0.00	0.00	0.00	0.00
	Liquor Drink, Daiquiri	60.0000	2.000	Fl Oz	0.06	0.06	4.08	111.60	0.00	0.00	0.00	0.01
	Liquor Drink, Daiquiri, Bottled	207.0000	6.800	Fl Oz	0.00	0.00	32.50	258.75	0.00	0.00	0.00	0.00
	Liquor Drink, Gin and Tonic	30.0000	1.000	Fl Oz	0.00	0.00	2.10	22.80	0.00	0.00	0.00	0.00
	Liquor Drink, Manhattan	28.5000	6.000	Fl Oz	0.03	0.00	0.91	63.84	0.00	0.00	0.00	0.00
	Liquor Drink, Margarita	29.5750	6.000	Fl Oz	0.00	0.00	4.50	28.75	0.00	0.00	0.00	0.00
	Liquor Drink, Martini	28.2000	6.000	Fl Oz	0.00	0.00	0.08	62.89	0.00	0.00	0.00	0.00
	Liquor Drink, Pina Colada	141.0000	4.500	Fl Oz	0.56	2.68	39.90	262.26	0.00	0.85	0.00	1.23
	Liquor Drink, Screwdriver	30.4000	6.000	Fl Oz	0.15	0.00	2.61	24.93	0.00	0.00	0.00	0.00
	Liquor Drink, Tom Collins	29.6000	1.000	Fl Oz	0.00	0.00	0.38	16.28	0.00	0.00	0.00	0.00
	Liquor Drink, Whiskey Sour	29.9000	1.000	Fl Oz	0.06	0.03	1.67	40.66	0.00	0.00	0.00	0.01
	Liquor, Distilled, All 100 Proof	42.0000	1.500	Fl Oz	0.00	0.00	0.00	123.90	0.00	0.00	0.00	0.00
	Liquor, Distilled, All 80 Proof	42.0000	1.500	Fl Oz	0.00	0.00	0.00	97.02	0.00	0.00	0.00	0.00
	Liquor, Distilled, All 86 Proof	42.0000	1.500	Fl Oz	0.00	0.00	0.04	105.00	0.00	0.00	0.00	0.00
	Liquor, Distilled, All 90 Proof	42.0000	1.000	Jigger	0.00	0.00	0.00	110.46	0.00	0.00	0.00	0.00
	Liquor, Distilled, All 94 Proof	42.0000	1.500	Fl Oz	0.00	0.00	0.00	115.50	0.00	0.00	0.00	0.00
	Liquor, Vodka, 80 Proof	42.0000	1.500	Fl Oz	0.00	0.00	0.00	97.02	0.00	0.00	0.00	0.00
	Punch Drink, Fruit, Cnd	248.0000	1.000	Cup	0.00	0.00	29.51	116.56	0.00	0.25	0.00	0.00
	Shake, Chocolate	458.0000	22.000	Fl Oz	15.57	16.95	93.89	581.66	13.74	3.66	59.54	10.58
	Shake, Chocolate, Thick	300.0000	1.330	Cup	9.15	8.10	63.45	355.83	6.00	0.90	31.50	5.04
	Shake, Strawberry	283.0000	10.000	Fl Oz	9.62	7.92	53.49	319.79	0.00	1.13	31.13	4.90
	Shake, Vanilla	458.0000	22.000	Fl Oz	16.03	13.74	81.98	508.38	0.00	1.83	50.38	8.52
	Shakes, Vanilla, Thick	313.0000	1.330	Cup	12.08	9.48	55.56	349.97	0.00	0.00	36.93	5.92
709	Snapple, cranberry raspberry	240.0000	8.000	Fl Oz	0.00	0.00	29.00	120.00	0.00	0.00	0.00	0.00
710	Snapple, cranberry raspberry, Diet	30.0000	8.000	Fl Oz	0.00	0.00	2.00	10.00	0.00	0.00	0.00	0.00
711	Snapple, grape, white, Diet	30.0000	8.000	Fl Oz	0.00	0.00	2.00	10.00	0.00	0.00	0.00	0.00
712	Snapple, grapeade	240.0000	8.000	Fl Oz	0.00	0.00	29.00	120.00	0.00	0.00	0.00	0.00
713	Snapple, kiwi strawberry	240.0000	8.000	Fl Oz	0.00	0.00	26.00	100.00	0.00	0.00	0.00	0.00

Page Key: A2 = Baby Food   A2 = Baked Goods   A8 = Beverages   A14 = Breads/Grains and Pasta   A18 = Breakfast Foods/Cereals   A26 = Dairy and Eggs   A40 = Fats and Oils   A42 = Fruits and Vegetables   A52 = Meats and Beans   A60 = Nuts and Seeds   A62 5 Frozen Entrees and Packaged Foods   A76 = Restaurant Chains–Fast Foods   A92 = Restaurant Chains–Other   A106 = Seafood and Fish   A110 = Snacks and Sweets   A120 = Soups   A122 = Supplements   A126 = Toppings and Sauces

Monounsaturated Fat (g)	Polyunsaturated Fat (g)	Vitamin D (mg)	Vitamin K (mg)	Vitamin E (mg)	Vitamin A (re)	Vitamin C (mg)	Thiamin (mg)	Riboflavin (mg)	Niacin (mg)	Vitamin B6 (mg)	Folate (mcg)	Vitamin B12 (mcg)	Calcium (mg)	Iron (mg)	Magnesium (mg)	Phosphorus (mg)	Potassium (mg)	Sodium (mg)	Zinc (mg)
0.02	0.02	0.00	0.00	0.47	19.92	96.86	0.20	0.05	0.50	0.10	109.06	0.00	22.41	0.25	24.90	39.84	473.10	2.49	0.12
0.02	0.03	0.00	0.00	0.00	19.89	96.70	0.20	0.04	0.50	0.11	108.88	0.00	298.31	0.25	24.86	39.77	472.32	2.49	0.12
0.02	0.07	0.00	0.00	0.12	177.84	73.61	0.00	0.32	3.61	0.12	17.29	0.00	9.88	0.59	41.99	32.11	686.66	14.82	0.12
0.05	0.27	0.00	0.00	0.12	595.27	44.95	0.00	0.25	5.53	0.15	19.76	0.00	9.88	0.89	41.99	61.75	686.66	14.82	0.15
0.03	0.08	0.00	0.00	0.05	0.00	26.75	0.15	0.05	0.65	0.25	57.75	0.00	42.50	0.65	32.50	20.00	335.00	2.50	0.28
0.05	0.03	0.00	0.00	0.03	0.00	10.50	0.05	0.18	2.02	0.56	1.02	0.00	30.72	3.02	35.84	64.00	706.56	10.24	0.54
0.05	0.07	0.00	0.00	0.22	104.58	54.78	0.15	0.05	0.25	0.07	11.45	0.00	44.82	0.50	19.92	34.86	443.22	2.49	0.07
0.10	0.10	0.00	0.00	0.22	103.74	76.57	0.15	0.05	0.25	0.10	11.36	0.00	44.46	0.49	19.76	34.58	439.66	2.47	0.07
0.02	0.05	0.00	0.00	2.21	136.08	44.47	0.12	0.07	1.63	0.27	48.36	0.00	21.87	1.41	26.73	46.17	534.60	877.23	0.34
0.02	0.05	0.00	0.00	2.21	136.08	44.47	0.12	0.07	1.63	0.27	48.36	0.00	21.87	1.41	26.73	46.17	534.60	24.30	0.34
0.00	0.00	0.00	0.00	0.00	2.47	108.43	0.02	0.02	0.05	0.02	2.22	0.00	9.88	0.22	4.94	2.47	32.11	9.88	0.10
0.00	0.00	0.00	0.00	0.00	0.00	0.00	0.00	0.00	0.00	0.00	0.00	0.00	0.00	0.00	0.00	0.00	0.00	25.00	0.00
0.00	0.00	0.00	0.00	0.00	0.00	0.00	0.00	0.00	0.00	0.00	0.00	0.00	0.00	0.00	0.00	0.00	0.00	10.00	0.00
0.00	0.00	0.00	0.00	0.00	0.00	0.00	0.00	0.00	0.00	0.00	0.00	0.00	0.00	0.00	0.00	0.00	0.00	20.00	0.00
0.00	0.00	0.00	0.00	0.00	62.50	39.00	0.04	0.05	0.00	0.00	0.00	0.00	31.00	1.20	0.00	0.00	439.00	41.00	0.00
0.02	0.10	0.00	0.00	0.77	283.14	67.03	0.10	0.07	1.77	0.34	51.06	0.00	26.62	1.02	26.62	41.14	467.06	653.40	0.48
0.00	0.00	0.00	0.00	0.00	0.00	6.00	0.00	0.00	0.00	0.00	0.00	0.00	15.00	0.00	0.00	8.00	1.00	8.00	0.00
0.00	0.00	0.00	0.00	0.00	0.00	34.05	0.00	0.00	0.00	0.00	0.00	0.00	29.26	0.05	2.66	2.66	2.66	18.62	0.08
0.00	0.00	0.00	0.00	0.00	0.00	5.93	0.00	0.00	0.00	0.00	0.24	0.00	49.77	0.09	2.37	23.70	0.00	7.11	0.07
0.00	0.02	0.00	0.07	0.00	0.00	9.63	0.02	0.05	0.05	0.02	5.43	0.00	7.41	0.40	4.94	4.94	37.05	7.41	0.10
0.00	0.02	0.00	0.00	0.00	4.96	9.67	0.02	0.05	0.05	0.02	5.46	0.00	7.44	0.40	4.96	4.96	37.20	7.44	0.10
2.10	0.31	0.00	0.00	0.12	20.21	0.00	0.00	0.03	0.04	0.01	0.00	0.06	7.52	0.06	0.94	23.50	15.04	43.24	0.08
0.01	0.06	0.00	0.00	0.00	0.00	0.00	0.00	0.01	0.07	0.00	0.00	0.00	0.52	0.03	1.56	3.12	15.60	4.16	0.02
0.01	0.06	0.00	0.00	0.00	0.00	0.00	0.00	0.01	0.07	0.00	0.00	0.00	0.52	0.03	1.56	3.12	15.60	4.16	0.02
0.01	0.09	0.00	0.00	0.00	0.00	0.00	0.00	0.00	0.00	0.00	0.00	0.00	0.00	0.04	0.00	0.00	0.00	2.50	0.02
0.00	0.00	0.00	0.00	0.00	0.00	0.00	0.00	0.00	0.01	0.00	0.00	0.00	0.87	0.01	0.29	0.58	0.58	4.06	0.02
0.01	0.01	0.00	0.00	0.00	0.00	0.96	0.01	0.00	0.02	0.01	1.20	0.00	1.80	0.09	1.20	3.60	12.60	3.00	0.04
0.00	0.00	0.00	0.00	0.00	0.00	2.69	0.00	0.00	0.02	0.00	1.66	0.00	0.00	0.02	2.07	4.14	22.77	82.80	0.06
0.00	0.00	0.00	0.00	0.00	0.00	0.12	0.00	0.00	0.00	0.00	0.15	0.00	0.60	0.01	0.30	0.30	1.50	1.20	0.02
0.00	0.00	0.00	0.00	0.00	0.00	0.00	0.00	0.00	0.03	0.00	0.03	0.00	0.57	0.03	0.57	2.00	7.41	0.86	0.01
0.00	0.00	0.00	0.00	0.00	0.00	0.00	0.00	0.00	0.00	0.00	0.00	0.00	0.00	0.00	0.00	0.00	0.00	11.88	0.00
0.00	0.00	0.00	0.00	0.00	0.00	0.00	0.00	0.00	0.06	0.00	0.00	0.00	0.56	0.00	0.56	0.85	5.08	0.85	0.01
0.23	0.49	0.00	0.00	0.00	0.00	6.63	0.04	0.01	0.17	0.07	14.38	0.00	11.28	0.31	11.28	9.87	100.11	8.46	0.18
0.00	0.00	0.00	0.00	0.00	1.82	9.48	0.02	0.00	0.05	0.01	10.67	0.00	2.13	0.02	2.43	4.26	46.51	0.30	0.01
0.00	0.00	0.00	0.00	0.00	0.00	0.50	0.00	0.00	0.00	0.00	0.21	0.00	1.18	0.00	0.30	0.30	2.37	5.03	0.02
0.00	0.01	0.00	0.00	0.00	0.30	3.77	0.06	0.00	0.04	0.01	1.55	0.00	1.79	0.02	1.20	2.09	15.85	3.29	0.01
0.00	0.00	0.00	0.00	0.00	0.00	0.00	0.00	0.00	0.00	0.00	0.00	0.00	0.00	0.02	0.00	1.68	0.84	0.42	0.02
0.00	0.00	0.00	0.00	0.00	0.00	0.00	0.00	0.00	0.00	0.00	0.00	0.00	0.00	0.02	0.00	1.68	0.84	0.42	0.02
0.00	0.00	0.00	0.00	0.00	0.00	0.00	0.00	0.00	0.00	0.00	0.00	0.00	0.00	0.02	0.00	1.68	0.84	0.42	0.02
0.00	0.00	0.00	0.00	0.00	0.00	0.00	0.00	0.00	0.00	0.00	0.00	0.00	0.00	0.02	0.00	1.68	0.84	0.42	0.02
0.00	0.00	0.00	0.00	0.00	0.00	0.00	0.00	0.00	0.00	0.00	0.00	0.00	0.00	0.00	0.00	2.10	0.42	0.42	0.00
0.00	0.00	0.00	0.00	0.00	2.48	73.41	0.05	0.05	0.05	0.00	3.22	0.00	19.84	0.52	4.96	2.48	62.00	54.56	0.30
4.95	0.64	1.83	0.00	0.32	105.34	1.83	0.27	1.15	0.73	0.23	16.03	1.56	517.54	1.42	77.86	467.16	916.00	444.26	1.88
2.34	0.30	0.00	0.00	0.30	63.00	0.00	0.15	0.66	0.36	0.09	14.70	0.96	396.00	0.93	48.00	378.00	672.00	333.00	1.44
0.00	0.00	0.57	0.00	0.00	82.07	2.26	0.14	0.57	0.51	0.11	8.49	0.88	319.79	0.31	36.79	283.00	515.06	234.89	1.02
3.94	0.50	0.92	0.00	0.27	146.56	3.66	0.23	0.82	0.87	0.23	15.11	1.65	558.76	0.41	54.96	467.16	796.92	375.56	1.65
2.75	0.34	0.00	0.00	0.31	87.64	0.00	0.09	0.63	0.47	0.13	20.66	1.63	457.29	0.31	36.81	360.58	571.85	298.60	1.22
0.00	0.00	0.00	0.00	0.00	0.00	0.00	0.00	0.00	0.00	0.00	0.00	0.00	0.00	0.00	0.00	0.00	0.00	10.00	0.00
0.00	0.00	0.00	0.00	0.00	0.00	0.00	0.00	0.00	0.00	0.00	0.00	0.00	0.00	0.00	0.00	0.00	0.00	10.00	0.00
0.00	0.00	0.00	0.00	0.00	0.00	0.00	0.00	0.00	0.00	0.00	0.00	0.00	0.00	0.00	0.00	0.00	0.00	10.00	0.00
0.00	0.00	0.00	0.00	0.00	0.00	0.00	0.00	0.00	0.00	0.00	0.00	0.00	0.00	0.00	0.00	0.00	0.00	10.00	0.00
0.00	0.00	0.00	0.00	0.00	0.00	0.00	0.00	0.00	0.00	0.00	0.00	0.00	0.00	0.00	0.00	0.00	0.00	10.00	0.00

USDA ID Code	Food Name	Weight in Grams*	Quantity of Units	Unit of Measure	Protein (g)	Fat (g)	Carbohydrate (g)	Kilocalories	Caffeine (g)	Fiber (g)	Cholesterol (mg)	Saturated Fat (g)
714	Snapple, mango madness	240.0000	8.000	Fl Oz	0.00	0.00	29.00	120.00	0.00	0.00	0.00	0.00
715	Snapple, pink lemonade	240.0000	8.000	Fl Oz	0.00	0.00	29.00	120.00	0.00	0.00	0.00	0.00
704	Snapple, Tea, Iced, lemon	240.0000	8.000	Fl Oz	0.00	0.00	25.00	100.00	0.00	0.00	0.00	0.00
705	Snapple, Tea, Iced, peach	240.0000	8.000	Fl Oz	0.00	0.00	26.00	100.00	0.00	0.00	0.00	0.00
706	Snapple, Tea, Iced, peach, Diet	30.0000	8.000	Fl Oz	0.00	0.00	1.00	0.00	0.00	0.00	0.00	0.00
707	Snapple, Tea, Iced, raspberry	240.0000	8.000	Fl Oz	0.00	0.00	26.00	100.00	0.00	0.00	0.00	0.00
708	Snapple, Tea, Iced, raspberry, Diet	30.0000	8.000	Fl Oz	0.00	0.00	1.00	0.00	0.00	0.00	0.00	0.00
	Soda, Club	474.0000	16.000	Fl Oz	0.00	0.00	0.00	0.00	0.00	0.00	0.00	0.00
	Soda, Cream	494.0000	16.000	Fl Oz	0.00	0.00	65.70	251.94	0.00	0.00	0.00	0.00
	Soda, Dr. Pepper	491.0000	16.000	Fl Oz	0.00	0.49	51.06	201.31	49.10	0.00	0.00	0.34
	Soda, Ginger Ale	488.0000	16.000	Fl Oz	0.00	0.00	42.46	165.92	0.00	0.00	0.00	0.00
	Soda, Ginger Ale, Diet	366.0000	12.000	Fl Oz	0.00	0.00	0.00	0.00	0.00	0.00	0.00	0.00
	Soda, Grape	372.0000	12.000	Fl Oz	0.00	0.00	41.66	159.96	0.00	0.00	0.00	0.00
	Soda, Grape Drink, Cnd	250.0000	1.000	Cup	0.00	0.00	28.75	112.50	0.00	0.00	0.00	0.00
716	Soda, Lemon-lime	355.0000	12.000	Fl Oz	0.00	0.00	38.40	149.00	0.00	0.00	0.00	0.00
	Soda, Lemon-lime, Diet	355.0000	12.000	Fl Oz	0.00	0.00	0.00	0.00	0.00	0.00	0.00	0.00
	Soda, Mountain Dew	360.0000	12.000	Fl Oz	0.00	0.00	44.40	179.00	54.00	0.00	0.00	0.00
	Soda, Orange Drink, Cnd	248.0000	1.000	Cup	0.00	0.00	31.99	126.48	0.00	0.25	0.00	0.00
	Soda, Root Beer	493.0000	16.000	Fl Oz	0.00	0.00	52.26	202.13	0.00	0.00	0.00	0.00
	Soda, Root Beer, Diet	355.0000	12.000	Fl Oz	0.00	0.00	0.36	0.00	0.00	0.00	0.00	0.00
719	Starbucks-Caffe Americano	340.8000	12.000	Fl Oz	0.00	0.00	2.00	10.00	0.00	0.00	0.00	0.00
720	Starbucks-Caffe Latte w/nonfat milk	340.8000	12.000	Fl Oz	12.00	0.50	17.00	120.00	0.00	0.00	0.00	0.00
721	Starbucks-Caffe Latte w/whole milk	340.8000	12.000	Fl Oz	11.00	11.00	17.00	210.00	0.00	0.00	0.00	0.00
722	Starbucks-Caffe Mocha w/nonfat milk	340.8000	12.000	Fl Oz	12.00	12.00	32.00	260.00	0.00	0.00	0.00	0.00
723	Starbucks-Caffe Mocha w/whole milk	340.8000	12.000	Fl Oz	12.00	21.00	31.00	340.00	0.00	0.00	0.00	0.00
724	Starbucks-Cappuccino w/nonfat milk	340.8000	12.000	Fl Oz	7.00	0.00	11.00	80.00	0.00	0.00	0.00	0.00
725	Starbucks-Cappuccino w/whole milk	340.8000	12.000	Fl Oz	7.00	7.00	11.00	140.00	0.00	0.00	0.00	0.00
726	Starbucks-Coffee Frappuccino	340.8000	12.000	Fl Oz	6.00	3.00	39.00	200.00	0.00	0.00	0.00	0.00
727	Starbucks-Coffee, Drip	340.8000	12.000	Fl Oz	1.00	0.00	1.00	10.00	0.00	0.00	0.00	0.00
	Tea, Brewed	237.0000	1.000	Cup	0.00	0.00	0.71	2.37	47.40	0.00	0.00	0.00
	Tea, Herb, Brewed	237.0000	1.000	Cup	0.00	0.00	0.47	2.37	0.00	0.00	0.00	0.00
	Tea, Iced, Bottled, All Flavors	236.6000	1.000	Cup	0.00	0.00	28.59	118.30	44.00	0.00	0.00	0.00
	Tea, Iced, Bottled, All Flavors,	236.6000	1.000	Cup	0.00	0.00	0.99	0.00	54.00	0.00	0.00	0.00
	Tea, Instant, Sweetened	259.0000	1.000	Cup	0.26	0.00	22.02	88.06	28.49	0.00	0.00	0.00
	Tea, Instant, Unsweetened	237.0000	1.000	Cup	0.00	0.00	0.47	2.37	30.81	0.00	0.00	0.00
	Tequila Sunrise	31.2000	6.000	Fl Oz	0.09	0.03	2.68	34.32	0.00	0.00	0.00	0.00
	Thirst Quencher Drink, Bottled	241.0000	1.000	Cup	0.00	0.00	15.18	60.25	0.00	0.00	0.00	0.00
	Water, Bottled, Perrier	192.0000	6.500	Fl Oz	0.00	0.00	0.00	0.00	0.00	0.00	0.00	0.00
	Water, Municipal	240.0000	8.000	Fl Oz	0.00	0.00	0.00	0.00	0.00	0.00	0.00	0.00
785	Water, Spring-Aquafina	240.0000	8.000	Fl Oz	0.00	0.00	0.00	0.00	0.00	0.00	0.00	0.00
786	Water, Spring-Avalon	240.0000	8.000	Fl Oz	0.00	0.00	0.00	0.00	0.00	0.00	0.00	0.00
787	Water, Spring-Dannon	240.0000	8.000	Fl Oz	0.00	0.00	0.00	0.00	0.00	0.00	0.00	0.00
788	Water, Spring-Deer Park	240.0000	8.000	Fl Oz	0.00	0.00	0.00	0.00	0.00	0.00	0.00	0.00
789	Water, Spring-Evian	240.0000	8.000	Fl Oz	0.00	0.00	0.00	0.00	0.00	0.00	0.00	0.00
790	Water, Spring-Naya	240.0000	8.000	Fl Oz	0.00	0.00	0.00	0.00	0.00	0.00	0.00	0.00
	Water, Tonic	488.0000	16.000	Fl Oz	0.00	0.00	42.94	165.92	0.00	0.00	0.00	0.00
	Wine, Dessert, Dry, 3.5 Oz Glass	103.0000	1.000	Glass	0.21	0.00	4.22	129.78	0.00	0.00	0.00	0.00
	Wine, Dessert, Sweet, 3.5 Oz Glass	103.0000	1.000	Glass	0.21	0.00	12.15	157.59	0.00	0.00	0.00	0.00
	Wine, Table, All, 3.5 Oz Glass	103.0000	1.000	Glass	0.21	0.00	1.44	72.10	0.00	0.00	0.00	0.00
	Wine, Table, Red, 3.5 Oz Glass	103.0000	1.000	Glass	0.21	0.00	1.75	74.16	0.00	0.00	0.00	0.00
	Wine, Table, Rose, 3.5 Oz Glass	103.0000	1.000	Glass	0.21	0.00	1.44	73.13	0.00	0.00	0.00	0.00
	Wine, Table, White, 3.5 Oz Glass	103.0000	1.000	Glass	0.10	0.00	0.82	70.04	0.00	0.00	0.00	0.00

Page Key: A2 = Baby Food   A2 = Baked Goods   A8 = Beverages   A14 = Breads/Grains and Pasta   A18 = Breakfast Foods/Cereals   A26 = Dairy and Eggs   A40 = Fats and Oils   A42 = Fruits and Vegetables   A52 = Meats and Beans   A60 = Nuts and Seeds   A62 5 Frozen Entrees and Packaged Foods   A76 = Restaurant Chains–Fast Foods   A92 = Restaurant Chains–Other   A106 = Seafood and Fish   A110 = Snacks and Sweets   A120 = Soups   A122 = Supplements   A126 = Toppings and Sauces

Monounsaturated Fat (g)	Polyunsaturated Fat (g)	Vitamin D (mg)	Vitamin K (mg)	Vitamin E (mg)	Vitamin A (re)	Vitamin C (mg)	Thiamin (mg)	Riboflavin (mg)	Niacin (mg)	Vitamin B_6 (mg)	Folate (mcg)	Vitamin B_{12} (mcg)	Calcium (mg)	Iron (mg)	Magnesium (mg)	Phosphorus (mg)	Potassium (mg)	Sodium (mg)	Zinc (mg)
0.00	0.00	0.00	0.00	0.00	0.00	0.00	0.00	0.00	0.00	0.00	0.00	0.00	0.00	0.00	0.00	0.00	0.00	10.00	0.00
0.00	0.00	0.00	0.00	0.00	0.00	0.00	0.00	0.00	0.00	0.00	0.00	0.00	0.00	0.00	0.00	0.00	0.00	10.00	0.00
0.00	0.00	0.00	0.00	0.00	0.00	0.00	0.00	0.00	0.00	0.00	0.00	0.00	0.00	0.00	0.00	0.00	0.00	0.00	0.00
0.00	0.00	0.00	0.00	0.00	0.00	0.00	0.00	0.00	0.00	0.00	0.00	0.00	0.00	0.00	0.00	0.00	0.00	0.00	0.00
0.00	0.00	0.00	0.00	0.00	0.00	0.00	0.00	0.00	0.00	0.00	0.00	0.00	0.00	0.00	0.00	0.00	0.00	10.00	0.00
0.00	0.00	0.00	0.00	0.00	0.00	0.00	0.00	0.00	0.00	0.00	0.00	0.00	0.00	0.00	0.00	0.00	0.00	0.00	0.00
0.00	0.00	0.00	0.00	0.00	0.00	0.00	0.00	0.00	0.00	0.00	0.00	0.00	0.00	0.00	0.00	0.00	0.00	10.00	0.00
0.00	0.00	0.00	0.00	0.00	0.00	0.00	0.00	0.00	0.00	0.00	0.00	0.00	23.70	0.05	4.74	0.00	9.48	99.54	0.47
0.00	0.00	0.00	0.00	0.00	0.00	0.00	0.00	0.00	0.00	0.00	0.00	0.00	24.70	0.25	4.94	0.00	4.94	59.28	0.35
0.00	0.00	0.00	0.00	0.00	0.00	0.00	0.00	0.00	0.00	0.00	0.00	0.00	14.73	0.20	0.00	54.01	4.91	49.10	0.20
0.00	0.00	0.00	0.05	0.00	0.00	0.00	0.00	0.00	0.00	0.00	0.00	0.00	14.64	0.88	4.88	0.00	4.88	34.16	0.24
0.00	0.00	0.00	0.00	0.00	0.00	0.00	0.00	0.00	0.00	0.00	0.00	0.00	0.00	0.00	0.00	0.00	0.00	2.50	0.00
0.00	0.00	0.00	0.00	0.00	0.00	0.00	0.00	0.00	0.00	0.00	0.00	0.00	11.16	0.30	3.72	0.00	3.72	55.80	0.26
0.00	0.00	0.00	0.00	0.00	0.00	85.25	0.00	0.00	0.08	0.03	0.75	0.00	7.50	0.43	5.00	2.50	12.50	15.00	0.28
0.00	0.00	0.00	0.00	0.00	0.00	0.00	0.00	0.00	0.10	0.00	0.00	0.00	9.00	0.25	2.00	1.00	4.00	41.00	0.18
0.00	0.00	0.00	0.00	0.00	0.00	0.00	0.00	0.00	0.00	0.00	0.00	0.00	0.00	0.00	0.00	0.00	0.00	2.50	0.00
0.00	0.00	0.00	0.00	0.00	0.00	0.00	0.00	0.00	0.00	0.00	0.00	0.00	0.00	0.00	0.00	0.00	10.00	31.00	0.00
0.00	0.00	0.00	0.00	0.00	4.96	84.57	0.02	0.00	0.07	0.02	5.46	0.00	14.88	0.69	4.96	2.48	44.64	39.68	0.22
0.00	0.00	0.00	0.00	0.00	0.00	0.00	0.00	0.00	0.00	0.00	0.00	0.00	24.65	0.25	4.93	0.00	4.93	64.09	0.35
0.00	0.00	0.00	0.00	0.00	0.00	0.00	0.00	0.00	0.00	0.00	0.00	0.00	0.00	0.00	0.00	0.00	0.00	2.50	0.00
0.00	0.00	0.00	0.00	0.00	0.00	0.00	0.00	0.00	0.00	0.00	0.00	0.00	0.00	0.00	0.00	0.00	0.00	105.00	0.00
0.00	0.00	0.00	0.00	0.00	0.00	0.00	0.00	0.00	0.00	0.00	0.00	0.00	0.00	0.00	0.00	0.00	0.00	170.00	0.00
0.00	0.00	0.00	0.00	0.00	0.00	0.00	0.00	0.00	0.00	0.00	0.00	0.00	0.00	0.00	0.00	0.00	0.00	160.00	0.00
0.00	0.00	0.00	0.00	0.00	0.00	0.00	0.00	0.00	0.00	0.00	0.00	0.00	0.00	0.00	0.00	0.00	0.00	170.00	0.00
0.00	0.00	0.00	0.00	0.00	0.00	0.00	0.00	0.00	0.00	0.00	0.00	0.00	0.00	0.00	0.00	0.00	0.00	160.00	0.00
0.00	0.00	0.00	0.00	0.00	0.00	0.00	0.00	0.00	0.00	0.00	0.00	0.00	0.00	0.00	0.00	0.00	0.00	110.00	0.00
0.00	0.00	0.00	0.00	0.00	0.00	0.00	0.00	0.00	0.00	0.00	0.00	0.00	0.00	0.00	0.00	0.00	0.00	105.00	0.00
0.00	0.00	0.00	0.00	0.00	0.00	0.00	0.00	0.00	0.00	0.00	0.00	0.00	0.00	0.00	0.00	0.00	0.00	170.00	0.00
0.00	0.00	0.00	0.00	0.00	0.00	0.00	0.00	0.00	0.00	0.00	0.00	0.00	0.00	0.00	0.00	0.00	0.00	10.00	0.00
0.00	0.00	0.00	0.12	0.00	0.00	0.00	0.00	0.02	0.00	0.00	12.32	0.00	0.00	0.05	7.11	2.37	87.69	7.11	0.05
0.00	0.02	0.00	0.00	0.00	0.00	0.00	0.02	0.00	0.00	0.00	1.42	0.00	4.74	0.19	2.37	0.00	21.33	2.37	0.09
0.00	0.00	0.00	0.00	0.00	0.00	0.00	0.00	0.00	0.00	0.00	0.00	0.00	0.00	0.00	0.00	0.00	0.00	9.86	0.00
0.00	0.03	0.00	0.00	0.00	0.00	0.00	0.00	0.05	0.10	0.00	9.58	0.00	5.18	0.05	5.18	2.59	49.21	7.77	0.08
0.00	0.00	0.00	0.00	0.00	0.00	0.00	0.00	0.00	0.09	0.00	0.71	0.00	4.74	0.05	4.74	2.37	47.40	7.11	0.07
0.01	0.01	0.00	0.00	0.00	3.12	6.02	0.01	0.00	0.06	0.02	3.31	0.00	1.87	0.09	2.18	3.12	32.45	1.25	0.02
0.00	0.00	0.00	0.00	0.00	0.00	0.00	0.00	0.02	0.00	0.00	0.00	0.00	0.00	0.12	2.41	21.69	26.51	96.40	0.05
0.00	0.00	0.00	0.00	0.00	0.00	0.00	0.00	0.00	0.00	0.00	0.00	0.00	26.88	0.00	0.00	0.00	0.00	1.92	0.00
0.00	0.00	0.00	0.00	0.00	0.00	0.00	0.00	0.00	0.00	0.00	0.00	0.00	0.00	0.00	0.00	0.00	0.00	0.00	0.00
0.00	0.00	0.00	0.00	0.00	0.00	0.00	0.00	0.00	0.00	0.00	0.00	0.00	0.00	0.00	0.00	0.00	0.00	0.00	0.00
0.00	0.00	0.00	0.00	0.00	0.00	0.00	0.00	0.00	0.00	0.00	0.00	0.00	0.00	0.00	0.00	0.00	0.00	0.00	0.00
0.00	0.00	0.00	0.00	0.00	0.00	0.00	0.00	0.00	0.00	0.00	0.00	0.00	0.00	0.00	0.00	0.00	0.00	0.00	0.00
0.00	0.00	0.00	0.00	0.00	0.00	0.00	0.00	0.00	0.00	0.00	0.00	0.00	0.00	0.00	0.00	0.00	0.00	0.00	0.00
0.00	0.00	0.00	0.00	0.00	0.00	0.00	0.00	0.00	0.00	0.00	0.00	0.00	4.88	0.05	0.00	0.00	0.00	19.52	0.49
0.00	0.00	0.00	0.00	0.00	0.00	0.00	0.02	0.02	0.22	0.00	0.41	0.00	8.24	0.25	9.27	9.27	94.76	9.27	0.07
0.00	0.00	0.00	0.00	0.00	0.00	0.00	0.02	0.02	0.22	0.00	0.41	0.00	8.24	0.25	9.27	9.27	94.76	9.27	0.07
0.00	0.00	0.00	0.00	0.00	0.00	0.00	0.00	0.02	0.07	0.02	1.13	0.01	8.24	0.42	10.30	14.42	91.67	8.24	0.07
0.00	0.00	0.00	0.00	0.00	0.00	0.00	0.01	0.03	0.08	0.03	2.06	0.01	8.24	0.44	13.39	14.42	115.36	5.15	0.09
0.00	0.00	0.00	0.00	0.00	0.00	0.00	0.00	0.02	0.07	0.02	1.13	0.01	8.24	0.39	10.30	15.45	101.97	5.15	0.06
0.00	0.00	0.00	0.00	0.00	0.00	0.00	0.00	0.01	0.07	0.01	0.21	0.00	9.27	0.33	10.30	14.42	82.40	5.15	0.07

Breads/Grains and Pasta

USDA ID Code	Food Name	Weight in Grams*	Quantity of Units	Unit of Measure	Protein (g)	Fat (g)	Carbohydrate (g)	Kilocalories	Caffeine (g)	Fiber (g)	Cholesterol (mg)	Saturated Fat (g)
	Barley, Cooked	184.0000	1.000	Cup	22.96	4.23	135.20	651.36	0.00	31.83	0.00	0.88
61	Bread Sticks, Plain	10.0000	1.000	Stick	1.20	0.95	6.84	41.20	0.00	0.00	0.00	0.14
	Bread Stuffing, Plain	232.0000	1.000	Cup	8.82	16.70	51.50	389.76	0.00	0.00	0.00	3.39
	Bread, Banana	60.0000	1.000	Slice	2.58	7.08	33.06	202.80	0.00	0.00	25.80	1.83
	Bread, Cornbread	28.3500	1.000	Slice	1.90	2.01	12.33	75.41	0.00	0.00	11.34	0.44
	Bread, Cracked-wheat	28.3500	1.000	Slice	2.47	1.11	14.03	73.71	0.00	1.56	0.00	0.26
	Bread, Cracked-wheat, Toasted	23.0000	1.000	Slice	2.19	0.97	12.37	65.09	0.00	0.00	0.00	0.23
	Bread, Dinner Roll, Egg	28.3500	1.000	Each	2.69	1.81	14.74	87.03	0.00	1.05	14.18	0.45
	Bread, Dinner Roll, French	28.3500	1.000	Each	2.44	1.22	14.23	78.53	0.00	0.91	0.00	0.27
	Bread, Dinner Roll, Oat Bran	28.3500	1.000	Each	2.69	1.30	11.40	66.91	0.00	1.16	0.00	0.18
	Bread, Dinner Roll, Plain	86.0000	1.000	Each	7.22	6.28	43.34	258.00	0.00	2.58	0.86	1.51
	Bread, Dinner Roll, Rye	43.0000	1.000	Large	4.43	1.46	22.83	122.98	0.00	2.09	0.00	0.26
	Bread, Dinner Roll, Wheat	28.3500	1.000	Each	2.44	1.79	13.04	77.40	0.00	1.07	0.00	0.43
	Bread, Dinner Roll, Whole-wheat	43.0000	1.000	Each	3.74	2.02	21.97	114.38	0.00	3.24	0.00	0.36
	Bread, Egg	28.3500	1.000	Slice	2.69	1.70	13.55	81.36	0.00	0.65	14.46	0.45
	Bread, Egg, Toasted	28.3500	1.000	Slice	2.98	1.87	14.91	89.30	0.00	0.71	15.88	0.46
	Bread, French or Vienna	28.3500	1.000	Slice	2.49	0.85	14.71	77.68	0.00	0.85	0.00	0.18
	Bread, French or Vienna, Toasted	28.3500	1.000	Slice	2.72	0.94	15.99	84.48	0.00	0.94	0.00	0.20
	Bread, Italian	28.3500	1.000	Slice	2.49	0.99	14.18	76.83	0.00	0.77	0.00	0.24
	Bread, Italian, Toasted	27.0000	1.000	Slice	2.62	1.05	14.85	80.46	0.00	0.00	0.00	0.25
	Bread, Lo Cal, Oat Bran	28.3500	1.000	Slice	2.27	0.91	11.71	56.98	0.00	3.40	0.00	0.13
	Bread, Lo Cal, Oat Bran, Toasted	28.3500	1.000	Slice	2.69	1.08	13.95	67.76	0.00	4.05	0.00	0.15
	Bread, Lo Cal, Oatmeal	28.3500	1.000	Slice	2.15	0.99	12.28	59.54	0.00	0.00	0.00	0.17
	Bread, Lo Cal, Oatmeal, Toasted	19.0000	1.000	Slice	1.71	0.80	9.79	47.69	0.00	0.00	0.00	0.14
	Bread, Lo Cal, Rye	28.3500	1.000	Slice	2.58	0.82	11.48	57.55	0.00	3.40	0.00	0.10
	Bread, Lo Cal, Rye, Toasted	19.0000	1.000	Slice	2.05	0.65	9.16	45.79	0.00	0.00	0.19	0.08
	Bread, Lo Cal, Wheat	28.3500	1.000	Slice	2.58	0.65	12.36	56.13	0.00	3.40	0.00	0.10
	Bread, Lo Cal, Wheat, Toasted	19.0000	1.000	Slice	2.05	0.51	9.86	44.84	0.00	0.00	0.00	0.08
	Bread, Lo Cal, White	28.3500	1.000	Slice	2.47	0.71	12.56	58.68	0.00	2.75	0.00	0.16
	Bread, Lo Cal, White, Toasted	19.0000	1.000	Slice	1.96	0.57	10.01	46.93	0.00	0.00	0.00	0.12
	Bread, Mixed-grain	28.3500	1.000	Slice	2.84	1.08	13.15	70.88	0.00	1.81	0.00	0.23
	Bread, Mixed-grain, Toasted	28.3500	1.000	Slice	3.09	1.16	14.29	77.11	0.00	1.87	0.00	0.25
	Bread, Oat Bran	28.3500	1.000	Slice	2.95	1.25	11.28	66.91	0.00	1.28	0.00	0.20
	Bread, Oat Bran, Toasted	28.3500	1.000	Slice	3.23	1.36	12.39	73.43	0.00	1.39	0.00	0.22
	Bread, Oatmeal	28.3500	1.000	Slice	2.38	1.25	13.75	76.26	0.00	1.13	0.00	0.20
	Bread, Oatmeal, Toasted	28.3500	1.000	Slice	2.61	1.36	14.94	82.78	0.00	1.22	0.00	0.22
	Bread, Pita, White, Enriched	60.0000	1.000	Pita	5.46	0.72	33.42	165.00	0.00	1.32	0.00	0.10
	Bread, Pita, Whole-wheat	64.0000	1.000	Pita	6.27	1.66	35.20	170.24	0.00	4.74	0.00	0.26
	Bread, Pumpernickel	28.3500	1.000	Slice	2.47	0.88	13.47	70.88	0.00	1.84	0.00	0.12
	Bread, Pumpernickel, Toasted	28.3500	1.000	Slice	2.69	0.96	14.80	77.96	0.00	2.01	0.00	0.14
	Bread, Pumpkin	60.0000	1.000	Slice	2.40	7.68	30.72	198.60	0.00	0.00	26.40	1.23
	Bread, Raisin	28.3500	1.000	Slice	2.24	1.25	14.83	77.68	0.00	1.22	0.00	0.31
	Bread, Raisin, Toasted	28.3500	1.000	Slice	2.44	1.36	16.13	84.20	0.00	1.33	0.00	0.33
	Bread, Rice Bran	28.3500	1.000	Slice	2.52	1.30	12.33	68.89	0.00	1.39	0.00	0.20
	Bread, Rice Bran, Toasted	28.3500	1.000	Slice	2.75	1.42	13.41	74.84	0.00	1.50	0.00	0.22
	Bread, Rolls, Hard (includes Kaiser)	28.3500	1.000	Each	2.81	1.22	14.94	83.07	0.00	0.65	0.00	0.17
	Bread, Rye	28.3500	1.000	Slice	2.41	0.94	13.69	73.43	0.00	1.64	0.00	0.18
	Bread, Rye, Toasted	28.3500	1.000	Slice	2.66	1.02	15.05	80.51	0.00	1.81	0.00	0.20
	Bread, Wheat (includes Wheat Berry)	28.3500	1.000	Slice	2.58	1.16	13.38	73.71	0.00	1.22	0.00	0.25
	Bread, Wheat Bran	28.3500	1.000	Slice	2.49	0.96	13.55	70.31	0.00	1.13	0.00	0.22
	Bread, Wheat Bran, Toasted	33.0000	1.000	Slice	3.20	1.22	17.33	90.09	0.00	0.00	0.00	0.28
	Bread, Wheat, Toasted	28.3500	1.000	Slice	2.81	1.25	14.54	79.95	0.00	1.50	0.00	0.27

Monounsaturated Fat (g)	Polyunsaturated Fat (g)	Vitamin D (mg)	Vitamin K (mg)	Vitamin E (mg)	Vitamin A (re)	Vitamin C (mg)	Thiamin (mg)	Riboflavin (mg)	Niacin (mg)	Vitamin B_6 (mg)	Folate (mcg)	Vitamin B_{12} (mcg)	Calcium (mg)	Iron (mg)	Magnesium (mg)	Phosphorus (mg)	Potassium (mg)	Sodium (mg)	Zinc (mg)
0.55	2.04	0.00	0.00	1.10	3.68	0.00	1.20	0.53	8.46	0.59	34.96	0.00	60.72	6.62	244.72	485.76	831.68	22.08	5.10
0.37	0.36	0.00	0.00	0.00	0.00	0.00	0.06	0.06	0.53	0.01	3.00	0.00	2.20	0.43	3.20	12.10	12.40	65.70	0.09
7.40	4.89	0.00	0.00	0.00	160.08	3.94	0.39	0.33	3.69	0.12	39.44	0.00	148.48	3.80	34.80	113.68	303.92	1069.52	0.74
3.02	1.77	0.00	0.00	0.00	14.40	1.02	0.10	0.12	0.87	0.09	6.60	0.05	10.80	0.84	8.40	33.60	78.60	118.80	0.22
0.52	0.91	0.00	0.00	0.00	15.31	0.09	0.08	0.08	0.64	0.03	18.14	0.04	70.59	0.71	7.09	47.91	41.67	186.54	0.17
0.54	0.19	0.00	0.00	0.17	0.00	0.00	0.10	0.07	1.04	0.09	17.29	0.01	12.19	0.80	14.74	43.38	50.18	152.52	0.35
0.48	0.17	0.00	0.00	0.00	0.00	0.00	0.07	0.05	0.83	0.07	6.90	0.01	10.81	0.70	13.11	38.18	44.16	134.55	0.31
0.83	0.32	0.00	0.00	0.20	2.27	0.00	0.15	0.15	0.93	0.01	29.77	0.07	16.73	1.00	7.09	28.63	29.48	154.51	0.32
0.56	0.24	0.00	0.00	0.13	0.00	0.00	0.15	0.09	1.23	0.01	26.93	0.00	25.80	0.77	5.67	23.81	32.32	172.65	0.26
0.42	0.45	0.00	0.00	0.20	0.00	0.00	0.13	0.08	1.40	0.01	26.93	0.00	24.10	1.17	9.36	32.60	34.30	117.09	0.29
3.18	1.04	0.00	0.00	0.76	0.00	0.09	0.42	0.28	3.47	0.04	81.70	0.05	102.34	2.69	19.78	99.76	114.38	448.06	0.66
0.53	0.31	0.00	0.00	0.15	0.43	0.00	0.16	0.12	1.68	0.03	36.98	0.00	12.90	1.16	23.22	68.37	77.40	383.56	0.42
0.88	0.31	0.00	0.00	0.27	0.00	0.00	0.12	0.08	1.15	0.02	14.46	0.00	49.90	1.01	10.21	29.48	32.60	96.39	0.26
0.52	0.93	0.00	0.00	0.58	0.00	0.00	0.11	0.12	1.58	0.09	12.90	0.00	45.58	1.04	36.55	96.32	116.96	205.54	0.86
0.65	0.31	0.00	0.00	0.17	6.52	0.00	0.12	0.12	1.37	0.02	29.77	0.03	26.37	0.86	5.39	30.05	32.60	139.48	0.22
0.85	0.33	0.00	0.00	0.24	6.52	0.00	0.11	0.12	1.36	0.02	25.23	0.03	28.92	0.95	5.95	33.17	35.72	153.09	0.24
0.35	0.20	0.00	0.00	0.08	0.00	0.00	0.15	0.09	1.35	0.01	26.93	0.00	21.26	0.72	7.65	29.77	32.04	172.65	0.25
0.37	0.21	0.00	0.00	0.07	0.00	0.00	0.13	0.09	1.32	0.01	22.96	0.00	22.96	0.78	8.51	32.32	34.59	187.39	0.27
0.23	0.39	0.00	0.00	0.10	0.00	0.00	0.13	0.08	1.24	0.01	26.93	0.00	22.11	0.83	7.65	29.20	31.19	165.56	0.24
0.24	0.41	0.00	0.00	0.00	0.00	0.00	0.11	0.08	1.17	0.01	6.21	0.00	22.95	0.87	8.10	30.78	32.67	173.34	0.26
0.19	0.47	0.00	0.00	0.13	0.00	0.00	0.10	0.06	1.07	0.03	18.71	0.00	16.16	0.89	15.59	39.41	28.92	99.51	0.30
0.23	0.56	0.00	0.00	0.15	0.00	0.00	0.10	0.06	1.14	0.03	15.88	0.00	19.28	1.06	15.59	40.82	34.59	118.50	0.34
0.23	0.38	0.00	0.00	0.00	0.28	0.06	0.10	0.08	0.86	0.01	15.59	0.03	32.60	0.65	6.80	28.35	35.15	110.00	0.24
0.19	0.31	0.00	0.00	0.00	0.19	0.04	0.06	0.06	0.62	0.01	5.32	0.03	26.03	0.52	6.46	24.58	34.58	87.78	0.21
0.19	0.21	0.00	0.00	0.07	0.00	0.11	0.10	0.07	0.72	0.02	13.61	0.01	21.55	0.88	6.24	22.11	27.78	114.82	0.19
0.15	0.17	0.00	0.00	0.00	0.00	0.02	0.07	0.05	0.51	0.01	3.61	0.02	17.29	0.70	3.99	18.81	22.23	91.77	0.17
0.07	0.27	0.00	0.00	0.03	0.00	0.03	0.12	0.09	1.10	0.04	20.13	0.00	22.68	0.84	11.06	28.92	34.59	144.87	0.32
0.06	0.22	0.00	0.00	0.00	0.00	0.02	0.08	0.06	0.79	0.03	4.37	0.01	18.24	0.67	6.46	20.71	27.93	115.52	0.19
0.31	0.16	0.00	0.00	0.04	0.28	0.14	0.12	0.08	1.03	0.01	26.93	0.08	26.65	0.90	6.52	34.30	21.55	128.43	0.38
0.24	0.13	0.00	0.00	0.00	0.19	0.08	0.07	0.06	0.74	0.01	5.51	0.06	21.28	0.72	5.89	30.21	17.29	102.41	0.30
0.43	0.26	0.00	0.00	0.19	0.00	0.09	0.12	0.10	1.24	0.09	22.68	0.02	25.80	0.98	15.03	49.90	57.83	138.06	0.36
0.47	0.28	0.00	0.00	0.19	0.00	0.09	0.10	0.09	1.21	0.09	19.28	0.02	28.07	1.07	16.44	54.15	62.94	150.26	0.39
0.45	0.48	0.00	0.00	0.18	0.00	0.00	0.14	0.10	1.37	0.02	22.96	0.00	18.43	0.88	9.92	39.97	41.67	115.38	0.25
0.50	0.53	0.00	0.00	0.12	0.00	0.00	0.12	0.10	1.36	0.01	19.56	0.00	20.13	0.97	9.64	32.89	34.87	127.01	0.30
0.45	0.48	0.00	0.00	0.17	0.57	0.00	0.11	0.07	0.89	0.02	17.58	0.01	18.71	0.77	10.49	35.72	40.26	169.82	0.29
0.49	0.52	0.00	0.00	0.10	0.57	0.09	0.10	0.07	0.87	0.02	15.03	0.01	20.41	0.83	11.62	38.84	43.66	184.56	0.31
0.07	0.32	0.00	0.00	0.02	0.00	0.00	0.36	0.02	2.78	0.02	57.00	0.02	51.60	1.57	15.60	58.20	72.00	321.60	0.50
0.22	0.68	0.00	0.00	0.58	0.00	0.00	0.22	0.05	1.82	0.17	22.40	0.00	9.60	1.96	44.16	115.20	108.80	340.48	0.97
0.26	0.35	0.00	0.00	0.12	0.00	0.00	0.09	0.09	0.88	0.04	22.68	0.00	19.28	0.81	15.31	50.46	58.97	190.23	0.42
0.29	0.39	0.00	0.00	0.17	0.00	0.00	0.08	0.09	0.87	0.03	19.28	0.00	20.98	0.89	17.01	55.28	64.64	209.22	0.46
1.85	4.11	0.00	0.00	0.00	334.20	0.60	0.09	0.10	0.79	0.02	6.60	0.05	10.80	0.99	7.80	31.80	55.20	187.80	0.20
0.65	0.19	0.00	0.00	0.14	0.00	0.03	0.10	0.11	0.98	0.02	24.66	0.00	18.71	0.82	7.37	30.90	64.35	110.57	0.20
0.71	0.21	0.00	0.00	0.23	0.00	0.11	0.08	0.11	0.96	0.02	20.98	0.00	20.41	0.89	7.94	33.45	69.74	120.20	0.22
0.47	0.50	0.00	0.00	0.24	0.00	0.00	0.18	0.09	1.93	0.08	18.43	0.00	19.56	1.02	22.68	50.46	60.95	124.74	0.37
0.51	0.54	0.00	0.00	0.22	0.00	0.00	0.16	0.08	1.89	0.06	15.59	0.00	21.26	1.11	21.55	49.33	60.10	135.51	0.39
0.32	0.49	0.00	0.00	0.09	0.00	0.00	0.14	0.10	1.20	0.01	26.93	0.00	26.93	0.93	7.65	28.35	30.62	154.22	0.27
0.37	0.23	0.00	0.00	0.10	0.28	0.11	0.12	0.10	1.08	0.02	24.38	0.00	20.70	0.80	11.34	35.44	47.06	187.11	0.32
0.41	0.25	0.00	0.00	0.17	0.00	0.06	0.11	0.09	1.07	0.02	20.70	0.00	22.68	0.88	12.19	39.12	51.88	205.54	0.35
0.49	0.26	0.00	0.00	0.15	0.00	0.00	0.12	0.08	1.17	0.03	21.83	0.00	29.77	0.94	13.04	42.53	56.98	150.26	0.29
0.46	0.18	0.00	0.00	0.13	0.00	0.00	0.11	0.08	1.25	0.05	19.56	0.00	20.98	0.87	22.96	52.45	64.35	137.78	0.38
0.59	0.24	0.00	0.00	0.00	0.00	0.00	0.12	0.09	1.44	0.06	6.60	0.00	26.73	1.11	29.37	67.32	82.17	176.22	0.49
0.53	0.28	0.00	0.00	0.17	0.00	0.00	0.10	0.08	1.14	0.03	18.43	0.00	32.32	1.02	14.18	46.21	61.80	163.30	0.32

USDA ID Code	Food Name	Weight in Grams*	Quantity of Units	Unit of Measure	Protein (g)	Fat (g)	Carbohydrate (g)	Kilocalories	Caffeine (g)	Fiber (g)	Cholesterol (mg)	Saturated Fat (g)
62	Bread, White	25.0000	1.000	Slice	2.05	0.90	12.38	66.75	0.00	0.58	0.25	0.20
63	Bread, White, Toasted	23.0000	1.000	Slice	2.07	0.92	12.51	67.39	0.00	0.00	0.23	0.21
	Bread, Whole Wheat	28.3500	1.000	Slice	2.75	1.19	13.07	69.74	0.00	1.96	0.00	0.26
	Bread, Whole Wheat, Toasted	28.3500	1.000	Slice	2.61	1.67	15.99	86.47	0.00	1.90	0.00	0.25
	Breadsticks, Sesame Sticks, Wheat	28.3500	1.000	Ounce	3.09	10.40	13.18	153.37	0.00	0.79	0.00	1.84
	Buns, Hamburger or Hot Dog, Mixed	28.3500	1.000	Each	5.44	3.40	25.25	149.12	0.00	2.16	0.00	0.78
	Buns, Hamburger or Hot Dog, Plain	28.3500	1.000	Each	4.82	2.90	28.52	162.16	0.00	1.54	0.00	0.68
	Cornstarch	128.0000	1.000	Cup	0.33	0.06	116.83	487.68	0.00	1.15	0.00	0.01
	Couscous, Cooked	157.0000	1.000	Cup	5.95	0.25	36.46	175.84	0.00	2.20	0.00	0.05
	Crackers, Cheese, Regular	62.0000	1.000	Cup	6.26	15.69	36.08	311.86	0.00	1.49	8.06	5.81
206	Crackers, Cheese, w/Peanut Butter	7.0000	1.000	Each	0.88	1.62	3.99	33.74	0.00	0.08	0.35	0.36
	Crackers, Crack Pepper, Fat Free	2.1400	7.000	Each	0.29	0.00	1.85	8.56	0.00	0.07	0.00	0.00
207	Crackers, Crispbread, Rye	10.0000	1.000	Each	0.79	0.13	8.22	36.60	0.00	1.62	0.00	0.01
	Crackers, Graham Snacks, Cinn.,	0.6700	20.000	Each	0.04	0.00	0.58	2.46	0.00	0.02	0.00	0.00
208	Crackers, Graham, Plain or Honey	7.0000	1.000	Each	0.48	0.71	5.38	29.61	0.00	0.19	0.00	0.18
	Crackers, Matzo, Egg	28.3500	1.000	Each	3.49	0.60	22.28	110.85	0.00	0.79	23.53	0.16
	Crackers, Matzo, Egg and Onion	28.3500	1.000	Each	2.84	1.11	21.86	110.85	0.00	1.42	12.76	0.27
	Crackers, Matzo, Plain	28.3500	1.000	Each	2.84	0.40	23.73	111.98	0.00	0.85	0.00	0.07
	Crackers, Matzo, Whole-wheat	28.3500	1.000	Each	3.71	0.43	22.37	99.51	0.00	3.35	0.00	0.07
	Crackers, Melba Toast, Plain	30.0000	1.000	Cup	3.63	0.96	22.98	117.00	0.00	1.89	0.00	0.14
209	Crackers, Melba Toast, Plain, w/	5.0000	1.000	Each	0.61	0.16	3.83	19.50	0.00	0.00	0.00	0.02
	Crackers, Melba Toast, Rye	14.1750	1.000	Each	1.64	0.48	10.96	55.14	0.00	1.13	0.00	0.06
	Crackers, Melba Toast, Wheat	14.1750	1.000	Each	1.83	0.33	10.83	53.01	0.00	1.05	0.00	0.05
	Crackers, Ritz	62.0000	1.000	Cup	4.59	15.69	37.82	311.24	0.00	0.99	0.00	2.34
	Crackers, Ritz, Low Sodium	62.0000	1.000	Cup	4.59	15.69	37.82	311.24	0.00	0.99	0.00	2.34
	Crackers, Rye, w/ Cheese Filling	14.1750	1.000	Each	1.30	3.16	8.62	68.18	0.00	0.51	1.28	0.85
210	Crackers, Rye, Wafers, Plain	25.0000	1.000	Each	2.40	0.23	20.10	83.50	0.00	0.00	0.00	0.03
	Crackers, Rye, Wafers, Seasoned	14.1750	1.000	Each	1.28	1.30	10.46	54.01	0.00	2.96	0.00	0.18
211	Crackers, Saltines	3.0000	1.000	Each	0.28	0.35	2.15	13.02	0.00	0.08	0.00	0.06
	Crackers, Saltines, Fat Free	3.0000	1.000	Each	0.40	0.00	2.40	12.00	0.00	0.00	0.00	0.00
212	Crackers, Saltines, Low Salt	3.0000	1.000	Each	0.28	0.35	2.15	13.02	0.00	0.00	0.00	0.06
	Crackers, w/ Cheese Filling, Snack	14.1750	1.000	Each	1.32	2.99	8.75	67.61	0.00	0.26	0.28	0.87
	Crackers, w/Peanut Butter Filling	14.1750	1.000	Each	1.57	3.39	8.32	69.17	0.00	0.39	0.00	0.79
	Crackers, Wheat, Fat Free-Snack	3.0000	5.000	Each	0.40	0.00	2.40	12.00	0.00	0.20	0.00	0.00
213	Crackers, Wheat, Low Salt	2.0000	1.000	Each	0.17	0.41	1.30	9.46	0.00	0.00	0.00	0.07
214	Crackers, Wheat, Regular	2.0000	1.000	Each	0.17	0.41	1.30	9.46	0.00	0.11	0.00	0.07
	Crackers, Wheat, w/ Cheese Filling	14.1750	1.000	Each	1.39	3.54	8.25	70.45	0.00	0.44	0.99	0.59
	Crackers, Wheat, w/ Peanut Butter	14.1750	1.000	Each	1.91	3.78	7.63	70.17	0.00	0.62	0.00	0.65
215	Crackers, Whole-wheat	4.0000	1.000	Each	0.35	0.69	2.74	17.72	0.00	0.42	0.00	0.12
216	Crackers, Whole-wheat, Low Salt	4.0000	1.000	Each	0.35	0.69	2.74	17.72	0.00	0.00	0.00	0.12
	Croutons, Plain	30.0000	1.000	Cup	3.57	1.98	22.05	122.10	0.00	1.53	0.00	0.45
	Croutons, Seasoned	40.0000	1.000	Cup	4.32	7.32	25.40	186.00	0.00	2.00	2.80	2.10
	English Muffins, Mixed-grain	56.7000	1.000	Each	5.16	1.02	26.26	133.24	0.00	1.58	0.00	0.14
	English Muffins, Mixed-grain, Toasted	56.7000	1.000	Each	5.62	1.08	28.52	144.58	0.00	1.72	0.00	0.14
	English Muffins, Plain	56.7000	1.000	Each	4.36	1.02	26.08	133.24	0.00	1.54	0.00	0.14
	English Muffins, Plain, Toasted	56.7000	1.000	Each	4.76	1.14	28.36	144.58	0.00	1.64	0.00	0.16
	English Muffins, Raisin-cinnamon	56.7000	1.000	Each	4.26	1.44	27.62	137.78	0.00	1.64	0.00	0.22
	English Muffins, Raisin-cinnamon	56.7000	1.000	Each	4.62	1.64	30.06	149.68	0.00	1.76	0.00	0.24
	English Muffins, Wheat	56.7000	1.000	Each	4.94	1.14	25.40	126.44	0.00	2.62	0.00	0.16
	English Muffins, Wheat, Toasted	56.7000	1.000	Each	5.32	1.20	27.62	137.78	0.00	2.86	0.00	0.18
	English Muffins, Whole-wheat	56.7000	1.000	Each	4.98	1.20	22.90	115.10	0.00	3.80	0.00	0.18
	English Muffins, Whole-wheat, Toasted	56.7000	1.000	Each	5.44	1.30	25.00	125.30	0.00	4.14	0.00	0.20
	Flour, White	125.0000	1.000	Cup	12.91	1.23	95.39	455.00	0.00	3.38	0.00	0.20

Page Key: A2 = Baby Food   A2 = Baked Goods   A8 = Beverages   A14 = Breads/Grains and Pasta   A18 = Breakfast Foods/Cereals   A26 = Dairy and Eggs   A40 = Fats and Oils   A42 = Fruits and Vegetables   A52 = Meats and Beans   A60 = Nuts and Seeds   A62 5 Frozen Entrees and Packaged Foods   A76 = Restaurant Chains–Fast Foods   A92 = Restaurant Chains–Other   A106 = Seafood and Fish   A110 = Snacks and Sweets   A120 = Soups   A122 = Supplements   A126 = Toppings and Sauces

Monounsaturated Fat (g)	Polyunsaturated Fat (g)	Vitamin D (mg)	Vitamin K (mg)	Vitamin E (mg)	Vitamin A (re)	Vitamin C (mg)	Thiamin (mg)	Riboflavin (mg)	Niacin (mg)	Vitamin B6 (mg)	Folate (mcg)	Vitamin B12 (mcg)	Calcium (mg)	Iron (mg)	Magnesium (mg)	Phosphorus (mg)	Potassium (mg)	Sodium (mg)	Zinc (mg)
0.40	0.19	0.00	0.00	0.00	0.00	0.00	0.12	0.09	0.99	0.02	8.50	0.00	27.00	0.76	6.00	23.50	29.75	134.50	0.16
0.41	0.19	0.00	0.00	0.00	0.00	0.00	0.10	0.08	0.90	0.01	5.98	0.00	27.37	0.77	5.98	23.69	30.13	136.16	0.16
0.48	0.28	0.00	0.00	0.24	0.00	0.00	0.10	0.06	1.09	0.05	14.18	0.00	20.41	0.94	24.38	64.92	71.44	149.40	0.55
0.36	0.92	0.00	0.00	0.45	0.00	0.00	0.08	0.07	1.12	0.06	16.16	0.00	10.21	0.96	25.23	58.12	97.81	108.01	0.47
3.09	4.94	0.00	0.00	1.11	2.55	0.00	0.03	0.02	0.44	0.03	6.24	0.00	48.20	0.21	12.76	39.12	50.18	421.85	0.33
1.62	0.66	0.00	0.00	0.32	0.00	0.00	0.26	0.18	2.54	0.06	53.86	0.00	53.86	2.24	24.94	69.18	90.72	259.68	0.60
0.48	1.42	0.00	0.00	0.88	0.00	0.06	0.28	0.18	2.22	0.02	53.86	0.04	78.82	1.80	11.34	49.84	79.94	317.52	0.36
0.02	0.03	0.00	0.00	0.00	0.00	0.00	0.00	0.00	0.00	0.00	0.00	0.00	2.56	0.60	3.84	16.64	3.84	11.52	0.08
0.04	0.10	0.00	0.00	0.02	0.00	0.00	0.10	0.04	1.54	0.08	23.55	0.00	12.56	0.60	12.56	34.54	91.06	7.85	0.41
7.51	1.53	0.00	0.00	1.64	18.60	0.00	0.35	0.27	2.90	0.34	49.60	0.29	93.62	2.96	22.32	135.16	89.90	616.90	0.70
0.85	0.31	0.00	0.00	0.00	0.00	0.00	0.03	0.02	0.46	0.10	1.75	0.00	5.53	0.20	4.06	22.68	17.15	69.44	0.08
0.00	0.00	0.00	0.00	0.00	0.00	0.00	0.00	0.00	0.00	0.00	0.00	0.00	3.42	0.06	0.00	0.00	0.00	21.40	0.00
0.02	0.06	0.00	0.00	0.00	0.00	0.00	0.02	0.01	0.10	0.02	2.20	0.00	3.10	0.24	7.80	26.90	31.90	26.40	0.24
0.00	0.00	0.00	0.00	0.00	0.00	0.00	0.00	0.00	0.00	0.00	0.00	0.00	0.00	0.01	0.00	0.00	0.00	2.01	0.00
0.35	0.11	0.00	0.00	0.00	0.00	0.00	0.02	0.02	0.29	0.00	1.19	0.00	1.68	0.26	2.10	7.28	9.45	42.35	0.06
0.17	0.13	0.00	0.00	0.00	3.69	0.03	0.22	0.18	1.44	0.01	33.17	0.05	11.34	0.77	6.80	41.96	42.53	5.95	0.21
0.28	0.28	0.00	0.00	0.00	1.98	0.06	0.16	0.12	1.39	0.03	44.79	0.06	10.21	1.24	8.51	25.23	23.53	80.80	0.21
0.04	0.17	0.00	0.00	0.02	0.00	0.00	0.11	0.08	1.10	0.03	33.17	0.00	3.69	0.90	7.09	25.23	31.75	0.57	0.19
0.05	0.18	0.00	0.00	0.38	0.00	0.00	0.10	0.08	1.53	0.05	9.92	0.00	6.52	1.32	37.99	86.47	89.59	0.57	0.74
0.23	0.38	0.00	0.00	0.02	0.00	0.00	0.12	0.08	1.23	0.03	37.20	0.00	27.90	1.11	17.70	58.80	60.60	248.70	0.60
0.04	0.06	0.00	0.00	0.00	0.00	0.00	0.02	0.01	0.21	0.00	1.30	0.00	4.65	0.19	2.95	9.80	10.10	0.95	0.10
0.13	0.19	0.00	0.00	0.09	0.00	0.00	0.07	0.04	0.67	0.01	12.05	0.00	11.06	0.52	5.53	25.94	27.36	127.43	0.19
0.08	0.13	0.00	0.00	0.00	0.00	0.00	0.06	0.04	0.72	0.01	18.71	0.00	6.10	0.64	7.94	23.39	20.98	118.64	0.21
6.60	5.92	0.00	0.00	2.80	0.00	0.00	0.25	0.21	2.51	0.03	47.74	0.00	74.40	2.23	16.74	141.36	82.46	525.14	0.42
6.60	5.92	0.00	0.00	2.80	0.00	0.00	0.25	0.21	2.51	0.03	47.74	0.00	74.40	2.23	16.74	141.36	220.10	231.26	0.42
1.74	0.41	0.00	0.00	0.00	5.53	0.06	0.09	0.07	0.51	0.01	11.48	0.02	31.47	0.35	5.24	48.05	48.48	147.99	0.10
0.04	0.10	0.00	0.00	0.00	0.50	0.03	0.11	0.07	0.40	0.07	11.25	0.00	10.00	1.49	30.25	83.50	123.75	198.50	0.70
0.46	0.51	0.00	0.00	0.00	0.14	0.01	0.05	0.03	0.35	0.03	7.37	0.00	6.24	0.43	15.03	43.52	64.35	125.73	0.36
0.19	0.06	0.00	0.00	0.00	0.00	0.00	0.02	0.01	0.16	0.00	0.93	0.00	3.57	0.16	0.81	3.15	3.84	39.06	0.02
0.00	0.00	0.00	0.00	0.00	0.00	0.00	0.00	0.00	0.00	0.00	0.00	0.00	0.00	0.12	0.00	0.00	25.60	36.00	0.00
0.19	0.06	0.00	0.00	0.00	0.00	0.00	0.02	0.01	0.16	0.00	0.93	0.00	3.57	0.16	0.81	3.15	21.72	19.08	0.02
1.59	0.36	0.00	0.00	0.37	2.69	0.01	0.06	0.10	0.53	0.01	11.91	0.01	36.43	0.34	5.10	57.55	60.81	198.59	0.09
1.79	0.62	0.00	0.00	0.53	0.00	0.00	0.06	0.05	0.83	0.02	11.91	0.00	13.75	0.43	7.51	34.16	31.61	133.53	0.15
0.00	0.00	0.00	0.00	0.00	0.00	0.00	0.00	0.00	0.00	0.00	0.00	0.00	4.80	0.08	0.00	0.00	9.00	34.00	0.00
0.23	0.06	0.00	0.00	0.00	0.00	0.00	0.01	0.01	0.10	0.00	0.36	0.00	0.98	0.09	1.24	4.40	4.06	5.66	0.03
0.23	0.06	0.00	0.00	0.00	0.00	0.00	0.01	0.01	0.10	0.00	0.36	0.00	0.98	0.09	1.24	4.40	3.66	15.90	0.03
1.47	1.30	0.00	0.00	0.00	1.28	0.21	0.05	0.06	0.45	0.04	9.07	0.02	28.92	0.37	7.65	54.15	43.38	129.42	0.12
1.67	1.26	0.00	0.00	0.00	0.00	0.06	0.04	0.83	0.02	9.92	0.00	24.10	0.38	5.39	49.19	42.10	114.39	0.12
0.38	0.11	0.00	0.00	0.00	0.00	0.00	0.01	0.00	0.18	0.01	1.12	0.00	2.00	0.12	3.96	11.80	11.88	26.36	0.09
0.38	0.11	0.00	0.00	0.00	0.00	0.00	0.01	0.00	0.18	0.01	1.12	0.00	2.00	0.12	3.96	11.80	11.88	9.88	0.09
0.92	0.38	0.00	0.00	0.00	0.00	0.00	0.19	0.08	1.63	0.01	39.60	0.00	22.80	1.22	9.30	34.50	37.20	209.40	0.27
3.80	0.95	0.00	0.00	0.87	4.00	0.00	0.20	0.17	1.86	0.03	35.20	0.06	38.40	1.13	16.80	56.00	72.40	495.20	0.38
0.48	0.32	0.00	0.00	0.16	0.00	0.00	0.24	0.18	2.02	0.02	45.36	0.00	111.14	1.72	23.24	45.92	88.46	235.88	0.78
0.52	0.54	0.00	0.00	0.70	0.56	0.00	0.20	0.18	2.00	0.06	37.98	0.00	120.78	1.86	27.22	91.86	95.82	256.86	0.60
0.18	0.50	0.00	0.00	0.10	0.00	0.00	0.24	0.16	2.20	0.02	45.92	0.02	98.66	1.42	11.90	75.42	74.28	263.08	0.40
0.18	0.54	0.00	0.00	0.10	0.00	0.06	0.22	0.16	2.16	0.02	41.96	0.02	107.16	1.54	12.48	82.22	81.08	285.76	0.44
0.28	0.78	0.00	0.00	0.24	0.00	0.18	0.22	0.16	2.02	0.04	45.92	0.00	83.34	1.38	8.50	39.12	117.94	253.44	0.56
0.32	0.82	0.00	0.00	0.10	0.00	0.18	0.18	0.16	3.96	0.04	39.12	0.00	90.16	1.50	9.64	47.62	128.14	275.56	0.62
0.16	0.48	0.00	0.00	0.28	0.00	0.00	0.24	0.16	1.90	0.06	31.18	0.00	100.92	1.62	20.98	60.66	105.46	216.60	0.60
0.18	0.52	0.00	0.00	0.20	0.00	0.00	0.22	0.16	1.86	0.06	26.04	0.00	109.44	1.76	23.82	70.88	114.54	235.30	0.70
0.28	0.48	0.00	0.00	0.40	0.00	0.00	0.18	0.08	1.94	0.10	27.78	0.00	150.26	1.38	40.26	159.90	119.08	361.18	0.90
0.32	0.52	0.00	0.00	0.44	0.00	0.00	0.14	0.08	1.90	0.10	20.98	0.00	163.12	1.50	43.66	174.06	129.28	392.36	0.98
0.11	0.51	0.00	0.63	0.08	0.00	0.00	0.99	0.61	7.38	0.05	192.50	0.00	18.75	5.80	27.50	135.00	133.75	2.50	0.88

USDA ID Code	Food Name	Weight in Grams*	Quantity of Units	Unit of Measure	Protein (g)	Fat (g)	Carbohydrate (g)	Kilocalories	Caffeine (g)	Fiber (g)	Cholesterol (mg)	Saturated Fat (g)
	Flour, Whole Grain	120.0000	1.000	Cup	16.44	2.24	87.08	406.80	0.00	14.64	0.00	0.38
	Grits	165.0000	1.000	Cup	2.44	1.45	23.53	118.80	0.00	4.13	0.00	0.20
	Hominy, Cnd, Yellow	160.0000	1.000	Cup	2.37	1.41	22.82	115.20	0.00	4.00	0.00	0.19
	Hush Puppies	152.0000	1.000	Cup	11.70	20.52	69.92	512.24	0.00	4.26	68.40	3.21
	Macaroni, Ckd, Enriched	140.0000	1.000	Cup	6.68	0.94	39.68	197.40	0.00	1.82	0.00	0.14
	Macaroni, Ckd, Unenriched	140.0000	1.000	Cup	6.68	0.94	39.68	197.40	0.00	1.82	0.00	0.14
	Macaroni, Vegetable, Ckd, Enriched	134.0000	1.000	Cup	6.07	0.15	35.66	171.52	0.00	5.76	0.00	0.03
	Macaroni, Whole-wheat, Ckd	140.0000	1.000	Cup	7.46	0.76	37.16	173.60	0.00	3.92	0.00	0.14
	Noodles, Chinese, Chow Mein	45.0000	1.000	Cup	3.77	13.84	25.89	237.15	0.00	1.76	0.00	1.97
	Noodles, Egg, Ckd, Enriched	160.0000	1.000	Cup	7.60	2.35	39.74	212.80	0.00	1.76	52.80	0.50
	Noodles, Egg, Ckd, Unenriched	160.0000	1.000	Cup	7.60	2.35	39.74	212.80	0.00	0.00	52.80	0.50
	Noodles, Egg, Spinach, Ckd, Enriched	160.0000	1.000	Cup	8.06	2.51	38.80	211.20	0.00	3.68	52.80	0.58
	Noodles, Japanese, Soba, Ckd	114.0000	1.000	Cup	5.77	0.11	24.44	112.86	0.00	0.00	0.00	0.02
	Noodles, Ramen	86.0000	1.000	Each	10.00	16.00	52.00	380.00	0.00	2.00	0.00	8.00
615	Noodles, Rice Stick	56.0000	2.000	Ounce	0.00	0.00	48.00	193.00	0.00	0.00	0.00	0.00
616	Noodles, Rice, dry	28.0000	0.500	Cup	2.30	3.00	21.40	121.00	0.00	0.40	0.00	0.60
	Pasta, Ckd, Enriched, w/ Added Salt	140.0000	1.000	Cup	6.68	0.94	39.68	197.40	0.00	2.38	0.00	0.14
	Pasta, Ckd, Enriched, w/o Added Salt	140.0000	1.000	Cup	6.68	0.94	39.68	197.40	0.00	2.38	0.00	0.14
	Pasta, Fresh-refrigerated, Plain	57.0000	2.000	Ounce	2.94	0.60	14.21	74.67	0.00	0.00	18.81	0.09
	Pasta, Fresh-refrigerated, Spina	57.0000	2.000	Ounce	2.88	0.54	14.27	74.10	0.00	0.00	18.81	0.13
	Pasta, Homemade, Made w/ Egg, Ckd	57.0000	2.000	Ounce	3.01	0.99	13.42	74.10	0.00	0.00	23.37	0.23
	Pasta, Homemade, Made w/o Egg, Ckd	57.0000	2.000	Ounce	2.49	0.56	14.32	70.68	0.00	0.00	0.00	0.08
	Pasta, Spinach, Ckd	140.0000	1.000	Cup	6.41	0.88	36.61	182.00	0.00	0.00	0.00	0.13
	Pasta, Whole-wheat, Ckd	140.0000	1.000	Cup	7.46	0.76	37.16	173.60	0.00	6.30	0.00	0.14
690	Rice, Basmati	45.0000	0.250	Cup	3.00	0.00	34.00	150.00	0.00	0.00	0.00	0.00
	Rice, Brown, Long-grain, Ckd	195.0000	1.000	Cup	5.03	1.76	44.77	216.45	0.00	3.51	0.00	0.35
	Rice, Brown, Medium-grain, Ckd	195.0000	1.000	Cup	4.52	1.62	45.84	218.40	0.00	3.51	0.00	0.33
691	Rice, Dirty Rice, mix	38.0000	3.000	Tbsp	3.00	0.00	29.00	130.00	0.00	0.00	0.00	0.00
693	Rice, Jasmine	45.0000	0.250	Cup	3.00	0.00	34.00	150.00	0.00	0.00	0.00	0.00
	Rice, w/ Red Beans	28.3500	2.000	Ounce	3.98	0.50	19.89	94.50	0.00	3.48	0.00	0.00
	Rice, White, Long-grain, Ckd	158.0000	1.000	Cup	4.25	0.44	44.51	205.40	0.00	0.63	0.00	0.13
	Rice, White, Long-grain, Instant	165.0000	1.000	Cup	3.40	0.26	35.10	161.70	0.00	0.99	0.00	0.07
	Rice, White, Medium-grain, Ckd	186.0000	1.000	Cup	4.43	0.39	53.18	241.80	0.00	0.56	0.00	0.11
	Rice, White, Short-grain, Ckd	186.0000	1.000	Cup	4.39	0.35	53.44	241.80	0.00	0.00	0.00	0.09
	Rice, White, w/ Pasta, Ckd	202.0000	1.000	Cup	5.13	5.70	43.29	246.44	0.00	5.05	2.02	1.09
	Rice, Wild, Ckd	164.0000	1.000	Cup	6.54	0.56	35.00	165.64	0.00	2.95	0.00	0.08
	Rice, Wild, Uncle Ben's	56.0000	1.000	Cup	6.00	0.50	41.00	190.00	0.00	1.00	0.00	0.00
	Sesame Breadsticks, Wheat-based,	28.3500	1.000	Ounce	3.09	10.40	13.18	153.37	0.00	0.00	0.00	1.84
	Tabouli	28.3500	1.000	Ounce	1.00	2.00	2.00	30.00	0.00	1.00	0.00	0.00
	Taco Shells, Baked	28.3500	1.000	Ounce	2.04	6.41	17.69	132.68	0.00	2.13	0.00	0.92
	Taco Shells, Baked, w/o Added Salt	28.3500	1.000	Ounce	2.04	6.41	17.69	132.68	0.00	2.13	0.00	0.92
739	Tempeh	166.0000	1.000	Cup	31.46	12.75	28.27	330.34	0.00	0.00	0.00	1.84
	Tortillas, Corn	28.3500	1.000	Each	1.62	0.71	13.21	62.94	0.00	1.47	0.00	0.09
	Tortillas, Corn, w/o Added Salt	28.3500	1.000	Each	1.62	0.71	13.21	62.94	0.00	1.47	0.00	0.09
	Tortillas, Flour	28.3500	1.000	Each	2.47	2.01	15.76	92.14	0.00	0.94	0.00	0.50
	Tortillas, Flour, w/o Added Salt	28.3500	1.000	Each	2.47	2.01	15.76	92.14	0.00	0.94	0.00	0.50

Breakfast Foods/Cereals

USDA ID Code	Food Name	Weight in Grams*	Quantity of Units	Unit of Measure	Protein (g)	Fat (g)	Carbohydrate (g)	Kilocalories	Caffeine (g)	Fiber (g)	Cholesterol (mg)	Saturated Fat (g)
	Biscuit	28.3500	1.000	Each	1.73	2.61	8.22	62.94	0.00	0.00	15.88	0.56
	Cereal, Bran 100%	66.0000	1.000	Cup	8.25	3.30	48.11	177.54	0.00	19.54	0.00	0.59
	Cereal, 100% Natural Cereal, Plain	48.0000	0.500	Cup	5.05	7.90	32.95	213.12	0.00	3.60	0.48	3.47
	Cereal, 100% Natural Cereal, w/	110.0000	1.000	Cup	11.22	20.35	72.38	496.10	0.00	7.26	0.00	13.68
	Cereal, 100% Natural Cereal, w/a	104.0000	1.000	Cup	10.71	19.55	69.78	477.36	0.00	6.86	0.00	15.46
	Cereal, 100% Natural Cereal, w/o	48.0000	0.500	Cup	5.05	7.90	32.95	213.12	0.00	3.60	0.48	3.47

Page Key: A2 = Baby Food   A2 = Baked Goods   A8 = Beverages   A14 = Breads/Grains and Pasta   A18 = Breakfast Foods/Cereals   A26 = Dairy and Eggs   A40 = Fats and Oils   A42 = Fruits and Vegetables   A52 = Meats and Beans   A60 = Nuts and Seeds   A62 5 Frozen Entrees and Packaged Foods   A76 = Restaurant Chains–Fast Foods   A92 = Restaurant Chains–Other   A106 = Seafood and Fish   A110 = Snacks and Sweets   A120 = Soups   A122 = Supplements   A126 = Toppings and Sauces

Monounsaturated Fat (g)	Polyunsaturated Fat (g)	Vitamin D (mg)	Vitamin K (mg)	Vitamin E (mg)	Vitamin A (re)	Vitamin C (mg)	Thiamin (mg)	Riboflavin (mg)	Niacin (mg)	Vitamin B₆ (mg)	Folate (mcg)	Vitamin B₁₂ (mcg)	Calcium (mg)	Iron (mg)	Magnesium (mg)	Phosphorus (mg)	Potassium (mg)	Sodium (mg)	Zinc (mg)
0.28	0.94	0.00	1.32	1.48	0.00	0.00	0.54	0.26	7.64	0.41	52.80	0.00	40.80	4.66	165.60	415.20	486.00	6.00	3.52
0.38	0.66	0.00	0.00	0.08	0.00	0.00	0.00	0.02	0.05	0.02	1.65	0.00	16.50	1.02	26.40	57.75	14.85	346.50	1.73
0.37	0.64	0.00	0.00	0.00	17.60	0.00	0.00	0.02	0.05	0.02	1.60	0.00	16.00	0.99	25.60	56.00	14.40	336.00	1.68
4.96	10.97	0.00	0.00	3.62	65.36	0.30	0.53	0.50	4.23	0.15	112.48	0.29	422.56	4.62	36.48	287.28	218.88	1015.36	1.00
0.11	0.38	0.00	0.00	0.04	0.00	0.00	0.28	0.14	2.34	0.06	98.00	0.00	9.80	1.96	25.20	75.60	43.40	1.40	0.74
0.11	0.38	0.00	0.00	0.04	0.00	0.00	0.03	0.03	0.56	0.06	9.80	0.00	9.80	0.70	25.20	75.60	43.40	1.40	0.74
0.01	0.05	0.00	0.00	0.05	6.70	0.00	0.15	0.08	1.43	0.03	87.10	0.00	14.74	0.66	25.46	67.00	41.54	8.04	0.59
0.11	0.29	0.00	0.00	0.14	0.00	0.00	0.15	0.07	0.99	0.11	7.00	0.00	21.00	1.48	42.00	124.60	61.60	4.20	1.13
3.46	7.80	0.00	0.00	0.07	4.05	0.00	0.26	0.19	2.68	0.05	40.50	0.00	9.00	2.13	23.40	72.45	54.00	197.55	0.63
0.69	0.66	0.00	0.00	0.00	9.60	0.00	0.30	0.13	2.38	0.06	102.40	0.14	19.20	2.54	30.40	110.40	44.80	264.00	0.99
0.69	0.66	0.00	0.00	0.00	9.60	0.00	0.05	0.03	0.64	0.06	11.20	0.14	19.20	0.96	30.40	110.40	44.80	264.00	0.99
0.78	0.56	0.00	0.00	0.08	22.40	0.00	0.40	0.19	2.35	0.18	102.40	0.22	30.40	1.74	38.40	91.20	59.20	19.20	1.01
0.03	0.03	0.00	0.00	0.00	0.00	0.00	0.10	0.03	0.58	0.05	7.98	0.00	4.56	0.55	10.26	28.50	39.90	68.40	0.14
0.00	0.00	0.00	0.00	0.00	0.00	0.00	0.00	0.00	0.00	0.00	0.00	0.00	0.00	1.60	0.00	0.00	0.00	1560.00	0.00
0.00	0.00	0.00	0.00	0.00	0.00	0.00	0.00	0.00	0.00	0.00	0.00	0.00	0.00	0.00	0.00	0.00	0.00	100.00	0.00
0.00	0.00	0.00	0.00	0.00	0.00	0.00	0.00	0.00	0.00	0.00	0.00	0.00	17.00	0.83	0.00	0.00	0.00	378.00	0.00
0.11	0.38	0.00	0.00	0.00	0.00	0.00	0.28	0.14	2.34	0.06	98.00	0.00	9.80	1.96	25.20	75.60	43.40	140.00	0.74
0.11	0.38	0.00	0.00	0.08	0.00	0.00	0.28	0.14	2.34	0.06	98.00	0.00	9.80	1.96	25.20	75.60	43.40	1.40	0.74
0.07	0.25	0.00	0.00	0.00	3.42	0.00	0.12	0.09	0.56	0.02	36.48	0.08	3.42	0.65	10.26	35.91	13.68	3.42	0.32
0.17	0.12	0.00	0.00	0.00	7.98	0.00	0.10	0.07	0.58	0.06	36.48	0.08	10.26	0.63	13.68	32.49	21.09	3.42	0.36
0.29	0.30	0.00	0.00	0.00	9.69	0.00	0.10	0.10	0.72	0.02	24.51	0.06	5.70	0.66	7.98	29.64	11.97	47.31	0.25
0.11	0.29	0.00	0.00	0.00	0.00	0.00	0.10	0.09	0.76	0.02	24.51	0.00	3.42	0.64	7.98	22.80	10.83	42.18	0.21
0.10	0.36	0.00	0.00	0.00	21.00	0.00	0.14	0.14	2.14	0.14	16.80	0.00	42.00	1.46	86.80	151.20	81.20	19.60	1.51
0.11	0.29	0.00	0.00	0.07	0.00	0.00	0.15	0.07	0.99	0.11	7.00	0.00	21.00	1.48	42.00	124.60	61.60	4.20	1.13
0.00	0.00	0.00	0.00	0.00	0.00	0.00	0.00	0.00	0.00	0.00	0.00	0.00	0.00	0.00	0.00	0.00	0.00	0.00	0.00
0.64	0.62	0.00	0.00	1.40	0.00	0.00	0.20	0.06	2.98	0.29	7.80	0.00	19.50	0.82	83.85	161.85	83.85	9.75	1.23
0.59	0.59	0.00	0.00	0.00	0.00	0.00	0.20	0.02	2.59	0.29	7.80	0.00	19.50	1.03	85.80	150.15	154.05	1.95	1.21
0.00	0.00	0.00	0.00	0.00	0.00	0.00	0.00	0.00	0.00	0.00	0.00	0.00	0.00	0.00	0.00	0.00	0.00	680.00	0.00
0.00	0.00	0.00	0.00	0.00	0.00	0.00	0.00	0.00	0.00	0.00	0.00	0.00	0.00	0.00	0.00	0.00	0.00	0.00	0.00
0.00	0.00	0.00	0.00	0.00	49.74	2.98	0.11	0.00	1.42	0.00	0.00	0.00	23.87	0.75	0.00	0.00	0.00	392.92	0.00
0.14	0.13	0.00	0.00	0.08	0.00	0.00	0.25	0.02	2.34	0.14	91.64	0.00	15.80	1.90	18.96	67.94	55.30	1.58	0.77
0.08	0.07	0.00	0.00	0.08	0.00	0.00	0.13	0.08	1.45	0.02	67.65	0.00	13.20	1.04	8.25	23.10	6.60	4.95	0.40
0.13	0.11	0.00	0.00	0.00	0.00	0.00	0.32	0.04	3.42	0.09	107.88	0.00	5.58	2.77	24.18	68.82	53.94	0.00	0.78
0.11	0.09	0.00	0.00	0.00	0.00	0.00	0.30	0.04	2.77	0.11	109.74	0.00	1.86	2.72	14.88	61.38	48.36	0.00	0.74
2.26	1.92	0.00	0.00	0.00	0.00	0.00	0.40	0.24	3.60	0.20	88.88	0.12	16.16	1.90	24.24	74.84	84.84	1147.36	0.57
0.08	0.34	0.00	0.00	0.38	0.00	0.00	0.08	0.15	2.12	0.23	42.64	0.00	4.92	0.98	52.48	134.48	165.64	4.92	2.20
0.00	0.00	0.00	0.00	0.00	0.00	2.40	0.00	0.00	0.00	0.00	0.00	0.00	24.00	1.00	0.00	0.00	0.00	620.00	0.00
3.09	4.94	0.00	0.00	0.00	2.55	0.00	0.03	0.02	0.44	0.03	6.24	0.00	48.20	0.21	12.76	39.12	50.18	8.22	0.33
0.00	0.00	0.00	0.00	0.00	100.00	12.00	0.00	0.00	0.00	0.00	0.00	0.00	0.00	0.40	0.00	0.00	0.00	75.00	0.00
2.53	2.41	0.00	0.00	1.03	0.00	0.00	0.07	0.01	0.38	0.09	29.77	0.00	45.36	0.71	29.77	70.31	50.75	104.04	0.40
2.53	2.41	0.00	0.00	1.03	0.00	0.00	0.07	0.01	0.38	0.09	29.77	0.00	45.36	0.71	29.77	70.31	50.75	4.25	0.40
2.81	7.19	0.00	0.00	0.00	114.54	0.00	0.22	0.18	7.69	0.50	86.32	1.66	154.38	3.75	116.20	341.96	609.22	9.96	3.01
0.18	0.32	0.00	0.00	0.04	0.00	0.00	0.03	0.02	0.43	0.06	32.32	0.00	49.61	0.40	18.43	89.02	43.66	45.64	0.27
0.18	0.32	0.00	0.00	0.04	0.00	0.00	0.03	0.02	0.43	0.06	32.32	0.00	49.61	0.40	18.43	89.02	43.66	3.12	0.27
1.07	0.30	0.00	0.00	0.26	0.00	0.00	0.15	0.08	1.01	0.01	34.87	0.00	35.44	0.94	7.37	35.15	37.14	135.51	0.20
1.07	0.30	0.00	0.00	0.26	0.00	0.00	0.15	0.08	1.01	0.01	34.87	0.00	11.06	0.94	7.37	35.15	37.14	135.51	0.20
0.66	1.18	0.00	0.00	0.00	14.46	0.62	0.06	0.08	0.43	0.01	10.21	0.06	58.40	0.49	4.54	42.81	39.12	116.80	0.15
0.57	1.87	0.00	0.00	1.53	0.00	62.70	1.58	1.78	20.92	2.11	46.86	6.27	46.20	8.12	312.18	801.24	652.08	457.38	5.74
3.48	1.04	0.00	0.00	0.55	0.48	0.14	0.17	0.08	0.85	0.09	12.00	0.05	46.08	1.44	50.40	148.80	210.72	12.96	1.15
3.72	1.71	0.00	0.00	0.77	6.60	0.00	0.31	0.65	2.09	0.17	45.10	0.15	159.50	3.12	124.30	347.60	537.90	47.30	2.11
1.83	1.33	0.00	0.00	0.73	6.24	1.04	0.33	0.57	1.87	0.11	16.64	0.30	157.04	2.89	71.76	350.48	513.76	52.00	2.00
3.48	1.04	0.00	0.00	0.55	0.48	0.14	0.17	0.08	0.85	0.09	12.00	0.05	46.08	1.44	50.40	148.80	210.72	12.96	1.15

USDA ID Code	Food Name	Weight in Grams*	Quantity of Units	Unit of Measure	Protein (g)	Fat (g)	Carbohydrate (g)	Kilocalories	Caffeine (g)	Fiber (g)	Cholesterol (mg)	Saturated Fat (g)
136	Cereal, 100% Natural Crl, w/oats	51.0000	0.500	Cup	4.84	7.28	35.83	218.28	0.00	3.67	0.51	3.19
	Cereal, All-bran	30.0000	0.500	Cup	3.66	0.93	22.77	79.20	0.00	9.69	0.00	0.21
137	Cereal, All-Bran with Extra Fiber	30.0000	0.500	Cup	3.69	0.93	22.68	52.80	0.00	15.33	0.00	0.17
	Cereal, Almond Crunch	55.0000	1.000	Cup	4.35	0.83	46.92	198.00	0.00	4.62	0.00	0.17
138	Cereal, Almond Crunch w/ Raisins	58.0000	1.000	Cup	5.00	2.50	46.00	210.00	0.00	5.00	0.00	0.00
	Cereal, Alpha-Bits	34.0000	1.000	Cup	2.58	0.78	29.44	133.28	0.00	1.46	0.00	0.13
139	Cereal, Apple Cinnamon Squares	55.0000	0.750	Cup	3.96	0.99	44.06	182.05	0.00	4.73	0.00	0.22
	Cereal, Apple Jacks	30.0000	1.000	Cup	1.44	0.39	26.84	115.50	0.00	0.57	0.00	0.09
	Cereal, Apple Raisin Crisp	55.0000	1.000	Cup	3.47	0.50	46.70	184.80	0.00	4.40	0.00	0.11
	Cereal, Basic 4	55.0000	1.000	Cup	4.18	2.84	41.97	200.75	0.00	3.36	0.00	0.42
	Cereal, Berry Berry-Kix	30.0000	0.750	Cup	1.31	1.16	26.13	120.00	0.00	0.18	0.00	0.20
	Cereal, Blueberry Squares	55.0000	0.750	Cup	4.18	0.99	43.78	181.50	0.00	4.84	0.00	0.22
140	Cereal, Boo Berry	30.0000	1.000	Cup	1.00	0.50	27.00	120.00	0.00	0.00	0.00	0.00
141	Cereal, Bran Buds	30.0000	0.330	Cup	2.82	0.72	23.97	82.80	0.00	11.97	0.00	0.12
	Cereal, Bran Flakes, 40%, Kellogg's	29.0000	0.750	Cup	3.02	0.64	23.16	94.83	0.00	4.61	0.00	0.12
	Cereal, Bran Flakes, 40%, Post	47.0000	1.000	Cup	5.31	0.75	37.27	152.28	0.00	9.17	0.00	0.00
	Cereal, Bran Flakes, 40%, Ralston	49.0000	1.000	Cup	5.64	0.69	39.10	158.76	0.00	6.91	0.00	0.00
	Cereal, Bran Flakes, Kellogg's	29.0000	0.750	Cup	3.02	0.64	23.16	94.83	0.00	4.61	0.00	0.12
	Cereal, Bran Flakes, Post	47.0000	1.000	Cup	5.31	0.75	37.27	152.28	0.00	9.17	0.00	0.12
142	Cereal, Bran, Frosted	30.0000	0.750	Cup	2.37	0.33	25.41	101.40	0.00	3.36	0.00	0.03
	Cereal, Brown Sugar Squares, Toa	55.0000	1.250	Cup	5.23	1.05	44.99	189.20	0.00	5.12	0.00	0.18
	Cereal, C.W. Post, Plain	97.0000	1.000	Cup	7.95	12.80	72.65	420.98	0.00	7.18	0.18	1.67
	Cereal, C.W. Post, w/ Raisins	103.0000	1.000	Cup	8.86	14.73	73.95	445.99	0.00	13.60	0.20	10.97
	Cereal, Cap'n Crunch	27.0000	0.750	Cup	1.35	1.37	23.04	107.19	0.00	0.86	0.00	0.37
	Cereal, Cap'n Crunch's Cruncher	26.0000	0.750	Cup	1.26	1.28	22.26	103.74	0.00	0.57	0.00	0.35
	Cereal, Cap'n Crunch's Peanut Butter	27.0000	0.750	Cup	1.95	2.32	21.51	112.32	0.00	0.78	0.00	0.52
	Cereal, Cheerios	30.0000	1.000	Cup	3.14	1.77	22.86	109.50	0.00	2.64	0.00	0.35
	Cereal, Cheerios, Apple Cinnamon	30.0000	0.750	Cup	1.86	1.63	25.05	117.90	0.00	1.59	0.00	0.30
143	Cereal, Cheerios, Frosted	30.0000	1.000	Cup	2.00	1.00	25.00	120.00	0.00	1.00	0.00	0.00
	Cereal, Cheerios, Honey Nut	30.0000	1.000	Cup	2.78	1.24	24.26	114.90	0.00	1.56	0.00	0.23
	Cereal, Cheerios, Multigrain	30.0000	1.000	Cup	2.56	1.09	24.45	111.90	0.00	1.92	0.00	0.25
	Cereal, Chex, Bran	49.0000	1.000	Cup	5.05	1.37	39.05	156.31	0.00	7.94	0.00	0.20
	Cereal, Chex, Corn	30.0000	1.000	Cup	2.18	0.37	25.61	112.80	0.00	0.54	0.00	0.07
	Cereal, Chex, Rice	31.0000	1.250	Cup	1.92	0.16	27.18	117.18	0.00	0.28	0.00	0.04
	Cereal, Chex, Wheat	30.0000	1.000	Cup	3.16	0.68	24.21	103.80	0.00	3.30	0.00	0.12
	Cereal, Cinnamon Mini Buns	30.0000	0.750	Cup	1.47	0.63	26.61	115.20	0.00	0.66	0.00	0.15
	Cereal, Cinnamon Oatmeal Squares	60.0000	1.000	Cup	7.57	2.57	47.15	231.60	0.00	4.56	0.00	0.50
	Cereal, Cinnamon Toast Crunch	30.0000	0.750	Cup	1.68	3.04	23.84	124.20	0.00	1.50	0.00	0.50
	Cereal, Cocoa Krispies	31.0000	0.750	Cup	1.55	0.81	27.25	120.28	1.24	0.40	0.00	0.59
	Cereal, Cocoa Puffs	30.0000	1.000	Cup	1.14	0.90	26.72	118.80	0.00	0.18	0.00	0.20
	Cereal, Cookie-crisp, Choc Chip	30.0000	1.000	Cup	1.53	1.08	26.25	120.00	0.60	0.42	0.00	0.60
	Cereal, Corn Bran	27.0000	0.750	Cup	1.86	0.89	22.73	89.91	0.00	4.81	0.00	0.21
144	Cereal, Corn Flakes, Country	30.0000	1.000	Cup	1.83	0.50	25.96	114.00	0.00	0.45	0.00	0.15
	Cereal, Corn Flakes, Honey and Nut	55.0000	1.250	Cup	4.02	2.48	45.98	222.75	0.00	0.88	0.00	0.50
145	Cereal, Corn Flakes, Honey Crunch	30.0000	0.750	Cup	5.00	1.00	44.00	190.00	0.00	5.00	0.00	0.00
	Cereal, Corn Flakes, Kellogg's	28.0000	1.000	Cup	1.84	0.20	24.22	102.20	0.00	0.78	0.00	0.06
	Cereal, Corn Flakes, Low Sodium	25.0000	1.000	Cup	1.93	0.08	22.20	99.75	0.00	0.28	0.00	0.01
	Cereal, Corn Flakes, Ralston Pur	25.0000	1.000	Cup	1.95	0.10	21.65	97.50	0.00	0.48	0.00	0.00
	Cereal, Corn Pops	31.0000	1.000	Cup	1.15	0.18	28.43	118.11	0.00	0.43	0.00	0.06
146	Cereal, Count Chocula	30.0000	1.000	Cup	1.00	1.00	26.00	120.00	0.00	0.00	0.00	0.00
	Cereal, Cracklin' Oat Bran	55.0000	0.750	Cup	4.61	6.97	40.10	224.95	0.00	6.55	0.00	2.92
	Cereal, Cream Of Rice, Ckd	244.0000	1.000	Cup	2.20	0.24	28.06	126.88	0.00	0.24	0.00	0.05
	Cereal, Cream Of Wheat, Instant	241.0000	1.000	Cup	4.34	0.48	31.57	154.24	0.00	2.89	0.00	0.07

Monounsaturated Fat (g)	Polyunsaturated Fat (g)	Vitamin D (mg)	Vitamin K (mg)	Vitamin E (mg)	Vitamin A (re)	Vitamin C (mg)	Thiamin (mg)	Riboflavin (mg)	Niacin (mg)	Vitamin B6 (mg)	Folate (mcg)	Vitamin B12 (mcg)	Calcium (mg)	Iron (mg)	Magnesium (mg)	Phosphorus (mg)	Potassium (mg)	Sodium (mg)	Zinc (mg)
3.17	0.82	0.00	0.00	0.51	0.51	0.31	0.14	0.09	0.77	0.08	11.73	0.05	38.76	1.67	47.94	149.94	213.69	11.22	1.08
0.18	0.54	0.03	0.00	0.55	225.30	15.00	0.39	0.42	5.01	0.51	90.00	1.50	105.90	4.50	128.70	294.00	341.70	60.90	3.75
0.18	0.58	0.00	0.00	0.64	259.80	17.31	0.42	0.48	5.76	0.57	120.00	1.74	115.50	5.19	119.70	287.40	300.00	126.90	4.32
0.22	0.44	0.00	0.00	3.00	47.30	0.00	0.52	0.59	7.00	0.69	99.00	2.10	26.40	5.99	48.95	129.80	170.50	284.35	1.43
1.50	1.00	0.05	0.00	3.00	500.00	0.00	0.53	0.60	7.00	0.70	0.10	2.10	20.00	6.30	60.00	150.00	200.00	230.00	1.50
0.26	0.29	0.00	0.00	0.02	450.16	0.00	0.44	0.51	5.98	0.61	120.02	1.80	9.86	3.23	20.06	61.54	65.96	215.90	1.80
0.28	0.50	0.00	0.00	0.59	0.00	0.00	0.39	0.44	5.00	0.50	110.00	1.49	20.90	16.23	48.40	154.00	166.00	19.80	1.49
0.12	0.18	0.00	0.00	0.05	225.30	15.00	0.39	0.42	5.01	0.51	105.90	0.00	3.30	4.50	8.70	30.00	31.80	134.40	3.75
0.17	0.22	0.00	0.00	0.46	233.75	0.00	0.39	0.44	5.17	0.50	110.00	1.54	14.85	1.87	9.90	85.80	85.25	373.45	1.54
0.99	1.10	0.00	0.00	0.68	375.10	14.96	0.37	0.42	5.00	0.50	99.55	0.00	309.65	4.50	40.15	231.55	161.70	322.85	3.75
0.46	0.06	0.00	0.00	0.17	225.30	15.00	0.38	0.43	5.00	0.50	99.90	0.00	66.00	4.50	5.70	37.20	23.70	184.50	3.75
0.22	0.55	0.00	0.00	0.85	0.00	0.00	0.39	0.44	5.12	0.50	110.00	1.54	19.25	16.50	51.15	161.70	183.15	20.35	1.54
0.00	0.00	0.00	0.00	0.00	0.00	15.00	0.38	0.43	5.00	0.50	100.00	0.00	20.00	4.50	0.00	20.00	15.00	210.00	3.75
0.15	0.45	0.00	0.00	0.48	225.30	15.00	0.39	0.42	5.01	0.51	90.00	0.00	20.10	4.50	83.40	166.20	269.70	199.80	6.45
0.12	0.41	0.03	0.00	5.37	362.79	14.99	0.38	0.44	5.00	0.49	102.37	1.45	13.92	8.12	60.03	149.93	175.16	226.20	3.75
0.00	0.00	0.00	0.00	0.54	622.28	0.00	0.61	0.70	8.27	0.85	165.91	2.49	20.68	7.47	101.52	296.10	250.51	430.99	2.49
0.00	0.00	0.00	0.00	0.00	648.76	25.97	0.64	0.74	8.62	0.88	172.97	2.60	22.54	7.79	117.60	272.93	286.16	456.19	2.04
0.12	0.41	0.00	0.00	5.37	362.79	14.99	0.38	0.44	5.00	0.49	102.37	1.45	13.92	8.12	60.03	149.93	175.16	226.20	3.75
0.11	0.37	0.00	0.00	0.54	622.28	0.00	0.61	0.71	8.27	0.85	165.91	2.49	20.68	13.44	101.52	296.10	250.51	430.99	2.49
0.09	0.21	0.00	0.00	0.23	217.80	14.52	0.36	0.42	4.83	0.48	90.00	1.44	9.30	4.35	37.80	92.40	122.10	206.40	3.63
0.15	0.43	0.00	0.00	3.00	51.15	0.00	0.55	0.61	7.15	0.72	110.00	2.15	18.70	6.44	59.40	194.15	213.95	1.65	1.54
6.00	4.66	0.00	0.00	0.68	1284.28	0.00	1.26	1.46	17.07	1.75	342.41	5.14	46.56	15.42	66.93	224.07	197.88	166.84	1.64
1.67	1.38	0.00	0.00	0.72	1363.72	0.00	1.34	1.55	18.13	1.85	363.59	5.46	50.47	16.38	74.16	231.75	260.59	160.68	1.64
0.27	0.19	0.00	0.00	0.14	3.51	0.00	0.38	0.42	5.00	0.50	100.17	0.00	5.40	4.50	9.45	28.62	34.56	208.44	3.75
0.26	0.20	0.00	0.00	0.18	4.68	0.03	0.37	0.42	5.00	0.50	100.10	0.01	6.50	4.50	9.88	29.64	36.66	190.32	4.01
0.82	0.53	0.00	0.00	0.15	3.78	0.00	0.38	0.42	5.00	0.50	100.17	0.00	2.70	4.50	18.63	51.84	62.10	203.85	3.75
0.64	0.22	0.03	0.00	0.21	375.30	15.00	0.38	0.43	5.00	0.50	99.90	0.00	55.20	8.10	32.70	114.00	88.50	284.10	3.75
0.64	0.21	0.00	0.00	0.30	225.30	15.00	0.38	0.43	5.00	0.50	99.90	0.00	35.40	4.50	20.10	65.10	60.00	150.30	3.75
0.00	0.00	0.00	0.00	0.00	750.00	15.00	0.38	0.43	5.00	0.50	100.00	0.00	20.00	4.50	16.00	60.00	60.00	210.00	3.75
0.48	0.19	0.03	0.00	0.31	225.30	15.00	0.38	0.43	5.00	0.50	99.90	0.00	20.40	4.50	29.40	102.90	85.20	258.90	3.75
0.30	0.15	0.00	0.00	0.19	225.30	15.00	0.38	0.43	5.00	0.50	99.90	0.00	57.00	8.10	29.70	114.30	97.20	254.10	3.75
0.25	0.67	0.00	0.00	0.56	10.78	25.97	0.64	0.26	8.62	0.88	172.97	2.60	29.40	13.99	69.09	172.97	216.09	345.45	6.48
0.09	0.20	0.00	0.00	0.10	0.00	6.00	0.38	0.00	5.00	0.50	99.90	1.50	100.20	9.00	8.40	21.60	32.40	288.90	0.37
0.05	0.05	0.00	0.00	0.00	0.00	6.01	0.38	0.02	5.00	0.50	99.82	1.50	103.54	9.00	9.30	35.34	35.96	291.40	0.00
0.11	0.28	0.00	0.00	0.44	0.00	3.60	0.23	0.04	3.00	0.30	60.00	0.90	60.00	9.00	33.60	109.50	116.10	268.50	0.74
0.18	0.30	0.00	0.00	0.05	225.30	15.00	0.39	0.42	5.01	0.51	90.00	0.00	3.90	4.50	11.10	24.00	36.60	207.60	3.75
0.86	1.07	0.00	0.00	2.22	165.00	6.60	0.41	0.46	5.48	0.55	109.80	0.00	41.40	14.55	70.20	181.80	250.20	266.40	4.11
0.93	0.53	0.00	0.00	0.28	225.30	15.00	0.38	0.43	5.00	0.50	99.90	0.00	42.30	4.50	13.50	74.40	44.10	210.30	3.75
0.09	0.12	0.00	0.00	0.14	225.06	15.00	0.37	0.43	4.99	0.50	93.00	0.00	4.03	1.80	11.47	29.45	60.14	210.18	1.49
0.35	0.05	0.00	0.00	0.14	0.00	15.00	0.38	0.43	5.00	0.50	99.90	0.00	33.00	4.50	6.60	42.60	52.20	180.60	3.75
0.22	0.16	0.00	0.00	0.08	0.00	0.00	0.39	0.27	5.28	0.54	105.90	1.59	5.70	4.77	8.40	24.00	29.40	206.70	3.17
0.23	0.27	0.00	0.00	0.14	3.78	0.00	0.08	0.42	5.00	0.50	100.17	0.00	20.52	7.56	14.31	35.64	56.16	253.26	3.75
0.09	0.03	0.00	0.00	0.08	225.30	15.00	0.38	0.43	5.00	0.50	99.90	0.00	53.40	8.10	7.20	39.30	40.50	283.80	3.75
1.16	0.83	1.25	0.00	0.14	225.50	15.02	0.39	0.44	5.01	0.50	110.00	0.00	5.50	4.51	4.95	36.30	59.95	370.15	0.39
0.50	0.00	0.05	0.00	3.00	500.00	0.00	0.53	0.60	7.00	0.70	0.10	2.10	0.00	6.30	60.00	200.00	210.00	5.00	1.50
0.03	0.11	0.02	0.00	0.04	210.28	14.00	0.36	0.39	4.68	0.48	98.84	0.00	1.12	8.68	3.36	10.92	25.48	297.92	0.17
0.02	0.03	0.00	0.00	0.03	9.50	0.00	0.00	0.05	0.11	0.02	1.75	0.00	10.75	0.56	3.25	12.25	18.25	2.50	0.07
0.00	0.00	0.00	0.00	0.00	9.50	0.00	0.13	0.03	1.05	0.02	1.75	0.00	1.75	0.63	2.75	9.75	22.00	239.00	0.06
0.06	0.03	0.00	0.00	0.03	232.81	15.50	0.40	0.43	5.18	0.53	109.43	0.00	2.48	1.86	2.48	6.51	22.63	123.07	1.55
0.00	0.00	0.00	0.00	0.00	0.00	15.00	0.38	0.43	5.00	0.50	100.00	1.50	20.00	4.50	0.00	20.00	65.00	190.00	3.75
3.25	0.75	0.05	0.00	0.36	253.00	16.83	0.42	0.48	5.61	0.56	152.90	0.00	24.75	2.04	76.45	186.45	254.65	195.25	1.65
0.00	0.00	0.00	0.00	0.00	0.00	0.00	0.00	0.00	0.98	0.07	7.32	0.00	7.32	0.49	7.32	41.48	48.80	422.12	0.39
0.00	0.00	0.00	0.00	0.00	0.00	0.00	0.24	0.00	1.69	0.02	149.42	0.00	60.25	12.05	14.46	43.38	48.20	363.91	0.41

USDA ID Code	Food Name	Weight in Grams*	Quantity of Units	Unit of Measure	Protein (g)	Fat (g)	Carbohydrate (g)	Kilocalories	Caffeine (g)	Fiber (g)	Cholesterol (mg)	Saturated Fat (g)
	Cereal, Cream Of Wheat, Quick	239.0000	1.000	Cup	3.59	0.48	26.77	129.06	0.00	1.20	0.00	0.07
	Cereal, Cream Of Wheat, Regular	251.0000	1.000	Cup	3.77	0.50	27.61	133.03	0.00	1.76	0.00	0.08
	Cereal, Crisp Rice, Low Sodium	26.0000	1.000	Cup	1.43	0.08	23.66	104.52	0.00	0.36	0.00	0.02
	Cereal, Crispex	29.0000	1.000	Cup	2.15	0.29	25.00	108.46	0.00	0.64	0.00	0.09
	Cereal, Crispy Rice	28.0000	1.000	Cup	1.79	0.11	24.81	110.88	0.00	0.34	0.00	0.03
	Cereal, Crispy Wheats 'n Raisins	55.0000	1.000	Cup	4.47	0.76	44.33	191.40	0.00	3.41	0.00	0.15
147	Cereal, Crunchy Pecan-Great Grains	53.0000	0.660	Cup	5.00	6.00	38.00	220.00	0.00	4.00	0.00	1.00
	Cereal, Fiber One	30.0000	0.500	Cup	2.78	0.84	24.01	61.50	0.00	14.25	0.00	0.13
	Cereal, Fortified Oat Flakes	48.0000	1.000	Cup	8.98	0.72	34.75	177.12	0.00	1.44	0.00	0.00
148	Cereal, Frankenberry	30.0000	1.000	Cup	1.00	1.00	27.00	120.00	0.00	0.00	0.00	0.00
149	Cereal, French Toast Crunch	30.0000	0.750	Cup	1.00	1.50	26.00	120.00	0.00	0.00	0.00	0.00
	Cereal, Frosted Flakes	31.0000	0.750	Cup	1.21	0.16	28.27	119.35	0.00	0.62	0.00	0.06
150	Cereal, Frosted Flakes, Cocoa-Kellogg's	31.0000	0.750	Cup	1.00	0.00	28.00	120.00	0.00	0.00	0.00	0.00
	Cereal, Frosted Mini-Wheats	55.0000	1.000	Cup	5.17	0.88	45.38	186.45	0.00	5.89	0.00	0.17
	Cereal, Fruit Loops	30.0000	1.000	Cup	1.47	0.87	26.46	117.30	0.00	0.57	0.00	0.39
	Cereal, Fruity Pebbles	32.0000	1.000	Cup	1.28	1.66	27.55	129.60	0.00	0.42	0.00	1.37
	Cereal, Golden Grahams	30.0000	0.750	Cup	1.60	1.08	25.69	115.50	0.00	0.93	0.00	0.18
	Cereal, Graham Crackos	30.0000	1.000	Cup	2.25	0.18	25.92	108.30	0.00	1.83	0.00	0.00
151	Cereal, Granola Low Fat w/ Raisin	60.0000	0.500	Cup	5.00	3.00	47.00	220.00	0.00	3.00	0.00	1.00
152	Cereal, Granola Low Fat-Kellogg's	50.0000	0.500	Cup	4.00	3.00	39.00	190.00	0.00	3.00	0.00	0.50
	Cereal, Granola w/ Almonds-Sun C	57.0000	0.500	Cup	6.71	10.27	38.30	266.19	0.00	2.96	0.00	1.27
	Cereal, Granola, Low Fat-Kellogg's	82.4590	1.000	Cup	7.50	4.50	64.47	314.84	0.00	4.50	0.00	1.50
	Cereal, Granola, Homemade	122.0000	1.000	Cup	17.93	30.01	64.66	569.74	0.00	12.81	0.00	5.80
	Cereal, Granola, w/ raisins, Low	55.0000	0.670	Cup	4.51	2.75	43.67	201.85	0.00	3.30	0.00	0.94
	Cereal, Granola, w/o raisins, L	55.0000	0.500	Cup	4.62	3.25	44.17	213.40	0.00	3.25	0.00	0.50
	Cereal, Granola, w/raisins & dates	31.0000	0.500	Cup	3.02	4.23	22.38	135.16	0.00	1.86	0.00	0.64
	Cereal, Granola-Nature Valley	55.0000	0.750	Cup	5.80	9.69	36.23	248.05	0.00	3.52	0.00	1.27
	Cereal, Grape-nuts	109.0000	1.000	Cup	12.75	0.44	89.38	389.13	0.00	10.90	0.00	0.06
	Cereal, Grape-nuts Flakes	39.0000	1.000	Cup	3.94	0.36	26.55	116.20	0.00	3.21	0.00	0.00
	Cereal, Great Grains	79.4600	1.000	Cup	1.13	9.00	56.97	329.84	0.00	6.00	0.00	1.50
	Cereal, Heartland Natural Cereal	115.0000	1.000	Cup	11.62	17.71	78.55	499.10	0.00	7.02	0.00	4.52
	Cereal, Heartland Natural Cereal	110.0000	1.000	Cup	10.67	15.62	75.90	467.50	0.00	6.05	0.00	3.98
	Cereal, Heartland Natural Cereal	105.0000	1.000	Cup	10.92	17.12	71.30	463.05	0.00	7.46	0.00	6.23
153	Cereal, Honey Bunches of Oats	30.0000	0.750	Cup	2.00	1.50	25.00	120.00	0.00	1.00	0.00	0.50
154	Cereal, Honey Bunches of Oats w/	31.0000	0.750	Cup	3.00	3.00	24.00	130.00	0.00	1.00	0.00	0.50
	Cereal, Honey Graham Oh!	27.0000	0.750	Cup	1.35	1.91	22.75	111.78	0.00	0.70	0.00	0.55
155	Cereal, Honey Nut Clusters	55.0000	1.000	Cup	4.00	2.50	46.00	210.00	0.00	3.00	0.00	0.00
	Cereal, Honeybran	35.0000	1.000	Cup	3.08	0.74	28.63	119.35	0.00	3.89	0.00	0.26
	Cereal, Honeycone	22.0000	1.000	Cup	1.28	0.40	19.60	86.02	0.00	0.62	0.00	0.00
	Cereal, Just Right	55.0000	1.000	Cup	4.24	1.49	46.04	204.05	0.00	2.81	0.00	0.11
	Cereal, Just Right, Fruit & Nut	55.0000	1.000	Cup	4.13	1.60	44.28	192.50	0.00	2.75	0.00	0.28
156	Cereal, King Vitamin	31.0000	1.500	Cup	2.30	1.10	26.10	120.00	0.00	1.20	0.00	0.30
	Cereal, Kix	30.0000	1.330	Cup	1.96	0.62	25.91	114.30	0.00	0.81	0.00	0.17
	Cereal, Life	32.0000	0.750	Cup	3.15	1.28	25.18	121.28	0.00	2.05	0.00	0.24
	Cereal, Life, Cinnamon	50.0000	1.000	Cup	4.36	1.74	40.40	189.50	0.00	2.95	0.00	0.33
	Cereal, Lucky Charms	30.0000	1.000	Cup	2.15	1.08	25.17	116.10	0.00	1.20	0.00	0.22
	Cereal, Malt-o-meal, Plain and C	240.0000	1.000	Cup	3.60	0.24	25.92	122.40	2.40	0.96	0.00	0.05
	Cereal, Maypo, Ckd w/ water, w/	240.0000	1.000	Cup	5.76	2.40	31.92	170.40	0.00	5.76	0.00	0.46
	Cereal, Maypo, Ckd w/ water, w/o	240.0000	1.000	Cup	5.76	2.40	31.92	170.40	0.00	5.76	0.00	0.43
157	Cereal, Mueslix Raisin & Almond Cr	55.0000	0.660	Cup	5.00	3.00	41.00	200.00	0.00	4.00	0.00	0.00
	Cereal, Mueslix, Apple & Almond	55.0000	0.750	Cup	5.39	4.95	40.87	210.65	0.00	4.68	0.00	1.05
	Cereal, Nut & Honey Crunch	55.0000	1.250	Cup	4.02	2.48	45.98	222.75	0.00	0.88	0.00	0.50
158	Cereal, Nutri-grain Almond Raisin	49.0000	1.250	Cup	4.00	2.50	38.00	180.00	0.00	4.00	0.00	0.00

Page Key: A2 = Baby Food   A2 = Baked Goods   A8 = Beverages   A14 = Breads/Grains and Pasta   A18 = Breakfast Foods/Cereals   A26 = Dairy and Eggs   A40 = Fats and Oils   A42 = Fruits and Vegetables   A52 = Meats and Beans   A60 = Nuts and Seeds   A62 5 Frozen Entrees and Packaged Foods   A76 = Restaurant Chains–Fast Foods   A92 = Restaurant Chains–Other   A106 = Seafood and Fish   A110 = Snacks and Sweets   A120 = Soups   A122 = Supplements   A126 = Toppings and Sauces

Monounsaturated Fat (g)	Polyunsaturated Fat (g)	Vitamin D (mg)	Vitamin K (mg)	Vitamin E (mg)	Vitamin A (re)	Vitamin C (mg)	Thiamin (mg)	Riboflavin (mg)	Niacin (mg)	Vitamin B6 (mg)	Folate (mcg)	Vitamin B12 (mcg)	Calcium (mg)	Iron (mg)	Magnesium (mg)	Phosphorus (mg)	Potassium (mg)	Sodium (mg)	Zinc (mg)
0.00	0.00	0.00	0.00	0.00	0.00	0.00	0.24	0.00	1.43	0.02	107.55	0.00	50.19	10.28	11.95	100.38	45.41	463.66	0.33
0.00	0.00	0.00	0.00	0.00	0.00	0.00	0.25	0.00	1.51	0.03	45.18	0.00	50.20	10.29	10.04	42.67	42.67	336.34	0.33
0.02	0.03	0.00	0.00	0.03	0.00	0.00	0.00	0.05	0.36	0.04	2.86	0.00	17.42	0.80	10.14	27.04	20.28	2.60	0.39
0.06	0.12	0.02	0.00	0.12	225.33	14.99	0.38	0.44	4.99	0.49	87.00	0.00	3.48	1.80	6.96	26.68	35.09	240.12	1.51
0.04	0.03	0.00	0.00	0.03	371.00	14.81	0.52	0.59	6.92	0.69	138.32	0.08	5.04	0.70	11.76	30.52	26.60	205.52	0.46
0.12	0.17	0.00	0.00	0.57	375.10	0.00	0.37	0.42	5.00	0.50	99.55	0.00	69.30	4.50	42.35	140.25	229.90	284.90	1.08
0.00	0.00	0.00	0.00	0.00	1250.00	0.00	0.38	0.43	5.00	0.50	100.00	1.50	20.00	2.70	40.00	150.00	120.00	150.00	1.20
0.14	0.06	0.00	0.00	0.33	0.00	9.00	0.38	0.43	5.00	0.50	99.90	0.00	58.50	4.50	68.10	168.30	216.90	142.50	1.24
0.00	0.00	0.00	0.00	0.34	635.52	0.00	0.62	0.72	8.45	0.86	169.44	2.54	68.16	13.73	57.60	176.16	343.20	429.12	1.50
0.50	0.00	0.00	0.00	0.00	0.00	15.00	0.38	0.43	5.00	0.50	100.00	1.50	20.00	4.50	0.00	20.00	15.00	210.00	3.75
0.00	0.00	0.00	0.00	0.00	750.00	15.00	0.38	0.43	5.00	0.50	100.00	0.00	60.00	4.50	0.00	40.00	20.00	170.00	3.75
0.03	0.09	0.03	0.00	0.04	225.06	15.00	0.37	0.43	4.99	0.50	93.00	0.00	0.62	4.50	2.79	8.06	20.46	199.95	0.16
0.00	0.00	0.00	0.00	0.03	750.00	15.00	0.38	0.43	5.00	0.50	0.10	1.50	0.00	4.50	0.00	0.00	20.00	210.00	0.00
0.11	0.61	0.00	0.00	0.50	0.00	0.00	0.39	0.44	5.01	0.50	102.30	1.49	19.80	61.23	55.55	159.50	183.15	1.65	1.49
0.21	0.27	0.03	0.00	0.11	211.20	14.07	0.39	0.42	5.01	0.51	90.00	0.00	3.30	4.23	8.70	20.70	31.50	140.70	3.75
0.10	0.08	0.00	0.00	0.03	423.68	0.00	0.42	0.48	5.63	0.58	112.96	1.70	3.84	2.02	9.28	18.88	24.32	177.60	1.70
0.28	0.16	0.03	0.00	0.23	225.30	15.00	0.38	0.43	5.00	0.50	99.90	0.00	14.40	4.50	9.30	36.00	52.80	274.50	3.75
0.00	0.00	0.00	0.00	0.02	397.20	15.90	0.39	0.45	5.28	0.54	105.90	0.00	13.80	1.89	24.90	65.70	108.30	195.90	1.59
0.50	1.50	0.03	0.00	8.00	750.00	3.60	0.38	0.43	5.00	0.50	0.10	1.50	20.00	1.80	40.00	150.00	170.00	150.00	3.75
0.50	2.00	0.03	0.00	0.00	750.00	2.40	0.38	0.43	5.00	0.50	0.10	1.50	20.00	1.80	40.00	100.00	120.00	120.00	3.75
3.33	1.81	0.00	0.00	1.19	0.00	0.06	0.18	0.10	0.54	0.07	19.38	0.04	49.02	2.48	51.87	167.58	221.16	18.81	1.14
0.00	0.00	0.02	0.00	0.00	224.89	0.00	0.56	0.64	7.12	0.75	74.96	0.75	35.98	1.50	52.47	179.91	254.87	202.40	5.62
9.60	12.90	0.00	0.00	15.71	4.88	1.71	0.90	0.34	2.50	0.39	104.92	0.00	98.82	5.12	217.16	563.64	656.36	29.28	4.95
0.66	1.16	0.00	0.00	5.53	206.25	0.00	0.33	0.39	4.57	0.44	110.00	1.38	24.20	1.93	45.65	127.05	155.65	123.75	3.47
0.66	2.09	0.00	0.00	5.53	253.00	0.00	0.44	0.50	5.61	0.55	110.00	1.71	22.55	2.04	46.75	134.75	137.50	134.75	4.24
1.42	0.80	0.00	0.00	0.48	0.00	0.12	0.09	0.07	0.26	0.04	9.61	0.06	23.87	1.29	26.04	91.76	132.68	7.75	0.50
6.49	1.87	0.00	0.00	3.88	0.00	0.00	0.17	0.06	0.61	0.08	8.25	0.00	41.25	1.72	52.25	160.05	182.60	89.10	1.11
0.06	0.19	1.00	0.00	0.27	1443.16	0.00	1.42	1.64	19.18	1.96	384.77	5.78	10.36	31.17	73.03	273.59	364.06	757.55	2.40
0.00	0.00	0.00	0.00	0.08	429.73	0.00	0.42	0.49	5.71	0.58	114.57	1.72	12.98	9.28	35.70	96.72	112.95	183.06	0.65
0.00	0.00	0.02	0.00	0.00	374.81	0.00	0.56	0.64	7.12	0.75	74.96	0.75	35.98	2.25	52.47	179.91	179.91	224.89	1.80
4.80	7.08	0.00	0.00	0.81	6.90	1.15	0.36	0.16	1.61	0.20	64.40	0.00	74.75	4.34	147.20	416.30	385.25	293.25	3.04
4.22	6.24	0.00	0.00	0.77	6.60	1.10	0.32	0.14	1.54	0.20	44.00	0.00	66.00	4.02	140.80	376.20	414.70	225.50	2.83
3.97	5.68	0.00	0.00	0.74	6.30	1.05	0.35	0.15	1.79	0.17	56.70	0.00	66.15	5.39	137.55	380.10	384.30	213.15	2.74
0.00	0.00	0.00	0.00	0.00	1250.00	0.00	0.38	0.43	5.00	0.50	100.00	1.50	0.00	2.70	16.00	40.00	50.00	190.00	0.30
0.00	0.00	0.00	0.00	0.00	1250.00	0.00	0.38	0.43	5.00	0.50	100.00	1.50	0.00	2.70	24.00	60.00	65.00	180.00	0.30
1.06	0.28	0.00	0.00	0.11	301.32	12.04	0.38	0.47	5.02	0.50	100.44	0.00	12.42	4.51	12.69	41.85	45.09	0.00	3.76
0.00	0.00	0.00	0.00	0.00	0.00	9.00	0.38	0.43	5.00	0.50	100.00	0.00	40.00	4.50	32.00	90.00	130.00	270.00	0.60
0.08	0.26	0.00	0.00	0.81	463.40	18.55	0.46	0.53	6.16	0.63	23.45	1.86	16.10	5.57	45.85	131.95	150.50	202.30	0.90
0.00	0.00	0.02	0.00	0.09	291.28	0.00	0.29	0.33	3.87	0.40	77.66	1.17	3.74	2.09	7.48	21.78	70.40	123.86	1.17
0.28	1.05	0.00	0.00	2.24	375.65	0.00	0.39	0.44	5.01	0.50	102.30	1.49	14.30	16.23	34.10	106.15	121.00	337.70	0.88
0.77	0.55	0.00	0.00	3.00	344.30	0.00	0.33	0.39	4.57	0.44	110.00	1.38	0.00	14.85	33.00	108.90	155.65	265.65	1.05
0.40	0.30	0.00	0.00	0.00	1044.00	13.00	0.39	0.44	5.20	0.52	104.00	1.57	4.00	8.74	26.00	79.00	86.00	260.00	3.91
0.15	0.04	0.03	0.00	0.08	375.30	15.00	0.38	0.43	5.00	0.50	99.90	0.00	43.50	8.10	9.30	42.00	41.10	263.10	3.75
0.41	0.56	0.00	0.00	0.16	1.28	0.00	0.40	0.45	5.33	0.53	106.88	0.00	97.60	8.96	31.04	135.68	79.04	174.40	4.00
0.57	0.77	0.00	0.00	0.23	1.50	0.10	0.63	0.71	8.38	0.84	167.50	0.00	134.50	74.54	41.50	181.00	113.00	220.00	6.29
0.39	0.15	0.03	0.00	0.13	225.30	15.00	0.38	0.43	5.00	0.50	99.90	0.00	32.40	4.50	19.50	75.60	54.00	203.10	3.75
0.00	0.00	0.00	0.00	0.00	0.00	0.00	0.48	0.24	5.76	0.02	4.80	0.00	4.80	9.60	4.80	24.00	31.20	324.00	0.17
0.00	0.00	0.00	0.00	0.00	703.20	28.80	0.72	0.72	9.36	0.96	9.60	2.88	124.80	8.40	50.40	247.20	211.20	259.20	1.49
0.74	0.89	0.00	0.00	1.68	703.20	28.80	0.72	0.72	9.36	0.96	9.60	2.88	124.80	8.40	50.40	247.20	211.20	9.60	1.49
2.00	1.00	0.20	0.00	8.00	200.00	20.00	0.38	0.43	5.00	0.50	0.10	1.50	20.00	4.50	40.00	150.00	240.00	160.00	3.75
2.59	1.05	0.00	0.00	5.78	233.75	0.00	0.39	0.44	5.17	0.50	110.00	1.27	33.55	4.68	62.70	175.45	209.00	270.05	3.14
1.16	0.83	0.00	0.00	0.14	225.50	15.02	0.39	0.44	5.01	0.50	110.00	0.00	5.50	4.51	4.95	36.30	59.95	370.15	0.39
1.00	1.50	0.00	0.00	8.00	0.00	0.00	0.38	0.43	5.00	0.50	0.10	1.50	150.00	1.40	16.00	200.00	190.00	170.00	3.75

USDA ID Code	Food Name	Weight in Grams*	Quantity of Units	Unit of Measure	Protein (g)	Fat (g)	Carbohydrate (g)	Kilocalories	Caffeine (g)	Fiber (g)	Cholesterol (mg)	Saturated Fat (g)
	Cereal, Nutri-grain, Barley	41.0000	1.000	Cup	4.47	0.33	33.95	152.52	0.00	2.38	0.00	0.00
	Cereal, Nutri-grain, Corn	42.0000	1.000	Cup	3.36	0.97	35.45	160.02	0.00	2.60	0.00	0.00
	Cereal, Nutri-grain, Rye	40.0000	1.000	Cup	3.48	0.28	33.88	143.60	0.00	2.56	0.00	0.00
	Cereal, Nutri-grain, Wheat	30.0000	0.750	Cup	3.03	0.99	24.00	100.50	0.00	3.78	0.00	0.06
	Cereal, Oat Bran Cereal	57.0000	1.250	Cup	8.54	2.95	41.39	212.61	0.00	5.99	0.00	0.54
	Cereal, Oat Flakes	48.0000	1.000	Cup	7.87	0.96	36.10	180.48	0.00	1.44	0.00	0.16
	Cereal, Oatmeal Cereal, Honey Nut	49.0000	1.000	Cup	4.89	2.71	38.96	190.61	0.00	3.33	0.49	0.52
	Cereal, Oatmeal Raisin Crisp	55.0000	1.000	Cup	4.35	2.45	43.70	204.05	0.00	3.52	0.00	0.39
	Cereal, Oatmeal Squares	56.0000	1.000	Cup	7.27	2.59	43.32	216.16	0.00	4.26	0.00	0.48
	Cereal, Oatmeal, Dry	2.5000	1.000	Tbsp	0.34	0.20	1.73	9.95	0.00	0.17	0.00	0.03
	Cereal, Oatmeal, Prepared	28.3500	1.000	Ounce	1.42	1.16	4.34	32.89	0.00	0.31	3.21	0.64
	Cereal, Oats Granola, Toasted	55.0000	0.750	Cup	5.80	9.69	36.23	238.05	0.00	3.52	0.00	1.27
	Cereal, Oats, Instant, Plain	234.0000	1.000	Cup	5.85	2.34	23.87	138.06	0.00	3.98	0.00	0.42
	Cereal, Oats, Instant, w/ apples	149.0000	1.000	Pkt.	3.19	1.42	26.15	125.16	0.00	2.53	0.00	0.30
	Cereal, Oats, Instant, w/ bran &	195.0000	1.000	Pkt.	4.88	1.95	30.42	157.95	0.00	5.46	0.00	0.35
	Cereal, Oats, Instant, w/ cinn a	240.0000	1.000	Cup	7.20	2.88	52.32	264.00	0.00	3.84	0.00	0.53
	Cereal, Oats, Instant, w/ maple	155.0000	1.000	Pkt.	4.17	1.78	31.40	153.45	0.00	2.64	0.00	0.36
	Cereal, Oats, Instant, w/ raisin	240.0000	1.000	Cup	6.48	2.64	48.48	244.80	0.00	3.36	0.00	0.50
	Cereal, Oats, Reg and Quick and	234.0000	1.000	Cup	6.08	2.34	25.27	145.08	0.00	3.98	0.00	0.42
159	Cereal, Organic Frst Ultra Mini	55.0000	0.750	Cup	4.00	1.00	46.00	190.00	0.00	7.00	0.00	0.00
160	Cereal, Organic Mini Cr Wheat-Ba	55.0000	0.750	Cup	5.00	1.00	45.00	190.00	0.00	8.00	0.00	0.00
	Cereal, Peanut Butter Puffs-Rees	30.0000	0.750	Cup	2.57	3.20	22.98	129.30	0.00	0.39	0.00	0.64
	Cereal, Product 19	30.0000	1.000	Cup	2.67	0.39	24.96	109.80	0.00	0.99	0.00	0.03
	Cereal, Puffed Rice	14.0000	1.000	Cup	0.98	0.13	12.29	53.62	0.00	0.20	0.00	0.05
	Cereal, Puffed Wheat	15.0000	1.250	Cup	2.44	0.32	11.46	54.90	0.00	1.14	0.00	0.02
161	Cereal, Puffins-Barbara	27.0000	0.750	Cup	2.00	1.00	23.00	90.00	0.00	5.00	0.00	0.00
	Cereal, Quisp	27.0000	1.000	Cup	1.35	1.49	22.97	108.81	0.00	0.68	0.00	0.41
	Cereal, Raisin Bran, Total-Gener	55.0000	1.000	Cup	4.00	1.01	42.75	178.20	0.00	5.01	0.00	0.23
	Cereal, Raisin Bran-Kellogg's	61.0000	1.000	Cup	5.61	1.46	47.09	186.05	0.00	8.17	0.00	0.00
	Cereal, Raisin Bran-Post	56.0000	1.000	Cup	5.21	1.06	42.34	171.92	0.00	7.90	0.00	0.18
	Cereal, Raisin Bran-Ralston Purina	56.0000	1.000	Cup	4.37	0.28	46.48	178.08	0.00	7.50	0.00	0.04
	Cereal, Raisin Nut Bran	55.0000	1.000	Cup	5.16	4.40	41.45	209.00	0.00	5.06	0.00	0.72
	Cereal, Raisin Squares	55.0000	0.750	Cup	4.40	1.54	42.90	187.00	0.00	5.17	0.00	0.17
162	Cereal, Raisins, Dates & Pecans-	54.0000	0.660	Cup	4.00	5.00	39.00	210.00	0.00	4.00	0.00	0.50
	Cereal, Raisins, Rice and Rye	46.0000	1.000	Cup	2.62	0.14	39.28	154.56	0.00	2.62	0.00	0.00
	Cereal, Rice Krispies	33.0000	1.250	Cup	2.08	0.36	28.55	124.41	0.00	0.36	0.00	0.13
163	Cereal, Rice Krispies, Apple-Cin	30.0000	0.750	Cup	1.53	0.51	26.70	111.90	0.00	0.45	0.00	0.00
	Cereal, Rice, Puffed	14.0000	1.000	Cup	0.88	0.07	12.57	56.28	0.00	0.24	0.00	0.02
	Cereal, Shredded Wheat, Large	23.6000	1.000	Biscuit	2.57	0.39	19.19	84.96	0.00	2.31	0.00	0.07
	Cereal, Shredded Wheat, Small	30.0000	1.000	Cup	3.30	0.50	24.12	107.10	0.00	2.94	0.00	0.08
164	Cereal, Smacks Kellogg's	27.0000	0.750	Cup	2.00	0.50	24.00	100.00	0.00	1.00	0.00	0.00
	Cereal, S'mores Grahams	30.0000	0.750	Cup	1.68	1.20	25.59	117.00	0.00	0.84	0.00	0.18
	Cereal, Special K	31.0000	1.000	Cup	6.36	0.28	22.44	114.70	0.00	0.96	0.00	0.00
	Cereal, Super Sugar Crisp	33.0000	1.000	Cup	2.15	0.30	29.77	123.42	0.00	0.50	0.00	0.05
	Cereal, Tasteeos	24.0000	1.000	Cup	3.07	0.67	18.98	94.32	0.00	2.54	0.00	0.23
	Cereal, Team	42.0000	1.000	Cup	2.69	0.76	36.04	164.22	0.00	0.55	0.00	0.00
165	Cereal, Temptations, Fr. Vanilla	30.0000	0.750	Cup	2.13	1.65	24.72	119.40	0.00	0.78	0.00	1.05
166	Cereal, Temptations, Honey Roast	30.0000	1.000	Cup	1.80	2.25	24.42	122.40	0.00	0.69	0.00	0.51
	Cereal, Toasties	23.0000	1.000	Cup	1.84	0.05	19.73	89.01	0.00	0.78	0.00	0.01
168	Cereal, Total	30.0000	0.750	Cup	2.99	0.70	23.88	105.30	0.00	2.64	0.00	0.18
	Cereal, Triples	30.0000	1.000	Cup	2.38	1.01	24.98	116.10	0.00	0.84	0.00	0.29
	Cereal, Trix	30.0000	1.000	Cup	0.95	1.71	26.04	122.40	0.00	0.72	0.00	0.41
	Cereal, Waffelos	30.0000	1.000	Cup	1.68	1.26	25.89	121.50	0.00	0.00	0.00	0.00

Monounsaturated Fat (g)	Polyunsaturated Fat (g)	Vitamin D (mg)	Vitamin K (mg)	Vitamin E (mg)	Vitamin A (re)	Vitamin C (mg)	Thiamin (mg)	Riboflavin (mg)	Niacin (mg)	Vitamin B6 (mg)	Folate (mcg)	Vitamin B12 (mcg)	Calcium (mg)	Iron (mg)	Magnesium (mg)	Phosphorus (mg)	Potassium (mg)	Sodium (mg)	Zinc (mg)
0.00	0.00	0.00	0.00	10.82	542.84	21.73	0.53	0.62	7.22	0.74	144.73	2.17	11.07	1.45	32.39	126.28	107.83	277.16	5.41
0.00	0.00	0.00	0.00	11.09	556.08	22.26	0.55	0.63	7.39	0.76	148.26	2.23	1.26	0.89	26.88	120.54	97.86	276.36	5.54
0.00	0.00	0.00	0.00	10.56	529.60	21.20	0.52	0.60	7.04	0.72	141.20	2.12	8.40	1.13	30.40	104.00	71.60	272.00	5.28
0.24	0.69	0.00	0.00	5.40	0.00	15.00	0.39	0.42	5.01	0.51	90.00	1.50	9.60	0.99	24.30	108.30	109.50	220.80	3.75
0.96	1.21	0.00	0.00	2.10	155.61	6.21	0.39	0.44	5.19	0.52	103.74	0.00	30.21	15.96	99.18	306.09	257.07	205.20	3.89
0.28	0.36	0.00	0.00	0.34	635.52	0.00	0.62	0.72	8.45	0.86	169.44	2.54	68.16	13.73	57.60	176.16	228.00	220.32	2.54
1.15	0.75	0.00	0.00	2.01	150.43	5.98	0.37	0.42	5.00	0.50	99.96	0.02	26.95	4.50	53.41	166.11	184.73	165.62	3.92
1.16	0.36	0.00	0.00	1.36	225.50	0.00	0.37	0.42	5.01	0.50	100.10	0.00	37.95	4.50	44.55	117.15	211.75	223.85	3.75
0.81	1.05	0.00	0.00	2.28	169.12	6.78	0.42	0.48	5.63	0.56	112.56	0.00	35.84	15.68	70.00	185.92	227.92	263.20	4.22
0.06	0.07	0.00	0.00	0.01	0.05	0.08	0.07	0.07	0.90	0.00	0.88	0.00	18.33	1.19	3.63	12.48	11.75	0.83	0.09
0.00	0.00	0.00	0.00	0.00	7.40	0.37	0.14	0.16	1.70	0.02	2.84	0.09	62.37	3.44	9.92	45.36	57.83	13.04	0.26
6.49	1.87	0.00	0.00	3.88	0.00	0.00	0.17	0.06	0.61	0.08	8.25	0.00	41.25	1.72	52.25	160.05	182.60	189.10	1.11
0.75	0.87	0.00	0.00	0.28	599.04	0.00	0.70	0.37	7.23	0.98	128.70	0.00	215.28	8.33	56.16	175.50	131.04	376.74	1.15
0.51	0.58	0.00	0.00	0.12	305.45	0.30	0.30	0.34	4.08	0.40	93.87	0.00	104.30	3.89	29.80	113.24	105.79	120.69	0.70
0.00	0.00	0.00	0.00	0.00	479.70	0.00	0.57	0.64	8.13	0.76	156.00	0.00	173.55	7.62	56.55	206.70	235.95	247.65	1.35
0.96	1.01	0.00	0.00	0.53	705.60	0.00	0.84	0.50	8.42	1.15	228.00	0.00	256.80	9.89	76.80	216.00	156.00	417.60	1.44
0.62	0.74	0.00	0.00	0.17	302.25	0.00	0.29	0.34	4.03	0.40	80.60	0.00	105.40	3.86	38.75	131.75	111.60	234.05	0.90
0.84	0.94	0.00	0.00	0.24	669.60	0.00	0.77	0.55	8.33	1.13	228.00	0.00	252.00	10.01	55.20	201.60	228.00	343.20	1.08
0.75	0.87	0.00	0.00	0.00	4.68	0.00	0.26	0.05	0.30	0.05	9.36	0.00	18.72	1.59	56.16	177.84	131.04	374.40	1.15
0.00	0.00	0.00	0.00	0.00	0.00	0.00	0.00	0.00	0.00	0.00	0.00	0.00	0.00	0.00	0.00	0.00	0.00	200.00	0.00
0.00	0.00	0.00	0.00	0.00	0.00	0.00	0.00	0.00	0.00	0.00	0.00	0.00	0.00	0.00	0.00	0.00	0.00	240.00	0.00
1.43	0.60	0.00	0.00	0.57	225.30	15.00	0.38	0.43	5.00	0.50	99.90	0.00	21.00	4.50	15.90	43.20	61.50	177.30	3.75
0.15	0.21	0.03	0.00	22.20	225.30	60.00	1.50	1.71	20.01	2.01	390.00	6.00	2.70	18.00	12.30	33.00	40.50	216.00	15.00
0.03	0.05	0.00	0.00	0.01	0.00	0.00	0.06	0.01	0.88	0.00	1.40	0.00	1.26	0.41	4.20	16.52	16.24	0.70	0.15
0.05	0.16	0.00	0.00	0.10	0.15	0.00	0.06	0.04	1.79	0.02	5.10	0.06	3.60	0.70	19.95	49.65	54.60	0.75	0.46
0.00	0.00	0.00	0.00	0.00	0.00	0.00	0.00	0.00	0.00	0.00	0.00	0.00	0.00	0.00	0.00	0.00	0.00	190.00	0.00
0.33	0.21	0.00	0.00	0.14	3.24	0.00	0.38	0.43	5.09	0.51	101.79	0.00	5.13	4.58	13.77	42.39	36.18	194.40	3.82
0.17	0.17	0.00	0.00	29.98	375.10	0.00	1.50	1.70	20.02	2.00	399.85	6.35	238.15	18.00	44.55	258.50	287.10	239.80	15.00
0.24	0.79	0.04	0.00	0.56	250.10	0.00	0.43	0.49	5.55	0.55	122.00	1.65	35.38	5.00	89.06	214.11	436.76	353.80	4.15
0.15	0.50	0.05	0.00	1.30	741.44	0.00	0.73	0.84	9.86	1.01	197.68	2.97	26.32	8.90	95.20	234.64	344.96	365.12	2.97
0.04	0.13	0.00	0.00	1.30	556.08	1.68	0.56	0.62	7.39	0.73	148.40	2.24	26.88	27.33	84.56	247.52	287.28	486.08	1.67
1.93	0.46	0.00	0.00	2.03	0.00	0.00	0.37	0.42	5.00	0.50	99.55	0.00	73.70	4.50	53.90	162.80	218.35	245.85	1.11
0.11	0.50	0.00	0.00	0.29	0.00	0.00	0.39	0.44	5.17	0.50	110.00	1.54	18.70	16.83	47.85	159.50	259.60	3.30	1.54
0.00	0.00	0.00	0.00	0.00	1500.00	0.00	0.45	0.51	6.00	0.60	120.00	1.80	20.00	3.60	40.00	150.00	150.00	150.00	1.20
0.00	0.00	0.00	0.00	0.25	467.82	0.46	0.46	0.55	6.26	0.64	124.66	1.89	10.12	5.61	19.78	49.68	143.52	349.60	4.69
0.10	0.17	0.03	0.00	0.04	247.83	16.50	0.43	0.46	5.51	0.56	116.49	0.00	3.30	1.98	15.84	43.56	42.24	353.76	0.60
0.00	0.51	0.00	0.00	0.13	233.10	15.51	0.39	0.45	5.16	0.51	90.00	0.00	2.10	1.86	7.80	24.90	30.90	222.90	0.33
0.00	0.00	0.00	0.00	0.00	0.00	0.00	0.36	0.25	4.94	0.01	2.66	0.00	0.84	4.44	3.50	13.72	15.82	0.42	0.14
0.06	0.21	0.00	0.00	0.13	0.00	0.00	0.07	0.07	1.08	0.06	11.80	0.00	9.68	0.74	40.12	85.67	77.17	0.47	0.59
0.08	0.26	0.00	0.00	0.16	0.00	0.00	0.08	0.08	1.58	0.08	15.00	0.00	11.40	1.27	39.60	105.90	108.30	3.00	0.99
0.00	0.00	0.03	0.00	0.00	750.00	15.00	0.38	0.43	5.00	0.50	0.10	1.50	0.00	1.80	8.00	40.00	40.00	50.00	0.30
0.39	0.15	0.00	0.00	0.22	225.30	15.00	0.38	0.43	5.00	0.50	99.90	0.00	14.40	4.50	10.80	40.50	48.00	212.40	3.75
0.00	0.22	1.25	0.00	0.08	225.06	15.00	0.53	0.59	7.01	0.71	93.00	0.00	4.65	8.71	17.67	50.84	54.56	249.86	3.75
0.06	0.12	0.00	0.00	0.12	436.92	0.00	0.43	0.50	5.81	0.59	116.49	1.75	6.93	2.08	19.80	43.89	47.85	50.82	1.75
0.17	0.18	0.00	0.00	0.17	317.76	12.72	0.31	0.36	4.22	0.43	84.72	1.27	11.04	6.86	26.16	95.76	71.04	182.88	0.69
0.00	0.00	0.00	0.00	0.10	556.08	22.26	0.55	0.63	7.39	0.76	6.72	2.23	6.30	2.57	18.48	65.10	70.98	259.56	0.58
0.36	0.24	0.00	0.00	0.83	259.80	17.31	0.42	0.48	5.76	0.57	120.00	0.00	10.80	5.19	6.90	20.40	40.80	207.00	0.21
1.17	0.57	0.00	0.00	0.14	232.80	15.51	0.39	0.45	5.16	0.51	90.00	0.00	0.60	4.65	2.70	7.50	28.80	248.40	0.12
0.01	0.02	0.00	0.00	0.06	304.52	0.00	0.30	0.35	4.05	0.41	81.91	1.22	0.92	0.61	3.45	10.12	26.68	241.04	0.07
0.14	0.08	0.03	0.00	23.49	375.30	60.00	1.50	1.70	20.10	2.00	399.90	7.67	258.30	18.00	32.10	210.90	96.90	198.60	15.00
0.27	0.03	0.00	0.00	0.14	375.30	15.00	0.38	0.43	5.00	0.50	99.90	0.00	41.10	8.10	6.90	35.40	30.60	191.40	3.75
0.90	0.29	0.03	0.00	0.60	225.30	15.00	0.38	0.43	5.00	0.50	99.90	0.00	32.10	4.50	3.60	26.10	17.70	196.80	3.75
0.00	0.00	0.00	0.00	0.00	397.20	15.90	0.39	0.45	5.28	0.54	3.30	1.59	8.40	4.77	6.30	244.50	26.40	124.80	0.24

USDA ID Code	Food Name	Weight in Grams*	Quantity of Units	Unit of Measure	Protein (g)	Fat (g)	Carbohydrate (g)	Kilocalories	Caffeine (g)	Fiber (g)	Cholesterol (mg)	Saturated Fat (g)
167	Cereal, Weetabix	35.0000	2.000	Biscuits	4.00	1.00	28.00	120.00	0.00	4.00	0.00	0.00
	Cereal, Wheat Germ, Toasted	28.3500	1.000	Ounce	8.25	3.03	14.06	108.30	0.00	3.66	0.00	0.52
	Cereal, Wheat 'n Raisin Chex	54.0000	1.000	Cup	5.08	0.43	42.98	185.22	0.00	3.56	0.00	0.00
	Cereal, Wheatena, Ckd w/ water	243.0000	1.000	Cup	4.86	1.22	28.67	136.08	0.00	6.56	0.00	0.19
	Cereal, Wheatena, Ckd w/ water,	243.0000	1.000	Cup	4.86	1.22	28.67	136.08	0.00	6.56	0.00	0.22
	Cereal, Wheaties	30.0000	1.000	Cup	3.24	0.93	23.79	110.10	0.00	2.10	0.00	0.20
	Cereal, Whole Wheat Hot Natural	242.0000	1.000	Cup	4.84	0.97	33.15	150.04	0.00	3.87	0.00	0.15
	French Toast, Frozen, Ready-to-h	28.3500	1.000	Slice	2.10	1.73	9.10	60.39	0.00	0.31	23.25	0.43
	French Toast, Made w/ Lowfat (2%)	28.3500	1.000	Slice	2.18	3.06	7.09	64.92	0.00	0.00	32.89	0.77
	French Toast, Made w/ Whole Milk	65.0000	1.000	Slice	5.01	7.35	16.19	150.80	0.00	0.00	76.05	1.95
546	Instant Breakfast, Caffe Mocha-Ca	37.0000	1.300	Ounce	4.50	0.50	28.00	130.00	0.40	0.00	3.00	0.00
547	Instant Breakfast, Choc Malt, No	20.0000	0.700	Ounce	4.50	1.50	11.00	70.00	0.00	1.00	3.00	1.00
548	Instant Breakfast, Choc, Creamy	37.0000	1.300	Ounce	4.50	1.00	28.00	130.00	0.00	1.00	2.00	0.00
549	Instant Breakfast, Choc, No Sugar	21.0000	0.720	Ounce	4.50	1.00	12.00	70.00	0.00	1.00	3.00	0.50
550	Instant Breakfast, Chocolate Malt	36.0000	1.250	Ounce	4.50	1.50	26.00	130.00	0.00	1.00	3.00	0.50
551	Instant Breakfast, Chocolate Malt	35.0000	1.200	Ounce	5.70	0.50	25.10	126.00	0.00	0.00	0.00	0.00
552	Instant Breakfast, Chocolate-Pil	35.0000	1.200	Ounce	5.70	0.50	25.70	130.00	0.00	0.00	0.00	0.00
553	Instant Breakfast, Strawberry, N	20.0000	0.700	Ounce	4.50	0.00	12.00	70.00	0.00	1.00	3.00	0.00
554	Instant Breakfast, Strawberry-Ca	36.0000	1.260	Ounce	4.50	0.00	28.00	130.00	0.00	0.00	3.00	0.00
555	Instant Breakfast, Strawberry-Pi	35.0000	1.200	Ounce	5.40	0.20	26.00	130.00	0.00	0.00	0.00	0.00
556	Instant Breakfast, Vanilla, French	36.0000	1.260	Ounce	4.50	0.00	27.00	130.00	0.00	0.00	3.00	0.00
557	Instant Breakfast, Vanilla-Pills	35.0000	1.200	Ounce	5.40	0.20	27.30	133.00	0.00	0.00	0.00	0.00
	Pancakes, Buttermilk	28.3500	1.000	Each	1.93	2.64	8.14	64.35	0.00	0.00	16.44	0.52
	Pancakes, Dietary	22.0000	1.000	3 In.	1.12	0.18	9.28	43.78	0.00	0.00	0.00	0.03
	Pancakes, Plain	28.3500	1.000	Each	1.81	2.75	8.02	64.35	0.00	0.00	16.73	0.60
	Pancakes, Plain, Frozen	28.3500	1.000	Each	1.47	0.94	12.36	64.92	0.00	0.51	2.55	0.22
	Pancakes, Whole-wheat	28.3500	1.000	Each	2.41	1.84	8.33	58.97	0.00	0.80	17.29	0.50
	Waffles, Buttermilk	75.0000	1.000	Each	6.23	10.20	24.75	216.75	0.00	0.00	50.25	1.88
	Waffles, Plain, Frozen, Toasted	28.3500	1.000	Each	1.76	2.32	11.54	74.84	0.00	0.65	6.80	0.41
	Waffles, Plain, Homemade	28.3500	1.000	Each	2.24	4.00	9.33	82.50	0.00	0.00	19.56	0.81

Dairy and Eggs

USDA ID Code	Food Name	Weight in Grams*	Quantity of Units	Unit of Measure	Protein (g)	Fat (g)	Carbohydrate (g)	Kilocalories	Caffeine (g)	Fiber (g)	Cholesterol (mg)	Saturated Fat (g)
	Cheese Spread, American, Past.	28.3500	1.000	Ounce	4.65	6.02	2.47	82.35	0.00	0.00	15.65	3.78
	Cheese, American, Pasteurized Pr	28.3500	1.000	Ounce	6.28	8.86	0.45	106.44	0.00	0.00	26.76	5.58
	Cheese, Blue	28.3500	1.500	Ounce	6.07	8.15	0.66	100.09	0.00	0.00	21.32	5.29
	Cheese, Brick	132.0000	1.000	Cup	30.68	39.18	3.68	489.61	0.00	0.00	124.61	24.76
	Cheese, Brie	240.0000	1.500	Cup	49.80	66.43	1.08	800.76	0.00	0.00	240.00	41.78
	Cheese, Caraway	28.3500	1.500	Ounce	7.14	8.28	0.87	106.60	0.00	0.00	26.37	5.27
	Cheese, Cheddar	132.0000	1.000	Cup	32.87	43.74	1.69	531.41	0.00	0.00	138.47	27.84
	Cheese, Cheddar, Non-Fat	28.3500	1.500	Ounce	8.10	0.00	2.03	45.56	0.00	0.00	4.05	0.00
	Cheese, Cheddar, Reduced Fat	28.3500	1.500	Ounce	8.00	5.00	1.00	80.00	0.00	0.00	15.00	3.00
	Cheese, Colby	132.0000	1.000	Cup	31.36	42.39	3.39	519.62	0.00	0.00	125.27	26.69
	Cheese, Cottage, Creamed	113.0000	4.000	Ounce	14.11	5.10	3.03	116.79	0.00	0.00	16.84	3.22
	Cheese, Cottage, Creamed, w/ Fruit	226.0000	1.000	Cup	22.37	7.68	30.06	279.40	0.00	0.00	25.31	4.86
	Cheese, Cottage, Fat Free	226.0000	0.500	Cup	26.00	0.00	0.00	140.00	0.00	0.00	20.00	0.00
	Cheese, Cottage, Lowfat, 1% Fat	226.0000	1.000	Cup	28.00	2.31	6.15	163.62	0.00	0.00	9.94	1.47
	Cheese, Cottage, Lowfat, 2% Fat	226.0000	1.000	Cup	31.05	4.36	8.20	202.68	0.00	0.00	18.98	2.76
	Cheese, Cottage, Uncreamed, Dry	145.0000	1.000	Cup	25.04	0.61	2.68	122.66	0.00	0.00	9.72	0.39
	Cheese, Cream	232.0000	1.000	Cup	17.52	80.90	6.17	809.77	0.00	0.00	254.50	50.97
	Cheese, Cream, Fat Free	17.5080	2.000	Tbsp	2.50	0.00	1.00	17.51	0.00	0.00	2.50	0.00
	Cheese, Cream, Light	16.0140	2.000	Tbsp	1.50	2.50	1.00	35.03	0.00	0.00	7.51	1.75
	Cheese, Cream, w/ Strawberry	30.0000	1.000	Ounce	4.00	0.00	2.00	35.00	0.00	0.00	3.00	0.00
	Cheese, Edam	28.3500	1.000	Ounce	7.08	7.88	0.41	101.10	0.00	0.00	25.29	4.98
	Cheese, Fat Free Slices, White	21.2630	1.000	Slice	5.00	0.00	2.00	30.00	0.00	0.00	0.00	0.00

Monounsaturated Fat (g)	Polyunsaturated Fat (g)	Vitamin D (mg)	Vitamin K (mg)	Vitamin E (mg)	Vitamin A (re)	Vitamin C (mg)	Thiamin (mg)	Riboflavin (mg)	Niacin (mg)	Vitamin B₆ (mg)	Folate (mcg)	Vitamin B₁₂ (mcg)	Calcium (mg)	Iron (mg)	Magnesium (mg)	Phosphorus (mg)	Potassium (mg)	Sodium (mg)	Zinc (mg)
0.00	0.00	0.00	0.00	0.00	0.00	0.00	0.00	0.00	0.00	0.00	0.00	0.00	0.00	0.00	0.00	0.00	120.00	130.00	0.00
0.43	1.88	0.00	0.00	5.14	0.00	1.70	0.47	0.23	1.59	0.28	99.79	0.00	12.76	2.58	90.72	324.89	268.48	1.13	4.73
0.00	0.00	0.00	0.00	0.31	0.00	1.62	0.54	0.59	7.13	0.70	143.10	2.16	24.30	7.72	52.92	163.08	226.80	305.64	1.19
0.17	0.61	0.00	0.00	0.90	0.00	0.00	0.02	0.05	1.34	0.05	17.01	0.00	9.72	1.36	48.60	145.80	187.11	4.86	1.68
0.00	0.00	0.00	0.00	0.00	0.00	0.00	0.02	0.05	1.34	0.05	17.01	0.00	9.72	1.36	48.60	145.80	187.11	578.34	1.68
0.22	0.15	0.03	0.00	0.37	225.30	15.00	0.38	0.43	5.00	0.50	99.90	0.00	54.60	8.10	31.80	95.40	104.10	222.30	0.71
0.00	0.00	0.00	0.00	0.00	0.00	0.00	0.17	0.12	2.15	0.17	26.62	0.00	16.94	1.50	53.24	166.98	171.82	563.86	1.16
0.58	0.35	0.00	0.00	0.19	15.31	0.09	0.08	0.11	0.77	0.14	14.74	0.48	30.33	0.63	4.82	39.41	37.99	140.33	0.22
1.28	0.73	0.00	0.00	0.00	37.42	0.09	0.06	0.09	0.46	0.02	12.19	0.09	28.35	0.47	4.82	33.17	37.99	135.80	0.19
3.03	1.70	0.00	0.00	0.00	80.60	0.20	0.13	0.21	1.06	0.05	14.95	0.20	64.35	1.09	11.05	76.05	86.45	310.70	0.44
0.00	0.00	0.00	0.00	0.00	1750.00	27.00	0.30	0.14	5.00	0.40	100.00	0.60	350.00	4.50	80.00	250.00	340.00	100.00	3.00
0.00	0.00	0.00	0.00	0.00	1750.00	27.00	0.30	0.10	5.00	0.40	100.00	0.60	250.00	4.50	80.00	250.00	290.00	115.00	3.00
0.00	0.00	0.00	0.00	0.00	1750.00	27.00	0.30	0.14	5.00	0.40	100.00	0.60	300.00	4.50	80.00	250.00	350.00	100.00	3.00
0.00	0.00	0.00	0.00	0.00	1750.00	27.00	0.30	0.10	5.00	0.40	100.00	0.60	300.00	4.50	80.00	250.00	350.00	95.00	3.00
0.00	0.00	0.00	0.00	0.00	1750.00	27.00	0.30	0.07	5.00	0.40	100.00	0.60	250.00	4.50	80.00	250.00	250.00	130.00	3.00
0.00	0.00	0.00	0.00	0.00	1684.00	23.00	0.47	0.41	5.80	0.00	0.00	0.00	335.00	5.60	0.00	125.00	263.00	119.00	0.00
0.00	0.00	0.00	0.00	0.00	1681.00	23.00	0.46	0.35	5.80	0.00	0.00	0.00	91.00	5.64	0.00	89.00	256.00	141.00	0.00
0.00	0.00	0.00	0.00	0.00	1750.00	27.00	0.30	0.14	5.00	0.40	100.00	0.60	350.00	4.50	80.00	250.00	250.00	95.00	3.00
0.00	0.00	0.00	0.00	0.00	1750.00	27.00	0.30	0.14	5.00	0.40	100.00	0.60	350.00	4.50	80.00	250.00	250.00	160.00	3.00
0.00	0.00	0.00	0.00	0.00	1681.00	23.00	0.44	0.32	5.80	0.00	0.00	0.00	91.00	5.40	0.00	70.00	250.00	130.00	0.00
0.00	0.00	0.00	0.00	0.00	1750.00	27.00	0.30	0.14	5.00	0.40	100.00	0.60	300.00	4.50	80.00	250.00	350.00	100.00	3.00
0.00	0.00	0.00	0.00	0.00	1686.00	23.00	0.33	0.23	4.70	0.00	0.00	0.00	79.00	5.10	0.00	111.00	229.00	198.00	0.00
0.67	1.27	0.00	0.00	0.00	8.51	0.11	0.06	0.08	0.45	0.01	10.77	0.05	44.51	0.48	4.25	39.41	41.11	147.99	0.18
0.03	0.08	0.00	0.00	0.00	2.20	0.04	0.04	0.02	0.37	0.00	1.10	0.00	12.76	0.39	5.94	74.80	84.92	57.64	0.15
0.70	1.26	0.00	0.00	0.00	15.31	0.09	0.06	0.08	0.45	0.01	10.77	0.06	62.09	0.51	4.54	45.08	37.42	124.46	0.16
0.34	0.27	0.00	0.00	0.11	8.22	0.09	0.11	0.13	1.14	0.02	14.18	0.05	17.58	0.99	3.97	105.46	20.70	144.30	0.19
0.49	0.68	0.00	0.00	0.00	18.14	0.14	0.06	0.15	0.65	0.03	8.22	0.08	70.88	0.88	13.04	105.75	79.10	162.16	0.29
2.52	5.09	0.00	0.00	0.00	26.25	0.38	0.20	0.27	1.55	0.04	11.25	0.16	136.50	1.63	13.50	123.75	128.25	450.75	0.56
0.91	0.79	0.00	0.00	0.24	103.19	0.00	0.11	0.14	1.26	0.26	12.76	0.71	65.77	1.27	6.24	119.07	36.29	223.11	0.16
1.00	1.92	0.00	0.00	0.00	18.43	0.11	0.07	0.10	0.59	0.02	13.04	0.07	72.29	0.65	5.39	53.87	45.08	144.87	0.19
1.76	0.18	0.00	0.00	0.00	53.58	0.00	0.01	0.12	0.04	0.03	1.98	0.11	159.30	0.09	8.09	248.06	68.58	460.69	0.73
2.54	0.28	0.00	0.00	0.00	82.22	0.00	0.01	0.10	0.02	0.02	2.21	0.20	174.49	0.11	6.31	125.87	45.93	184.28	0.85
2.21	0.23	0.00	0.00	0.18	64.64	0.00	0.01	0.11	0.29	0.05	10.32	0.35	149.57	0.09	6.50	109.83	72.66	395.57	0.75
11.35	1.03	0.00	0.00	0.66	398.64	0.00	0.01	0.46	0.16	0.09	26.80	1.66	889.28	0.57	32.10	595.32	179.26	738.67	3.43
19.22	1.99	0.00	0.00	1.58	436.80	0.00	0.17	1.25	0.91	0.58	156.00	3.96	441.60	1.20	48.00	451.20	364.80	1510.56	5.71
2.35	0.24	0.00	0.00	0.00	81.93	0.00	0.01	0.13	0.05	0.02	5.16	0.08	190.88	0.18	6.27	138.92	26.37	195.62	0.83
12.39	1.24	0.40	0.00	0.48	366.96	0.00	0.04	0.50	0.11	0.09	24.02	1.10	952.12	0.90	36.67	675.97	129.89	819.06	4.11
0.00	0.00	0.00	0.00	0.00	60.75	0.00	0.00	0.00	0.00	0.00	0.00	0.00	243.00	0.00	0.00	0.00	0.00	283.50	0.00
0.00	0.00	0.00	0.00	0.00	60.00	0.00	0.00	0.00	0.00	0.00	0.00	0.00	240.00	0.00	0.00	0.00	23.00	180.00	0.00
12.25	1.25	0.00	0.00	0.46	363.00	0.00	0.03	0.50	0.12	0.11	24.02	1.10	903.67	1.00	34.08	602.58	166.98	797.54	4.05
1.46	0.16	0.00	0.00	0.14	54.24	0.00	0.02	0.18	0.15	0.08	13.79	0.70	67.80	0.16	5.94	148.93	95.26	457.42	0.42
2.19	0.25	0.00	0.00	0.20	81.36	0.00	0.05	0.29	0.23	0.11	21.92	1.11	107.58	0.25	9.42	236.17	151.19	914.85	0.66
0.00	0.00	0.00	0.00	0.00	0.00	0.00	0.00	0.00	0.00	0.00	0.00	0.00	240.00	0.00	0.00	0.00	0.00	840.00	0.00
0.66	0.07	0.00	0.00	0.25	24.86	0.00	0.05	0.38	0.29	0.16	28.02	1.42	137.63	0.32	12.07	302.39	193.23	917.56	0.86
1.24	0.14	0.00	0.00	0.14	45.20	0.00	0.05	0.43	0.32	0.18	29.61	1.60	154.81	0.36	13.56	340.13	217.41	917.56	0.95
0.16	0.03	0.00	0.00	0.16	11.60	0.00	0.04	0.20	0.23	0.12	21.46	1.20	45.97	0.33	5.71	150.80	46.98	18.56	0.68
22.83	2.95	0.00	0.00	2.18	886.24	0.00	0.05	0.46	0.23	0.12	30.62	0.97	185.37	2.78	14.94	242.21	277.01	685.56	1.25
0.00	0.00	0.00	0.00	0.00	50.02	0.00	0.00	0.00	0.00	0.00	0.00	0.00	60.03	0.00	0.00	0.00	0.00	90.04	0.00
0.00	0.00	0.00	0.00	0.00	40.03	0.00	0.00	0.00	0.00	0.00	0.00	0.00	24.02	0.00	0.00	0.00	0.00	75.06	0.00
0.00	0.00	0.00	0.00	0.00	10.00	0.00	0.00	0.00	0.00	0.00	0.00	0.00	24.00	0.00	0.00	0.00	0.00	200.00	0.00
2.30	0.19	0.26	0.00	0.21	71.73	0.00	0.01	0.11	0.02	0.02	4.59	0.44	207.24	0.12	8.44	151.84	53.21	273.58	1.06
0.00	0.00	0.00	0.00	0.00	40.00	0.00	0.00	0.00	0.00	0.00	0.00	0.00	120.00	0.00	0.00	0.00	18.00	310.00	0.00

USDA ID Code	Food Name	Weight in Grams*	Quantity of Units	Unit of Measure	Protein (g)	Fat (g)	Carbohydrate (g)	Kilocalories	Caffeine (g)	Fiber (g)	Cholesterol (mg)	Saturated Fat (g)
	Cheese, Fat Free Slices, Yellow	21.2630	1.000	Slice	5.00	0.00	2.00	30.00	0.00	0.00	0.00	0.00
	Cheese, Feta	150.0000	1.000	Cup	21.32	31.92	6.14	395.34	0.00	0.00	133.50	22.43
	Cheese, Fontina	132.0000	1.000	Cup	33.79	41.10	2.05	513.52	0.00	0.00	153.12	25.34
	Cheese, Goat, Hard Type	28.3500	1.000	Ounce	8.65	10.09	0.62	128.14	0.00	0.00	29.77	6.98
	Cheese, Goat, Semisoft Type	28.3500	1.000	Ounce	6.12	8.46	0.72	103.19	0.00	0.00	22.40	5.85
	Cheese, Goat, Soft Type	28.3500	1.000	Ounce	5.25	5.98	0.25	75.98	0.00	0.00	13.04	4.13
	Cheese, Gouda	28.3500	1.500	Ounce	7.07	7.78	0.63	101.01	0.00	0.00	32.32	4.99
	Cheese, Gruyere	132.0000	1.000	Cup	39.35	42.69	0.48	545.09	0.00	0.00	145.20	24.96
	Cheese, Limburger	134.0000	1.000	Cup	26.87	36.52	0.66	438.23	0.00	0.00	120.60	22.45
	Cheese, Monterey	132.0000	1.000	Cup	32.31	39.97	0.90	492.78	0.00	0.00	117.48	25.17
	Cheese, Monterey, Reduced Fat	28.3500	1.500	Ounce	8.00	5.00	1.00	80.00	0.00	0.00	15.00	3.00
	Cheese, Mozzarella, Part Skim Milk	28.3500	1.500	Ounce	6.88	4.51	0.79	72.08	0.00	0.00	16.39	2.87
	Cheese, Mozzarella, Part Skim Milk	132.0000	1.000	Cup	36.26	22.60	4.14	369.51	0.00	0.00	71.28	14.36
	Cheese, Mozzarella, Stick	28.0000	1.000	Each	8.00	5.00	0.00	80.00	0.00	0.00	15.00	3.00
	Cheese, Mozzarella, Substitute	113.0000	1.000	Cup	12.96	13.81	26.75	280.24	0.00	0.00	0.00	4.19
	Cheese, Mozzarella, Whole Milk	112.0000	1.000	Cup	21.75	24.19	2.49	315.15	0.00	0.00	87.81	14.73
	Cheese, Mozzarella, Whole Milk,	28.3500	1.000	Ounce	6.12	6.99	0.70	90.26	0.00	0.00	25.34	4.41
	Cheese, Muenster	132.0000	1.000	Cup	30.90	39.65	1.48	486.22	0.00	0.00	126.19	25.23
	Cheese, Parmesan, Grated	100.0000	1.000	Cup	41.56	30.02	3.74	455.81	0.00	0.00	78.70	19.07
	Cheese, Parmesan, Grated, Fat Free	5.0020	1.000	Tbsp	0.67	0.00	0.67	5.00	0.00	0.00	1.67	0.00
	Cheese, Parmesan, Piece	28.3500	1.000	Ounce	10.14	7.32	0.91	111.18	0.00	0.00	19.19	4.65
	Cheese, Parmesan, Shredded	5.0000	1.000	Tbsp	1.89	1.37	0.17	20.75	0.00	0.00	3.60	0.87
	Cheese, Pepper	132.0000	1.000	Cup	32.31	39.97	0.90	492.78	0.00	0.00	117.48	25.17
	Cheese, Provolone	132.0000	1.000	Cup	33.77	35.14	2.82	463.98	0.00	0.00	90.95	22.55
	Cheese, Ricotta, Part Skim Milk	246.0000	1.000	Cup	28.02	19.46	12.64	339.63	0.00	0.00	75.77	12.13
	Cheese, Ricotta, Whole Milk	246.0000	1.000	Cup	27.70	31.93	7.48	427.89	0.00	0.00	124.48	20.42
	Cheese, Romano	28.3500	1.000	Ounce	9.02	7.64	1.03	109.61	0.00	0.00	29.48	4.85
	Cheese, Roquefort	28.3500	1.000	Ounce	6.11	8.69	0.57	104.62	0.00	0.00	25.52	5.46
	Cheese, Swiss, Domestic	132.0000	1.000	Cup	37.53	36.23	4.46	496.00	0.00	0.00	121.04	23.47
	Cheese, Swiss, Pasteurized Proce	140.0000	1.000	Cup	34.62	35.01	2.94	466.98	0.00	0.00	118.72	22.47
	Cream Substitute, Non-dairy, Liq	240.0000	1.000	Cup	2.40	23.93	27.31	325.56	0.00	0.00	0.00	4.66
	Cream Substitute, Non-dairy, Pow	94.0000	1.000	Cup	4.50	33.35	51.59	513.69	0.00	0.00	0.00	30.58
	Cream, Half and Half, Cream and	242.0000	1.000	Cup	7.16	27.83	10.41	315.50	0.00	0.00	89.30	17.33
	Cream, Light, Coffee or Table	240.0000	1.000	Cup	6.48	46.34	8.78	469.03	0.00	0.00	158.64	28.85
	Cream, Medium, 25% Fat	15.0000	1.000	Tbsp	0.37	3.75	0.52	36.56	0.00	0.00	13.12	2.33
	Cream, Whipped, Pressurized	60.0000	1.000	Cup	1.92	13.33	7.49	154.39	0.00	0.00	45.60	8.30
	Cream, Whipping, Heavy	119.5000	1.000	Cup	2.45	44.22	3.33	412.01	0.00	0.00	163.83	27.52
	Cream, Whipping, Light	120.0000	1.000	Cup	2.60	37.09	3.55	350.90	0.00	0.00	133.20	23.21
	Dessert Topping, Non-dairy	75.0000	1.000	Cup	0.94	18.98	17.29	238.71	0.00	0.00	0.00	16.34
	Egg Substitute, Frozen	240.0000	1.000	Cup	27.10	26.66	7.68	383.57	0.00	0.00	4.80	4.63
	Egg Substitute, Liquid	251.0000	1.000	Cup	30.12	8.31	1.61	210.99	0.00	0.00	2.51	1.66
	Egg White Only, w/o Yolk	243.0000	1.000	Cup	25.56	0.00	2.50	121.50	0.00	0.00	0.00	0.00
	Eggnog	254.0000	1.000	Cup	9.68	19.00	34.39	341.91	0.00	0.00	149.10	11.28
	Eggnog, Reduced Fat	246.0000	1.000	Cup	12.00	8.00	48.00	320.00	0.00	0.00	90.00	5.00
	Eggs, Chicken, Whole, Ckd, Fried	46.0000	1.000	Large	6.23	6.90	0.63	91.54	0.00	0.00	211.14	1.92
	Eggs, Chicken, Whole, Ckd, Hard-	136.0000	1.000	Cup	17.11	14.43	1.52	210.80	0.00	0.00	576.64	4.45
	Eggs, Chicken, Whole, Ckd, Omelet	15.2000	1.000	Tbsp	1.57	1.74	0.16	23.10	0.00	0.00	53.20	0.48
	Eggs, Chicken, Whole, Ckd, Poach	50.0000	1.000	Large	6.22	4.99	0.61	74.50	0.00	0.00	211.50	1.55
	Eggs, Chicken, Whole, Ckd, Scram	220.0000	1.000	Cup	24.40	26.86	4.84	365.20	0.00	0.00	774.40	8.10
264	Eggs, Chicken, Whole, Fresh, and	50.0000	1.000	Large	6.25	5.01	0.61	74.50	0.00	0.00	212.50	1.55
	Frozen Yogurt	148.0000	0.500	Cup	6.00	12.00	48.00	320.00	0.00	0.00	20.00	4.00
444	Frozen Yogurt Bar, Banana/Straw-	71.0000	1.000	Each	2.00	0.00	20.00	90.00	0.00	0.00	0.00	0.00
445	Frozen Yogurt Bar, Rasp/Vanilla-	71.0000	1.000	Each	2.00	0.00	20.00	90.00	0.00	0.00	0.00	0.00

Page Key: A2 = Baby Food   A2 = Baked Goods   A8 = Beverages   A14 = Breads/Grains and Pasta   A18 = Breakfast Foods/Cereals   A26 = Dairy and Eggs   A40 = Fats and Oils   A42 = Fruits and Vegetables   A52 = Meats and Beans   A60 = Nuts and Seeds   A62 5 Frozen Entrees and Packaged Foods   A76 = Restaurant Chains–Fast Foods   A92 = Restaurant Chains–Other   A106 = Seafood and Fish   A110 = Snacks and Sweets   A120 = Soups   A122 = Supplements   A126 = Toppings and Sauces

Monounsaturated Fat (g)	Polyunsaturated Fat (g)	Vitamin D (mg)	Vitamin K (mg)	Vitamin E (mg)	Vitamin A (re)	Vitamin C (mg)	Thiamin (mg)	Riboflavin (mg)	Niacin (mg)	Vitamin B6 (mg)	Folate (mcg)	Vitamin B12 (mcg)	Calcium (mg)	Iron (mg)	Magnesium (mg)	Phosphorus (mg)	Potassium (mg)	Sodium (mg)	Zinc (mg)
0.00	0.00	0.00	0.00	0.00	40.00	0.00	0.00	0.00	0.00	0.00	0.00	0.00	120.00	0.00	0.00	0.00	18.00	310.00	0.00
6.93	0.89	0.00	0.00	0.05	192.00	0.00	0.23	1.26	1.49	0.63	48.00	2.54	738.75	0.98	28.82	505.80	92.70	1674.15	4.32
11.47	2.18	0.00	0.00	0.46	382.80	0.00	0.03	0.26	0.20	0.11	7.92	2.22	726.00	0.30	18.48	457.12	83.82	1056.00	4.62
2.30	0.24	0.00	0.00	0.22	135.23	0.00	0.04	0.34	0.68	0.02	1.13	0.03	253.73	0.53	15.31	206.67	13.61	98.09	0.45
1.93	0.20	0.00	0.00	0.18	113.40	0.00	0.02	0.19	0.33	0.02	0.57	0.06	84.48	0.46	8.22	106.31	44.79	146.00	0.19
1.36	0.14	0.00	0.00	0.13	80.23	0.00	0.02	0.11	0.12	0.07	3.40	0.05	39.69	0.54	4.54	72.58	7.37	104.33	0.26
2.20	0.19	0.00	0.00	0.10	49.33	0.00	0.01	0.09	0.02	0.02	5.93	0.44	198.39	0.07	8.22	154.88	34.16	232.27	1.11
13.25	2.28	0.00	0.00	0.46	397.32	0.00	0.08	0.37	0.15	0.11	13.73	2.11	1334.52	0.22	47.40	799.00	106.92	443.52	5.15
11.54	0.67	0.00	0.00	0.86	423.44	0.00	0.11	0.67	0.21	0.12	77.05	1.39	665.58	0.17	28.14	526.62	171.52	1072.00	2.81
11.55	1.19	0.00	0.00	0.45	333.96	0.00	0.03	0.51	0.12	0.11	24.02	1.10	985.25	0.95	35.65	586.08	106.52	707.92	3.96
0.00	0.00	0.00	0.00	0.00	60.00	0.00	0.00	0.00	0.00	0.00	0.00	0.00	240.00	0.00	0.00	0.00	18.00	180.00	0.00
1.28	0.13	0.00	0.00	0.12	50.18	0.00	0.01	0.09	0.03	0.02	2.49	0.23	183.06	0.06	6.58	131.26	23.73	132.11	0.78
6.40	0.67	0.00	0.00	0.61	252.12	0.00	0.03	0.45	0.16	0.11	13.07	1.23	965.32	0.33	34.68	691.81	125.19	696.56	4.13
0.00	0.00	0.00	0.00	0.00	40.00	0.00	0.00	0.00	0.00	0.00	0.00	0.00	240.00	0.00	0.00	0.00	0.00	170.00	0.00
7.05	1.97	0.00	0.00	2.24	493.81	0.11	0.03	0.50	0.36	0.06	12.43	0.92	689.30	0.45	46.33	658.79	514.15	774.05	2.17
7.36	0.86	0.00	0.00	0.39	269.92	0.00	0.02	0.27	0.09	0.07	7.84	0.73	579.04	0.20	20.81	415.18	75.15	417.87	2.48
1.99	0.22	0.00	0.00	0.19	77.68	0.00	0.01	0.08	0.03	0.02	2.21	0.21	162.98	0.06	5.86	116.89	21.15	117.65	0.70
11.50	0.87	0.00	0.00	0.62	417.12	0.00	0.01	0.42	0.13	0.08	15.97	1.94	946.84	0.54	36.10	617.36	177.41	828.56	3.71
8.73	0.66	0.00	0.00	0.80	173.00	0.00	0.05	0.39	0.32	0.11	8.00	1.40	1375.70	0.95	50.80	807.10	107.10	1861.50	3.19
0.00	0.00	0.00	0.00	0.00	0.00	0.00	0.00	0.00	0.00	0.00	0.00	0.00	16.01	0.00	0.00	0.00	10.00	15.01	0.00
2.13	0.16	0.20	0.00	0.23	42.24	0.00	0.01	0.09	0.08	0.03	1.96	0.34	335.52	0.23	12.39	196.86	26.14	454.03	0.78
0.44	0.03	0.00	0.00	0.00	8.65	0.00	0.00	0.02	0.01	0.01	0.40	0.07	62.65	0.04	2.54	36.75	4.85	84.80	0.16
11.55	1.19	0.00	0.00	0.45	333.96	0.00	0.03	0.51	0.12	0.11	24.02	1.10	985.25	0.95	35.65	586.08	106.52	707.92	3.96
9.75	1.02	0.00	0.00	0.46	348.48	0.00	0.03	0.42	0.21	0.09	13.73	1.93	997.79	0.69	36.41	654.85	182.56	1155.66	4.26
5.68	0.64	0.00	0.00	0.52	277.98	0.00	0.05	0.47	0.20	0.05	32.23	0.71	669.12	1.08	36.33	449.20	307.50	306.76	3.30
8.93	0.96	0.00	0.00	0.86	329.64	0.00	0.02	0.49	0.25	0.10	30.01	0.84	509.22	0.93	27.80	388.93	257.32	206.89	2.85
2.22	0.17	0.00	0.00	0.21	39.97	0.00	0.01	0.10	0.02	0.03	1.93	0.32	301.59	0.22	11.60	215.46	24.47	340.20	0.73
2.40	0.37	0.00	0.00	0.00	84.77	0.00	0.01	0.17	0.21	0.03	13.89	0.18	187.62	0.16	8.37	111.16	25.71	512.85	0.59
9.60	1.28	1.45	0.00	0.66	333.96	0.00	0.03	0.49	0.12	0.11	8.45	2.22	1268.39	0.22	47.40	798.07	146.12	343.20	5.15
9.87	0.87	0.00	0.00	0.95	320.60	0.00	0.01	0.39	0.06	0.06	8.26	1.72	1080.66	0.85	40.77	1066.10	301.70	1918.42	5.05
18.12	0.07	0.00	0.00	3.89	21.60	0.00	0.00	0.00	0.00	0.00	0.00	0.00	22.32	0.07	0.79	154.08	457.20	190.08	0.05
0.91	0.01	0.00	0.00	0.25	18.80	0.00	0.00	0.16	0.00	0.00	0.00	0.00	20.96	1.08	3.82	396.68	763.09	170.23	0.48
8.03	1.04	0.00	0.00	0.27	258.94	2.08	0.10	0.36	0.19	0.10	6.05	0.80	253.86	0.17	24.61	230.38	313.63	98.49	1.23
13.39	1.73	0.00	0.00	0.36	436.80	1.82	0.07	0.36	0.14	0.07	5.52	0.53	230.88	0.10	20.76	191.76	292.08	95.04	0.65
1.08	0.14	0.00	0.00	0.09	34.80	0.11	0.00	0.02	0.01	0.00	0.34	0.03	13.53	0.01	1.26	10.59	17.17	5.55	0.04
3.85	0.50	0.00	0.00	0.36	124.20	0.00	0.02	0.04	0.04	0.02	1.56	0.17	60.60	0.03	6.47	53.58	88.38	78.00	0.22
12.77	1.64	0.35	0.00	0.75	503.10	0.69	0.02	0.13	0.05	0.04	4.42	0.22	77.20	0.04	8.40	74.57	90.10	44.93	0.27
10.91	1.06	0.00	0.00	0.72	354.00	0.73	0.02	0.16	0.05	0.04	4.44	0.24	83.28	0.04	8.68	73.32	116.16	41.16	0.30
1.22	0.39	0.00	0.00	0.14	64.50	0.00	0.00	0.00	0.00	0.00	0.00	0.00	4.73	0.09	1.34	5.78	13.65	18.98	0.02
5.86	14.98	0.00	0.00	5.06	324.00	1.13	0.29	0.94	0.34	0.31	39.36	0.82	174.72	4.75	35.90	172.08	511.92	478.56	2.35
2.26	4.02	0.00	0.00	1.23	542.16	0.00	0.28	0.75	0.28	0.00	37.40	0.75	133.03	5.27	21.89	303.71	828.30	444.27	3.26
0.00	0.00	0.00	0.05	0.00	0.00	0.00	0.02	1.09	0.22	0.00	7.29	0.49	14.58	0.07	26.73	31.59	347.49	398.52	0.02
5.66	0.86	0.00	0.00	0.58	203.20	3.81	0.08	0.48	0.28	0.13	2.29	1.14	330.20	0.51	46.99	277.88	419.61	138.18	1.17
0.00	0.00	0.00	0.00	0.00	160.00	2.40	0.00	0.00	0.00	0.00	0.00	0.00	480.00	0.40	0.00	0.00	0.00	280.00	0.00
2.75	1.28	0.00	0.00	0.75	114.08	0.00	0.03	0.24	0.04	0.06	17.48	0.42	25.30	0.72	5.06	89.24	60.72	162.38	0.55
5.55	1.92	0.00	0.00	1.43	228.48	0.00	0.10	0.69	0.08	0.16	59.84	1.51	68.00	1.62	13.60	233.92	171.36	168.64	1.43
0.69	0.32	0.00	0.00	0.20	28.42	0.00	0.01	0.06	0.01	0.02	4.41	0.11	6.38	0.18	1.37	22.50	15.35	41.04	0.14
1.90	0.68	0.00	0.00	0.53	95.00	0.00	0.03	0.22	0.03	0.06	17.50	0.40	24.50	0.72	5.00	88.50	60.00	140.00	0.55
10.49	4.73	0.00	0.00	2.88	429.00	0.44	0.11	0.97	0.18	0.26	66.00	1.69	156.20	2.64	26.40	374.00	303.60	616.00	2.20
1.90	0.68	0.02	25.00	1.03	95.50	0.00	0.03	0.25	0.04	0.07	23.50	0.50	24.50	0.72	5.00	89.00	60.50	63.00	0.55
0.00	0.00	0.00	0.00	0.00	40.00	0.00	0.00	0.00	0.00	0.00	0.00	0.00	192.00	0.00	0.00	0.00	0.00	100.00	0.00
0.00	0.00	0.00	0.00	0.00	0.00	0.00	0.00	0.00	0.00	0.00	0.00	0.00	0.00	0.00	0.00	0.00	0.00	15.00	0.00
0.00	0.00	0.00	0.00	0.00	0.00	0.00	0.00	0.00	0.00	0.00	0.00	0.00	0.00	0.00	0.00	0.00	0.00	15.00	0.00

USDA ID Code	Food Name	Weight in Grams*	Quantity of Units	Unit of Measure	Protein (g)	Fat (g)	Carbohydrate (g)	Kilocalories	Caffeine (g)	Fiber (g)	Cholesterol (mg)	Saturated Fat (g)
446	Frozen Yogurt Bar, Straw Daiquir	70.0000	1.000	Each	2.00	1.00	18.00	90.00	0.00	0.00	15.00	0.50
447	Frozen Yogurt Bar, Toc/Cherry-Ha	71.0000	1.000	Each	3.00	0.00	21.00	100.00	0.00	0.00	0.00	0.00
448	Frozen Yogurt Bar, Toc/Vanilla-H	71.0000	1.000	Each	3.00	0.00	20.00	90.00	0.00	0.00	0.00	0.00
449	Frozen Yogurt, Capp., No Fat-Ben	95.0000	0.500	Cup	4.00	0.00	26.00	120.00	0.00	0.00	0.00	0.00
450	Frozen Yogurt, Cherry Garcia-Ben	95.0000	0.500	Cup	4.00	2.50	27.00	140.00	0.00	0.00	5.00	2.00
451	Frozen Yogurt, Cherry Vanilla-Ha	93.0000	0.500	Cup	6.00	0.00	30.00	140.00	0.00	0.00	0.00	0.00
452	Frozen Yogurt, Choc Chip Cookie	95.0000	0.500	Cup	4.00	3.00	34.00	180.00	0.00	0.00	10.00	2.00
453	Frozen Yogurt, Choc Fudge Brownie	95.0000	0.500	Cup	4.00	1.00	32.00	150.00	0.00	0.00	0.00	0.00
454	Frozen Yogurt, Chocolate, No Fat	95.0000	0.500	Cup	4.00	0.00	25.00	120.00	0.00	0.00	0.00	0.00
	Frozen Yogurt, Chocolate, Soft-s	72.0000	0.500	Cup	2.88	4.32	17.93	115.20	2.16	1.58	3.60	2.61
455	Frozen Yogurt, Chocolate-Haagen-	93.0000	0.500	Cup	6.00	0.00	28.00	140.00	0.00	0.00	0.00	0.00
456	Frozen Yogurt, Coffee Fudge, No	95.0000	0.500	Cup	4.00	0.00	25.00	120.00	0.00	0.00	0.00	0.00
457	Frozen Yogurt, Coffee-Haagen-Daz	93.0000	0.500	Cup	6.00	0.00	29.00	140.00	0.00	0.00	0.00	0.00
	Frozen Yogurt, Fat Free	133.9160	0.500	Cup	7.99	0.00	43.97	199.87	0.00	0.00	0.00	0.00
	Frozen Yogurt, Low Fat	148.0000	0.500	Cup	6.00	6.00	48.00	280.00	0.00	0.00	20.00	4.00
458	Frozen Yogurt, Low Fat-Ben & Jer	106.0000	0.500	Cup	4.00	3.00	31.00	170.00	0.00	0.00	10.00	2.00
459	Frozen Yogurt, Peach Melba, Tang	95.0000	0.500	Cup	3.00	0.00	29.00	130.00	0.00	0.00	0.00	0.00
460	Frozen Yogurt, Raspberry, Black,	95.0000	0.500	Cup	3.00	0.00	27.00	120.00	0.00	1.00	0.00	0.00
461	Frozen Yogurt, Vanilla Fudge, No	95.0000	0.500	Cup	4.00	0.00	31.00	140.00	0.00	1.00	0.00	0.00
462	Frozen Yogurt, Vanilla Fudge-Haa	93.0000	0.500	Cup	6.00	0.00	34.00	160.00	0.00	0.00	0.00	0.00
463	Frozen Yogurt, Vanilla Rasp Swir	96.0000	0.500	Cup	4.00	0.00	28.00	130.00	0.00	0.00	0.00	0.00
464	Frozen Yogurt, Vanilla w/ Heath	95.0000	0.500	Cup	4.00	5.00	29.00	180.00	0.00	0.00	10.00	2.50
465	Frozen Yogurt, Vanilla, No Fat-B	95.0000	0.500	Cup	4.00	0.00	26.00	120.00	0.00	0.00	0.00	0.00
	Frozen Yogurt, Vanilla, Soft-ser	72.0000	0.500	Cup	2.88	4.03	17.42	114.48	0.00	0.00	1.44	2.46
466	Frozen Yogurt, Vanilla-Haagen-Da	93.0000	0.500	Cup	6.00	0.00	29.00	140.00	0.00	0.00	0.00	0.00
	Ice Cream-fat free	72.0000	0.500	Cup	4.00	0.00	23.00	100.00	0.00	0.00	0.00	0.00
469	Ice Cream Bar, Choc/Dark Choc-Ha	102.0000	1.000	Each	5.00	24.00	28.00	350.00	0.00	2.00	85.00	15.00
470	Ice Cream Bar, Coffee/Almond Cru	106.0000	1.000	Each	5.00	26.00	27.00	360.00	0.00	1.00	100.00	15.00
471	Ice Cream Bar, Straw/White Choc-	97.0000	1.000	Each	4.00	23.00	24.00	320.00	0.00	0.00	70.00	14.00
472	Ice Cream Bar, Vanilla & Almonds	106.0000	1.000	Each	6.00	27.00	26.00	370.00	0.00	1.00	90.00	14.00
473	Ice Cream Bar, Vanilla/Dark Choc	102.0000	1.000	Each	5.00	24.00	27.00	350.00	0.00	1.00	85.00	15.00
474	Ice Cream Bar, Vanilla/Milk Choc	100.0000	1.000	Each	5.00	24.00	24.00	330.00	0.00	0.00	90.00	14.00
	Ice Cream Cones, Cake or Wafer-t	28.3500	1.000	Ounce	2.30	1.96	22.40	118.22	0.00	0.85	0.00	0.35
	Ice Cream Cones, Sugar, Rolled-t	28.3500	1.000	Ounce	2.24	1.08	23.84	113.97	0.00	0.47	0.00	0.16
	Ice Cream Sandwich	63.0000	1.000	Each	3.00	6.00	27.00	170.00	0.00	1.00	10.00	3.00
476	Ice Cream Sandwich, Vanilla/Choc	80.0000	1.000	Each	4.00	13.00	31.00	260.00	0.00	1.00	65.00	8.00
477	Ice Cream Sandwich, Vanilla/Dark	83.0000	1.000	Each	4.00	20.00	23.00	290.00	0.00	2.00	70.00	12.00
475	Ice Cream Sandwich, Vanilla-Haag	80.0000	1.000	Each	4.00	13.00	32.00	260.00	0.00	0.00	65.00	8.00
478	Ice Cream, Bailey's Irish Cream-	102.0000	0.500	Cup	5.00	17.00	23.00	270.00	0.00	0.00	115.00	10.00
479	Ice Cream, Brownies a la Mode-Ha	99.0000	0.500	Cup	4.00	18.00	26.00	280.00	0.00	0.00	100.00	11.00
480	Ice Cream, Butter Pecan-Ben & Je	106.0000	0.500	Cup	4.00	21.00	15.00	250.00	0.00	1.00	80.00	9.00
481	Ice Cream, Butter Pecan-Haagen-D	106.0000	0.500	Cup	5.00	23.00	20.00	310.00	0.00	0.00	110.00	11.00
482	Ice Cream, Cappuccino Choc Chunk	106.0000	0.500	Cup	3.00	15.00	22.00	220.00	0.00	1.00	65.00	10.00
483	Ice Cream, Cappuccino Commotion-	103.0000	0.500	Cup	5.00	21.00	25.00	310.00	0.00	1.00	100.00	12.00
484	Ice Cream, Caramel Cone Explosio	103.0000	0.500	Cup	5.00	20.00	27.00	310.00	0.00	0.00	95.00	12.00
485	Ice Cream, Cherry Garcia-Ben & J	106.0000	0.500	Cup	3.00	13.00	21.00	200.00	0.00	0.00	65.00	8.00
486	Ice Cream, Cherry Vanilla-Haagen	101.0000	0.500	Cup	4.00	15.00	23.00	240.00	0.00	0.00	100.00	9.00
487	Ice Cream, Choc Chip Cookie Doug	106.0000	0.500	Cup	4.00	14.00	27.00	230.00	0.00	0.00	65.00	8.00
488	Ice Cream, Choc Choc Chip-Haagen	106.0000	0.500	Cup	5.00	20.00	26.00	300.00	0.00	2.00	100.00	12.00
489	Ice Cream, Choc Choc, Belgian-Ha	102.0000	0.500	Cup	5.00	21.00	29.00	330.00	0.00	3.00	85.00	12.00
490	Ice Cream, Choc Fudge Brownie, L	92.0000	0.500	Cup	7.00	2.50	34.00	190.00	0.00	1.00	8.00	1.50
491	Ice Cream, Choc Fudge Brownie-Be	106.0000	0.500	Cup	4.00	11.00	27.00	220.00	0.00	2.00	40.00	7.00
492	Ice Cream, Choc Mint Chip-Haagen	106.0000	0.500	Cup	5.00	20.00	25.00	300.00	0.00	4.00	95.00	11.00

Page Key: A2 = Baby Food   A2 = Baked Goods   A8 = Beverages   A14 = Breads/Grains and Pasta   A18 = Breakfast Foods/Cereals   A26 = Dairy and Eggs   A40 = Fats and Oils   A42 = Fruits and Vegetables   A52 = Meats and Beans   A60 = Nuts and Seeds   A62 5 Frozen Entrees and Packaged Foods   A76 = Restaurant Chains–Fast Foods   A92 = Restaurant Chains–Other   A106 = Seafood and Fish   A110 = Snacks and Sweets   A120 = Soups   A122 = Supplements   A126 = Toppings and Sauces

Monounsaturated Fat (g)	Polyunsaturated Fat (g)	Vitamin D (mg)	Vitamin K (mg)	Vitamin E (mg)	Vitamin A (re)	Vitamin C (mg)	Thiamin (mg)	Riboflavin (mg)	Niacin (mg)	Vitamin B6 (mg)	Folate (mcg)	Vitamin B12 (mcg)	Calcium (mg)	Iron (mg)	Magnesium (mg)	Phosphorus (mg)	Potassium (mg)	Sodium (mg)	Zinc (mg)
0.00	0.00	0.00	0.00	0.00	0.00	0.00	0.00	0.00	0.00	0.00	0.00	0.00	0.00	0.00	0.00	0.00	0.00	20.00	0.00
0.00	0.00	0.00	0.00	0.00	0.00	0.00	0.00	0.00	0.00	0.00	0.00	0.00	0.00	0.00	0.00	0.00	0.00	40.00	0.00
0.00	0.00	0.00	0.00	0.00	0.00	0.00	0.00	0.00	0.00	0.00	0.00	0.00	0.00	0.00	0.00	0.00	0.00	45.00	0.00
0.00	0.00	0.00	0.00	0.00	0.00	0.00	0.00	0.00	0.00	0.00	0.00	0.00	0.00	0.00	0.00	0.00	0.00	65.00	0.00
0.00	0.00	0.00	0.00	0.00	0.00	0.00	0.00	0.00	0.00	0.00	0.00	0.00	0.00	0.00	0.00	0.00	0.00	65.00	0.00
0.00	0.00	0.00	0.00	0.00	0.00	0.00	0.00	0.00	0.00	0.00	0.00	0.00	0.00	0.00	0.00	0.00	0.00	40.00	0.00
0.00	0.00	0.00	0.00	0.00	0.00	0.00	0.00	0.00	0.00	0.00	0.00	0.00	0.00	0.00	0.00	0.00	0.00	110.00	0.00
0.00	0.00	0.00	0.00	0.00	0.00	0.00	0.00	0.00	0.00	0.00	0.00	0.00	0.00	0.00	0.00	0.00	0.00	80.00	0.00
0.00	0.00	0.00	0.00	0.00	0.00	0.00	0.00	0.00	0.00	0.00	0.00	0.00	0.00	0.00	0.00	0.00	0.00	65.00	0.00
1.26	0.16	0.00	0.00	0.10	30.96	0.22	0.03	0.15	0.22	0.05	7.92	0.21	105.84	0.90	19.44	100.08	187.92	70.56	0.35
0.00	0.00	0.00	0.00	0.00	0.00	0.00	0.00	0.00	0.00	0.00	0.00	0.00	0.00	0.00	0.00	0.00	0.00	45.00	0.00
0.00	0.00	0.00	0.00	0.00	0.00	0.00	0.00	0.00	0.00	0.00	0.00	0.00	0.00	0.00	0.00	0.00	0.00	65.00	0.00
0.00	0.00	0.00	0.00	0.00	39.97	0.00	0.00	0.00	0.00	0.00	0.00	0.00	191.88	0.00	0.00	0.00	0.00	139.91	0.00
0.00	0.00	0.00	0.00	0.00	40.00	0.00	0.00	0.00	0.00	0.00	0.00	0.00	192.00	0.00	0.00	0.00	0.00	100.00	0.00
0.00	0.00	0.00	0.00	0.00	0.00	1.20	0.00	0.00	0.00	0.00	0.00	0.00	120.00	0.20	0.00	0.00	0.00	70.00	0.00
0.00	0.00	0.00	0.00	0.00	0.00	0.00	0.00	0.00	0.00	0.00	0.00	0.00	0.00	0.00	0.00	0.00	0.00	55.00	0.00
0.00	0.00	0.00	0.00	0.00	0.00	0.00	0.00	0.00	0.00	0.00	0.00	0.00	0.00	0.00	0.00	0.00	0.00	50.00	0.00
0.00	0.00	0.00	0.00	0.00	0.00	0.00	0.00	0.00	0.00	0.00	0.00	0.00	0.00	0.00	0.00	0.00	0.00	75.00	0.00
0.00	0.00	0.00	0.00	0.00	0.00	0.00	0.00	0.00	0.00	0.00	0.00	0.00	0.00	0.00	0.00	0.00	0.00	100.00	0.00
0.00	0.00	0.00	0.00	0.00	0.00	0.00	0.00	0.00	0.00	0.00	0.00	0.00	0.00	0.00	0.00	0.00	0.00	30.00	0.00
0.00	0.00	0.00	0.00	0.00	0.00	0.00	0.00	0.00	0.00	0.00	0.00	0.00	0.00	0.00	0.00	0.00	0.00	100.00	0.00
0.00	0.00	0.00	0.00	0.00	0.00	0.00	0.00	0.00	0.00	0.00	0.00	0.00	0.00	0.00	0.00	0.00	0.00	65.00	0.00
1.14	0.15	0.00	0.00	0.04	41.04	0.58	0.03	0.16	0.21	0.06	4.32	0.21	102.96	0.22	10.08	92.88	151.92	62.64	0.30
0.00	0.00	0.00	0.00	0.00	0.00	0.00	0.00	0.00	0.00	0.00	0.00	0.00	0.00	0.00	0.00	0.00	0.00	45.00	0.00
0.00	0.00	0.00	0.00	0.00	0.00	0.00	0.00	0.00	0.00	0.00	0.00	0.00	120.00	0.00	0.00	0.00	0.00	65.00	0.00
0.00	0.00	0.00	0.00	0.00	0.00	0.00	0.00	0.00	0.00	0.00	0.00	0.00	0.00	0.00	0.00	0.00	0.00	60.00	0.00
0.00	0.00	0.00	0.00	0.00	0.00	0.00	0.00	0.00	0.00	0.00	0.00	0.00	0.00	0.00	0.00	0.00	0.00	85.00	0.00
0.00	0.00	0.00	0.00	0.00	0.00	0.00	0.00	0.00	0.00	0.00	0.00	0.00	0.00	0.00	0.00	0.00	0.00	75.00	0.00
0.00	0.00	0.00	0.00	0.00	0.00	0.00	0.00	0.00	0.00	0.00	0.00	0.00	0.00	0.00	0.00	0.00	0.00	80.00	0.00
0.00	0.00	0.00	0.00	0.00	0.00	0.00	0.00	0.00	0.00	0.00	0.00	0.00	0.00	0.00	0.00	0.00	0.00	65.00	0.00
0.00	0.00	0.00	0.00	0.00	0.00	0.00	0.00	0.00	0.00	0.00	0.00	0.00	0.00	0.00	0.00	0.00	0.00	75.00	0.00
0.52	0.92	0.00	0.00	0.49	0.00	0.00	0.07	0.10	1.26	0.01	28.92	0.00	7.09	1.02	7.37	27.50	31.75	40.54	0.19
0.42	0.41	0.00	0.00	0.13	0.00	0.00	0.14	0.12	1.44	0.01	23.53	0.00	12.47	1.26	8.79	29.20	41.11	90.72	0.21
0.00	0.00	0.00	0.00	0.00	20.00	0.00	0.00	0.00	0.00	0.00	0.00	0.00	48.00	0.40	0.00	0.00	0.00	140.00	0.00
0.00	0.00	0.00	0.00	0.00	0.00	0.00	0.00	0.00	0.00	0.00	0.00	0.00	0.00	0.00	0.00	0.00	0.00	120.00	0.00
0.00	0.00	0.00	0.00	0.00	0.00	0.00	0.00	0.00	0.00	0.00	0.00	0.00	0.00	0.00	0.00	0.00	0.00	45.00	0.00
0.00	0.00	0.00	0.00	0.00	0.00	0.00	0.00	0.00	0.00	0.00	0.00	0.00	0.00	0.00	0.00	0.00	0.00	125.00	0.00
0.00	0.00	0.00	0.00	0.00	0.00	0.00	0.00	0.00	0.00	0.00	0.00	0.00	0.00	0.00	0.00	0.00	0.00	85.00	0.00
0.00	0.00	0.00	0.00	0.00	0.00	0.00	0.00	0.00	0.00	0.00	0.00	0.00	0.00	0.00	0.00	0.00	0.00	115.00	0.00
0.00	0.00	0.00	0.00	0.00	0.00	0.00	0.00	0.00	0.00	0.00	0.00	0.00	0.00	0.00	0.00	0.00	0.00	135.00	0.00
0.00	0.00	0.00	0.00	0.00	0.00	0.00	0.00	0.00	0.00	0.00	0.00	0.00	0.00	0.00	0.00	0.00	0.00	160.00	0.00
0.00	0.00	0.00	0.00	0.00	0.00	0.00	0.00	0.00	0.00	0.00	0.00	0.00	0.00	0.00	0.00	0.00	0.00	50.00	0.00
0.00	0.00	0.00	0.00	0.00	0.00	0.00	0.00	0.00	0.00	0.00	0.00	0.00	0.00	0.00	0.00	0.00	0.00	105.00	0.00
0.00	0.00	0.00	0.00	0.00	0.00	0.00	0.00	0.00	0.00	0.00	0.00	0.00	0.00	0.00	0.00	0.00	0.00	130.00	0.00
0.00	0.00	0.00	0.00	0.00	0.00	0.00	0.00	0.00	0.00	0.00	0.00	0.00	0.00	0.00	0.00	0.00	0.00	50.00	0.00
0.00	0.00	0.00	0.00	0.00	0.00	0.00	0.00	0.00	0.00	0.00	0.00	0.00	0.00	0.00	0.00	0.00	0.00	75.00	0.00
0.00	0.00	0.00	0.00	0.00	0.00	0.00	0.00	0.00	0.00	0.00	0.00	0.00	0.00	0.00	0.00	0.00	0.00	85.00	0.00
0.00	0.00	0.00	0.00	0.00	0.00	0.00	0.00	0.00	0.00	0.00	0.00	0.00	0.00	0.00	0.00	0.00	0.00	70.00	0.00
0.00	0.00	0.00	0.00	0.00	0.00	0.00	0.00	0.00	0.00	0.00	0.00	0.00	0.00	0.00	0.00	0.00	0.00	60.00	0.00
0.00	0.00	0.00	0.00	0.00	0.00	0.00	0.00	0.00	0.00	0.00	0.00	0.00	0.00	0.00	0.00	0.00	0.00	110.00	0.00
0.00	0.00	0.00	0.00	0.00	0.00	0.00	0.00	0.00	0.00	0.00	0.00	0.00	0.00	0.00	0.00	0.00	0.00	75.00	0.00
0.00	0.00	0.00	0.00	0.00	0.00	0.00	0.00	0.00	0.00	0.00	0.00	0.00	0.00	0.00	0.00	0.00	0.00	65.00	0.00

USDA ID Code	Food Name	Weight in Grams*	Quantity of Units	Unit of Measure	Protein (g)	Fat (g)	Carbohydrate (g)	Kilocalories	Caffeine (g)	Fiber (g)	Cholesterol (mg)	Saturated Fat (g)
493	Ice Cream, Choc PB, Deep-Haagen-	102.0000	0.500	Cup	8.00	24.00	26.00	350.00	0.00	4.00	80.00	11.00
494	Ice Cream, Choc Peanut Butter Do	106.0000	0.500	Cup	4.00	16.00	23.00	240.00	0.00	1.00	50.00	6.00
495	Ice Cream, Choc Raspberry Swirl-	106.0000	0.500	Cup	3.00	11.00	28.00	220.00	0.00	2.00	35.00	7.00
496	Ice Cream, Choc, Deep Dark, Egg	106.0000	0.500	Cup	3.00	12.00	24.00	200.00	0.00	2.00	45.00	7.00
	Ice Cream, Chocolate	58.0000	3.500	Fl Oz	2.20	6.38	16.36	125.28	1.74	0.70	19.72	3.94
497	Ice Cream, Chocolate, Low Fat-Ha	92.0000	0.500	Cup	7.00	2.50	29.00	170.00	0.00	0.00	8.00	4.00
498	Ice Cream, Chocolate-Haagen-Daz	106.0000	0.500	Cup	5.00	18.00	22.00	270.00	0.00	1.00	115.00	11.00
499	Ice Cream, Chubby Hubby-Ben & Je	106.0000	0.500	Cup	6.00	17.00	24.00	260.00	0.00	2.00	50.00	8.00
500	Ice Cream, Chunky Monkey-Ben & J	106.0000	0.500	Cup	3.00	16.00	24.00	240.00	0.00	1.00	55.00	8.00
501	Ice Cream, Coconut Almond Fudge	106.0000	0.500	Cup	5.00	20.00	19.00	260.00	0.00	2.00	60.00	11.00
502	Ice Cream, Coffee Fudge, Low Fat	92.0000	0.500	Cup	5.00	2.50	32.00	170.00	0.00	0.00	25.00	1.50
503	Ice Cream, Coffee Mocha Chip-Haa	106.0000	0.500	Cup	4.00	19.00	25.00	290.00	0.00	0.00	110.00	12.00
504	Ice Cream, Coffee Ole-Ben & Jerr	106.0000	0.500	Cup	3.00	13.00	18.00	180.00	0.00	0.00	70.00	8.00
505	Ice Cream, Coffee w/ Heath Crunc	106.0000	0.500	Cup	3.00	16.00	24.00	240.00	0.00	0.00	60.00	9.00
506	Ice Cream, Coffee-Haagen-Daz	106.0000	0.500	Cup	5.00	18.00	21.00	270.00	0.00	0.00	120.00	11.00
507	Ice Cream, Cookie Dough Dynamo-H	103.0000	0.500	Cup	4.00	19.00	29.00	300.00	0.00	0.00	95.00	12.00
508	Ice Cream, Cookie, Sweet Cream-B	106.0000	0.500	Cup	3.00	14.00	22.00	220.00	0.00	1.00	65.00	8.00
509	Ice Cream, Cookies & Cream, Midn	102.0000	0.500	Cup	5.00	18.00	29.00	300.00	0.00	1.00	90.00	11.00
510	Ice Cream, Cookies & Cream-Haage	102.0000	0.500	Cup	5.00	17.00	23.00	270.00	0.00	1.00	110.00	11.00
511	Ice Cream, Cool Britannia-Ben &	106.0000	0.500	Cup	3.00	12.00	23.00	200.00	0.00	0.00	55.00	8.00
512	Ice Cream, De Leche Caramel-Haag	106.0000	0.500	Cup	5.00	17.00	28.00	290.00	0.00	0.00	100.00	10.00
513	Ice Cream, DiSaronno Amaretto-Ha	103.0000	0.500	Cup	4.00	15.00	26.00	260.00	0.00	0.00	95.00	9.00
514	Ice Cream, Fudge Chunk, NY Super	106.0000	0.500	Cup	4.00	17.00	23.00	240.00	0.00	2.00	40.00	9.00
	Ice Cream, Light	67.0000	0.500	Cup	3.00	4.50	18.00	130.00	0.00	0.00	35.00	2.50
	Ice Cream, Low Fat-Haagen Daz	92.0000	0.500	Cup	7.00	2.50	29.00	170.00	0.00	0.00	0.00	0.00
	Ice Cream, Low Fat-Starbucks	99.0000	0.500	Cup	5.00	3.00	31.00	170.00	0.00	0.00	10.00	1.50
515	Ice Cream, Macadamia Nut Brittle	106.0000	0.500	Cup	4.00	20.00	25.00	300.00	0.00	0.00	110.00	11.00
516	Ice Cream, Malted Milk Ball-Ben	106.0000	0.500	Cup	3.00	14.00	22.00	220.00	0.00	0.00	65.00	9.00
517	Ice Cream, Maple Walnut-Ben & Je	106.0000	0.500	Cup	4.00	18.00	18.00	240.00	0.00	1.00	60.00	8.00
518	Ice Cream, Mint Chip-Haagen-Daz	106.0000	0.500	Cup	4.00	19.00	26.00	290.00	0.00	0.00	105.00	12.00
519	Ice Cream, Mint Choc Chunk-Ben &	106.0000	0.500	Cup	3.00	15.00	22.00	220.00	0.00	1.00	65.00	10.00
520	Ice Cream, Mint Choc Cookie-Ben	106.0000	0.500	Cup	3.00	14.00	23.00	220.00	0.00	1.00	65.00	8.00
521	Ice Cream, Mocha Fudge-Ben & Jer	106.0000	0.500	Cup	3.00	13.00	22.00	200.00	0.00	1.00	60.00	7.00
522	Ice Cream, Peanut Butter Cup-Ben	106.0000	0.500	Cup	5.00	18.00	21.00	260.00	0.00	1.00	60.00	9.00
523	Ice Cream, Pistachio Pistachio-B	106.0000	0.500	Cup	4.00	17.00	16.00	220.00	0.00	1.00	70.00	8.00
524	Ice Cream, Praline Pecan-Ben & J	106.0000	0.500	Cup	3.00	17.00	26.00	250.00	0.00	0.00	70.00	8.00
525	Ice Cream, Pralines & Cream-Haag	102.0000	0.500	Cup	4.00	18.00	27.00	290.00	0.00	0.00	95.00	9.00
526	Ice Cream, Rainforest Crunch-Ben	106.0000	0.500	Cup	4.00	18.00	19.00	240.00	0.00	0.00	70.00	9.00
527	Ice Cream, Rum Raisin-Haagen-Daz	106.0000	0.500	Cup	4.00	17.00	22.00	270.00	0.00	0.00	110.00	10.00
	Ice Cream, Strawberry	58.0000	3.500	Fl Oz	1.86	4.87	16.01	111.36	0.00	0.17	16.82	3.01
528	Ice Cream, Strawberry Cheesecake	103.0000	0.500	Cup	4.00	16.00	27.00	270.00	0.00	0.00	100.00	10.00
529	Ice Cream, Strawberry, Low Fat-H	92.0000	0.500	Cup	5.00	2.00	28.00	150.00	0.00	0.00	15.00	1.00
530	Ice Cream, Strawberry-Ben & Jerr	106.0000	0.500	Cup	2.00	10.00	19.00	170.00	0.00	1.00	55.00	6.00
531	Ice Cream, Strawberry-Haagen-Daz	106.0000	0.500	Cup	4.00	16.00	23.00	250.00	0.00	0.00	95.00	10.00
	Ice Cream, Vanilla	58.0000	3.500	Fl Oz	2.03	6.38	13.69	116.58	0.00	0.00	25.52	3.94
532	Ice Cream, Vanilla Bean-Ben & J	106.0000	0.500	Cup	3.00	13.00	18.00	190.00	0.00	0.00	75.00	8.00
533	Ice Cream, Vanilla Caramel Fudge	106.0000	0.500	Cup	2.00	12.00	24.00	180.00	0.00	0.00	70.00	7.00
534	Ice Cream, Vanilla Caramel, Low	92.0000	0.500	Cup	6.00	2.50	32.00	180.00	0.00	0.00	20.00	1.50
535	Ice Cream, Vanilla Choc Chip-Haa	106.0000	0.500	Cup	5.00	20.00	26.00	310.00	0.00	0.00	105.00	12.00
536	Ice Cream, Vanilla Choc Chunk-Be	106.0000	0.500	Cup	3.00	15.00	22.00	220.00	0.00	1.00	65.00	10.00
537	Ice Cream, Vanilla Fudge Brownie	106.0000	0.500	Cup	4.00	12.00	23.00	210.00	0.00	0.00	60.00	7.00
538	Ice Cream, Vanilla Fudge-Haagen-	106.0000	0.500	Cup	5.00	18.00	26.00	290.00	0.00	0.00	100.00	12.00
539	Ice Cream, Vanilla Swiss Almond-	106.0000	0.500	Cup	6.00	21.00	23.00	310.00	0.00	1.00	105.00	11.00

Page Key: A2 = Baby Food   A2 = Baked Goods   A8 = Beverages   A14 = Breads/Grains and Pasta   A18 = Breakfast Foods/Cereals   A26 = Dairy and Eggs   A40 = Fats and Oils   A42 = Fruits and Vegetables   A52 = Meats and Beans   A60 = Nuts and Seeds   A62 5 Frozen Entrees and Packaged Foods   A76 = Restaurant Chains–Fast Foods   A92 = Restaurant Chains–Other   A106 = Seafood and Fish   A110 = Snacks and Sweets   A120 = Soups   A122 = Supplements   A126 = Toppings and Sauces

Monounsaturated Fat (g)	Polyunsaturated Fat (g)	Vitamin D (mg)	Vitamin K (mg)	Vitamin E (mg)	Vitamin A (re)	Vitamin C (mg)	Thiamin (mg)	Riboflavin (mg)	Niacin (mg)	Vitamin B$_6$ (mg)	Folate (mcg)	Vitamin B$_{12}$ (mcg)	Calcium (mg)	Iron (mg)	Magnesium (mg)	Phosphorus (mg)	Potassium (mg)	Sodium (mg)	Zinc (mg)
0.00	0.00	0.00	0.00	0.00	0.00	0.00	0.00	0.00	0.00	0.00	0.00	0.00	0.00	0.00	0.00	0.00	0.00	100.00	0.00
0.00	0.00	0.00	0.00	0.00	0.00	0.00	0.00	0.00	0.00	0.00	0.00	0.00	0.00	0.00	0.00	0.00	0.00	65.00	0.00
0.00	0.00	0.00	0.00	0.00	0.00	0.00	0.00	0.00	0.00	0.00	0.00	0.00	0.00	0.00	0.00	0.00	0.00	35.00	0.00
0.00	0.00	0.00	0.00	0.00	0.00	0.00	0.00	0.00	0.00	0.00	0.00	0.00	0.00	0.00	0.00	0.00	0.00	35.00	0.00
1.86	0.24	0.00	0.00	0.19	69.02	0.41	0.02	0.11	0.13	0.03	9.28	0.17	63.22	0.54	16.82	62.06	144.42	44.08	0.34
0.00	0.00	0.00	0.00	0.00	0.00	0.00	0.00	0.00	0.00	0.00	0.00	0.00	0.00	0.00	0.00	0.00	0.00	50.00	0.00
0.00	0.00	0.00	0.00	0.00	0.00	0.00	0.00	0.00	0.00	0.00	0.00	0.00	0.00	0.00	0.00	0.00	0.00	75.00	0.00
0.00	0.00	0.00	0.00	0.00	0.00	0.00	0.00	0.00	0.00	0.00	0.00	0.00	0.00	0.00	0.00	0.00	0.00	140.00	0.00
0.00	0.00	0.00	0.00	0.00	0.00	0.00	0.00	0.00	0.00	0.00	0.00	0.00	0.00	0.00	0.00	0.00	0.00	40.00	0.00
0.00	0.00	0.00	0.00	0.00	0.00	0.00	0.00	0.00	0.00	0.00	0.00	0.00	0.00	0.00	0.00	0.00	0.00	70.00	0.00
0.00	0.00	0.00	0.00	0.00	0.00	0.00	0.00	0.00	0.00	0.00	0.00	0.00	0.00	0.00	0.00	0.00	0.00	95.00	0.00
0.00	0.00	0.00	0.00	0.00	0.00	0.00	0.00	0.00	0.00	0.00	0.00	0.00	0.00	0.00	0.00	0.00	0.00	90.00	0.00
0.00	0.00	0.00	0.00	0.00	0.00	0.00	0.00	0.00	0.00	0.00	0.00	0.00	0.00	0.00	0.00	0.00	0.00	45.00	0.00
0.00	0.00	0.00	0.00	0.00	0.00	0.00	0.00	0.00	0.00	0.00	0.00	0.00	0.00	0.00	0.00	0.00	0.00	110.00	0.00
0.00	0.00	0.00	0.00	0.00	0.00	0.00	0.00	0.00	0.00	0.00	0.00	0.00	0.00	0.00	0.00	0.00	0.00	85.00	0.00
0.00	0.00	0.00	0.00	0.00	0.00	0.00	0.00	0.00	0.00	0.00	0.00	0.00	0.00	0.00	0.00	0.00	0.00	140.00	0.00
0.00	0.00	0.00	0.00	0.00	0.00	0.00	0.00	0.00	0.00	0.00	0.00	0.00	0.00	0.00	0.00	0.00	0.00	110.00	0.00
0.00	0.00	0.00	0.00	0.00	0.00	0.00	0.00	0.00	0.00	0.00	0.00	0.00	0.00	0.00	0.00	0.00	0.00	140.00	0.00
0.00	0.00	0.00	0.00	0.00	0.00	0.00	0.00	0.00	0.00	0.00	0.00	0.00	0.00	0.00	0.00	0.00	0.00	115.00	0.00
0.00	0.00	0.00	0.00	0.00	0.00	0.00	0.00	0.00	0.00	0.00	0.00	0.00	0.00	0.00	0.00	0.00	0.00	55.00	0.00
0.00	0.00	0.00	0.00	0.00	0.00	0.00	0.00	0.00	0.00	0.00	0.00	0.00	0.00	0.00	0.00	0.00	0.00	110.00	0.00
0.00	0.00	0.00	0.00	0.00	0.00	0.00	0.00	0.00	0.00	0.00	0.00	0.00	0.00	0.00	0.00	0.00	0.00	80.00	0.00
0.00	0.00	0.00	0.00	0.00	0.00	0.00	0.00	0.00	0.00	0.00	0.00	0.00	0.00	0.00	0.00	0.00	0.00	50.00	0.00
0.00	0.00	0.00	0.00	0.00	0.00	0.00	0.00	0.00	0.00	0.00	0.00	0.00	80.00	0.00	0.00	0.00	0.00	50.00	0.00
0.00	0.00	0.00	0.00	0.00	0.00	0.00	0.00	0.00	0.00	0.00	0.00	0.00	160.00	0.00	0.00	0.00	0.00	50.00	0.00
0.00	0.00	0.00	0.00	0.00	0.00	0.00	0.00	0.00	0.00	0.00	0.00	0.00	80.00	0.00	0.00	0.00	0.00	65.00	0.00
0.00	0.00	0.00	0.00	0.00	0.00	0.00	0.00	0.00	0.00	0.00	0.00	0.00	0.00	0.00	0.00	0.00	0.00	120.00	0.00
0.00	0.00	0.00	0.00	0.00	0.00	0.00	0.00	0.00	0.00	0.00	0.00	0.00	0.00	0.00	0.00	0.00	0.00	60.00	0.00
0.00	0.00	0.00	0.00	0.00	0.00	0.00	0.00	0.00	0.00	0.00	0.00	0.00	0.00	0.00	0.00	0.00	0.00	40.00	0.00
0.00	0.00	0.00	0.00	0.00	0.00	0.00	0.00	0.00	0.00	0.00	0.00	0.00	0.00	0.00	0.00	0.00	0.00	105.00	0.00
0.00	0.00	0.00	0.00	0.00	0.00	0.00	0.00	0.00	0.00	0.00	0.00	0.00	0.00	0.00	0.00	0.00	0.00	50.00	0.00
0.00	0.00	0.00	0.00	0.00	0.00	0.00	0.00	0.00	0.00	0.00	0.00	0.00	0.00	0.00	0.00	0.00	0.00	110.00	0.00
0.00	0.00	0.00	0.00	0.00	0.00	0.00	0.00	0.00	0.00	0.00	0.00	0.00	0.00	0.00	0.00	0.00	0.00	45.00	0.00
0.00	0.00	0.00	0.00	0.00	0.00	0.00	0.00	0.00	0.00	0.00	0.00	0.00	0.00	0.00	0.00	0.00	0.00	95.00	0.00
0.00	0.00	0.00	0.00	0.00	0.00	0.00	0.00	0.00	0.00	0.00	0.00	0.00	0.00	0.00	0.00	0.00	0.00	70.00	0.00
0.00	0.00	0.00	0.00	0.00	0.00	0.00	0.00	0.00	0.00	0.00	0.00	0.00	0.00	0.00	0.00	0.00	0.00	90.00	0.00
0.00	0.00	0.00	0.00	0.00	0.00	0.00	0.00	0.00	0.00	0.00	0.00	0.00	0.00	0.00	0.00	0.00	0.00	180.00	0.00
0.00	0.00	0.00	0.00	0.00	0.00	0.00	0.00	0.00	0.00	0.00	0.00	0.00	0.00	0.00	0.00	0.00	0.00	105.00	0.00
0.00	0.00	0.00	0.00	0.00	0.00	0.00	0.00	0.00	0.00	0.00	0.00	0.00	0.00	0.00	0.00	0.00	0.00	75.00	0.00
0.00	0.00	0.00	0.00	0.00	45.24	4.47	0.03	0.15	0.10	0.03	6.96	0.17	69.60	0.12	8.12	58.00	109.04	34.80	0.20
0.00	0.00	0.00	0.00	0.00	0.00	0.00	0.00	0.00	0.00	0.00	0.00	0.00	0.00	0.00	0.00	0.00	0.00	150.00	0.00
0.00	0.00	0.00	0.00	0.00	0.00	0.00	0.00	0.00	0.00	0.00	0.00	0.00	0.00	0.00	0.00	0.00	0.00	40.00	0.00
0.00	0.00	0.00	0.00	0.00	0.00	0.00	0.00	0.00	0.00	0.00	0.00	0.00	0.00	0.00	0.00	0.00	0.00	35.00	0.00
0.00	0.00	0.00	0.00	0.00	0.00	0.00	0.00	0.00	0.00	0.00	0.00	0.00	0.00	0.00	0.00	0.00	0.00	80.00	0.00
1.84	0.24	0.00	0.00	0.00	67.86	0.35	0.02	0.14	0.07	0.03	2.90	0.23	74.24	0.05	8.12	60.90	115.42	46.40	0.40
0.00	0.00	0.00	0.00	0.00	0.00	0.00	0.00	0.00	0.00	0.00	0.00	0.00	0.00	0.00	0.00	0.00	0.00	45.00	0.00
0.00	0.00	0.00	0.00	0.00	0.00	0.00	0.00	0.00	0.00	0.00	0.00	0.00	0.00	0.00	0.00	0.00	0.00	50.00	0.00
0.00	0.00	0.00	0.00	0.00	0.00	0.00	0.00	0.00	0.00	0.00	0.00	0.00	0.00	0.00	0.00	0.00	0.00	120.00	0.00
0.00	0.00	0.00	0.00	0.00	0.00	0.00	0.00	0.00	0.00	0.00	0.00	0.00	0.00	0.00	0.00	0.00	0.00	90.00	0.00
0.00	0.00	0.00	0.00	0.00	0.00	0.00	0.00	0.00	0.00	0.00	0.00	0.00	0.00	0.00	0.00	0.00	0.00	50.00	0.00
0.00	0.00	0.00	0.00	0.00	0.00	0.00	0.00	0.00	0.00	0.00	0.00	0.00	0.00	0.00	0.00	0.00	0.00	80.00	0.00
0.00	0.00	0.00	0.00	0.00	0.00	0.00	0.00	0.00	0.00	0.00	0.00	0.00	0.00	0.00	0.00	0.00	0.00	110.00	0.00
0.00	0.00	0.00	0.00	0.00	0.00	0.00	0.00	0.00	0.00	0.00	0.00	0.00	0.00	0.00	0.00	0.00	0.00	90.00	0.00

USDA ID Code	Food Name	Weight in Grams*	Quantity of Units	Unit of Measure	Protein (g)	Fat (g)	Carbohydrate (g)	Kilocalories	Caffeine (g)	Fiber (g)	Cholesterol (mg)	Saturated Fat (g)
540	Ice Cream, Vanilla w/ Heath Crun	106.0000	0.500	Cup	3.00	17.00	24.00	240.00	0.00	0.00	65.00	9.00
541	Ice Cream, Vanilla, French, Coff	106.0000	0.500	Cup	5.00	18.00	21.00	270.00	0.00	0.00	120.00	11.00
	Ice Cream, Vanilla, French, Soft	86.0000	0.500	Cup	3.53	11.18	19.09	184.90	0.00	0.00	78.26	6.43
543	Ice Cream, Vanilla, Low Fat-Haag	92.0000	0.500	Cup	7.00	2.50	29.00	170.00	0.00	0.00	20.00	1.50
	Ice Cream, Vanilla, Rich	74.0000	0.500	Cup	2.59	11.99	16.58	178.34	0.00	0.00	45.14	7.38
542	Ice Cream, Vanilla-Haagen-Daz	106.0000	0.500	Cup	5.00	18.00	21.00	270.00	0.00	0.00	120.00	11.00
544	Ice Cream, Wavy Gravy-Ben & Jerr	106.0000	0.500	Cup	5.00	19.00	22.00	260.00	0.00	2.00	55.00	7.00
545	Ice Cream, White Russian-Ben & J	106.0000	0.500	Cup	3.00	13.00	18.00	190.00	0.00	0.00	70.00	8.00
	Ice Cream-Starbucks	99.0000	0.500	Cup	4.00	13.00	30.00	250.00	0.00	0.00	60.00	8.00
	Milk Substitutes, Fluid w/ hydr	244.0000	1.000	Cup	4.27	8.32	15.03	149.96	0.00	0.00	0.49	1.88
	Milk Substitutes, Fluid, w/ laur	244.0000	1.000	Cup	4.27	8.32	15.03	149.96	0.00	0.00	0.49	7.42
	Milk, Buttermilk	245.0000	1.000	Cup	8.11	2.16	11.74	99.00	0.00	0.00	8.57	1.35
	Milk, Chocolate Drink, Lowfat, 1	250.0000	1.000	Cup	8.10	2.50	26.10	157.58	5.00	1.25	7.25	1.55
	Milk, Chocolate Drink, Lowfat, 2	250.0000	1.000	Cup	8.03	5.00	26.00	178.85	5.00	1.25	17.00	3.10
	Milk, Chocolate Drink, Whole	250.0000	1.000	Cup	7.93	8.48	25.85	208.38	5.00	2.00	30.50	5.25
	Milk, Chocolate Homemade Hot Coc	250.0000	1.000	Cup	9.78	5.83	29.48	192.50	5.00	2.00	20.00	3.60
	Milk, Condensed, Sweetened, Cnd	306.0000	1.000	Cup	24.20	26.62	166.46	981.59	0.00	0.00	103.73	16.80
	Milk, Evaporated, Cnd	31.5000	1.000	Fl Oz	2.15	2.38	3.16	42.33	0.00	0.00	9.26	1.45
	Milk, Evaporated, Skim, Cnd	256.0000	1.000	Cup	19.33	0.51	29.06	199.48	0.00	0.00	9.22	0.31
	Milk, Light, 1% Fat	244.0000	1.000	Cup	8.03	2.59	11.66	102.14	0.00	0.00	9.76	1.61
	Milk, Malted, Beverage	265.0000	1.000	Cup	10.34	9.81	27.30	235.85	0.00	0.00	37.10	5.95
	Milk, Malted, Chocolate Flavor,	265.0000	1.000	Cup	9.01	9.01	29.95	227.90	7.95	0.00	34.45	5.53
	Milk, Non-Fat, Skim	245.0000	1.000	Cup	8.35	0.44	11.88	85.53	0.00	0.00	4.41	0.29
	Milk, Reduced, 2% Fat	244.0000	1.000	Cup	8.13	4.68	11.71	121.19	0.00	0.00	18.30	2.93
583	Milk, Rice, Enriched Brown-Rice	240.0000	8.000	Fl Oz	1.00	2.00	25.00	120.00	0.00	0.00	0.00	0.00
584	Milk, Soy	240.0000	1.000	Cup	6.60	4.58	4.34	79.00	0.00	3.12	0.00	0.51
	Milk, Whole, 3.3% Fat	244.0000	1.000	Cup	8.03	8.15	11.37	149.91	0.00	0.00	33.18	5.08
	Milk, Whole, 3.7% Fat	244.0000	1.000	Cup	8.00	8.93	11.35	156.57	0.00	0.00	34.89	5.56
	Sour Cream	230.0000	1.000	Cup	7.27	48.21	9.82	492.80	0.00	0.00	102.12	30.02
	Sour Cream, Fat Free	16.0140	1.000	Tbsp	0.50	0.00	2.50	12.51	0.00	0.00	2.50	0.00
	Sour Cream, Imitation, Non-dairy	230.0000	1.000	Cup	5.52	44.90	15.25	479.46	0.00	0.00	0.00	40.92
	Sour Cream, Light	16.0140	1.000	Tbsp	0.92	1.14	0.92	16.01	0.00	0.00	4.58	0.69
	Sour Cream, Non-Fat	16.0000	2.000	Tbsp	0.50	0.00	2.50	12.50	0.00	0.00	2.50	0.00
	Yogurt, 99% Fat Free-Dannon	227.0000	8.000	Ounce	9.00	3.00	45.00	240.00	0.00	0.00	15.00	1.50
834	Yogurt, Apl Cin., Non Fat, Chunk	170.0000	6.000	Ounce	7.00	0.00	33.00	160.00	0.00	0.00	5.00	0.00
835	Yogurt, Apple Cin, Fruit on Bott	227.0000	8.000	Ounce	9.00	3.00	46.00	240.00	0.00	1.00	15.00	1.50
836	Yogurt, Apple Cobbler, Smooth &	227.0000	8.000	Ounce	8.00	2.00	46.00	230.00	0.00	0.00	20.00	1.00
837	Yogurt, Apple Pie a la Mode, Non	227.0000	8.000	Ounce	7.00	0.00	22.00	120.00	0.00	0.00	10.00	0.00
838	Yogurt, Ban Crm/Straw, Double De	170.0000	6.000	Ounce	7.00	1.00	32.00	160.00	0.00	0.00	10.00	0.50
839	Yogurt, Banana Cream Pie, Light-	227.0000	8.000	Ounce	8.00	0.00	16.00	100.00	0.00	0.00	5.00	0.00
840	Yogurt, Bav Crm/Rasp, Double Del	170.0000	6.000	Ounce	7.00	1.00	34.00	170.00	0.00	0.00	10.00	0.50
841	Yogurt, Bavarian & Peach, Light	170.0000	6.000	Ounce	5.00	0.00	18.00	90.00	0.00	0.00	0.00	0.00
842	Yogurt, Berries, Mixed, Fruit on	227.0000	8.000	Ounce	9.00	3.00	45.00	240.00	0.00	1.00	15.00	1.50
843	Yogurt, Berry Banana Split, Non	227.0000	8.000	Ounce	8.00	0.00	21.00	120.00	0.00	0.00	10.00	0.00
844	Yogurt, Berry, Mixed, Fruit on B	125.0000	4.400	Ounce	5.00	1.50	25.00	130.00	0.00	0.00	10.00	1.00
845	Yogurt, Berry, Mixed, Lowfat-Bre	227.0000	8.000	Ounce	9.00	2.50	43.00	230.00	0.00	0.00	15.00	1.50
846	Yogurt, Berry, Tropical, Non Fat	170.0000	6.000	Ounce	7.00	0.00	32.00	160.00	0.00	0.00	5.00	0.00
847	Yogurt, Blackberry Pie, Light-Da	227.0000	8.000	Ounce	8.00	0.00	16.00	100.00	0.00	0.00	5.00	0.00
848	Yogurt, Blueberries N' Cream, No	227.0000	8.000	Ounce	8.00	0.00	23.00	120.00	0.00	0.00	10.00	0.00
849	Yogurt, Blueberries/Crm, Smooth	227.0000	8.000	Ounce	9.00	2.00	46.00	240.00	0.00	0.00	20.00	1.00
850	Yogurt, Blueberry, Blended-Breye	125.0000	4.400	Ounce	4.00	1.00	25.00	130.00	0.00	0.00	10.00	0.50
851	Yogurt, Blueberry, Danimals-Dann	125.0000	4.400	Ounce	6.00	1.00	24.00	130.00	0.00	0.00	5.00	0.50
852	Yogurt, Blueberry, Fruit on Bott	227.0000	8.000	Ounce	9.00	3.00	46.00	240.00	0.00	1.00	15.00	1.50

Page Key: A2 = Baby Food   A2 = Baked Goods   A8 = Beverages   A14 = Breads/Grains and Pasta   A18 = Breakfast Foods/Cereals   A26 = Dairy and Eggs   A40 = Fats and Oils   A42 = Fruits and Vegetables   A52 = Meats and Beans   A60 = Nuts and Seeds   A62 5 Frozen Entrees and Packaged Foods   A76 = Restaurant Chains–Fast Foods   A92 = Restaurant Chains–Other   A106 = Seafood and Fish   A110 = Snacks and Sweets   A120 = Soups   A122 = Supplements   A126 = Toppings and Sauces

Monounsaturated Fat (g)	Polyunsaturated Fat (g)	Vitamin D (mg)	Vitamin K (mg)	Vitamin E (mg)	Vitamin A (re)	Vitamin C (mg)	Thiamin (mg)	Riboflavin (mg)	Niacin (mg)	Vitamin B$_6$ (mg)	Folate (mcg)	Vitamin B$_{12}$ (mcg)	Calcium (mg)	Iron (mg)	Magnesium (mg)	Phosphorus (mg)	Potassium (mg)	Sodium (mg)	Zinc (mg)
0.00	0.00	0.00	0.00	0.00	0.00	0.00	0.00	0.00	0.00	0.00	0.00	0.00	0.00	0.00	0.00	0.00	0.00	110.00	0.00
0.00	0.00	0.00	0.00	0.00	0.00	0.00	0.00	0.00	0.00	0.00	0.00	0.00	0.00	0.00	0.00	0.00	0.00	85.00	0.00
3.00	0.39	0.00	0.00	0.32	132.44	0.69	0.04	0.15	0.09	0.04	7.74	0.43	112.66	0.18	10.32	99.76	152.22	52.46	0.45
0.00	0.00	0.00	0.00	0.00	0.00	0.00	0.00	0.00	0.00	0.00	0.00	0.00	0.00	0.00	0.00	0.00	0.00	50.00	0.00
3.45	0.44	0.00	0.00	0.00	136.16	0.52	0.03	0.12	0.06	0.03	3.70	0.27	86.58	0.04	8.14	70.30	117.66	41.44	0.30
0.00	0.00	0.00	0.00	0.00	0.00	0.00	0.00	0.00	0.00	0.00	0.00	0.00	0.00	0.00	0.00	0.00	0.00	85.00	0.00
0.00	0.00	0.00	0.00	0.00	0.00	0.00	0.00	0.00	0.00	0.00	0.00	0.00	0.00	0.00	0.00	0.00	0.00	90.00	0.00
0.00	0.00	0.00	0.00	0.00	0.00	0.00	0.00	0.00	0.00	0.00	0.00	0.00	0.00	0.00	0.00	0.00	0.00	45.00	0.00
0.00	0.00	0.00	0.00	0.00	0.00	0.00	0.00	0.00	0.00	0.00	0.00	0.00	120.00	0.00	0.00	0.00	0.00	15.00	0.00
4.88	1.20	0.00	0.00	2.56	0.00	0.00	0.02	0.22	0.00	0.00	0.00	0.00	79.30	0.95	15.57	181.05	278.89	191.05	2.88
0.44	0.02	0.00	0.00	0.00	0.00	0.00	0.02	0.22	0.00	0.00	0.00	0.00	79.30	0.95	15.57	181.05	278.89	191.05	2.88
0.61	0.07	0.00	0.00	0.15	19.60	2.40	0.07	0.37	0.15	0.07	12.25	0.54	285.18	0.12	26.83	218.54	370.69	257.01	1.03
0.75	0.10	2.50	0.00	0.08	147.50	2.33	0.10	0.43	0.33	0.10	12.00	0.85	286.75	0.60	33.33	256.50	425.50	151.75	1.03
1.48	0.18	2.50	0.00	0.13	142.50	2.30	0.10	0.40	0.33	0.10	12.00	0.85	284.00	0.60	33.00	254.25	422.00	150.50	1.03
2.48	0.30	2.50	0.00	0.23	72.50	2.28	0.10	0.40	0.33	0.10	11.75	0.83	280.25	0.60	32.58	251.25	417.25	149.00	1.03
1.70	0.23	0.00	0.00	0.25	137.50	2.50	0.10	0.43	0.38	0.13	15.00	0.93	315.00	1.15	70.00	292.50	500.00	127.50	1.48
7.44	1.04	0.00	0.00	0.64	247.86	7.96	0.28	1.29	0.64	0.15	34.27	1.35	867.51	0.58	78.49	775.10	1136.48	388.62	2.88
0.74	0.08	0.00	0.00	0.00	17.01	0.59	0.02	0.10	0.06	0.02	2.49	0.05	82.15	0.06	7.62	63.79	95.48	33.33	0.24
0.15	0.03	5.12	0.00	0.03	299.52	3.17	0.13	0.79	0.44	0.15	22.02	0.61	741.12	0.74	69.12	498.94	848.64	294.40	2.30
0.76	0.10	2.44	0.00	0.10	143.96	2.37	0.10	0.41	0.22	0.10	12.44	0.90	300.12	0.12	33.72	234.73	380.88	123.22	0.95
2.78	0.56	0.00	0.00	0.00	95.40	2.92	0.20	0.59	1.31	0.19	21.73	1.03	355.10	0.27	53.00	302.10	530.00	222.60	1.14
2.57	0.38	0.00	0.00	0.00	79.50	2.65	0.13	0.44	0.63	0.14	16.43	0.93	304.75	0.61	47.70	265.00	498.20	172.25	1.09
0.12	0.02	2.45	9.80	0.10	149.45	2.40	0.10	0.34	0.22	0.10	12.74	0.93	302.33	0.10	27.83	247.21	405.72	126.18	0.98
1.37	0.17	2.44	0.00	0.17	139.08	2.32	0.10	0.41	0.22	0.10	12.44	0.88	296.70	0.12	33.35	232.04	376.74	121.76	0.95
0.00	0.00	0.00	0.00	0.00	0.00	0.00	0.00	0.00	0.00	0.00	0.00	0.00	0.00	0.00	0.00	0.00	0.00	90.00	0.00
0.78	1.90	0.00	0.00	0.00	23.06	0.00	0.38	0.16	0.35	0.09	3.60	0.00	9.60	1.39	45.60	117.60	338.40	28.80	0.55
2.37	0.29	2.44	9.76	0.24	75.64	2.29	0.10	0.39	0.20	0.10	12.20	0.88	291.34	0.12	32.79	227.90	369.66	119.56	0.93
2.59	0.34	0.00	0.00	0.24	82.96	3.59	0.10	0.39	0.20	0.10	12.20	0.88	290.36	0.12	32.70	227.16	368.44	119.07	0.93
13.92	1.79	0.00	0.00	1.31	448.50	1.98	0.09	0.35	0.16	0.05	24.84	0.69	267.72	0.14	25.83	195.27	331.20	122.59	0.62
0.00	0.00	0.00	0.00	0.00	30.03	0.00	0.00	0.00	0.00	0.00	0.00	0.00	36.03	0.00	0.00	0.00	0.00	17.51	0.00
1.36	0.14	0.00	0.00	0.35	0.00	0.00	0.00	0.00	0.00	0.00	0.00	0.00	5.75	0.90	14.67	102.35	369.15	234.60	2.71
0.00	0.00	0.00	0.00	0.00	18.30	0.00	0.00	0.00	0.00	0.00	0.00	0.00	21.96	0.00	0.00	0.00	27.45	9.15	0.00
0.00	0.00	0.00	0.00	0.00	30.00	0.00	0.00	0.00	0.00	0.00	0.00	0.00	36.00	0.00	0.00	0.00	0.00	17.50	0.00
0.00	0.00	0.00	0.00	0.00	0.00	12.00	0.00	0.00	0.00	0.00	0.00	0.00	280.00	0.00	0.00	0.00	0.00	140.00	0.00
0.00	0.00	0.00	0.00	0.00	0.00	0.00	0.00	0.00	0.00	0.00	0.00	0.00	0.00	0.00	0.00	0.00	320.00	100.00	0.00
0.00	0.00	0.00	0.00	0.00	0.00	0.00	0.00	0.00	0.00	0.00	0.00	0.00	0.00	0.00	0.00	0.00	460.00	140.00	0.00
0.00	0.00	0.00	0.00	0.00	0.00	0.00	0.00	0.00	0.00	0.00	0.00	0.00	0.00	0.00	0.00	0.00	390.00	140.00	0.00
0.00	0.00	0.00	0.00	0.00	0.00	0.00	0.00	0.00	0.00	0.00	0.00	0.00	0.00	0.00	0.00	0.00	300.00	105.00	0.00
0.00	0.00	0.00	0.00	0.00	0.00	0.00	0.00	0.00	0.00	0.00	0.00	0.00	0.00	0.00	0.00	0.00	330.00	100.00	0.00
0.00	0.00	0.00	0.00	0.00	0.00	0.00	0.00	0.00	0.00	0.00	0.00	0.00	0.00	0.00	0.00	0.00	360.00	130.00	0.00
0.00	0.00	0.00	0.00	0.00	0.00	0.00	0.00	0.00	0.00	0.00	0.00	0.00	0.00	0.00	0.00	0.00	330.00	125.00	0.00
0.00	0.00	0.00	0.00	0.00	0.00	0.00	0.00	0.00	0.00	0.00	0.00	0.00	0.00	0.00	0.00	0.00	240.00	75.00	0.00
0.00	0.00	0.00	0.00	0.00	0.00	0.00	0.00	0.00	0.00	0.00	0.00	0.00	0.00	0.00	0.00	0.00	450.00	150.00	0.00
0.00	0.00	0.00	0.00	0.00	0.00	0.00	0.00	0.00	0.00	0.00	0.00	0.00	0.00	0.00	0.00	0.00	320.00	105.00	0.00
0.00	0.00	0.00	0.00	0.00	0.00	0.00	0.00	0.00	0.00	0.00	0.00	0.00	0.00	0.00	0.00	0.00	250.00	80.00	0.00
0.00	0.00	0.00	0.00	0.00	0.00	0.00	0.00	0.00	0.00	0.00	0.00	0.00	0.00	0.00	0.00	0.00	440.00	125.00	0.00
0.00	0.00	0.00	0.00	0.00	0.00	0.00	0.00	0.00	0.00	0.00	0.00	0.00	0.00	0.00	0.00	0.00	340.00	110.00	0.00
0.00	0.00	0.00	0.00	0.00	0.00	0.00	0.00	0.00	0.00	0.00	0.00	0.00	0.00	0.00	0.00	0.00	360.00	135.00	0.00
0.00	0.00	0.00	0.00	0.00	0.00	0.00	0.00	0.00	0.00	0.00	0.00	0.00	0.00	0.00	0.00	0.00	310.00	100.00	0.00
0.00	0.00	0.00	0.00	0.00	0.00	0.00	0.00	0.00	0.00	0.00	0.00	0.00	0.00	0.00	0.00	0.00	380.00	125.00	0.00
0.00	0.00	0.00	0.00	0.00	0.00	0.00	0.00	0.00	0.00	0.00	0.00	0.00	0.00	0.00	0.00	0.00	180.00	60.00	0.00
0.00	0.00	0.00	0.00	0.00	0.00	0.00	0.00	0.00	0.00	0.00	0.00	0.00	0.00	0.00	0.00	0.00	270.00	100.00	0.00
0.00	0.00	0.00	0.00	0.00	0.00	0.00	0.00	0.00	0.00	0.00	0.00	0.00	0.00	0.00	0.00	0.00	460.00	140.00	0.00

USDA ID Code	Food Name	Weight in Grams*	Quantity of Units	Unit of Measure	Protein (g)	Fat (g)	Carbohydrate (g)	Kilocalories	Caffeine (g)	Fiber (g)	Cholesterol (mg)	Saturated Fat (g)
853	Yogurt, Blueberry, Light-Dannon	227.0000	8.000	Ounce	8.00	0.00	18.00	100.00	0.00	0.00	5.00	0.00
854	Yogurt, Blueberry, Lowfat-Breye	227.0000	8.000	Ounce	9.00	2.50	43.00	230.00	0.00	0.00	15.00	1.50
855	Yogurt, Blueberry, Non Fat, Blen	125.0000	4.400	Ounce	5.00	0.00	25.00	120.00	0.00	0.00	5.00	0.00
856	Yogurt, Blueberry, Non Fat, Chun	170.0000	6.000	Ounce	7.00	0.00	32.00	160.00	0.00	0.00	5.00	0.00
857	Yogurt, Boysenberry, Fruit on B	227.0000	8.000	Ounce	9.00	3.00	45.00	240.00	0.00	1.00	15.00	1.50
858	Yogurt, Cappuccino, Light-Dannon	227.0000	8.000	Ounce	8.00	0.00	16.00	100.00	0.00	0.00	5.00	0.00
859	Yogurt, Car Apl Cinn, Double Del	170.0000	6.000	Ounce	7.00	1.00	47.00	220.00	0.00	0.00	10.00	0.50
860	Yogurt, Car Praline, Double Deli	170.0000	6.000	Ounce	7.00	1.00	47.00	200.00	0.00	0.00	10.00	0.50
861	Yogurt, Caramel Apple Crunch, Li	227.0000	8.000	Ounce	8.00	0.00	25.00	140.00	0.00	0.00	5.00	0.00
862	Yogurt, Cheesck/Straw, Double De	170.0000	6.000	Ounce	7.00	1.00	33.00	170.00	0.00	0.00	10.00	0.50
863	Yogurt, Cheescke/Cher, Double De	170.0000	6.000	Ounce	7.00	1.00	34.00	170.00	0.00	0.00	10.00	0.50
864	Yogurt, Cheeseck & Cherry, Light	170.0000	6.000	Ounce	5.00	0.00	18.00	90.00	0.00	0.00	0.00	0.00
865	Yogurt, Cheeseck & Straw, Light	170.0000	6.000	Ounce	5.00	0.00	17.00	90.00	0.00	0.00	0.00	0.00
866	Yogurt, Cherr Van, Sprinklin' Ra	116.0000	4.000	Ounce	5.00	1.50	24.00	130.00	0.00	0.00	5.00	0.00
867	Yogurt, Cherry Bon-Bon, Non Fat-	227.0000	8.000	Ounce	8.00	0.00	22.00	120.00	0.00	0.00	10.00	0.00
868	Yogurt, Cherry Van, Non Fat, Chu	170.0000	6.000	Ounce	7.00	0.00	31.00	160.00	0.00	0.00	5.00	0.00
869	Yogurt, Cherry Vanilla Crm, Non	227.0000	8.000	Ounce	8.00	0.00	22.00	120.00	0.00	0.00	10.00	0.00
870	Yogurt, Cherry Vanilla, Light-Da	227.0000	8.000	Ounce	8.00	0.00	18.00	100.00	0.00	0.00	5.00	0.00
871	Yogurt, Cherry, Black Jubilee, N	227.0000	8.000	Ounce	8.00	0.00	23.00	120.00	0.00	0.00	10.00	0.00
872	Yogurt, Cherry, Black, Lowfat-Br	227.0000	8.000	Ounce	9.00	2.50	44.00	240.00	0.00	0.00	15.00	1.50
873	Yogurt, Cherry, Danimals-Dannon	125.0000	4.400	Ounce	6.00	1.00	23.00	120.00	0.00	0.00	5.00	0.50
874	Yogurt, Cherry, Fruit on Bottom-	227.0000	8.000	Ounce	9.00	3.00	45.00	240.00	0.00	0.00	15.00	1.50
875	Yogurt, Cherry, Non Fat, Blended	125.0000	4.400	Ounce	5.00	0.00	23.00	110.00	0.00	0.00	5.00	0.00
876	Yogurt, Choc Chscake, Double Deli	170.0000	6.000	Ounce	8.00	1.00	45.00	220.00	0.00	0.00	10.00	0.50
877	Yogurt, Choc Éclair, Double Del	170.0000	6.000	Ounce	8.00	1.00	45.00	220.00	0.00	0.00	10.00	0.50
878	Yogurt, Choc, White & Rasp, Ligh	170.0000	6.000	Ounce	5.00	0.00	17.00	90.00	0.00	0.00	0.00	0.00
879	Yogurt, Choc, White, Rasp, Light	227.0000	8.000	Ounce	8.00	0.00	16.00	100.00	0.00	0.00	5.00	0.00
880	Yogurt, Choc/Straw, Double Delig	170.0000	6.000	Ounce	8.00	1.00	45.00	210.00	0.00	0.00	10.00	0.50
881	Yogurt, Coconut Crm Pie, Light-D	227.0000	8.000	Ounce	8.00	0.00	16.00	100.00	0.00	0.00	5.00	0.00
882	Yogurt, Coffee, Lowfat-Dannon	227.0000	8.000	Ounce	10.00	3.00	36.00	210.00	0.00	0.00	15.00	2.00
883	Yogurt, Cookies 'N Cream, Light-	227.0000	8.000	Ounce	8.00	0.00	24.00	130.00	0.00	0.00	5.00	0.00
884	Yogurt, Cranberry Raspberry, Low	227.0000	8.000	Ounce	10.00	3.00	36.00	210.00	0.00	0.00	15.00	2.00
885	Yogurt, Creme Caramel, Light-Dan	227.0000	8.000	Ounce	8.00	0.00	16.00	100.00	0.00	0.00	5.00	0.00
	Yogurt, Fruit, Fat Free	247.9570	1.000	Cup	10.21	0.00	48.13	233.37	0.00	0.00	7.29	0.00
	Yogurt, Fruit, Fat Free, Light	247.9570	1.000	Cup	10.00	0.00	19.00	109.98	0.00	0.00	5.00	0.00
	Yogurt, Fruit, Lowfat, 10 Gm Pro	245.0000	1.000	Cup	10.71	2.65	46.67	249.61	0.00	0.00	10.29	1.72
	Yogurt, Fruit, Lowfat, 11 Gm Pro	227.0000	1.000	Cup	11.03	3.20	42.22	238.65	0.00	0.00	12.49	2.07
	Yogurt, Fruit, Lowfat, 9 Gm Prot	245.0000	1.000	Cup	9.75	2.82	45.67	243.14	0.00	0.00	11.03	1.81
886	Yogurt, Key Lime Pie, Non Fat-Br	227.0000	8.000	Ounce	8.00	0.00	22.00	120.00	0.00	0.00	10.00	0.00
887	Yogurt, Lem Mer Pie, Double Deli	170.0000	6.000	Ounce	6.00	1.00	37.00	180.00	0.00	0.00	10.00	0.50
888	Yogurt, Lemon Blueberry Cobbler,	227.0000	8.000	Ounce	8.00	0.00	24.00	140.00	0.00	0.00	5.00	0.00
889	Yogurt, Lemon Chiffon, Light Non	227.0000	8.000	Ounce	7.00	0.00	22.00	120.00	0.00	0.00	10.00	0.00
890	Yogurt, Lemon Chiffon, Light-Dan	227.0000	8.000	Ounce	8.00	0.00	16.00	100.00	0.00	0.00	5.00	0.00
891	Yogurt, Lemon Ice, Danimals-Dann	125.0000	4.400	Ounce	6.00	1.00	22.00	120.00	0.00	0.00	5.00	0.50
892	Yogurt, Lemon, Lowfat-Dannon	227.0000	8.000	Ounce	10.00	3.00	36.00	210.00	0.00	0.00	15.00	2.00
893	Yogurt, Light, Strawberry Kiwi-D	227.0000	8.000	Ounce	8.00	0.00	17.00	100.00	0.00	0.00	5.00	0.00
	Yogurt, Light-Dannon	227.0000	8.000	Ounce	9.00	0.00	45.00	240.00	0.00	0.00	15.00	1.50
	Yogurt, No Sugar w/ Granola, Non	227.0000	8.000	Ounce	9.00	0.00	26.00	140.00	0.00	0.00	5.00	0.00
894	Yogurt, Orange Van, Smooth & Crm	227.0000	8.000	Ounce	9.00	2.00	45.00	230.00	0.00	0.00	20.00	1.00
895	Yogurt, Orange, Fruit on Bottom-	227.0000	8.000	Ounce	9.00	3.00	45.00	240.00	0.00	0.00	15.00	1.50
896	Yogurt, Peach, Blended-Breyer's	125.0000	4.400	Ounce	4.00	1.00	26.00	130.00	0.00	0.00	10.00	0.50
897	Yogurt, Peach, Fruit on Bottom-D	227.0000	8.000	Ounce	9.00	3.00	45.00	240.00	0.00	0.00	15.00	1.50
898	Yogurt, Peach, Light-Dannon	227.0000	8.000	Ounce	8.00	0.00	18.00	100.00	0.00	0.00	5.00	0.00

Page Key: A2 = Baby Food   A2 = Baked Goods   A8 = Beverages   A14 = Breads/Grains and Pasta   A18 = Breakfast Foods/Cereals   A26 = Dairy and Eggs   A40 = Fats and Oils   A42 = Fruits and Vegetables   A52 = Meats and Beans   A60 = Nuts and Seeds   A62 5 Frozen Entrees and Packaged Foods   A76 = Restaurant Chains–Fast Foods   A92 = Restaurant Chains–Other   A106 = Seafood and Fish   A110 = Snacks and Sweets   A120 = Soups   A122 = Supplements   A126 = Toppings and Sauces

Monounsaturated Fat (g)	Polyunsaturated Fat (g)	Vitamin D (mg)	Vitamin K (mg)	Vitamin E (mg)	Vitamin A (re)	Vitamin C (mg)	Thiamin (mg)	Riboflavin (mg)	Niacin (mg)	Vitamin B$_6$ (mg)	Folate (mcg)	Vitamin B$_{12}$ (mcg)	Calcium (mg)	Iron (mg)	Magnesium (mg)	Phosphorus (mg)	Potassium (mg)	Sodium (mg)	Zinc (mg)
0.00	0.00	0.00	0.00	0.00	0.00	0.00	0.00	0.00	0.00	0.00	0.00	0.00	0.00	0.00	0.00	0.00	370.00	130.00	0.00
0.00	0.00	0.00	0.00	0.00	0.00	0.00	0.00	0.00	0.00	0.00	0.00	0.00	0.00	0.00	0.00	0.00	430.00	125.00	0.00
0.00	0.00	0.00	0.00	0.00	0.00	0.00	0.00	0.00	0.00	0.00	0.00	0.00	0.00	0.00	0.00	0.00	260.00	105.00	0.00
0.00	0.00	0.00	0.00	0.00	0.00	0.00	0.00	0.00	0.00	0.00	0.00	0.00	0.00	0.00	0.00	0.00	310.00	110.00	0.00
0.00	0.00	0.00	0.00	0.00	0.00	0.00	0.00	0.00	0.00	0.00	0.00	0.00	0.00	0.00	0.00	0.00	450.00	150.00	0.00
0.00	0.00	0.00	0.00	0.00	0.00	0.00	0.00	0.00	0.00	0.00	0.00	0.00	0.00	0.00	0.00	0.00	350.00	135.00	0.00
0.00	0.00	0.00	0.00	0.00	0.00	0.00	0.00	0.00	0.00	0.00	0.00	0.00	0.00	0.00	0.00	0.00	330.00	200.00	0.00
0.00	0.00	0.00	0.00	0.00	0.00	0.00	0.00	0.00	0.00	0.00	0.00	0.00	0.00	0.00	0.00	0.00	330.00	200.00	0.00
0.00	0.00	0.00	0.00	0.00	0.00	0.00	0.00	0.00	0.00	0.00	0.00	0.00	0.00	0.00	0.00	0.00	350.00	170.00	0.00
0.00	0.00	0.00	0.00	0.00	0.00	0.00	0.00	0.00	0.00	0.00	0.00	0.00	0.00	0.00	0.00	0.00	340.00	100.00	0.00
0.00	0.00	0.00	0.00	0.00	0.00	0.00	0.00	0.00	0.00	0.00	0.00	0.00	0.00	0.00	0.00	0.00	340.00	100.00	0.00
0.00	0.00	0.00	0.00	0.00	0.00	0.00	0.00	0.00	0.00	0.00	0.00	0.00	0.00	0.00	0.00	0.00	250.00	75.00	0.00
0.00	0.00	0.00	0.00	0.00	0.00	0.00	0.00	0.00	0.00	0.00	0.00	0.00	0.00	0.00	0.00	0.00	250.00	75.00	0.00
0.00	0.00	0.00	0.00	0.00	0.00	0.00	0.00	0.00	0.00	0.00	0.00	0.00	0.00	0.00	0.00	0.00	250.00	85.00	0.00
0.00	0.00	0.00	0.00	0.00	0.00	0.00	0.00	0.00	0.00	0.00	0.00	0.00	0.00	0.00	0.00	0.00	300.00	105.00	0.00
0.00	0.00	0.00	0.00	0.00	0.00	0.00	0.00	0.00	0.00	0.00	0.00	0.00	0.00	0.00	0.00	0.00	360.00	100.00	0.00
0.00	0.00	0.00	0.00	0.00	0.00	0.00	0.00	0.00	0.00	0.00	0.00	0.00	0.00	0.00	0.00	0.00	320.00	105.00	0.00
0.00	0.00	0.00	0.00	0.00	0.00	0.00	0.00	0.00	0.00	0.00	0.00	0.00	0.00	0.00	0.00	0.00	380.00	130.00	0.00
0.00	0.00	0.00	0.00	0.00	0.00	0.00	0.00	0.00	0.00	0.00	0.00	0.00	0.00	0.00	0.00	0.00	330.00	100.00	0.00
0.00	0.00	0.00	0.00	0.00	0.00	0.00	0.00	0.00	0.00	0.00	0.00	0.00	0.00	0.00	0.00	0.00	450.00	125.00	0.00
0.00	0.00	0.00	0.00	0.00	0.00	0.00	0.00	0.00	0.00	0.00	0.00	0.00	0.00	0.00	0.00	0.00	270.00	95.00	0.00
0.00	0.00	0.00	0.00	0.00	0.00	0.00	0.00	0.00	0.00	0.00	0.00	0.00	0.00	0.00	0.00	0.00	480.00	140.00	0.00
0.00	0.00	0.00	0.00	0.00	0.00	0.00	0.00	0.00	0.00	0.00	0.00	0.00	0.00	0.00	0.00	0.00	250.00	75.00	0.00
0.00	0.00	0.00	0.00	0.00	0.00	0.00	0.00	0.00	0.00	0.00	0.00	0.00	0.00	0.00	0.00	0.00	350.00	150.00	0.00
0.00	0.00	0.00	0.00	0.00	0.00	0.00	0.00	0.00	0.00	0.00	0.00	0.00	0.00	0.00	0.00	0.00	350.00	150.00	0.00
0.00	0.00	0.00	0.00	0.00	0.00	0.00	0.00	0.00	0.00	0.00	0.00	0.00	0.00	0.00	0.00	0.00	230.00	80.00	0.00
0.00	0.00	0.00	0.00	0.00	0.00	0.00	0.00	0.00	0.00	0.00	0.00	0.00	0.00	0.00	0.00	0.00	360.00	135.00	0.00
0.00	0.00	0.00	0.00	0.00	0.00	0.00	0.00	0.00	0.00	0.00	0.00	0.00	0.00	0.00	0.00	0.00	350.00	150.00	0.00
0.00	0.00	0.00	0.00	0.00	0.00	0.00	0.00	0.00	0.00	0.00	0.00	0.00	0.00	0.00	0.00	0.00	350.00	130.00	0.00
0.00	0.00	0.00	0.00	0.00	0.00	0.00	0.00	0.00	0.00	0.00	0.00	0.00	0.00	0.00	0.00	0.00	510.00	160.00	0.00
0.00	0.00	0.00	0.00	0.00	0.00	0.00	0.00	0.00	0.00	0.00	0.00	0.00	0.00	0.00	0.00	0.00	350.00	150.00	0.00
0.00	0.00	0.00	0.00	0.00	0.00	0.00	0.00	0.00	0.00	0.00	0.00	0.00	0.00	0.00	0.00	0.00	510.00	160.00	0.00
0.00	0.00	0.00	0.00	0.00	0.00	0.00	0.00	0.00	0.00	0.00	0.00	0.00	0.00	0.00	0.00	0.00	370.00	135.00	0.00
0.00	0.00	0.00	0.00	0.00	0.00	0.00	0.00	0.00	0.00	0.00	0.00	0.00	437.57	0.00	0.00	0.00	422.99	153.15	0.00
0.00	0.00	0.00	0.00	0.00	0.00	15.00	0.00	0.00	0.00	0.00	0.00	0.00	419.93	0.20	0.00	0.00	509.91	159.97	0.00
0.74	0.07	0.00	0.00	0.07	26.95	1.62	0.10	0.44	0.25	0.10	22.79	1.15	372.16	0.17	35.70	292.53	476.53	143.08	1.81
0.89	0.09	0.00	0.00	0.00	34.05	1.68	0.09	0.45	0.25	0.11	23.61	1.18	383.40	0.16	36.77	301.23	491.00	147.32	1.86
0.78	0.07	0.00	0.00	0.07	29.40	1.47	0.07	0.39	0.22	0.10	20.83	1.05	338.84	0.15	32.51	266.32	433.90	130.34	1.64
0.00	0.00	0.00	0.00	0.00	0.00	0.00	0.00	0.00	0.00	0.00	0.00	0.00	0.00	0.00	0.00	0.00	300.00	100.00	0.00
0.00	0.00	0.00	0.00	0.00	0.00	0.00	0.00	0.00	0.00	0.00	0.00	0.00	0.00	0.00	0.00	0.00	300.00	170.00	0.00
0.00	0.00	0.00	0.00	0.00	0.00	0.00	0.00	0.00	0.00	0.00	0.00	0.00	0.00	0.00	0.00	0.00	360.00	140.00	0.00
0.00	0.00	0.00	0.00	0.00	0.00	0.00	0.00	0.00	0.00	0.00	0.00	0.00	0.00	0.00	0.00	0.00	310.00	100.00	0.00
0.00	0.00	0.00	0.00	0.00	0.00	0.00	0.00	0.00	0.00	0.00	0.00	0.00	0.00	0.00	0.00	0.00	360.00	130.00	0.00
0.00	0.00	0.00	0.00	0.00	0.00	0.00	0.00	0.00	0.00	0.00	0.00	0.00	0.00	0.00	0.00	0.00	270.00	100.00	0.00
0.00	0.00	0.00	0.00	0.00	0.00	0.00	0.00	0.00	0.00	0.00	0.00	0.00	0.00	0.00	0.00	0.00	510.00	160.00	0.00
0.00	0.00	0.00	0.00	0.00	0.00	0.00	0.00	0.00	0.00	0.00	0.00	0.00	0.00	0.00	0.00	0.00	380.00	140.00	0.00
0.00	0.00	0.00	0.00	0.00	0.00	12.00	0.00	0.00	0.00	0.00	0.00	0.00	280.00	0.00	0.00	0.00	0.00	130.00	0.00
0.00	0.00	0.00	0.00	0.00	0.00	2.40	0.00	0.00	0.00	0.00	0.00	0.00	280.00	0.40	0.00	0.00	0.00	125.00	0.00
0.00	0.00	0.00	0.00	0.00	0.00	0.00	0.00	0.00	0.00	0.00	0.00	0.00	0.00	0.00	0.00	0.00	380.00	125.00	0.00
0.00	0.00	0.00	0.00	0.00	0.00	0.00	0.00	0.00	0.00	0.00	0.00	0.00	0.00	0.00	0.00	0.00	470.00	135.00	0.00
0.00	0.00	0.00	0.00	0.00	0.00	0.00	0.00	0.00	0.00	0.00	0.00	0.00	0.00	0.00	0.00	0.00	180.00	65.00	0.00
0.00	0.00	0.00	0.00	0.00	0.00	0.00	0.00	0.00	0.00	0.00	0.00	0.00	0.00	0.00	0.00	0.00	450.00	140.00	0.00
0.00	0.00	0.00	0.00	0.00	0.00	0.00	0.00	0.00	0.00	0.00	0.00	0.00	0.00	0.00	0.00	0.00	370.00	130.00	0.00

USDA ID Code	Food Name	Weight in Grams*	Quantity of Units	Unit of Measure	Protein (g)	Fat (g)	Carbohydrate (g)	Kilocalories	Caffeine (g)	Fiber (g)	Cholesterol (mg)	Saturated Fat (g)
901	Yogurt, Peach, Lowfat-Breyer's	227.0000	8.000	Ounce	9.00	2.50	43.00	240.00	0.00	0.00	15.00	1.50
899	Yogurt, Peach, Non Fat, Blended-	125.0000	4.400	Ounce	5.00	0.00	23.00	110.00	0.00	0.00	5.00	0.00
900	Yogurt, Peach, Non Fat, Chunky F	170.0000	6.000	Ounce	7.00	0.00	33.00	160.00	0.00	0.00	5.00	0.00
902	Yogurt, Peaches N' Crm, Light No	227.0000	8.000	Ounce	8.00	0.00	22.00	120.00	0.00	0.00	10.00	0.00
903	Yogurt, Peaches/Crm, Smooth & Cr	227.0000	8.000	Ounce	9.00	2.00	45.00	230.00	0.00	0.00	20.00	1.00
904	Yogurt, Pina Co, Non Fat, Chunky	170.0000	6.000	Ounce	7.00	0.00	32.00	160.00	0.00	0.00	5.00	0.00
905	Yogurt, Pineapple, Lowfat-Breyer	227.0000	8.000	Ounce	9.00	2.50	45.00	240.00	0.00	0.00	15.00	1.50
906	Yogurt, Plain Lowfat-Dannon	227.0000	8.000	Ounce	12.00	4.00	16.00	140.00	0.00	0.00	20.00	2.50
907	Yogurt, Plain Non Fat-Dannon	227.0000	8.000	Ounce	12.00	0.00	16.00	110.00	0.00	0.00	5.00	0.00
	Yogurt, Plain, Fat Free	247.9570	1.000	Cup	13.00	0.00	17.00	119.98	0.00	0.00	5.00	0.00
	Yogurt, Plain, Lowfat, 12 Gm Pro	245.0000	1.000	Cup	12.86	3.80	17.25	155.06	0.00	0.00	14.95	2.45
	Yogurt, Plain, Skim Milk, 13 Gm	245.0000	1.000	Cup	14.04	0.44	18.82	136.64	0.00	0.00	4.41	0.29
	Yogurt, Plain, Whole Milk, 8 Gm	245.0000	1.000	Cup	8.50	7.96	11.42	150.48	0.00	0.00	31.12	5.15
908	Yogurt, Rasp N' Cream, Light Non	227.0000	8.000	Ounce	8.00	0.00	22.00	120.00	0.00	0.00	10.00	0.00
909	Yogurt, Rasp/Cream, Smooth & Crm	227.0000	8.000	Ounce	9.00	2.00	45.00	230.00	0.00	0.00	20.00	1.00
910	Yogurt, Raspberry w/Granola, Lig	227.0000	8.000	Ounce	8.00	0.00	25.00	140.00	0.00	0.00	5.00	0.00
911	Yogurt, Raspberry, Fruit on Bott	227.0000	8.000	Ounce	9.00	3.00	45.00	240.00	0.00	1.00	15.00	1.50
912	Yogurt, Raspberry, Light-Dannon	227.0000	8.000	Ounce	8.00	0.00	17.00	100.00	0.00	0.00	5.00	0.00
913	Yogurt, Raspberry, Non Fat, Blen	125.0000	4.400	Ounce	5.00	0.00	24.00	110.00	0.00	0.00	5.00	0.00
914	Yogurt, Raspberry, Red, Lowfat-B	227.0000	8.000	Ounce	9.00	2.50	43.00	230.00	0.00	0.00	15.00	1.50
915	Yogurt, Raspberry, Wild, Danimal	125.0000	4.400	Ounce	6.00	1.00	22.00	120.00	0.00	0.00	5.00	0.50
916	Yogurt, Smooth & Crmy, Black Che	227.0000	8.000	Ounce	9.00	2.00	46.00	240.00	0.00	0.00	20.00	1.00
917	Yogurt, Straw Ban Spl, Smooth &	227.0000	8.000	Ounce	8.00	2.00	48.00	240.00	0.00	0.00	20.00	1.00
918	Yogurt, Straw Cheesck, Light Non	227.0000	8.000	Ounce	8.00	0.00	22.00	120.00	0.00	0.00	10.00	0.00
919	Yogurt, Straw Chscke, Smooth & C	227.0000	8.000	Ounce	9.00	2.00	46.00	240.00	0.00	0.00	20.00	1.00
920	Yogurt, Straw Sundae, Light Duet	170.0000	6.000	Ounce	5.00	0.00	17.00	90.00	0.00	0.00	0.00	0.00
924	Yogurt, Straw/Ban, Sprinklin' Ra	116.0000	4.000	Ounce	5.00	1.50	24.00	130.00	0.00	0.00	5.00	0.50
921	Yogurt, Straw-Ban, Fruit on Bot	227.0000	8.000	Ounce	9.00	3.00	43.00	240.00	0.00	1.00	15.00	1.50
922	Yogurt, Straw-Ban, Non Fat, Blen	125.0000	4.400	Ounce	5.00	0.00	23.00	110.00	0.00	0.00	5.00	0.00
923	Yogurt, Straw-Ban, Non Fat, Chun	170.0000	6.000	Ounce	7.00	0.00	32.00	160.00	0.00	0.00	5.00	0.00
925	Yogurt, Strawberry Banana, Light	227.0000	8.000	Ounce	8.00	0.00	17.00	100.00	0.00	0.00	5.00	0.00
926	Yogurt, Strawberry Banana, Lowfat	227.0000	8.000	Ounce	9.00	2.50	44.00	240.00	0.00	0.00	15.00	1.50
927	Yogurt, Strawberry, Blended-Brey	125.0000	4.400	Ounce	4.00	1.00	26.00	130.00	0.00	0.00	10.00	0.50
928	Yogurt, Strawberry, Danimals-Dan	125.0000	4.400	Ounce	6.00	1.00	24.00	130.00	0.00	0.00	5.00	0.50
929	Yogurt, Strawberry, Fruit on Bot	227.0000	8.000	Ounce	9.00	3.00	45.00	240.00	0.00	1.00	15.00	1.50
931	Yogurt, Strawberry, Light-Dannon	227.0000	8.000	Ounce	8.00	0.00	17.00	100.00	0.00	0.00	5.00	0.00
932	Yogurt, Strawberry, Lowfat-Breye	227.0000	8.000	Ounce	9.00	2.50	43.00	230.00	0.00	0.00	15.00	1.50
933	Yogurt, Strawberry, Non Fat, Ble	125.0000	4.400	Ounce	5.00	0.00	23.00	110.00	0.00	0.00	5.00	0.00
934	Yogurt, Strawberry, Non Fat, Chu	170.0000	6.000	Ounce	7.00	0.00	32.00	160.00	0.00	0.00	5.00	0.00
937	Yogurt, Strawberry, Non Fat-Brey	227.0000	8.000	Ounce	8.00	0.00	22.00	120.00	0.00	0.00	10.00	0.00
935	Yogurt, Strawberry, Smooth & Crm	227.0000	8.000	Ounce	9.00	2.00	45.00	230.00	0.00	0.00	20.00	1.00
936	Yogurt, Strawberry, Sprinklin' R	116.0000	4.000	Ounce	5.00	1.50	24.00	130.00	0.00	0.00	5.00	0.50
938	Yogurt, Tangerine Chiffon, Light	227.0000	8.000	Ounce	8.00	0.00	16.00	100.00	0.00	0.00	5.00	0.00
939	Yogurt, Tropical Punch, Danimals	125.0000	4.400	Ounce	6.00	1.00	25.00	130.00	0.00	0.00	5.00	0.50
940	Yogurt, Van/Cherry, Magic Crysta	116.0000	4.000	Ounce	5.00	1.00	21.00	110.00	0.00	0.00	5.00	0.50
941	Yogurt, Van/Orange, Magic Crysta	116.0000	4.000	Ounce	5.00	1.00	21.00	110.00	0.00	0.00	5.00	0.50
942	Yogurt, Van/Peach/Apr, Double De	170.0000	6.000	Ounce	7.00	1.00	33.00	170.00	0.00	0.00	10.00	0.50
943	Yogurt, Vanilla, Danimals-Dannon	125.0000	4.000	Ounce	6.00	1.00	23.00	120.00	0.00	0.00	5.00	0.50
944	Yogurt, Vanilla, Light-Dannon	227.0000	8.000	Ounce	8.00	0.00	16.00	100.00	0.00	0.00	5.00	0.00
	Yogurt, Vanilla, Lowfat, 11 Gm P	245.0000	1.000	Cup	12.08	3.06	33.81	209.33	0.00	0.00	12.01	1.98
945	Yogurt, Vanilla, Lowfat-Breyer's	227.0000	8.000	Ounce	10.00	3.00	38.00	220.00	0.00	0.00	20.00	2.00
946	Yogurt, Vanilla, Lowfat-Dannon	227.0000	8.000	Ounce	10.00	3.00	36.00	210.00	0.00	0.00	15.00	2.00
947	Yogurt, Vanilla/Straw, Double De	170.0000	6.000	Ounce	7.00	1.00	33.00	170.00	0.00	0.00	10.00	0.50

Page Key: A2 = Baby Food   A2 = Baked Goods   A8 = Beverages   A14 = Breads/Grains and Pasta   A18 = Breakfast Foods/Cereals   A26 = Dairy and Eggs   A40 = Fats and Oils   A42 = Fruits and Vegetables   A52 = Meats and Beans   A60 = Nuts and Seeds   A62 5 Frozen Entrees and Packaged Foods   A76 = Restaurant Chains–Fast Foods   A92 = Restaurant Chains–Other   A106 = Seafood and Fish   A110 = Snacks and Sweets   A120 = Soups   A122 = Supplements   A126 = Toppings and Sauces

Monounsaturated Fat (g)	Polyunsaturated Fat (g)	Vitamin D (mg)	Vitamin K (mg)	Vitamin E (mg)	Vitamin A (re)	Vitamin C (mg)	Thiamin (mg)	Riboflavin (mg)	Niacin (mg)	Vitamin B6 (mg)	Folate (mcg)	Vitamin B12 (mcg)	Calcium (mg)	Iron (mg)	Magnesium (mg)	Phosphorus (mg)	Potassium (mg)	Sodium (mg)	Zinc (mg)
0.00	0.00	0.00	0.00	0.00	0.00	0.00	0.00	0.00	0.00	0.00	0.00	0.00	0.00	0.00	0.00	0.00	440.00	125.00	0.00
0.00	0.00	0.00	0.00	0.00	0.00	0.00	0.00	0.00	0.00	0.00	0.00	0.00	0.00	0.00	0.00	0.00	240.00	75.00	0.00
0.00	0.00	0.00	0.00	0.00	0.00	0.00	0.00	0.00	0.00	0.00	0.00	0.00	0.00	0.00	0.00	0.00	330.00	100.00	0.00
0.00	0.00	0.00	0.00	0.00	0.00	0.00	0.00	0.00	0.00	0.00	0.00	0.00	0.00	0.00	0.00	0.00	340.00	115.00	0.00
0.00	0.00	0.00	0.00	0.00	0.00	0.00	0.00	0.00	0.00	0.00	0.00	0.00	0.00	0.00	0.00	0.00	390.00	125.00	0.00
0.00	0.00	0.00	0.00	0.00	0.00	0.00	0.00	0.00	0.00	0.00	0.00	0.00	0.00	0.00	0.00	0.00	330.00	110.00	0.00
0.00	0.00	0.00	0.00	0.00	0.00	0.00	0.00	0.00	0.00	0.00	0.00	0.00	0.00	0.00	0.00	0.00	430.00	125.00	0.00
0.00	0.00	0.00	0.00	0.00	0.00	0.00	0.00	0.00	0.00	0.00	0.00	0.00	0.00	0.00	0.00	0.00	590.00	170.00	0.00
0.00	0.00	0.00	0.00	0.00	0.00	0.00	0.00	0.00	0.00	0.00	0.00	0.00	0.00	0.00	0.00	0.00	550.00	150.00	0.00
0.00	0.00	0.00	0.00	0.00	0.00	3.60	0.00	0.25	0.00	0.00	0.00	0.00	479.92	0.00	0.00	0.21	599.90	169.97	0.00
1.05	0.10	0.00	0.00	0.10	39.20	1.96	0.10	0.51	0.27	0.12	27.44	1.37	447.37	0.20	42.75	351.58	572.81	171.99	2.18
0.12	0.02	0.00	0.00	0.02	4.90	2.13	0.12	0.56	0.29	0.12	29.89	1.49	487.80	0.22	46.80	383.43	624.51	187.43	2.38
2.18	0.22	0.00	0.00	0.22	73.50	1.30	0.07	0.34	0.20	0.07	18.13	0.91	295.72	0.12	28.37	232.51	378.77	113.68	1.45
0.00	0.00	0.00	0.00	0.00	0.00	0.00	0.00	0.00	0.00	0.00	0.00	0.00	0.00	0.00	0.00	0.00	330.00	105.00	0.00
0.00	0.00	0.00	0.00	0.00	0.00	0.00	0.00	0.00	0.00	0.00	0.00	0.00	0.00	0.00	0.00	0.00	400.00	135.00	0.00
0.00	0.00	0.00	0.00	0.00	0.00	0.00	0.00	0.00	0.00	0.00	0.00	0.00	0.00	0.00	0.00	0.00	380.00	150.00	0.00
0.00	0.00	0.00	0.00	0.00	0.00	0.00	0.00	0.00	0.00	0.00	0.00	0.00	0.00	0.00	0.00	0.00	460.00	150.00	0.00
0.00	0.00	0.00	0.00	0.00	0.00	0.00	0.00	0.00	0.00	0.00	0.00	0.00	0.00	0.00	0.00	0.00	370.00	150.00	0.00
0.00	0.00	0.00	0.00	0.00	0.00	0.00	0.00	0.00	0.00	0.00	0.00	0.00	0.00	0.00	0.00	0.00	250.00	75.00	0.00
0.00	0.00	0.00	0.00	0.00	0.00	0.00	0.00	0.00	0.00	0.00	0.00	0.00	0.00	0.00	0.00	0.00	450.00	125.00	0.00
0.00	0.00	0.00	0.00	0.00	0.00	0.00	0.00	0.00	0.00	0.00	0.00	0.00	0.00	0.00	0.00	0.00	270.00	90.00	0.00
0.00	0.00	0.00	0.00	0.00	0.00	0.00	0.00	0.00	0.00	0.00	0.00	0.00	0.00	0.00	0.00	0.00	390.00	130.00	0.00
0.00	0.00	0.00	0.00	0.00	0.00	0.00	0.00	0.00	0.00	0.00	0.00	0.00	0.00	0.00	0.00	0.00	390.00	125.00	0.00
0.00	0.00	0.00	0.00	0.00	0.00	0.00	0.00	0.00	0.00	0.00	0.00	0.00	0.00	0.00	0.00	0.00	320.00	100.00	0.00
0.00	0.00	0.00	0.00	0.00	0.00	0.00	0.00	0.00	0.00	0.00	0.00	0.00	0.00	0.00	0.00	0.00	400.00	125.00	0.00
0.00	0.00	0.00	0.00	0.00	0.00	0.00	0.00	0.00	0.00	0.00	0.00	0.00	0.00	0.00	0.00	0.00	250.00	75.00	0.00
0.00	0.00	0.00	0.00	0.00	0.00	0.00	0.00	0.00	0.00	0.00	0.00	0.00	0.00	0.00	0.00	0.00	250.00	80.00	0.00
0.00	0.00	0.00	0.00	0.00	0.00	0.00	0.00	0.00	0.00	0.00	0.00	0.00	0.00	0.00	0.00	0.00	480.00	140.00	0.00
0.00	0.00	0.00	0.00	0.00	0.00	0.00	0.00	0.00	0.00	0.00	0.00	0.00	0.00	0.00	0.00	0.00	240.00	75.00	0.00
0.00	0.00	0.00	0.00	0.00	0.00	0.00	0.00	0.00	0.00	0.00	0.00	0.00	0.00	0.00	0.00	0.00	350.00	105.00	0.00
0.00	0.00	0.00	0.00	0.00	0.00	0.00	0.00	0.00	0.00	0.00	0.00	0.00	0.00	0.00	0.00	0.00	380.00	140.00	0.00
0.00	0.00	0.00	0.00	0.00	0.00	0.00	0.00	0.00	0.00	0.00	0.00	0.00	0.00	0.00	0.00	0.00	470.00	125.00	0.00
0.00	0.00	0.00	0.00	0.00	0.00	0.00	0.00	0.00	0.00	0.00	0.00	0.00	0.00	0.00	0.00	0.00	180.00	60.00	0.00
0.00	0.00	0.00	0.00	0.00	0.00	0.00	0.00	0.00	0.00	0.00	0.00	0.00	0.00	0.00	0.00	0.00	270.00	90.00	0.00
0.00	0.00	0.00	0.00	0.00	0.00	0.00	0.00	0.00	0.00	0.00	0.00	0.00	0.00	0.00	0.00	0.00	460.00	140.00	0.00
0.00	0.00	0.00	0.00	0.00	0.00	0.00	0.00	0.00	0.00	0.00	0.00	0.00	0.00	0.00	0.00	0.00	380.00	140.00	0.00
0.00	0.00	0.00	0.00	0.00	0.00	0.00	0.00	0.00	0.00	0.00	0.00	0.00	0.00	0.00	0.00	0.00	440.00	125.00	0.00
0.00	0.00	0.00	0.00	0.00	0.00	0.00	0.00	0.00	0.00	0.00	0.00	0.00	0.00	0.00	0.00	0.00	230.00	80.00	0.00
0.00	0.00	0.00	0.00	0.00	0.00	0.00	0.00	0.00	0.00	0.00	0.00	0.00	0.00	0.00	0.00	0.00	360.00	115.00	0.00
0.00	0.00	0.00	0.00	0.00	0.00	0.00	0.00	0.00	0.00	0.00	0.00	0.00	0.00	0.00	0.00	0.00	320.00	100.00	0.00
0.00	0.00	0.00	0.00	0.00	0.00	0.00	0.00	0.00	0.00	0.00	0.00	0.00	0.00	0.00	0.00	0.00	400.00	125.00	0.00
0.00	0.00	0.00	0.00	0.00	0.00	0.00	0.00	0.00	0.00	0.00	0.00	0.00	0.00	0.00	0.00	0.00	250.00	85.00	0.00
0.00	0.00	0.00	0.00	0.00	0.00	0.00	0.00	0.00	0.00	0.00	0.00	0.00	0.00	0.00	0.00	0.00	360.00	130.00	0.00
0.00	0.00	0.00	0.00	0.00	0.00	0.00	0.00	0.00	0.00	0.00	0.00	0.00	0.00	0.00	0.00	0.00	270.00	95.00	0.00
0.00	0.00	0.00	0.00	0.00	0.00	0.00	0.00	0.00	0.00	0.00	0.00	0.00	0.00	0.00	0.00	0.00	240.00	85.00	0.00
0.00	0.00	0.00	0.00	0.00	0.00	0.00	0.00	0.00	0.00	0.00	0.00	0.00	0.00	0.00	0.00	0.00	240.00	85.00	0.00
0.00	0.00	0.00	0.00	0.00	0.00	0.00	0.00	0.00	0.00	0.00	0.00	0.00	0.00	0.00	0.00	0.00	330.00	100.00	0.00
0.00	0.00	0.00	0.00	0.00	0.00	0.00	0.00	0.00	0.00	0.00	0.00	0.00	0.00	0.00	0.00	0.00	270.00	90.00	0.00
0.00	0.00	0.00	0.00	0.00	0.00	0.00	0.00	0.00	0.00	0.00	0.00	0.00	0.00	0.00	0.00	0.00	350.00	130.00	0.00
0.83	0.10	0.00	0.00	0.07	31.85	1.84	0.10	0.49	0.27	0.12	25.73	1.30	419.69	0.17	40.25	329.77	537.29	161.21	2.03
0.00	0.00	0.00	0.00	0.00	0.00	0.00	0.00	0.00	0.00	0.00	0.00	0.00	0.00	0.00	0.00	0.00	480.00	135.00	0.00
0.00	0.00	0.00	0.00	0.00	0.00	0.00	0.00	0.00	0.00	0.00	0.00	0.00	0.00	0.00	0.00	0.00	510.00	160.00	0.00
0.00	0.00	0.00	0.00	0.00	0.00	0.00	0.00	0.00	0.00	0.00	0.00	0.00	0.00	0.00	0.00	0.00	340.00	100.00	0.00

Fats and Oils

USDA ID Code	Food Name	Weight in Grams*	Quantity of Units	Unit of Measure	Protein (g)	Fat (g)	Carbohydrate (g)	Kilocalories	Caffeine (g)	Fiber (g)	Cholesterol (mg)	Saturated Fat (g)
	Butter, w/ Salt	5.0000	1.000	Pat	0.05	4.06	0.01	35.85	0.00	0.00	10.95	2.53
	Butter, w/o Salt	5.0000	1.000	Pat	0.04	4.06	0.00	35.85	0.00	0.00	10.95	2.52
	Butter, Whipped	3.8000	1.000	Pat	0.03	3.08	0.00	27.24	0.00	0.00	8.32	1.92
	Lard	12.8000	1.000	Tbsp	0.00	12.80	0.00	115.46	0.00	0.00	12.16	5.02
	Margarine, Hard, Corn & soybn	4.7000	1.000	Tbsp	0.04	3.78	0.04	33.78	0.00	0.00	0.00	0.71
	Margarine, Hard, Corn (hydr)	4.7000	1.000	Tbsp	0.04	3.78	0.04	33.78	0.00	0.00	0.00	0.62
	Margarine, Imitation (appx 40% Fat)	4.8000	1.000	Tbsp	0.02	1.86	0.02	16.57	0.00	0.00	0.00	0.37
	Margarine, Regular, w/ Salt Added	4.7000	1.000	Tbsp	0.04	3.78	0.04	33.78	0.00	0.00	0.00	0.74
	Margarine, Regular, w/o Added Salt	4.7000	1.000	Tbsp	0.02	3.77	0.02	33.56	0.00	0.00	0.00	0.71
	Margarine, Soft, w/ Salt Added	227.0000	1.000	Cup	1.82	182.51	1.14	1626.23	0.00	0.00	0.00	31.33
	Margarine, Soft, w/o Added Salt	4.7000	1.000	Tbsp	0.04	3.77	0.04	33.67	0.00	0.00	0.00	0.65
	Mayonnaise	14.7000	1.000	Tbsp	0.13	4.91	3.51	57.29	0.00	0.00	3.82	0.72
	Mayonnaise, Fat Free	15.0070	1.000	Tbsp	0.00	0.00	3.00	10.00	0.00	0.00	0.00	0.00
	Mayonnaise, Light	15.0070	1.000	Tbsp	0.00	2.00	1.00	25.01	0.00	0.00	5.00	0.00
	Oil, Olive	13.5000	1.000	Tbsp	0.00	13.50	0.00	119.34	0.00	0.00	0.00	1.82
	Oil, Peanut	13.5000	1.000	Tbsp	0.00	13.50	0.00	119.34	0.00	0.00	0.00	2.28
	Oil, Sesame	13.6000	1.000	Tbsp	0.00	13.60	0.00	120.22	0.00	0.00	0.00	1.93
	Oil, Soybean	13.6000	1.000	Tbsp	0.00	13.60	0.00	120.22	0.00	0.00	0.00	1.96
	Oil, Soybean, (hydr)	13.6000	1.000	Tbsp	0.00	13.60	0.00	120.22	0.00	0.00	0.00	2.03
	Oil, Soybean, (hydr) & cottonsee	13.6000	1.000	Tbsp	0.00	13.60	0.00	120.22	0.00	0.00	0.00	2.45
	Oil, Vegetable Corn	13.6000	1.000	Tbsp	0.00	13.60	0.00	120.22	0.00	0.00	0.00	1.73
	Oil, Vegetable, Canola	14.0000	1.000	Tbsp	0.00	14.00	0.00	123.76	0.00	0.00	0.00	0.99
	Oil, Vegetable, Cocoa Butter	13.6000	1.000	Tbsp	0.00	13.60	0.00	120.22	0.00	0.00	0.00	8.12
	Oil, Vegetable, Cottonseed	13.6000	1.000	Tbsp	0.00	13.60	0.00	120.22	0.00	0.00	0.00	3.52
	Oil, Vegetable, Palm	13.6000	1.000	Tbsp	0.00	13.60	0.00	120.22	0.00	0.00	0.00	6.70
	Oil, Vegetable, Palm Kernel	13.6000	1.000	Tbsp	0.00	13.60	0.00	117.23	0.00	0.00	0.00	11.08
	Oil, Vegetable, Safflower, Linol	13.6000	1.000	Tbsp	0.00	13.60	0.00	120.22	0.00	0.00	0.00	0.84
	Oil, Vegetable, Safflower, Oleic	13.6000	1.000	Tbsp	0.00	13.60	0.00	120.22	0.00	0.00	0.00	0.84
	Oil, Vegetable, Sunflower	14.0000	1.000	Tbsp	0.00	14.00	0.00	123.76	0.00	0.00	0.00	1.37
	Salad Dressing, Blue Cheese	16.0140	2.000	Tbsp	0.50	3.50	2.50	45.04	0.00	0.00	5.00	2.00
	Salad Dressing, Blue Cheese, Fat Free	17.5080	2.000	Tbsp	0.25	0.00	6.00	25.01	0.00	0.00	0.00	0.00
	Salad Dressing, Ceasar	17.1200	2.000	Tbsp	0.17	17.12	1.31	155.00	0.00	0.00	1.11	3.22
	Salad Dressing, French	12.3000	1.000	Pkt	0.07	5.04	2.15	52.85	0.00	0.00	0.00	1.17
	Salad Dressing, French, Fat Free	17.5080	2.000	Tbsp	0.00	0.00	6.00	25.01	0.00	0.00	0.00	0.00
	Salad Dressing, French, Low Fat	16.3000	1.000	Tbsp	0.03	0.95	3.54	21.87	0.00	0.00	0.00	0.13
	Salad Dressing, Honey Mustard	31.2000	2.000	Tbsp	0.05	6.33	14.22	102.11	0.00	0.23	0.00	1.33
	Salad Dressing, Italian	14.7000	1.000	Tbsp	0.10	7.10	1.50	68.69	0.00	0.00	0.00	1.03
	Salad Dressing, Italian, Creamy	29.4000	2.000	Tbsp	0.03	16.12	2.33	147.43	0.00	0.00	1.22	2.43
	Salad Dressing, Italian, Fat Free	15.5100	2.000	Tbsp	0.00	0.00	1.00	5.00	0.00	0.00	0.00	0.00
	Salad Dressing, Italian, Low Cal	15.0000	1.000	Tbsp	0.02	1.47	0.74	15.81	0.00	0.02	0.90	0.20
	Salad Dressing, Peppercorn	26.8000	2.000	Tbsp	0.02	16.22	1.10	151.22	0.00	0.00	13.11	3.11
	Salad Dressing, Poppy Seed	29.4000	2.000	Tbsp	0.02	12.31	6.41	130.44	0.00	0.00	0.00	2.33
	Salad Dressing, Ranch	14.5190	2.000	Tbsp	0.00	9.01	1.00	85.11	0.00	0.00	2.50	1.50
	Salad Dressing, Ranch, Fat Free	17.5080	2.000	Tbsp	0.00	0.00	5.50	25.01	0.00	0.00	0.00	0.00
	Salad Dressing, Raspberry Vinegar	14.7000	2.000	Tbsp	0.10	7.10	1.50	68.69	0.00	0.00	0.00	1.03
	Salad Dressing, Russian	15.3000	1.000	Tbsp	0.24	7.77	1.59	75.58	0.00	0.00	2.75	1.12
	Salad Dressing, Russian, Low Cal	16.3000	1.000	Tbsp	0.08	0.65	4.50	23.05	0.00	0.05	0.98	0.10
	Salad Dressing, Sesame Seed	15.3000	1.000	Tbsp	0.47	6.92	1.32	67.79	0.00	0.15	0.00	0.95
	Salad Dressing, Thousand Island	15.6000	1.000	Tbsp	0.14	5.57	2.37	58.86	0.00	0.00	4.06	0.94
	Salad Dressing, Thousand Island,	17.5080	2.000	Tbsp	0.00	0.00	5.50	22.51	0.00	0.00	0.00	0.00
	Salad Dressing, Thousand Island,	15.3000	1.000	Tbsp	0.12	1.64	2.48	24.27	0.00	0.18	2.30	0.24
	Salad Dressing, Vinegar and Oil	15.6000	1.000	Tbsp	0.00	7.82	0.39	70.01	0.00	0.00	0.00	1.42

Monounsaturated Fat (g)	Polyunsaturated Fat (g)	Vitamin D (mg)	Vitamin K (mg)	Vitamin E (mg)	Vitamin A (re)	Vitamin C (mg)	Thiamin (mg)	Riboflavin (mg)	Niacin (mg)	Vitamin B₆ (mg)	Folate (mcg)	Vitamin B₁₂ (mcg)	Calcium (mg)	Iron (mg)	Magnesium (mg)	Phosphorus (mg)	Potassium (mg)	Sodium (mg)	Zinc (mg)
1.17	0.15	0.00	0.00	0.08	37.70	0.00	0.00	0.00	0.00	0.00	0.15	0.01	1.20	0.01	0.10	1.15	1.30	41.30	0.00
1.17	0.15	0.00	0.00	0.08	37.70	0.00	0.00	0.00	0.00	0.00	0.14	0.01	1.18	0.01	0.10	1.14	1.30	0.55	0.00
0.89	0.11	0.00	0.00	0.06	28.65	0.00	0.00	0.00	0.00	0.00	0.11	0.00	0.89	0.01	0.08	0.87	0.99	31.41	0.00
5.77	1.43	0.00	0.00	0.15	0.00	0.00	0.00	0.00	0.00	0.00	0.00	0.00	0.01	0.00	0.00	0.00	0.00	0.00	0.01
1.73	1.18	0.00	0.00	0.52	37.55	0.01	0.00	0.00	0.00	0.00	0.06	0.00	1.41	0.00	0.12	1.08	1.99	44.34	0.00
2.15	0.85	0.00	0.00	0.55	37.55	0.01	0.00	0.00	0.00	0.00	0.06	0.00	1.41	0.00	0.12	1.08	1.99	44.34	0.00
0.75	0.66	0.00	0.00	0.11	38.35	0.00	0.00	0.00	0.00	0.00	0.03	0.00	0.85	0.00	0.07	0.66	1.21	46.06	0.00
1.68	1.19	0.00	0.00	0.60	37.55	0.01	0.00	0.00	0.00	0.00	0.06	0.00	1.41	0.00	0.12	1.08	1.99	44.34	0.00
1.72	1.18	0.00	0.00	0.60	37.55	0.00	0.00	0.00	0.00	0.00	0.03	0.00	0.82	0.00	0.07	0.63	1.16	0.10	0.00
64.69	78.54	0.00	0.00	27.24	1813.73	0.32	0.02	0.07	0.05	0.02	2.38	0.18	60.16	0.00	5.24	46.08	85.58	2448.54	0.00
1.75	1.21	0.00	0.00	0.41	37.55	0.01	0.00	0.00	0.00	0.00	0.05	0.00	1.25	0.00	0.11	0.95	1.77	1.29	0.00
1.32	2.65	0.00	0.00	0.59	12.35	0.00	0.00	0.00	0.00	0.00	0.92	0.03	2.06	0.03	0.29	3.82	1.32	104.48	0.03
0.00	0.00	0.00	0.00	0.00	0.00	0.00	0.00	0.00	0.00	0.00	0.00	0.00	0.00	0.00	0.00	0.00	10.00	105.05	0.00
0.00	0.00	0.00	0.00	0.00	0.00	0.00	0.00	0.00	0.00	0.00	0.00	0.00	0.00	0.00	0.00	0.00	5.00	130.06	0.00
9.95	1.13	0.00	7.83	1.67	0.00	0.00	0.00	0.00	0.00	0.00	0.00	0.00	0.02	0.05	0.00	0.16	0.00	0.01	0.01
6.24	4.32	0.00	0.27	1.74	0.00	0.00	0.00	0.00	0.00	0.00	0.00	0.00	0.01	0.00	0.01	0.00	0.00	0.01	0.00
5.40	5.67	0.00	1.63	0.56	0.00	0.00	0.00	0.00	0.00	0.00	0.00	0.00	0.00	0.00	0.00	0.00	0.00	0.00	0.00
3.17	7.87	0.00	0.00	2.47	0.00	0.00	0.00	0.00	0.00	0.00	0.00	0.00	0.01	0.00	0.00	0.03	0.00	0.00	0.00
5.85	5.11	0.00	0.00	2.47	0.00	0.00	0.00	0.00	0.00	0.00	0.00	0.00	0.00	0.00	0.00	0.00	0.00	0.00	0.00
4.01	6.54	0.00	0.00	3.84	0.00	0.00	0.00	0.00	0.00	0.00	0.00	0.00	0.00	0.00	0.00	0.00	0.00	0.00	0.00
3.29	7.98	0.00	0.68	2.87	0.00	0.00	0.00	0.00	0.00	0.00	0.00	0.00	0.00	0.00	0.00	0.00	0.00	0.00	0.00
8.25	4.14	0.00	116.20	2.93	0.00	0.00	0.00	0.00	0.00	0.00	0.00	0.00	0.00	0.00	0.00	0.00	0.00	0.00	0.00
4.47	0.41	0.00	0.00	0.24	0.00	0.00	0.00	0.00	0.00	0.00	0.00	0.00	0.00	0.00	0.00	0.00	0.00	0.00	0.00
2.42	7.06	0.00	0.00	5.20	0.00	0.00	0.00	0.00	0.00	0.00	0.00	0.00	0.00	0.00	0.00	0.00	0.00	0.00	0.00
5.03	1.26	0.00	1.09	2.96	0.00	0.00	0.00	0.00	0.00	0.00	0.00	0.00	0.00	0.00	0.02	0.00	0.00	0.00	0.00
1.55	0.22	0.00	0.00	0.52	0.00	0.00	0.00	0.00	0.00	0.00	0.00	0.00	0.00	0.00	0.00	0.00	0.00	0.00	0.00
1.95	10.15	0.00	0.95	5.86	0.00	0.00	0.00	0.00	0.00	0.00	0.00	0.00	0.00	0.00	0.00	0.00	0.00	0.00	0.00
10.15	1.95	0.00	0.00	4.68	0.00	0.00	0.00	0.00	0.00	0.00	0.00	0.00	0.00	0.00	0.00	0.00	0.00	0.00	0.00
11.70	0.53	0.00	0.00	0.00	0.00	0.00	0.00	0.00	0.00	0.00	0.00	0.00	0.00	0.00	0.00	0.00	0.00	0.00	0.00
0.00	0.00	0.00	0.00	0.00	0.00	0.00	0.00	0.00	0.00	0.00	0.00	0.00	12.01	0.00	0.00	0.00	0.00	235.20	0.00
0.00	0.00	0.00	0.00	0.20	0.00	0.00	0.00	0.00	0.00	0.00	0.00	0.00	0.00	0.00	0.00	0.00	0.00	170.08	0.00
2.22	5.89	0.00	0.00	0.77	0.44	0.00	0.00	0.00	0.00	0.00	0.00	0.00	12.01	0.00	0.00	0.00	0.00	317.33	0.00
0.98	2.67	0.00	0.00	1.04	15.99	0.00	0.00	0.00	0.00	0.00	0.52	0.02	1.35	0.05	0.00	1.72	9.72	168.51	0.01
0.00	0.00	0.00	0.00	0.00	50.02	0.00	0.00	0.00	0.00	0.00	0.00	0.00	0.00	0.00	0.00	0.00	0.00	150.07	0.00
0.23	0.55	0.00	0.00	0.19	21.19	0.00	0.00	0.00	0.00	0.00	0.00	0.00	1.79	0.07	0.00	2.28	12.88	128.28	0.03
1.64	3.22	0.00	0.00	0.98	0.00	0.30	0.00	0.00	0.00	0.00	0.00	0.00	10.11	0.11	0.00	0.00	0.00	74.33	0.00
1.65	4.12	0.00	0.00	1.52	3.53	0.00	0.00	0.00	0.00	0.00	0.72	0.02	1.47	0.03	0.09	0.74	2.21	115.69	0.02
1.77	4.13	0.00	0.00	0.43	9.77	0.00	0.00	0.00	0.00	0.00	0.00	0.00	0.74	0.05	0.00	0.00	0.00	2.33	0.00
0.00	0.00	0.00	0.00	0.00	0.00	0.00	0.00	0.00	0.00	0.00	0.00	0.00	0.00	0.00	0.00	0.00	0.00	145.10	0.00
0.30	0.90	0.00	0.00	0.23	0.00	0.00	0.00	0.00	0.00	0.00	0.00	0.00	0.30	0.03	0.00	0.75	2.25	118.05	0.02
1.77	4.11	0.00	0.00	0.00	0.00	0.30	0.00	0.00	0.00	0.00	0.00	0.00	0.22	0.02	0.00	0.00	0.00	285.32	0.00
1.33	2.88	0.00	0.00	0.00	0.00	0.30	0.00	0.00	0.00	0.00	0.00	0.00	0.22	0.02	0.00	0.00	0.00	127.11	0.00
0.00	0.00	0.00	0.00	0.00	0.00	0.00	0.00	0.00	0.00	0.00	0.00	0.00	0.00	0.00	0.00	0.00	0.00	135.18	0.00
0.00	0.00	0.00	0.00	0.30	0.00	0.00	0.00	0.00	0.00	0.00	0.00	0.00	0.00	0.00	0.00	0.00	0.00	155.07	0.00
1.65	4.12	0.00	0.00	1.52	3.53	0.00	0.00	0.00	0.00	0.00	0.72	0.02	1.47	0.03	0.09	0.73	2.20	115.69	0.02
1.81	4.50	0.00	0.00	1.56	31.67	0.92	0.01	0.01	0.09	0.00	1.59	0.05	2.91	0.09	0.23	5.66	24.02	132.80	0.07
0.15	0.37	0.00	0.00	0.12	2.61	0.98	0.00	0.00	0.00	0.00	0.57	0.02	3.10	0.10	0.07	6.03	25.59	141.48	0.02
1.82	3.84	0.00	0.00	0.77	31.67	0.00	0.00	0.00	0.00	0.00	0.00	0.00	2.91	0.09	0.00	5.66	24.02	153.00	0.02
1.29	3.09	0.00	0.00	0.18	14.98	0.00	0.00	0.00	0.00	0.00	0.98	0.03	1.72	0.09	0.31	2.65	17.63	109.20	0.02
0.00	0.00	0.00	0.00	0.00	0.00	0.00	0.00	0.00	0.00	0.00	0.00	0.00	0.00	0.00	0.00	0.00	0.00	150.07	0.00
0.37	0.95	0.00	0.00	0.18	14.69	0.00	0.00	0.00	0.00	0.00	0.85	0.03	1.68	0.09	0.11	2.60	17.29	153.00	0.02
2.31	3.76	0.00	0.00	1.37	0.00	0.00	0.00	0.00	0.00	0.00	0.00	0.00	0.00	0.00	0.00	0.00	1.17	0.08	0.00

USDA ID Code	Food Name	Weight in Grams*	Quantity of Units	Unit of Measure	Protein (g)	Fat (g)	Carbohydrate (g)	Kilocalories	Caffeine (g)	Fiber (g)	Cholesterol (mg)	Saturated Fat (g)
Fruits and Vegetables												
	Apples, Cnd, Sweetened	204.0000	1.000	Cup	0.37	1.00	34.07	136.68	0.00	3.47	0.00	0.16
	Apples, Dehydrated, Sulfured	60.0000	0.250	Cup	0.79	0.35	56.12	207.60	0.00	7.44	0.00	0.06
	Apples, Fresh, w/ Skin	125.0000	1.000	Cup	0.24	0.45	19.06	73.75	0.00	3.38	0.00	0.08
	Apples, Fresh, w/o Skin	110.0000	1.000	Cup	0.17	0.34	16.32	62.70	0.00	2.09	0.00	0.06
	Applesauce, Sweetened	255.0000	1.000	Cup	0.46	0.46	50.77	193.80	0.00	3.06	0.00	0.08
	Applesauce, Unsweetened	244.0000	1.000	Cup	0.41	0.12	27.55	104.92	0.00	2.93	0.00	0.02
	Apricots, Cnd, Heavy Syrup Pack	258.0000	1.000	Cup	1.32	0.23	55.34	214.14	0.00	4.13	0.00	0.03
	Apricots, Cnd, Juice Pack	244.0000	1.000	Cup	1.54	0.10	30.11	117.12	0.00	3.90	0.00	0.00
	Apricots, Cnd, Light Syrup Pack	253.0000	1.000	Cup	1.34	0.13	41.72	159.39	0.00	4.05	0.00	0.00
	Apricots, Cnd, Water Pack	243.0000	1.000	Cup	1.73	0.39	15.53	65.61	0.00	3.89	0.00	0.02
	Apricots, Dehydrated, Sulfured	119.0000	0.500	Cup	5.83	0.74	98.64	380.80	0.00	0.00	0.00	0.05
	Apricots, Dried, Sulfured	130.0000	1.000	Cup	4.75	0.60	80.28	309.40	0.00	11.70	0.00	0.04
	Apricots, Fresh	155.0000	1.000	Cup	2.17	0.60	17.24	74.40	0.00	3.72	0.00	0.05
	Apricots, Frozen, Sweetened	242.0000	1.000	Cup	1.69	0.24	60.74	237.16	0.00	5.32	0.00	0.02
	Artichoke, Boiled, Hearts w/ Salt	84.0000	0.500	Cup	2.92	0.13	9.39	42.00	0.00	4.54	0.00	0.03
	Artichoke, Boiled, Hearts w/o Salt	84.0000	0.500	Cup	2.92	0.13	9.39	42.00	0.00	4.54	0.00	0.03
	Asparagus, Ckd	90.0000	0.500	Cup	2.33	0.28	3.81	21.60	0.00	1.89	0.00	0.06
	Asparagus, Cnd	242.0000	1.000	Cup	5.18	1.57	6.00	45.98	0.00	3.87	0.00	0.36
	Asparagus, Fresh	134.0000	1.000	Cup	3.06	0.27	6.08	30.82	0.00	2.81	0.00	0.07
	Asparagus, Frz, Ckd	180.0000	1.000	Cup	5.31	0.76	8.77	50.40	0.00	2.88	0.00	0.18
	Avocados, Fresh	150.0000	1.000	Cup	2.97	22.98	11.09	241.50	0.00	7.50	0.00	3.66
	Bamboo Shoots, Cnd	131.0000	1.000	Cup	2.25	0.52	4.22	24.89	0.00	1.83	0.00	0.12
	Bamboo Shoots, Fresh	151.0000	1.000	Cup	3.93	0.45	7.85	40.77	0.00	3.32	0.00	0.11
	Banana, Dehydrated, Chips	100.0000	1.000	Cup	3.89	1.81	88.28	346.00	0.00	7.50	0.00	0.70
	Bananas, Fresh	225.0000	1.000	Cup	2.32	1.08	52.72	207.00	0.00	5.40	0.00	0.43
	Bean Sprouts	133.3330	0.500	Cup	17.47	9.47	12.53	166.67	0.00	0.00	0.00	0.00
	Beans, Green, Cnd	135.0000	1.000	Cup	1.55	0.14	6.08	27.00	0.00	2.57	0.00	0.03
	Beans, Green, Fresh	110.0000	1.000	Cup	2.00	0.13	7.85	34.10	0.00	3.74	0.00	0.03
	Beans, Green, Fzn	135.0000	1.000	Cup	2.01	0.23	8.71	37.80	0.00	4.05	0.00	0.05
	Beans, Lima, Fzn	311.0000	1.250	Cup	20.68	0.93	60.49	326.55	0.00	18.66	0.00	0.22
	Beans, Yellow, Cnd	135.0000	1.000	Cup	1.55	0.14	6.08	27.00	0.00	1.76	0.00	0.03
	Beans, Yellow, Fresh	110.0000	1.000	Cup	2.00	0.13	7.85	34.10	0.00	3.74	0.00	0.03
	Beets, Ckd	85.0000	0.500	Cup	1.43	0.15	8.47	37.40	0.00	1.70	0.00	0.03
	Blueberries, Cnd, Heavy Syrup	256.0000	1.000	Cup	1.66	0.84	56.47	225.28	0.00	3.84	0.00	0.08
	Blueberries, Fresh	145.0000	1.000	Cup	0.97	0.55	20.49	81.20	0.00	3.92	0.00	0.04
	Blueberries, Frozen, Sweetened	230.0000	1.000	Cup	0.92	0.30	50.49	186.30	0.00	4.83	0.00	0.02
	Blueberries, Frozen, Unsweetened	155.0000	1.000	Cup	0.65	0.99	18.86	79.05	0.00	4.19	0.00	0.08
	Broccoli, Ckd	280.0000	1.000	Cup	8.34	0.98	14.17	78.40	0.00	8.12	0.00	0.14
	Broccoli, Flower Clusters, Fresh	71.0000	1.000	Cup	2.12	0.25	3.72	19.88	0.00	0.00	0.00	0.04
	Broccoli, Frz, Chopped, Ckd	184.0000	1.000	Cup	5.70	0.22	9.84	51.52	0.00	5.52	0.00	0.04
	Brussels Sprouts, Ckd	21.0000	1.000	Each	0.54	0.11	1.82	8.19	0.00	0.55	0.00	0.02
	Cabbage, Chinese (pak-choi)	70.0000	1.000	Cup	1.05	0.14	1.56	9.10	0.00	0.70	0.00	0.02
	Cabbage, Ckd		1.000	Head	12.87	5.43	56.29	277.64	0.00	29.03	0.00	0.63
	Cabbage, Fresh	908.0000	1.000	Head	10.99	1.63	48.76	217.92	0.00	20.88	0.00	0.18
	Carrots, Baby, Fresh	15.0000	1.000	Large	0.13	0.08	1.22	5.70	0.00	0.27	0.00	0.01
135	Carrots, Ckd	156.0000	1.000	Cup	1.70	0.28	16.35	70.20	0.00	5.15	0.00	0.05
	Carrots, Cnd, Reg Pk	228.0000	1.000	Cup	1.46	0.43	12.63	57.00	0.00	3.42	0.00	0.09
	Carrots, Fresh	128.0000	1.000	Cup	1.32	0.24	12.98	55.04	0.00	3.84	0.00	0.04
	Carrots, Frz, Ckd	146.0000	0.500	Cup	1.74	0.16	12.05	52.56	0.00	5.11	0.00	0.03
	Cauliflower, Ckd, Boiled	62.0000	0.500	Cup	1.14	0.28	2.55	14.26	0.00	1.67	0.00	0.04
	Cauliflower, Fresh	100.0000	0.500	Cup	1.98	0.21	5.20	25.00	0.00	2.50	0.00	0.03
	Cauliflower, Frz, Ckd	180.0000	1.000	Cup	2.90	0.40	6.75	34.20	0.00	4.86	0.00	0.05

Page Key: A2 = Baby Food   A2 = Baked Goods   A8 = Beverages   A14 = Breads/Grains and Pasta   A18 = Breakfast Foods/Cereals   A26 = Dairy and Eggs   A40 = Fats and Oils   A42 = Fruits and Vegetables   A52 = Meats and Beans   A60 = Nuts and Seeds   A62 5 Frozen Entrees and Packaged Foods   A76 = Restaurant Chains–Fast Foods   A92 = Restaurant Chains–Other   A106 = Seafood and Fish   A110 = Snacks and Sweets   A120 = Soups   A122 = Supplements   A126 = Toppings and Sauces

Monounsaturated Fat (g)	Polyunsaturated Fat (g)	Vitamin D (mg)	Vitamin K (mg)	Vitamin E (mg)	Vitamin A (re)	Vitamin C (mg)	Thiamin (mg)	Riboflavin (mg)	Niacin (mg)	Vitamin B6 (mg)	Folate (mcg)	Vitamin B12 (mcg)	Calcium (mg)	Iron (mg)	Magnesium (mg)	Phosphorus (mg)	Potassium (mg)	Sodium (mg)	Zinc (mg)
0.04	0.29	0.00	0.00	0.02	10.20	0.82	0.02	0.02	0.14	0.08	0.61	0.00	8.16	0.47	4.08	10.20	138.72	6.12	0.06
0.01	0.10	0.00	0.00	2.15	4.80	1.32	0.03	0.08	0.41	0.17	0.60	0.00	11.40	1.20	13.20	33.00	384.00	74.40	0.17
0.03	0.14	0.00	5.00	0.40	6.25	7.13	0.03	0.01	0.10	0.06	3.50	0.00	8.75	0.23	6.25	8.75	143.75	0.00	0.05
0.01	0.10	0.00	0.51	0.09	4.40	4.40	0.02	0.01	0.10	0.06	0.44	0.00	4.40	0.08	3.30	7.70	124.30	0.00	0.04
0.03	0.13	0.00	0.00	0.03	2.55	4.34	0.03	0.08	0.48	0.08	1.53	0.00	10.20	0.89	7.65	17.85	155.55	7.65	0.10
0.00	0.02	0.00	0.00	0.02	7.32	2.93	0.02	0.07	0.46	0.07	1.46	0.00	7.32	0.29	7.32	17.08	183.00	4.88	0.07
0.10	0.05	0.00	0.00	0.00	319.92	7.22	0.05	0.05	1.08	0.13	4.39	0.00	23.22	1.11	20.64	33.54	345.72	28.38	0.26
0.05	0.02	0.00	0.00	2.17	412.36	11.96	0.05	0.05	0.83	0.12	4.15	0.00	29.28	0.73	24.40	48.80	402.60	9.76	0.27
0.05	0.03	0.00	0.00	2.25	333.96	6.83	0.05	0.05	0.76	0.13	4.30	0.00	27.83	0.99	20.24	32.89	349.14	10.12	0.28
0.17	0.07	0.00	0.00	2.16	313.47	8.26	0.05	0.05	0.97	0.12	4.13	0.00	19.44	0.78	17.01	31.59	466.56	7.29	0.27
0.32	0.14	0.00	0.00	0.00	72.59	11.31	0.05	0.18	4.26	0.62	5.24	0.00	72.59	7.51	74.97	186.83	2201.50	15.47	1.19
0.26	0.12	0.00	0.00	1.95	941.20	3.12	0.01	0.20	3.90	0.21	13.39	0.00	58.50	6.11	61.10	152.10	1791.40	13.00	0.96
0.26	0.12	0.00	0.00	1.38	404.55	15.50	0.05	0.06	0.93	0.08	13.33	0.00	21.70	0.84	12.40	29.45	458.80	1.55	0.40
0.10	0.05	0.00	0.00	2.15	406.56	21.78	0.05	0.10	1.94	0.15	4.11	0.00	24.20	2.18	21.78	45.98	554.18	9.68	0.24
0.00	0.06	0.00	0.00	0.16	15.12	8.40	0.06	0.06	0.84	0.09	42.84	0.00	37.80	1.08	50.40	72.24	297.36	278.04	0.41
0.00	0.06	0.00	0.00	0.16	15.12	8.40	0.06	0.06	0.84	0.09	42.84	0.00	37.80	1.08	50.40	72.24	297.36	79.80	0.41
0.01	0.13	0.00	0.00	0.00	48.60	9.72	0.11	0.12	0.97	0.11	131.40	0.00	18.00	0.66	9.00	48.60	144.00	216.00	0.38
0.05	0.68	0.00	0.00	1.04	128.26	44.53	0.15	0.24	2.30	0.27	231.35	0.00	38.72	4.43	24.20	104.06	416.24	694.54	0.97
0.01	0.12	0.00	52.26	2.68	77.72	17.69	0.19	0.17	1.57	0.17	171.52	0.00	28.14	1.17	24.12	75.04	365.82	2.68	0.62
0.02	0.32	0.00	0.00	2.25	147.60	43.92	0.13	0.18	1.87	0.04	242.46	0.00	41.40	1.15	23.40	99.00	392.40	7.20	1.01
14.42	2.94	0.00	0.00	2.01	91.50	11.85	0.17	0.18	2.88	0.42	92.85	0.00	16.50	1.53	58.50	61.50	898.50	15.00	0.63
0.01	0.24	0.00	0.00	0.50	1.31	1.44	0.04	0.04	0.18	0.18	4.19	0.00	10.48	0.42	5.24	32.75	104.80	9.17	0.85
0.02	0.20	0.00	0.00	1.51	3.02	6.04	0.23	0.11	0.91	0.36	10.72	0.00	19.63	0.76	4.53	89.09	804.83	6.04	1.66
0.15	0.34	0.00	0.00	0.00	31.00	7.00	0.18	0.24	2.80	0.44	14.00	0.00	22.00	1.15	108.00	74.00	1491.00	3.00	0.61
0.09	0.20	0.00	1.13	0.61	18.00	20.48	0.11	0.23	1.22	1.31	42.98	0.00	13.50	0.70	65.25	45.00	891.00	2.25	0.36
0.00	0.00	0.00	0.00	0.00	2.67	16.00	0.56	0.25	1.47	0.22	169.87	0.00	109.33	0.53	128.00	288.00	756.00	333.33	2.80
0.00	0.07	0.00	0.00	0.19	47.25	6.48	0.03	0.08	0.27	0.05	42.93	0.00	35.10	1.22	17.55	25.65	147.15	353.70	0.39
0.01	0.07	0.00	30.80	0.45	73.70	17.93	0.09	0.12	0.83	0.08	40.15	0.00	40.70	1.14	27.50	41.80	229.90	6.60	0.26
0.01	0.11	0.00	0.00	0.19	54.00	5.54	0.05	0.12	0.51	0.08	31.05	0.00	66.15	1.19	32.40	41.85	170.10	12.15	0.65
0.06	0.47	0.00	0.00	1.99	52.87	18.04	0.22	0.19	2.39	0.37	48.21	0.00	87.08	6.10	174.16	348.32	1278.21	90.19	1.71
0.00	0.07	0.00	0.00	0.39	14.85	6.48	0.03	0.08	0.27	0.05	42.93	0.00	35.10	1.22	17.55	25.65	147.15	338.85	0.39
0.01	0.07	0.00	0.00	0.00	12.10	17.93	0.09	0.12	0.83	0.08	40.15	0.00	40.70	1.14	27.50	41.80	229.90	6.60	0.26
0.03	0.05	0.00	0.00	0.26	3.40	3.06	0.03	0.03	0.28	0.06	68.00	0.00	13.60	0.67	19.55	32.30	259.25	65.45	0.30
0.13	0.36	0.00	1.28	2.56	15.36	2.82	0.08	0.13	0.28	0.10	4.10	0.00	12.80	0.84	10.24	25.60	102.40	7.68	0.18
0.07	0.25	0.00	0.00	1.45	14.50	18.85	0.07	0.07	0.52	0.06	9.28	0.00	8.70	0.25	7.25	14.50	129.05	8.70	0.16
0.05	0.14	0.00	0.00	1.63	9.20	2.30	0.05	0.12	0.58	0.14	15.41	0.00	13.80	0.90	4.60	16.10	138.00	2.30	0.14
0.14	0.43	0.00	0.00	1.55	12.40	3.88	0.05	0.06	0.81	0.09	10.39	0.00	12.40	0.28	7.75	17.05	83.70	1.55	0.11
0.06	0.48	0.00	0.00	4.73	389.20	208.88	0.17	0.31	1.60	0.39	140.00	0.00	128.80	2.35	67.20	165.20	817.60	72.80	1.06
0.01	0.12	0.00	0.00	1.18	213.00	66.17	0.05	0.09	0.45	0.11	50.41	0.00	34.08	0.62	17.75	46.86	230.75	19.17	0.28
0.02	0.11	0.00	0.00	3.04	347.76	73.78	0.11	0.15	0.85	0.24	103.78	0.00	93.84	1.12	36.80	101.20	331.20	44.16	0.55
0.01	0.05	0.00	0.00	0.18	15.12	13.02	0.02	0.02	0.13	0.04	12.60	0.00	7.56	0.25	4.20	11.76	66.57	4.41	0.07
0.01	0.07	0.00	0.00	0.08	210.00	31.50	0.03	0.05	0.35	0.14	45.99	0.00	73.50	0.56	13.30	25.90	176.40	45.50	0.13
0.38	2.52	0.00	0.00	1.39	164.06	253.66	0.76	0.76	3.53	1.39	252.40	0.00	391.22	2.15	100.96	189.30	1224.14	100.96	1.14
0.09	0.82	0.00	0.00	0.00	118.04	463.08	0.45	0.27	2.72	0.91	514.84	0.00	426.76	5.08	136.20	208.84	2233.68	163.44	1.63
0.00	0.04	0.00	0.00	0.00	225.15	1.26	0.00	0.01	0.13	0.01	4.95	0.00	3.45	0.12	1.80	5.70	41.85	5.25	0.02
0.01	0.14	0.00	0.00	0.66	3829.80	3.59	0.05	0.09	0.79	0.38	21.68	0.00	48.36	0.97	20.28	46.80	354.12	102.96	0.47
0.02	0.21	0.00	0.00	0.96	3139.56	6.16	0.05	0.07	1.25	0.25	20.98	0.00	57.00	1.46	18.24	54.72	408.12	551.76	0.59
0.01	0.10	0.00	16.64	0.59	3600.64	11.90	0.13	0.08	1.19	0.19	17.92	0.00	34.56	0.64	19.20	56.32	413.44	44.80	0.26
0.01	0.07	0.00	0.00	0.61	2584.20	4.09	0.04	0.06	0.64	0.19	15.77	0.00	40.88	0.69	14.60	37.96	230.68	86.14	0.35
0.02	0.14	0.00	0.00	0.02	1.24	27.47	0.02	0.03	0.25	0.11	27.28	0.00	9.92	0.20	5.58	19.84	88.04	9.30	0.11
0.01	0.10	0.00	191.00	0.04	2.00	46.40	0.06	0.06	0.53	0.22	57.00	0.00	22.00	0.44	15.00	44.00	303.00	30.00	0.28
0.04	0.18	0.00	0.00	0.07	3.60	56.34	0.07	0.09	0.56	0.16	73.80	0.00	30.60	0.74	16.20	43.20	250.20	32.40	0.23

USDA ID Code	Food Name	Weight in Grams*	Quantity of Units	Unit of Measure	Protein (g)	Fat (g)	Carbohydrate (g)	Kilocalories	Caffeine (g)	Fiber (g)	Cholesterol (mg)	Saturated Fat (g)
	Celery, Ckd	150.0000	1.000	Cup	1.25	0.24	6.02	27.00	0.00	2.40	0.00	0.06
	Celery, Fresh	120.0000	1.000	Cup	0.90	0.17	4.38	19.20	0.00	2.04	0.00	0.05
	Cherries, Sour, Red, Cnd, Heavy	256.0000	1.000	Cup	1.87	0.26	59.57	232.96	0.00	2.82	0.00	0.05
	Cherries, Sour, Red, Cnd, Light	252.0000	1.000	Cup	1.86	0.25	48.64	189.00	0.00	2.02	0.00	0.05
	Cherries, Sour, Red, Cnd, Water	244.0000	1.000	Cup	1.88	0.24	21.81	87.84	0.00	2.68	0.00	0.05
	Cherries, Sour, Red, Cnd, X-heav	261.0000	1.000	Cup	1.85	0.23	76.29	297.54	0.00	2.09	0.00	0.05
	Cherries, Sour, Red, Fresh	155.0000	1.000	Cup	1.55	0.47	18.88	77.50	0.00	2.48	0.00	0.11
	Cherries, Sweet, Cnd, Heavy Syrup	253.0000	1.000	Cup	1.52	0.38	53.81	209.99	0.00	3.80	0.00	0.08
	Cherries, Sweet, Cnd, Juice Pack	250.0000	1.000	Cup	2.28	0.05	34.53	135.00	0.00	3.75	0.00	0.00
	Cherries, Sweet, Cnd, Light Syrup	252.0000	1.000	Cup	1.54	0.38	43.57	168.84	0.00	3.78	0.00	0.08
	Cherries, Sweet, Cnd, Water Pack	248.0000	1.000	Cup	1.91	0.32	29.16	114.08	0.00	3.72	0.00	0.07
	Cherries, Sweet, Cnd, X-heavy Sy	261.0000	1.000	Cup	1.54	0.39	68.46	266.22	0.00	3.92	0.00	0.08
	Cherries, Sweet, Fresh	117.0000	1.000	Cup	1.40	1.12	19.36	84.24	0.00	2.69	0.00	0.26
	Cherries, Sweet, Frozen, Sweeten	259.0000	1.000	Cup	2.98	0.34	57.91	230.51	0.00	5.44	0.00	0.08
	Chives, Raw	1.0000	1.000	Tsp	0.03	0.01	0.04	0.30	0.00	0.03	0.00	0.00
	Coleslaw	8.0000	1.000	Tbsp	0.10	0.21	0.99	5.52	0.00	0.12	0.64	0.03
	Collards, Ckd	190.0000	1.000	Cup	4.01	0.68	9.31	49.40	0.00	5.32	0.00	0.10
	Collards, Fresh	36.0000	1.000	Cup	0.88	0.15	2.05	10.80	0.00	1.30	0.00	0.02
	Collards, Frz, Chopped, Ckd	170.0000	1.000	Cup	5.05	0.70	12.09	61.20	0.00	4.76	0.00	0.10
	Corn, Ckd	140.0000	1.000	Cup	3.68	1.02	39.07	176.40	0.00	6.72	0.00	0.14
	Corn, Sweet, White, Ckd	77.0000	1.000	Cup	2.56	0.99	19.33	83.16	0.00	2.08	0.00	0.15
	Corn, Sweet, White, Cnd	164.0000	1.000	Cup	4.30	1.64	30.49	132.84	0.00	3.28	0.00	0.25
	Corn, Sweet, White, Cnd, Cream S	256.0000	1.000	Cup	4.45	1.08	46.41	184.32	0.00	3.07	0.00	0.18
	Corn, Sweet, White, Fresh	154.0000	1.000	Cup	4.96	1.82	29.29	132.44	0.00	4.16	0.00	0.28
	Corn, Sweet, Yellow, Ckd	164.0000	1.000	Cup	5.44	2.10	41.18	177.12	0.00	4.59	0.00	0.33
	Corn, Sweet, Yellow, Cnd, Brine	164.0000	1.000	Cup	4.30	1.64	30.49	132.84	0.00	3.28	0.00	0.25
	Corn, Sweet, Yellow, Cnd, Cream	256.0000	1.000	Cup	4.45	1.08	46.41	184.32	0.00	3.07	0.00	0.18
	Corn, Sweet, Yellow, Fresh	154.0000	1.000	Cup	4.96	1.82	29.29	132.44	0.00	4.16	0.00	0.28
	Crabapples, Fresh	110.0000	1.000	Cup	0.44	0.33	21.95	83.60	0.00	0.00	0.00	0.06
	Cranberries, Fresh	110.0000	1.000	Cup	0.43	0.22	13.95	53.90	0.00	4.62	0.00	0.02
	Cranberry Sauce, Cnd, Sweetened	277.0000	1.000	Cup	0.55	0.42	107.75	418.27	0.00	2.77	0.00	0.03
	Cranberry-orange Relish, Cnd	275.0000	1.000	Cup	0.83	0.28	127.05	489.50	0.00	0.00	0.00	0.03
	Cucumber, Fresh	52.0000	0.500	Cup	0.36	0.07	1.44	6.76	0.00	0.42	0.00	0.02
	Dates, Domestic, Natural and Dry	178.0000	1.000	Cup	3.51	0.80	130.85	489.50	0.00	13.35	0.00	0.34
	Eggplant, Ckd	99.0000	1.000	Cup	0.82	0.23	6.57	27.72	0.00	2.48	0.00	0.04
	Eggplant, Fresh	82.0000	1.000	Cup	0.84	0.15	4.98	21.32	0.00	2.05	0.00	0.02
	Endive, Raw	25.0000	0.500	Cup	0.31	0.05	0.84	4.25	0.00	0.78	0.00	0.01
	Fruit Salad, Heavy Syrup	255.0000	1.000	Cup	0.87	0.18	48.73	186.15	0.00	2.55	0.00	0.03
	Fruit Salad, Juice Pack	249.0000	1.000	Cup	1.27	0.07	32.49	124.50	0.00	2.49	0.00	0.00
	Fruit Salad, Light Syrup	252.0000	1.000	Cup	0.86	0.18	38.15	146.16	0.00	2.52	0.00	0.03
	Fruit Salad, Water Pack	245.0000	1.000	Cup	0.86	0.17	19.28	73.50	0.00	2.45	0.00	0.02
	Fruit, Heavy Syrup	248.0000	1.000	Cup	0.97	0.17	46.90	181.04	0.00	2.48	0.00	0.02
	Fruit, Juice Pack	237.0000	1.000	Cup	1.09	0.02	28.11	109.02	0.00	2.37	0.00	0.00
	Fruit, Light Syrup	242.0000	1.000	Cup	0.97	0.17	36.13	137.94	0.00	2.42	0.00	0.02
	Fruit, Mixed, Dried	293.0000	1.250	Cup	7.21	1.44	187.70	711.99	0.00	22.85	0.00	0.12
	Fruit, Mixed, Frzn, Swtnd, Thawd	250.0000	1.000	Cup	3.55	0.45	60.58	245.00	0.00	4.75	0.00	0.08
	Fruit, Mixed, Hvy Syrup	255.0000	1.000	Cup	0.94	0.26	47.84	183.60	0.00	2.55	0.00	0.03
	Fruit, Water Pack	237.0000	1.000	Cup	1.00	0.12	20.17	75.84	0.00	2.37	0.00	0.02
	Garlic, Raw	3.0000	1.000	Clove	0.19	0.02	0.99	4.47	0.00	0.06	0.00	0.00
	Grapefruit, Fresh, Pink & Red	230.0000	1.000	Cup	1.27	0.23	17.66	69.00	0.00	0.00	0.00	0.02
	Grapefruit, Fresh, White	230.0000	1.000	Cup	1.59	0.23	19.34	75.90	0.00	2.53	0.00	0.02
	Grapefruit, Sections, Cnd, Juice	249.0000	1.000	Cup	1.74	0.22	22.93	92.13	0.00	1.00	0.00	0.02
	Grapefruit, Sections, Cnd, Light	254.0000	1.000	Cup	1.42	0.25	39.22	152.40	0.00	1.02	0.00	0.03

Page Key: A2 = Baby Food   A2 = Baked Goods   A8 = Beverages   A14 = Breads/Grains and Pasta   A18 = Breakfast Foods/Cereals   A26 = Dairy and Eggs   A40 = Fats and Oils   A42 = Fruits and Vegetables   A52 = Meats and Beans   A60 = Nuts and Seeds   A62 5 Frozen Entrees and Packaged Foods   A76 = Restaurant Chains–Fast Foods   A92 = Restaurant Chains–Other   A106 = Seafood and Fish   A110 = Snacks and Sweets   A120 = Soups   A122 = Supplements   A126 = Toppings and Sauces

Monounsaturated Fat (g)	Polyunsaturated Fat (g)	Vitamin D (mg)	Vitamin K (mg)	Vitamin E (mg)	Vitamin A (re)	Vitamin C (mg)	Thiamin (mg)	Riboflavin (mg)	Niacin (mg)	Vitamin B_6 (mg)	Folate (mcg)	Vitamin B_{12} (mcg)	Calcium (mg)	Iron (mg)	Magnesium (mg)	Phosphorus (mg)	Potassium (mg)	Sodium (mg)	Zinc (mg)
0.05	0.12	0.00	0.00	0.54	19.50	9.15	0.06	0.08	0.48	0.14	33.00	0.00	63.00	0.63	18.00	37.50	426.00	136.50	0.21
0.04	0.08	0.00	0.00	0.43	15.60	8.40	0.06	0.06	0.38	0.11	33.60	0.00	48.00	0.48	13.20	30.00	344.40	104.40	0.16
0.08	0.08	0.00	0.00	0.33	181.76	5.12	0.05	0.10	0.44	0.10	19.46	0.00	25.60	3.33	15.36	25.60	238.08	17.92	0.15
0.08	0.08	0.00	0.00	0.00	183.96	5.04	0.05	0.10	0.43	0.10	19.40	0.00	25.20	3.33	15.12	25.20	239.40	17.64	0.18
0.07	0.07	0.00	0.00	0.32	183.00	5.12	0.05	0.10	0.44	0.10	19.52	0.00	26.84	3.34	14.64	24.40	239.12	17.08	0.17
0.08	0.08	0.00	0.00	0.00	182.70	4.96	0.05	0.10	0.42	0.10	19.31	0.00	26.10	3.29	13.05	23.49	237.51	18.27	0.16
0.12	0.14	0.00	0.00	0.20	198.40	15.50	0.05	0.06	0.62	0.06	11.63	0.00	24.80	0.50	13.95	23.25	268.15	4.65	0.16
0.10	0.13	0.00	0.00	0.15	37.95	9.11	0.05	0.10	1.01	0.08	10.63	0.00	22.77	0.89	22.77	45.54	366.85	7.59	0.25
0.03	0.03	0.00	0.00	0.25	32.50	6.25	0.05	0.05	1.03	0.08	10.50	0.00	35.00	1.45	30.00	55.00	327.50	7.50	0.25
0.10	0.13	0.00	0.00	0.33	40.32	9.32	0.05	0.10	1.01	0.08	10.58	0.00	22.68	0.91	22.68	45.36	372.96	7.56	0.25
0.07	0.10	0.00	0.00	0.32	39.68	5.46	0.05	0.10	1.02	0.07	10.42	0.00	27.28	0.89	22.32	37.20	324.88	2.48	0.20
0.10	0.13	0.00	0.00	0.00	39.15	9.40	0.05	0.10	1.02	0.08	10.96	0.00	23.49	0.91	20.88	44.37	370.62	7.83	0.26
0.30	0.34	0.00	0.00	0.15	24.57	8.19	0.06	0.07	0.47	0.05	4.91	0.00	17.55	0.46	12.87	22.23	262.08	0.00	0.07
0.10	0.10	0.00	0.00	0.34	49.21	2.59	0.08	0.13	0.47	0.10	10.88	0.00	31.08	0.91	25.90	41.44	515.41	2.59	0.10
0.00	0.00	0.00	0.00	0.00	4.35	0.58	0.00	0.00	0.01	0.00	1.05	0.00	0.92	0.02	0.42	0.58	2.96	0.03	0.01
0.06	0.11	0.00	0.00	0.00	6.56	2.62	0.01	0.00	0.02	0.01	2.12	0.00	3.60	0.05	0.80	2.56	14.48	1.84	0.02
0.06	0.32	0.00	0.00	1.67	594.70	34.58	0.08	0.21	1.10	0.25	176.70	0.00	226.10	0.87	32.30	49.40	494.00	17.10	0.80
0.01	0.07	0.00	0.00	0.81	137.52	12.71	0.02	0.05	0.27	0.06	59.76	0.00	52.20	0.07	3.24	3.60	60.84	7.20	0.05
0.03	0.36	0.00	0.00	0.85	1016.60	44.88	0.09	0.20	1.09	0.19	129.37	0.00	357.00	1.90	51.00	45.90	426.70	85.00	0.46
0.27	0.46	0.00	0.00	0.46	8.40	0.00	0.07	0.03	0.78	0.08	8.40	0.00	1.40	0.35	50.40	106.40	43.40	0.00	0.88
0.28	0.46	0.00	0.00	0.07	0.00	4.77	0.17	0.05	1.24	0.05	35.73	0.00	1.54	0.47	24.64	79.31	191.73	13.09	0.37
0.48	0.77	0.00	0.00	0.15	0.00	13.94	0.05	0.13	1.97	0.08	79.70	0.00	8.20	1.41	32.80	106.60	319.80	529.72	0.64
0.31	0.51	0.00	0.00	0.23	0.00	11.78	0.08	0.13	2.46	0.15	114.69	0.00	7.68	0.97	43.52	130.56	343.04	729.60	1.36
0.54	0.86	0.00	0.00	0.14	0.00	10.47	0.31	0.09	2.62	0.09	70.53	0.00	3.08	0.80	56.98	137.06	415.80	23.10	0.69
0.61	0.98	0.00	0.00	0.15	36.08	10.17	0.36	0.11	2.64	0.10	76.10	0.00	3.28	1.00	52.48	168.92	408.36	27.88	0.79
0.48	0.77	0.00	0.00	0.25	26.24	13.94	0.05	0.13	1.97	0.08	79.70	0.00	8.20	1.41	32.80	106.60	319.80	350.96	0.64
0.31	0.51	0.00	0.00	0.23	25.60	11.78	0.08	0.13	2.46	0.15	114.69	0.00	7.68	0.97	43.52	130.56	343.04	729.60	1.36
0.54	0.86	0.00	10.78	0.14	43.12	10.47	0.31	0.09	2.62	0.09	70.53	0.00	3.08	0.80	56.98	137.06	415.80	23.10	0.69
0.01	0.10	0.00	0.00	0.00	4.40	8.80	0.03	0.02	0.11	0.00	0.00	0.00	19.80	0.40	7.70	16.50	213.40	1.10	0.00
0.03	0.10	0.00	0.00	0.11	5.50	14.85	0.03	0.02	0.11	0.08	1.87	0.00	7.70	0.22	5.50	9.90	78.10	1.10	0.14
0.06	0.19	0.00	3.88	0.28	5.54	5.54	0.06	0.06	0.28	0.03	2.77	0.00	11.08	0.61	8.31	16.62	72.02	80.33	0.14
0.00	0.00	0.00	0.00	0.00	19.25	49.50	0.08	0.06	0.28	0.00	0.00	0.00	30.25	0.55	11.00	22.00	104.50	88.00	0.00
0.00	0.03	0.00	2.60	0.04	10.92	2.76	0.01	0.01	0.11	0.02	6.76	0.00	7.28	0.34	5.72	10.40	74.88	1.04	0.10
0.27	0.05	0.00	0.00	0.18	8.90	0.00	0.16	0.18	3.92	0.34	22.43	0.00	56.96	2.05	62.30	71.20	1160.56	5.34	0.52
0.02	0.09	0.00	0.00	0.03	5.94	1.29	0.08	0.02	0.59	0.09	14.26	0.00	5.94	0.35	12.87	21.78	245.52	2.97	0.15
0.02	0.07	0.00	0.00	0.02	6.56	1.39	0.04	0.02	0.49	0.07	15.58	0.00	5.74	0.22	11.48	18.04	177.94	2.46	0.11
0.00	0.02	0.00	0.00	0.11	51.25	1.63	0.02	0.02	0.10	0.01	35.50	0.00	13.00	0.21	3.75	7.00	78.50	5.50	0.20
0.03	0.08	0.00	0.00	1.17	127.50	6.12	0.05	0.05	0.89	0.08	6.38	0.00	15.30	0.71	12.75	22.95	204.00	15.30	0.18
0.02	0.02	0.00	0.00	0.00	149.40	8.22	0.02	0.02	0.90	0.07	6.47	0.00	27.39	0.62	19.92	34.86	288.84	12.45	0.35
0.03	0.08	0.00	0.00	0.00	108.36	6.30	0.03	0.05	0.93	0.08	6.55	0.00	17.64	0.73	12.60	22.68	206.64	15.12	0.18
0.02	0.07	0.00	0.00	0.00	107.80	4.66	0.05	0.05	0.91	0.07	6.37	0.00	17.15	0.74	12.25	22.05	191.10	7.35	0.20
0.02	0.07	0.00	0.00	0.72	49.60	4.71	0.05	0.05	0.92	0.12	6.45	0.00	14.88	0.72	12.40	27.28	218.24	14.88	0.20
0.00	0.00	0.00	0.00	0.47	73.47	6.40	0.02	0.05	0.95	0.12	5.93	0.00	18.96	0.50	16.59	33.18	225.15	9.48	0.21
0.02	0.07	0.00	0.00	0.70	50.82	4.60	0.05	0.05	0.92	0.12	6.53	0.00	14.52	0.70	12.10	26.62	215.38	14.52	0.22
0.67	0.32	0.00	0.00	0.00	714.92	11.13	0.12	0.47	5.65	0.47	11.43	0.00	111.34	7.94	114.27	225.61	2332.28	52.74	1.47
0.08	0.20	0.00	0.00	0.00	80.00	187.50	0.05	0.10	1.00	0.08	19.00	0.00	17.50	0.70	15.00	30.00	327.50	7.50	0.13
0.05	0.10	0.00	0.00	0.00	48.45	175.95	0.05	0.10	1.53	0.10	7.65	0.00	2.55	0.92	12.75	25.50	214.20	10.20	0.18
0.02	0.05	0.00	0.00	0.69	59.25	4.98	0.05	0.02	0.85	0.12	6.40	0.00	11.85	0.59	16.59	26.07	222.78	9.48	0.21
0.00	0.01	0.00	0.00	0.00	0.00	0.94	0.01	0.00	0.02	0.04	0.09	0.00	5.43	0.05	0.75	4.59	12.03	0.51	0.04
0.02	0.05	0.00	0.00	0.00	59.80	87.63	0.07	0.05	0.44	0.09	28.06	0.00	25.30	0.28	18.40	20.70	296.70	0.00	0.16
0.02	0.05	0.00	0.00	0.58	2.30	76.59	0.09	0.05	0.62	0.09	23.00	0.00	27.60	0.14	20.70	18.40	340.40	0.00	0.16
0.02	0.05	0.00	0.00	0.62	0.00	84.41	0.07	0.05	0.62	0.05	21.91	0.00	37.35	0.52	27.39	29.88	420.81	17.43	0.20
0.03	0.05	0.00	0.00	0.64	0.00	54.10	0.10	0.05	0.61	0.05	21.59	0.00	35.56	1.02	25.40	25.40	327.66	5.08	0.20

USDA ID Code	Food Name	Weight in Grams*	Quantity of Units	Unit of Measure	Protein (g)	Fat (g)	Carbohydrate (g)	Kilocalories	Caffeine (g)	Fiber (g)	Cholesterol (mg)	Saturated Fat (g)
	Grapefruit, Sections, Cnd, Water	244.0000	1.000	Cup	1.42	0.24	22.33	87.84	0.00	0.98	0.00	0.02
	Grapes, Fresh	92.0000	1.000	Cup	0.58	0.32	15.78	61.64	0.00	0.92	0.00	0.10
	Kiwifruit, Fresh	177.0000	1.000	Cup	1.75	0.78	26.34	107.97	0.00	6.02	0.00	0.05
	Leeks, Ckd	124.0000	1.000	Leek	1.00	0.25	9.45	38.44	0.00	1.24	0.00	0.04
	Leeks, Fresh	89.0000	1.000	Cup	1.34	0.27	12.59	54.29	0.00	1.60	0.00	0.04
	Lemons, Fresh, w/o Peel	212.0000	1.000	Cup	2.33	0.64	19.76	61.48	0.00	5.94	0.00	0.08
	Lettuce, Butterhead, Fresh	55.0000	1.000	Cup	0.71	0.12	1.28	7.15	0.00	0.55	0.00	0.02
	Lettuce, Iceberg, Fresh	55.0000	1.000	Cup	0.56	0.10	1.15	6.60	0.00	0.77	0.00	0.02
	Lettuce, Looseleaf, Fresh	10.0000	1.000	Leaf	0.13	0.03	0.35	1.80	0.00	0.19	0.00	0.00
	Lettuce, Romaine, Fresh	10.0000	1.000	Leaf	0.16	0.02	0.24	1.40	0.00	0.17	0.00	0.00
	Lime, Raw	7.0000	1.000	Medium	0.47	0.13	7.06	20.10	0.00	1.88	0.00	0.02
	Mangos, Fresh	165.0000	0.500	Cup	0.84	0.45	28.05	107.25	0.00	2.97	0.00	0.12
	Melon Balls, Frozen, Unthawed	173.0000	1.000	Cup	1.45	0.43	13.74	57.09	0.00	1.21	0.00	0.10
	Melons, Cantaloupe, Fresh	177.0000	1.000	Cup	1.56	0.50	14.80	61.95	0.00	1.42	0.00	0.12
	Melons, Casaba, Fresh	170.0000	1.000	Cup	1.53	0.17	10.54	44.20	0.00	1.36	0.00	0.05
	Melons, Honeydew, Fresh	177.0000	1.000	Cup	0.81	0.18	16.25	61.95	0.00	1.06	0.00	0.05
	Mushrooms, Ckd	156.0000	1.000	Cup	3.39	0.73	8.02	42.12	0.00	3.43	0.00	0.09
	Mushrooms, Cnd, Drained Solids	156.0000	1.000	Cup	2.92	0.45	7.74	37.44	0.00	3.74	0.00	0.06
	Mushrooms, Enoki, Fresh	5.0000	1.000	Large	0.12	0.02	0.35	1.70	0.00	0.13	0.00	0.00
	Mushrooms, Fresh	70.0000	1.000	Cup	2.03	0.23	2.86	17.50	0.00	0.84	0.00	0.04
	Mushrooms, Shiitake, Ckd	145.0000	1.000	Cup	2.26	0.32	20.71	79.75	0.00	3.05	0.00	0.09
	Mushrooms, Shiitake, Dried	3.6000	1.000	Medium	0.34	0.04	2.71	10.66	0.00	0.41	0.00	0.01
	Nectar, Apricot, Cnd, w/ Added V	251.0000	1.000	Cup	0.93	0.23	36.12	140.56	0.00	1.51	0.00	0.03
	Nectar, Apricot, Cnd, w/o Vit C	251.0000	1.000	Cup	0.93	0.23	36.12	140.56	0.00	1.51	0.00	0.03
	Nectar, Papaya, Cnd.	250.0000	1.000	Cup	0.43	0.38	36.28	142.50	0.00	1.50	0.00	0.13
	Nectar, Peach, Cnd, wo/ Added Vi	249.0000	1.000	Cup	0.67	0.05	34.66	134.46	0.00	1.49	0.00	0.00
	Nectarine, Raw	136.0000	1.000	Medium	1.28	0.63	16.02	66.64	0.00	2.18	0.00	0.07
	Okra, Ckd	80.0000	0.500	Cup	1.50	0.14	5.77	25.60	0.00	2.00	0.00	0.04
	Okra, Fresh	100.0000	1.000	Cup	2.00	0.10	7.63	33.00	0.00	3.20	0.00	0.03
	Okra, Frz, Ckd	255.0000	1.250	Cup	5.30	0.77	14.66	71.40	0.00	7.14	0.00	0.20
	Okra, Frz, Unprepared	284.0000	1.250	Cup	4.80	0.71	18.86	85.20	0.00	6.25	0.00	0.20
	Olives, Green	3.0000	5.000	Each	0.00	0.50	0.00	5.00	0.00	0.00	0.00	0.00
	Olives, Ripe, Canned (jumbo-super)	8.3000	1.000	Jumbo	0.08	0.57	0.47	6.72	0.00	0.21	0.00	0.08
	Olives, Ripe, Canned (small-extra)	8.4000	1.000	Tbsp	0.07	0.90	0.53	9.66	0.00	0.27	0.00	0.12
	Onions, Ckd	210.0000	1.000	Cup	2.86	0.40	21.32	92.40	0.00	2.94	0.00	0.06
	Onions, Cnd, Solid & Liquid	63.0000	1.000	Onion	0.54	0.06	2.53	11.97	0.00	0.76	0.00	0.01
	Onions, Fresh	160.0000	1.000	Cup	1.86	0.26	13.81	60.80	0.00	2.88	0.00	0.05
	Oranges, Fresh	180.0000	1.000	Cup	1.69	0.22	21.15	84.60	0.00	4.32	0.00	0.04
	Papayas, Fresh	140.0000	1.000	Cup	0.85	0.20	13.73	54.60	0.00	2.52	0.00	0.06
	Parsnips, Ckd, w/ Salt	78.0000	0.500	Cup	1.03	0.23	15.23	63.18	0.00	3.12	0.00	0.04
	Parsnips, Ckd, w/o Salt	78.0000	0.500	Cup	1.03	0.23	15.23	63.18	0.00	3.12	0.00	0.04
	Parsnips, Fresh	133.0000	1.000	Cup	1.60	0.40	23.93	99.75	0.00	6.52	0.00	0.07
	Peaches, Cnd, Heavy Syrup Pack	262.0000	1.000	Cup	1.18	0.26	52.24	193.88	0.00	3.41	0.00	0.03
	Peaches, Cnd, Juice Pack	250.0000	1.000	Cup	1.58	0.08	28.93	110.00	0.00	3.25	0.00	0.00
	Peaches, Cnd, Light Syrup Pack	251.0000	1.000	Cup	1.13	0.08	36.52	135.54	0.00	3.26	0.00	0.00
	Peaches, Cnd, Water Pack	244.0000	1.000	Cup	1.07	0.15	14.91	58.56	0.00	3.17	0.00	0.02
	Peaches, Cnd, X-heavy Syrup Pack	262.0000	1.000	Cup	1.23	0.08	68.28	251.52	0.00	2.62	0.00	0.00
	Peaches, Cnd, X-light Syrup	247.0000	1.000	Cup	0.99	0.25	27.42	103.74	0.00	2.47	0.00	0.02
	Peaches, Dehydrated, Sulfured	116.0000	1.000	Cup	5.67	1.19	96.49	377.00	0.00	0.00	0.00	0.13
	Peaches, Dried, Sulfured	160.0000	1.000	Cup	5.78	1.22	98.13	382.40	0.00	13.12	0.00	0.13
	Peaches, Fresh	170.0000	1.000	Cup	1.19	0.15	18.87	73.10	0.00	3.40	0.00	0.02
	Peaches, Frozen, Sliced, Sweeten	250.0000	1.000	Cup	1.58	0.33	59.95	235.00	0.00	4.50	0.00	0.03
	Pears, Asian, Fresh	122.0000	1.000	Medium	0.61	0.28	12.99	51.24	0.00	4.39	0.00	0.01

Page Key: A2 = Baby Food   A2 = Baked Goods   A8 = Beverages   A14 = Breads/Grains and Pasta   A18 = Breakfast Foods/Cereals   A26 = Dairy and Eggs   A40 = Fats and Oils   A42 = Fruits and Vegetables   A52 = Meats and Beans   A60 = Nuts and Seeds   A62 5 Frozen Entrees and Packaged Foods   A76 = Restaurant Chains–Fast Foods   A92 = Restaurant Chains–Other   A106 = Seafood and Fish   A110 = Snacks and Sweets   A120 = Soups   A122 = Supplements   A126 = Toppings and Sauces

Monounsaturated Fat (g)	Polyunsaturated Fat (g)	Vitamin D (mg)	Vitamin K (mg)	Vitamin E (mg)	Vitamin A (re)	Vitamin C (mg)	Thiamin (mg)	Riboflavin (mg)	Niacin (mg)	Vitamin B6 (mg)	Folate (mcg)	Vitamin B12 (mcg)	Calcium (mg)	Iron (mg)	Magnesium (mg)	Phosphorus (mg)	Potassium (mg)	Sodium (mg)	Zinc (mg)
0.02	0.05	0.00	0.00	0.61	0.00	53.19	0.10	0.05	0.61	0.05	21.47	0.00	36.60	1.00	24.40	24.40	322.08	4.88	0.22
0.01	0.09	0.00	0.00	0.31	9.20	3.68	0.08	0.06	0.28	0.10	3.59	0.00	12.88	0.27	4.60	9.20	175.72	1.84	0.04
0.07	0.42	0.00	0.00	1.98	31.86	173.46	0.04	0.09	0.89	0.16	67.26	0.00	46.02	0.73	53.10	70.80	587.64	8.85	0.30
0.00	0.14	0.00	0.00	0.00	6.20	5.21	0.04	0.02	0.25	0.14	30.13	0.00	37.20	1.36	17.36	21.08	107.88	12.40	0.07
0.00	0.15	0.00	0.00	0.82	8.90	10.68	0.05	0.03	0.36	0.20	57.05	0.00	52.51	1.87	24.92	31.15	160.20	17.80	0.11
0.02	0.19	0.00	0.00	0.51	6.36	112.36	0.08	0.04	0.21	0.17	22.47	0.00	55.12	1.27	16.96	33.92	292.56	4.24	0.13
0.01	0.07	0.00	0.00	0.24	53.35	4.40	0.03	0.03	0.17	0.03	40.32	0.00	17.60	0.17	7.15	12.65	141.35	2.75	0.09
0.01	0.06	0.00	62.15	0.15	18.15	2.15	0.03	0.02	0.10	0.02	30.80	0.00	10.45	0.28	4.95	11.00	86.90	4.95	0.12
0.00	0.02	0.00	0.00	0.04	19.00	1.80	0.01	0.01	0.04	0.01	4.98	0.00	6.80	0.14	1.10	2.50	26.40	0.90	0.03
0.00	0.01	0.00	0.00	0.04	26.00	2.40	0.01	0.01	0.05	0.01	13.57	0.00	3.60	0.11	0.60	4.50	29.00	0.80	0.03
0.01	0.04	0.00	0.00	0.16	0.67	19.49	0.02	0.01	0.13	0.03	5.49	0.00	22.11	0.40	4.02	12.06	68.34	1.34	0.07
0.17	0.08	0.00	0.00	1.85	641.85	45.71	0.10	0.10	0.96	0.21	23.10	0.00	16.50	0.21	14.85	18.15	257.40	3.30	0.07
0.02	0.17	0.00	0.00	0.26	306.21	10.73	0.29	0.03	1.11	0.19	44.46	0.00	17.30	0.50	24.22	20.76	484.40	53.63	0.29
0.02	0.19	0.00	0.00	0.27	569.94	74.69	0.07	0.04	1.01	0.21	30.09	0.00	19.47	0.37	19.47	30.09	546.93	15.93	0.28
0.00	0.07	0.00	0.00	0.26	5.10	27.20	0.10	0.03	0.68	0.20	28.90	0.00	8.50	0.68	13.60	11.90	357.00	20.40	0.27
0.00	0.07	0.00	0.00	0.27	7.08	43.90	0.14	0.04	1.06	0.11	10.62	0.00	10.62	0.12	12.39	17.70	479.67	17.70	0.12
0.02	0.28	0.00	0.00	0.19	0.00	6.24	0.11	0.47	6.96	0.16	28.39	0.00	9.36	2.71	18.72	135.72	555.36	3.12	1.36
0.02	0.17	0.00	0.00	0.19	0.00	0.00	0.14	0.03	2.48	0.09	19.19	0.00	17.16	1.23	23.40	102.96	201.24	663.00	1.12
0.00	0.01	0.00	0.00	0.00	0.05	0.60	0.00	0.01	0.18	0.00	1.50	0.00	0.05	0.04	0.80	5.65	19.05	0.15	0.03
0.01	0.10	1.33	5.60	0.08	0.00	1.61	0.06	0.29	2.83	0.07	8.40	0.03	3.50	0.73	7.00	72.80	259.00	2.80	0.51
0.10	0.04	0.00	0.00	0.17	0.00	0.44	0.06	0.25	2.18	0.23	30.31	0.00	4.35	0.64	20.30	42.05	169.65	5.80	1.93
0.01	0.01	1.49	0.00	0.00	0.00	0.13	0.01	0.05	0.51	0.03	5.88	0.00	0.40	0.06	4.75	10.58	55.22	0.47	0.28
0.10	0.05	0.00	0.00	0.00	331.32	136.54	0.03	0.03	0.65	0.05	3.26	0.00	17.57	0.95	12.55	22.59	286.14	7.53	0.23
0.10	0.05	0.00	0.00	0.20	331.32	1.51	0.03	0.03	0.65	0.05	3.26	0.00	17.57	0.95	12.55	22.59	286.14	7.53	0.23
0.10	0.10	0.00	0.00	0.05	27.50	7.50	0.03	0.03	0.38	0.03	5.25	0.00	25.00	0.85	7.50	0.00	77.50	12.50	0.38
0.02	0.02	0.00	0.00	0.02	64.74	13.20	0.00	0.02	0.72	0.02	3.49	0.00	12.45	0.47	9.96	14.94	99.60	17.43	0.20
0.24	0.31	0.00	0.00	1.21	100.64	7.34	0.02	0.06	1.35	0.03	5.03	0.00	6.80	0.10	10.88	21.76	288.32	0.00	0.12
0.02	0.04	0.00	0.00	0.55	46.40	13.04	0.10	0.05	0.70	0.15	36.56	0.00	50.40	0.36	45.60	44.80	257.60	4.00	0.44
0.02	0.03	0.00	0.00	0.69	66.00	21.10	0.20	0.06	1.00	0.22	87.80	0.00	81.00	0.80	57.00	63.00	303.00	8.00	0.60
0.13	0.20	0.00	0.00	1.76	130.05	31.11	0.26	0.31	2.01	0.13	371.28	0.00	244.80	1.71	130.05	117.30	596.70	7.65	1.58
0.11	0.20	0.00	0.00	1.96	130.64	35.22	0.26	0.31	2.02	0.11	419.18	0.00	230.04	1.62	122.12	119.28	599.24	8.52	1.51
0.00	0.00	0.00	0.00	0.00	0.00	0.00	0.00	0.00	0.00	0.00	0.00	0.00	0.00	0.00	0.00	0.00	0.00	13.00	0.00
0.42	0.05	0.00	0.00	0.25	2.91	0.12	0.00	0.00	0.00	0.00	0.00	0.00	7.80	0.28	0.33	0.25	0.75	74.53	0.02
0.66	0.08	0.00	0.00	0.25	3.36	0.08	0.00	0.00	0.00	0.00	0.00	0.00	7.39	0.28	0.34	0.25	0.67	73.25	0.02
0.06	0.15	0.00	0.00	0.27	0.00	10.92	0.08	0.04	0.36	0.27	31.50	0.00	46.20	0.50	23.10	73.50	348.60	6.30	0.44
0.01	0.03	0.00	0.00	0.04	0.00	2.71	0.02	0.01	0.04	0.09	6.11	0.00	28.35	0.08	3.78	17.64	69.93	233.73	0.18
0.03	0.10	0.00	0.83	0.21	0.00	10.24	0.06	0.03	0.24	0.19	30.40	0.00	32.00	0.35	16.00	52.80	251.20	4.80	0.30
0.04	0.05	0.00	2.43	0.43	37.80	95.76	0.16	0.07	0.50	0.11	54.54	0.00	72.00	0.18	18.00	25.20	325.80	0.00	0.13
0.06	0.04	0.00	0.00	1.57	39.20	86.52	0.04	0.04	0.48	0.03	53.20	0.00	33.60	0.14	14.00	7.00	359.80	4.20	0.10
0.09	0.04	0.00	0.00	0.00	0.00	10.14	0.06	0.04	0.56	0.07	45.40	0.00	28.86	0.45	22.62	53.82	286.26	191.88	0.20
0.09	0.04	0.00	0.00	0.78	0.00	10.14	0.06	0.04	0.56	0.07	45.40	0.00	28.86	0.45	22.62	53.82	286.26	7.80	0.20
0.15	0.07	0.00	0.00	0.00	0.00	22.61	0.12	0.07	0.93	0.12	88.84	0.00	47.88	0.78	38.57	94.43	498.75	13.30	0.78
0.10	0.13	0.00	0.00	2.33	86.46	7.34	0.03	0.05	1.60	0.05	8.38	0.00	7.86	0.71	13.10	28.82	241.04	15.72	0.24
0.03	0.05	0.00	7.50	3.75	95.00	9.00	0.03	0.05	1.45	0.05	8.50	0.00	15.00	0.68	17.50	42.50	320.00	10.00	0.28
0.03	0.05	0.00	0.00	2.23	87.85	6.02	0.03	0.08	1.48	0.05	8.28	0.00	7.53	0.90	12.55	27.61	243.47	12.55	0.23
0.05	0.07	0.00	0.00	2.17	129.32	7.08	0.02	0.05	1.27	0.05	8.30	0.00	4.88	0.78	12.20	24.40	241.56	7.32	0.22
0.03	0.03	0.00	0.00	0.00	34.06	3.14	0.03	0.05	1.36	0.05	8.12	0.00	7.86	0.76	13.10	28.82	217.46	20.96	0.24
0.10	0.12	0.00	0.00	0.00	66.69	7.41	0.05	0.05	1.98	0.05	8.15	0.00	12.35	0.74	12.35	27.17	182.78	12.35	0.22
0.44	0.58	0.00	0.00	0.00	164.72	12.30	0.05	0.13	5.60	0.19	7.66	0.00	44.08	6.39	66.12	187.92	1567.16	11.60	0.90
0.45	0.59	0.00	0.00	0.00	345.60	7.68	0.00	0.34	7.01	0.11	0.48	0.00	44.80	6.50	67.20	190.40	1593.60	11.20	0.91
0.05	0.09	0.00	0.00	1.19	91.80	11.22	0.03	0.07	1.68	0.03	5.78	0.00	8.50	0.19	11.90	20.40	334.90	0.00	0.24
0.13	0.15	0.00	0.00	2.23	70.00	235.50	0.03	0.10	1.63	0.05	8.00	0.00	7.50	0.93	12.50	27.50	325.00	15.00	0.13
0.06	0.07	0.00	0.00	0.61	0.00	4.64	0.01	0.01	0.27	0.02	9.76	0.00	4.88	0.00	9.76	13.42	147.62	0.00	0.02

USDA ID Code / Food Name	Weight in Grams*	Quantity of Units	Unit of Measure	Protein (g)	Fat (g)	Carbohydrate (g)	Kilocalories	Caffeine (g)	Fiber (g)	Cholesterol (mg)	Saturated Fat (g)
Pears, Cnd, Heavy Syrup Pack	266.0000	1.000	Cup	0.53	0.35	50.99	196.84	0.00	4.26	0.00	0.03
Pears, Cnd, Juice Pack	248.0000	1.000	Cup	0.84	0.17	32.09	124.00	0.00	3.97	0.00	0.00
Pears, Cnd, Light Syrup Pack	251.0000	1.000	Cup	0.48	0.08	38.08	143.07	0.00	4.02	0.00	0.00
Pears, Cnd, Water Pack	244.0000	1.000	Cup	0.46	0.07	19.06	70.76	0.00	3.90	0.00	0.00
Pears, Cnd, X-heavy Syrup Pack	266.0000	1.000	Cup	0.51	0.35	67.17	258.02	0.00	4.26	0.00	0.03
Pears, Cnd, X-light Syrup Pack	247.0000	1.000	Cup	0.74	0.25	30.13	116.09	0.00	3.95	0.00	0.02
Pears, Fresh	165.0000	1.000	Cup	0.64	0.66	24.93	97.35	0.00	3.96	0.00	0.03
Peas and Carrots, Cnd	255.0000	1.000	Cup	5.53	0.69	21.62	96.90	0.00	5.10	0.00	0.13
Peas and Carrots, Frz, Ckd	278.0000	1.250	Cup	8.59	1.17	28.13	133.44	0.00	8.62	0.00	0.22
Peas and Onions, Cnd	120.0000	1.000	Cup	3.94	0.46	10.28	61.20	0.00	2.76	0.00	0.08
Peas and Onions, Frz, Ckd	180.0000	1.000	Cup	4.57	0.36	15.53	81.00	0.00	3.96	0.00	0.07
Peas, Edible-podded, Fresh	98.0000	1.000	Cup	2.74	0.20	7.41	41.16	0.00	2.55	0.00	0.04
Peas, Green, Ckd	160.0000	1.000	Cup	8.58	0.35	25.02	134.40	0.00	8.80	0.00	0.06
Peas, Green, Cnd	170.0000	1.000	Cup	7.51	0.60	21.39	117.30	0.00	6.97	0.00	0.10
Peas, Green, Cnd, Seasoned	227.0000	1.000	Cup	7.01	0.61	21.00	113.50	0.00	4.54	0.00	0.11
Peas, Green, Fresh	145.0000	1.000	Cup	7.86	0.58	20.97	117.45	0.00	7.40	0.00	0.10
Peas, Green, Frz, Ckd	253.0000	1.250	Cup	13.03	0.68	36.08	197.34	0.00	13.92	0.00	0.13
Peppers, Hot Chili, Green, Cnd	73.0000	1.000	Each	0.66	0.07	3.72	15.33	0.00	0.95	0.00	0.01
Peppers, Hot Chili, Green, Fresh	45.0000	1.000	Each	0.90	0.09	4.26	18.00	0.00	0.68	0.00	0.01
Peppers, Hot Chili, Red, Cnd	73.0000	1.000	Each	0.66	0.07	3.72	15.33	0.00	0.95	0.00	0.01
Peppers, Hot Chili, Red, Fresh	45.0000	1.000	Each	0.90	0.09	4.26	18.00	0.00	0.68	0.00	0.01
Peppers, Jalapeno, Cnd	136.0000	1.000	Cup	1.25	1.28	6.42	36.72	0.00	3.54	0.00	0.14
Peppers, Sweet, Green, Fresh	149.0000	1.000	Cup	1.33	0.28	9.58	40.23	0.00	2.68	0.00	0.04
Peppers, Sweet, Red, Fresh	149.0000	1.000	Cup	1.33	0.28	9.58	40.23	0.00	2.98	0.00	0.04
Peppers, Sweet, Yellow, Fresh	186.0000	1.000	Large	1.86	0.39	11.76	50.22	0.00	1.67	0.00	0.06
Persimmon, Japanese, Raw	168.0000	1.000	Medium	0.97	0.32	31.23	117.60	0.00	6.05	0.00	0.03
Pickle, Cucumber, Sour	155.0000	1.000	Cup	0.51	0.31	3.49	17.05	0.00	1.86	0.00	0.08
Pickle, Cucumber, Dill	143.0000	1.000	Cup	0.89	0.27	5.91	25.74	0.00	1.72	0.00	0.07
Pickle, Cucumber, Dill, Low Sodium	65.0000	1.000	Slice	0.40	0.12	2.68	11.70	0.00	0.78	0.00	0.03
Pickle, Cucumber, Sour, Low Sodium	143.0000	1.000	Cup	0.47	0.29	3.22	15.73	0.00	1.72	0.00	0.07
Pickle, Cucumber, Sweet	160.0000	1.000	Cup	0.59	0.42	50.90	187.20	0.00	1.76	0.00	0.11
Pickle, Cucumber, Sweet, Low Sodium	160.0000	1.000	Cup	0.59	0.42	50.90	187.20	0.00	1.76	0.00	0.11
Pineapple, Cnd, Heavy Syrup Pack	254.0000	1.000	Cup	0.89	0.28	51.31	198.12	0.00	2.03	0.00	0.03
Pineapple, Cnd, Juice Pack	249.0000	1.000	Cup	1.05	0.20	39.09	149.40	0.00	1.99	0.00	0.02
Pineapple, Cnd, Light Syrup Pack	252.0000	1.000	Cup	0.91	0.30	33.89	131.04	0.00	2.02	0.00	0.03
Pineapple, Cnd, Water Pack	246.0000	1.000	Cup	1.06	0.22	20.42	78.72	0.00	1.97	0.00	0.02
Pineapple, Cnd, X-heavy Syrup Pack	260.0000	1.000	Cup	0.88	0.29	55.90	215.80	0.00	2.08	0.00	0.03
Pineapple, Fresh	155.0000	1.000	Cup	0.60	0.67	19.20	75.95	0.00	1.86	0.00	0.05
Plantain, Raw	179.0000	1.000	Medium	2.33	0.66	57.08	218.38	0.00	4.12	0.00	0.26
Plums, Cnd, Purple, Heavy Syrup	258.0000	1.000	Cup	0.93	0.26	59.96	229.62	0.00	2.58	0.00	0.03
Plums, Cnd, Purple, Juice Pack	252.0000	1.000	Cup	1.29	0.05	38.18	146.16	0.00	2.52	0.00	0.00
Plums, Cnd, Purple, Light Syrup	252.0000	1.000	Cup	0.93	0.25	41.03	158.76	0.00	2.52	0.00	0.03
Plums, Cnd, Purple, Water Pack	249.0000	1.000	Cup	0.97	0.02	27.46	102.09	0.00	2.49	0.00	0.00
Plums, Cnd, Purple, X-heavy Syrup	261.0000	1.000	Cup	0.94	0.26	68.67	263.61	0.00	2.61	0.00	0.03
Plums, Fresh	165.0000	0.500	Cup	1.30	1.02	21.47	90.75	0.00	2.48	0.00	0.08
Potato Pancakes, Home-prepared	76.0000	1.000	Each	4.68	11.58	21.77	206.72	0.00	1.52	72.96	2.31
Potato Puffs, Frz, Prepared	128.0000	1.000	Cup	4.29	13.73	39.01	284.16	0.00	4.10	0.00	6.53
Potato Salad	250.0000	1.000	Cup	6.70	20.50	27.93	357.50	0.00	3.25	170.00	3.58
Potatoes, Au Gratin, Home-prepar	245.0000	1.000	Cup	12.40	18.60	27.61	323.40	0.00	4.41	36.75	8.65
Potatoes, Baked w/o Skin	61.0000	0.500	Cup	1.20	0.06	13.15	56.73	0.00	0.92	0.00	0.02
Potatoes, Baked, Skin only	58.0000	1.000	Each	2.49	0.06	26.72	114.84	0.00	4.58	0.00	0.02
Potatoes, Baked, w/ Skin	202.0000	1.000	Medium	4.65	0.20	50.96	220.18	0.00	4.85	0.00	0.06
Potatoes, Boiled, Ckd In Skin w/	78.0000	0.500	Cup	1.46	0.08	15.70	67.86	0.00	1.40	0.00	0.02

Monounsaturated Fat (g)	Polyunsaturated Fat (g)	Vitamin D (mg)	Vitamin K (mg)	Vitamin E (mg)	Vitamin A (re)	Vitamin C (mg)	Thiamin (mg)	Riboflavin (mg)	Niacin (mg)	Vitamin B_6 (mg)	Folate (mcg)	Vitamin B_{12} (mcg)	Calcium (mg)	Iron (mg)	Magnesium (mg)	Phosphorus (mg)	Potassium (mg)	Sodium (mg)	Zinc (mg)
0.08	0.08	0.00	0.00	1.33	0.00	2.93	0.03	0.05	0.64	0.03	3.19	0.00	13.30	0.59	10.64	18.62	172.90	13.30	0.21
0.02	0.05	0.00	1.14	1.24	2.48	3.97	0.02	0.02	0.50	0.02	2.98	0.00	22.32	0.72	17.36	29.76	238.08	9.92	0.22
0.03	0.03	0.00	0.00	1.26	0.00	1.76	0.03	0.05	0.38	0.03	3.01	0.00	12.55	0.70	10.04	17.57	165.66	12.55	0.20
0.02	0.02	0.00	0.00	1.22	0.00	2.44	0.02	0.02	0.12	0.02	2.93	0.00	9.76	0.51	9.76	17.08	129.32	4.88	0.22
0.08	0.08	0.00	0.00	0.00	0.00	2.93	0.03	0.05	0.64	0.03	3.19	0.00	13.30	0.59	10.64	18.62	170.24	13.30	0.21
0.05	0.05	0.00	0.00	0.00	0.00	4.94	0.02	0.05	0.99	0.02	2.96	0.00	17.29	0.49	12.35	17.29	111.15	4.94	0.17
0.13	0.15	0.00	0.00	0.83	3.30	6.60	0.03	0.07	0.17	0.03	12.05	0.00	18.15	0.41	9.90	18.15	206.25	0.00	0.20
0.05	0.33	0.00	0.00	0.00	1471.35	16.83	0.18	0.13	1.48	0.23	46.67	0.00	58.65	1.91	35.70	117.30	255.00	663.00	1.48
0.11	0.56	0.00	0.00	0.89	2157.28	22.52	0.64	0.17	3.20	0.25	72.28	0.00	63.94	2.61	44.48	136.22	439.24	189.04	1.25
0.05	0.22	0.00	0.00	0.00	19.20	3.60	0.12	0.08	1.54	0.23	31.92	0.00	20.40	1.04	19.20	61.20	115.20	530.40	0.70
0.04	0.16	0.00	0.00	0.27	63.00	12.42	0.27	0.13	1.87	0.16	35.82	0.00	25.20	1.69	23.40	61.20	210.60	66.60	0.52
0.02	0.09	0.00	0.00	0.38	13.72	58.80	0.15	0.08	0.59	0.16	40.87	0.00	42.14	2.04	23.52	51.94	196.00	3.92	0.26
0.03	0.16	0.00	0.00	0.62	96.00	22.72	0.42	0.24	3.23	0.35	101.28	0.00	43.20	2.46	62.40	187.20	433.60	4.80	1.90
0.05	0.27	0.00	0.00	0.65	130.90	16.32	0.20	0.14	1.24	0.10	75.31	0.00	34.00	1.62	28.90	113.90	294.10	428.40	1.21
0.05	0.30	0.00	0.00	0.00	97.61	26.11	0.23	0.16	1.57	0.23	64.92	0.00	34.05	2.72	34.05	122.58	276.94	576.58	1.48
0.06	0.28	0.00	0.00	0.57	92.80	58.00	0.39	0.19	3.03	0.25	94.25	0.00	36.25	2.13	47.85	156.60	353.80	7.25	1.80
0.05	0.33	0.00	0.00	0.43	169.51	25.05	0.71	0.25	3.74	0.28	148.26	0.00	60.72	3.97	73.37	227.70	425.04	220.11	2.38
0.01	0.04	0.00	0.00	0.50	44.53	49.64	0.01	0.04	0.58	0.11	7.30	0.00	5.11	0.37	10.22	12.41	136.51	856.29	0.12
0.00	0.05	0.00	0.00	0.31	34.65	109.13	0.04	0.04	0.43	0.13	10.53	0.00	8.10	0.54	11.25	20.70	153.00	3.15	0.14
0.01	0.04	0.00	0.00	0.50	867.97	49.64	0.01	0.04	0.58	0.11	7.30	0.00	5.11	0.37	10.22	12.41	136.51	856.29	0.12
0.00	0.05	0.00	0.00	0.31	483.75	109.13	0.04	0.04	0.43	0.13	10.53	0.00	8.10	0.54	11.25	20.70	153.00	3.15	0.14
0.07	0.69	0.00	0.00	0.94	231.20	13.60	0.05	0.05	0.54	0.26	19.04	0.00	31.28	2.56	20.40	24.48	262.48	2272.56	0.46
0.01	0.15	0.00	0.00	1.03	93.87	133.06	0.10	0.04	0.76	0.37	32.78	0.00	13.41	0.69	14.90	28.31	263.73	2.98	0.18
0.01	0.15	0.00	0.00	1.03	849.30	283.10	0.10	0.04	0.76	0.37	32.78	0.00	13.41	0.69	14.90	28.31	263.73	2.98	0.18
0.00	0.00	0.00	0.00	0.00	44.64	341.31	0.06	0.06	1.66	0.32	48.36	0.00	20.46	0.86	22.32	44.64	394.32	3.72	0.32
0.06	0.07	0.00	0.00	0.99	364.56	12.60	0.05	0.03	0.17	0.17	12.60	0.00	13.44	0.25	15.12	28.56	270.48	1.68	0.19
0.00	0.12	0.00	0.00	0.25	23.25	1.55	0.00	0.02	0.00	0.02	1.10	0.00	0.00	0.62	6.20	21.70	35.65	1872.40	0.03
0.00	0.11	0.00	0.00	0.23	47.19	2.72	0.01	0.04	0.09	0.01	1.43	0.00	12.87	0.76	15.73	30.03	165.88	1833.26	0.20
0.00	0.05	0.00	0.00	0.00	21.45	1.24	0.01	0.02	0.04	0.01	0.65	0.00	5.85	0.34	7.15	13.65	75.40	11.70	0.09
0.00	0.11	0.00	0.00	0.07	21.45	1.43	0.00	0.01	0.00	0.01	1.02	0.00	0.00	0.57	5.72	20.02	32.89	25.74	0.03
0.00	0.18	0.00	0.00	0.26	20.80	1.92	0.02	0.05	0.27	0.03	1.60	0.00	6.40	0.94	6.40	19.20	51.20	1502.40	0.13
0.00	0.18	0.00	0.00	0.26	20.80	1.92	0.02	0.05	0.27	0.03	1.60	0.00	6.40	0.94	6.40	19.20	51.20	28.80	0.13
0.03	0.10	0.00	0.00	0.25	2.54	18.80	0.23	0.08	0.74	0.18	11.68	0.00	35.56	0.97	40.64	17.78	264.16	2.54	0.30
0.02	0.07	0.00	0.00	0.25	9.96	23.66	0.25	0.05	0.70	0.17	11.95	0.00	34.86	0.70	34.86	14.94	303.78	2.49	0.25
0.03	0.10	0.00	0.00	0.25	2.52	18.90	0.23	0.08	0.73	0.18	11.84	0.00	35.28	0.98	40.32	17.64	264.60	2.52	0.30
0.02	0.07	0.00	0.00	0.25	4.92	18.94	0.22	0.07	0.74	0.17	11.81	0.00	36.90	0.98	44.28	9.84	312.42	2.46	0.30
0.03	0.10	0.00	0.00	0.00	2.60	18.98	0.23	0.08	0.73	0.18	11.96	0.00	36.40	0.99	39.00	18.20	265.20	2.60	0.29
0.08	0.23	0.00	0.00	0.16	3.10	23.87	0.14	0.06	0.65	0.14	16.43	0.00	10.85	0.57	21.70	10.85	175.15	1.55	0.12
0.06	0.12	0.00	0.00	0.48	202.27	32.94	0.09	0.10	1.23	0.54	39.38	0.00	5.37	1.07	66.23	60.86	893.21	7.16	0.25
0.18	0.05	0.00	0.00	1.81	67.08	1.03	0.05	0.10	0.75	0.08	6.45	0.00	23.22	2.17	12.90	33.54	234.78	49.02	0.18
0.03	0.03	0.00	0.00	1.76	254.52	7.06	0.05	0.15	1.18	0.08	6.55	0.00	25.20	0.86	20.16	37.80	388.08	2.52	0.28
0.18	0.05	0.00	0.00	1.76	65.52	1.01	0.05	0.10	0.76	0.08	6.55	0.00	22.68	2.17	12.60	32.76	234.36	50.40	0.20
0.02	0.00	0.00	0.00	1.74	226.59	6.72	0.05	0.10	0.92	0.07	6.47	0.00	17.43	0.40	12.45	32.37	313.74	2.49	0.20
0.18	0.05	0.00	0.00	0.00	65.25	1.04	0.05	0.10	0.76	0.08	6.53	0.00	23.49	2.14	13.05	31.32	232.29	49.59	0.18
0.68	0.21	0.00	0.00	0.99	52.80	15.68	0.07	0.17	0.83	0.13	3.63	0.00	6.60	0.17	11.55	16.50	283.80	0.00	0.17
3.53	4.97	0.00	0.00	0.00	10.64	16.72	0.11	0.13	1.63	0.29	17.48	0.14	18.24	1.19	25.08	84.36	597.36	386.08	0.63
5.58	1.02	0.00	0.00	0.06	2.56	8.83	0.26	0.09	2.76	0.29	21.12	0.00	38.40	2.00	24.32	61.44	486.40	954.88	0.38
6.20	9.35	0.00	0.00	0.00	82.50	25.00	0.20	0.15	2.23	0.35	16.75	0.00	47.50	1.63	37.50	130.00	635.00	1322.50	0.78
6.35	2.65	0.00	0.00	0.00	93.10	24.26	0.15	0.29	2.43	0.42	26.95	0.00	291.55	1.57	49.00	276.85	970.20	1060.85	1.69
0.00	0.02	0.00	0.13	0.02	0.00	7.81	0.07	0.01	0.85	0.18	5.55	0.00	3.05	0.21	15.25	30.50	238.51	3.05	0.18
0.00	0.02	0.00	0.00	0.02	0.00	7.83	0.07	0.06	1.78	0.35	12.53	0.00	19.72	4.08	24.94	58.58	332.34	12.18	0.28
0.00	0.08	0.00	1.07	0.10	0.00	26.06	0.22	0.06	3.33	0.71	22.22	0.00	20.20	2.75	54.54	115.14	844.36	16.16	0.65
0.00	0.03	0.00	0.00	0.04	0.00	10.14	0.09	0.02	1.12	0.23	7.80	0.00	3.90	0.24	17.16	34.32	295.62	3.12	0.23

USDA ID Code	Food Name	Weight in Grams*	Quantity of Units	Unit of Measure	Protein (g)	Fat (g)	Carbohydrate (g)	Kilocalories	Caffeine (g)	Fiber (g)	Cholesterol (mg)	Saturated Fat (g)
	Potatoes, Boiled, Ckd w/o Skin	78.0000	0.500	Cup	1.33	0.08	15.61	67.08	0.00	1.40	0.00	0.02
	Potatoes, Boiled, Skin only	34.0000	1.000	Each	0.97	0.03	5.85	26.52	0.00	1.12	0.00	0.01
	Potatoes, Cnd, Drained Solids	180.0000	1.000	Cup	2.54	0.38	24.50	108.00	0.00	4.14	0.00	0.09
	Potatoes, Cnd, Solids and Liquid	300.0000	1.000	Cup	3.60	0.33	29.67	132.00	0.00	4.20	0.00	0.09
	Potatoes, Hashed Brown	156.0000	1.000	Cup	3.78	21.70	33.26	326.04	0.00	3.12	0.00	8.47
	Potatoes, Mashed, Home-prepared	210.0000	1.000	Cup	4.07	1.24	36.86	161.70	0.00	4.20	4.20	0.69
	Potatoes, Mashed, Prepared From	210.0000	1.000	Cup	3.99	11.76	31.54	237.30	0.00	4.83	8.40	3.07
	Potatoes, Microwaved w/o Skin	78.0000	0.500	Cup	1.64	0.08	18.16	78.00	0.00	1.25	0.00	0.02
	Potatoes, Microwaved, Skin only	58.0000	1.000	Each	2.55	0.06	17.19	76.56	0.00	3.19	0.00	0.02
	Potatoes, Microwaved, w/ Skin	202.0000	1.000	Medium	4.93	0.20	48.74	212.10	0.00	4.65	0.00	0.06
	Potatoes, O'brien, Home-prepared	194.0000	1.000	Cup	4.56	2.48	30.01	157.14	0.00	0.00	7.76	1.55
	Potatoes, Scalloped	245.0000	1.000	Cup	7.03	9.02	26.41	210.70	0.00	4.66	14.70	3.38
	Prunes, Dehydrated	132.0000	1.000	Cup	4.88	0.96	117.57	447.48	0.00	0.00	0.00	0.08
	Prunes, Dried, Stewed, w/ Added	248.0000	1.000	Cup	2.70	0.55	81.54	307.52	0.00	9.42	0.00	0.05
	Prunes, Dried, Stewed, w/o Added	248.0000	1.000	Cup	2.90	0.57	69.64	265.36	0.00	16.37	0.00	0.05
	Prunes, Dried, Uncooked	170.0000	1.000	Cup	4.44	0.88	106.64	406.30	0.00	12.07	0.00	0.07
	Pumpkin, Ckd	245.0000	1.000	Cup	1.76	0.17	11.98	49.00	0.00	2.70	0.00	0.10
	Pumpkin, Cnd, w/o Salt	245.0000	1.000	Cup	2.70	0.69	19.80	83.30	0.00	7.11	0.00	0.37
	Radishes, Fresh	116.0000	1.000	Cup	0.70	0.63	4.16	23.20	0.00	1.86	0.00	0.03
	Radishes, Oriental, Ckd	147.0000	0.500	Cup	0.98	0.35	5.04	24.99	0.00	2.35	0.00	0.10
	Radishes, Oriental, Dried	116.0000	1.000	Cup	9.16	0.84	73.51	314.36	0.00	0.00	0.00	0.26
	Radishes, Oriental, Fresh	338.0000	1.000	Each	2.03	0.34	13.89	60.84	0.00	5.41	0.00	0.10
	Radishes, White Icicle, Fresh	50.0000	0.500	Cup	0.55	0.05	1.32	7.00	0.00	0.70	0.00	0.02
	Raisins, Golden Seedless	165.0000	1.000	Cup	5.59	0.76	131.21	498.30	0.00	6.60	0.00	0.25
	Raisins, Seeded	165.0000	1.000	Cup	4.16	0.89	129.48	488.40	0.00	11.22	0.00	0.30
	Raisins, Seedless	165.0000	1.000	Cup	5.31	0.76	130.56	495.00	0.00	6.60	0.00	0.25
	Raspberries, Cnd, Red, Heavy Syrup	256.0000	1.000	Cup	2.12	0.31	59.80	232.96	0.00	8.45	0.00	0.03
	Raspberries, Fresh	123.0000	1.000	Cup	1.12	0.68	14.23	60.27	0.00	8.36	0.00	0.02
	Raspberries, Frozen, Red, Sweete	250.0000	1.000	Cup	1.75	0.40	65.40	257.50	0.00	11.00	0.00	0.03
	Sauerkraut, Cnd, Solid & Liquid	142.0000	1.000	Cup	1.29	0.20	6.08	26.98	0.00	3.55	0.00	0.06
	Shallots, Freeze-dried	0.9000	1.000	Tbsp	0.11	0.00	0.73	3.13	0.00	0.00	0.00	0.00
	Shallots, Fresh	10.0000	1.000	Tbsp	0.25	0.01	1.68	7.20	0.00	0.00	0.00	0.00
	Spinach, Ckd	180.0000	1.000	Cup	5.35	0.47	6.75	41.40	0.00	4.32	0.00	0.07
	Spinach, Cnd, Drained Solids	214.0000	1.000	Cup	6.01	1.07	7.28	49.22	0.00	5.14	0.00	0.17
	Spinach, Cnd, Reg Pk, Solid & Li	234.0000	1.000	Cup	4.94	0.87	6.83	44.46	0.00	3.74	0.00	0.14
	Spinach, Fresh	30.0000	1.000	Cup	0.86	0.11	1.05	6.60	0.00	0.81	0.00	0.02
	Spinach, Frz, Ckd	220.0000	1.250	Cup	6.91	0.46	11.75	61.60	0.00	6.60	0.00	0.07
	Spinach, Frz, Unprepared	156.0000	1.000	Cup	4.56	0.48	6.24	37.44	0.00	4.68	0.00	0.08
	Squash, Acorn, Ckd, w/o Salt	205.0000	1.000	Cup	2.30	0.29	29.89	114.80	0.00	9.02	0.00	0.06
	Squash, Butternut, Ckd, w/o Salt	205.0000	1.000	Cup	1.85	0.18	21.50	82.00	0.00	0.00	0.00	0.04
	Squash, Spaghetti, Ckd. w/o Salt	155.0000	1.000	Cup	1.02	0.40	10.01	41.85	0.00	2.17	0.00	0.09
	Squash, Summer, Ckd	180.0000	0.500	Cup	1.64	0.56	7.76	36.00	0.00	2.52	0.00	0.11
	Squash, Summer, Fresh	113.0000	0.500	Cup	1.33	0.24	4.92	22.60	0.00	2.15	0.00	0.05
	Squash, Winter, Baked	205.0000	1.000	Cup	1.82	1.29	17.94	79.95	0.00	5.74	0.00	0.27
	Squash, Winter, Fresh	116.0000	1.000	Cup	1.68	0.27	10.21	42.92	0.00	1.74	0.00	0.06
	Squash, Zucchini, Baby, Fresh	16.0000	1.000	Large	0.43	0.06	0.50	3.36	0.00	0.18	0.00	0.01
	Strawberries, Fresh	152.0000	1.000	Cup	0.93	0.56	10.67	45.60	0.00	3.50	0.00	0.03
	Strawberries, Frozen, Sweetened	255.0000	1.000	Cup	1.35	0.33	66.10	244.80	0.00	4.85	0.00	0.03
	Strawberries, Frozen, Unsweetened	221.0000	1.000	Cup	0.95	0.24	20.18	77.35	0.00	4.64	0.00	0.02
	Sweet Potatoes, Baked In Skin	200.0000	1.000	Cup	3.44	0.22	48.54	206.00	0.00	6.00	0.00	0.04
	Sweet Potatoes, Boiled, w/o Skin	328.0000	1.000	Cup	5.41	0.98	79.64	344.40	0.00	5.90	0.00	0.20
	Sweet Potatoes, Candied	105.0000	1.000	Piece	0.91	3.41	29.25	143.85	0.00	2.52	8.40	1.42
	Sweet Potatoes, Mashed	255.0000	1.000	Cup	5.05	0.51	59.16	257.55	0.00	4.34	0.00	0.10

Page Key: A2 = Baby Food   A2 = Baked Goods   A8 = Beverages   A14 = Breads/Grains and Pasta   A18 = Breakfast Foods/Cereals   A26 = Dairy and Eggs   A40 = Fats and Oils
A42 = Fruits and Vegetables   A52 = Meats and Beans   A60 = Nuts and Seeds   A62 5 Frozen Entrees and Packaged Foods   A76 = Restaurant Chains–Fast Foods
A92 = Restaurant Chains–Other   A106 = Seafood and Fish   A110 = Snacks and Sweets   A120 = Soups   A122 = Supplements   A126 = Toppings and Sauces

Monounsaturated Fat (g)	Polyunsaturated Fat (g)	Vitamin D (mg)	Vitamin K (mg)	Vitamin E (mg)	Vitamin A (re)	Vitamin C (mg)	Thiamin (mg)	Riboflavin (mg)	Niacin (mg)	Vitamin B₆ (mg)	Folate (mcg)	Vitamin B₁₂ (mcg)	Calcium (mg)	Iron (mg)	Magnesium (mg)	Phosphorus (mg)	Potassium (mg)	Sodium (mg)	Zinc (mg)
0.00	0.03	0.00	0.00	0.04	0.00	5.77	0.08	0.02	1.02	0.21	6.94	0.00	6.24	0.24	15.60	31.20	255.84	3.90	0.21
0.00	0.01	0.00	0.00	0.00	0.00	1.77	0.01	0.01	0.41	0.08	3.30	0.00	15.30	2.06	10.20	18.36	138.38	4.76	0.15
0.02	0.16	0.00	0.00	0.09	0.00	9.18	0.13	0.02	1.66	0.34	11.16	0.00	9.00	2.27	25.20	50.40	412.20	394.20	0.50
0.00	0.15	0.00	0.00	0.12	0.00	22.80	0.09	0.06	2.67	0.42	13.50	0.00	117.00	2.16	42.00	66.00	615.00	651.00	1.17
9.69	2.50	0.00	0.00	0.30	0.00	8.89	0.11	0.03	3.12	0.44	12.01	0.00	12.48	1.26	31.20	65.52	500.76	37.44	0.47
0.32	0.13	0.00	0.00	0.11	12.60	14.07	0.19	0.08	2.35	0.48	17.22	0.00	54.60	0.57	37.80	100.80	627.90	636.30	0.61
4.85	3.26	0.00	0.00	0.00	44.10	20.37	0.23	0.11	1.41	0.02	15.54	0.00	102.90	0.46	37.80	117.60	489.30	697.20	0.38
0.00	0.03	0.00	0.00	0.00	0.00	11.78	0.10	0.02	1.27	0.25	9.67	0.00	3.90	0.32	19.50	85.02	320.58	5.46	0.26
0.00	0.02	0.00	0.00	0.00	0.00	8.87	0.04	0.05	1.29	0.28	9.63	0.00	26.68	3.45	21.46	47.56	377.00	9.28	0.30
0.00	0.08	0.00	0.00	0.00	0.00	30.50	0.24	0.06	3.45	0.69	24.24	0.00	22.22	2.50	54.54	212.10	902.94	16.16	0.73
0.68	0.12	0.00	0.00	0.00	110.58	32.40	0.16	0.12	1.96	0.41	16.10	0.00	69.84	0.91	34.92	97.00	516.04	420.98	0.58
3.31	1.84	0.00	0.00	0.00	46.55	25.97	0.17	0.22	2.57	0.44	26.95	0.00	139.65	1.40	46.55	154.35	926.10	820.75	0.98
0.63	0.21	0.00	0.00	0.00	232.32	0.00	0.16	0.22	3.96	0.99	2.51	0.00	95.04	4.65	84.48	147.84	1396.56	6.60	0.99
0.35	0.12	0.00	0.00	0.00	71.92	6.70	0.05	0.22	1.69	0.50	0.25	0.00	52.08	2.58	47.12	81.84	773.76	4.96	0.55
0.37	0.12	0.00	0.00	0.00	76.88	7.19	0.05	0.25	1.79	0.55	0.25	0.00	57.04	2.75	49.60	86.80	828.32	4.96	0.60
0.58	0.19	0.00	0.00	2.47	338.30	5.61	0.14	0.27	3.33	0.44	6.29	0.00	86.70	4.22	76.50	134.30	1266.50	6.80	0.90
0.02	0.00	0.00	0.00	2.60	264.60	11.52	0.07	0.20	1.00	0.10	20.83	0.00	36.75	1.40	22.05	73.50	563.50	2.45	0.56
0.10	0.05	0.00	36.75	2.60	5404.70	10.29	0.05	0.12	0.91	0.15	30.14	0.00	63.70	3.41	56.35	85.75	504.70	12.25	0.42
0.02	0.06	0.00	0.00	0.00	1.16	26.45	0.01	0.06	0.35	0.08	31.32	0.00	24.36	0.34	10.44	20.88	269.12	27.84	0.35
0.06	0.16	0.00	0.00	0.00	0.00	22.20	0.00	0.03	0.22	0.06	25.58	0.00	24.99	0.22	13.23	35.28	418.95	19.11	0.19
0.14	0.38	0.00	0.00	0.00	0.00	0.00	0.31	0.79	3.94	0.72	341.85	0.00	729.64	7.81	197.20	236.64	4053.04	322.48	2.47
0.07	0.17	0.00	0.00	0.00	0.00	74.36	0.07	0.07	0.68	0.17	95.32	0.00	91.26	1.35	54.08	77.74	767.26	70.98	0.51
0.01	0.03	0.00	0.00	0.00	0.00	14.50	0.02	0.01	0.15	0.04	7.00	0.00	13.50	0.40	4.50	14.00	140.00	8.00	0.07
0.03	0.23	0.00	0.00	1.16	6.60	5.28	0.02	0.31	1.88	0.53	5.45	0.00	87.45	2.95	57.75	189.75	1230.90	19.80	0.53
0.03	0.26	0.00	0.00	1.16	0.00	8.91	0.18	0.30	1.83	0.31	5.45	0.00	46.20	4.27	49.50	123.75	1361.25	46.20	0.30
0.03	0.23	0.00	0.00	1.16	1.65	5.45	0.26	0.15	1.35	0.41	5.45	0.00	80.85	3.43	54.45	160.05	1239.15	19.80	0.45
0.03	0.18	0.00	0.00	1.15	7.68	22.27	0.05	0.08	1.13	0.10	26.88	0.00	28.16	1.08	30.72	23.04	240.64	7.68	0.41
0.06	0.38	0.00	0.00	0.55	15.99	30.75	0.04	0.11	1.11	0.07	31.98	0.00	27.06	0.70	22.14	14.76	186.96	0.00	0.57
0.05	0.23	0.00	0.00	1.13	15.00	41.25	0.05	0.13	0.58	0.08	65.00	0.00	37.50	1.63	32.50	42.50	285.00	2.50	0.45
0.01	0.09	0.00	0.00	0.14	2.84	20.87	0.03	0.03	0.20	0.18	33.65	0.00	42.60	2.09	18.46	28.40	241.40	938.62	0.27
0.00	0.00	0.00	0.00	0.00	50.49	0.35	0.00	0.00	0.01	0.02	1.05	0.00	1.65	0.05	0.94	2.66	14.85	0.53	0.02
0.00	0.00	0.00	0.00	0.00	11.90	0.80	0.01	0.00	0.02	0.04	3.42	0.00	3.70	0.12	2.10	6.00	33.40	1.20	0.04
0.02	0.20	0.00	0.00	1.73	1474.20	17.64	0.18	0.43	0.88	0.43	262.44	0.00	244.80	6.43	156.60	100.80	838.80	126.00	1.37
0.02	0.45	0.00	0.00	2.78	1878.92	30.60	0.04	0.30	0.83	0.21	209.29	0.00	271.78	4.92	162.64	94.16	740.44	57.78	0.98
0.02	0.37	0.00	0.00	2.50	1504.62	31.59	0.05	0.26	0.63	0.19	135.72	0.00	194.22	3.70	131.04	74.88	538.20	746.46	0.98
0.00	0.05	0.00	79.80	0.57	201.60	8.43	0.02	0.06	0.22	0.06	58.32	0.00	29.70	0.81	23.70	14.70	167.40	23.70	0.16
0.02	0.20	0.00	0.00	2.11	1711.60	27.06	0.13	0.37	0.92	0.33	236.50	0.00	321.20	3.34	151.80	105.60	655.60	189.20	1.54
0.02	0.20	0.00	215.28	1.50	1210.56	37.91	0.12	0.23	0.69	0.22	186.58	0.00	173.16	3.20	90.48	63.96	503.88	115.44	0.69
0.02	0.12	0.00	0.00	0.00	88.15	22.14	0.35	0.02	1.80	0.39	38.34	0.00	90.20	1.91	88.15	92.25	895.85	8.20	0.35
0.02	0.08	0.00	0.00	0.00	1435.00	30.96	0.14	0.04	1.99	0.25	39.36	0.00	84.05	1.23	59.45	55.35	582.20	8.20	0.27
0.03	0.20	0.00	0.00	0.19	17.05	5.43	0.06	0.03	1.26	0.16	12.40	0.00	32.55	0.53	17.05	21.70	181.35	27.90	0.31
0.04	0.23	0.00	0.00	0.22	52.20	9.90	0.07	0.07	0.92	0.13	36.18	0.00	48.60	0.65	43.20	70.20	345.60	1.80	0.70
0.02	0.10	0.00	0.00	0.14	22.60	16.72	0.07	0.05	0.62	0.12	28.93	0.00	22.60	0.52	25.99	39.55	220.35	2.26	0.29
0.10	0.55	0.00	0.00	0.25	729.80	19.68	0.18	0.04	1.44	0.14	57.40	0.00	28.70	0.68	16.40	41.00	895.85	2.05	0.53
0.02	0.10	0.00	0.00	0.14	470.96	14.27	0.12	0.03	0.93	0.09	25.17	0.00	35.96	0.67	24.36	37.12	406.00	4.64	0.15
0.00	0.03	0.00	0.00	0.00	7.84	5.46	0.01	0.01	0.11	0.02	3.20	0.00	3.36	0.13	5.28	14.88	73.44	0.48	0.13
0.08	0.29	0.00	21.28	0.21	4.56	86.18	0.03	0.11	0.35	0.09	86.40	0.00	21.28	0.58	15.20	28.88	252.32	1.52	0.20
0.05	0.15	0.00	0.00	0.36	5.10	105.57	0.05	0.13	1.02	0.08	38.00	0.00	28.05	1.50	17.85	33.15	249.90	7.65	0.15
0.04	0.11	0.00	0.00	0.60	8.84	91.05	0.04	0.09	1.02	0.07	37.13	0.00	35.36	1.66	24.31	28.73	327.08	4.42	0.29
0.00	0.10	0.00	0.00	0.56	4364.00	49.20	0.14	0.26	1.20	0.48	45.20	0.00	56.00	0.90	40.00	110.00	696.00	20.00	0.58
0.03	0.43	0.00	0.00	0.92	5592.40	56.09	0.16	0.46	2.10	0.79	36.41	0.00	68.88	1.84	32.80	88.56	603.52	42.64	0.89
0.66	0.16	0.00	0.00	0.00	439.95	7.04	0.02	0.04	0.41	0.04	11.97	0.00	27.30	1.19	11.55	27.30	198.45	73.50	0.16
0.03	0.23	0.00	0.00	0.69	3858.15	13.26	0.08	0.23	2.45	0.61	27.29	0.00	76.50	3.39	61.20	132.60	535.50	191.25	0.54

USDA ID Code	Food Name	Weight in Grams*	Quantity of Units	Unit of Measure	Protein (g)	Fat (g)	Carbohydrate (g)	Kilocalories	Caffeine (g)	Fiber (g)	Cholesterol (mg)	Saturated Fat (g)
	Sweet Potatoes, Syrup Pack, Drai	196.0000	1.000	Cup	2.51	0.63	49.71	211.68	0.00	5.88	0.00	0.14
	Tangerines, Cnd, Juice Pack	249.0000	1.000	Cup	1.54	0.07	23.83	92.13	0.00	1.74	0.00	0.00
	Tangerines, Cnd, Light Syrup Pack	252.0000	1.000	Cup	1.13	0.25	40.80	153.72	0.00	1.76	0.00	0.03
	Tangerines, Fresh	195.0000	1.000	Cup	1.23	0.37	21.82	85.80	0.00	4.48	0.00	0.04
	Tator Tots	2.8350	10.000	Each	0.30	0.50	2.00	14.00	0.00	0.30	0.00	0.10
	Tomatillos, Fresh	34.0000	1.000	Slice	0.33	0.35	1.98	10.88	0.00	0.65	0.00	0.05
	Tomatoes, Cherry	149.0000	1.000	Cup	1.27	0.49	6.91	31.29	0.00	1.64	0.00	0.07
	Tomatoes, Ckd, Boiled	240.0000	1.000	Cup	2.57	0.98	13.99	64.80	0.00	2.40	0.00	0.14
	Tomatoes, Ckd, Stewed	101.0000	1.000	Cup	1.98	2.71	13.18	79.79	0.00	1.72	0.00	0.53
	Tomatoes, Cnd, Stewed	255.0000	1.000	Cup	2.42	0.33	17.29	71.40	0.00	2.55	0.00	0.05
	Tomatoes, Cnd, w/ Green Chilies	241.0000	1.000	Cup	1.66	0.19	8.72	36.15	0.00	0.00	0.00	0.02
	Tomatoes, Cnd, Wedges In Tomato	261.0000	1.000	Cup	2.06	0.42	16.47	67.86	0.00	0.00	0.00	0.05
	Tomatoes, Cnd, Whole, Reg Pk	240.0000	1.000	Cup	2.21	0.31	10.49	45.60	0.00	2.40	0.00	0.05
	Tomatoes, Fresh	149.0000	1.000	Cup	1.27	0.49	6.91	31.29	0.00	1.64	0.00	0.07
	Tomatoes, Green, Fresh	180.0000	1.000	Cup	2.16	0.36	9.18	43.20	0.00	1.98	0.00	0.05
	Tomatoes, Sun-dried	54.0000	0.250	Cup	7.62	1.60	30.11	139.32	0.00	6.64	0.00	0.23
	Tomatoes, Sun-dried, Packed In 0	110.0000	1.000	Cup	5.57	15.49	25.66	234.30	0.00	6.38	0.00	2.08
	Turnips, Ckd	156.0000	1.000	Cup	1.11	0.12	7.64	32.76	0.00	3.12	0.00	0.02
	Turnips, Fresh	130.0000	1.000	Cup	1.17	0.13	8.10	35.10	0.00	2.34	0.00	0.01
	Vegetables, Mixed, Cnd	163.0000	1.000	Cup	4.22	0.41	15.09	76.61	0.00	4.89	0.00	0.08
	Vegetables, Mixed, Frz	275.0000	1.250	Cup	7.87	0.41	36.00	162.25	0.00	12.10	0.00	0.08
	Veggie Burger	90.0000	1.000	Each	18.00	4.00	8.00	140.00	0.00	5.00	0.00	1.50
	Watercress, Raw	2.5000	1.000	Sprig	0.06	0.00	0.03	0.28	0.00	0.04	0.00	0.00
	Watermelon	154.0000	1.000	Cup	0.95	0.66	11.06	49.28	0.00	0.77	0.00	0.08
	Yam, Baked	136.0000	1.000	Cup	2.03	0.19	37.54	157.76	0.00	5.30	0.00	0.04

Meats and Beans

USDA ID Code	Food Name	Weight in Grams*	Quantity of Units	Unit of Measure	Protein (g)	Fat (g)	Carbohydrate (g)	Kilocalories	Caffeine (g)	Fiber (g)	Cholesterol (mg)	Saturated Fat (g)
	Bacon	19.0000	3.000	Slice	5.79	9.36	0.11	109.44	0.00	0.00	16.15	3.31
	Bacon, Canadian-style Bacon, Gri	46.5000	2.000	Slice	11.27	3.92	0.63	86.03	0.00	0.00	26.97	1.32
	Bacon, Turkey	14.0000	1.000	Slice	3.00	2.00	0.00	25.00	0.00	0.00	10.00	0.50
	Barbecue Loaf, Lunch Meat	23.0000	1.000	Slice	3.64	2.05	1.47	39.79	0.00	0.00	8.51	0.73
	Beans, Baked, Cnd, Vegetarian	254.0000	1.000	Cup	12.17	1.14	52.10	236.22	0.00	12.70	0.00	0.30
	Beans, Baked, Cnd, w/ Beef	266.0000	1.000	Cup	16.97	9.18	44.98	321.86	0.00	0.00	58.52	4.47
	Beans, Baked, Cnd, w/ Franks	259.0000	1.000	Cup	17.48	17.02	39.86	367.78	0.00	17.87	15.54	6.09
	Beans, Baked, Cnd, w/ Pork	253.0000	1.000	Cup	13.13	3.92	50.55	268.18	0.00	13.92	17.71	1.52
	Beans, Baked, Home Prepared	253.0000	1.000	Cup	14.02	13.03	54.12	382.03	0.00	13.92	12.65	4.93
	Beans, Black, Ckd	172.0000	1.000	Cup	15.24	0.93	40.78	227.04	0.00	14.96	0.00	0.24
	Beans, Garbanzo, Cnd	240.0000	1.000	Cup	11.88	2.74	54.29	285.60	0.00	10.56	0.00	0.29
	Beans, Kidney, Cnd	256.0000	1.000	Cup	13.31	0.79	38.09	207.36	0.00	8.96	0.00	0.13
1	Beans, Lentils	198.0000	1.000	Cup	17.87	0.74	39.87	231.00	0.00	5.46	0.00	0.11
	Beans, Lima, Cnd	241.0000	1.000	Cup	11.88	0.41	35.93	190.39	0.00	11.57	0.00	0.10
	Beans, Navy, Cnd	262.0000	1.000	Cup	19.73	1.13	53.58	296.06	0.00	13.36	0.00	0.29
	Beans, Pinto, Cnd	240.0000	1.000	Cup	11.66	1.94	36.60	206.40	0.00	11.04	0.00	0.41
	Beans, Refried, Cnd	15.8000	1.000	Tbsp	0.87	0.20	2.45	14.85	0.00	0.84	1.26	0.07
	Beans, Refried, Lowfat, Cnd	268.0000	0.500	Cup	16.00	0.00	42.00	240.00	0.00	14.00	0.00	0.00
2	Beans, Refried, No Fat	128.0000	0.500	Cup	7.30	0.50	19.50	92.00	0.00	6.20	0.00	0.00
	Beef, Corned, Brisket, Ckd	85.0000	3.000	Ounce	15.44	16.13	0.40	213.35	0.00	0.00	83.30	5.39
	Beef, Corned, Loaf, Jellied	28.3500	1.000	Slice	6.49	1.73	0.00	43.38	0.00	0.00	13.32	0.74
	Beef, Cured, Lunch Meat, Jellied	28.3500	1.000	Slice	5.39	0.94	0.00	31.47	0.00	0.00	9.64	0.40
	Beef, Cured, Smoked, Chopped Beef	28.3500	1.000	Slice	5.72	1.25	0.53	37.71	0.00	0.00	13.04	0.51
	Beef, Cured, Thin-sliced	21.0000	5.000	Slice	5.90	0.81	1.20	37.17	0.00	0.00	8.61	0.35
	Beef, Filet, Tenderloin, Broiled	85.0000	3.000	Ounce	23.55	9.75	0.00	188.70	0.00	0.00	70.55	3.68
	Beef, Ground, Extra Lean, Broiled	85.0000	3.000	Ounce	21.59	13.88	0.00	217.60	0.00	0.00	71.40	5.46
	Beef, Ground, Extra Lean, Pan-fried	85.0000	3.000	Ounce	21.22	13.96	0.00	216.75	0.00	0.00	68.85	5.48

Page Key: A2 = Baby Food   A2 = Baked Goods   A8 = Beverages   A14 = Breads/Grains and Pasta   A18 = Breakfast Foods/Cereals   A26 = Dairy and Eggs   A40 = Fats and Oils   A42 = Fruits and Vegetables   A52 = Meats and Beans   A60 = Nuts and Seeds   A62 5 Frozen Entrees and Packaged Foods   A76 = Restaurant Chains–Fast Foods   A92 = Restaurant Chains–Other   A106 = Seafood and Fish   A110 = Snacks and Sweets   A120 = Soups   A122 = Supplements   A126 = Toppings and Sauces

Monounsaturated Fat (g)	Polyunsaturated Fat (g)	Vitamin D (mg)	Vitamin K (mg)	Vitamin E (mg)	Vitamin A (re)	Vitamin C (mg)	Thiamin (mg)	Riboflavin (mg)	Niacin (mg)	Vitamin B6 (mg)	Folate (mcg)	Vitamin B12 (mcg)	Calcium (mg)	Iron (mg)	Magnesium (mg)	Phosphorus (mg)	Potassium (mg)	Sodium (mg)	Zinc (mg)
0.02	0.27	0.00	0.00	0.55	1403.36	21.17	0.06	0.08	0.67	0.12	15.48	0.00	33.32	1.86	23.52	49.00	378.28	76.44	0.31
0.02	0.02	0.00	0.00	1.25	211.65	85.16	0.20	0.07	1.12	0.10	11.45	0.00	27.39	0.67	27.39	24.90	331.17	12.45	1.27
0.05	0.05	0.00	0.00	0.86	211.68	49.90	0.13	0.10	1.13	0.10	11.59	0.00	17.64	0.93	20.16	25.20	196.56	15.12	0.60
0.06	0.08	0.00	0.00	0.47	179.40	60.06	0.21	0.04	0.31	0.14	39.78	0.00	27.30	0.20	23.40	19.50	306.15	1.95	0.47
0.00	0.00	0.00	0.00	0.00	0.00	0.00	0.00	0.00	0.00	0.00	0.00	0.00	0.00	0.00	0.00	0.00	24.00	24.00	0.00
0.05	0.14	0.00	0.00	0.13	3.74	3.98	0.01	0.01	0.63	0.02	2.38	0.00	2.38	0.21	6.80	13.26	91.12	0.34	0.07
0.07	0.21	0.00	0.00	0.57	92.38	38.74	0.09	0.07	0.94	0.12	22.35	0.00	7.45	0.67	16.39	35.76	330.78	13.41	0.13
0.14	0.41	0.00	0.00	0.91	177.60	54.72	0.17	0.14	1.80	0.24	31.20	0.00	14.40	1.34	33.60	74.40	669.60	26.40	0.26
1.06	0.89	0.00	0.00	1.28	67.67	18.38	0.11	0.08	1.12	0.09	11.11	0.00	26.26	1.07	15.15	38.38	249.47	459.55	0.18
0.05	0.13	0.00	0.00	0.97	137.70	29.07	0.13	0.10	1.81	0.05	13.77	0.00	84.15	1.86	30.60	51.00	606.90	563.55	0.43
0.02	0.07	0.00	0.00	0.00	93.99	14.94	0.07	0.05	1.54	0.24	21.93	0.00	48.20	0.63	26.51	33.74	257.87	966.41	0.31
0.05	0.18	0.00	0.00	0.00	151.38	38.63	0.16	0.08	1.77	0.31	26.36	0.00	67.86	1.20	28.71	60.03	655.11	566.37	0.42
0.05	0.12	0.00	0.00	0.77	144.00	34.08	0.12	0.07	1.78	0.22	18.72	0.00	72.00	1.32	28.80	45.60	530.40	355.20	0.38
0.07	0.21	0.00	34.27	0.57	92.38	28.46	0.09	0.07	0.94	0.12	22.35	0.00	7.45	0.67	16.39	35.76	330.78	13.41	0.13
0.05	0.14	0.00	84.60	0.68	115.20	42.12	0.11	0.07	0.90	0.14	15.84	0.00	23.40	0.92	18.00	50.40	367.20	23.40	0.13
0.26	0.60	0.00	0.00	0.01	46.98	21.17	0.29	0.26	4.89	0.18	36.72	0.00	59.40	4.91	104.76	192.24	1850.58	1131.30	1.07
9.53	2.27	0.00	0.00	0.00	141.90	111.98	0.21	0.42	3.99	0.35	25.30	0.00	51.70	2.95	89.10	152.90	1721.50	292.60	0.86
0.02	0.06	0.00	0.00	0.05	0.00	18.10	0.05	0.03	0.47	0.11	14.35	0.00	34.32	0.34	12.48	29.64	210.60	78.00	0.31
0.01	0.07	0.00	0.00	0.04	0.00	27.30	0.05	0.04	0.52	0.12	18.85	0.00	39.00	0.39	14.30	35.10	248.30	87.10	0.35
0.03	0.20	0.00	0.00	0.98	1898.95	8.15	0.08	0.08	0.95	0.13	38.47	0.00	44.01	1.71	26.08	68.46	474.33	242.87	0.67
0.03	0.19	0.00	0.00	0.99	1177.00	8.80	0.19	0.33	2.34	0.19	52.25	0.00	68.75	2.26	60.50	140.25	464.75	96.25	1.35
0.00	0.50	0.00	0.00	0.00	0.00	0.00	0.25	0.00	4.00	0.00	0.00	0.00	96.00	1.50	0.00	0.00	0.00	380.00	7.50
0.00	0.00	0.00	0.00	0.03	0.00	11.75	1.08	0.00	0.01	0.00	0.23	0.00	3.00	0.01	0.53	1.50	8.25	1.03	0.00
0.17	0.23	0.00	0.00	0.23	56.98	14.78	0.12	0.03	0.31	0.22	3.39	0.00	12.32	0.26	16.94	13.86	178.64	3.08	0.11
0.01	0.00	0.00	0.00	0.22	0.00	16.46	0.14	0.04	0.75	0.31	21.76	0.00	19.04	0.71	24.48	66.64	911.20	10.88	0.27
4.50	1.10	0.00	0.00	0.10	0.00	0.00	0.13	0.06	1.39	0.05	0.95	0.33	2.28	0.31	4.56	63.84	92.34	303.24	0.62
1.88	0.38	0.00	0.00	0.12	0.00	0.00	0.38	0.09	3.22	0.21	1.86	0.36	4.65	0.38	9.77	137.64	181.35	718.89	0.79
0.00	0.00	0.00	0.00	0.00	0.00	0.00	0.00	0.00	0.00	0.00	0.00	0.00	0.00	0.00	0.00	0.00	0.00	170.00	0.00
0.95	0.19	0.21	0.00	0.00	1.61	0.00	0.08	0.06	0.52	0.06	2.07	0.39	12.65	0.27	3.91	30.36	75.67	306.82	0.57
0.10	0.48	0.00	0.00	1.35	43.18	7.87	0.38	0.15	1.09	0.33	60.71	0.00	127.00	0.74	81.28	264.16	751.84	1008.38	3.56
3.70	0.56	0.00	0.00	0.00	55.86	4.79	0.13	0.13	2.50	0.24	115.44	0.00	119.70	4.26	66.50	215.46	851.20	1263.50	3.19
7.33	2.18	0.00	0.00	1.22	38.85	5.96	0.16	0.16	2.33	0.13	77.70	0.00	124.32	4.48	72.52	269.36	608.65	1113.70	4.84
1.70	0.51	0.00	0.00	0.00	45.54	5.06	0.13	0.10	1.14	0.15	91.84	0.00	134.09	4.30	86.02	273.24	781.77	1047.42	3.69
5.39	1.87	0.00	0.00	0.00	0.00	2.78	0.35	0.13	1.04	0.23	122.45	0.00	154.33	5.03	108.79	275.77	905.74	1067.66	1.85
0.09	0.40	0.00	0.00	0.00	1.72	0.00	0.41	0.10	0.88	0.12	255.94	0.00	46.44	3.61	120.40	240.80	610.60	407.64	1.93
0.62	1.22	0.00	0.00	0.00	4.80	9.12	0.07	0.07	0.34	1.13	160.32	0.00	76.80	3.24	69.60	216.00	412.80	717.60	2.54
0.05	0.44	0.00	0.00	0.00	0.00	3.07	0.28	0.18	1.28	0.18	125.95	0.00	69.12	3.15	79.36	268.80	657.92	888.32	1.41
0.13	0.35	0.00	0.00	0.00	2.00	2.90	0.34	0.15	2.10	0.35	357.90	0.00	37.00	6.59	71.00	356.00	731.00	4.00	2.50
0.05	0.17	0.00	0.00	0.00	0.00	0.00	0.14	0.07	0.63	0.22	121.46	0.00	50.61	4.36	93.99	178.34	530.20	809.76	1.57
0.10	0.50	0.00	0.00	1.00	0.00	1.83	0.37	0.16	1.28	0.26	163.23	0.00	123.14	4.85	123.14	351.08	754.56	1173.76	2.02
0.38	0.70	0.00	0.00	2.26	4.80	2.16	0.24	0.14	0.70	0.17	144.48	0.00	103.20	3.50	64.80	220.80	583.20	705.60	1.66
0.09	0.02	0.00	0.00	0.00	0.00	0.95	0.00	0.00	0.05	0.02	1.74	0.00	5.53	0.26	5.21	13.59	42.19	47.24	0.18
0.00	0.00	0.00	0.00	0.00	0.00	0.00	0.00	0.00	0.00	0.00	0.00	0.00	0.00	2.00	0.00	0.00	0.00	960.00	0.00
0.00	0.00	0.00	0.00	0.00	0.00	0.00	0.00	0.00	0.00	0.00	0.00	0.00	43.00	1.92	0.00	0.00	0.00	480.00	0.00
7.84	0.57	0.00	0.00	0.14	0.00	0.00	0.03	0.14	2.58	0.20	5.10	1.39	6.80	1.58	10.20	106.25	123.25	963.90	3.89
0.76	0.09	0.00	0.00	0.05	0.00	0.00	0.00	0.03	0.50	0.03	2.27	0.36	3.12	0.58	3.12	20.70	28.63	270.18	1.16
0.41	0.05	0.00	0.00	0.00	0.00	0.00	0.04	0.08	1.37	0.07	1.98	1.46	2.84	0.98	5.10	39.41	113.97	374.79	1.01
0.52	0.07	0.00	0.00	0.00	0.00	0.00	0.02	0.05	1.30	0.10	2.27	0.49	2.27	0.81	5.95	51.31	106.88	356.64	1.11
0.35	0.04	0.00	0.00	0.03	0.00	0.00	0.02	0.04	1.11	0.07	2.31	0.54	2.31	0.57	3.99	35.28	90.09	302.19	0.84
3.81	0.44	0.00	0.00	0.00	0.00	0.00	0.09	0.26	2.90	0.25	7.65	2.30	5.95	3.13	22.95	203.15	332.35	51.85	4.07
6.08	0.52	0.00	0.00	0.15	0.00	0.00	0.05	0.23	4.22	0.23	7.65	1.84	5.95	2.00	17.85	136.85	266.05	59.50	4.63
6.11	0.52	0.00	0.00	0.15	0.00	0.00	0.05	0.22	4.00	0.23	7.65	1.70	5.95	2.01	17.85	136.00	265.20	59.50	4.61

USDA ID Code	Food Name	Weight in Grams*	Quantity of Units	Unit of Measure	Protein (g)	Fat (g)	Carbohydrate (g)	Kilocalories	Caffeine (g)	Fiber (g)	Cholesterol (mg)	Saturated Fat (g)
	Beef, Ground, Lean, Broiled	85.0000	3.000	Ounce	21.01	15.69	0.00	231.20	0.00	0.00	73.95	6.16
	Beef, Ground, Lean, Pan-fried	85.0000	3.000	Ounce	20.60	16.20	0.00	233.75	0.00	0.00	71.40	6.37
	Beef, Ground, Regular, Broiled	85.0000	3.000	Ounce	20.46	17.59	0.00	245.65	0.00	0.00	76.50	6.91
	Beef, Ground, Regular, Pan-fried	85.0000	3.000	Ounce	20.33	19.18	0.00	260.10	0.00	0.00	75.65	7.53
	Beef, Liver, Ckd, Braised	85.0000	3.000	Ounce	20.72	4.16	2.90	136.85	0.00	0.00	330.65	1.62
	Beef, Liver, Ckd, Pan-fried	85.0000	3.000	Ounce	22.71	6.80	6.67	184.45	0.00	0.00	409.70	2.27
	Beef, Loaved, Lunch Meat	28.3500	1.000	Slice	4.08	7.43	0.82	87.32	0.00	0.00	18.14	3.17
	Beef, Steaks and Roasts, Ckd, 1/	28.3500	3.000	Ounce	7.07	7.62	0.00	98.94	0.00	0.00	25.80	3.15
	Beef, Steaks and Roasts, Ckd, Fa	85.0000	3.000	Ounce	23.23	14.76	0.00	232.05	0.00	0.00	73.95	5.82
	Beef, Steaks and Roasts, Ckd., 1	85.0000	3.000	Ounce	22.05	18.31	0.00	259.25	0.00	0.00	74.80	7.26
	Beef, Thin Sliced	21.0000	5.000	Slice	5.90	0.81	1.20	37.17	0.00	0.00	8.61	0.35
	Bologna, Beef, Lunch Meat	23.0000	1.000	Slice	2.81	6.56	0.18	71.76	0.00	0.00	13.34	2.78
	Bologna, Lunch Meat	23.0000	1.000	Slice	3.52	4.57	0.17	56.81	0.00	0.00	13.57	1.58
	Bologna, Turkey	21.0000	1.000	Slice	2.88	3.19	0.20	41.79	0.00	0.00	20.79	1.06
	Buffalo (Chicken) Wings	22.7500	4.000	Each	4.50	3.00	0.50	47.50	0.00	0.00	25.00	0.75
	Chicken Roll, Light Meat	28.3500	3.000	Ounce	5.54	2.09	0.69	45.08	0.00	0.00	14.18	0.57
	Chicken Salad Sandwich Spread	28.3500	3.000	Ounce	3.30	3.83	2.10	56.70	0.00	0.00	8.51	0.98
	Chicken Spread, Cnd	28.3500	3.000	Ounce	4.37	3.32	1.53	54.43	0.00	0.00	14.74	0.96
	Chicken, Back, Meat & Skin, Ckd,	72.0000	3.000	Ounce	15.82	15.78	7.38	238.32	0.00	0.00	63.36	4.20
	Chicken, Back, Meat & Skin, Ckd,	44.0000	3.000	Ounce	12.23	9.13	2.86	145.64	0.00	0.00	39.16	2.47
	Chicken, Back, Meat & Skin, Ckd,	32.0000	3.000	Ounce	8.30	6.71	0.00	96.00	0.00	0.00	28.16	1.86
	Chicken, Back, Meat & Skin, Ckd,	36.0000	3.000	Ounce	7.98	6.53	0.00	92.88	0.00	0.00	28.08	1.81
	Chicken, Back, Meat Only, Ckd, F	35.0000	3.000	Ounce	10.50	5.36	1.99	100.80	0.00	0.00	32.55	1.44
	Chicken, Back, Meat Only, Ckd, R	24.0000	3.000	Ounce	6.77	3.16	0.00	57.36	0.00	0.00	21.60	0.86
	Chicken, Back, Meat Only, Ckd, S	26.0000	3.000	Ounce	6.58	2.91	0.00	54.34	0.00	0.00	22.10	0.79
	Chicken, Breast, Meat & Skin, Ck	84.0000	3.000	Ounce	20.87	11.09	7.55	218.40	0.00	0.25	71.40	2.96
	Chicken, Breast, Meat & Skin, Ck	59.0000	3.000	Ounce	18.79	5.23	0.97	130.98	0.00	0.06	52.51	1.45
	Chicken, Breast, Meat & Skin, Ck	58.0000	3.000	Ounce	17.28	4.51	0.00	114.26	0.00	0.00	48.72	1.27
	Chicken, Breast, Meat & Skin, Ck	66.0000	3.000	Ounce	18.08	4.90	0.00	121.44	0.00	0.00	49.50	1.37
	Chicken, Breast, Meat Only, Ckd,	52.0000	3.000	Ounce	17.39	2.45	0.27	97.24	0.00	0.00	47.32	0.67
	Chicken, Breast, Meat Only, Ckd,	52.0000	3.000	Ounce	16.13	1.86	0.00	85.80	0.00	0.00	44.20	0.53
	Chicken, Breast, Meat Only, Ckd,	57.0000	3.000	Ounce	16.52	1.73	0.00	86.07	0.00	0.00	43.89	0.48
	Chicken, Cnd	142.0000	5.000	Fl Oz	30.91	11.29	0.00	234.30	0.00	0.00	88.04	3.12
	Chicken, Dark Meat, Meat & Skin,	167.0000	3.000	Ounce	36.49	31.13	15.66	497.66	0.00	0.00	148.63	8.27
	Chicken, Dark Meat, Meat & Skin,	110.0000	3.000	Ounce	29.94	18.60	4.49	313.50	0.00	0.00	101.20	5.04
	Chicken, Dark Meat, Meat & Skin,	101.0000	3.000	Ounce	26.23	15.94	0.00	255.53	0.00	0.00	91.91	4.41
	Chicken, Dark Meat, Meat & Skin,	110.0000	3.000	Ounce	25.85	16.13	0.00	256.30	0.00	0.00	90.20	4.47
	Chicken, Dark Meat, Meat Only, C	91.0000	3.000	Ounce	26.38	10.57	2.36	217.49	0.00	0.00	87.36	2.84
	Chicken, Dark Meat, Meat Only, C	81.0000	3.000	Ounce	22.17	7.88	0.00	166.05	0.00	0.00	75.33	2.15
	Chicken, Dark Meat, Meat Only, C	86.0000	3.000	Ounce	22.33	7.72	0.00	165.12	0.00	0.00	75.68	2.11
	Chicken, Drumstick, Meat & Skin,	43.0000	3.000	Ounce	9.44	6.77	3.56	115.24	0.00	0.13	36.98	1.78
	Chicken, Drumstick, Meat & Skin,	29.0000	3.000	Ounce	7.82	3.98	0.47	71.05	0.00	0.03	26.10	1.06
	Chicken, Drumstick, Meat & Skin,	31.0000	3.000	Ounce	8.38	3.46	0.00	66.96	0.00	0.00	28.21	0.95
	Chicken, Drumstick, Meat & Skin,	34.0000	3.000	Ounce	8.61	3.62	0.00	69.36	0.00	0.00	28.22	0.99
	Chicken, Drumstick, Meat Only, C	25.0000	3.000	Ounce	7.16	2.02	0.00	48.75	0.00	0.00	23.50	0.53
	Chicken, Drumstick, Meat Only, C	26.0000	3.000	Ounce	7.36	1.47	0.00	44.72	0.00	0.00	24.18	0.38
	Chicken, Drumstick, Meat Only, C	28.0000	3.000	Ounce	7.70	1.60	0.00	47.32	0.00	0.00	24.64	0.42
	Chicken, Giblets, Ckd, Fried	13.0000	3.000	Ounce	4.23	1.75	0.57	36.01	0.00	0.00	57.98	0.49
	Chicken, Giblets, Ckd, Simmered	14.0000	3.000	Ounce	3.62	0.67	0.13	21.98	0.00	0.00	55.02	0.21
	Chicken, Heart, Ckd, Simmered	1.0000	3.000	Ounce	0.26	0.08	0.00	1.85	0.00	0.00	2.42	0.02
	Chicken, Leg, Meat & Skin, Ckd,	95.0000	3.000	Ounce	20.68	15.36	8.28	259.35	0.00	0.29	85.50	4.07
	Chicken, Leg, Meat & Skin, Ckd,	67.0000	3.000	Ounce	17.98	9.67	1.68	170.18	0.00	0.07	62.98	2.61
	Chicken, Leg, Meat & Skin, Ckd,	69.0000	3.000	Ounce	17.91	9.29	0.00	160.08	0.00	0.00	63.48	2.57

Monounsaturated Fat (g)	Polyunsaturated Fat (g)	Vitamin D (mg)	Vitamin K (mg)	Vitamin E (mg)	Vitamin A (re)	Vitamin C (mg)	Thiamin (mg)	Riboflavin (mg)	Niacin (mg)	Vitamin B6 (mg)	Folate (mcg)	Vitamin B12 (mcg)	Calcium (mg)	Iron (mg)	Magnesium (mg)	Phosphorus (mg)	Potassium (mg)	Sodium (mg)	Zinc (mg)
6.87	0.59	0.00	0.00	0.17	0.00	0.00	0.04	0.18	4.39	0.22	7.65	2.00	9.35	1.79	17.85	134.30	255.85	65.45	4.56
7.09	0.60	0.00	0.00	0.17	0.00	0.00	0.04	0.19	4.07	0.24	7.65	1.93	8.50	1.85	17.00	135.15	254.15	65.45	4.42
7.70	0.65	0.00	0.00	0.20	0.00	0.00	0.03	0.16	4.90	0.23	7.65	2.49	9.35	2.07	17.00	144.50	248.20	70.55	4.40
8.40	0.71	0.00	0.00	0.20	0.00	0.00	0.03	0.17	4.96	0.20	7.65	2.30	9.35	2.08	17.00	145.35	255.00	71.40	4.31
0.55	0.91	0.00	0.00	0.00	9011.70	19.55	0.17	3.48	9.11	0.77	184.45	60.35	5.95	5.75	17.00	343.40	199.75	59.50	5.16
1.38	1.45	0.00	0.00	0.54	9119.65	19.55	0.18	3.52	12.27	1.22	187.00	95.03	9.35	5.34	19.55	391.85	309.40	90.10	4.63
3.47	0.25	0.00	0.00	0.06	0.00	0.00	0.03	0.06	1.04	0.05	1.42	1.10	3.12	0.66	3.97	33.74	58.97	376.77	0.72
3.41	0.29	0.00	0.00	0.00	0.00	0.00	0.02	0.06	0.98	0.09	1.98	0.68	2.84	0.74	5.95	54.72	81.36	16.73	1.56
6.30	0.54	0.00	0.00	0.15	0.00	0.00	0.07	0.19	3.13	0.28	5.95	2.13	7.65	2.32	19.55	179.35	274.55	52.70	5.15
7.84	0.66	0.00	0.00	0.17	0.00	0.00	0.07	0.18	3.09	0.28	5.95	2.07	8.50	2.23	18.70	172.55	266.05	52.70	4.97
0.35	0.04	0.00	0.00	0.04	0.00	0.00	0.02	0.04	1.11	0.07	2.31	0.54	2.31	0.57	3.99	35.28	90.09	302.19	0.84
3.17	0.25	0.16	0.00	0.04	0.00	0.00	0.01	0.03	0.55	0.03	1.15	0.33	2.76	0.38	2.76	20.24	36.11	225.63	0.50
2.25	0.49	0.00	0.00	0.06	0.00	8.12	0.12	0.04	0.90	0.06	1.15	0.21	2.53	0.18	3.22	31.97	64.63	272.32	0.47
1.01	0.90	0.00	0.00	0.00	0.00	0.00	0.01	0.03	0.74	0.05	1.47	0.06	17.64	0.32	2.94	27.51	41.79	184.38	0.37
0.00	0.00	0.00	0.00	0.00	15.00	0.30	0.00	0.00	0.00	0.00	0.00	0.00	6.00	0.10	0.00	0.00	0.00	225.00	0.00
0.84	0.45	0.00	0.00	0.08	6.80	0.00	0.02	0.04	1.50	0.06	0.57	0.04	12.19	0.27	5.39	44.51	64.64	165.56	0.20
0.92	1.76	0.00	0.00	0.00	11.91	0.34	0.01	0.02	0.47	0.03	1.42	0.11	2.84	0.17	2.84	9.36	51.88	106.88	0.29
1.38	0.71	0.00	0.00	0.00	7.09	0.00	0.00	0.03	0.78	0.04	0.85	0.04	35.44	0.66	3.40	25.23	30.05	109.43	0.33
6.42	3.74	0.00	0.00	0.00	25.92	0.00	0.09	0.15	4.20	0.17	14.40	0.19	18.72	1.07	13.68	98.64	129.60	228.24	1.41
3.60	2.12	0.00	0.00	0.00	16.28	0.00	0.05	0.11	3.21	0.13	6.60	0.12	10.56	0.71	10.12	73.04	99.44	39.60	1.09
2.65	1.48	0.00	0.00	0.09	31.68	0.00	0.02	0.06	2.15	0.09	1.92	0.09	6.72	0.45	6.40	49.28	67.20	27.84	0.72
2.57	1.44	0.00	0.00	0.10	31.68	0.00	0.01	0.05	1.56	0.05	1.80	0.06	6.48	0.44	5.76	43.20	52.20	23.04	0.69
2.01	1.27	0.00	0.00	0.00	10.15	0.00	0.04	0.09	2.69	0.12	3.15	0.11	9.10	0.58	8.75	61.60	87.85	34.65	0.98
1.16	0.73	0.00	0.00	0.06	6.72	0.00	0.02	0.05	1.70	0.08	1.68	0.07	5.76	0.33	5.28	39.60	56.88	23.04	0.64
1.05	0.68	0.00	0.00	0.07	7.02	0.00	0.01	0.04	1.19	0.05	1.82	0.05	5.46	0.33	4.42	33.80	41.08	17.42	0.70
4.59	2.59	0.00	0.00	0.89	16.80	0.00	0.10	0.13	8.84	0.36	12.60	0.25	16.80	1.05	20.16	155.40	168.84	231.00	0.80
2.07	1.16	0.00	0.00	0.00	8.85	0.00	0.05	0.08	8.11	0.34	3.54	0.20	9.44	0.70	17.70	137.47	152.81	44.84	0.65
1.76	0.96	0.00	0.00	0.16	15.66	0.00	0.04	0.07	7.37	0.32	2.32	0.19	8.12	0.62	15.66	124.12	142.10	41.18	0.59
1.91	1.04	0.00	0.00	0.18	15.84	0.00	0.03	0.08	5.15	0.19	1.98	0.14	8.58	0.61	14.52	102.96	117.48	40.92	0.64
0.89	0.56	0.00	0.00	0.22	3.64	0.00	0.04	0.07	7.69	0.33	2.08	0.19	8.32	0.59	16.12	127.92	143.52	41.08	0.56
0.64	0.40	0.00	0.00	0.14	3.12	0.00	0.04	0.06	7.13	0.31	2.08	0.18	7.80	0.54	15.08	118.56	133.12	38.48	0.52
0.59	0.38	0.00	0.00	0.15	3.42	0.00	0.02	0.07	4.83	0.19	1.71	0.13	7.41	0.50	13.68	94.05	106.59	35.91	0.55
4.47	2.49	0.00	0.00	0.30	48.28	2.84	0.03	0.18	8.99	0.50	5.68	0.41	19.88	2.24	17.04	157.62	195.96	714.26	2.00
12.66	7.40	0.00	0.00	0.00	51.77	0.00	0.20	0.37	9.37	0.42	30.06	0.45	35.07	2.40	33.40	242.15	308.95	492.65	3.47
7.33	4.30	0.00	0.00	0.00	34.10	0.00	0.11	0.26	7.52	0.35	12.10	0.33	18.70	1.65	26.40	193.60	253.00	97.90	2.86
6.25	3.52	0.00	0.00	0.00	58.58	0.00	0.07	0.21	6.42	0.31	7.07	0.29	15.15	1.37	22.22	169.68	222.20	87.87	2.51
6.33	3.56	0.00	0.00	0.00	59.40	0.00	0.06	0.20	4.96	0.19	6.60	0.22	15.40	1.44	19.80	146.30	182.60	77.00	2.49
3.93	2.52	0.00	0.00	0.00	21.84	0.00	0.08	0.23	6.43	0.34	8.19	0.30	16.38	1.36	22.75	170.17	230.23	88.27	2.65
2.88	1.83	0.00	0.00	0.22	17.82	0.00	0.06	0.19	5.31	0.29	6.48	0.26	12.15	1.08	18.63	144.99	194.40	75.33	2.27
2.80	1.80	0.00	0.00	0.23	18.06	0.00	0.05	0.17	4.08	0.18	6.02	0.19	12.04	1.17	17.20	122.98	155.66	63.64	2.29
2.76	1.63	0.00	0.00	0.00	11.18	0.00	0.05	0.09	2.19	0.12	7.74	0.12	7.31	0.58	8.60	63.21	79.98	115.67	1.00
1.57	0.94	0.00	0.00	0.00	7.25	0.00	0.02	0.07	1.75	0.10	2.90	0.09	3.48	0.39	6.67	51.04	66.41	25.81	0.84
1.32	0.78	0.00	0.00	0.08	9.30	0.00	0.02	0.07	1.86	0.11	2.48	0.10	3.72	0.41	7.13	54.25	70.99	27.90	0.89
1.38	0.81	0.00	0.00	0.09	9.18	0.00	0.02	0.06	1.43	0.06	2.38	0.07	3.74	0.45	6.80	47.94	62.56	25.84	0.90
0.74	0.49	0.00	0.00	0.12	4.50	0.00	0.02	0.06	1.54	0.10	2.25	0.09	3.00	0.33	6.00	46.50	62.25	24.00	0.81
0.49	0.36	0.00	0.00	0.07	4.68	0.00	0.02	0.06	1.58	0.10	2.34	0.09	3.12	0.34	6.24	47.84	63.96	24.70	0.83
0.54	0.38	0.00	0.00	0.08	4.76	0.00	0.01	0.06	1.20	0.06	2.24	0.07	3.08	0.38	5.88	42.00	55.72	22.40	0.85
0.57	0.44	0.00	0.00	0.00	465.27	1.13	0.01	0.20	1.43	0.08	49.27	1.73	2.34	1.34	3.25	37.18	42.90	14.69	0.82
0.17	0.15	0.00	0.00	0.18	312.06	1.12	0.01	0.13	0.57	0.05	52.64	1.42	1.68	0.90	2.80	32.06	22.12	8.12	0.64
0.02	0.02	0.00	0.00	0.00	0.09	0.02	0.00	0.01	0.03	0.00	0.80	0.07	0.19	0.09	0.20	1.99	1.32	0.48	0.07
6.25	3.66	0.00	0.00	0.00	25.65	0.00	0.11	0.21	5.16	0.26	17.10	0.27	17.10	1.33	19.00	144.40	179.55	265.05	2.06
3.81	2.23	0.00	0.00	0.00	18.76	0.00	0.06	0.16	4.39	0.23	7.37	0.21	8.71	0.96	16.08	121.94	156.11	58.96	1.80
3.62	2.07	0.00	0.00	0.19	26.91	0.00	0.05	0.14	4.28	0.23	4.83	0.21	8.28	0.92	15.87	120.06	155.25	60.03	1.79

USDA ID Code	Food Name	Weight in Grams*	Quantity of Units	Unit of Measure	Protein (g)	Fat (g)	Carbohydrate (g)	Kilocalories	Caffeine (g)	Fiber (g)	Cholesterol (mg)	Saturated Fat (g)
	Chicken, Leg, Meat & Skin, Ckd,	75.0000	3.000	Ounce	18.13	9.69	0.00	165.00	0.00	0.00	63.00	2.68
	Chicken, Leg, Meat Only, Ckd, Fr	56.0000	3.000	Ounce	15.89	5.22	0.36	116.48	0.00	0.00	55.44	1.39
	Chicken, Leg, Meat Only, Ckd, Ro	57.0000	3.000	Ounce	15.41	4.81	0.00	108.87	0.00	0.00	53.58	1.31
	Chicken, Leg, Meat Only, Ckd, St	60.0000	3.000	Ounce	15.76	4.84	0.00	111.00	0.00	0.00	53.40	1.32
	Chicken, Liver, Ckd, Simmered	6.0000	3.000	Ounce	1.46	0.33	0.05	9.42	0.00	0.00	37.86	0.11
	Chicken, Meat Only, Ckd, Fried	140.0000	1.000	Cup	42.80	12.77	2.37	306.60	0.00	0.14	131.60	3.44
	Chicken, Meat Only, Roasted	8.7000	1.000	Tbsp	2.52	0.64	0.00	16.53	0.00	0.00	7.74	0.18
	Chicken, Meat Only, Stewed	8.7000	1.000	Tbsp	2.37	0.58	0.00	15.40	0.00	0.00	7.22	0.16
	Chicken, Thigh, Meat & Skin, Ckd	52.0000	3.000	Ounce	11.24	8.60	4.72	144.04	0.00	0.16	48.36	2.29
	Chicken, Thigh, Meat & Skin, Ckd	38.0000	3.000	Ounce	10.17	5.69	1.21	99.56	0.00	0.04	36.86	1.55
	Chicken, Thigh, Meat & Skin, Ckd	37.0000	3.000	Ounce	9.27	5.73	0.00	91.39	0.00	0.00	34.41	1.60
	Chicken, Thigh, Meat & Skin, Ckd	41.0000	3.000	Ounce	9.54	6.04	0.00	95.12	0.00	0.00	34.44	1.69
	Chicken, Thigh, Meat Only, Ckd,	31.0000	3.000	Ounce	8.74	3.19	0.37	67.58	0.00	0.00	31.62	0.86
	Chicken, Thigh, Meat Only, Ckd,	31.0000	3.000	Ounce	8.04	3.37	0.00	64.79	0.00	0.00	29.45	0.94
	Chicken, Thigh, Meat Only, Ckd,	33.0000	3.000	Ounce	8.25	3.23	0.00	64.35	0.00	0.00	29.70	0.89
	Chicken, Wing, Meat & Skin, Ckd,	29.0000	3.000	Ounce	5.76	6.32	3.17	93.96	0.00	0.09	22.91	1.69
	Chicken, Wing, Meat & Skin, Ckd,	19.0000	3.000	Ounce	4.96	4.21	0.45	60.99	0.00	0.02	15.39	1.15
	Chicken, Wing, Meat & Skin, Ckd,	21.0000	3.000	Ounce	5.64	4.09	0.00	60.90	0.00	0.00	17.64	1.14
	Chicken, Wing, Meat & Skin, Ckd,	24.0000	3.000	Ounce	5.47	4.04	0.00	59.76	0.00	0.00	16.80	1.13
	Chicken, Wing, Meat Only, Ckd, F	12.0000	3.000	Ounce	3.62	1.10	0.00	25.32	0.00	0.00	10.08	0.30
	Chicken, Wing, Meat Only, Ckd, R	13.0000	3.000	Ounce	3.96	1.06	0.00	26.39	0.00	0.00	11.05	0.29
	Chicken, Wing, Meat Only, Ckd, S	14.0000	3.000	Ounce	3.81	1.01	0.00	25.34	0.00	0.00	10.36	0.28
189	Chili w/ Beans, Cnd	255.0000	0.500	Cup	14.56	14.00	30.37	285.60	0.00	11.22	43.35	6.00
	Cornish Game Hen	110.0000	0.500	Bird	25.63	4.26	0.00	147.40	0.00	0.00	116.60	1.09
	Duck, Domesticated, Meat & Skin,	140.0000	1.000	Cup	26.59	39.69	0.00	471.80	0.00	0.00	117.60	13.54
	Duck, Domesticated, Meat Only, R	100.0000	3.000	Ounce	23.48	11.20	0.00	201.00	0.00	0.00	89.00	4.17
	Gardenburger	90.0000	1.000	Each	18.00	4.00	8.00	140.00	0.00	5.00	0.00	2.00
	Ham and Cheese Loaf (or Roll), Lu	28.3500	1.000	Slice	4.71	5.73	0.41	73.43	0.00	0.00	16.16	2.13
	Ham and Cheese Spread, Lunch Meat	15.0000	1.000	Tbsp	2.43	2.78	0.34	36.75	0.00	0.00	9.15	1.29
	Ham Salad Spread	15.0000	1.000	Tbsp	1.30	2.33	1.60	32.40	0.00	0.00	5.55	0.76
	Ham, Approx 11% Fat, Sliced	28.3500	1.000	Slice	4.98	3.00	0.88	51.60	0.00	0.00	16.16	0.96
	Ham, Chopped, Not Cnd	21.0000	1.000	Slice	3.60	3.62	0.00	48.09	0.00	0.00	10.71	1.20
	Ham, Chopped, Spiced, Cnd	21.0000	1.000	Slice	3.37	3.95	0.06	50.19	0.00	0.00	10.29	1.32
	Ham, Extra Lean, Appx 5% Fat	28.3500	1.000	Slice	5.49	1.41	0.27	37.14	0.00	0.00	13.32	0.46
	Ham, Minced	21.0000	1.000	Slice	3.42	4.34	0.39	55.23	0.00	0.00	14.70	1.51
	Hamburger Patty, Meatless	90.0000	1.000	Each	18.00	4.00	8.00	140.00	0.00	5.00	0.00	1.50
	Hot Dog, Beef	45.0000	1.000	Each	5.40	12.83	0.81	141.75	0.00	0.00	27.45	5.42
	Hot Dog, Chicken	28.3500	1.000	Ounce	3.67	5.52	1.92	72.86	0.00	0.00	28.63	1.57
	Hot Dog, Fat Free	50.0000	1.000	Each	7.00	0.00	2.00	40.00	0.00	0.00	15.00	0.00
	Hot Dog, Turkey	28.3500	1.000	Ounce	4.05	5.02	0.42	64.07	0.00	0.00	30.33	1.67
	Hummus, Fresh	15.0000	1.000	Tbsp	0.74	1.27	3.03	25.65	0.00	0.77	0.00	0.19
	Lamb, Ground, Ckd, Broiled	85.0000	3.000	Ounce	21.04	16.70	0.00	240.55	0.00	0.00	82.45	6.90
	Lamb, Leg, Shank, Meat and Fat,	85.0000	3.000	Ounce	22.45	10.58	0.00	191.25	0.00	0.00	76.50	4.33
	Lamb, Leg, Shank, Meat Only, Ckd	85.0000	3.000	Ounce	23.94	5.67	0.00	153.00	0.00	0.00	73.95	2.02
	Lamb, Leg, Sirloin, Meat and Fat	85.0000	3.000	Ounce	20.94	17.57	0.00	248.20	0.00	0.00	82.45	7.43
	Lamb, Leg, Sirloin, Meat Only, C	85.0000	3.000	Ounce	24.10	7.79	0.00	173.40	0.00	0.00	78.20	2.79
	Lamb, Leg, Whole, Meat and Fat,	85.0000	3.000	Ounce	21.72	14.01	0.00	219.30	0.00	0.00	79.05	5.86
	Lamb, Leg, Whole, Meat Only, Ckd	85.0000	3.000	Ounce	24.06	6.58	0.00	162.35	0.00	0.00	75.65	2.35
	Lamb, Loin, Meat and Fat, Ckd, B	64.0000	3.000	Ounce	16.11	14.77	0.00	202.24	0.00	0.00	64.00	6.29
	Lamb, Loin, Meat and Fat, Ckd, R	85.0000	3.000	Ounce	19.17	20.05	0.00	262.65	0.00	0.00	80.75	8.70
	Lamb, Loin, Meat Only, Ckd, Broi	46.0000	3.000	Ounce	13.80	4.48	0.00	99.36	0.00	0.00	43.70	1.60
	Lamb, Loin, Meat Only, Ckd, Roas	85.0000	3.000	Ounce	22.60	8.30	0.00	171.70	0.00	0.00	73.95	3.16
	Lamb, Meat and Fat, Ckd	85.0000	3.000	Ounce	20.84	17.80	0.00	249.90	0.00	0.00	82.45	7.51

Page Key: A2 = Baby Food   A2 = Baked Goods   A8 = Beverages   A14 = Breads/Grains and Pasta   A18 = Breakfast Foods/Cereals   A26 = Dairy and Eggs   A40 = Fats and Oils
A42 = Fruits and Vegetables   A52 = Meats and Beans   A60 = Nuts and Seeds   A62 5 Frozen Entrees and Packaged Foods   A76 = Restaurant Chains–Fast Foods
A92 = Restaurant Chains–Other   A106 = Seafood and Fish   A110 = Snacks and Sweets   A120 = Soups   A122 = Supplements   A126 = Toppings and Sauces

Monounsaturated Fat (g)	Polyunsaturated Fat (g)	Vitamin D (mg)	Vitamin K (mg)	Vitamin E (mg)	Vitamin A (re)	Vitamin C (mg)	Thiamin (mg)	Riboflavin (mg)	Niacin (mg)	Vitamin B6 (mg)	Folate (mcg)	Vitamin B12 (mcg)	Calcium (mg)	Iron (mg)	Magnesium (mg)	Phosphorus (mg)	Potassium (mg)	Sodium (mg)	Zinc (mg)
3.78	2.15	0.00	0.00	0.20	27.00	0.00	0.04	0.14	3.44	0.14	4.50	0.15	8.25	1.01	15.00	104.25	132.00	54.75	1.82
1.92	1.24	0.00	0.00	0.00	11.20	0.00	0.04	0.14	3.75	0.22	5.04	0.19	7.28	0.78	14.00	108.08	142.24	53.76	1.67
1.74	1.12	0.00	0.00	0.15	10.83	0.00	0.05	0.13	3.60	0.21	4.56	0.18	6.84	0.75	13.68	104.31	137.94	51.87	1.63
1.76	1.13	0.00	0.00	0.16	10.80	0.00	0.04	0.13	2.88	0.13	4.80	0.14	6.60	0.84	12.60	89.40	114.00	46.80	1.67
0.08	0.05	0.00	0.00	0.09	294.78	0.95	0.01	0.11	0.27	0.03	46.20	1.16	0.84	0.51	1.26	18.72	8.40	3.06	0.26
4.69	3.01	0.00	0.00	0.64	25.20	0.00	0.13	0.28	13.52	0.67	9.80	0.48	23.80	1.89	37.80	287.00	359.80	127.40	3.14
0.23	0.15	0.00	0.00	0.02	1.39	0.00	0.01	0.02	0.80	0.04	0.52	0.03	1.31	0.11	2.18	16.97	21.14	7.48	0.18
0.21	0.13	0.00	0.00	0.02	1.31	0.00	0.00	0.01	0.53	0.02	0.52	0.02	1.22	0.10	1.83	13.05	15.66	6.09	0.17
3.48	2.03	0.00	0.00	0.00	15.08	0.00	0.06	0.12	2.97	0.14	9.88	0.15	9.36	0.75	10.92	80.60	99.84	149.76	1.06
2.23	1.30	0.00	0.00	0.00	11.02	0.00	0.03	0.09	2.64	0.13	4.56	0.11	5.32	0.57	9.50	71.06	90.06	33.44	0.96
2.28	1.27	0.00	0.00	0.10	17.76	0.00	0.03	0.08	2.36	0.11	2.59	0.11	4.44	0.50	8.14	64.38	82.14	31.08	0.87
2.39	1.33	0.00	0.00	0.11	18.04	0.00	0.02	0.08	2.00	0.07	2.46	0.10	4.51	0.56	7.79	56.99	69.70	29.11	0.92
1.18	0.75	0.00	0.00	0.00	6.51	0.00	0.03	0.08	2.21	0.12	2.79	0.10	4.03	0.45	8.06	61.69	80.29	29.45	0.86
1.29	0.77	0.00	0.00	0.08	6.20	0.00	0.02	0.07	2.02	0.11	2.48	0.10	3.72	0.41	7.44	56.73	73.78	27.28	0.80
1.22	0.74	0.00	0.00	0.09	6.27	0.00	0.02	0.07	1.72	0.07	2.31	0.07	3.63	0.47	6.93	49.17	60.39	24.75	0.85
2.60	1.47	0.00	0.00	0.00	9.86	0.00	0.03	0.04	1.53	0.09	5.22	0.07	5.80	0.37	4.64	35.09	40.02	92.80	0.40
1.69	0.94	0.00	0.00	0.00	7.22	0.00	0.01	0.03	1.27	0.08	1.14	0.05	2.85	0.24	3.61	28.50	33.63	14.63	0.33
1.60	0.87	0.00	0.00	0.06	9.87	0.00	0.01	0.03	1.40	0.09	0.63	0.06	3.15	0.27	3.99	31.71	38.64	17.22	0.38
1.58	0.86	0.00	0.00	0.06	9.60	0.00	0.01	0.02	1.11	0.05	0.72	0.04	2.88	0.27	3.84	29.04	33.36	16.08	0.39
0.37	0.25	0.00	0.00	0.00	2.16	0.00	0.01	0.02	0.87	0.07	0.48	0.04	1.80	0.14	2.52	19.68	24.96	10.92	0.25
0.34	0.23	0.00	0.00	0.0<	2.34	0.00	0.01	0.02	0.95	0.08	0.52	0.04	2.08	0.15	2.73	21.58	27.30	11.96	0.28
0.32	0.22	0.00	0.00	0.04	2.24	0.00	0.01	0.02	0.73	0.04	0.42	0.03	1.82	0.16	2.52	18.76	21.42	10.22	0.28
5.95	0.92	0.00	0.00	1.87	86.70	4.34	0.12	0.27	0.91	0.34	57.89	0.00	119.85	8.75	114.75	392.70	930.75	1331.10	5.10
1.36	1.03	0.00	0.00	0.29	22.00	0.66	0.08	0.25	6.90	0.39	2.20	0.33	14.30	0.85	20.90	163.90	275.00	69.30	1.68
18.06	5.11	0.00	0.00	0.98	88.20	0.00	0.24	0.38	6.76	0.25	8.40	0.42	15.40	3.78	22.40	218.40	285.60	82.60	2.60
3.70	1.43	0.00	0.00	0.70	23.00	0.00	0.26	0.47	5.10	0.25	10.00	0.40	12.00	2.70	20.00	203.00	252.00	65.00	2.60
0.00	1.00	0.00	0.00	0.00	0.00	0.00	0.00	0.00	4.00	0.00	0.00	0.00	96.00	2.00	0.00	0.00	0.00	380.00	8.00
2.63	0.62	0.31	0.00	0.08	6.52	0.00	0.17	0.05	0.98	0.07	0.85	0.23	16.44	0.26	4.54	71.73	83.35	380.74	0.57
1.06	0.21	0.00	0.00	0.00	13.65	0.00	0.05	0.03	0.32	0.02	0.45	0.11	32.55	0.11	2.70	74.25	24.30	179.55	0.34
1.08	0.41	0.00	0.00	0.26	0.00	0.00	0.07	0.02	0.32	0.02	0.15	0.11	1.20	0.09	1.50	18.00	22.50	136.80	0.17
1.40	0.34	0.00	0.00	0.08	0.00	0.00	0.24	0.07	1.49	0.10	0.85	0.24	1.98	0.28	5.39	70.02	94.12	373.37	0.61
1.72	0.44	0.00	0.00	0.00	0.00	0.00	0.13	0.04	0.81	0.07	0.21	0.19	1.47	0.17	3.36	32.55	66.99	287.91	0.41
1.93	0.43	0.00	0.00	0.05	0.00	0.42	0.11	0.04	0.67	0.07	0.21	0.15	1.47	0.20	2.73	29.19	59.64	286.65	0.38
0.67	0.14	0.00	0.00	0.08	0.00	0.00	0.26	0.06	1.37	0.13	1.13	0.21	1.98	0.22	4.82	61.80	99.22	405.12	0.55
2.01	0.52	0.00	0.00	0.00	0.00	0.00	0.15	0.04	0.87	0.05	0.21	0.20	2.10	0.17	3.36	32.97	65.31	261.45	0.40
0.00	0.50	0.00	0.00	0.00	0.00	0.00	0.25	0.00	4.00	0.00	0.00	0.00	96.00	1.50	0.00	0.00	0.00	380.00	7.50
6.13	0.62	0.41	0.00	0.09	0.00	0.00	0.02	0.05	1.09	0.05	1.80	0.69	9.00	0.64	1.35	39.15	74.70	461.70	0.98
2.40	1.15	0.00	0.00	0.06	10.77	0.00	0.02	0.03	0.88	0.09	1.13	0.07	26.93	0.57	2.84	30.33	23.81	388.40	0.29
0.00	0.00	0.00	0.00	0.00	0.00	0.00	0.00	0.00	0.00	0.00	0.00	0.00	0.00	0.20	0.00	0.00	0.00	460.00	0.00
1.58	1.42	0.00	0.00	0.18	0.00	0.00	0.01	0.05	1.17	0.07	2.27	0.08	30.05	0.52	3.97	37.99	50.75	404.27	0.88
0.53	0.48	0.00	0.00	0.15	0.30	1.19	0.01	0.01	0.06	0.06	8.91	0.00	7.50	0.24	4.35	16.80	26.10	36.60	0.17
7.07	1.19	0.00	0.00	0.21	0.00	0.00	0.09	0.21	5.70	0.12	16.15	2.22	18.70	1.52	20.40	170.85	288.15	68.85	3.97
4.50	0.75	0.00	0.00	0.14	0.00	0.00	0.09	0.23	5.57	0.14	18.70	2.27	8.50	1.68	21.25	168.30	277.10	55.25	3.96
2.48	0.37	0.00	0.00	0.15	0.00	0.00	0.09	0.24	5.43	0.14	20.40	2.30	6.80	1.75	22.10	176.80	290.70	56.10	4.27
7.40	1.27	0.00	0.00	0.11	0.00	0.00	0.09	0.24	5.63	0.12	14.45	2.15	9.35	1.70	18.70	155.55	255.85	57.80	3.51
3.42	0.51	0.00	0.00	0.14	0.00	0.00	0.10	0.26	5.33	0.14	17.85	2.19	6.80	1.87	21.25	172.55	283.05	60.35	4.12
5.92	1.00	0.00	0.00	0.13	0.00	0.00	0.09	0.23	5.60	0.13	17.00	2.20	9.35	1.68	20.40	162.35	266.05	56.10	3.74
2.88	0.43	0.00	0.00	0.15	0.00	0.00	0.09	0.24	5.39	0.14	19.55	2.24	6.80	1.80	22.10	175.10	287.30	57.80	4.20
6.21	1.08	0.00	0.00	0.08	0.00	0.00	0.06	0.16	4.54	0.08	11.52	1.58	12.80	1.16	15.36	125.44	209.28	49.28	2.23
8.23	1.59	0.00	0.00	0.09	0.00	0.00	0.09	0.20	6.04	0.09	16.15	1.88	15.30	1.80	19.55	153.00	209.10	54.40	2.90
1.96	0.29	0.00	0.00	0.07	0.00	0.00	0.05	0.13	3.15	0.07	11.04	1.16	8.74	0.92	12.88	103.96	172.96	38.64	1.90
3.36	0.73	0.00	0.00	0.14	0.00	0.00	0.09	0.23	5.81	0.14	21.25	1.84	14.45	2.07	22.95	175.10	226.95	56.10	3.45
7.50	1.28	0.00	0.00	0.12	0.00	0.00	0.09	0.21	5.66	0.11	15.30	2.17	14.45	1.60	19.55	159.80	263.50	61.20	3.79

USDA ID Code	Food Name	Weight in Grams*	Quantity of Units	Unit of Measure	Protein (g)	Fat (g)	Carbohydrate (g)	Kilocalories	Caffeine (g)	Fiber (g)	Cholesterol (mg)	Saturated Fat (g)
	Lamb, Meat Only, Ckd	85.0000	3.000	Ounce	23.99	8.09	0.00	175.10	0.00	0.00	78.20	2.89
	Lamb, Rib, Meat and Fat, Ckd, Br	85.0000	3.000	Ounce	18.81	25.15	0.00	306.85	0.00	0.00	84.15	10.80
	Lamb, Rib, Meat and Fat, Ckd, Ro	85.0000	3.000	Ounce	17.95	25.35	0.00	305.15	0.00	0.00	82.45	10.85
	Lamb, Rib, Meat Only, Ckd, Broil	85.0000	3.000	Ounce	23.58	11.01	0.00	199.75	0.00	0.00	77.35	3.95
	Lamb, Rib, Meat Only, Ckd, Roast	85.0000	3.000	Ounce	22.24	11.31	0.00	197.20	0.00	0.00	74.80	4.05
	Lunch Meat, Dutch Brand Loaf	28.3500	1.000	Slice	3.80	5.05	1.58	68.04	0.00	0.00	13.32	1.80
	Lunch Meat, Honey Loaf	28.3500	1.000	Slice	4.47	1.27	1.51	36.29	0.00	0.00	9.64	0.41
	Lunch Meat, Olive Loaf	28.3500	1.000	Slice	3.36	4.68	2.60	66.62	0.00	0.00	10.77	1.66
	Lunch Meat, Olive Loaf, Pork	28.3500	1.000	Slice	3.35	4.68	2.61	66.62	0.00	0.00	10.77	1.66
	Lunch Meat, Pickle and Pimento L	28.3500	1.000	Slice	3.26	5.98	1.67	74.28	0.00	0.00	10.49	2.23
	Lunch Meat, Pickle and Pimiento	28.3500	1.000	Slice	3.26	5.98	1.67	74.28	0.00	0.00	10.49	2.22
	Lunch Meat, Picnic Loaf	28.3500	1.000	Slice	4.23	4.72	1.35	65.77	0.00	0.00	10.77	1.72
	Pastrami, Beef, Cured	28.3500	1.000	Slice	4.89	8.27	0.86	98.94	0.00	0.00	26.37	2.95
	Pastrami, Turkey	28.3500	1.000	Slice	5.21	1.76	0.47	39.97	0.00	0.00	15.31	0.51
	Pork, Backribs	85.0000	3.000	Ounce	20.62	25.14	0.00	314.50	0.00	0.00	100.30	9.34
	Pork, Braunschweiger	28.3500	3.000	Ounce	3.83	9.10	0.89	101.78	0.00	0.00	44.23	3.09
	Pork, Cnd, Lunch Meat	21.0000	1.000	Slice	2.63	6.36	0.44	70.14	0.00	0.00	13.02	2.27
	Pork, Ground, Ckd	85.0000	3.000	Ounce	21.84	17.65	0.00	252.45	0.00	0.00	79.90	6.56
	Pork, Ham and Cheese Loaf or Rol	28.3500	3.000	Ounce	4.71	5.73	0.41	73.43	0.00	0.00	16.16	2.13
	Pork, Ham Patties, Grilled	59.5000	3.000	Ounce	7.91	18.36	1.01	203.49	0.00	0.00	42.84	6.60
	Pork, Ham Salad Spread	28.3500	3.000	Ounce	2.46	4.40	3.02	61.24	0.00	0.00	10.49	1.43
	Pork, Ham, Chopped, Cnd	28.3500	3.000	Ounce	4.55	5.34	0.08	67.76	0.00	0.00	13.89	1.78
	Pork, Ham, Cnd, Extra Lean (appx	85.0000	3.000	Ounce	17.99	4.15	0.44	115.60	0.00	0.00	25.50	1.36
	Pork, Ham, Cnd, Extra Lean and R	85.0000	3.000	Ounce	17.80	7.17	0.42	141.95	0.00	0.00	34.85	2.39
	Pork, Ham, Cnd, Extra Lean and R	28.3500	1.000	Ounce	5.09	2.11	0.00	40.82	0.00	0.00	10.77	0.69
	Pork, Ham, Cnd, Regular (approx	85.0000	3.000	Ounce	17.45	12.92	0.36	192.10	0.00	0.00	52.70	4.28
	Pork, Ham, Extra Lean (5% Fat),	85.0000	3.000	Ounce	17.79	4.70	1.28	123.25	0.00	0.00	45.05	1.54
	Pork, Ham, Extra Lean (5% Fat),	28.3500	3.000	Ounce	5.49	1.41	0.27	37.14	0.00	0.00	13.32	0.46
	Pork, Ham, Extra Lean and Reg, R	85.0000	3.000	Ounce	18.67	6.51	0.43	140.25	0.00	0.00	48.45	2.22
	Pork, Ham, Extra Lean and Reg, U	28.3500	1.000	Slice	5.18	2.38	0.65	45.93	0.00	0.00	15.03	0.77
	Pork, Ham, Meat and Fat, Roasted	85.0000	3.000	Ounce	18.33	14.25	0.00	206.55	0.00	0.00	52.70	5.08
	Pork, Ham, Meat Only, Roasted	85.0000	3.000	Ounce	21.29	4.68	0.00	133.45	0.00	0.00	46.75	1.56
	Pork, Ham, Regular (11% Fat), Ro	85.0000	3.000	Ounce	19.23	7.67	0.00	151.30	0.00	0.00	50.15	2.65
	Pork, Ham, Regular (11% Fat), Un	28.3500	3.000	Ounce	4.98	3.00	0.88	51.60	0.00	0.00	16.16	0.96
	Pork, Spareribs, Meat and Fat, C	85.0000	3.000	Ounce	24.70	25.76	0.00	337.45	0.00	0.00	102.85	9.45
	Pork, Tenderloin, Meat and Fat,	76.0000	3.000	Ounce	22.69	6.16	0.00	152.76	0.00	0.00	71.44	2.23
	Pork, Tenderloin, Meat Only, Ckd	73.0000	3.000	Ounce	22.21	4.62	0.00	136.51	0.00	0.00	68.62	1.64
	Salami, Turkey	28.3500	1.000	Slice	4.64	3.91	0.16	55.57	0.00	0.00	23.25	1.14
	Sausage, Beerwurst, Pork	6.0000	1.000	Slice	0.85	1.13	0.12	14.28	0.00	0.00	3.54	0.38
	Sausage, Bockwurst	28.3500	1.000	Ounce	3.78	7.82	0.14	87.03	0.00	0.00	16.73	2.87
	Sausage, Bratwurst	28.3500	1.000	Ounce	3.99	7.33	0.59	85.33	0.00	0.00	17.01	2.64
	Sausage, Italian, Ckd	67.0000	1.000	Link	13.42	17.22	1.01	216.41	0.00	0.00	52.26	6.08
	Sausage, Kielbasa, Kolbassy	26.0000	1.000	Slice	3.45	7.06	0.56	80.60	0.00	0.00	17.42	2.58
	Sausage, Knockwurst	28.3500	1.000	Ounce	3.37	7.87	0.50	87.32	0.00	0.00	16.44	2.89
	Sausage, Link, Pork and Beef	16.0000	1.000	Small	2.14	4.85	0.23	53.76	0.00	0.00	11.36	1.70
	Sausage, Pepperoni	5.5000	1.000	Slice	1.15	2.42	0.16	27.34	0.00	0.00	4.35	0.89
	Sausage, Polish-style	28.3500	1.000	Ounce	4.00	8.14	0.46	92.42	0.00	0.00	19.85	2.93
	Sausage, Pork, Links or Bulk, Ck	13.0000	1.000	Link	2.55	4.05	0.13	47.97	0.00	0.00	10.79	1.41
	Sausage, Pork, Smoked Link, Gril	28.3500	3.000	Ounce	6.29	9.00	0.60	110.28	0.00	0.00	19.28	3.21
	Sausage, Salami, Beef and Pork,	10.0000	1.000	Slice	2.29	3.44	0.26	41.80	0.00	0.00	7.90	1.22
	Sausage, Salami, Beef, Ckd	23.0000	1.000	Slice	3.46	4.76	0.65	60.26	0.00	0.00	14.95	2.07
	Sausage, Smoked Link, Pork	16.0000	1.000	Small	3.55	5.07	0.34	62.24	0.00	0.00	10.88	1.81
	Sausage, Smoked, Beef, Cured,	28.3500	1.000	Ounce	4.00	7.63	0.69	88.45	0.00	0.00	18.99	3.24

Page Key: A2 = Baby Food   A2 = Baked Goods   A8 = Beverages   A14 = Breads/Grains and Pasta   A18 = Breakfast Foods/Cereals   A26 = Dairy and Eggs   A40 = Fats and Oils
A42 = Fruits and Vegetables   A52 = Meats and Beans   A60 = Nuts and Seeds   A62 5 Frozen Entrees and Packaged Foods   A76 = Restaurant Chains–Fast Foods
A92 = Restaurant Chains–Other   A106 = Seafood and Fish   A110 = Snacks and Sweets   A120 = Soups   A122 = Supplements   A126 = Toppings and Sauces

Monounsaturated Fat (g)	Polyunsaturated Fat (g)	Vitamin D (mg)	Vitamin K (mg)	Vitamin E (mg)	Vitamin A (re)	Vitamin C (mg)	Thiamin (mg)	Riboflavin (mg)	Niacin (mg)	Vitamin B₆ (mg)	Folate (mcg)	Vitamin B₁₂ (mcg)	Calcium (mg)	Iron (mg)	Magnesium (mg)	Phosphorus (mg)	Potassium (mg)	Sodium (mg)	Zinc (mg)
3.54	0.53	0.00	0.00	0.16	0.00	0.00	0.09	0.24	5.37	0.14	19.55	2.22	12.75	1.74	22.10	178.50	292.40	64.60	4.48
10.30	2.01	0.00	0.00	0.10	0.00	0.00	0.08	0.19	5.95	0.09	11.90	2.16	16.15	1.60	19.55	151.30	229.50	64.60	3.40
10.64	1.84	0.00	0.00	0.09	0.00	0.00	0.08	0.18	5.74	0.09	12.75	1.90	18.70	1.36	17.00	141.10	230.35	62.05	2.97
4.43	1.00	0.00	0.00	0.15	0.00	0.00	0.09	0.21	5.57	0.13	17.85	2.24	13.60	1.88	24.65	181.05	266.05	72.25	4.48
4.96	0.74	0.00	0.00	0.13	0.00	0.00	0.08	0.20	5.24	0.13	18.70	1.84	17.85	1.50	19.55	165.75	267.75	68.85	3.80
2.36	0.54	0.28	0.00	0.06	0.00	0.00	0.09	0.08	0.68	0.07	0.57	0.37	23.81	0.35	5.95	45.93	106.60	354.38	0.49
0.57	0.13	0.26	0.00	0.06	0.00	0.00	0.14	0.07	0.89	0.09	2.27	0.31	4.82	0.38	4.82	40.54	97.24	374.22	0.69
2.23	0.55	0.00	0.00	0.00	5.67	2.49	0.08	0.07	0.52	0.07	0.57	0.36	30.90	0.15	5.39	36.00	84.20	420.71	0.39
2.23	0.55	0.31	0.00	0.07	5.67	0.00	0.09	0.07	0.52	0.07	0.57	0.36	30.90	0.15	5.39	36.00	84.20	420.71	0.39
2.72	0.73	0.00	0.00	0.00	1.98	3.83	0.08	0.07	0.58	0.05	1.42	0.33	26.93	0.29	5.10	39.69	96.39	393.78	0.40
2.72	0.73	0.31	0.00	0.07	1.98	0.00	0.08	0.07	0.58	0.05	1.42	0.33	26.93	0.29	5.10	39.69	96.39	393.78	0.40
2.18	0.54	0.34	0.00	0.00	0.00	0.00	0.10	0.07	0.65	0.09	0.57	0.43	13.32	0.29	4.25	35.44	75.69	329.99	0.62
4.10	0.28	0.00	0.00	0.07	0.00	0.00	0.03	0.05	1.44	0.05	1.98	0.50	2.55	0.54	5.10	42.53	64.64	347.85	1.21
0.58	0.45	0.00	0.00	0.06	0.00	0.00	0.02	0.07	1.00	0.08	1.42	0.07	2.55	0.47	3.97	56.70	73.71	296.26	0.61
11.44	1.97	0.00	0.00	0.00	2.55	0.26	0.37	0.17	3.02	0.26	2.55	0.54	38.25	1.17	17.85	165.75	267.75	85.85	2.86
4.23	1.06	0.00	0.00	0.00	1196.37	2.72	0.07	0.43	2.37	0.09	12.47	5.70	2.55	2.65	3.12	47.63	56.42	324.04	0.80
3.00	0.75	0.00	0.00	0.05	0.00	0.21	0.08	0.04	0.66	0.04	1.26	0.19	1.26	0.15	2.10	17.22	45.15	270.69	0.31
7.86	1.59	0.00	0.00	0.22	1.70	0.60	0.60	0.19	3.58	0.33	5.10	0.46	18.70	1.10	20.40	192.10	307.70	62.05	2.73
2.63	0.62	0.00	0.00	0.00	6.52	7.12	0.17	0.05	0.98	0.07	0.85	0.23	16.44	0.26	4.54	71.73	83.35	380.74	0.57
8.73	1.98	0.00	0.00	0.15	0.00	0.00	0.21	0.11	1.93	0.10	1.79	0.42	5.36	0.96	5.95	60.10	145.18	632.49	1.13
2.04	0.77	0.00	0.00	0.00	0.00	1.70	0.12	0.03	0.59	0.04	0.28	0.22	2.27	0.17	2.84	34.02	42.53	258.55	0.31
2.60	0.58	0.00	0.00	0.00	0.00	0.51	0.15	0.05	0.91	0.09	0.28	0.20	1.98	0.27	3.69	39.41	80.51	386.98	0.52
2.12	0.37	0.00	0.00	0.22	0.00	0.00	0.88	0.21	4.16	0.38	4.25	0.60	5.10	0.78	17.85	177.65	295.80	964.75	1.90
3.45	0.77	0.00	0.00	0.22	0.00	0.00	0.82	0.21	4.28	0.34	4.25	0.71	5.95	0.91	17.00	187.85	298.35	907.80	1.97
1.01	0.22	0.00	0.00	0.07	0.00	0.00	0.25	0.07	1.30	0.13	1.70	0.23	1.70	0.26	4.54	58.68	94.69	361.75	0.52
6.01	1.51	0.00	0.00	0.00	0.00	11.90	0.70	0.22	4.51	0.26	4.25	0.90	6.80	1.16	14.45	206.55	303.45	799.85	2.13
2.23	0.46	0.00	0.00	0.22	0.00	0.00	0.64	0.17	3.42	0.34	2.55	0.55	6.80	1.26	11.90	166.60	243.95	1022.55	2.45
0.67	0.14	0.00	0.00	0.07	0.00	7.46	0.26	0.06	1.37	0.13	1.13	0.21	1.98	0.22	4.82	61.80	99.23	405.12	0.55
3.18	0.91	0.00	0.00	0.22	0.00	0.00	0.63	0.24	4.52	0.30	2.55	0.58	6.80	1.19	16.15	210.80	307.70	1177.25	2.24
1.12	0.26	0.00	0.00	0.07	0.00	0.00	0.25	0.07	1.44	0.11	0.85	0.23	1.98	0.26	5.10	66.91	84.20	362.31	0.58
6.70	1.54	0.00	0.00	0.22	0.00	0.00	0.51	0.19	3.79	0.32	2.55	0.54	5.95	0.74	16.15	181.90	243.10	1008.95	1.97
2.15	0.54	0.00	0.00	0.22	0.00	0.00	0.58	0.21	4.27	0.40	3.40	0.60	5.95	0.80	18.70	192.95	268.60	1127.95	2.18
3.77	1.20	0.00	0.00	0.22	0.00	0.00	0.62	0.28	5.23	0.26	2.55	0.60	6.80	1.14	18.70	238.85	347.65	1275.00	2.10
1.40	0.34	0.00	0.00	0.07	0.00	7.85	0.24	0.07	1.49	0.10	0.85	0.24	1.98	0.28	5.39	70.02	94.12	373.37	0.61
11.46	2.32	0.00	0.00	0.22	2.55	0.00	0.35	0.32	4.66	0.30	3.40	0.92	39.95	1.57	20.40	221.85	272.00	79.05	3.91
2.54	0.56	0.00	0.00	0.00	1.52	0.76	0.74	0.29	3.84	0.40	4.56	0.74	3.80	1.06	26.60	220.40	337.44	48.64	2.20
1.88	0.41	0.00	0.00	0.00	1.46	0.73	0.72	0.28	3.75	0.39	4.38	0.73	3.65	1.04	26.28	215.35	329.23	47.45	2.15
1.29	1.00	0.00	0.00	0.00		0.00	0.02	0.05	1.00	0.07	1.13	0.06	5.67	0.46	4.25	30.05	69.17	284.63	0.51
0.54	0.14	0.05	0.00	0.00	0.00	0.00	0.03	0.01	0.20	0.02	0.18	0.05	0.48	0.05	0.78	6.18	15.18	74.40	0.10
3.69	0.84	0.00	0.00	0.04	1.70	0.00	0.12	0.05	1.17	0.07	1.70	0.23	4.54	0.18	5.10	41.39	76.55	313.27	0.44
3.46	0.78	0.31	0.00	0.07	0.00	0.28	0.14	0.05	0.91	0.06	0.57	0.27	12.47	0.37	4.25	42.24	60.10	157.91	0.65
8.01	2.20	0.00	0.00	0.17	0.00	1.34	0.42	0.15	2.79	0.22	3.35	0.87	16.08	1.01	12.06	113.90	203.68	617.74	1.60
3.36	0.80	0.00	0.00	0.06	0.00	0.00	0.06	0.05	0.75	0.05	1.30	0.42	11.44	0.38	4.16	38.48	70.46	279.76	0.53
3.63	0.83	0.00	0.00	0.16	0.00	0.00	0.10	0.04	0.77	0.05	0.57	0.33	3.12	0.26	3.12	27.78	56.42	286.34	0.47
2.27	0.52	0.20	0.00	0.04	0.00	0.00	0.04	0.03	0.52	0.03	0.32	0.24	1.60	0.23	1.92	17.12	30.24	151.20	0.34
1.16	0.24	0.00	0.00	0.01	0.00	0.00	0.02	0.01	0.27	0.01	0.22	0.14	0.55	0.08	0.88	6.55	19.09	112.20	0.14
3.83	0.87	0.00	0.00	0.00		0.28	0.14	0.04	0.98	0.05	0.57	0.28	3.40	0.41	3.97	38.56	67.19	248.35	0.55
1.81	0.50	0.00	0.00	0.02		0.26	0.10	0.03	0.59	0.04	0.26	0.22	4.16	0.21	3.04	23.92	46.93	168.22	0.33
4.15	1.07	0.00	0.00	0.09		0.51	0.20	0.07	1.28	0.10	1.42	0.46	8.51	0.33	5.39	45.93	95.26	425.25	0.80
1.71	0.32	0.00	0.00	0.03			0.06	0.03	0.49	0.05	0.20	0.19	0.80	0.15	1.70	14.20	37.80	186.00	0.32
2.17	0.24	0.28	0.00	0.04	0.00	0.00	0.02	0.04	0.75	0.04	0.46	0.70	2.07	0.50	3.22	25.99	51.52	270.48	0.50
2.34	0.60	0.00	0.00	0.04	0.00	0.32	0.11	0.04	0.72	0.06	0.80	0.26	4.80	0.19	3.04	25.92	53.76	240.00	0.45
3.68	0.30	0.00	0.00	0.00		0.00	0.01	0.04	0.90	0.03	1.13	0.53	1.98	0.50	3.69	29.77	49.90	320.64	0.79

USDA ID Code	Food Name	Weight in Grams*	Quantity of Units	Unit of Measure	Protein (g)	Fat (g)	Carbohydrate (g)	Kilocalories	Caffeine (g)	Fiber (g)	Cholesterol (mg)	Saturated Fat (g)
	Sausage, Turkey	28.3500	3.000	Ounce	4.00	2.50	1.50	45.00	0.00	0.00	15.00	1.25
743	Tofu Pups-Light Life	42.0000	1.000	Each	8.00	2.50	2.00	60.00	0.00	0.00	0.00	1.00
744	Tofu Rella, Garlic Herb	28.0000	1.000	Ounce	6.00	5.00	3.00	80.00	0.00	0.00	0.00	1.00
745	Tofu Rella, Monterey Style	28.0000	1.000	Ounce	6.00	5.00	3.00	80.00	0.00	0.00	0.00	1.00
746	Tofu Wieners-Yves	38.0000	1.000	Each	9.00	0.50	2.00	45.00	0.00	0.00	0.00	0.00
	Turkey Breast Meat	21.0000	1.000	Slice	4.73	0.33	0.00	23.10	0.00	0.00	8.61	0.10
	Turkey Burger, Breaded, Battered	28.0000	3.000	Ounce	3.92	5.04	4.40	79.24	0.00	0.14	17.36	1.31
749	Turkey Burger, Grilled	82.0000	3.000	Ounce	22.44	10.78	0.00	192.70	0.00	0.00	83.64	2.78
	Turkey Lunch Meat	28.3500	1.000	Slice	5.37	1.44	0.10	36.29	0.00	0.00	15.88	0.48
	Turkey Roast, Roasted	135.0000	1.000	Cup	28.78	7.80	4.14	209.25	0.00	0.00	71.55	2.57
	Turkey Roll, Light and Dark Meat	28.3500	3.000	Ounce	5.14	1.98	0.60	42.24	0.00	0.00	15.59	0.58
	Turkey Roll, Light Meat	28.3500	3.000	Ounce	5.30	2.05	0.15	41.67	0.00	0.00	12.19	0.57
	Turkey Sticks, Breaded, Battered	64.0000	2.250	Ounce	9.09	10.82	10.88	178.56	0.00	0.00	40.96	2.80
	Turkey Thigh, Prebasted, Meat &	314.0000	3.000	Ounce	59.03	26.82	0.00	492.98	0.00	0.00	194.68	8.32
	Turkey, Back, Meat & Skin, Ckd,	34.0000	3.000	Ounce	9.04	4.89	0.00	82.62	0.00	0.00	30.94	1.42
	Turkey, Breast, Meat & Skin, Ckd	112.0000	3.000	Ounce	32.16	8.30	0.00	211.68	0.00	0.00	82.88	2.35
	Turkey, Ckd, Roasted, Meat & Ski	260.0000	3.000	Ounce	72.75	24.57	0.18	533.00	0.00	0.00	247.00	7.20
	Turkey, Dark Meat, Ckd, Roasted	91.0000	3.000	Ounce	26.00	6.57	0.00	170.17	0.00	0.00	77.35	2.20
	Turkey, Dark Meat, Meat & Skin,	104.0000	3.000	Ounce	28.59	12.00	0.00	229.84	0.00	0.00	92.56	3.63
	Turkey, Giblets, Ckd, Simmered,	10.0000	3.000	Ounce	2.66	0.51	0.21	16.70	0.00	0.00	41.80	0.15
	Turkey, Ground, Ckd	82.0000	3.000	Ounce	22.44	10.78	0.00	192.70	0.00	0.00	83.64	2.78
	Turkey, Leg, Meat & Skin, Ckd, R	71.0000	3.000	Ounce	19.79	6.97	0.00	147.68	0.00	0.00	60.35	2.17
	Turkey, Light Meat, Ckd, Roasted	117.0000	3.000	Ounce	34.98	3.77	0.00	183.69	0.00	0.00	80.73	1.21
	Turkey, Light Meat, Meat & Skin,	136.0000	3.000	Ounce	38.86	11.33	0.00	267.92	0.00	0.00	103.36	3.18
	Turkey, Meat & Skin, Ckd, Roaste	140.0000	1.000	Cup	39.34	13.62	0.00	291.20	0.00	0.00	114.80	3.98
	Turkey, Meat Only, Ckd, Roasted	140.0000	1.000	Cup	41.05	6.96	0.00	238.00	0.00	0.00	106.40	2.30
	Turkey, Thin Sliced	28.3500	3.000	Ounce	6.38	0.45	0.00	31.19	0.00	0.00	11.62	0.14
	Turkey, Wing, Meat & Skin, Ckd,	24.0000	3.000	Ounce	6.57	2.98	0.00	54.96	0.00	0.00	19.44	0.81
	Veal, Meat and Fat, Ckd	85.0000	3.000	Ounce	25.59	9.68	0.00	196.35	0.00	0.00	96.90	3.64
	Veal, Meat Only, Ckd	85.0000	3.000	Ounce	27.12	5.59	0.00	166.60	0.00	0.00	100.30	1.56
	Venison, Ckd, Roasted	85.0000	3.000	Ounce	25.68	2.71	0.00	134.30	0.00	0.00	95.20	1.06
Nuts and Seeds												
	Alfalfa Seeds, Sprouted, Fresh	3.0000	1.000	Tbsp	0.12	0.02	0.11	0.87	0.00	0.08	0.00	0.00
	Almond Butter, w/ salt	16.0000	1.000	Tbsp	2.43	9.46	3.40	101.28	0.00	0.59	0.00	0.90
	Almond Butter, w/o salt	16.0000	1.000	Tbsp	2.43	9.46	3.40	101.28	0.00	0.59	0.00	0.90
	Almonds, Toasted, Unblanched	141.9600	0.500	Cup	28.93	72.07	32.52	836.14	0.00	15.90	0.00	6.83
	Brazil Nuts, Dried, Unblanched	28.3500	1.000	Ounce	4.07	18.77	3.63	185.98	0.00	1.53	0.00	4.58
	Cashews, Dry Roasted	28.3500	1.000	Ounce	4.34	13.14	9.27	162.73	0.00	0.85	0.00	2.60
	Cashews, Oil Roasted	28.3500	1.000	Ounce	4.58	13.67	8.09	163.30	0.00	1.08	0.00	2.70
467	Hazelnuts, Dry Roasted	28.0000	1.000	Ounce	2.80	18.80	5.10	188.00	0.00	2.00	0.00	1.40
468	Hazelnuts, Oil Roasted	28.0000	1.000	Ounce	4.00	18.00	5.40	187.00	0.00	1.80	0.00	1.30
	Macadamias, Dried	28.3500	1.000	Ounce	2.24	21.48	3.92	203.55	0.00	2.44	0.00	3.42
	Macadamias, Oil Roasted	112.0000	0.500	Cup	9.60	83.60	15.60	769.00	0.00	10.40	0.00	13.60
	Peanut Butter, Chunk Style, w/ S	32.0000	2.000	Tbsp	7.70	15.98	6.91	188.48	0.00	2.11	0.00	3.07
	Peanut Butter, Chunk Style, w/o	32.0000	2.000	Tbsp	7.70	15.98	6.91	188.48	0.00	2.11	0.00	3.07
	Peanut Butter, Reduced Fat, Crea	18.0000	2.000	Tbsp	4.00	6.00	7.50	95.00	0.00	1.00	0.00	1.25
638	Peanut Butter, Reduced Fat, Crun	18.0000	2.000	Tbsp	4.00	6.00	7.50	95.00	0.00	1.00	0.00	1.25
	Peanut Butter, Smooth Style, w/	32.0000	2.000	Tbsp	8.07	16.33	6.17	189.76	0.00	1.89	0.00	3.31
	Peanut Butter, Smooth Style, w/o	32.0000	2.000	Tbsp	8.07	16.33	6.17	189.76	0.00	1.89	0.00	3.31
	Peanut Kernels, Oil Roasted	112.0000	0.500	Cup	37.94	70.99	27.26	836.64	0.00	12.67	0.00	9.85
	Peanuts, All Types, Ckd, Boiled,	28.0000	33.000	Each	3.78	6.16	5.95	89.04	0.00	2.46	0.00	0.86
	Peanuts, All Types, Dry-roasted,	1.0000	1.000	Each	0.24	0.50	0.22	5.85	0.00	0.08	0.00	0.07
	Peanuts, All Types, Dry-roasted,	1.0000	1.000	Each	0.24	0.50	0.22	5.85	0.00	0.08	0.00	0.07

Monounsaturated Fat (g)	Polyunsaturated Fat (g)	Vitamin D (mg)	Vitamin K (mg)	Vitamin E (mg)	Vitamin A (re)	Vitamin C (mg)	Thiamin (mg)	Riboflavin (mg)	Niacin (mg)	Vitamin B₆ (mg)	Folate (mcg)	Vitamin B₁₂ (mcg)	Calcium (mg)	Iron (mg)	Magnesium (mg)	Phosphorus (mg)	Potassium (mg)	Sodium (mg)	Zinc (mg)
0.00	0.00	0.00	0.00	0.00	10.00	6.00	0.00	0.00	0.00	0.00	0.00	0.00	12.00	1.75	0.00	0.00	0.00	300.00	0.00
0.00	0.00	0.00	0.00	0.00	0.00	0.00	0.00	0.00	0.00	0.00	0.00	0.00	0.00	0.00	0.00	0.00	0.00	140.00	0.00
0.00	0.00	0.00	0.00	0.00	0.00	0.00	0.00	0.00	0.00	0.00	0.00	0.00	0.00	0.00	0.00	0.00	0.00	280.00	0.00
0.00	0.00	0.00	0.00	0.00	0.00	0.00	0.00	0.00	0.00	0.00	0.00	0.00	0.00	0.00	0.00	0.00	0.00	280.00	0.00
0.00	0.00	0.00	0.00	0.00	0.00	0.00	0.00	0.00	0.00	0.00	0.00	0.00	0.00	0.00	0.00	0.00	0.00	240.00	0.00
0.09	0.06	0.00	0.00	0.02	0.00	0.00	0.01	0.02	1.75	0.08	0.84	0.42	1.47	0.08	4.20	48.09	58.38	300.51	0.24
2.09	1.32	0.00	0.00	0.67	3.08	0.00	0.03	0.05	0.64	0.06	7.84	0.06	3.92	0.62	4.20	75.60	77.00	224.00	0.40
4.01	2.65	0.00	0.00	0.28	0.00	0.00	0.04	0.14	3.95	0.32	5.74	0.27	20.50	1.58	19.68	160.72	221.40	87.74	2.35
0.33	0.43	0.00	0.00	0.18	0.00	0.00	0.01	0.07	1.00	0.07	1.70	0.07	2.84	0.78	4.54	54.15	92.14	282.37	0.83
1.62	2.24	0.00	0.00	0.51	0.00	0.00	0.07	0.22	8.46	0.36	6.75	2.05	6.75	2.20	29.70	329.40	402.30	918.00	3.43
0.65	0.50	0.00	0.00	0.10	0.00	0.00	0.03	0.08	1.36	0.08	1.42	0.07	9.07	0.38	5.10	47.63	76.55	166.13	0.57
0.71	0.49	0.00	0.00	0.00	0.00	0.00	0.03	0.06	1.98	0.09	1.13	0.00	11.34	0.36	4.54	51.88	71.16	138.63	0.44
4.43	2.81	0.00	0.00	0.00	7.68	0.00	0.06	0.12	1.34	0.13	18.56	0.15	8.96	1.41	9.60	149.76	166.40	536.32	0.93
7.94	7.38	0.00	0.00	0.00	0.00	0.00	0.25	0.82	7.57	0.72	18.84	0.75	25.12	4.74	53.38	536.94	756.74	1372.18	12.94
1.70	1.26	0.00	0.00	0.20	0.00	0.00	0.02	0.07	1.17	0.10	2.72	0.12	11.22	0.74	7.48	64.26	88.40	24.82	1.33
2.74	2.02	0.00	0.00	0.00	0.00	0.00	0.07	0.15	7.13	0.54	6.72	0.40	23.52	1.57	30.24	235.20	322.56	70.56	2.27
7.93	6.29	0.00	0.00	0.00	176.80	0.26	0.16	0.55	12.84	1.04	52.00	3.33	67.60	5.23	62.40	520.00	707.20	174.20	8.19
1.49	1.97	0.00	0.00	0.58	0.00	0.00	0.05	0.23	3.32	0.33	8.19	0.34	29.12	2.12	21.84	185.64	263.90	71.89	4.06
3.80	3.21	0.00	0.00	0.63	0.00	0.00	0.06	0.25	3.67	0.33	9.36	0.37	34.32	2.36	23.92	203.84	284.96	79.04	4.33
0.12	0.12	0.00	0.00	0.15	179.50	0.17	0.01	0.09	0.45	0.03	34.50	2.40	1.30	0.67	1.70	20.40	20.00	5.90	0.37
4.01	2.65	0.00	0.00	0.28	0.00	0.00	0.04	0.14	3.95	0.32	5.74	0.27	20.50	1.58	19.68	160.72	221.40	87.74	2.35
2.04	1.93	0.00	0.00	0.44	0.00	0.00	0.04	0.17	2.53	0.23	6.39	0.26	22.72	1.63	16.33	141.29	198.80	54.67	3.03
0.66	1.01	0.00	0.00	0.11	0.00	0.00	0.07	0.15	8.00	0.63	7.02	0.43	22.23	1.58	32.76	256.23	356.85	74.88	2.39
3.86	2.73	0.00	0.00	0.18	0.00	0.00	0.08	0.18	8.55	0.64	8.16	0.48	28.56	1.92	35.36	282.88	387.60	85.68	2.77
4.47	3.47	0.00	0.00	0.48	0.00	0.00	0.08	0.25	7.13	0.57	9.80	0.49	36.40	2.51	35.00	284.20	392.00	95.20	4.14
1.44	2.00	0.00	0.00	0.46	0.00	0.00	0.08	0.25	7.62	0.64	9.80	0.52	35.00	2.49	36.40	298.20	417.20	98.00	4.34
0.13	0.08	0.00	0.00	0.03	0.00	0.00	0.01	0.03	2.36	0.10	1.13	0.57	1.98	0.11	5.67	64.92	78.81	405.69	0.32
1.12	0.71	0.00	0.00	0.04	0.00	0.00	0.01	0.03	1.38	0.10	1.44	0.08	5.76	0.35	6.00	47.28	63.84	14.64	0.50
3.74	0.68	0.00	0.00	0.34	0.00	0.00	0.05	0.27	6.77	0.26	12.75	1.33	18.70	0.98	22.10	203.15	276.25	73.95	4.05
2.00	0.50	0.00	0.00	0.36	0.00	0.00	0.05	0.29	7.16	0.28	13.60	1.40	20.40	0.99	23.80	212.50	287.30	75.65	4.33
0.75	0.53	0.00	0.00	0.00	0.00	0.00	0.15	0.51	5.70	0.00	0.00	0.00	5.95	3.80	20.40	192.10	284.75	45.90	2.34
0.00	0.01	0.00	0.00	0.00	0.48	0.25	0.00	0.51	0.01	0.00	1.08	0.00	0.96	0.03	0.81	2.10	2.37	0.18	0.03
6.14	1.98	0.00	0.00	3.24	0.00	0.11	0.02	0.10	0.46	0.01	10.43	0.00	43.20	0.59	48.48	83.68	121.28	72.00	0.49
6.14	1.98	0.00	0.00	3.25	0.00	0.11	0.02	0.10	0.46	0.01	10.43	0.00	43.20	0.59	48.48	83.68	121.28	1.76	0.49
46.80	15.12	0.00	0.00	22.71	0.00	0.99	0.19	0.85	4.02	0.11	91.00	0.00	401.75	6.98	432.98	780.78	1097.35	15.62	6.98
6.53	6.84	0.00	0.00	2.15	0.00	0.20	0.28	0.03	0.46	0.07	1.13	0.00	49.90	0.96	63.79	170.10	170.10	0.57	1.30
7.75	2.22	0.00	0.00	0.16	0.00	0.00	0.06	0.06	0.40	0.07	19.62	0.00	12.76	1.70	73.71	138.92	160.18	181.44	1.59
8.06	2.31	0.00	0.00	0.44	0.00	0.00	0.12	0.05	0.51	0.07	19.19	0.00	11.62	1.16	72.29	120.77	150.26	177.47	1.35
14.70	1.80	0.00	0.00	0.00	20.00	0.00	0.06	0.06	0.80	0.18	21.00	0.00	55.00	0.96	84.00	92.00	131.00	1.00	0.71
14.10	1.70	0.00	0.00	0.00	20.00	0.00	0.06	0.06	0.80	0.18	21.00	0.00	56.00	0.97	84.00	92.00	132.00	1.00	0.71
16.69	0.43	0.00	0.00	0.15	0.00	0.34	0.34	0.05	0.70	0.08	3.12	0.00	24.10	1.05	36.86	53.30	104.33	1.42	0.37
66.00	1.77	0.00	0.00	0.55	0.00	0.00	0.40	0.15	2.71	0.27	16.00	0.00	80.00	2.41	156.78	156.00	440.86	8.00	1.47
7.54	4.53	0.00	0.00	0.00	0.00	0.00	0.04	0.04	4.38	0.14	29.44	0.00	13.12	0.61	50.88	101.44	239.04	155.52	0.89
7.54	4.53	0.00	0.00	3.20	0.00	0.00	0.04	0.04	4.38	0.14	29.44	0.00	13.12	0.61	50.88	101.44	239.04	5.44	0.89
0.00	0.00	0.00	0.00	0.00	0.00	0.00	0.00	0.00	2.38	0.06	6.00	0.00	0.00	0.20	26.25	0.00	360.50	125.00	0.45
0.00	0.00	0.00	0.00	0.00	0.00	0.00	0.00	0.00	2.38	0.06	6.00	0.00	0.00	0.20	26.25	0.00	360.50	110.00	0.45
7.77	4.41	0.00	0.04	3.20	0.00	0.00	0.03	0.04	4.29	0.14	23.68	0.00	12.16	0.59	50.88	118.08	214.08	149.44	0.93
7.77	4.41	0.00	0.00	3.20	0.00	0.00	0.03	0.04	4.29	0.14	23.68	0.00	12.16	0.59	50.88	118.08	214.08	5.44	0.93
35.23	22.44	0.00	0.00	10.67	0.00	0.00	0.36	0.16	20.56	0.37	181.01	0.00	126.72	2.64	266.40	744.48	982.08	623.52	9.55
3.06	1.95	0.00	0.00	0.89	0.00	0.00	0.07	0.02	1.47	0.04	20.89	0.00	15.40	0.28	28.56	55.44	50.40	210.28	0.51
0.25	0.16	0.00	0.00	0.07	0.00	0.00	0.00	0.00	0.14	0.00	1.45	0.00	0.54	0.02	1.76	3.58	6.58	8.13	0.03
0.25	0.16	0.00	0.00	0.08	0.00	0.00	0.00	0.00	0.14	0.00	1.45	0.00	0.54	0.02	1.76	3.58	6.58	0.06	0.03

USDA ID Code	Food Name	Weight in Grams*	Quantity of Units	Unit of Measure	Protein (g)	Fat (g)	Carbohydrate (g)	Kilocalories	Caffeine (g)	Fiber (g)	Cholesterol (mg)	Saturated Fat (g)
	Peanuts, All Types, Fresh	28.3500	1.000	Ounce	7.31	13.96	4.58	160.74	0.00	2.41	0.00	1.94
	Peanuts, All Types, Oil-roasted,	0.9000	1.000	Each	0.24	0.44	0.17	5.23	0.00	0.08	0.00	0.06
	Peanuts, All Types, Oil-roasted,	28.0000	32.000	Each	7.38	13.80	5.30	162.68	0.00	1.93	0.00	1.92
	Peanuts, Dry Roasted	28.3500	1.000	Ounce	4.90	14.59	7.19	168.40	0.00	2.55	0.00	1.96
	Peanuts, Oil Roasted	28.3500	1.000	Ounce	4.40	15.92	6.31	174.35	0.00	1.56	0.00	2.58
	Peanuts, Spanish, Fresh	28.3500	1.000	Ounce	7.41	14.06	4.48	161.60	0.00	2.69	0.00	2.17
	Peanuts, Spanish, Oil-roasted, w	28.3500	1.000	Ounce	7.94	13.90	4.95	164.15	0.00	2.52	0.00	2.14
	Peanuts, Spanish, Oil-roasted, w	28.3500	1.000	Ounce	7.94	13.90	4.95	164.15	0.00	2.52	0.00	2.14
	Peanuts, Valencia, Fresh	28.3500	1.000	Ounce	7.11	13.49	5.93	161.60	0.00	2.47	0.00	2.08
	Peanuts, Valencia, Oil-roasted,	28.3500	1.000	Ounce	7.67	14.53	4.62	166.98	0.00	2.52	0.00	2.24
	Peanuts, Valencia, Oil-roasted,	28.3500	1.000	Ounce	7.67	14.53	4.62	166.98	0.00	2.52	0.00	2.24
	Peanuts, Virginia, Fresh	28.3500	1.000	Ounce	7.14	13.82	4.69	159.61	0.00	2.41	0.00	1.80
	Peanuts, Virginia, Oil-roasted,	28.3500	1.000	Ounce	7.33	13.78	5.63	163.86	0.00	2.52	0.00	1.80
	Peanuts, Virginia, Oil-roasted,	28.3500	1.000	Ounce	7.33	13.78	5.63	163.86	0.00	2.52	0.00	1.80
	Pecans, Dried	28.3500	1.000	Ounce	2.60	20.40	3.93	195.90	0.00	2.72	0.00	1.75
	Pine Nuts	1.8000	10.000	Each	0.43	0.91	0.26	10.19	0.00	0.08	0.00	0.14
	Pistachios, Dried	18.0000	30.000	Each	3.69	7.77	5.25	99.18	0.00	1.80	0.00	0.95
	Pistachios, Dry Roasted	28.3500	1.000	Ounce	6.02	12.96	7.69	160.74	0.00	2.92	0.00	1.57
	Sausage, Meatless	25.0000	1.000	Link	4.63	4.54	2.46	64.00	0.00	0.70	0.00	0.73
	Seeds, Sesame, Toasted, w/o salt	28.3500	1.000	Ounce	4.81	13.61	7.38	160.75	0.00	4.79	0.00	1.91
	Seeds, Sesame, Toasted, w/salt	28.3500	1.000	Ounce	4.81	13.61	7.38	160.75	0.00	4.79	0.00	1.91
	Seeds, Sunflower, Dried	46.0000	1.000	Cup	10.48	22.80	8.63	262.20	0.00	4.83	0.00	2.39
	Seeds, Sunflower, Dry Roasted, w	28.3500	1.000	Ounce	5.48	14.12	6.82	165.00	0.00	2.55	0.00	1.48
	Seeds, Sunflower, Dry Roasted, w	28.3500	1.000	Ounce	5.48	14.12	6.82	165.00	0.00	3.15	0.00	1.48
	Seeds, Sunflower, Oil Roasted, w	28.3500	1.000	Ounce	6.06	16.29	4.18	174.35	0.00	1.93	0.00	1.71
	Seeds, Sunflower, Oil Roasted, w	28.3500	1.000	Ounce	6.06	16.29	4.18	174.35	0.00	1.93	0.00	1.71
	Seeds, Sunflower, Toasted, w/ Sa	28.3500	1.000	Ounce	4.88	16.10	5.84	175.49	0.00	3.26	0.00	1.69
	Seeds, Sunflower, Toasted, w/o S	28.3500	1.000	Ounce	4.88	16.10	5.84	175.49	0.00	3.26	0.00	1.69
	Sesame Butter, Tahini, Toasted	15.0000	1.000	Tbsp	2.55	8.06	3.18	89.25	0.00	1.40	0.00	1.13
	Soybeans, Boiled	10.7000	1.000	Tbsp	1.78	0.96	1.06	18.51	0.00	0.64	0.00	0.14
	Soybeans, Dry Roasted	172.0000	1.000	Cup	68.08	37.19	56.28	774.00	0.00	13.93	0.00	5.38
	Tofu, Fresh, Firm	81.0000	1.000	Ounce	6.51	3.61	2.41	62.37	0.00	0.32	0.00	0.53
	Tofu, Fresh, Regular	17.6000	1.000	Ounce	1.15	0.65	0.32	10.74	0.00	0.04	0.00	0.09
	Tofu, Fried	13.0000	1.000	Piece	2.23	2.62	1.37	35.23	0.00	0.51	0.00	0.38
	Tofu, Fried, Prepared w/ Calcium	13.0000	1.000	Piece	2.23	2.62	1.37	35.23	0.00	0.51	0.00	0.38
	Tofu, Okara	122.0000	1.000	Cup	3.93	2.11	15.30	93.94	0.00	0.00	0.00	0.23
	Tofu, Salted and Fermented (fuyu	11.0000	1.000	Block	0.90	0.88	0.57	12.76	0.00	0.00	0.00	0.13
	Walnuts, Black, Dried	7.8000	1.000	Tbsp	1.90	4.41	0.94	47.35	0.00	0.39	0.00	0.28
	Walnuts, English, Dried	28.0000	0.500	Cup	4.26	18.26	3.84	183.12	0.00	1.88	0.00	1.72

Frozen Entrees and Packaged Foods

USDA ID Code	Food Name	Weight in Grams*	Quantity of Units	Unit of Measure	Protein (g)	Fat (g)	Carbohydrate (g)	Kilocalories	Caffeine (g)	Fiber (g)	Cholesterol (mg)	Saturated Fat (g)
	Apples, Escalloped-Stouffer's	170.0960	1.000	Each	0.00	4.00	41.00	200.00	0.00	0.00	0.00	0.00
	Bean, Green, Mushroom Casserole-	134.6590	1.000	Each	5.00	10.00	13.00	160.00	0.00	0.00	0.00	0.00
	Beef Ribs w/Barbecue Sauce, Bone	311.8430	1.000	Each	28.00	6.00	40.00	330.00	0.00	0.00	70.00	2.00
	Beef Roast, Tender, Top Shelf-Ho	283.4930	1.000	Each	28.00	6.00	19.00	240.00	0.00	0.00	60.00	2.00
	Beef Sirloin Tips w/ Mushroom Gr	269.3190	1.000	Each	22.00	5.00	43.00	310.00	0.00	0.00	35.00	2.00
	Beef Sirloin Tips-Healthy Choice	318.9300	1.000	Each	22.00	7.00	29.00	270.00	0.00	0.00	65.00	3.00
	Beef Stew, Micro Cup-Hormel	212.6200	1.000	Each	13.00	15.00	11.00	230.00	0.00	0.00	45.00	5.00
	Beef Stroganoff w/ Parsley Noodle	276.4060	1.000	Each	24.00	20.00	28.00	390.00	0.00	0.00	0.00	5.00
	Beef, Chipped, Creamed-Stouffer's	28.3500	1.000	Ounce	2.10	3.30	1.60	45.00	0.00	0.00	13.00	0.00
	Beef, Oriental, w/ Veg., Lean Cu	244.5130	1.000	Each	20.00	9.00	31.00	290.00	0.00	0.00	40.00	2.00
	Beef, Pot Roast, Yankee-Healthy	311.8430	1.000	Each	19.00	4.00	36.00	260.00	0.00	0.00	55.00	2.00
	Beef, Sirloin, w/ Barbecue Sauce	311.8430	1.000	Each	17.00	4.00	44.00	280.00	0.00	0.00	25.00	2.00
	Burritos, Beef and Bean (medium)	148.8340	1.000	Each	12.00	7.00	42.00	270.00	0.00	0.00	15.00	3.00

Monounsaturated Fat (g)	Polyunsaturated Fat (g)	Vitamin D (mg)	Vitamin K (mg)	Vitamin E (mg)	Vitamin A (re)	Vitamin C (mg)	Thiamin (mg)	Riboflavin (mg)	Niacin (mg)	Vitamin B6 (mg)	Folate (mcg)	Vitamin B12 (mcg)	Calcium (mg)	Iron (mg)	Magnesium (mg)	Phosphorus (mg)	Potassium (mg)	Sodium (mg)	Zinc (mg)
6.93	4.41	0.00	0.00	2.59	0.00	0.00	0.18	0.04	3.42	0.10	67.98	0.00	26.08	1.30	47.63	106.60	199.87	5.10	0.93
0.22	0.14	0.00	0.00	0.07	0.00	0.00	0.00	0.00	0.13	0.00	1.13	0.00	0.79	0.02	1.67	4.65	6.14	3.90	0.06
6.85	4.36	0.00	0.00	2.07	0.00	0.00	0.07	0.03	4.00	0.07	35.20	0.00	24.64	0.51	51.80	144.76	190.96	1.68	1.86
8.90	3.05	0.00	0.00	1.70	0.28	0.11	0.06	0.06	1.33	0.09	14.29	0.00	19.85	1.05	63.79	123.32	169.25	189.66	1.08
9.40	3.25	0.00	0.00	1.70	0.57	0.14	0.14	0.14	0.56	0.15	15.99	0.00	30.05	0.73	71.16	127.29	154.22	198.45	1.32
6.33	4.88	0.00	0.00	0.00	0.00	0.00	0.19	0.04	4.52	0.10	68.04	0.00	30.05	1.11	53.30	110.00	210.92	6.24	0.60
6.26	4.82	0.00	0.00	0.00	0.00	0.00	0.09	0.03	4.23	0.07	35.69	0.00	28.35	0.65	47.63	109.71	220.00	122.76	0.57
6.26	4.82	0.00	0.00	0.00	0.00	0.00	0.09	0.03	4.23	0.07	35.69	0.00	28.35	0.65	47.63	109.71	220.00	1.70	0.57
6.07	4.68	0.00	0.00	0.00	0.00	0.00	0.18	0.09	3.65	0.10	69.60	0.00	17.58	0.59	52.16	95.26	94.12	0.28	0.95
6.54	5.04	0.00	0.00	0.00	0.00	0.00	0.03	0.04	4.07	0.07	35.58	0.00	15.31	0.47	45.36	90.44	173.50	218.86	0.87
6.54	5.04	0.00	0.00	0.00	0.00	0.00	0.03	0.04	4.07	0.07	35.58	0.00	15.31	0.47	45.36	90.44	173.50	1.70	0.87
7.17	4.17	0.00	0.00	0.00	0.00	0.00	0.18	0.04	3.51	0.10	67.67	0.00	25.23	0.72	48.48	107.73	195.62	2.84	1.26
7.15	4.16	0.00	0.00	0.00	0.00	0.00	0.08	0.03	4.17	0.07	35.55	0.00	24.38	0.47	53.30	143.45	184.84	122.76	1.88
7.15	4.16	0.00	0.00	0.00	0.00	0.00	0.08	0.03	4.17	0.07	35.55	0.00	24.38	0.47	53.30	143.45	184.84	1.70	1.88
11.56	6.12	0.00	0.00	1.04	2.27	0.31	0.19	0.04	0.33	0.06	6.24	0.00	19.85	0.72	34.30	78.53	116.24	0.00	1.28
0.34	0.38	0.00	0.00	0.06	0.05	0.03	0.01	0.01	0.06	0.00	1.03	0.00	0.47	0.17	4.19	9.14	10.78	0.07	0.08
4.08	2.35	0.00	0.00	0.83	9.90	0.90	0.16	0.03	0.23	0.31	9.18	0.00	19.26	0.77	21.78	88.20	175.86	0.18	0.40
6.83	3.92	0.00	0.00	1.21	15.03	0.65	0.24	0.05	0.41	0.48	14.18	0.00	30.62	1.19	34.02	137.50	292.86	120.77	0.65
1.13	2.32	0.00	0.00	0.53	16.00	0.00	0.59	0.10	2.80	0.21	6.50	0.00	15.75	0.93	9.00	56.25	57.75	222.00	0.37
5.14	5.97	0.00	0.00	0.64	1.99	0.00	0.34	0.13	1.54	0.04	27.16	0.00	37.14	2.21	98.09	219.43	115.10	11.06	2.90
5.14	5.97	0.00	0.00	0.64	1.99	0.00	0.34	0.13	1.54	0.04	27.16	0.00	37.14	2.21	98.09	219.43	115.10	166.70	2.90
4.35	15.06	0.00	0.00	23.12	2.30	0.64	1.05	0.12	2.07	0.35	104.60	0.00	53.36	3.11	162.84	324.30	316.94	1.38	2.33
2.70	9.32	0.00	0.00	14.25	0.00	0.40	0.03	0.07	2.00	0.23	67.30	0.00	19.85	1.08	36.57	327.44	240.98	221.13	1.50
2.70	9.32	0.00	0.00	14.25	0.00	0.40	0.03	0.07	2.00	0.23	67.30	0.00	19.85	1.08	36.57	327.44	240.98	0.85	1.50
3.11	10.76	0.00	0.00	11.34	1.42	0.40	0.09	0.08	1.17	0.22	66.34	0.00	15.88	1.90	36.00	322.91	136.93	170.95	1.48
3.11	10.76	0.00	0.00	14.25	1.42	0.40	0.09	0.08	1.17	0.22	66.34	0.00	15.88	1.90	36.00	322.91	136.93	0.85	1.48
3.07	10.63	0.00	0.00	0.00	0.00	0.40	0.09	0.08	1.19	0.23	67.42	0.00	16.16	1.93	36.57	328.29	139.20	173.79	1.50
3.07	10.63	0.00	0.00	0.00	0.00	0.40	0.09	0.08	1.19	0.23	67.42	0.00	16.16	1.93	36.57	328.29	139.20	0.85	1.50
3.05	3.54	0.00	0.00	0.34	1.05	0.00	0.18	0.07	0.82	0.02	14.66	0.00	63.90	1.34	14.25	109.80	62.10	17.25	0.69
0.21	0.54	0.00	0.00	0.21	0.11	0.18	0.02	0.03	0.04	0.02	5.76	0.00	10.91	0.55	9.20	26.22	55.11	0.11	0.12
8.22	21.00	0.00	0.00	0.00	3.44	7.91	0.74	1.31	1.82	0.40	351.91	0.00	240.80	6.79	392.16	1116.28	2346.08	3.44	8.20
0.80	2.04	0.00	0.00	0.00	0.81	0.16	0.07	0.08	0.01	0.05	26.73	0.00	131.22	1.17	37.26	119.07	142.56	6.48	0.82
0.14	0.37	0.00	0.00	0.00	0.18	0.04	0.01	0.01	0.10	0.01	7.74	0.00	19.54	0.20	4.75	16.19	21.12	1.41	0.11
0.58	1.48	0.00	0.00	0.00	0.00	0.00	0.02	0.01	0.01	0.01	3.48	0.00	48.36	0.63	7.80	37.31	18.98	2.08	0.26
0.58	1.48	0.00	0.00	0.00	0.00	0.00	0.02	0.01	0.01	0.01	3.48	0.00	124.93	0.63	12.35	37.31	18.98	2.08	0.26
0.37	0.93	0.00	0.00	0.00	0.00	0.00	0.02	0.02	0.12	0.15	32.21	0.00	97.60	1.59	31.72	73.20	259.86	10.98	0.68
0.19	0.50	0.00	0.00	0.00	1.87	0.02	0.02	0.01	0.04	0.01	3.20	0.00	5.06	0.22	5.72	8.03	8.25	316.03	0.17
0.99	2.92	0.00	0.00	0.20	2.34	0.25	0.02	0.01	0.05	0.04	5.11	0.00	4.52	0.24	15.76	36.19	40.87	0.08	0.27
2.50	13.21	0.00	0.00	0.82	1.12	0.36	0.10	0.04	0.53	0.15	27.44	0.00	29.12	0.81	44.24	96.88	123.48	0.56	0.87
0.00	0.00	0.00	0.00	0.00	0.00	30.00	0.03	0.00	0.00	0.00	0.00	0.00	0.00	0.00	0.00	0.00	90.00	15.00	0.00
0.00	0.00	0.00	0.00	0.00	40.00	2.40	0.06	0.17	0.38	0.00	0.00	0.00	64.00	0.20	0.00	0.00	200.00	550.00	0.00
0.00	2.00	0.00	0.00	0.00	60.00	4.80	0.23	0.26	2.85	0.00	0.00	0.00	48.00	1.00	0.00	220.00	670.00	530.00	0.00
2.00	1.00	0.00	0.00	0.00	400.00	2.40	0.75	0.43	5.70	0.00	0.00	0.00	16.00	1.50	42.00	0.00	933.00	880.00	4.50
0.00	0.00	0.00	0.00	0.00	60.00	2.40	0.00	0.03	0.38	0.00	0.00	0.00	0.00	0.20	0.00	0.00	80.00	500.00	0.00
0.00	2.00	0.00	0.00	0.00	700.00	42.00	0.15	0.17	2.85	0.00	0.00	0.00	16.00	1.00	0.00	190.00	520.00	360.00	0.00
4.00	0.00	0.00	0.00	0.28	320.00	2.40	0.05	0.10	2.28	0.00	0.00	0.00	16.00	0.90	21.00	0.00	487.00	1140.00	2.40
0.00	0.00	0.00	0.00	0.00	40.00	1.20	0.12	0.34	2.85	0.00	0.00	0.00	48.00	1.50	0.00	0.00	300.00	1090.00	0.00
0.00	0.00	0.00	0.00	0.00	0.00	0.00	0.00	0.00	0.21	0.00	0.00	0.00	184.00	0.02	0.00	0.00	57.00	176.00	0.00
0.00	0.00	0.00	0.00	0.00	150.00	1.20	0.09	0.17	2.85	0.00	0.00	0.00	16.00	1.00	0.00	0.00	400.00	590.00	0.00
0.00	0.00	0.00	0.00	0.00	100.00	9.00	0.15	0.17	1.52	0.00	0.00	0.00	32.00	1.00	0.00	150.00	350.00	400.00	0.00
0.00	1.00	0.00	0.00	0.00	0.00	0.00	0.00	0.00	0.00	0.00	0.00	0.00	0.00	0.00	0.00	190.00	630.00	240.00	0.00
0.00	3.00	0.00	0.00	0.00	20.00	3.60	0.38	0.17	1.90	0.00	0.00	0.00	48.00	1.50	0.00	180.00	270.00	520.00	0.00

USDA ID Code	Food Name	Weight in Grams*	Quantity of Units	Unit of Measure	Protein (g)	Fat (g)	Carbohydrate (g)	Kilocalories	Caffeine (g)	Fiber (g)	Cholesterol (mg)	Saturated Fat (g)
	Burritos, Beef and Bean (mild)-H	148.8340	1.000	Each	11.00	5.00	45.00	250.00	0.00	0.00	10.00	1.00
	Burritos, Chicken Con Queso (mil	148.8340	1.000	Each	15.00	8.00	40.00	280.00	0.00	0.00	20.00	2.00
	Cabbage, Stuffed, no Sauce-Stouf	28.3500	1.000	Ounce	2.00	2.10	3.10	39.00	0.00	0.00	5.00	0.00
	Cabbage, Stuffed, w/ Meat, Lean	269.3190	1.000	Each	13.00	6.00	26.00	210.00	0.00	0.00	30.00	2.00
	Cabbage, Stuffed-Stouffer's	28.3500	1.000	Ounce	1.40	1.40	2.70	29.00	0.00	0.00	4.00	0.00
	Cacciatore, Chicken, Lean Cuisin	308.2990	1.000	Each	22.00	7.00	31.00	280.00	0.00	0.00	45.00	2.00
	Cacciatore, Chicken, Top Shelf-H	283.4930	1.000	Each	21.00	3.00	25.00	210.00	0.00	0.00	50.00	0.00
	Cannelloni, Beef, w/ Sauce, Lean	272.8620	1.000	Each	14.00	3.00	28.00	200.00	0.00	0.00	25.00	1.00
	Cannelloni, Cheese, Lean Cuisine	258.6880	1.000	Each	23.00	8.00	27.00	270.00	0.00	0.00	25.00	4.00
	Chicken a la King w/ Rice-Stouff	269.3190	1.000	Each	18.00	5.00	38.00	270.00	0.00	0.00	0.00	0.00
	Chicken a la King, Top Shelf-Hor	5283.4930	1.000	Each	18.00	10.00	49.00	360.00	0.00	0.00	37.00	4.00
	Chicken a la King-Swanson	250.0000	1.000	Each	16.80	20.16	15.12	319.15	0.00	0.00	0.00	0.00
	Chicken a la Orange, Lean Cuisin	226.7950	1.000	Each	27.00	4.00	33.00	280.00	0.00	0.00	55.00	1.00
	Chicken a la Orange-Healthy Choi	255.1440	1.000	Each	20.00	2.00	36.00	240.00	0.00	0.00	45.00	2.00
	Chicken and Dumplings-Stouffer's	220.0000	1.000	Each	14.74	16.30	24.06	302.65	0.00	0.00	69.84	0.00
	Chicken and Dumplings-Swanson	200.0000	1.000	Each	10.35	10.35	17.87	206.94	0.00	0.00	0.00	0.00
	Chicken and Pasta Divan-Healthy	340.1920	1.000	Each	25.00	4.00	41.00	300.00	0.00	0.00	50.00	2.00
	Chicken and Veg. Oriental-Stouff	220.0000	1.000	Each	11.64	9.31	13.97	186.25	0.00	0.00	31.04	0.00
	Chicken and Veg. w/ Vermicelli,	333.1050	1.000	Each	18.00	5.00	30.00	240.00	0.00	0.00	30.00	1.00
	Chicken and Vegetables-Healthy C	326.0170	1.000	Each	20.00	1.00	31.00	210.00	0.00	0.00	35.00	0.00
	Chicken Classica-Stouffer's	28.3500	1.000	Ounce	1.80	0.70	2.30	22.00	0.00	0.00	5.00	0.00
	Chicken Dijon-Healthy Choice	311.8430	1.000	Each	21.00	3.00	40.00	250.00	0.00	0.00	40.00	1.00
	Chicken Divan-Stouffer's	226.7950	1.000	Each	24.00	10.00	11.00	220.00	0.00	0.00	0.00	0.00
	Chicken in BBQ Sauce, Lean Cuisi	248.0570	1.000	Each	20.00	6.00	32.00	260.00	0.00	0.00	50.00	1.00
	Chicken Italiano, Lean Cuisine-S	255.1440	1.000	Each	22.00	6.00	33.00	270.00	0.00	0.00	40.00	1.00
	Chicken Italienne-Stouffer's	28.3500	1.000	Ounce	2.20	0.90	1.20	22.00	0.00	0.00	7.00	0.00
	Chicken Oriental, Lean Cuisine-S	255.1440	1.000	Each	22.00	7.00	31.00	280.00	0.00	0.00	35.00	2.00
	Chicken Oriental-Healthy Choice	318.9300	1.000	Each	19.00	1.00	32.00	200.00	0.00	0.00	35.00	0.00
	Chicken Parmigiana-Healthy Choic	326.0170	1.000	Each	22.00	4.00	45.00	280.00	0.00	0.00	45.00	2.00
186	Chicken Piccata, Lemon Herb-Smar	238.0000	8.500	Ounce	11.00	2.00	34.00	200.00	0.00	3.00	25.00	0.50
	Chicken Stir Fry w/ Broccoli-Hea	340.1920	1.000	Each	21.00	6.00	35.00	280.00	0.00	0.00	55.00	3.00
	Chicken Tenderloins, Lean Cuisin	269.3190	1.000	Each	29.00	5.00	19.00	240.00	0.00	0.00	60.00	2.00
	Chicken w/ Barbecue Sauce-Health	361.4540	1.000	Each	24.00	6.00	65.00	410.00	0.00	0.00	55.00	2.00
	Chicken w/ Spanish Rice, Breast	283.4930	1.000	Each	27.00	15.00	38.00	400.00	0.00	0.00	75.00	7.00
	Chicken, Breast, Glazed, Top She	283.4930	1.000	Each	19.00	2.00	19.00	170.00	0.00	0.00	35.00	1.00
	Chicken, Creamed-Stouffer's	28.3500	1.000	Ounce	2.80	3.50	1.20	48.00	0.00	0.00	14.00	0.00
	Chicken, Escalloped, and Noodles	283.4930	1.000	Each	21.00	24.00	30.00	420.00	0.00	0.00	0.00	0.00
	Chicken, Fiesta-Weight Watchers	240.9750	1.000	Each	12.00	2.00	38.00	220.00	0.00	5.00	25.00	0.50
	Chicken, Glazed, w/ Veg. Lean Cu	240.9690	1.000	Each	21.00	7.00	24.00	250.00	0.00	0.00	50.00	2.00
	Chicken, Glazed-Healthy Choice	240.9690	1.000	Each	21.00	3.00	27.00	220.00	0.00	0.00	45.00	1.00
	Chicken, Glazed-Stouffer's	28.3500	1.000	Ounce	2.90	1.10	1.00	26.00	0.00	0.00	9.00	0.00
	Chicken, Herb Roasted-Healthy C	347.2790	1.000	Each	22.00	5.00	50.00	300.00	0.00	0.00	40.00	2.00
	Chicken, Honey Mustard, Lean Cui	212.6200	1.000	Each	18.00	4.00	30.00	230.00	0.00	0.00	40.00	1.00
	Chicken, Honey Mustard-Healthy C	269.3190	1.000	Each	26.00	4.00	41.00	310.00	0.00	0.00	45.00	1.00
187	Chicken, Honey Mustard-Smart One	238.0000	8.500	Ounce	11.00	2.00	37.00	200.00	0.00	3.00	30.00	0.50
	Chicken, Mandarin-Healthy Choice	311.8430	1.000	Each	23.00	2.00	39.00	260.00	0.00	0.00	50.00	0.00
	Chicken, Mexicali-Stouffer's	28.3500	1.000	Ounce	1.40	0.80	1.80	20.00	0.00	0.00	5.00	0.00
	Chicken, Oriental, w/ Spicy Pean	269.3190	1.000	Each	33.00	5.00	40.00	340.00	0.00	0.00	45.00	1.00
	Chicken, Oven Baked, Lean Cuisin	226.7950	1.000	Each	17.00	5.00	21.00	200.00	0.00	0.00	35.00	2.00
	Chicken, Salsa-Healthy Choice	318.9300	1.000	Each	20.00	2.00	36.00	240.00	0.00	0.00	50.00	1.00
	Chicken, Southwestern Style-Heal	354.3670	1.000	Each	25.00	5.00	51.00	340.00	0.00	0.00	60.00	2.00
	Chicken, Sweet and Sour-Healthy	326.0170	1.000	Each	20.00	2.00	52.00	280.00	0.00	0.00	35.00	0.00
188	Chicken, Szechwan Veg, Spicy & H	252.0000	9.000	Ounce	11.00	2.00	39.00	220.00	0.00	3.00	10.00	0.50

Page Key: A2 = Baby Food   A2 = Baked Goods   A8 = Beverages   A14 = Breads/Grains and Pasta   A18 = Breakfast Foods/Cereals   A26 = Dairy and Eggs   A40 = Fats and Oils   A42 = Fruits and Vegetables   A52 = Meats and Beans   A60 = Nuts and Seeds   A62 5 Frozen Entrees and Packaged Foods   A76 = Restaurant Chains–Fast Foods   A92 = Restaurant Chains–Other   A106 = Seafood and Fish   A110 = Snacks and Sweets   A120 = Soups   A122 = Supplements   A126 = Toppings and Sauces

Monounsaturated Fat (g)	Polyunsaturated Fat (g)	Vitamin D (mg)	Vitamin K (mg)	Vitamin E (mg)	Vitamin A (re)	Vitamin C (mg)	Thiamin (mg)	Riboflavin (mg)	Niacin (mg)	Vitamin B6 (mg)	Folate (mcg)	Vitamin B12 (mcg)	Calcium (mg)	Iron (mg)	Magnesium (mg)	Phosphorus (mg)	Potassium (mg)	Sodium (mg)	Zinc (mg)
0.00	2.00	0.00	0.00	0.00	20.00	1.20	0.38	0.17	2.85	0.00	0.00	0.00	32.00	2.00	0.00	130.00	330.00	450.00	0.00
0.00	3.00	0.00	0.00	0.00	20.00	6.00	0.45	0.34	2.85	0.00	0.00	0.00	80.00	1.50	0.00	170.00	260.00	500.00	0.00
0.00	0.00	0.00	0.00	0.00	0.00	0.60	0.00	0.00	0.08	0.00	0.00	0.00	72.00	0.04	0.00	0.00	48.00	150.00	0.00
0.00	1.00	0.00	0.00	0.00	80.00	6.00	0.12	0.17	3.80	0.00	0.00	0.00	64.00	1.50	0.00	0.00	600.00	560.00	0.00
0.00	0.00	0.00	0.00	0.00	0.00	3.00	0.00	0.00	0.06	0.00	0.00	0.00	48.00	0.02	0.00	0.00	51.00	145.00	0.00
0.00	1.00	0.00	0.00	0.00	100.00	9.00	0.23	0.17	5.70	0.00	0.00	0.00	32.00	0.80	0.00	0.00	560.00	570.00	0.00
0.00	0.00	0.00	0.00	0.46	100.00	2.40	0.15	0.26	6.65	0.00	0.00	0.00	80.00	1.00	0.00	0.00	0.00	810.00	0.00
0.00	0.00	0.00	0.00	0.00	350.00	6.00	0.12	0.17	2.85	0.00	0.00	0.00	120.00	1.50	0.00	0.00	800.00	490.00	0.00
0.00	0.00	0.00	0.00	0.00	60.00	21.00	0.12	0.26	1.52	0.00	0.00	0.00	240.00	0.40	0.00	0.00	400.00	590.00	0.00
0.00	0.00	0.00	0.00	0.00	20.00	1.20	0.09	0.17	2.85	0.00	0.00	0.00	160.00	0.80	0.00	32.00	260.00	800.00	0.00
4.00	2.00	0.00	0.00	0.17	250.00	1.20	0.12	0.17	8.55	0.00	0.00	0.00	48.00	0.20	28.00	0.00	476.00	890.00	1.20
0.00	0.00	0.00	0.00	0.00	0.00	0.00	0.05	0.23	3.19	0.00	0.00	0.00	53.75	0.34	0.00	0.00	0.00	1159.01	0.00
0.00	0.00	0.00	0.00	0.00	80.00	12.00	0.23	0.17	9.50	0.00	0.00	0.00	32.00	0.40	0.00	0.00	490.00	290.00	0.00
0.00	0.00	0.00	0.00	0.00	150.00	27.00	0.15	0.10	5.70	0.00	0.00	0.00	16.00	0.80	0.00	230.00	430.00	220.00	0.00
0.00	0.00	0.00	0.00	0.00	0.00	0.00	0.00	0.01	0.44	0.00	0.00	0.00	1.06	0.16	0.00	0.00	248.33	659.63	0.00
0.00	0.00	0.00	0.00	0.00	75.25	0.00	0.03	0.10	1.79	0.00	0.00	0.00	15.05	0.38	0.00	0.00	0.00	921.83	0.00
0.00	1.00	0.00	0.00	0.00	800.00	72.00	0.38	0.26	4.75	0.00	0.00	0.00	120.00	1.00	0.00	270.00	500.00	520.00	0.00
0.00	0.00	0.00	0.00	0.00	0.00	4.66	0.00	0.00	0.59	0.00	0.00	0.00	372.49	0.08	0.00	0.00	349.21	1078.68	0.00
0.00	1.00	0.00	0.00	0.00	150.00	6.00	0.30	0.26	5.70	0.00	0.00	0.00	64.00	1.00	0.00	0.00	500.00	500.00	0.00
0.00	0.00	0.00	0.00	0.00	150.00	9.00	0.30	0.17	3.80	0.00	0.00	0.00	32.00	1.50	0.00	190.00	390.00	490.00	0.00
0.00	0.00	0.00	0.00	0.00	0.00	1.20	0.00	0.00	0.10	0.00	0.00	0.00	112.00	0.01	0.00	0.00	50.00	83.00	0.00
0.00	0.00	0.00	0.00	0.00	100.00	9.00	0.23	0.14	9.50	0.00	0.00	0.00	16.00	1.00	0.00	300.00	350.00	470.00	0.00
0.00	0.00	0.00	0.00	0.00	60.00	3.60	0.45	0.17	3.80	0.00	0.00	0.00	200.00	2.00	0.00	32.00	490.00	610.00	0.00
0.00	2.00	0.00	0.00	0.00	250.00	18.00	0.15	0.17	5.70	0.00	0.00	0.00	48.00	0.80	0.00	0.00	650.00	500.00	0.00
0.00	2.00	0.00	0.00	0.00	100.00	24.00	0.30	0.26	5.70	0.00	0.00	0.00	80.00	0.80	0.00	0.00	600.00	590.00	0.00
0.00	0.00	0.00	0.00	0.00	0.00	1.20	0.00	0.00	0.10	0.00	0.00	0.00	48.00	0.01	0.00	0.00	57.00	128.00	0.00
0.00	2.00	0.00	0.00	0.00	40.00	6.00	0.23	0.17	6.65	0.00	0.00	0.00	32.00	1.00	0.00	0.00	470.00	480.00	0.00
0.00	0.00	0.00	0.00	0.00	250.00	36.00	0.15	0.14	7.60	0.00	0.00	0.00	32.00	0.80	0.00	200.00	400.00	440.00	0.00
0.00	0.00	0.00	0.00	0.00	900.00	12.00	0.15	0.17	9.50	0.00	0.00	0.00	80.00	1.00	0.00	260.00	500.00	370.00	0.00
0.00	0.00	0.00	0.00	0.00	0.00	0.00	0.00	0.00	0.00	0.00	0.00	0.00	0.00	0.00	0.00	0.00	0.00	460.00	0.00
0.00	0.00	0.00	0.00	0.00	20.00	0.00	0.23	0.34	2.85	0.00	0.00	0.00	48.00	1.50	0.00	260.00	630.00	500.00	0.00
0.00	1.00	0.00	0.00	0.00	200.00	4.80	0.23	0.34	7.60	0.00	0.00	0.00	120.00	0.40	0.00	0.00	750.00	490.00	0.00
0.00	2.00	0.00	0.00	0.00	100.00	12.00	0.12	0.14	8.55	0.00	0.00	0.00	48.00	1.50	0.00	250.00	670.00	550.00	0.00
4.00	3.00	0.00	0.00	0.07	100.00	3.60	0.09	0.26	7.60	0.00	0.00	0.00	80.00	0.40	35.00	0.00	584.00	810.00	1.65
1.00	1.00	0.00	0.00	0.76	400.00	3.60	0.06	0.17	7.60	0.00	0.00	0.00	32.00	0.40	35.00	0.00	804.00	780.00	1.05
0.00	0.00	0.00	0.00	0.00	0.00	0.00	0.00	0.00	0.10	0.00	0.00	0.00	352.00	0.01	0.00	0.00	37.00	119.00	0.00
0.00	0.00	0.00	0.00	0.00	20.00	0.00	0.15	0.34	3.80	0.00	0.00	0.00	80.00	0.80	0.00	0.00	300.00	840.00	0.00
0.00	0.00	0.00	0.00	0.00	450.00	42.00	0.00	0.00	0.00	0.00	0.00	0.00	72.00	1.50	0.00	0.00	490.00	480.00	0.00
0.00	4.00	0.00	0.00	0.00	20.00	3.60	0.15	0.17	7.60	0.00	0.00	0.00	16.00	0.20	0.00	0.00	580.00	590.00	0.00
0.00	1.00	0.00	0.00	0.00	0.00	1.20	0.15	0.14	6.65	0.00	0.00	0.00	0.00	0.60	0.00	240.00	370.00	510.00	0.00
0.00	0.00	0.00	0.00	0.00	0.00	0.00	0.00	0.00	0.23	0.00	0.00	0.00	24.00	0.01	0.00	0.00	45.00	105.00	0.00
0.00	1.00	0.00	0.00	0.00	250.00	24.00	0.15	0.14	7.60	0.00	0.00	0.00	32.00	0.80	0.00	280.00	370.00	560.00	0.00
0.00	1.00	0.00	0.00	0.00	200.00	2.40	0.15	0.17	3.80	0.00	0.00	0.00	16.00	0.40	0.00	0.00	340.00	540.00	0.00
0.00	0.00	0.00	0.00	0.00	100.00	3.60	0.15	0.03	1.52	0.00	0.00	0.00	16.00	0.80	0.00	0.00	110.00	520.00	0.00
0.00	0.00	0.00	0.00	0.00	0.00	0.00	0.00	0.00	0.00	0.00	0.00	0.00	0.00	0.00	0.00	0.00	0.00	370.00	0.00
0.00	0.00	0.00	0.00	0.00	250.00	9.00	0.15	0.17	4.75	0.00	0.00	0.00	16.00	1.00	0.00	200.00	400.00	400.00	0.00
0.00	0.00	0.00	0.00	0.00	0.00	4.20	0.00	0.00	0.11	0.00	0.00	0.00	88.00	0.02	0.00	0.00	68.00	48.00	0.00
0.00	1.00	0.00	0.00	0.00	0.00	2.40	0.00	0.00	0.38	0.00	0.00	0.00	0.00	0.20	0.00	0.00	50.00	470.00	0.00
0.00	0.00	0.00	0.00	0.00	350.00	6.00	0.15	0.17	7.60	0.00	0.00	0.00	16.00	0.80	0.00	0.00	550.00	480.00	0.00
0.00	0.00	0.00	0.00	0.00	200.00	66.00	0.23	0.17	3.80	0.00	0.00	0.00	64.00	0.60	0.00	200.00	540.00	450.00	0.00
0.00	2.00	0.00	0.00	0.00	0.00	0.00	0.00	0.00	0.00	0.00	0.00	0.00	0.00	0.00	0.00	260.00	560.00	550.00	0.00
0.00	0.00	0.00	0.00	0.00	250.00	30.00	0.15	0.17	8.55	0.00	0.00	0.00	32.00	1.00	0.00	220.00	480.00	320.00	0.00
0.00	0.00	0.00	0.00	0.00	0.00	0.00	0.00	0.00	0.00	0.00	0.00	0.00	0.00	0.00	0.00	0.00	0.00	730.00	0.00

USDA ID Code	Food Name	Weight in Grams*	Quantity of Units	Unit of Measure	Protein (g)	Fat (g)	Carbohydrate (g)	Kilocalories	Caffeine (g)	Fiber (g)	Cholesterol (mg)	Saturated Fat (g)
	Chicken, Teriyaki-Healthy Choice	347.2790	1.000	Each	24.00	4.00	39.00	290.00	0.00	0.00	55.00	1.00
	Chili Beef Soup-Healthy Choice	212.6200	1.000	Each	11.00	1.00	22.00	150.00	0.00	0.00	15.00	0.00
	Chili Con Carne w/ Beans-Stouffe	248.0570	1.000	Each	20.00	10.00	28.00	280.00	0.00	0.00	0.00	0.00
	Chili Mac, Micro Cup-Hormel	212.6200	1.000	Each	10.00	9.00	18.00	192.00	0.00	0.00	22.00	4.00
	Chili no Beans, Micro Cup-Hormel	209.0760	1.000	Each	18.00	17.00	15.00	290.00	0.00	0.00	60.00	8.00
	Chili w/ Beans Soup-Stouffer's	283.9200	1.000	Cup	14.02	9.01	25.04	240.36	0.00	0.00	30.04	0.00
	Chili w/ Beans, Chunky-Hormel	253.1620	1.000	Cup	17.86	16.67	29.77	345.30	0.00	0.00	59.53	0.00
	Chili w/ Beans, Micro Cup-Hormel	209.0760	1.000	Each	15.00	11.00	23.00	250.00	0.00	0.00	49.00	4.00
	Chili w/ Beans-Hormel	253.1620	1.000	Cup	17.86	17.86	32.15	357.20	0.00	0.00	65.49	5.95
	Chili w/o Beans-Hormel	253.1620	1.000	Cup	19.05	32.15	16.67	428.64	0.00	0.00	71.44	13.10
	Chili, Fat Free	240.0000	0.500	Cup	14.00	0.00	30.00	160.00	0.00	14.00	0.00	0.00
	Chili, Hot, no Beans-Hormel	212.6200	1.000	Each	16.00	27.00	14.00	360.00	0.00	0.00	60.00	11.00
	Chili, Hot, w/ Beans, Micro Cup-	209.0760	1.000	Each	15.00	11.00	24.00	250.00	0.00	0.00	49.00	4.00
	Chili, Hot, w/ Beans-Hormel	212.6200	1.000	Each	15.00	15.00	27.00	300.00	0.00	0.00	55.00	5.00
	Chili, Three Bean-Stouffer's	283.9200	1.000	Cup	10.02	5.01	32.05	210.32	0.00	0.00	20.03	0.00
	Chow Mein w/ Rice, Chicken, Lean	255.1440	1.000	Each	14.00	5.00	34.00	240.00	0.00	0.00	30.00	1.00
	Chow Mein w/ Rice, Chicken-Stouf	304.7550	1.000	Each	13.00	5.00	39.00	250.00	0.00	0.00	0.00	0.00
	Chow Mein, Beef	247.0000	1.000	Cup	10.00	1.50	15.00	110.00	0.00	4.00	10.00	1.00
	Chow Mein, Chicken-Weight Watch	255.1500	1.000	Each	12.00	2.00	34.00	200.00	0.00	3.00	25.00	0.50
	Chow Mein, Chicken-Healthy Choic	240.9690	1.000	Each	18.00	3.00	31.00	220.00	0.00	0.00	45.00	1.00
190	Chow Mein, Chicken-Smart Ones	252.0000	9.000	Ounce	12.00	2.00	34.00	200.00	0.00	3.00	25.00	0.50
	Chow Mein, Vegetable-Stouffer's	28.3500	1.000	Ounce	0.30	0.70	1.60	14.00	0.00	0.00	0.00	0.00
	Corn Pudding-Stouffer's	28.3500	1.000	Ounce	1.20	1.70	4.50	38.00	0.00	0.00	15.00	0.00
	Corn Souffle-Stouffer's	170.0960	1.000	Each	7.00	11.00	27.00	240.00	0.00	0.00	0.00	0.00
	Corned Beef Hash-Hormel	253.1620	1.000	Cup	26.79	26.79	17.86	419.71	0.00	0.00	80.37	8.93
	Egg Roll	85.0000	1.000	Each	7.00	5.00	21.00	160.00	0.00	2.00	10.00	1.00
	Enchiladas, Beef and Bean, Lean	262.2310	1.000	Each	15.00	6.00	32.00	240.00	0.00	0.00	45.00	3.00
	Enchiladas, Beef-Healthy Choice	379.1720	1.000	Each	15.00	5.00	66.00	370.00	0.00	0.00	30.00	2.00
	Enchiladas, Cheese-Stouffer's	276.4060	1.000	Each	23.00	29.00	33.00	490.00	0.00	0.00	0.00	0.00
	Enchiladas, Chicken Suiza-Weight	255.1500	1.000	Each	15.00	8.00	28.00	250.00	0.00	4.00	25.00	3.00
	Enchiladas, Chicken, Lean Cuisine	279.9500	1.000	Each	17.00	9.00	34.00	290.00	0.00	0.00	55.00	3.00
	Enchiladas, Chicken, Nacho Grand	255.1500	1.000	Each	15.00	8.00	42.00	290.00	0.00	4.00	20.00	2.50
	Enchiladas, Chicken-Healthy Choice	269.3190	1.000	Each	14.00	9.00	44.00	310.00	0.00	0.00	35.00	3.00
	Enchiladas, Chicken-Stouffer's	283.4930	1.000	Each	21.00	31.00	31.00	490.00	0.00	0.00	0.00	0.00
	Fajitas, Chicken-Healthy Choice	198.4450	1.000	Each	17.00	3.00	25.00	200.00	0.00	0.00	35.00	1.00
442	Fettuccini Alfredo w/Broccoli-Sm	238.0000	8.500	Ounce	10.00	6.00	34.00	230.00	0.00	3.00	20.00	3.00
443	Fettuccini, Chicken-Smart Ones	280.0000	10.000	Ounce	19.00	7.00	39.00	290.00	0.00	4.00	50.00	2.00
	Fettucini Alfredo with Broccoli-	240.9750	1.000	Each	15.00	6.00	24.00	220.00	0.00	6.00	15.00	2.50
	Fettucini Alfredo, Lean Cuisine-	255.1440	1.000	Each	14.00	7.00	41.00	280.00	0.00	0.00	15.00	3.00
	Fettucini Alfredo-Stouffer's	141.7460	1.000	Each	8.00	14.00	22.00	245.00	0.00	0.00	0.00	0.00
	Fettucini Primavera, Lean Cuisine	283.4930	1.000	Each	14.00	8.00	32.00	260.00	0.00	0.00	45.00	3.00
	Fettucini Sauce (Alfredo Style)-	283.9200	1.000	Cup	14.02	67.10	11.02	701.05	0.00	0.00	180.27	0.00
	Fettucini w/ Turkey and Vegetable	354.3670	1.000	Each	29.00	6.00	45.00	350.00	0.00	0.00	60.00	3.00
	Fettucini, Chicken-Weight Watch	233.8900	1.000	Each	22.00	9.00	25.00	280.00	0.00	2.00	40.00	3.00
	Fettucini, Chicken, Lean Cuisine	255.1440	1.000	Each	23.00	6.00	33.00	280.00	0.00	0.00	35.00	3.00
	Fettucini, Chicken-Healthy Choice	240.9690	1.000	Each	19.00	7.00	39.00	240.00	0.00	0.00	45.00	2.00
	Fish Divan, Filet of, Lean Cuisine	294.1240	1.000	Each	27.00	5.00	13.00	210.00	0.00	0.00	65.00	2.00
	Fish Florentine, Filet of, Lean	272.8620	1.000	Each	26.00	7.00	13.00	220.00	0.00	0.00	65.00	3.00
	Fish, Breaded-Healthy Choice	9.7450	1.000	Stick	1.00	0.50	1.75	15.00	0.00	0.00	2.50	0.00
	Fish, Lemon Pepper-Healthy Choice	304.7550	1.000	Each	13.00	5.00	52.00	300.00	0.00	0.00	40.00	1.00
	Ham and Asparagus Bake-Stouffer'	269.3190	1.000	Each	18.00	35.00	32.00	520.00	0.00	0.00	0.00	0.00
	Hamburger Helper, Beef Noodle	220.0000	1.000	Cup	4.00	10.50	23.00	260.00	0.00	1.00	5.00	4.00
	Hamburger Helper, Cheesy Italian	220.0000	1.000	Cup	5.00	21.00	30.00	330.00	0.00	1.00	5.00	2.00

Page Key: A2 = Baby Food   A2 = Baked Goods   A8 = Beverages   A14 = Breads/Grains and Pasta   A18 = Breakfast Foods/Cereals   A26 = Dairy and Eggs   A40 = Fats and Oils
A42 = Fruits and Vegetables   A52 = Meats and Beans   A60 = Nuts and Seeds   A62 = Frozen Entrees and Packaged Foods   A76 = Restaurant Chains–Fast Foods
A92 = Restaurant Chains–Other   A106 = Seafood and Fish   A110 = Snacks and Sweets   A120 = Soups   A122 = Supplements   A126 = Toppings and Sauces

Monounsaturated Fat (g)	Polyunsaturated Fat (g)	Vitamin D (mg)	Vitamin K (mg)	Vitamin E (mg)	Vitamin A (re)	Vitamin C (mg)	Thiamin (mg)	Riboflavin (mg)	Niacin (mg)	Vitamin B6 (mg)	Folate (mcg)	Vitamin B12 (mcg)	Calcium (mg)	Iron (mg)	Magnesium (mg)	Phosphorus (mg)	Potassium (mg)	Sodium (mg)	Zinc (mg)
0.00	2.00	0.00	0.00	0.00	20.00	6.00	0.09	0.10	7.60	0.00	0.00	0.00	32.00	0.80	0.00	250.00	520.00	560.00	0.00
0.00	0.00	0.00	0.00	0.00	20.00	6.00	0.09	0.03	0.38	0.00	0.00	0.00	16.00	0.60	0.00	0.00	290.00	560.00	0.00
0.00	0.00	0.00	0.00	0.00	200.00	15.00	0.15	0.26	2.85	0.00	0.00	0.00	64.00	2.00	0.00	0.00	700.00	910.00	0.00
4.00	0.00	0.00	0.00	0.17	210.00	0.00	0.08	0.17	2.09	0.00	0.00	0.00	0.00	1.50	35.00	0.00	443.00	977.00	2.10
8.00	1.00	0.00	0.00	0.01	400.00	0.00	0.08	0.24	2.47	0.00	0.00	0.00	48.00	1.60	35.00	0.00	507.00	830.00	3.90
0.00	0.00	0.00	0.00	0.00	0.00	0.00	0.00	0.00	0.57	0.00	0.00	0.00	0.00	0.30	0.00	0.00	711.07	991.49	0.00
0.00	0.00	0.00	0.00	0.00	0.00	0.00	0.00	0.00	0.00	0.00	0.00	0.00	0.00	0.00	0.00	0.00	0.00	928.73	0.00
4.00	0.00	0.00	0.00	18.90	190.00	0.00	0.14	0.15	1.71	0.00	0.00	0.00	48.00	1.90	45.50	0.00	677.00	977.00	2.70
7.14	1.19	0.00	0.00	0.01	250.04	0.00	0.11	0.20	2.04	0.00	0.00	0.00	57.15	1.91	58.34	0.00	913.25	1226.40	2.50
15.48	1.19	0.00	0.00	0.60	785.85	0.00	0.11	0.26	2.94	0.00	0.00	0.00	47.63	1.67	41.67	0.00	591.77	1023.98	3.21
0.00	0.00	0.00	0.00	0.00	2000.00	24.00	0.00	0.00	0.00	0.00	0.00	0.00	48.00	2.00	0.00	0.00	0.00	320.00	0.00
13.00	1.00	0.00	0.00	10.56	330.00	0.00	0.05	0.22	2.47	0.00	0.00	0.00	40.00	1.40	35.00	0.00	497.00	860.00	2.70
4.00	0.00	0.00	0.00	1.95	190.00	0.00	0.14	0.15	1.71	0.00	0.00	0.00	48.00	1.90	45.50	0.00	677.00	977.00	2.70
6.00	1.00	0.00	0.00	0.00	210.00	0.00	0.09	0.17	1.71	0.00	0.00	0.00	48.00	1.80	49.00	0.00	777.00	1030.00	2.25
0.00	0.00	0.00	0.00	0.00	0.00	6.01	0.00	0.01	0.57	0.00	0.00	0.00	1.20	0.40	0.00	0.00	891.34	861.29	0.00
0.00	1.00	0.00	0.00	0.00	60.00	6.00	0.15	0.17	4.75	0.00	0.00	0.00	32.00	0.60	0.00	0.00	350.00	530.00	0.00
0.00	0.00	0.00	0.00	0.00	80.00	12.00	0.03	0.17	1.90	0.00	0.00	0.00	16.00	0.40	0.00	0.00	340.00	720.00	0.00
0.00	0.00	0.00	0.00	0.00	40.00	12.00	0.00	0.00	7.00	0.00	0.00	0.00	24.00	0.40	0.00	0.00	0.00	760.00	0.00
0.00	0.00	0.00	0.00	0.00	300.00	36.00	0.00	0.00	0.00	0.00	0.00	0.00	48.00	0.40	0.00	0.00	360.00	570.00	0.00
0.00	1.00	0.00	0.00	0.00	80.00	3.60	0.15	0.14	3.80	0.00	0.00	0.00	16.00	0.80	0.00	290.00	290.00	440.00	0.00
0.00	0.00	0.00	0.00	0.00	0.00	0.00	0.00	0.00	0.00	0.00	0.00	0.00	0.00	0.00	0.00	0.00	0.00	570.00	0.00
0.00	0.00	0.00	0.00	0.00	0.00	0.60	0.00	0.00	0.02	0.00	0.00	0.00	24.00	0.01	0.00	0.00	26.00	156.00	0.00
0.00	0.00	0.00	0.00	0.00	0.00	0.60	0.00	0.00	0.06	0.00	0.00	0.00	88.00	0.02	0.00	0.00	51.00	125.00	0.00
0.00	0.00	0.00	0.00	0.00	60.00	0.00	0.15	0.26	1.14	0.00	0.00	0.00	48.00	0.40	0.00	0.00	200.00	760.00	0.00
17.86	0.00	0.00	0.00	0.43	0.00	0.00	0.00	0.15	3.39	0.00	0.00	0.00	71.44	1.79	31.26	0.00	625.11	991.24	4.02
0.00	0.00	0.00	0.00	0.00	100.00	1.20	0.00	0.00	0.00	0.00	0.00	0.00	24.00	0.20	0.00	0.00	0.00	350.00	0.00
0.00	1.00	0.00	0.00	0.00	80.00	6.00	0.23	0.26	1.90	0.00	0.00	0.00	80.00	1.00	0.00	0.00	470.00	480.00	0.00
0.00	2.00	0.00	0.00	0.00	250.00	24.00	0.30	0.26	1.90	0.00	0.00	0.00	120.00	1.00	0.00	260.00	600.00	450.00	0.00
0.00	0.00	0.00	0.00	0.00	150.00	6.00	0.09	0.34	1.52	0.00	0.00	0.00	480.00	0.80	0.00	0.00	400.00	550.00	0.00
0.00	0.00	0.00	0.00	0.00	40.00	1.20	0.00	0.00	0.00	0.00	0.00	0.00	360.00	0.80	0.00	0.00	470.00	570.00	0.00
0.00	2.00	0.00	0.00	0.00	250.00	6.00	0.23	0.34	2.85	0.00	0.00	0.00	120.00	1.50	0.00	0.00	450.00	500.00	0.00
0.00	0.00	0.00	0.00	0.00	300.00	12.00	0.00	0.00	0.00	0.00	0.00	0.00	360.00	0.60	0.00	0.00	600.00	560.00	0.00
0.00	1.00	0.00	0.00	0.00	80.00	21.00	0.15	0.17	4.75	0.00	0.00	0.00	80.00	0.80	0.00	160.00	380.00	480.00	0.00
0.00	0.00	0.00	0.00	0.00	60.00	2.40	0.09	0.34	2.85	0.00	0.00	0.00	240.00	0.60	0.00	0.00	420.00	860.00	0.00
0.00	1.00	0.00	0.00	0.00	150.00	9.00	0.23	0.17	3.80	0.00	0.00	0.00	64.00	1.50	0.00	210.00	360.00	310.00	0.00
0.00	0.00	0.00	0.00	0.00	0.00	0.00	0.00	0.00	0.00	0.00	0.00	0.00	0.00	0.00	0.00	0.00	0.00	450.00	0.00
0.00	0.00	0.00	0.00	0.00	0.00	0.00	0.00	0.00	0.00	0.00	0.00	0.00	0.00	0.00	0.00	0.00	0.00	590.00	0.00
0.00	0.00	0.00	0.00	0.00	60.00	1.20	0.00	0.00	0.00	0.00	0.00	0.00	300.00	1.50	0.00	0.00	510.00	540.00	0.00
0.00	0.00	0.00	0.00	0.00	0.00	0.00	0.30	0.43	1.52	0.00	0.00	0.00	200.00	0.00	0.00	0.00	270.00	570.00	0.00
0.00	0.00	0.00	0.00	0.00	0.00	0.00	0.15	0.26	0.95	0.00	0.00	0.00	120.00	0.40	0.00	0.00	100.00	400.00	0.00
0.00	0.00	0.00	0.00	0.00	400.00	18.00	0.30	0.43	1.52	0.00	0.00	0.00	240.00	0.80	0.00	0.00	400.00	510.00	0.00
0.00	0.00	0.00	0.00	0.00	0.00	0.00	0.00	0.01	0.00	0.00	0.00	0.00	2.72	0.00	0.00	0.00	340.51	1812.72	0.00
0.00	2.00	0.00	0.00	0.00	150.00	0.00	0.45	0.51	3.80	0.00	0.00	0.00	120.00	1.50	0.00	310.00	450.00	480.00	0.00
0.00	0.00	0.00	0.00	0.00	40.00	0.00	0.00	0.00	0.00	0.00	0.00	0.00	240.00	1.00	0.00	0.00	730.00	590.00	0.00
0.00	0.00	0.00	0.00	0.00	0.00	0.00	0.30	0.43	5.70	0.00	0.00	0.00	120.00	0.80	0.00	0.00	420.00	500.00	0.00
0.00	2.00	0.00	0.00	0.00	0.00	0.00	0.23	0.17	2.85	0.00	0.00	0.00	64.00	1.00	0.00	210.00	190.00	370.00	0.00
0.00	1.00	0.00	0.00	0.00	20.00	27.00	0.15	0.34	1.90	0.00	0.00	0.00	120.00	0.40	0.00	0.00	800.00	490.00	0.00
0.00	2.00	0.00	0.00	0.00	500.00	1.20	0.15	0.34	1.90	0.00	0.00	0.00	120.00	0.40	0.00	0.00	780.00	590.00	0.00
0.00	0.13	0.00	0.00	0.00	0.00	0.00	0.01	0.02	0.10	0.00	0.00	0.00	0.00	0.10	0.00	0.00	20.00	31.25	0.00
0.00	2.00	0.00	0.00	0.00	80.00	48.00	0.23	0.14	1.14	0.00	0.00	0.00	32.00	0.60	0.00	180.00	410.00	370.00	0.00
0.00	0.00	0.00	0.00	0.00	60.00	36.00	0.53	0.51	2.85	0.00	0.00	0.00	160.00	0.80	0.00	0.00	360.00	1100.00	0.00
0.00	0.00	0.00	0.00	0.00	60.00	0.00	0.23	0.17	3.80	0.00	0.00	0.00	24.00	1.00	0.00	0.00	240.00	900.00	0.00
0.00	0.00	0.00	0.00	0.00	60.00	0.00	0.30	0.34	3.80	0.00	0.00	0.00	120.00	1.50	0.00	0.00	400.00	900.00	0.00

USDA ID Code	Food Name	Weight in Grams*	Quantity of Units	Unit of Measure	Protein (g)	Fat (g)	Carbohydrate (g)	Kilocalories	Caffeine (g)	Fiber (g)	Cholesterol (mg)	Saturated Fat (g)
	Hamburger Helper, Chili Mac	220.0000	1.000	Cup	3.00	16.00	30.00	290.00	0.00	1.00	4.00	4.00
	Heartland Medley-Stouffer's	28.3500	1.000	Ounce	1.40	0.40	1.80	17.00	0.00	0.00	3.00	0.00
580	Lasagna Florentine-Smart Ones	280.0000	10.000	Ounce	10.00	2.00	34.00	200.00	0.00	5.00	10.00	0.00
	Lasagna Florentine-Weight Watche	283.5000	1.000	Each	13.00	2.00	37.00	210.00	0.00	5.00	10.00	0.50
	Lasagna w/ Meat Sauce, Lean Cuis	290.5810	1.000	Each	20.00	6.00	36.00	280.00	0.00	0.00	25.00	3.00
	Lasagna w/ Meat Sauce-Healthy Ch	283.4930	1.000	Each	18.00	5.00	37.00	260.00	0.00	0.00	20.00	2.00
581	Lasagna w/ Meat Sauce-Smart Ones	252.0000	9.000	Ounce	13.00	2.00	43.00	240.00	0.00	4.00	10.00	0.50
	Lasagna w/ Meat Sauce-Weight Wat	290.5900	1.000	Each	24.00	7.00	34.00	290.00	0.00	7.00	15.00	2.50
	Lasagna, Cheese, Italian-Weight	311.8500	1.000	Each	29.00	8.00	28.00	300.00	0.00	7.00	25.00	3.00
	Lasagna, Italian, Top Shelf-Horm	283.4930	1.000	Each	23.00	16.00	30.00	350.00	0.00	0.00	60.00	8.00
	Lasagna, Micro Cup-Hormel	212.6200	1.000	Each	8.00	13.00	25.00	250.00	0.00	0.00	23.00	6.00
	Lasagna, Vegetable-Stouffer's	274.0420	1.000	Each	23.00	20.00	33.00	400.00	0.00	0.00	0.00	0.00
	Lasagna, Zucchini, Lean Cuisine-	311.8430	1.000	Each	17.00	6.00	34.00	260.00	0.00	0.00	20.00	2.00
	Lasagna, Zucchini-Healthy Choice	326.0170	1.000	Each	14.00	3.00	41.00	250.00	0.00	0.00	15.00	2.00
	Lasagna-Stouffer's	283.4930	1.000	Each	18.00	12.00	40.00	340.00	0.00	0.00	0.00	0.00
	Linguini w/ Clam Sauce, Lean Cui	272.8620	1.000	Each	17.00	8.00	36.00	280.00	0.00	0.00	30.00	2.00
	Macaroni and Beef in Sauce, Lean	283.4930	1.000	Each	14.00	6.00	35.00	250.00	0.00	0.00	25.00	1.00
	Macaroni and Beef w/ Tomatoes-St	326.0170	1.000	Each	21.00	12.00	38.00	340.00	0.00	0.00	0.00	0.00
	Macaroni and Beef-Healthy Choice	240.9690	1.000	Each	12.00	3.00	32.00	200.00	0.00	0.00	15.00	1.00
	Macaroni and Cheese	111.9120	1.000	Cup	1.00	12.99	43.97	359.72	0.00	15.99	39.97	7.99
	Macaroni and Cheese, Deluxe Ligh	90.0000	1.000	Serving	14.00	4.50	48.00	290.00	0.00	0.00	15.00	2.50
	Macaroni and Cheese, Kraft	70.0000	1.000	Serving	12.00	18.50	50.00	420.00	0.00	0.00	15.00	5.00
	Macaroni and Cheese, Lean Cuisine	255.1440	1.000	Each	15.00	9.00	37.00	290.00	0.00	0.00	30.00	4.00
	Macaroni and Cheese, Micro Cup-H	212.6200	1.000	Each	12.00	11.00	28.00	260.00	0.00	0.00	45.00	6.00
	Macaroni and Cheese, Nacho-Healt	255.1440	1.000	Each	13.00	5.00	44.00	280.00	0.00	0.00	20.00	3.00
	Macaroni and Cheese-Healthy Choi	255.1440	1.000	Each	12.00	6.00	45.00	280.00	0.00	0.00	20.00	3.00
	Macaroni and Cheese-Stouffer's	170.0960	1.000	Each	11.00	13.00	23.00	250.00	0.00	0.00	0.00	0.00
	Macaroni and Cheese-Weight Watch	255.1500	1.000	Each	11.00	7.00	49.00	300.00	0.00	7.00	20.00	2.00
	Manicotti, Cheese-Healthy Choice	262.2310	1.000	Each	15.00	3.00	34.00	220.00	0.00	0.00	30.00	2.00
	Manicotti, Cheese-Stouffer's	28.3500	1.000	Ounce	1.60	1.30	2.60	29.00	0.00	0.00	4.00	0.00
	Meatballs, Swedish, w/ Pasta, Le	258.6880	1.000	Each	23.00	8.00	31.00	290.00	0.00	0.00	55.00	3.00
	Meatballs, Swedish, w/ Pasta-Sto	262.2310	1.000	Each	24.00	21.00	32.00	420.00	0.00	0.00	0.00	0.00
582	Meatballs, Swedish-Smart Ones	252.0000	9.000	Ounce	19.00	10.00	33.00	300.00	0.00	2.00	50.00	4.00
	Meatloaf w/ Mac. and Cheese, Lea	265.7750	1.000	Each	26.00	8.00	26.00	280.00	0.00	0.00	55.00	3.00
	Meatloaf-Healthy Choice	340.1920	1.000	Each	17.00	8.00	48.00	340.00	0.00	0.00	40.00	3.00
	Meatloaf-Stouffer's	28.3500	1.000	Ounce	4.40	3.40	2.10	57.00	0.00	0.00	15.00	0.00
585	Morningstar Farms-Buffalo Wings	85.0000	5.000	Each	13.00	9.00	16.00	200.00	0.00	3.00	0.00	1.50
586	Morningstar Farms-Burger, Bean,	78.0000	1.000	Each	11.00	1.00	16.00	110.00	0.00	5.00	0.00	0.00
587	Morningstar Farms-Burger, Veggi	67.0000	1.000	Each	14.00	8.00	40.00	120.00	0.00	2.00	0.00	3.50
588	Morningstar Farms-Burger/Cheese	128.0000	1.000	Each	14.00	8.00	40.00	290.00	0.00	2.00	0.00	3.50
589	Morningstar Farms-Burgers, Bett	78.0000	1.000	Each	13.00	0.00	8.00	80.00	0.00	3.00	0.00	0.00
590	Morningstar Farms-Chik Nuggets	86.0000	4.000	Each	13.00	4.00	17.00	160.00	0.00	5.00	0.00	0.50
591	Morningstar Farms-Chik Patties	71.0000	1.000	Each	9.00	6.00	15.00	150.00	0.00	2.00	0.00	1.00
592	Morningstar Farms-Corn Dogs, Me	71.0000	1.000	Each	7.00	4.00	22.00	150.00	0.00	3.00	0.00	0.50
593	Morningstar Farms-Corn Dogs, Mi	71.0000	1.000	Each	11.00	4.50	21.00	150.00	0.00	1.00	0.00	0.50
594	Morningstar Farms-Crumbles, Bur	55.0000	0.660	Cup	10.00	2.50	4.00	80.00	0.00	2.00	0.00	0.00
595	Morningstar Farms-Crumbles, Sau	55.0000	0.660	Cup	11.00	3.00	5.00	90.00	0.00	2.00	0.00	0.00
596	Morningstar Farms-Eggs, Better'	57.0000	0.250	Cup	5.00	0.00	0.00	20.00	0.00	0.00	0.00	0.00
597	Morningstar Farms-Garden Grille	71.0000	1.000	Each	6.00	2.50	18.00	120.00	0.00	4.00	0.00	1.00
598	Morningstar Farms-Grillers	64.0000	1.000	Each	15.00	6.00	5.00	140.00	0.00	2.00	0.00	1.00
599	Morningstar Farms-Ham/Cheese Sd	128.0000	1.000	Each	15.00	7.00	25.00	300.00	0.00	1.00	0.00	2.50
600	Morningstar Farms-Harvest Burge	90.0000	1.000	Each	17.00	4.50	8.00	140.00	0.00	5.00	0.00	1.50
601	Morningstar Farms-Harvest Burge	90.0000	1.000	Each	18.00	4.00	8.00	140.00	0.00	5.00	0.00	1.50

Page Key: A2 = Baby Food   A2 = Baked Goods   A8 = Beverages   A14 = Breads/Grains and Pasta   A18 = Breakfast Foods/Cereals   A26 = Dairy and Eggs   A40 = Fats and Oils   A42 = Fruits and Vegetables   A52 = Meats and Beans   A60 = Nuts and Seeds   A62 = Frozen Entrees and Packaged Foods   A76 = Restaurant Chains–Fast Foods   A92 = Restaurant Chains–Other   A106 = Seafood and Fish   A110 = Snacks and Sweets   A120 = Soups   A122 = Supplements   A126 = Toppings and Sauces

Monounsaturated Fat (g)	Polyunsaturated Fat (g)	Vitamin D (mg)	Vitamin K (mg)	Vitamin E (mg)	Vitamin A (re)	Vitamin C (mg)	Thiamin (mg)	Riboflavin (mg)	Niacin (mg)	Vitamin B6 (mg)	Folate (mcg)	Vitamin B12 (mcg)	Calcium (mg)	Iron (mg)	Magnesium (mg)	Phosphorus (mg)	Potassium (mg)	Sodium (mg)	Zinc (mg)
0.00	0.00	0.00	0.00	0.00	200.00	0.00	0.30	0.26	4.75	0.00	0.00	0.00	24.00	1.50	0.00	0.00	0.00	900.00	0.00
0.00	0.00	0.00	0.00	0.00	0.00	0.60	0.00	0.00	0.06	0.00	0.00	0.00	40.00	0.02	0.00	0.00	60.00	85.00	0.00
0.00	0.00	0.00	0.00	0.00	0.00	0.00	0.00	0.00	0.00	0.00	0.00	0.00	0.00	0.00	0.00	0.00	0.00	590.00	0.00
0.00	0.00	0.00	0.00	0.00	300.00	15.00	0.00	0.00	0.00	0.00	0.00	0.00	300.00	1.50	0.00	0.00	440.00	420.00	0.00
0.00	0.00	0.00	0.00	0.00	100.00	6.00	0.15	0.26	2.85	0.00	0.00	0.00	120.00	1.00	0.00	0.00	700.00	560.00	0.00
0.00	1.00	0.00	0.00	0.00	150.00	2.40	0.30	0.26	1.90	0.00	0.00	0.00	80.00	1.50	0.00	210.00	500.00	420.00	0.00
0.00	0.00	0.00	0.00	0.00	0.00	0.00	0.00	0.00	0.00	0.00	0.00	0.00	0.00	0.00	0.00	0.00	0.00	520.00	0.00
0.00	0.00	0.00	0.00	0.00	250.00	12.00	0.00	0.00	0.00	0.00	0.00	0.00	480.00	1.50	0.00	0.00	720.00	580.00	0.00
0.00	0.00	0.00	0.00	0.00	350.00	15.00	0.00	0.00	0.00	0.00	0.00	0.00	780.00	1.50	0.00	0.00	720.00	560.00	0.00
5.00	1.00	0.00	0.00	0.70	100.00	2.40	0.30	0.51	3.80	0.00	0.00	0.00	240.00	1.50	49.00	0.00	728.00	840.00	3.15
4.00	2.00	0.00	0.00	0.00	100.00	1.80	0.12	0.20	1.90	0.00	0.00	0.00	40.00	0.80	24.50	0.00	331.00	949.00	1.05
0.00	0.00	0.00	0.00	0.00	250.00	0.00	0.12	0.43	0.76	0.00	0.00	0.00	160.00	0.60	0.00	0.00	350.00	760.00	0.00
0.00	0.00	0.00	0.00	0.00	150.00	6.00	0.15	0.26	1.90	0.00	0.00	0.00	200.00	0.80	0.00	0.00	650.00	520.00	0.00
0.00	0.00	0.00	0.00	0.00	350.00	6.00	0.38	0.26	1.90	0.00	0.00	0.00	200.00	1.50	0.00	250.00	830.00	400.00	0.00
0.00	0.00	0.00	0.00	0.00	150.00	6.00	0.15	0.34	6.65	0.00	0.00	0.00	200.00	1.00	0.00	0.00	570.00	840.00	0.00
0.00	2.00	0.00	0.00	0.00	0.00	0.00	0.30	0.17	1.90	0.00	0.00	0.00	32.00	1.50	0.00	0.00	90.00	560.00	0.00
0.00	1.00	0.00	0.00	0.00	100.00	3.60	0.15	0.17	2.85	0.00	0.00	0.00	48.00	1.50	0.00	0.00	450.00	540.00	0.00
0.00	0.00	0.00	0.00	0.00	60.00	6.00	0.06	0.10	1.90	0.00	0.00	0.00	32.00	0.80	0.00	0.00	300.00	1440.00	0.00
0.00	0.00	0.00	0.00	0.00	200.00	15.00	0.30	0.26	0.00	0.00	0.00	0.00	32.00	1.00	0.00	0.00	530.00	420.00	0.00
0.00	0.00	0.00	0.00	0.00	99.92	0.00	0.00	0.00	0.00	0.00	0.00	0.00	239.81	1.50	0.00	0.00	0.00	1029.19	0.00
0.00	0.00	0.00	0.00	0.00	0.00	0.00	0.00	0.00	0.00	0.00	0.00	0.00	160.00	1.50	0.00	0.00	0.00	810.00	0.00
0.00	0.00	0.00	0.00	0.00	0.00	0.00	0.00	0.00	0.00	0.00	0.00	0.00	120.00	1.50	0.00	0.00	0.00	760.00	0.00
0.00	0.00	0.00	0.00	0.00	0.00	0.00	0.30	0.43	1.52	0.00	0.00	0.00	200.00	0.80	0.00	0.00	160.00	550.00	0.00
3.00	1.00	0.00	0.00	0.00	80.00	6.00	0.09	0.26	1.14	0.00	0.00	0.00	80.00	0.60	24.50	0.00	209.00	650.00	1.05
0.00	0.00	0.00	0.00	0.00	0.00	0.00	0.60	0.51	0.00	0.00	0.00	0.00	160.00	0.80	0.00	0.00	420.00	560.00	0.00
0.00	1.00	0.00	0.00	0.00	0.00	0.00	0.30	0.26	1.14	0.00	0.00	0.00	120.00	1.00	0.00	230.00	220.00	520.00	0.00
0.00	0.00	0.00	0.00	0.00	20.00	0.00	0.15	0.26	0.38	0.00	0.00	0.00	160.00	0.40	0.00	0.00	140.00	640.00	0.00
0.00	0.00	0.00	0.00	0.00	100.00	0.00	0.00	0.00	0.00	0.00	0.00	0.00	300.00	1.00	0.00	0.00	410.00	570.00	0.00
0.00	0.00	0.00	0.00	0.00	250.00	6.00	0.30	0.26	1.90	0.00	0.00	0.00	120.00	1.50	0.00	210.00	590.00	310.00	0.00
0.00	0.00	0.00	0.00	0.00	0.00	2.40	0.00	0.00	0.04	0.00	0.00	0.00	296.01	0.02	0.00	0.00	45.00	108.00	0.00
0.00	1.00	0.00	0.00	0.00	20.00	0.00	0.23	0.34	3.80	0.00	0.00	0.00	48.00	1.50	0.00	0.00	450.00	550.00	0.00
0.00	0.00	0.00	0.00	0.00	20.00	1.20	0.15	0.26	2.85	0.00	0.00	0.00	48.00	1.50	0.00	0.00	350.00	740.00	0.00
0.00	0.00	0.00	0.00	0.00	0.00	0.00	0.00	0.00	0.00	0.00	0.00	0.00	0.00	0.00	0.00	0.00	0.00	510.00	0.00
0.00	1.00	0.00	0.00	0.00	60.00	9.00	0.23	0.43	3.80	0.00	0.00	0.00	120.00	2.00	0.00	0.00	550.00	540.00	0.00
0.00	1.00	0.00	0.00	0.00	0.00	0.00	0.00	0.00	0.00	0.00	0.00	0.00	0.00	0.00	0.00	240.00	690.00	560.00	0.00
0.00	0.00	0.00	0.00	0.00	0.00	0.00	0.13	0.00	0.00	0.00	0.00	0.00	48.00	0.06	0.00	0.00	4.40	193.00	0.00
2.50	5.00	0.00	0.00	0.00	0.00	0.00	1.05	0.17	3.00	0.20	0.00	1.20	40.00	2.70	0.00	0.00	390.00	730.00	0.00
0.00	0.00	0.00	0.00	0.00	0.00	0.00	0.00	0.00	0.00	0.00	0.00	0.00	40.00	1.80	0.00	0.00	350.00	470.00	0.00
3.00	1.50	0.00	0.00	0.00	0.00	0.00	0.00	0.00	0.00	0.00	0.00	0.00	100.00	1.08	0.00	0.00	130.00	400.00	0.00
3.00	1.50	0.00	0.00	0.00	0.00	0.00	0.00	0.00	0.00	0.00	0.00	0.00	60.00	1.08	0.00	0.00	130.00	400.00	0.00
0.00	0.00	0.00	0.00	0.00	0.00	0.00	0.00	0.00	0.00	0.00	0.00	0.00	20.00	1.80	0.00	0.00	390.00	360.00	0.00
1.00	2.50	0.00	0.00	0.00	0.00	0.00	0.90	0.17	2.00	0.20	0.00	1.50	20.00	1.80	0.00	0.00	330.00	670.00	0.00
1.50	3.50	0.00	0.00	0.00	0.00	0.00	0.60	0.10	0.40	0.16	0.00	0.90	0.00	0.72	0.00	0.00	150.00	570.00	0.00
1.00	2.50	0.00	0.00	0.00	0.00	0.00	0.00	0.00	0.00	0.00	0.00	0.00	0.00	1.08	0.00	0.00	60.00	500.00	0.00
2.50	1.50	0.00	0.00	0.00	0.00	0.00	0.00	0.00	0.00	0.00	0.00	0.00	0.00	1.08	0.00	0.00	90.00	580.00	0.00
0.50	2.00	0.00	0.00	0.00	0.00	0.00	0.30	0.10	4.00	0.30	0.00	1.80	20.00	1.80	0.00	0.00	120.00	210.00	0.00
0.50	2.00	0.00	0.00	0.00	0.00	0.00	1.80	0.17	4.00	0.40	0.00	1.80	20.00	1.80	0.00	0.00	80.00	370.00	0.00
0.00	0.00	0.60	0.00	1.20	225.00	0.00	0.03	0.34	0.00	0.08	0.02	0.60	20.00	0.72	0.00	0.00	75.00	90.00	0.60
1.00	0.50	0.00	0.00	0.00	0.00	0.00	0.00	0.00	0.00	0.00	0.00	0.00	60.00	1.80	0.00	0.00	130.00	280.00	0.00
2.00	3.00	0.00	0.00	0.00	0.00	0.00	1.80	0.17	2.00	0.40	0.00	2.70	40.00	1.08	0.00	0.00	130.00	260.00	0.00
3.00	1.50	0.00	0.00	0.00	0.00	0.00	0.00	0.00	0.00	0.00	0.00	0.00	60.00	1.08	0.00	0.00	100.00	520.00	0.00
0.50	0.50	0.00	0.00	0.00	0.00	0.00	0.30	0.14	4.00	0.30	0.00	1.50	80.00	2.70	0.00	0.00	440.00	370.00	6.75
0.00	0.50	0.00	0.00	0.00	0.00	0.00	0.30	0.14	4.00	0.30	0.00	1.50	80.00	2.70	0.00	0.00	430.00	370.00	7.50

USDA ID Code	Food Name	Weight in Grams*	Quantity of Units	Unit of Measure	Protein (g)	Fat (g)	Carbohydrate (g)	Kilocalories	Caffeine (g)	Fiber (g)	Cholesterol (mg)	Saturated Fat (g)
602	Morningstar Farms-Harvest Burge	90.0000	1.000	Each	16.00	4.00	9.00	140.00	0.00	5.00	0.00	1.50
603	Morningstar Farms-Links, Breakf	45.0000	2.000	Each	8.00	2.00	2.00	60.00	0.00	2.00	0.00	0.50
604	Morningstar Farms-Meatless, Gro	55.0000	0.500	Cup	10.00	0.00	4.00	60.00	0.00	2.00	0.00	0.00
605	Morningstar Farms-Patties, Brea	38.0000	1.000	Each	10.00	0.00	3.00	38.00	0.00	2.00	0.00	0.50
606	Morningstar Farms-Patties, Gard	67.0000	1.000	Each	10.00	2.50	9.00	100.00	0.00	4.00	0.00	0.50
607	Morningstar Farms-Pizza, Pepper	128.0000	1.000	Each	12.00	7.00	42.00	280.00	0.00	5.00	0.00	3.00
608	Morningstar Farms-Quarter Prime	96.0000	1.000	Each	24.00	2.00	6.00	140.00	0.00	3.00	0.00	0.00
609	Morningstar Farms-Scramblers	57.0000	0.250	Cup	6.00	0.00	2.00	35.00	0.00	0.00	0.00	0.00
610	Morningstar Farms-Strips, Break	16.0000	2.000	Each	2.00	4.50	2.00	60.00	0.00	1.00	0.00	0.50
611	Morningstar Farms-Veggie Dog	57.0000	1.000	Each	11.00	0.50	6.00	57.00	0.00	1.00	0.00	0.00
	Muffin, Banana Nut-Healthy Choice	70.8730	1.000	Each	3.00	6.00	32.00	180.00	0.00	0.00	0.00	0.00
	Muffin, English, Sandwich-Healthy	120.4840	1.000	Each	16.00	3.00	30.00	200.00	0.00	0.00	20.00	1.00
	Noodles and Chicken, Micro Cup-H	212.6200	1.000	Each	7.00	7.00	19.00	174.00	0.00	0.00	29.00	2.00
	Noodles Romanoff-Stouffer's	283.9200	1.000	Cup	17.03	25.04	36.05	440.66	0.00	0.00	40.06	0.00
614	Noodles, Kung Pao & Veg-Smart On	280.0000	10.000	Ounce	8.00	10.00	35.00	260.00	0.00	5.00	5.00	1.50
	Omelet, Turkey Sausage, on Engli	134.6590	1.000	Each	16.00	4.00	30.00	210.00	0.00	0.00	20.00	2.00
	Omelet, Western Style, on Englis	134.6590	1.000	Each	16.00	3.00	29.00	200.00	0.00	0.00	15.00	2.00
624	Pasta Accents, White Cheddar Sce	181.0000	1.750	Cup	9.00	9.00	37.00	270.00	0.00	3.00	10.00	2.50
625	Pasta Accents-Alfredo	160.0000	2.000	Cup	9.00	8.00	25.00	210.00	0.00	4.00	5.00	2.50
626	Pasta Accents-Crmy Cheddar	190.0000	2.330	Cup	9.00	8.00	36.00	250.00	0.00	5.00	15.00	3.00
627	Pasta Accents-Florentine	206.0000	2.000	Cup	13.00	9.00	44.00	310.00	0.00	5.00	20.00	3.00
628	Pasta Accents-Garden Herb	195.0000	2.000	Cup	9.00	7.00	32.00	230.00	0.00	7.00	15.00	4.00
629	Pasta Accents-Garlic Seasoning	188.0000	2.000	Cup	7.00	10.00	36.00	260.00	0.00	3.00	15.00	5.00
630	Pasta Accents-Lasagna Style	188.0000	2.000	Cup	9.00	10.00	33.00	260.00	0.00	4.00	10.00	3.00
631	Pasta Accents-Oriental Style	201.0000	2.500	Cup	8.00	10.00	35.00	260.00	0.00	4.00	20.00	4.00
632	Pasta Accents-Primavera	200.0000	2.250	Cup	12.00	9.00	39.00	290.00	0.00	4.00	5.00	2.50
	Pasta Accents-Primavera	175.0000	1.000	Serving	9.00	10.00	27.00	230.00	0.00	0.00	0.00	0.00
633	Pasta and Spinach Romano-Smart O	291.0000	10.400	Ounce	11.00	8.00	32.00	240.00	0.00	4.00	5.00	3.50
	Pasta Florentine-Stouffer's	283.9200	0.500	Cup	16.02	21.03	32.05	380.57	0.00	0.00	50.07	0.00
	Pasta Italiano, Vegetable-Health	283.4930	1.000	Each	7.00	1.00	46.00	220.00	0.00	0.00	0.00	0.00
	Pasta Italiano-Healthy Choice	340.1920	1.000	Each	16.00	5.00	59.00	350.00	0.00	0.00	30.00	2.00
	Pasta Roma-Stouffer's	283.9200	0.500	Cup	16.02	7.01	31.05	260.39	0.00	0.00	30.04	0.00
	Pasta Shells w/ Tomato Sauce-Hea	340.1920	1.000	Each	24.00	3.00	53.00	330.00	0.00	0.00	35.00	2.00
	Pasta Shells, Cheese w/ Sauce-St	262.2310	1.000	Each	17.00	13.00	28.00	300.00	0.00	0.00	0.00	0.00
	Pasta w/ Chicken, Cacciatore-Hea	354.3670	1.000	Each	26.00	3.00	47.00	310.00	0.00	0.00	35.00	0.00
	Pasta w/ Chicken, Teriyaki-Healt	357.9100	1.000	Each	24.00	3.00	58.00	350.00	0.00	0.00	45.00	1.00
634	Pasta w/ Tomato Basil Sauce-Smar	268.8000	9.600	Ounce	12.00	9.00	33.00	260.00	0.00	5.00	10.00	3.50
	Pasta, Angel Hair, Lean Cuisine-	283.4930	1.000	Each	10.00	5.00	38.00	240.00	0.00	0.00	10.00	1.00
635	Pasta, Bowtie & Mushroom Marsala	270.0000	9.650	Ounce	13.00	9.00	36.00	280.00	0.00	5.00	10.00	3.50
636	Pasta, Crmy Rigatoni w/ Brocc &	252.0000	9.000	Ounce	14.00	2.00	40.00	230.00	0.00	4.00	20.00	0.50
637	Pasta, Penne w/ Sun-dried Tomato	280.0000	10.000	Ounce	12.00	9.00	41.00	290.00	0.00	4.00	15.00	3.00
639	Penne Pollo-Smart Ones	280.0000	10.000	Ounce	22.00	5.00	40.00	290.00	0.00	3.00	35.00	2.00
640	Penne, Spicy, & Ricotta-Smart On	285.6000	10.200	Ounce	12.00	6.00	45.00	280.00	0.00	5.00	5.00	2.00
	Pepper, Stuffed, Single Serving-	283.4930	1.000	Each	10.00	8.00	28.00	220.00	0.00	0.00	0.00	0.00
	Peppers, Stuffed Green-Stouffer'	219.7070	1.000	Each	9.00	8.00	22.00	200.00	0.00	0.00	0.00	0.00
654	Pizza Combo, Deluxe-Smart Ones	184.0000	6.570	Ounce	23.00	11.00	47.00	380.00	0.00	6.00	40.00	3.50
	Pizza, Cheese, 4-DiGiorno	139.0000	1.000	Slice	16.00	11.00	39.00	320.00	0.00	3.11	25.10	6.10
	Pizza, Cheese, Microwave for One	104.0000	1.000	Each	10.00	11.00	25.00	240.00	0.00	1.00	15.00	3.50
	Pizza, Cheese, Party-Totino's	277.0000	1.000	Slice	15.00	5.00	33.00	320.00	0.00	2.00	20.00	5.00
	Pizza, French Bread, Cheese-Heal	159.4650	1.000	Each	19.00	4.00	46.00	290.00	0.00	0.00	15.00	2.00
	Pizza, French Bread, Cheese-Stou	145.2900	1.000	Each	16.00	14.00	40.00	350.00	0.00	0.00	0.00	0.00
	Pizza, French Bread, Deluxe-Heal	180.7270	1.000	Each	23.00	7.00	41.00	330.00	0.00	0.00	35.00	3.00
	Pizza, French Bread, Deluxe-Stou	173.6390	1.000	Each	21.00	19.00	40.00	420.00	0.00	0.00	0.00	0.00

Monounsaturated Fat (g)	Polyunsaturated Fat (g)	Vitamin D (mg)	Vitamin K (mg)	Vitamin E (mg)	Vitamin A (re)	Vitamin C (mg)	Thiamin (mg)	Riboflavin (mg)	Niacin (mg)	Vitamin B6 (mg)	Folate (mcg)	Vitamin B12 (mcg)	Calcium (mg)	Iron (mg)	Magnesium (mg)	Phosphorus (mg)	Potassium (mg)	Sodium (mg)	Zinc (mg)
0.00	0.50	0.00	0.00	0.00	0.00	0.00	0.30	0.14	4.00	0.30	0.00	1.20	80.00	2.70	0.00	0.00	450.00	370.00	6.75
0.50	1.00	0.00	0.00	0.00	0.00	0.00	1.80	0.14	2.00	0.30	0.00	3.60	0.00	1.44	0.00	0.00	60.00	340.00	0.00
0.00	0.00	0.00	0.00	0.00	0.00	0.00	0.45	0.14	3.00	0.30	0.00	1.80	20.00	1.80	0.00	0.00	100.00	260.00	0.00
0.50	2.00	0.00	0.00	0.00	0.00	0.00	1.80	0.10	2.00	0.20	0.00	1.50	0.00	1.80	0.00	0.00	110.00	270.00	0.00
0.50	1.50	0.00	0.00	0.00	60.04	0.00	0.00	0.00	0.00	0.00	0.00	0.00	40.00	0.72	0.00	0.00	180.00	350.00	0.00
2.50	1.50	0.00	0.00	0.00	0.00	0.00	0.00	0.00	0.00	0.00	0.00	0.00	40.00	1.80	0.00	0.00	180.00	420.00	0.00
1.00	1.00	0.00	0.00	0.00	0.00	9.00	0.75	0.34	2.00	0.50	0.00	5.40	60.00	2.70	0.00	0.00	210.00	370.00	0.00
0.00	0.00	0.40	0.00	0.00	225.00	0.00	0.30	0.34	0.00	0.12	0.00	1.80	20.00	1.08	0.00	0.00	60.00	95.00	0.60
1.00	3.00	0.00	0.00	0.00	0.00	0.00	0.75	0.03	0.04	0.08	0.00	0.24	0.00	0.36	0.00	0.00	15.00	220.00	0.00
0.00	0.00	0.00	0.00	0.00	0.00	0.00	0.00	0.00	0.00	0.00	0.00	0.00	0.00	0.72	0.00	0.00	60.00	580.00	0.00
0.00	3.00	0.00	0.00	0.00	0.00	0.00	0.15	0.14	0.76	0.00	0.00	0.00	80.00	1.00	0.00	160.00	250.00	80.00	0.00
0.00	1.00	0.00	0.00	0.00	60.00	3.60	0.45	0.43	2.85	0.00	0.00	0.00	120.00	2.00	0.00	220.00	200.00	510.00	0.00
3.00	2.00	0.00	0.00	0.00	270.00	8.40	0.08	0.12	1.71	0.00	0.00	0.00	32.00	0.70	21.00	0.00	254.00	1009.00	0.75
0.00	0.00	0.00	0.00	0.00	0.00	0.00	0.00	0.01	0.19	0.00	0.00	0.00	1.60	0.20	0.00	0.00	260.39	1992.99	0.00
0.00	0.00	0.00	0.00	0.00	0.00	0.00	0.00	0.00	0.00	0.00	0.00	0.00	0.00	0.00	0.00	0.00	0.00	690.00	0.00
0.00	1.00	0.00	0.00	0.00	60.00	0.00	0.38	0.51	2.85	0.00	0.00	0.00	160.00	2.00	0.00	250.00	590.00	470.00	0.00
0.00	0.00	0.00	0.00	0.00	100.00	3.60	0.45	0.51	1.90	0.00	0.00	0.00	160.00	2.00	0.00	240.00	220.00	480.00	0.00
0.00	0.00	0.00	0.00	0.00	0.00	0.00	0.00	0.00	0.00	0.00	0.00	0.00	0.00	0.00	0.00	0.00	0.00	750.00	0.00
0.00	0.00	0.00	0.00	0.00	0.00	0.00	0.00	0.00	0.00	0.00	0.00	0.00	0.00	0.00	0.00	0.00	0.00	480.00	0.00
0.00	0.00	0.00	0.00	0.00	0.00	0.00	0.00	0.00	0.00	0.00	0.00	0.00	0.00	0.00	0.00	0.00	0.00	700.00	0.00
0.00	0.00	0.00	0.00	0.00	0.00	0.00	0.00	0.00	0.00	0.00	0.00	0.00	0.00	0.00	0.00	0.00	0.00	910.00	0.00
0.00	0.00	0.00	0.00	0.00	0.00	0.00	0.00	0.00	0.00	0.00	0.00	0.00	0.00	0.00	0.00	0.00	0.00	750.00	0.00
0.00	0.00	0.00	0.00	0.00	0.00	0.00	0.00	0.00	0.00	0.00	0.00	0.00	0.00	0.00	0.00	0.00	0.00	640.00	0.00
0.00	0.00	0.00	0.00	0.00	0.00	0.00	0.00	0.00	0.00	0.00	0.00	0.00	0.00	0.00	0.00	0.00	0.00	540.00	0.00
0.00	0.00	0.00	0.00	0.00	0.00	0.00	0.00	0.00	0.00	0.00	0.00	0.00	0.00	0.00	0.00	0.00	0.00	580.00	0.00
0.00	0.00	0.00	0.00	0.00	0.00	0.00	0.00	0.00	0.00	0.00	0.00	0.00	0.00	0.00	0.00	0.00	0.00	530.00	0.00
0.00	0.00	0.00	0.00	0.00	0.00	20.00	0.00	0.00	0.00	0.00	0.00	0.00	160.00	1.20	0.00	0.00	0.00	450.00	0.00
0.00	0.00	0.00	0.00	0.00	0.00	0.00	0.00	0.00	0.00	0.00	0.00	0.00	0.00	0.00	0.00	0.00	0.00	510.00	0.00
0.00	0.00	0.00	0.00	0.00	0.00	0.54	0.00	0.01	0.19	0.00	0.00	0.00	3.45	0.10	0.00	0.00	400.60	891.34	0.00
0.00	0.00	0.00	0.00	0.00	250.00	0.00	0.45	0.26	1.52	0.00	0.00	0.00	32.00	2.50	0.00	0.00	380.00	330.00	0.00
0.00	3.00	0.00	0.00	0.00	60.00	0.00	0.53	0.51	2.85	0.00	0.00	0.00	48.00	2.00	0.00	180.00	540.00	530.00	0.00
0.00	0.00	0.00	0.00	0.00	0.00	6.01	0.11	0.01	0.95	0.00	0.00	0.00	1.04	0.30	0.00	0.00	600.90	781.17	0.00
0.00	0.00	0.00	0.00	0.00	100.00	21.00	0.53	0.43	2.85	0.00	0.00	0.00	320.00	1.50	0.00	240.00	640.00	470.00	0.00
0.00	0.00	0.00	0.00	0.00	150.00	9.00	0.12	0.26	1.90	0.00	0.00	0.00	280.00	1.00	0.00	0.00	480.00	820.00	0.00
0.00	1.00	0.00	0.00	0.00	100.00	6.00	0.45	0.43	6.65	0.00	0.00	0.00	32.00	1.50	0.00	250.00	660.00	430.00	0.00
0.00	2.00	0.00	0.00	0.00	100.00	6.00	0.30	0.34	3.80	0.00	0.00	0.00	48.00	1.50	0.00	200.00	390.00	370.00	0.00
0.00	0.00	0.00	0.00	0.00	0.00	0.00	0.00	0.00	0.00	0.00	0.00	0.00	0.00	0.00	0.00	0.00	0.00	360.00	0.00
0.00	1.00	0.00	0.00	0.00	250.00	6.00	0.30	0.34	2.85	0.00	0.00	0.00	80.00	1.50	0.00	0.00	500.00	410.00	0.00
0.00	0.00	0.00	0.00	0.00	0.00	0.00	0.00	0.00	0.00	0.00	0.00	0.00	0.00	0.00	0.00	0.00	0.00	560.00	0.00
0.00	0.00	0.00	0.00	0.00	0.00	0.00	0.00	0.00	0.00	0.00	0.00	0.00	0.00	0.00	0.00	0.00	0.00	670.00	0.00
0.00	0.00	0.00	0.00	0.00	0.00	0.00	0.00	0.00	0.00	0.00	0.00	0.00	0.00	0.00	0.00	0.00	0.00	560.00	0.00
0.00	0.00	0.00	0.00	0.00	0.00	0.00	0.00	0.00	0.00	0.00	0.00	0.00	0.00	0.00	0.00	0.00	0.00	620.00	0.00
0.00	0.00	0.00	0.00	0.00	0.00	0.00	0.00	0.00	0.00	0.00	0.00	0.00	0.00	0.00	0.00	0.00	0.00	370.00	0.00
0.00	0.00	0.00	0.00	0.00	20.00	6.00	0.23	0.17	2.85	0.00	0.00	0.00	32.00	1.00	0.00	0.00	400.00	1010.00	0.00
0.00	0.00	0.00	0.00	0.00	60.00	6.00	0.12	0.14	2.85	0.00	0.00	0.00	32.00	0.80	0.00	0.00	380.00	650.00	0.00
0.00	0.00	0.00	0.00	0.00	0.00	0.00	0.00	0.00	0.00	0.00	0.00	0.00	0.00	0.00	0.00	0.00	0.00	550.00	0.00
0.00	1.00	0.00	0.00	0.00	138.30	0.00	0.50	0.30	3.00	0.00	0.00	0.00	350.00	0.90	0.00	200.00	330.00	870.00	0.00
0.00	0.00	0.00	0.00	0.00	0.00	0.00	0.00	0.00	0.00	0.00	0.00	0.00	220.00	1.50	0.00	180.00	290.00	530.00	0.00
0.00	1.00	0.00	0.00	0.00	0.00	0.00	0.00	0.00	0.00	0.00	0.00	0.00	300.00	1.50	0.00	200.00	330.00	630.00	0.00
0.00	1.00	0.00	0.00	0.00	20.00	0.00	0.45	0.26	2.85	0.00	0.00	0.00	240.00	2.00	0.00	240.00	310.00	390.00	0.00
0.00	0.00	0.00	0.00	0.00	60.00	3.60	0.45	0.34	2.85	0.00	0.00	0.00	200.00	1.50	0.00	0.00	300.00	630.00	0.00
0.00	1.00	0.00	0.00	0.00	80.00	0.00	0.45	0.34	3.80	0.00	0.00	0.00	200.00	2.50	0.00	280.00	350.00	500.00	0.00
0.00	0.00	0.00	0.00	0.00	100.00	6.00	0.45	0.43	3.80	0.00	0.00	0.00	160.00	1.50	0.00	0.00	350.00	950.00	0.00

USDA ID Code	Food Name	Weight in Grams*	Quantity of Units	Unit of Measure	Protein (g)	Fat (g)	Carbohydrate (g)	Kilocalories	Caffeine (g)	Fiber (g)	Cholesterol (mg)	Saturated Fat (g)
	Pizza, French Bread, Double Chee	166.5520	1.000	Each	22.00	18.00	43.00	420.00	0.00	0.00	0.00	0.00
	Pizza, French Bread, Hamburger-S	173.6390	1.000	Each	23.00	18.00	39.00	410.00	0.00	0.00	0.00	0.00
	Pizza, French Bread, Pepperoni-H	170.0960	1.000	Each	20.00	7.00	38.00	310.00	0.00	0.00	30.00	3.00
	Pizza, French Bread, Pepperoni-S	159.4650	1.000	Each	19.00	19.00	39.00	400.00	0.00	0.00	0.00	0.00
	Pizza, French Bread, Sausage-Sto	170.0960	1.000	Each	20.00	21.00	40.00	430.00	0.00	0.00	0.00	0.00
	Pizza, French Bread, Vegetable D	180.7270	1.000	Each	18.00	20.00	41.00	420.00	0.00	0.00	0.00	0.00
	Pizza, Meat, 3-DiGiorno	154.0000	1.000	Slice	19.00	16.00	40.00	380.00	0.00	3.11	40.00	8.00
	Pizza, Pepperoni	154.0000	1.000	Slice	19.00	24.00	40.00	450.00	0.00	2.00	35.00	9.00
	Pizza, Pepperoni-Weight Watcher	157.6260	1.000	Each	23.00	12.00	46.00	390.00	0.00	4.00	45.00	4.00
	Pizza, Pepperoni, Microwave for	104.0000	1.000	Each	10.00	16.00	25.00	280.00	0.00	1.00	15.00	3.50
	Pizza, Pepperoni, Party-Totino	289.0000	1.000	Slice	14.00	21.00	33.00	380.00	0.00	2.00	20.00	5.00
	Pizza, Sausage & Pepperoni-Tom	132.0000	1.000	Slice	19.00	19.00	25.00	340.00	0.00	2.00	45.00	9.00
	Pizza, Sausage & Pepperoni, Supr	122.0000	1.000	Slice	13.00	20.00	28.00	340.00	0.00	2.00	25.00	7.00
	Pizza, Special Deluxe-Red Baron	129.0000	1.000	Slice	13.00	18.00	32.00	340.00	0.00	2.00	25.00	7.00
	Pizza, Supreme, Party-Totino's	309.0000	1.000	Slice	15.00	20.00	34.00	380.00	0.00	2.00	20.00	4.50
	Pizzas, French Bread, Bacon, Can	163.0080	1.000	Each	18.00	15.00	40.00	370.00	0.00	0.00	0.00	0.00
	Pot Pie, Beef-Swanson	198.4450	1.000	Each	12.00	19.00	36.00	370.00	0.00	0.00	0.00	0.00
	Pot Pie, Beef-Stouffer's	283.4930	1.000	Each	18.00	27.00	37.00	460.00	0.00	0.00	0.00	0.00
	Pot Pie, Chicken-Swanson	198.4450	1.000	Each	11.00	22.00	35.00	380.00	0.00	0.00	0.00	0.00
	Pot Pie, Chicken-Stouffer's	283.4930	1.000	Each	16.00	27.00	32.00	440.00	0.00	0.00	0.00	0.00
	Pot Pie, Macaroni and Cheese-Sw	198.4450	1.000	Each	7.00	8.00	24.00	200.00	0.00	0.00	0.00	0.00
	Pot Pie, Turkey-Swanson	198.0000	1.000	Each	5.54	10.58	18.14	191.49	0.00	0.00	0.00	0.00
	Pot Pie, Turkey-Stouffer's	283.4930	1.000	Each	16.00	24.00	33.00	410.00	0.00	0.00	0.00	0.00
	Potato Casserole, Garden-Healthy	262.2310	1.000	Each	12.00	4.00	23.00	180.00	0.00	2.00	20.00	2.00
	Potato, Baked, Broccoli and Chee	283.5000	1.000	Each	12.00	7.00	34.00	230.00	0.00	6.00	10.00	2.00
	Potato, Baked, w/ Sour Cream, Le	294.1240	1.000	Each	9.00	5.00	38.00	230.00	0.00	0.00	15.00	2.00
672	Potato, Bkd, Broccoli & Chse-Sm	280.0000	10.000	Ounce	12.00	7.00	35.00	250.00	0.00	6.00	15.00	2.00
	Potatoes Au Gratin-Stouffer's	163.0080	1.000	Each	5.00	9.00	17.00	170.00	0.00	0.00	0.00	0.00
	Potatoes, Scalloped, and Ham, Mi	212.6200	1.000	Each	8.00	16.00	21.00	260.00	0.00	0.00	33.00	6.00
	Potatoes, Scalloped-Stouffer's	163.0080	1.000	Each	4.00	6.00	16.00	130.00	0.00	0.00	0.00	0.00
	Primavera, Chicken-Stouffer's	28.3500	1.000	Ounce	1.60	0.60	1.20	17.00	0.00	0.00	5.00	0.00
689	Ravioli Florentine-Smart Ones	238.0000	8.500	Ounce	9.00	2.00	43.00	220.00	0.00	4.00	5.00	0.50
	Ravioli, Baked Cheese, Lean Cuis	240.9690	1.000	Each	13.00	8.00	30.00	240.00	0.00	0.00	55.00	3.00
	Ravioli, Baked Cheese-Healthy Ch	255.1440	1.000	Each	14.00	2.00	44.00	250.00	0.00	0.00	20.00	1.00
	Ravioli, Beef	243.9350	1.000	Cup	9.00	5.00	35.99	229.94	0.00	4.00	19.99	2.50
	Ravioli, Beef, Micro Cup-Hormel	212.6200	1.000	Each	9.00	11.00	34.00	270.00	0.00	0.00	20.00	4.00
	Ravioli, Cheese	243.9350	1.000	Cup	9.00	3.00	37.99	219.94	0.00	4.00	15.00	1.50
	Ravioli, Cheese-Stouffer's	28.3500	1.000	Ounce	2.80	1.90	6.40	54.00	0.00	0.00	14.00	0.00
	Rice, Confetti-Stouffer's	28.3500	1.000	Ounce	0.50	0.30	4.80	24.00	0.00	0.00	1.00	0.00
692	Rice, Hunan & Vegetables-Smart O	289.5000	10.340	Ounce	7.00	7.00	39.00	250.00	0.00	8.00	5.00	2.00
694	Rice, Sante Fe and Beans-Smart O	280.0000	10.000	Ounce	12.00	9.00	41.00	290.00	0.00	10.00	5.00	4.00
	Rice, Wild-Rice-a-Roni	56.0000	1.000	Cup	5.00	1.00	43.00	240.00	0.00	1.00	0.00	0.00
	Rigatoni Bake, Lean Cuisine-Stou	276.4060	1.000	Each	18.00	8.00	27.00	250.00	0.00	0.00	25.00	3.00
	Rigatoni in Meat Sauce-Healthy C	269.3190	1.000	Each	16.00	6.00	34.00	260.00	0.00	0.00	30.00	2.00
	Rigatoni w/ Meat Sauce-Stouffer'	283.9200	0.500	Cup	16.02	11.02	31.05	290.44	0.00	0.00	30.04	0.00
695	Risotto w/Cheese & Mushrooms-Sma	280.0000	10.000	Ounce	11.00	8.00	44.00	290.00	0.00	4.00	20.00	4.00
	Sauce, Cheddar Cheese-Stouffer's	283.9200	1.000	Cup	26.04	60.09	22.03	731.10	0.00	0.00	130.20	0.00
	Sauce, Marinara-Stouffer's	283.9200	1.000	Cup	3.00	11.02	18.03	180.27	0.00	0.00	0.00	0.00
	Sauce, Newburg, Supreme-Stouffer	283.9200	1.000	Cup	7.01	41.06	20.03	480.72	0.00	0.00	120.18	0.00
	Sauce, Pesto-Stouffer's	283.9200	0.250	Cup	35.05	61.09	21.03	771.16	0.00	0.00	70.11	0.00
	Sauce, Veloute, Supreme-Stouffer	307.5800	1.000	Cup	8.68	49.91	20.61	564.18	0.00	0.00	97.65	0.00
	Shells, Cheese Stuffed-Stouffer'	28.3500	1.000	Ounce	1.50	0.90	3.40	28.00	0.00	0.00	3.00	0.00
	Shrimp Marinara-Healthy Choice	297.6680	1.000	Each	10.00	1.00	51.00	260.00	0.00	0.00	60.00	0.00

Monounsaturated Fat (g)	Polyunsaturated Fat (g)	Vitamin D (mg)	Vitamin K (mg)	Vitamin E (mg)	Vitamin A (re)	Vitamin C (mg)	Thiamin (mg)	Riboflavin (mg)	Niacin (mg)	Vitamin B_6 (mg)	Folate (mcg)	Vitamin B_{12} (mcg)	Calcium (mg)	Iron (mg)	Magnesium (mg)	Phosphorus (mg)	Potassium (mg)	Sodium (mg)	Zinc (mg)
0.00	0.00	0.00	0.00	0.00	40.00	6.00	0.45	0.51	3.80	0.00	0.00	0.00	360.00	1.50	0.00	0.00	320.00	850.00	0.00
0.00	0.00	0.00	0.00	0.00	60.00	6.00	0.38	0.34	3.80	0.00	0.00	0.00	160.00	1.50	0.00	0.00	340.00	650.00	0.00
0.00	1.00	0.00	0.00	0.00	150.00	0.00	0.53	0.34	3.80	0.00	0.00	0.00	160.00	2.50	0.00	240.00	350.00	470.00	0.00
0.00	0.00	0.00	0.00	0.00	100.00	6.00	0.53	0.43	3.80	0.00	0.00	0.00	160.00	1.50	0.00	0.00	300.00	880.00	0.00
0.00	0.00	0.00	0.00	0.00	80.00	6.00	0.60	0.43	3.80	0.00	0.00	0.00	160.00	1.50	0.00	0.00	340.00	840.00	0.00
0.00	0.00	0.00	0.00	0.00	250.00	3.60	0.45	0.43	3.80	0.00	0.00	0.00	280.00	1.50	0.00	0.00	230.00	830.00	0.00
0.00	1.00	0.00	0.00	0.00	138.30	0.00	0.50	0.30	3.00	0.00	0.00	0.00	330.00	1.00	0.00	200.00	330.00	1100.00	0.00
0.00	1.00	0.00	0.00	0.00	90.00	0.00	0.00	0.00	0.00	0.00	0.00	0.00	330.00	1.90	0.00	200.00	330.00	920.00	0.00
0.00	1.00	0.00	0.00	0.00	80.00	4.80	0.00	0.00	0.00	0.00	0.00	0.00	540.00	1.00	0.00	0.00	320.00	650.00	0.00
0.00	1.00	0.00	0.00	0.00	0.00	0.00	0.00	0.00	0.00	0.00	0.00	0.00	200.00	1.50	0.00	180.00	290.00	710.00	0.00
0.00	1.00	0.00	0.00	0.00	0.00	0.00	0.00	0.00	0.00	0.00	0.00	0.00	280.00	1.50	0.00	200.00	330.00	920.00	0.00
0.00	1.00	0.00	0.00	0.00	150.00	1.20	0.00	0.00	0.00	0.00	0.00	0.00	350.00	0.90	0.00	200.00	330.00	820.00	0.00
0.00	1.00	0.00	0.00	0.00	40.00	2.40	0.00	0.00	0.00	0.00	0.00	0.00	200.00	1.50	0.00	200.00	330.00	610.00	0.00
0.00	1.00	0.00	0.00	0.00	78.00	0.00	0.00	0.00	0.00	0.00	0.00	0.00	220.00	2.70	0.00	200.00	330.00	690.00	0.00
0.00	1.00	0.00	0.00	0.00	0.00	0.00	0.00	0.00	0.00	0.00	0.00	0.00	280.00	1.50	0.00	200.00	330.00	890.00	0.00
0.00	0.00	0.00	0.00	0.00	80.00	6.00	0.60	0.43	3.80	0.00	0.00	0.00	160.00	1.00	0.00	0.00	300.00	1070.00	0.00
0.00	0.00	0.00	0.00	0.00	250.00	0.00	0.23	0.17	2.85	0.00	0.00	0.00	16.00	1.50	0.00	0.00	0.00	730.00	0.00
0.00	0.00	0.00	0.00	0.00	700.00	2.40	0.30	0.43	3.80	0.00	0.00	0.00	32.00	1.50	0.00	0.00	300.00	1130.00	0.00
0.00	0.00	0.00	0.00	0.00	400.00	0.00	0.23	0.17	2.85	0.00	0.00	0.00	16.00	1.00	0.00	0.00	0.00	760.00	0.00
0.00	0.00	0.00	0.00	0.00	500.00	1.20	0.30	0.43	4.75	0.00	0.00	0.00	80.00	1.00	0.00	0.00	320.00	750.00	0.00
0.00	0.00	0.00	0.00	0.00	80.00	0.00	0.09	0.17	0.76	0.00	0.00	0.00	120.00	0.60	0.00	0.00	0.00	740.00	0.00
0.00	0.00	0.00	0.00	0.00	176.37	0.00	0.11	0.09	1.44	0.00	0.00	0.00	8.06	0.50	0.00	0.00	0.00	362.82	0.00
0.00	0.00	0.00	0.00	0.00	250.00	0.00	0.30	0.43	3.80	0.00	0.00	0.00	80.00	1.00	0.00	0.00	290.00	750.00	0.00
0.00	0.00	0.00	0.00	0.00	0.00	0.00	0.00	0.00	0.00	0.00	0.00	0.00	0.00	0.00	0.00	0.00	600.00	360.00	0.00
0.00	0.00	0.00	0.00	0.00	200.00	9.00	0.00	0.00	0.00	0.00	0.00	0.00	300.00	0.80	0.00	0.00	830.00	510.00	0.00
0.00	0.00	0.00	0.00	0.00	350.00	30.00	0.23	0.26	1.14	0.00	0.00	0.00	160.00	0.60	0.00	0.00	900.00	570.00	0.00
0.00	0.00	0.00	0.00	0.00	0.00	0.00	0.00	0.00	0.00	0.00	0.00	0.00	0.00	0.00	0.00	0.00	0.00	590.00	0.00
0.00	0.00	0.00	0.00	0.00	20.00	3.60	0.00	0.10	0.76	0.00	0.00	0.00	48.00	0.80	0.00	0.00	260.00	670.00	0.00
8.00	2.00	0.00	0.00	0.39	0.00	11.40	0.09	0.10	2.09	0.00	0.00	0.00	32.00	0.40	21.00	0.00	425.00	768.00	0.90
0.00	0.00	0.00	0.00	0.00	0.00	2.40	0.03	0.14	0.76	0.00	0.00	0.00	80.00	0.20	0.00	0.00	375.00	610.00	0.00
0.00	0.00	0.00	0.00	0.00	0.00	1.20	0.00	0.00	0.06	0.00	0.00	0.00	48.00	0.01	0.00	0.00	40.00	119.00	0.00
0.00	0.00	0.00	0.00	0.00	0.00	0.00	0.00	0.00	0.00	0.00	0.00	0.00	0.00	0.00	0.00	0.00	0.00	490.00	0.00
0.00	0.00	0.00	0.00	0.00	60.00	36.00	0.06	0.26	1.14	0.00	0.00	0.00	160.00	0.80	0.00	0.00	380.00	590.00	0.00
0.00	0.00	0.00	0.00	0.00	500.00	4.80	0.30	0.26	1.90	0.00	0.00	0.00	200.00	1.50	0.00	240.00	590.00	420.00	0.00
0.00	0.00	0.00	0.00	0.00	149.96	2.40	0.00	0.00	0.00	0.00	0.00	0.00	0.00	1.50	0.00	0.00	0.00	1149.69	0.00
5.00	1.00	0.00	0.00	0.50	100.00	11.40	0.15	0.27	2.47	0.00	0.00	0.00	48.00	0.90	28.00	0.00	359.00	920.00	1.05
0.00	0.00	0.00	0.00	0.00	59.98	1.20	0.00	0.00	0.00	0.00	0.00	0.00	23.99	1.50	0.00	0.00	0.00	1279.66	0.00
0.00	0.00	0.00	0.00	0.00	0.00	0.00	0.00	0.00	0.02	0.00	0.00	0.00	336.01	0.01	0.00	0.00	16.00	52.00	0.00
0.00	0.00	0.00	0.00	0.00	0.00	0.00	0.00	0.00	0.04	0.00	0.00	0.00	24.00	0.00	0.00	0.00	14.00	136.00	0.00
0.00	0.00	0.00	0.00	0.00	0.00	0.00	0.00	0.00	0.00	0.00	0.00	0.00	0.00	0.00	0.00	0.00	0.00	630.00	0.00
0.00	0.00	0.00	0.00	0.00	0.00	0.00	0.00	0.00	0.00	0.00	0.00	0.00	0.00	0.00	0.00	0.00	0.00	670.00	0.00
0.00	0.00	0.00	0.00	0.00	80.00	6.00	0.15	0.10	1.52	0.00	0.00	0.00	48.00	0.80	0.00	0.00	0.00	1110.00	0.00
0.00	1.00	0.00	0.00	0.00	200.00	6.00	0.23	0.34	3.80	0.00	0.00	0.00	160.00	1.50	0.00	0.00	620.00	430.00	0.00
0.00	0.00	0.00	0.00	0.00	200.00	2.40	0.30	0.26	2.85	0.00	0.00	0.00	120.00	1.50	0.00	200.00	700.00	540.00	0.00
0.00	0.00	0.00	0.00	0.00	0.00	48.07	0.00	0.01	0.76	0.00	0.00	0.00	2.08	0.30	0.00	0.00	620.93	851.28	0.00
0.00	0.00	0.00	0.00	0.00	0.00	0.00	0.00	0.00	0.00	0.00	0.00	0.00	0.00	0.00	0.00	0.00	0.00	540.00	0.00
0.00	0.00	0.00	0.00	0.00	0.00	0.00	0.00	0.01	0.00	0.00	0.00	0.00	6.33	0.10	0.00	240.00	340.51	1392.09	0.00
0.00	0.00	0.00	0.00	0.00	0.00	66.10	0.00	0.00	0.38	0.00	0.00	0.00	1.84	0.20	0.00	0.00	681.02	1221.83	0.00
0.00	0.00	0.00	0.00	0.00	0.00	12.02	0.00	0.02	0.38	0.00	0.00	0.00	5.69	0.30	0.00	0.00	620.93	1362.04	0.00
0.00	0.00	0.00	0.00	0.00	0.00	0.00	0.00	0.01	0.00	0.00	0.00	0.00	2.26	0.00	0.00	0.00	368.89	1410.45	0.00
0.00	0.00	0.00	0.00	0.00	0.00	0.60	0.00	0.00	0.06	0.00	0.00	0.00	248.01	0.02	0.00	0.00	53.00	59.00	0.00
0.00	0.00	0.00	0.00	0.00	100.00	114.00	0.23	0.14	1.14	0.00	0.00	0.00	48.00	1.50	0.00	130.00	390.00	320.00	0.00

USDA ID Code	Food Name	Weight in Grams*	Quantity of Units	Unit of Measure	Protein (g)	Fat (g)	Carbohydrate (g)	Kilocalories	Caffeine (g)	Fiber (g)	Cholesterol (mg)	Saturated Fat (g)
697	Shrimp Marinara-Smart Ones	252.0000	9.000	Ounce	9.00	2.00	35.00	190.00	0.00	4.00	40.00	0.50
	Shrimp Marinara-Weight Watchers	255.1500	1.000	Each	9.00	2.00	35.00	190.00	0.00	4.00	40.00	0.50
717	Spaghetti Marinara-Smart Ones	252.0000	9.000	Ounce	9.00	7.00	46.00	280.00	0.00	5.00	5.00	1.50
	Spaghetti w/ Meat Sauce, Lean Cu	326.0170	1.000	Each	15.00	6.00	45.00	290.00	0.00	0.00	20.00	2.00
	Spaghetti w/ Meat Sauce, Top She	283.4930	1.000	Each	14.00	6.00	37.00	260.00	0.00	0.00	20.00	2.00
	Spaghetti w/ Meat Sauce-Healthy	283.4930	1.000	Each	14.00	6.00	42.00	280.00	0.00	0.00	20.00	2.00
718	Spaghetti w/ Meat Sauce-Smart On	280.0000	10.000	Ounce	17.00	6.00	41.00	290.00	0.00	4.00	15.00	2.00
	Spaghetti w/ Meat Sauce-Stouffer	364.9980	1.000	Each	16.00	12.00	38.00	320.00	0.00	0.00	0.00	0.00
	Spaghetti w/ Meatballs, Micro Cu	212.6200	1.000	Each	10.00	7.00	27.00	210.00	0.00	0.00	20.00	3.00
	Spaghetti w/ Meatballs-Stouffer'	276.4060	1.000	Each	14.00	9.00	37.00	290.00	0.00	0.00	0.00	0.00
	Spinach Souffle-Stouffer's	170.0960	1.000	Each	9.00	15.00	11.00	220.00	0.00	0.00	0.00	0.00
	Spinach, Creamed-Stouffer's	127.5720	1.000	Each	4.00	16.00	8.00	190.00	0.00	0.00	0.00	0.00
	Steak, Green Pepper, w/ Rice-Sto	297.6680	1.000	Each	20.00	10.00	35.00	310.00	0.00	0.00	0.00	0.00
	Steak, Green Pepper-Stouffer's	28.3500	1.000	Ounce	2.60	1.40	1.30	28.00	0.00	0.00	7.00	0.00
728	Steak, Pepper-Smart Ones	280.0000	10.000	Ounce	18.00	4.50	33.00	240.00	0.00	4.00	35.00	1.50
	Steak, Salisbury, Grilled-Weigh	240.9750	1.000	Each	19.00	9.00	24.00	250.00	0.00	4.00	30.00	3.00
	Steak, Salisbury, Top Shelf-Horm	283.4930	1.000	Each	25.00	15.00	22.00	320.00	0.00	0.00	70.00	7.00
	Steak, Salisbury, w/ Mushroom Gr	311.8430	1.000	Each	21.00	6.00	35.00	280.00	0.00	0.00	55.00	3.00
	Stew, Beef, Dinty Moore-Hormel	253.1620	1.000	Cup	12.28	14.51	17.86	245.58	0.00	0.00	33.49	6.70
	Stew, Chicken, Dinty Moore-Horm	253.1620	1.000	Cup	13.10	21.43	17.86	309.58	0.00	0.00	95.25	4.76
	Stew, Meatball, Dinty Moore-Hor	253.1620	1.000	Cup	12.28	17.86	15.63	267.90	0.00	0.00	33.49	7.81
	Stew, Vegetable, Dinty Moore-Ho	253.1620	1.000	Cup	5.58	6.70	22.33	173.02	0.00	0.00	15.63	2.23
	Stuff'n, Old-Fashion-Stouffer's	283.9200	0.500	Cup	11.02	37.06	61.09	620.93	0.00	0.00	10.02	0.00
	Sweet Potatoes, Whipped-Stouffer	283.9200	1.000	Cup	3.00	18.03	60.09	410.61	0.00	0.00	60.09	0.00
	Taco Shells, Chi-Chi's-Hormel	20.0000	1.000	Each	1.41	4.94	11.99	98.77	0.00	0.00	0.00	0.00
	Tetrazzini, Turkey-Healthy Choice	357.9100	1.000	Each	23.00	6.00	49.00	340.00	0.00	0.00	40.00	3.00
	Tetrazzini, Turkey-Stouffer's	283.4930	1.000	Each	22.00	23.00	26.00	400.00	0.00	0.00	0.00	0.00
	Tortellini w/ Egg Pasta, Cheese-	145.2900	1.000	Each	11.29	8.47	22.22	211.64	0.00	0.00	63.49	0.00
	Tortellini w/ Egg Pasta, Chicken	28.3500	1.000	Ounce	3.10	1.50	6.20	51.00	0.00	0.00	20.00	0.00
	Tortellini w/ Spinach Pasta, Che	28.3500	1.000	Ounce	3.00	2.40	5.70	56.00	0.00	0.00	19.00	0.00
	Tortellini, Beef	257.8940	1.000	Cup	5.00	1.00	45.98	229.91	0.00	9.00	14.99	0.00
	Tortellini, Cheese in Alfredo Sa	251.6000	1.000	Each	26.00	37.00	35.00	580.00	0.00	0.00	0.00	0.00
	Tortellini, Cheese w/ Tomato Sau	262.2310	1.000	Each	18.00	15.00	39.00	360.00	0.00	0.00	0.00	0.00
747	Tuna Noodle Casserole-Smart Ones	266.0000	9.500	Ounce	13.00	7.00	39.00	270.00	0.00	4.00	40.00	3.50
	Tuna Noodle Casserole-Stouffer's	283.4930	1.000	Each	17.00	15.00	33.00	280.00	0.00	0.00	0.00	0.00
	Turkey and Gravy-Stouffer's	255.0000	1.000	Each	11.99	2.47	2.12	77.60	0.00	0.00	23.28	0.00
	Turkey Breast, Sliced, w/ Gravy	283.4930	1.000	Each	27.00	4.00	30.00	270.00	0.00	0.00	50.00	2.00
	Turkey Breast, Sliced, w/ Gravy-	340.1920	1.000	Each	19.00	3.00	46.00	290.00	0.00	0.00	20.00	1.00
748	Turkey Breast, Stuffed-Smart One	280.0000	10.000	Ounce	13.00	7.00	37.00	260.00	0.00	5.00	20.00	2.00
	Turkey Dijon, Lean Cuisine-Stouf	269.3190	1.000	Each	20.00	6.00	20.00	210.00	0.00	0.00	45.00	2.00
	Turkey Dijonnaise-Stouffer's	260.0000	1.000	Each	8.47	5.29	7.05	112.88	0.00	0.00	28.22	0.00
	Turkey Medallions, Roast-Weight	240.9750	1.000	Each	10.00	2.00	34.00	190.00	0.00	4.00	20.00	0.50
750	Turkey Medallions, Rst, /Mush-Sm	238.0000	8.500	Ounce	10.00	2.00	32.00	190.00	0.00	2.00	20.00	0.50
	Turkey, Breast of-Healthy Choice	297.6680	1.000	Each	21.00	5.00	39.00	290.00	0.00	0.00	45.00	2.00
	Turkey, Homestyle w/ Vegetables-	269.3190	1.000	Each	26.00	2.00	34.00	260.00	0.00	0.00	30.00	0.00
	Turkey, Roasted, and Mushrooms i	240.9690	1.000	Each	18.00	3.00	26.00	200.00	0.00	0.00	40.00	1.00
	Turkey, Sliced, w/ Dressing, Lea	223.2510	1.000	Each	16.00	5.00	23.00	200.00	0.00	0.00	25.00	1.00
	Vegetables, Italian Style-Stouff	28.3500	1.000	Ounce	0.30	0.30	1.60	10.00	0.00	0.00	0.00	0.00
	Welsh Rarebit-Stouffer's	141.7460	1.000	Each	13.00	20.00	9.00	270.00	0.00	0.00	0.00	0.00
791	Worthington-Beef, Smoked, Meatl	57.0000	6.000	Slices	11.00	6.00	6.00	120.00	0.00	3.00	0.00	1.00
792	Worthington-Bolono	57.0000	3.000	Slices	10.00	3.50	2.00	80.00	0.00	2.00	0.00	1.00
793	Worthington-Burger, Vegetarian	55.0000	0.250	Cup	9.00	2.00	2.00	60.00	0.00	1.00	0.00	0.00
795	Worthington-Chicken Roll, Meatl	55.0000	1.000	Slice	9.00	4.50	1.00	80.00	0.00	1.00	0.00	1.00

Page Key: A2 = Baby Food   A2 = Baked Goods   A8 = Beverages   A14 = Breads/Grains and Pasta   A18 = Breakfast Foods/Cereals   A26 = Dairy and Eggs   A40 = Fats and Oils   A42 = Fruits and Vegetables   A52 = Meats and Beans   A60 = Nuts and Seeds   A62 = Frozen Entrees and Packaged Foods   A76 = Restaurant Chains–Fast Foods   A92 = Restaurant Chains–Other   A106 = Seafood and Fish   A110 = Snacks and Sweets   A120 = Soups   A122 = Supplements   A126 = Toppings and Sauces

Monounsaturated Fat (g)	Polyunsaturated Fat (g)	Vitamin D (mg)	Vitamin K (mg)	Vitamin E (mg)	Vitamin A (re)	Vitamin C (mg)	Thiamin (mg)	Riboflavin (mg)	Niacin (mg)	Vitamin B6 (mg)	Folate (mcg)	Vitamin B12 (mcg)	Calcium (mg)	Iron (mg)	Magnesium (mg)	Phosphorus (mg)	Potassium (mg)	Sodium (mg)	Zinc (mg)
0.00	0.00	0.00	0.00	0.00	0.00	0.00	0.00	0.00	0.00	0.00	0.00	0.00	0.00	0.00	0.00	0.00	0.00	470.00	0.00
0.00	0.00	0.00	0.00	0.00	150.00	6.00	0.00	0.00	0.00	0.00	0.00	0.00	120.00	1.00	0.00	0.00	440.00	400.00	0.00
0.00	0.00	0.00	0.00	0.00	0.00	0.00	0.00	0.00	0.00	0.00	0.00	0.00	0.00	0.00	0.00	0.00	0.00	690.00	0.00
0.00	2.00	0.00	0.00	0.00	100.00	6.00	0.30	0.34	3.80	0.00	0.00	0.00	48.00	2.00	0.00	0.00	500.00	500.00	0.00
2.00	1.00	0.00	0.00	0.11	100.00	2.40	0.23	0.26	3.80	0.00	0.00	0.00	48.00	1.50	45.50	0.00	879.00	980.00	2.40
0.00	2.00	0.00	0.00	0.00	250.00	4.80	0.38	0.26	1.90	0.00	0.00	0.00	48.00	2.00	0.00	160.00	540.00	480.00	0.00
0.00	0.00	0.00	0.00	0.00	0.00	0.00	0.00	0.00	0.00	0.00	0.00	0.00	0.00	0.00	0.00	0.00	0.00	560.00	0.00
0.00	12.00	0.00	0.00	0.00	150.00	6.00	0.15	0.17	3.80	0.00	0.00	0.00	80.00	1.50	0.00	0.00	800.00	560.00	0.00
3.00	1.00	0.00	0.00	0.00	140.00	3.60	0.12	0.26	2.28	0.00	0.00	0.00	32.00	1.10	24.50	0.00	341.00	930.00	1.05
0.00	0.00	0.00	0.00	0.00	100.00	6.00	0.30	0.26	3.80	0.00	0.00	0.00	64.00	1.50	0.00	0.00	550.00	790.00	0.00
0.00	0.00	0.00	0.00	0.00	200.00	6.00	0.12	0.34	0.38	0.00	0.00	0.00	120.00	0.40	0.00	0.00	345.00	820.00	0.00
0.00	0.00	0.00	0.00	0.00	400.00	6.00	0.03	0.17	0.00	0.00	0.00	0.00	80.00	0.40	0.00	0.00	400.00	400.00	0.00
0.00	0.00	0.00	0.00	0.00	40.00	6.00	0.15	0.17	3.80	0.00	0.00	0.00	16.00	1.00	0.00	0.00	410.00	700.00	0.00
0.00	0.00	0.00	0.00	0.00	0.00	3.60	0.00	0.00	0.10	0.00	0.00	0.00	48.00	0.02	0.00	0.00	51.00	164.00	0.00
0.00	0.00	0.00	0.00	0.00	0.00	0.00	0.00	0.00	0.00	0.00	0.00	0.00	0.00	0.00	0.00	0.00	0.00	690.00	0.00
0.00	0.00	0.00	0.00	0.00	60.00	0.00	0.00	0.00	0.00	0.00	0.00	0.00	120.00	1.50	0.00	0.00	450.00	590.00	0.00
8.00	1.00	0.00	0.00	0.03	0.00	3.60	0.03	0.26	4.75	0.00	0.00	0.00	16.00	1.50	35.00	0.00	801.00	910.00	5.70
0.00	0.00	0.00	0.00	0.00	0.00	0.00	0.00	0.00	0.00	0.00	0.00	0.00	0.00	0.00	0.00	260.00	630.00	500.00	0.00
5.58	1.12	0.00	0.00	0.00	814.87	2.68	0.03	0.13	2.55	0.00	0.00	0.00	26.79	1.00	23.44	0.00	588.27	971.15	2.85
7.14	8.33	0.00	0.00	0.00	476.27	2.14	0.05	0.28	3.62	0.00	0.00	0.00	38.10	0.71	25.00	0.00	609.63	1012.08	1.25
7.81	1.12	0.00	0.00	2.59	279.06	1.34	0.07	0.15	3.18	0.00	0.00	0.00	26.79	1.23	27.35	0.00	586.04	1093.93	2.68
1.12	2.23	0.00	0.00	0.60	714.41	2.01	0.08	0.09	1.70	0.00	0.00	0.00	35.72	0.67	31.26	0.00	509.01	948.82	0.84
0.00	0.00	0.00	0.00	0.00	0.00	0.84	0.01	0.01	0.74	0.00	0.00	0.00	0.00	0.33	0.00	0.00	200.30	1121.68	0.00
0.00	0.00	0.00	0.00	0.00	0.00	0.00	0.00	0.00	0.19	0.00	0.00	0.00	0.00	0.10	0.00	0.00	400.60	1111.67	0.00
0.00	0.00	0.00	0.00	0.09	0.00	0.00	0.06	0.07	0.54	0.00	0.00	0.00	0.00	0.14	0.00	0.00	0.00	3.53	0.00
0.00	2.00	0.00	0.00	0.00	0.00	72.00	0.23	0.34	3.80	0.00	0.00	0.00	80.00	1.00	0.00	250.00	510.00	490.00	0.00
0.00	0.00	0.00	0.00	0.00	20.00	0.00	0.15	0.43	2.85	0.00	0.00	0.00	80.00	0.80	0.00	0.00	300.00	960.00	0.00
0.00	0.00	0.00	0.00	0.00	0.00	0.00	0.00	0.00	0.20	0.00	0.00	0.00	1.52	0.07	0.00	0.00	70.55	271.61	0.00
0.00	0.00	0.00	0.00	0.00	0.00	0.00	0.00	0.00	0.13	0.00	0.00	0.00	72.00	0.03	0.00	0.00	31.00	57.00	0.00
0.00	0.00	0.00	0.00	0.00	0.00	0.00	0.00	0.00	0.06	0.00	0.00	0.00	0.00	0.02	0.00	0.00	26.00	79.00	0.00
0.00	0.00	0.00	0.00	0.00	149.94	3.60	0.00	0.00	0.00	0.00	0.00	0.00	95.96	1.50	0.00	0.00	0.00	769.68	0.00
0.00	0.00	0.00	0.00	0.00	40.00	3.60	0.30	0.51	1.90	0.00	0.00	0.00	320.00	0.80	0.00	0.00	270.00	830.00	0.00
0.00	0.00	0.00	0.00	0.00	150.00	6.00	0.23	0.34	1.90	0.00	0.00	0.00	240.00	1.00	0.00	0.00	420.00	720.00	0.00
0.00	0.00	0.00	0.00	0.00	0.00	0.00	0.00	0.00	0.00	0.00	0.00	0.00	0.00	0.00	0.00	0.00	0.00	670.00	0.00
0.00	0.00	0.00	0.00	0.00	20.00	0.00	0.15	0.34	3.80	0.00	0.00	0.00	120.00	0.60	0.00	0.00	380.00	1090.00	0.00
0.00	0.00	0.00	0.00	0.00	0.00	0.42	0.00	0.00	0.87	0.00	0.00	0.00	84.66	0.03	0.00	0.00	405.65	296.30	0.00
0.00	1.00	0.00	0.00	0.00	150.00	0.00	0.30	0.34	7.60	0.00	0.00	0.00	48.00	1.00	0.00	310.00	590.00	530.00	0.00
0.00	1.00	0.00	0.00	0.00	150.00	27.00	0.15	0.10	1.52	0.00	0.00	0.00	16.00	0.60	0.00	0.00	360.00	520.00	0.00
0.00	0.00	0.00	0.00	0.00	0.00	0.00	0.00	0.00	0.00	0.00	0.00	0.00	0.00	0.00	0.00	0.00	0.00	680.00	0.00
0.00	0.00	0.00	0.00	0.00	400.00	2.40	0.23	0.34	4.75	0.00	0.00	0.00	120.00	0.40	0.00	0.00	640.00	590.00	0.00
0.00	0.00	0.00	0.00	0.00	0.00	0.63	0.00	0.00	0.27	0.00	0.00	0.00	0.00	0.07	0.00	0.00	176.37	356.27	0.00
0.00	0.00	0.00	0.00	0.00	100.00	4.80	0.00	0.00	0.00	0.00	0.00	0.00	24.00	1.00	0.00	0.00	220.00	530.00	0.00
0.00	0.00	0.00	0.00	0.00	0.00	0.00	0.00	0.00	0.00	0.00	0.00	0.00	0.00	0.00	0.00	0.00	0.00	530.00	0.00
0.00	0.00	0.00	0.00	0.00	40.00	48.00	0.45	0.26	5.70	0.00	0.00	0.00	32.00	1.00	0.00	270.00	540.00	420.00	0.00
0.00	0.00	0.00	0.00	0.00	100.00	4.80	0.03	0.07	0.00	0.00	0.00	0.00	32.00	0.00	0.00	0.00	100.00	550.00	0.00
0.00	1.00	0.00	0.00	0.00	200.00	0.00	0.12	0.14	2.85	0.00	0.00	0.00	16.00	0.80	0.00	150.00	260.00	380.00	0.00
0.00	2.00	0.00	0.00	0.00	500.00	6.00	0.23	0.26	4.75	0.00	0.00	0.00	32.00	0.80	0.00	0.00	400.00	590.00	0.00
0.00	0.00	0.00	0.00	0.00	0.00	1.80	0.00	0.00	0.02	0.00	0.00	0.00	72.00	0.01	0.00	0.00	62.00	147.00	0.00
0.00	0.00	0.00	0.00	0.00	40.00	0.00	0.03	0.34	0.00	0.00	0.00	0.00	280.00	0.20	0.00	0.00	140.00	460.00	0.00
2.50	2.50	0.00	0.00	0.00	0.00	0.00	1.80	0.14	3.00	0.30	0.00	1.80	0.00	1.08	0.00	0.00	150.00	730.00	0.00
1.00	1.50	0.00	0.00	0.00	0.00	0.00	0.60	0.14	0.40	0.40	0.00	0.90	40.00	1.80	0.00	0.00	120.00	720.00	0.00
0.50	1.00	0.00	0.00	0.00	0.00	0.00	0.12	0.07	1.60	0.20	0.00	1.20	0.00	1.80	0.00	0.00	25.00	270.00	0.00
1.00	2.50	0.00	0.00	0.00	0.00	0.00	0.30	0.14	1.20	2.00	0.00	0.90	0.00	1.80	0.00	0.00	270.00	360.00	0.00

USDA ID Code	Food Name	Weight in Grams*	Quantity of Units	Unit of Measure	Protein (g)	Fat (g)	Carbohydrate (g)	Kilocalories	Caffeine (g)	Fiber (g)	Cholesterol (mg)	Saturated Fat (g)
796	Worthington-Chicken Slices, Mea	57.0000	2.000	Slices	9.00	4.50	1.00	80.00	0.00	1.00	0.00	1.00
797	Worthington-Chicken, Diced, Mea	55.0000	0.250	Cup	10.00	0.00	2.00	50.00	0.00	1.00	0.00	0.00
794	Worthington-Chic-Ketts	55.0000	2.000	Slices	13.00	7.00	2.00	120.00	0.00	2.00	0.00	1.00
798	Worthington-Chik Patties, Crisp	71.0000	1.000	Each	8.00	6.00	15.00	150.00	0.00	2.00	0.00	1.00
799	Worthington-Chik Stiks	47.0000	1.000	Each	9.00	7.00	3.00	110.00	0.00	2.00	0.00	1.00
800	Worthington-Chik, Diced	55.0000	0.250	Cup	7.00	0.00	1.00	40.00	0.00	1.00	0.00	0.00
801	Worthington-Chik, Sliced	90.0000	3.000	Slices	14.00	0.50	2.00	70.00	0.00	2.00	0.00	0.00
802	Worthington-Chili	230.0000	1.000	Cup	19.00	15.00	21.00	290.00	0.00	9.00	0.00	2.50
803	Worthington-Chili, Low Fat	230.0000	1.000	Cup	18.00	1.00	21.00	170.00	0.00	11.00	0.00	0.00
804	Worthington-Choplets	92.0000	2.000	Slices	17.00	1.50	3.00	90.00	0.00	2.00	0.00	1.00
805	Worthington-Choplets, Multigrai	92.0000	2.000	Slices	15.00	2.00	5.00	100.00	0.00	4.00	0.00	0.50
806	Worthington-Corned Beef, Meatle	57.0000	4.000	Slices	10.00	9.00	5.00	140.00	0.00	2.00	0.00	1.00
807	Worthington-Croquettes, Golden	85.0000	4.000	Each	14.00	10.00	14.00	210.00	0.00	3.00	0.00	1.50
808	Worthington-Fillets	85.0000	2.000	Each	16.00	10.00	8.00	180.00	0.00	4.00	0.00	2.00
809	Worthington-FriChik	90.0000	2.000	Each	10.00	8.00	1.00	120.00	0.00	1.00	0.00	1.00
810	Worthington-FriChik, Low Fat	85.0000	2.000	Each	10.00	3.00	2.00	80.00	0.00	1.00	0.00	0.00
811	Worthington-FriPats	64.0000	1.000	Each	14.00	6.00	4.00	130.00	0.00	3.00	0.00	1.00
812	Worthington-Leanies	40.0000	1.000	Each	7.00	7.00	2.00	100.00	0.00	1.00	0.00	1.00
813	Worthington-Links, Super	48.0000	1.000	Each	7.00	8.00	2.00	110.00	0.00	1.00	0.00	1.00
814	Worthington-Links, Veja	31.0000	1.000	Each	5.00	3.00	1.00	50.00	0.00	0.00	0.00	0.50
815	Worthington-Numete	55.0000	1.000	Slice	6.00	10.00	5.00	130.00	0.00	3.00	0.00	2.50
816	Worthington-Prosage Links	45.0000	2.000	Each	8.00	2.50	2.00	60.00	0.00	2.00	0.00	0.50
817	Worthington-Prosage Patties	38.0000	1.000	Each	9.00	3.00	3.00	80.00	0.00	1.00	0.00	0.50
818	Worthington-Prosage Roll, Frozen	55.0000	1.000	Slice	10.00	10.00	2.00	140.00	0.00	2.00	0.00	2.00
819	Worthington-Protose	55.0000	1.000	Slice	13.00	7.00	5.00	130.00	0.00	3.00	0.00	1.00
820	Worthington-Roast, Dinner	85.0000	1.000	Slice	12.00	12.00	5.00	180.00	0.00	3.00	0.00	1.50
821	Worthington-Salami, Meatless	57.0000	3.000	Slices	12.00	8.00	2.00	130.00	0.00	2.00	0.00	1.00
822	Worthington-Saucettes	38.0000	1.000	Each	6.00	6.00	1.00	90.00	0.00	1.00	0.00	1.00
823	Worthington-Skallops, Vegetable	85.0000	0.500	Cup	15.00	1.50	3.00	90.00	0.00	3.00	0.00	0.50
824	Worthington-Slices, Savory	84.0000	3.000	Slices	10.00	9.00	6.00	150.00	0.00	3.00	0.00	3.50
825	Worthington-Stakelets	71.0000	1.000	Each	12.00	8.00	6.00	140.00	0.00	2.00	0.00	1.00
826	Worthington-Stakes, Prime	92.0000	1.000	Each	10.00	7.00	4.00	120.00	0.00	4.00	0.00	1.00
827	Worthington-Steaks, Vegetable	72.0000	2.000	Slices	15.00	1.50	3.00	80.00	0.00	3.00	0.00	0.50
828	Worthington-Stew, Country	240.0000	1.000	Cup	13.00	9.00	20.00	210.00	0.00	5.00	0.00	1.00
829	Worthington-Stripples	16.0000	2.000	Each	2.00	4.50	2.00	60.00	0.00	1.00	0.00	0.50
830	Worthington-Tuno	55.0000	0.500	Cup	6.00	6.00	2.00	80.00	0.00	1.00	0.00	1.00
831	Worthington-Turkee Slices	94.0000	3.000	Slices	13.00	12.00	3.00	170.00	0.00	2.00	0.00	1.50
832	Worthington-Turkey, Smoked, Mea	57.0000	3.000	Slices	10.00	0.00	3.00	140.00	0.00	2.00	0.00	2.00
833	Worthington-Wham	45.0000	2.000	Slices	7.00	5.00	1.00	80.00	0.00	0.00	0.00	1.00
948	Ziti Mozzarella-Smart Ones	252.0000	9.000	Ounce	11.00	6.00	45.00	280.00	0.00	4.00	5.00	1.50

Restaurant Chains–Fast Foods

USDA ID Code	Food Name	Weight in Grams*	Quantity of Units	Unit of Measure	Protein (g)	Fat (g)	Carbohydrate (g)	Kilocalories	Caffeine (g)	Fiber (g)	Cholesterol (mg)	Saturated Fat (g)
	Arby's-Beef, Roast, Regular	155.9210	1.000	Each	24.68	15.70	38.14	388.12	0.00	1.12	58.33	4.04
	Arby's-Beef, Roast, Super	240.9690	1.000	Each	25.74	22.66	51.49	515.92	0.00	1.65	41.19	8.75
	Arby's-Beef 'N Cheddar Sandwich	194.0000	1.000	Each	35.27	19.84	29.76	443.11	0.00	1.21	84.88	9.92
	Arby's-Chicken BBQ, Grilled	201.0000	1.000	Each	23.00	13.00	47.00	388.00	0.00	2.00	43.00	3.00
	Arby's-Chicken Breast Fillet San	204.0000	1.000	Each	25.50	27.72	53.22	546.59	0.00	1.77	100.89	5.65
	Arby's-Chicken Cordon Bleu	240.0000	1.000	Each	38.00	33.00	46.00	623.00	0.00	5.00	77.00	5.65
	Arby's-Chicken Fingers	102.0000	1.000	Each	16.00	16.00	20.00	290.00	0.00	0.50	32.00	2.00
	Arby's-Chicken, Grilled, Delux	230.0000	1.000	Each	23.00	20.00	47.00	430.00	0.00	3.00	61.00	4.00
	Arby's-Chicken, Roast, Delux	195.0000	1.000	Each	20.00	6.00	33.00	276.00	0.00	4.00	33.00	2.00
	Arby's-Chowder, Clam, Boston	226.7950	1.000	Each	10.00	11.00	18.00	207.00	0.00	1.40	28.00	4.00
	Arby's-Fish Fillet Sandwich	221.0000	1.000	Each	23.00	27.00	50.00	526.00	0.00	0.00	43.80	7.00
	Arby's-French Fries	70.8730	1.000	Order	2.10	13.20	29.80	246.00	0.00	0.00	0.00	3.00

Page Key: A2 = Baby Food   A2 = Baked Goods   A8 = Beverages   A14 = Breads/Grains and Pasta   A18 = Breakfast Foods/Cereals   A26 = Dairy and Eggs   A40 = Fats and Oils   A42 = Fruits and Vegetables   A52 = Meats and Beans   A60 = Nuts and Seeds   A62 = Frozen Entrees and Packaged Foods   A76 = Restaurant Chains–Fast Foods   A92 = Restaurant Chains–Other   A106 = Seafood and Fish   A110 = Snacks and Sweets   A120 = Soups   A122 = Supplements   A126 = Toppings and Sauces

Monounsaturated Fat (g)	Polyunsaturated Fat (g)	Vitamin D (mg)	Vitamin K (mg)	Vitamin E (mg)	Vitamin A (re)	Vitamin C (mg)	Thiamin (mg)	Riboflavin (mg)	Niacin (mg)	Vitamin B6 (mg)	Folate (mcg)	Vitamin B12 (mcg)	Calcium (mg)	Iron (mg)	Magnesium (mg)	Phosphorus (mg)	Potassium (mg)	Sodium (mg)	Zinc (mg)
1.00	2.50	0.00	0.00	0.00	0.00	0.00	0.30	0.14	1.20	0.20	0.00	0.90	0.00	1.80	0.00	0.00	280.00	370.00	0.00
0.00	0.00	0.00	0.00	0.00	0.00	0.00	0.15	0.14	2.00	0.20	0.00	0.90	0.00	1.44	0.00	0.00	200.00	400.00	0.00
1.50	4.00	0.00	0.00	0.00	0.00	0.00	0.43	0.14	0.80	0.12	0.00	1.20	0.00	1.80	0.00	0.00	30.00	390.00	0.00
1.50	3.50	0.00	0.00	0.00	0.00	0.00	1.20	0.10	0.40	0.20	0.00	0.60	0.00	0.72	0.00	0.00	200.00	600.00	0.00
2.50	3.50	0.00	0.00	0.00	0.00	0.00	0.30	0.03	2.00	0.30	0.00	2.10	0.00	0.72	0.00	0.00	60.00	360.00	0.00
0.00	0.00	0.00	0.00	0.00	0.00	0.00	0.06	0.10	4.00	0.08	0.00	0.24	0.00	1.08	0.00	0.00	100.00	270.00	0.00
0.00	0.00	0.00	0.00	0.00	0.00	0.00	0.12	0.26	7.00	0.12	0.00	0.48	20.00	1.80	0.00	0.00	170.00	430.00	0.00
3.50	9.00	0.00	0.00	0.00	0.00	0.00	0.06	0.07	2.00	0.70	0.00	1.50	40.00	3.60	0.00	0.00	420.00	1130.00	0.00
0.00	0.00	0.00	0.00	0.00	150.00	0.00	0.00	0.00	0.00	0.00	0.00	0.00	40.00	1.80	0.00	0.00	480.00	870.00	0.00
0.00	0.00	0.00	0.00	0.00	0.00	0.00	0.00	0.00	0.00	0.00	0.00	0.00	0.00	0.36	0.00	0.00	40.00	500.00	0.00
0.50	1.00	0.00	0.00	0.00	0.00	0.00	0.00	0.00	0.00	0.00	0.00	0.00	0.00	0.72	0.00	0.00	30.00	390.00	0.00
2.00	6.00	0.00	0.00	0.00	0.00	0.00	1.80	0.07	1.20	0.30	0.00	1.80	0.00	1.08	0.00	0.00	60.00	520.00	0.00
2.50	6.00	0.00	0.00	0.00	0.00	0.00	0.45	0.07	2.00	0.30	0.00	2.70	40.00	1.44	0.00	0.00	190.00	600.00	0.00
3.50	4.50	0.00	0.00	0.00	0.00	0.00	0.68	0.14	0.80	0.40	0.00	2.70	0.00	1.80	0.00	0.00	130.00	750.00	0.00
2.00	5.00	0.00	0.00	0.00	0.00	0.00	0.09	0.14	0.80	0.16	0.00	2.40	0.00	1.08	0.00	0.00	150.00	430.00	0.00
1.00	2.00	0.00	0.00	0.00	0.00	0.00	0.09	0.14	0.80	0.16	0.00	2.40	0.00	1.08	0.00	0.00	150.00	430.00	0.00
1.50	3.50	0.00	0.00	0.00	0.00	0.00	1.80	0.17	3.00	0.60	0.00	1.20	60.00	1.08	0.00	0.00	125.00	320.00	0.00
1.50	4.50	0.00	0.00	0.00	0.00	0.00	0.23	0.14	0.80	0.20	0.00	0.90	20.00	0.72	0.00	0.00	40.00	430.00	0.00
2.00	4.50	0.00	0.00	0.00	0.00	0.00	0.09	0.10	0.80	0.12	0.00	1.20	0.00	0.00	0.00	0.00	30.00	350.00	0.00
1.50	1.00	0.00	0.00	0.00	0.00	0.00	0.12	0.10	1.60	0.16	0.00	0.48	0.00	0.72	0.00	0.00	20.00	190.00	0.00
4.50	2.50	0.00	0.00	0.00	0.00	0.00	0.09	0.07	0.40	0.20	0.00	0.60	0.00	1.08	0.00	0.00	160.00	270.00	0.00
0.50	1.50	0.00	0.00	0.00	0.00	0.00	1.80	0.14	2.00	0.30	0.00	3.60	0.00	1.44	0.00	0.00	60.00	340.00	0.00
0.50	2.00	0.00	0.00	0.00	0.00	0.00	0.45	0.10	0.40	0.30	0.00	1.50	0.00	1.08	0.00	0.00	100.00	300.00	0.00
3.50	4.50	0.00	0.00	0.00	0.00	0.00	1.05	0.17	1.60	0.20	0.00	0.90	0.00	1.80	0.00	0.00	80.00	390.00	0.00
3.00	2.50	0.00	0.00	0.00	0.00	0.00	0.15	0.14	1.20	0.20	0.00	1.20	0.00	1.80	0.00	0.00	50.00	280.00	0.00
5.00	5.00	0.00	0.00	0.00	0.00	0.00	1.80	0.23	6.00	0.60	0.00	1.50	40.00	0.36	0.00	0.00	55.00	580.00	0.00
1.00	6.00	0.00	0.00	0.00	0.00	0.00	0.75	0.14	1.20	0.20	0.00	0.60	20.00	1.44	0.00	0.00	95.00	930.00	0.00
1.50	3.50	0.00	0.00	0.00	0.00	0.00	0.60	0.07	4.00	0.12	0.00	0.36	0.00	1.08	0.00	0.00	25.00	200.00	0.00
0.50	0.00	0.00	0.00	0.00	0.00	0.00	0.00	0.00	0.00	0.00	0.00	0.00	0.00	0.72	0.00	0.00	10.00	410.00	0.00
4.00	1.50	0.00	0.00	0.00	0.00	0.00	0.23	0.17	1.60	0.30	0.00	1.50	0.00	1.44	0.00	0.00	40.00	540.00	0.00
5.00	2.00	0.00	0.00	0.00	0.00	0.00	1.50	0.14	3.00	0.30	0.00	1.50	40.00	1.08	0.00	0.00	95.00	480.00	0.00
1.50	4.00	0.00	0.00	0.00	0.00	0.00	0.12	0.14	2.00	0.40	0.00	0.90	0.00	0.36	0.00	0.00	80.00	440.00	0.00
0.00	0.00	0.00	0.00	0.00	0.00	0.00	0.53	0.10	4.00	0.20	0.00	3.00	0.00	3.60	0.00	0.00	20.00	300.00	0.00
2.00	5.00	0.00	0.00	0.00	675.45	0.00	1.80	0.23	4.00	0.90	0.00	3.60	60.00	5.40	0.00	0.00	270.00	830.00	0.00
1.00	2.50	0.00	0.00	0.00	0.00	0.00	0.75	0.03	0.40	0.08	0.00	0.24	0.00	0.36	0.00	0.00	15.00	220.00	0.00
1.50	3.00	0.00	0.00	0.00	0.00	0.00	0.15	0.03	1.20	0.30	0.00	2.10	20.00	1.08	0.00	0.00	35.00	290.00	0.00
2.50	8.00	0.00	0.00	0.00	0.00	0.00	1.80	0.14	1.20	0.20	0.00	1.50	0.00	1.44	0.00	0.00	45.00	580.00	0.00
3.50	4.00	0.00	0.00	0.00	0.00	0.00	1.80	0.17	2.00	0.30	0.00	2.10	0.00	1.80	0.00	0.00	70.00	620.00	0.00
1.00	3.00	0.00	0.00	0.00	0.00	0.00	1.80	0.14	1.60	0.20	0.00	1.20	0.00	1.08	0.00	0.00	90.00	430.00	0.00
0.00	0.00	0.00	0.00	0.00	0.00	0.00	0.00	0.00	0.00	0.00	0.00	0.00	0.00	0.00	0.00	0.00	0.00	430.00	0.00
7.63	1.91	0.00	0.00	0.22	70.67	2.24	0.43	0.35	6.62	0.30	44.87	1.37	60.57	4.71	34.77	268.09	354.47	888.41	3.81
8.44	5.56	0.00	0.00	0.41	0.00	0.00	0.65	0.62	9.68	0.49	42.22	4.42	118.42	6.59	59.73	413.97	517.98	821.77	11.02
4.08	3.86	0.00	0.00	0.44	63.93	1.32	0.42	0.51	6.50	0.37	45.19	2.26	201.72	5.62	44.09	442.01	380.28	1801.11	5.95
2.00	1.00	0.00	0.00	0.00	16.63	0.00	0.50	0.43	16.41	0.72	35.48	0.38	123.07	3.88	51.00	321.52	365.87	1002.00	1.88
10.64	11.42	0.00	0.00	2.88	16.63	0.00	0.50	0.43	16.41	0.72	35.48	0.38	123.07	3.88	51.00	321.52	365.87	1129.76	1.88
10.64	11.42	0.00	0.00	2.88	16.63	0.00	0.50	0.43	16.41	0.72	35.48	0.38	123.07	3.88	51.00	321.52	365.87	1594.00	1.88
4.00	4.10	0.00	0.00	1.40	2.60	0.00	0.00	0.00	0.00	0.09	17.00	0.19	92.00	1.90	22.00	140.00	190.00	677.00	0.30
2.00	1.00	0.00	0.00	0.00	16.63	0.00	0.50	0.43	16.41	0.72	35.48	0.38	123.07	3.88	51.00	321.52	365.87	848.00	1.88
2.00	1.00	0.00	0.00	0.00	16.63	0.00	0.50	0.43	16.41	0.72	35.48	0.38	123.07	3.88	51.00	321.52	365.87	777.00	1.88
5.00	2.00	0.00	0.00	0.10	100.00	4.00	0.06	0.22	0.90	0.12	9.00	9.38	170.00	1.40	20.00	143.00	319.00	1157.00	0.70
9.20	10.60	0.00	0.00	0.00	0.00	1.20	0.35	0.31	5.32	0.00	0.00	0.00	72.00	2.10	0.00	0.00	450.00	872.00	0.00
5.50	4.70	0.00	0.00	0.00	0.00	3.60	0.06	0.00	1.90	0.00	0.00	0.00	0.00	0.60	0.00	0.00	240.00	114.00	0.00

USDA ID Code	Food Name	Weight in Grams*	Quantity of Units	Unit of Measure	Protein (g)	Fat (g)	Carbohydrate (g)	Kilocalories	Caffeine (g)	Fiber (g)	Cholesterol (mg)	Saturated Fat (g)
	Arby's-French Fries, Curly	99.2230	1.000	Order	4.20	17.70	43.20	337.00	0.00	0.00	0.00	7.40
	Arby's-Ham 'N Cheese Sandwich	170.0960	1.000	Each	24.47	18.64	38.45	411.26	0.00	1.17	67.57	7.46
	Arby's-Soup, Broccoli, Cream Of	226.7950	1.000	Each	9.00	8.00	19.00	180.00	0.00	1.80	3.00	5.00
	Arby's-Soup, Cheese, Wisconsin	226.7950	1.000	Each	9.00	19.00	19.00	287.00	0.00	1.80	31.00	8.00
	Arby's-Turkey Sub	277.0000	1.000	Each	32.86	28.17	53.99	598.60	0.00	0.00	82.16	6.22
10	Boston Market-Apples, Cinnamon,	181.0000	0.750	Cup	0.00	4.50	56.00	250.00	0.00	3.00	0.00	0.00
11	Boston Market-Beans, BBQ Baked	201.0000	0.750	Cup	11.00	9.00	53.00	330.00	0.00	9.00	10.00	0.00
12	Boston Market-Brownie	95.0000	1.000	Each	6.00	27.00	47.00	450.00	0.00	3.00	80.00	0.00
13	Boston Market-Caesar, no dressing	225.0000	8.000	Ounce	19.00	13.00	14.00	240.00	0.00	4.00	25.00	0.00
14	Boston Market-Chicken Salad Sand	327.0000	1.000	Each	38.00	33.00	63.00	680.00	0.00	5.00	145.00	0.00
15	Boston Market-Chicken Salad, Chu	158.0000	0.750	Cup	27.00	30.00	3.00	390.00	0.00	1.00	145.00	0.00
16	Boston Market-Chicken Sandwich w	352.0000	1.000	Each	46.00	32.00	71.00	760.00	0.00	12.00	160.00	0.00
17	Boston Market-Chicken Sandwich,	281.0000	1.000	Each	39.00	3.50	61.00	430.00	0.00	11.00	95.00	0.00
18	Boston Market-Chicken, Dark Meat	125.0000	1.000	Each	31.00	22.00	2.00	330.00	0.00	1.00	180.00	0.00
19	Boston Market-Chicken, Dark Meat	95.0000	1.000	Each	28.00	10.00	1.00	210.00	0.00	1.00	150.00	0.00
22	Boston Market-Chicken, w/ skin,	227.0000	1.000	Each	74.00	37.00	2.00	630.00	0.00	2.00	370.00	0.00
20	Boston Market-Chicken, White Mea	140.0000	1.000	Each	31.00	3.50	0.00	160.00	0.00	0.00	95.00	0.00
21	Boston Market-Chicken, White Mea	152.0000	1.000	Each	43.00	17.00	2.00	330.00	0.00	1.00	175.00	0.00
23	Boston Market-Coleslaw	184.0000	0.750	Cup	2.00	16.00	32.00	280.00	0.00	3.00	25.00	0.00
24	Boston Market-Cookie, Chocolate	79.0000	1.000	Each	4.00	17.00	48.00	340.00	0.00	1.00	25.00	0.00
25	Boston Market-Cookie, Oatmeal Ra	79.0000	1.000	Each	4.00	13.00	48.00	320.00	0.00	1.00	25.00	0.00
26	Boston Market-Corn Bread	68.0000	1.000	Each	3.00	6.00	33.00	200.00	0.00	1.00	25.00	0.00
27	Boston Market-Corn, Buttered	146.0000	0.750	Cup	6.00	4.00	39.00	190.00	0.00	4.00	0.00	0.00
28	Boston Market-Cranberry Relish	225.0000	0.750	Cup	2.00	5.00	84.00	370.00	0.00	5.00	0.00	0.00
29	Boston Market-Fruit Salad	156.0000	0.750	Cup	1.00	0.50	17.00	70.00	0.00	2.00	0.00	0.00
30	Boston Market-Gravy, Chicken	28.0000	1.000	Ounce	0.00	1.00	2.00	15.00	0.00	0.00	0.00	0.00
31	Boston Market-Ham Sandwich w/ Ch	337.0000	1.000	Each	38.00	35.00	71.00	760.00	0.00	5.00	100.00	0.00
32	Boston Market-Ham Sandwich, plai	266.0000	1.000	Each	25.00	9.00	66.00	450.00	0.00	4.00	45.00	0.00
33	Boston Market-Ham, Hearth Honey	142.0000	5.000	Ounce	25.00	9.00	9.00	210.00	0.00	0.00	75.00	0.00
34	Boston Market-Ham/Turkey Club w/	379.0000	1.000	Each	47.00	43.00	79.00	890.00	0.00	4.00	150.00	0.00
35	Boston Market-Ham/Turkey Club, p	266.0000	1.000	Each	29.00	6.00	64.00	430.00	0.00	4.00	55.00	0.00
36	Boston Market-Macaroni & Cheese	192.0000	0.750	Cup	12.00	10.00	36.00	280.00	0.00	1.00	20.00	0.00
37	Boston Market-Meatloaf Sandwich	383.0000	1.000	Each	46.00	33.00	95.00	860.00	0.00	6.00	165.00	0.00
38	Boston Market-Meatloaf w/ Brown	198.0000	7.000	Ounce	30.00	22.00	19.00	390.00	0.00	1.00	120.00	0.00
39	Boston Market-Meatloaf, plain	351.0000	1.000	Each	40.00	21.00	86.00	690.00	0.00	6.00	120.00	0.00
40	Boston Market-Meatloaf/Chunky To	227.0000	8.000	Ounce	30.00	18.00	22.00	370.00	0.00	5.00	120.00	0.00
41	Boston Market-Pot Pie, Chicken,	425.0000	1.000	Each	34.00	34.00	78.00	750.00	0.00	6.00	115.00	0.00
42	Boston Market-Potatoes, Mashed	161.0000	0.660	Cup	3.00	8.00	25.00	180.00	0.00	4.00	25.00	0.00
43	Boston Market-Potatoes, Mashed &	189.0000	0.750	Cup	3.00	9.00	27.00	200.00	0.00	4.00	25.00	0.00
44	Boston Market-Potatoes, New	131.0000	0.750	Cup	3.00	3.00	25.00	140.00	0.00	2.00	0.00	0.00
45	Boston Market-Rice Pilaf	145.0000	0.660	Cup	5.00	5.00	32.00	180.00	0.00	2.00	0.00	0.00
46	Boston Market-Salad, Caesar, Chi	369.0000	13.000	Ounce	45.00	47.00	16.00	670.00	0.00	3.00	120.00	0.00
47	Boston Market-Salad, Caesar, Ent	283.0000	10.000	Ounce	20.00	43.00	16.00	520.00	0.00	3.00	40.00	0.00
48	Boston Market-Salad, Caesar, Sid	113.0000	4.000	Ounce	8.00	17.00	6.00	210.00	0.00	1.00	20.00	0.00
49	Boston Market-Salad, Pasta, Med.	156.0000	0.750	Cup	4.00	10.00	16.00	170.00	0.00	2.00	10.00	0.00
50	Boston Market-Salad, Tortellini	156.0000	0.750	Cup	14.00	24.00	29.00	380.00	0.00	2.00	90.00	0.00
51	Boston Market-Soup, Chicken	257.0000	1.000	Cup	9.00	3.00	4.00	80.00	0.00	2.00	25.00	0.00
52	Boston Market-Soup, Chicken Tort	238.0000	1.000	Cup	10.00	11.00	19.00	220.00	0.00	2.00	35.00	0.00
53	Boston Market-Spinach, Creamed	181.0000	0.750	Cup	10.00	24.00	13.00	300.00	0.00	2.00	75.00	0.00
54	Boston Market-Squash, Butternut	193.0000	0.750	Cup	2.00	6.00	25.00	160.00	0.00	3.00	15.00	0.00
55	Boston Market-Stuffing	174.0000	0.750	Cup	6.00	12.00	44.00	310.00	0.00	3.00	0.00	0.00
56	Boston Market-Turkey Breast, Rot	142.0000	5.000	Ounce	36.00	1.00	1.00	170.00	0.00	0.00	100.00	0.00
57	Boston Market-Turkey Sandwich w/	337.0000	1.000	Each	45.00	28.00	68.00	710.00	0.00	4.00	110.00	0.00

Page Key: A2 = Baby Food   A2 = Baked Goods   A8 = Beverages   A14 = Breads/Grains and Pasta   A18 = Breakfast Foods/Cereals   A26 = Dairy and Eggs   A40 = Fats and Oils   A42 = Fruits and Vegetables   A52 = Meats and Beans   A60 = Nuts and Seeds   A62 = Frozen Entrees and Packaged Foods   A76 = Restaurant Chains–Fast Foods   A92 = Restaurant Chains–Other   A106 = Seafood and Fish   A110 = Snacks and Sweets   A120 = Soups   A122 = Supplements   A126 = Toppings and Sauces

Monounsaturated Fat (g)	Polyunsaturated Fat (g)	Vitamin D (mg)	Vitamin K (mg)	Vitamin E (mg)	Vitamin A (re)	Vitamin C (mg)	Thiamin (mg)	Riboflavin (mg)	Niacin (mg)	Vitamin B6 (mg)	Folate (mcg)	Vitamin B12 (mcg)	Calcium (mg)	Iron (mg)	Magnesium (mg)	Phosphorus (mg)	Potassium (mg)	Sodium (mg)	Zinc (mg)
7.60	1.50	0.00	0.00	0.00	0.00	0.00	0.06	0.07	1.90	0.00	0.00	0.00	16.00	0.80	0.00	0.00	724.00	167.00	0.00
7.81	1.63	0.00	0.00	1.28	111.84	3.50	0.36	0.57	3.15	0.23	82.72	0.63	151.46	3.84	18.64	177.09	337.86	899.41	1.63
2.00	1.00	0.00	0.00	1.40	50.00	9.00	0.11	0.42	0.80	0.18	46.00	0.59	237.00	0.80	55.00	193.00	455.00	1113.00	0.70
8.00	3.00	0.00	0.00	0.40	90.00	2.00	0.03	0.24	0.70	0.05	7.00	0.00	252.00	1.30	7.00	241.00	441.00	1129.00	1.10
7.04	8.22	0.00	0.00	0.00	0.00	0.00	0.53	0.40	9.39	0.00	0.00	0.00	93.90	3.17	0.00	0.00	0.00	1431.95	0.00
0.00	0.00	0.00	0.00	0.00	0.00	0.00	0.00	0.00	0.00	0.00	0.00	0.00	0.00	0.00	0.00	0.00	0.00	45.00	0.00
0.00	0.00	0.00	0.00	0.00	0.00	0.00	0.00	0.00	0.00	0.00	0.00	0.00	0.00	0.00	0.00	0.00	0.00	630.00	0.00
0.00	0.00	0.00	0.00	0.00	0.00	0.00	0.00	0.00	0.00	0.00	0.00	0.00	0.00	0.00	0.00	0.00	0.00	190.00	0.00
0.00	0.00	0.00	0.00	0.00	0.00	0.00	0.00	0.00	0.00	0.00	0.00	0.00	0.00	0.00	0.00	0.00	0.00	780.00	0.00
0.00	0.00	0.00	0.00	0.00	0.00	0.00	0.00	0.00	0.00	0.00	0.00	0.00	0.00	0.00	0.00	0.00	0.00	1350.00	0.00
0.00	0.00	0.00	0.00	0.00	0.00	0.00	0.00	0.00	0.00	0.00	0.00	0.00	0.00	0.00	0.00	0.00	0.00	790.00	0.00
0.00	0.00	0.00	0.00	0.00	0.00	0.00	0.00	0.00	0.00	0.00	0.00	0.00	0.00	0.00	0.00	0.00	0.00	1810.00	0.00
0.00	0.00	0.00	0.00	0.00	0.00	0.00	0.00	0.00	0.00	0.00	0.00	0.00	0.00	0.00	0.00	0.00	0.00	860.00	0.00
0.00	0.00	0.00	0.00	0.00	0.00	0.00	0.00	0.00	0.00	0.00	0.00	0.00	0.00	0.00	0.00	0.00	0.00	460.00	0.00
0.00	0.00	0.00	0.00	0.00	0.00	0.00	0.00	0.00	0.00	0.00	0.00	0.00	0.00	0.00	0.00	0.00	0.00	320.00	0.00
0.00	0.00	0.00	0.00	0.00	0.00	0.00	0.00	0.00	0.00	0.00	0.00	0.00	0.00	0.00	0.00	0.00	0.00	960.00	0.00
0.00	0.00	0.00	0.00	0.00	0.00	0.00	0.00	0.00	0.00	0.00	0.00	0.00	0.00	0.00	0.00	0.00	0.00	350.00	0.00
0.00	0.00	0.00	0.00	0.00	0.00	0.00	0.00	0.00	0.00	0.00	0.00	0.00	0.00	0.00	0.00	0.00	0.00	530.00	0.00
0.00	0.00	0.00	0.00	0.00	0.00	0.00	0.00	0.00	0.00	0.00	0.00	0.00	0.00	0.00	0.00	0.00	0.00	520.00	0.00
0.00	0.00	0.00	0.00	0.00	0.00	0.00	0.00	0.00	0.00	0.00	0.00	0.00	0.00	0.00	0.00	0.00	0.00	240.00	0.00
0.00	0.00	0.00	0.00	0.00	0.00	0.00	0.00	0.00	0.00	0.00	0.00	0.00	0.00	0.00	0.00	0.00	0.00	260.00	0.00
0.00	0.00	0.00	0.00	0.00	0.00	0.00	0.00	0.00	0.00	0.00	0.00	0.00	0.00	0.00	0.00	0.00	0.00	390.00	0.00
0.00	0.00	0.00	0.00	0.00	0.00	0.00	0.00	0.00	0.00	0.00	0.00	0.00	0.00	0.00	0.00	0.00	0.00	130.00	0.00
0.00	0.00	0.00	0.00	0.00	0.00	0.00	0.00	0.00	0.00	0.00	0.00	0.00	0.00	0.00	0.00	0.00	0.00	5.00	0.00
0.00	0.00	0.00	0.00	0.00	0.00	0.00	0.00	0.00	0.00	0.00	0.00	0.00	0.00	0.00	0.00	0.00	0.00	10.00	0.00
0.00	0.00	0.00	0.00	0.00	0.00	0.00	0.00	0.00	0.00	0.00	0.00	0.00	0.00	0.00	0.00	0.00	0.00	170.00	0.00
0.00	0.00	0.00	0.00	0.00	0.00	0.00	0.00	0.00	0.00	0.00	0.00	0.00	0.00	0.00	0.00	0.00	0.00	1880.00	0.00
0.00	0.00	0.00	0.00	0.00	0.00	0.00	0.00	0.00	0.00	0.00	0.00	0.00	0.00	0.00	0.00	0.00	0.00	1600.00	0.00
0.00	0.00	0.00	0.00	0.00	0.00	0.00	0.00	0.00	0.00	0.00	0.00	0.00	0.00	0.00	0.00	0.00	0.00	1490.00	0.00
0.00	0.00	0.00	0.00	0.00	0.00	0.00	0.00	0.00	0.00	0.00	0.00	0.00	0.00	0.00	0.00	0.00	0.00	2310.00	0.00
0.00	0.00	0.00	0.00	0.00	0.00	0.00	0.00	0.00	0.00	0.00	0.00	0.00	0.00	0.00	0.00	0.00	0.00	1330.00	0.00
0.00	0.00	0.00	0.00	0.00	0.00	0.00	0.00	0.00	0.00	0.00	0.00	0.00	0.00	0.00	0.00	0.00	0.00	760.00	0.00
0.00	0.00	0.00	0.00	0.00	0.00	0.00	0.00	0.00	0.00	0.00	0.00	0.00	0.00	0.00	0.00	0.00	0.00	2270.00	0.00
0.00	0.00	0.00	0.00	0.00	0.00	0.00	0.00	0.00	0.00	0.00	0.00	0.00	0.00	0.00	0.00	0.00	0.00	1040.00	0.00
0.00	0.00	0.00	0.00	0.00	0.00	0.00	0.00	0.00	0.00	0.00	0.00	0.00	0.00	0.00	0.00	0.00	0.00	1610.00	0.00
0.00	0.00	0.00	0.00	0.00	0.00	0.00	0.00	0.00	0.00	0.00	0.00	0.00	0.00	0.00	0.00	0.00	0.00	1170.00	0.00
0.00	0.00	0.00	0.00	0.00	0.00	0.00	0.00	0.00	0.00	0.00	0.00	0.00	0.00	0.00	0.00	0.00	0.00	2380.00	0.00
0.00	0.00	0.00	0.00	0.00	0.00	0.00	0.00	0.00	0.00	0.00	0.00	0.00	0.00	0.00	0.00	0.00	0.00	390.00	0.00
0.00	0.00	0.00	0.00	0.00	0.00	0.00	0.00	0.00	0.00	0.00	0.00	0.00	0.00	0.00	0.00	0.00	0.00	560.00	0.00
0.00	0.00	0.00	0.00	0.00	0.00	0.00	0.00	0.00	0.00	0.00	0.00	0.00	0.00	0.00	0.00	0.00	0.00	100.00	0.00
0.00	0.00	0.00	0.00	0.00	0.00	0.00	0.00	0.00	0.00	0.00	0.00	0.00	0.00	0.00	0.00	0.00	0.00	600.00	0.00
0.00	0.00	0.00	0.00	0.00	0.00	0.00	0.00	0.00	0.00	0.00	0.00	0.00	0.00	0.00	0.00	0.00	0.00	1860.00	0.00
0.00	0.00	0.00	0.00	0.00	0.00	0.00	0.00	0.00	0.00	0.00	0.00	0.00	0.00	0.00	0.00	0.00	0.00	1420.00	0.00
0.00	0.00	0.00	0.00	0.00	0.00	0.00	0.00	0.00	0.00	0.00	0.00	0.00	0.00	0.00	0.00	0.00	0.00	560.00	0.00
0.00	0.00	0.00	0.00	0.00	0.00	0.00	0.00	0.00	0.00	0.00	0.00	0.00	0.00	0.00	0.00	0.00	0.00	490.00	0.00
0.00	0.00	0.00	0.00	0.00	0.00	0.00	0.00	0.00	0.00	0.00	0.00	0.00	0.00	0.00	0.00	0.00	0.00	530.00	0.00
0.00	0.00	0.00	0.00	0.00	0.00	0.00	0.00	0.00	0.00	0.00	0.00	0.00	0.00	0.00	0.00	0.00	0.00	470.00	0.00
0.00	0.00	0.00	0.00	0.00	0.00	0.00	0.00	0.00	0.00	0.00	0.00	0.00	0.00	0.00	0.00	0.00	0.00	1410.00	0.00
0.00	0.00	0.00	0.00	0.00	0.00	0.00	0.00	0.00	0.00	0.00	0.00	0.00	0.00	0.00	0.00	0.00	0.00	790.00	0.00
0.00	0.00	0.00	0.00	0.00	0.00	0.00	0.00	0.00	0.00	0.00	0.00	0.00	0.00	0.00	0.00	0.00	0.00	580.00	0.00
0.00	0.00	0.00	0.00	0.00	0.00	0.00	0.00	0.00	0.00	0.00	0.00	0.00	0.00	0.00	0.00	0.00	0.00	1140.00	0.00
0.00	0.00	0.00	0.00	0.00	0.00	0.00	0.00	0.00	0.00	0.00	0.00	0.00	0.00	0.00	0.00	0.00	0.00	850.00	0.00
0.00	0.00	0.00	0.00	0.00	0.00	0.00	0.00	0.00	0.00	0.00	0.00	0.00	0.00	0.00	0.00	0.00	0.00	1390.00	0.00

USDA ID Code	Food Name	Weight in Grams*	Quantity of Units	Unit of Measure	Protein (g)	Fat (g)	Carbohydrate (g)	Kilocalories	Caffeine (g)	Fiber (g)	Cholesterol (mg)	Saturated Fat (g)
58	Boston Market-Turkey Sandwich, p	266.0000	1.000	Each	32.00	3.50	61.00	400.00	0.00	4.00	60.00	0.00
59	Boston Market-Vegetables, Steame	105.0000	0.660	Cup	2.00	0.50	7.00	35.00	0.00	3.00	0.00	0.00
60	Boston Market-Zucchini Marinara	146.0000	0.750	Cup	2.00	4.00	10.00	80.00	0.00	2.00	0.00	0.00
	Burger King-Biscuit With Bacon,	171.0000	1.000	Each	19.00	31.00	39.00	280.00	0.00	1.00	225.00	10.00
	Burger King-Biscuit with Sausage	151.0000	1.000	Each	16.00	40.00	41.00	360.00	0.00	1.00	45.00	13.00
	Burger King-Cheeseburger	138.0000	1.000	Each	23.00	16.00	28.00	380.00	0.00	1.00	65.00	9.00
	Burger King-Cheeseburger, Bacon	218.0000	1.000	Each	44.00	39.00	28.00	640.00	0.00	1.00	145.00	18.00
	Burger King-Cheeseburger, Double	210.0000	1.000	Each	41.00	36.00	28.00	600.00	0.00	1.00	135.00	17.00
	Burger King-Chicken Salad, Broil	302.0000	1.000	Each	21.00	10.00	7.00	90.00	0.00	3.00	60.00	4.00
	Burger King-Chicken Sandwich	229.0000	1.000	Each	26.00	43.00	54.00	710.00	0.00	2.00	60.00	9.00
	Burger King-Chicken Sandwich-BK	248.0000	1.000	Each	30.00	29.00	41.00	550.00	0.00	2.00	80.00	6.00
	Burger King-Chicken Tenders-8	117.0000	1.000	Each	21.00	17.00	19.00	310.00	0.00	3.00	50.00	4.00
	Burger King-Coca Cola Classic-	360.0000	1.000	Each	0.00	0.00	70.00	280.00	3.08	0.00	0.00	0.00
	Burger King-Coke, Diet-medium	360.0000	1.000	Each	0.00	0.00	0.00	1.00	3.08	0.00	0.00	0.00
	Burger King-Croissan'Wich, w/ sa	176.0000	1.000	Each	22.00	46.00	25.00	600.00	0.00	1.00	260.00	16.00
	Burger King-Dressing, French	30.0000	1.000	Each	0.00	10.00	11.00	140.00	0.00	0.00	0.00	2.00
	Burger King-Dressing, Italian, R	30.0000	1.000	Each	0.00	0.50	3.00	15.00	0.00	0.00	0.00	0.00
	Burger King-Dressing, Ranch	30.0000	1.000	Each	0.00	19.00	2.00	180.00	0.00	0.00	10.00	4.00
	Burger King-Dressing, Thousand I	30.0000	1.000	Each	0.00	12.00	7.00	140.00	0.00	0.00	15.00	3.00
	Burger King-Fish Sandwich, BK Bi	255.0000	1.000	Each	26.00	41.00	56.00	700.00	0.00	3.00	90.00	6.00
	Burger King-French Fries, Coated	102.0000	1.000	Each	3.00	17.00	43.00	340.00	0.00	3.00	0.00	5.00
	Burger King-French Fries, Medium	116.0000	1.000	Each	5.00	20.00	43.00	180.00	0.00	3.00	0.00	5.00
	Burger King-French Toast Sticks	141.0000	1.000	Each	4.00	27.00	60.00	500.00	0.00	1.00	0.00	27.00
	Burger King-Hamburger	126.0000	1.000	Each	20.00	15.00	28.00	330.00	0.00	1.00	55.00	6.00
	Burger King-Hash Browns	71.0000	1.000	Each	2.00	12.00	25.00	110.00	0.00	2.00	0.00	3.00
	Burger King-Jam, Grape	12.0000	1.000	Each	0.00	0.00	8.00	30.00	0.00	0.00	0.00	0.00
	Burger King-Jam, Strawberry	12.0000	1.000	Each	0.00	0.00	8.00	30.00	0.00	0.00	0.00	0.00
	Burger King-Ketchup	14.0000	1.000	Each	0.00	0.00	4.00	15.00	0.00	0.00	0.00	0.00
	Burger King-Onion Rings	124.0000	1.000	Each	4.00	14.00	41.00	310.00	0.00	6.00	0.00	2.00
	Burger King-Pie, Apple, Dutch	113.0000	1.000	Each	3.00	15.00	39.00	300.00	0.00	2.00	0.00	3.00
	Burger King-Salad w/ 1000 Island	176.0000	1.000	Each	2.00	12.00	9.00	145.00	0.00	0.00	17.00	0.00
	Burger King-Salad w/ Bleu Cheese	176.0000	1.000	Each	3.00	16.00	7.00	184.00	0.00	0.00	22.00	0.00
	Burger King-Salad w/ Dressing, H	176.0000	1.000	Each	3.00	13.00	8.00	159.00	0.00	0.00	11.00	0.00
	Burger King-Salad w/ French	176.0000	1.000	Each	2.00	11.00	13.00	152.00	0.00	0.00	0.00	0.00
	Burger King-Salad w/ Italian, Go	176.0000	1.000	Each	2.00	14.00	7.00	162.00	0.00	0.00	0.00	0.00
	Burger King-Salad w/ Italian, Re	176.0000	1.000	Each	2.00	1.00	7.00	42.00	0.00	0.00	0.00	0.00
	Burger King-Salad, Garden	255.0000	1.000	Each	6.00	5.00	8.00	100.00	0.00	4.00	15.00	3.00
	Burger King-Salad, Side	133.0000	1.000	Each	3.00	3.00	4.00	60.00	0.00	2.00	5.00	2.00
	Burger King-Sauce, Dipping, Barb	28.0000	1.000	Each	0.00	0.00	9.00	35.00	0.00	0.00	0.00	0.00
	Burger King-Sauce, Dipping, Hone	28.0000	1.000	Each	0.00	0.00	21.00	80.00	0.00	0.00	0.00	0.00
	Burger King-Sauce, Dipping, Swee	28.0000	1.000	Each	0.00	0.00	11.00	45.00	0.00	0.00	0.00	0.00
	Burger King-Shake, Chocolate, Me	397.0000	1.000	Each	12.00	10.00	75.00	440.00	0.00	4.00	30.00	6.00
	Burger King-Shake, Vanilla, Medi	397.0000	1.000	Each	13.00	9.00	73.00	430.00	0.00	2.00	30.00	5.00
	Burger King-Whopper	270.0000	1.000	Each	27.00	39.00	45.00	640.00	0.00	3.00	90.00	11.00
	Burger King-Whopper Jr.	164.0000	1.000	Each	21.00	24.00	29.00	420.00	0.00	2.00	60.00	8.00
	Burger King-Whopper Jr. w/ chees	177.0000	1.000	Each	23.00	28.00	29.00	460.00	0.00	2.00	75.00	10.00
	Burger King-Whopper w/ Cheese, D	375.0000	1.000	Each	52.00	63.00	46.00	960.00	0.00	3.00	195.00	24.00
	Burger King-Whopper, Double	351.0000	1.000	Each	33.00	46.00	46.00	730.00	0.00	3.00	115.00	16.00
177	Chick-fil-A-Chicken Club, Chargr	232.0000	1.000	Each	33.00	12.00	38.00	390.00	0.00	2.00	70.00	5.00
178	Chick-fil-A-Chicken Salad Sandwi	167.0000	1.000	Each	25.00	5.00	42.00	320.00	0.00	1.00	10.00	2.00
179	Chick-fil-A-Chicken Sandwich	167.0000	1.000	Each	24.00	9.00	27.00	290.00	0.00	1.00	50.00	0.00
180	Chick-fil-A-Chicken, Chargrilled	150.0000	1.000	Each	27.00	3.00	36.00	280.00	0.00	1.00	40.00	1.00
176	Chick-fil-A-Chick-n-Strips	119.0000	4.000	Each	29.00	8.00	10.00	230.00	0.00	1.00	20.00	2.00

Page Key: A2 = Baby Food   A2 = Baked Goods   A8 = Beverages   A14 = Breads/Grains and Pasta   A18 = Breakfast Foods/Cereals   A26 = Dairy and Eggs   A40 = Fats and Oils   A42 = Fruits and Vegetables   A52 = Meats and Beans   A60 = Nuts and Seeds   A62 = Frozen Entrees and Packaged Foods   A76 = Restaurant Chains–Fast Foods   A92 = Restaurant Chains–Other   A106 = Seafood and Fish   A110 = Snacks and Sweets   A120 = Soups   A122 = Supplements   A126 = Toppings and Sauces

Monounsaturated Fat (g)	Polyunsaturated Fat (g)	Vitamin D (mg)	Vitamin K (mg)	Vitamin E (mg)	Vitamin A (re)	Vitamin C (mg)	Thiamin (mg)	Riboflavin (mg)	Niacin (mg)	Vitamin B$_6$ (mg)	Folate (mcg)	Vitamin B$_{12}$ (mcg)	Calcium (mg)	Iron (mg)	Magnesium (mg)	Phosphorus (mg)	Potassium (mg)	Sodium (mg)	Zinc (mg)
0.00	0.00	0.00	0.00	0.00	0.00	0.00	0.00	0.00	0.00	0.00	0.00	0.00	0.00	0.00	0.00	0.00	0.00	1070.00	0.00
0.00	0.00	0.00	0.00	0.00	0.00	0.00	0.00	0.00	0.00	0.00	0.00	0.00	0.00	0.00	0.00	0.00	0.00	35.00	0.00
0.00	0.00	0.00	0.00	0.00	0.00	0.00	0.00	0.00	0.00	0.00	0.00	0.00	0.00	0.00	0.00	0.00	0.00	470.00	0.00
0.00	0.00	0.00	0.00	0.00	0.00	0.00	0.00	0.00	0.00	0.00	0.00	0.00	0.00	0.00	0.00	0.00	0.00	1530.00	0.00
0.00	0.00	0.00	0.00	0.00	0.00	0.00	0.00	0.00	0.00	0.00	0.00	0.00	0.00	0.00	0.00	0.00	0.00	1390.00	0.00
0.00	0.00	0.00	0.00	0.00	0.00	0.00	0.00	0.00	0.00	0.00	0.00	0.00	0.00	0.00	0.00	0.00	0.00	770.00	0.00
14.50	6.22	0.00	0.00	1.55	73.54	8.29	0.31	0.40	8.39	0.38	32.11	3.36	161.59	4.14	39.36	386.37	479.59	1240.00	6.63
12.24	2.23	0.00	0.00	2.00	111.25	6.68	0.24	0.34	5.45	0.27	34.49	2.01	210.27	3.34	34.49	339.33	382.72	1060.00	4.45
0.00	0.00	0.00	0.00	0.00	0.00	0.00	0.00	0.00	0.00	0.00	0.00	0.00	0.00	0.00	0.00	0.00	0.00	110.00	0.00
0.00	0.00	0.00	0.00	0.00	0.00	0.00	0.00	0.00	0.00	0.00	0.00	0.00	0.00	0.00	0.00	0.00	0.00	1400.00	0.00
0.00	0.00	0.00	0.00	0.00	0.00	0.00	0.00	0.00	0.00	0.00	0.00	0.00	0.00	0.00	0.00	0.00	0.00	4803.00	0.00
0.00	0.00	0.00	0.00	0.00	0.00	0.00	0.00	0.00	0.00	0.00	0.00	0.00	0.00	0.00	0.00	0.00	0.00	710.00	0.00
0.00	0.00	0.00	0.00	0.00	0.00	0.00	0.00	0.00	0.00	0.00	0.00	0.00	0.00	0.00	0.00	0.00	0.00	0.00	0.00
0.00	0.00	0.00	0.00	0.00	0.00	0.00	0.00	0.00	0.00	0.00	0.00	0.00	0.00	0.00	0.00	0.00	0.00	1140.00	0.00
0.00	0.00	0.00	0.00	0.00	0.00	0.00	0.00	0.00	0.00	0.00	0.00	0.00	0.00	0.00	0.00	0.00	0.00	190.00	0.00
0.00	0.00	0.00	0.00	0.00	0.00	0.00	0.00	0.00	0.00	0.00	0.00	0.00	0.00	0.00	0.00	0.00	0.00	50.00	0.00
0.00	0.00	0.00	0.00	0.00	0.00	0.00	0.00	0.00	0.00	0.00	0.00	0.00	0.00	0.00	0.00	0.00	0.00	170.00	0.00
0.00	0.00	0.00	0.00	0.00	0.00	0.00	0.00	0.00	0.00	0.00	0.00	0.00	0.00	0.00	0.00	0.00	0.00	190.00	0.00
0.00	0.00	0.00	0.00	0.00	0.00	0.00	0.00	0.00	0.00	0.00	0.00	0.00	0.00	0.00	0.00	0.00	0.00	980.00	0.00
0.00	0.00	0.00	0.00	0.00	0.00	0.00	0.00	0.00	0.00	0.00	0.00	0.00	0.00	0.00	0.00	0.00	0.00	680.00	0.00
0.00	0.00	0.00	0.00	0.00	0.00	0.00	0.00	0.00	0.00	0.00	0.00	0.00	0.00	0.00	0.00	0.00	0.00	240.00	0.00
0.00	0.00	0.00	0.00	0.00	0.00	0.00	0.00	0.00	0.00	0.00	0.00	0.00	0.00	0.00	0.00	0.00	0.00	490.00	0.00
0.00	0.00	0.00	0.00	0.00	0.00	0.00	0.00	0.00	0.00	0.00	0.00	0.00	0.00	0.00	0.00	0.00	0.00	530.00	0.00
0.00	0.00	0.00	0.00	0.00	0.00	0.00	0.00	0.00	0.00	0.00	0.00	0.00	0.00	0.00	0.00	0.00	0.00	320.00	0.00
0.00	0.00	0.00	0.00	0.00	0.00	0.00	0.00	0.00	0.00	0.00	0.00	0.00	0.00	0.00	0.00	0.00	0.00	0.00	0.00
0.00	0.00	0.00	0.00	0.00	0.00	0.00	0.00	0.00	0.00	0.00	0.00	0.00	0.00	0.00	0.00	0.00	0.00	5.00	0.00
0.00	0.00	0.00	0.00	0.00	0.00	0.00	0.00	0.00	0.00	0.00	0.00	0.00	0.00	0.00	0.00	0.00	0.00	180.00	0.00
0.00	0.00	0.00	0.00	0.00	0.00	0.00	0.00	0.00	0.00	0.00	0.00	0.00	0.00	0.00	0.00	0.00	0.00	810.00	0.00
0.00	0.00	0.00	0.00	0.00	0.00	0.00	0.00	0.00	0.00	0.00	0.00	0.00	0.00	0.00	0.00	0.00	0.00	230.00	0.00
0.00	0.00	0.00	0.00	0.00	0.00	25.80	0.00	0.00	0.19	0.00	0.00	0.00	336.00	0.14	98.00	528.00	405.00	251.00	0.08
0.00	0.00	0.00	0.00	0.00	0.00	25.20	0.00	0.00	0.19	0.00	0.00	0.00	528.00	0.13	101.50	664.00	382.00	333.00	0.09
0.00	0.00	0.00	0.00	0.00	0.00	25.20	0.00	0.00	0.19	0.00	0.00	0.00	352.00	0.13	94.50	592.00	402.00	293.00	0.08
0.00	0.00	0.00	0.00	0.00	0.00	25.80	0.00	0.00	0.19	0.00	0.00	0.00	320.00	0.14	98.00	480.00	410.00	330.00	0.07
0.00	0.00	0.00	0.00	0.00	0.00	5.20	0.00	0.00	0.19	0.00	0.00	0.00	320.00	0.13	98.00	480.00	389.00	292.00	0.06
0.00	0.00	0.00	0.00	0.00	0.00	25.20	0.00	0.00	0.19	0.00	0.00	0.00	320.00	0.14	105.00	472.00	390.00	430.00	0.06
0.00	0.00	0.00	0.00	0.00	0.00	0.00	0.00	0.00	0.00	0.00	0.00	0.00	0.00	0.00	0.00	0.00	0.00	115.00	0.00
0.00	0.00	0.00	0.00	0.00	0.00	0.00	0.00	0.00	0.00	0.00	0.00	0.00	0.00	0.00	0.00	0.00	0.00	55.00	0.00
0.00	0.00	0.00	0.00	0.00	0.00	0.00	0.00	0.00	0.00	0.00	0.00	0.00	0.00	0.00	0.00	0.00	0.00	400.00	0.00
0.00	0.00	0.00	0.00	0.00	0.00	0.00	0.00	0.00	0.00	0.00	0.00	0.00	0.00	0.00	0.00	0.00	0.00	20.00	0.00
0.00	0.00	0.00	0.00	0.00	0.00	0.00	0.00	0.00	0.00	0.00	0.00	0.00	0.00	0.00	0.00	0.00	0.00	50.00	0.00
0.00	0.00	0.00	0.00	0.00	0.00	0.00	0.00	0.00	0.00	0.00	0.00	0.00	0.00	0.00	0.00	0.00	0.00	330.00	0.00
0.00	0.00	0.00	0.00	0.00	0.00	0.00	0.00	0.00	0.00	0.00	0.00	0.00	0.00	0.00	0.00	0.00	0.00	330.00	0.00
14.99	2.39	0.00	0.00	4.24	208.55	14.12	0.02	0.03	5.65	0.34	33.67	3.05	112.96	6.52	54.31	338.89	564.81	870.00	5.76
0.00	0.00	0.00	0.00	0.00	0.00	0.00	0.00	0.00	0.00	0.00	0.00	0.00	0.00	0.00	0.00	0.00	0.00	530.00	0.00
0.00	0.00	0.00	0.00	0.00	0.00	0.00	0.00	0.00	0.00	0.00	0.00	0.00	0.00	0.00	0.00	0.00	0.00	770.00	0.00
0.00	0.00	0.00	0.00	0.00	0.00	0.00	0.00	0.00	0.00	0.00	0.00	0.00	0.00	0.00	0.00	0.00	0.00	1420.00	0.00
0.00	0.00	0.00	0.00	0.00	0.00	0.00	0.00	0.00	0.00	0.00	0.00	0.00	0.00	0.00	0.00	0.00	0.00	1350.00	0.00
0.00	0.00	0.00	0.00	0.00	0.00	0.00	0.00	0.00	0.00	0.00	0.00	0.00	0.00	0.00	0.00	0.00	0.00	980.00	0.00
0.00	0.00	0.00	0.00	0.00	0.00	0.00	0.00	0.00	0.00	0.00	0.00	0.00	0.00	0.00	0.00	0.00	0.00	810.00	0.00
0.00	0.00	0.00	0.00	0.00	0.00	0.00	0.00	0.00	0.00	0.00	0.00	0.00	0.00	0.00	0.00	0.00	0.00	870.00	0.00
0.00	0.00	0.00	0.00	0.00	0.00	0.00	0.00	0.00	0.00	0.00	0.00	0.00	0.00	0.00	0.00	0.00	0.00	640.00	0.00
0.00	0.00	0.00	0.00	0.00	0.00	0.00	0.00	0.00	0.00	0.00	0.00	0.00	0.00	0.00	0.00	0.00	0.00	810.00	0.00

USDA ID Code	Food Name	Weight in Grams*	Quantity of Units	Unit of Measure	Protein (g)	Fat (g)	Carbohydrate (g)	Kilocalories	Caffeine (g)	Fiber (g)	Cholesterol (mg)	Saturated Fat (g)
181	Chick-fil-A-Nuggets	110.0000	8.000	Each	28.00	14.00	12.00	290.00	0.00	0.00	60.00	3.00
182	Chick-fil-A-Salad, Ceasar, Chick	241.0000	1.000	Serving	33.00	10.00	5.00	240.00	0.00	2.00	90.00	7.00
184	Chick-fil-A-Salad, Garden w/ Chi	289.0000	1.000	Serving	30.00	8.00	7.00	200.00	0.00	3.00	80.00	3.00
183	Chick-fil-A-Salad, Garden w/ Chi	334.0000	1.000	Serving	32.00	17.00	21.00	370.00	0.00	4.00	113.00	6.00
185	Chick-fil-A-Soup, Chicken Breast	215.0000	1.000	Serving	16.00	1.00	10.00	110.00	0.00	1.00	45.00	0.00
	Fast Food-Beef, Roast Sandwich w	176.0000	1.000	Each	32.23	18.00	45.37	473.44	0.00	0.00	77.44	9.03
	Fast Food-Beef, Roast Sandwich,	139.0000	1.000	Each	21.50	13.76	33.44	346.11	0.00	0.00	51.43	3.60
	Fast Food-Biscuit w/ Egg	136.0000	1.000	Each	11.12	20.20	24.17	315.52	0.00	0.00	232.56	6.17
	Fast Food-Biscuit w/ Egg and Bac	150.0000	1.000	Each	17.00	31.10	28.59	457.50	0.00	0.75	352.50	7.95
	Fast Food-Biscuit w/ Egg and Ham	192.0000	1.000	Each	20.43	27.03	30.32	441.60	0.00	0.77	299.52	5.91
	Fast Food-Biscuit w/ Egg and Sau	180.0000	1.000	Each	19.15	38.70	41.15	581.40	0.00	0.90	302.40	14.98
	Fast Food-Biscuit w/ Egg, Cheese	144.0000	1.000	Each	16.26	31.39	33.42	476.64	0.00	0.00	260.64	11.40
	Fast Food-Biscuit w/ Ham	113.0000	1.000	Each	13.39	18.42	43.79	386.46	0.00	0.79	24.86	11.41
	Fast Food-Biscuit w/ Sausage	124.0000	1.000	Each	12.11	31.78	40.04	484.84	0.00	1.36	34.72	14.22
	Fast Food-Biscuit w/ Steak	141.0000	1.000	Each	13.10	25.99	44.39	455.43	0.00	0.00	25.38	6.94
	Fast Food-Biscuit, Plain	74.0000	1.000	Each	4.31	13.35	34.43	276.02	0.00	0.00	5.18	8.74
	Fast Food-Brownie	60.0000	1.000	Each	2.74	10.10	38.97	243.00	1.20	0.00	9.60	3.13
	Fast Food-Burrito w/ Beans	217.0000	2.000	Each	14.06	13.50	71.44	447.02	0.00	0.00	4.34	6.88
	Fast Food-Burrito w/ Beans and C	186.0000	2.000	Each	15.07	11.70	54.96	377.58	0.00	0.00	27.90	6.84
	Fast Food-Burrito w/ Beans and C	204.0000	2.000	Each	16.38	14.67	58.08	412.08	0.00	0.00	32.64	7.61
	Fast Food-Burrito w/ Beans and M	231.0000	2.000	Each	22.48	17.81	66.02	508.20	0.00	0.00	48.51	8.32
	Fast Food-Burrito w/ Beans, Chee	336.0000	2.000	Each	33.30	22.98	85.18	661.92	0.00	0.00	157.92	11.19
	Fast Food-Burrito w/ Beans, Chee	203.0000	2.000	Each	14.58	13.30	39.69	330.89	0.00	0.00	123.83	7.15
	Fast Food-Burrito w/ Beef	220.0000	2.000	Each	26.60	20.81	58.52	523.60	0.00	0.00	63.80	10.45
	Fast Food-Burrito w/ Beef and Ch	201.0000	2.000	Each	21.51	16.54	49.45	426.12	0.00	0.00	54.27	8.00
	Fast Food-Burrito w/ Beef, Chees	304.0000	2.000	Each	40.92	24.78	63.72	632.32	0.00	0.00	170.24	10.40
	Fast Food-Burrito w/ Fruit (Appl	74.0000	1.000	Each	2.50	9.52	34.98	230.88	0.00	0.00	3.70	4.57
	Fast Food-Cheeseburger, Large, D	258.0000	1.000	Each	37.98	43.65	39.65	704.34	0.00	0.00	141.90	17.67
	Fast Food-Cheeseburger, Large, S	185.0000	1.000	Each	30.14	32.99	47.42	608.65	0.00	0.00	96.20	14.84
	Fast Food-Cheeseburger, Large, S	195.0000	1.000	Each	32.00	36.76	37.13	608.40	0.00	0.00	111.15	16.24
	Fast Food-Cheeseburger, Large, S	219.0000	1.000	Each	28.19	32.94	38.39	562.83	0.00	0.00	87.60	15.05
	Fast Food-Cheeseburger, Regular,	228.0000	1.000	Each	29.73	35.27	53.12	649.80	0.00	0.00	93.48	12.77
	Fast Food-Cheeseburger, Regular,	102.0000	1.000	Each	14.77	15.15	31.75	319.26	0.00	0.00	49.98	6.47
	Fast Food-Cheeseburger, Regular,	154.0000	1.000	Each	17.83	19.79	28.14	358.82	0.00	0.00	52.36	9.19
	Fast Food-Cheeseburger, Triple P	304.0000	1.000	Each	56.06	50.95	26.69	796.48	0.00	0.00	161.12	21.71
	Fast Food-Chicken Fillet Sandwic	228.0000	1.000	Each	29.41	38.76	41.59	631.56	0.00	0.00	77.52	12.45
	Fast Food-Chicken Fillet Sandwic	182.0000	1.000	Each	24.12	29.45	38.69	515.06	0.00	0.00	60.06	8.54
	Fast Food-Chicken Nuggets, Plain	17.7000	1.000	Piece	3.01	3.44	2.55	53.28	0.00	0.00	10.27	0.78
	Fast Food-Chicken Nuggets, w/ Ba	130.0000	6.000	Each	17.15	17.97	25.03	330.20	0.00	0.00	61.10	5.58
	Fast Food-Chicken Nuggets, w/ Ho	115.0000	6.000	Each	16.77	17.54	26.88	328.90	0.00	0.00	60.95	5.50
	Fast Food-Chicken Nuggets, w/ Mu	130.0000	6.000	Each	17.42	18.94	20.85	322.40	0.00	0.00	61.10	5.72
	Fast Food-Chicken Nuggets, w/ Sw	130.0000	6.000	Each	16.95	17.95	28.95	345.80	0.00	0.00	61.10	5.51
	Fast Food-Chili Con Carne	253.0000	1.000	Cup	24.62	8.27	21.94	255.53	0.00	0.00	134.09	3.44
	Fast Food-Chimichanga, w/ Beef	174.0000	1.000	Each	19.61	19.68	42.80	424.56	0.00	0.00	8.70	8.51
	Fast Food-Chimichanga, w/ Beef a	183.0000	1.000	Each	20.06	23.44	39.33	442.86	0.00	0.00	51.24	11.18
	Fast Food-Clams, Breaded and Fri	115.0000	0.750	Cup	12.82	26.40	38.81	450.80	0.00	0.00	87.40	6.60
	Fast Food-Cookies, Chocolate Chi	55.0000	1.000	Box	2.89	12.14	36.22	232.65	6.05	0.00	11.55	5.34
	Fast Food-Corn On The Cob w/ But	146.0000	1.000	Each	4.47	3.43	31.94	154.76	0.00	0.00	5.84	1.65
	Fast Food-Crab, Soft-shell, Frie	125.0000	1.000	Each	10.99	17.86	31.20	333.75	0.00	0.00	45.00	4.40
	Fast Food-Croissant w/Egg and Ch	127.0000	1.000	Each	12.79	24.70	24.31	368.30	0.00	0.00	215.90	14.07
	Fast Food-Croissant w/Egg, Cheese	160.0000	1.000	Each	20.30	38.16	24.72	523.20	0.00	0.00	216.00	18.22
	Fast Food-Croissant w/Egg, Cheese	129.0000	1.000	Each	16.23	28.35	23.65	412.80	0.00	0.00	215.43	15.43
	Fast Food-Croissant w/Egg, Cheese	152.0000	1.000	Each	18.92	33.58	24.20	474.24	0.00	0.00	212.80	17.48

Page Key: A2 = Baby Food   A2 = Baked Goods   A8 = Beverages   A14 = Breads/Grains and Pasta   A18 = Breakfast Foods/Cereals   A26 = Dairy and Eggs   A40 = Fats and Oils   A42 = Fruits and Vegetables   A52 = Meats and Beans   A60 = Nuts and Seeds   A62 = Frozen Entrees and Packaged Foods   A76 = Restaurant Chains–Fast Foods   A92 = Restaurant Chains–Other   A106 = Seafood and Fish   A110 = Snacks and Sweets   A120 = Soups   A122 = Supplements   A126 = Toppings and Sauces

Monounsaturated Fat (g)	Polyunsaturated Fat (g)	Vitamin D (mg)	Vitamin K (mg)	Vitamin E (mg)	Vitamin A (re)	Vitamin C (mg)	Thiamin (mg)	Riboflavin (mg)	Niacin (mg)	Vitamin B6 (mg)	Folate (mcg)	Vitamin B12 (mcg)	Calcium (mg)	Iron (mg)	Magnesium (mg)	Phosphorus (mg)	Potassium (mg)	Sodium (mg)	Zinc (mg)
0.00	0.00	0.00	0.00	0.00	0.00	0.00	0.00	0.00	0.00	0.00	0.00	0.00	0.00	0.00	0.00	0.00	0.00	770.00	0.00
0.00	0.00	0.00	0.00	0.00	700.00	6.00	0.00	0.00	0.00	0.00	0.00	0.00	350.00	2.70	0.00	0.00	0.00	990.00	0.00
0.00	0.00	0.00	0.00	0.00	1100.00	18.00	0.00	0.00	0.00	0.00	0.00	0.00	170.00	0.90	0.00	0.00	0.00	790.00	0.00
0.00	0.00	0.00	0.00	0.00	1200.00	15.00	0.00	0.00	0.00	0.00	0.00	0.00	170.00	0.72	0.00	0.00	0.00	725.00	0.00
0.00	0.00	0.00	0.00	0.00	0.00	0.00	0.00	0.00	0.00	0.00	0.00	0.00	0.00	0.00	0.00	0.00	0.00	760.00	0.00
3.66	3.50	0.00	0.00	0.00	45.76	0.00	0.39	0.46	5.90	0.33	63.36	2.06	183.04	5.05	40.48	401.28	344.96	1633.28	5.37
6.81	1.71	0.00	0.00	0.00	20.85	2.09	0.38	0.31	5.87	0.26	56.99	1.22	54.21	4.23	30.58	239.08	315.53	792.30	3.39
8.19	4.22	0.00	0.00	0.00	178.16	0.00	0.34	0.34	0.71	0.08	61.20	0.75	153.68	3.13	20.40	184.96	160.48	654.16	1.10
13.44	7.47	0.00	0.00	2.12	52.50	2.70	0.14	0.23	2.40	0.14	60.00	1.04	189.00	3.74	24.00	238.50	250.50	999.00	1.64
10.96	7.70	0.00	0.00	2.21	240.00	0.00	0.67	0.60	2.00	0.27	65.28	1.19	220.80	4.55	30.72	316.80	318.72	1382.40	2.23
16.40	4.45	0.00	0.00	2.77	163.80	0.00	0.50	0.45	3.60	0.20	64.80	1.37	154.80	3.96	25.20	489.60	320.40	1141.20	2.16
14.23	3.50	0.00	0.00	0.00	165.60	1.58	0.30	0.43	2.30	0.10	53.28	1.05	164.16	2.55	20.16	459.36	230.40	1260.00	1.54
4.84	1.04	0.00	0.00	2.24	33.90	0.11	0.51	0.32	3.48	0.14	38.42	0.03	160.46	2.72	22.60	553.70	196.62	1432.84	1.65
12.82	3.03	0.00	0.00	3.08	13.64	0.12	0.40	0.29	3.27	0.11	45.88	0.51	127.72	2.58	19.84	446.40	198.40	1071.36	1.55
11.08	6.42	0.00	0.00	0.00	15.51	0.14	0.35	0.39	4.16	0.16	63.45	0.94	115.62	4.30	26.79	204.45	234.06	795.24	2.66
3.41	0.52	0.00	0.00	0.00	24.42	0.00	0.27	0.18	1.62	0.03	5.92	0.10	89.54	1.63	8.88	260.48	86.58	583.86	0.29
3.83	2.64	0.00	0.00	0.00	2.40	3.18	0.07	0.13	0.58	0.02	17.40	0.16	25.20	1.29	16.20	87.60	83.40	153.00	0.55
4.73	1.19	0.00	0.00	0.00	32.55	1.95	0.63	0.61	4.06	0.30	86.80	1.09	112.84	4.51	86.80	97.65	653.17	985.18	1.52
2.49	1.79	0.00	0.00	0.00	238.08	1.67	0.22	0.71	3.57	0.24	74.40	0.89	213.90	2.27	79.98	180.42	496.62	1166.22	1.64
5.37	0.96	0.00	0.00	0.00	20.40	1.22	0.45	0.71	4.39	0.29	95.88	1.16	99.96	4.55	71.40	114.24	579.36	1044.48	3.41
7.02	1.22	0.00	0.00	0.00	64.68	1.85	0.53	0.83	5.41	0.37	115.50	1.73	106.26	4.90	83.16	140.91	656.04	1335.18	3.83
8.47	1.28	0.00	0.00	0.00	383.04	6.72	0.54	1.21	7.69	0.40	164.64	1.98	288.96	7.69	97.44	285.60	809.76	2059.68	6.08
4.47	1.02	0.00	0.00	0.00	150.22	5.08	0.30	0.71	3.86	0.22	75.11	1.10	129.92	3.74	50.75	140.07	410.06	990.64	2.35
7.41	0.86	0.00	0.00	0.00	28.60	1.10	0.24	0.92	6.45	0.31	129.80	1.96	83.60	6.09	81.40	173.80	739.20	1491.60	4.73
6.07	0.98	0.00	0.00	0.00	46.23	1.61	0.40	0.80	5.09	0.30	96.48	1.29	86.43	4.44	60.30	140.70	498.48	1115.55	4.32
9.94	2.22	0.00	0.00	0.00	112.48	3.65	0.61	1.25	8.33	0.36	139.84	2.07	221.92	7.81	69.92	316.16	665.76	2091.52	7.90
3.42	1.06	0.00	0.00	0.00	37.00	0.74	0.17	0.18	1.86	0.07	24.42	0.51	15.54	1.07	7.40	14.80	104.34	211.64	0.40
17.36	4.70	0.00	0.00	0.00	54.18	1.03	0.36	0.49	7.25	0.41	74.82	3.41	239.94	5.91	51.60	394.74	595.98	1148.10	6.68
12.75	2.44	0.56	0.00	0.00	148.00	0.00	0.48	0.57	11.17	0.28	74.00	2.53	90.65	5.46	38.85	421.80	643.80	1589.15	5.55
14.49	2.71	0.00	0.00	0.00	79.95	2.15	0.31	0.41	6.63	0.31	85.80	2.34	161.85	4.74	44.85	399.75	331.50	1043.25	6.83
12.61	2.04	0.00	0.00	1.18	129.21	7.88	0.39	0.46	7.38	0.28	81.03	2.56	205.86	4.66	43.80	310.98	444.57	1108.14	4.60
12.63	6.36	0.00	0.00	1.98	84.36	2.74	0.57	0.43	8.34	0.27	91.20	2.07	168.72	4.72	36.48	348.84	389.88	921.12	4.13
5.77	1.54	0.31	0.00	0.00	36.72	0.00	0.40	0.40	3.70	0.09	54.06	0.97	140.76	2.44	21.42	195.84	164.22	499.80	2.37
7.16	1.48	0.00	0.00	0.00	70.84	2.31	0.32	0.23	6.38	0.15	64.68	1.23	181.72	2.65	26.18	215.60	229.46	976.36	2.62
21.52	3.16	0.00	0.00	0.00	85.12	2.74	0.61	0.64	11.46	0.61	69.92	5.90	282.72	8.30	60.80	541.12	820.80	1212.96	10.88
13.66	9.94	0.00	0.00	0.00	127.68	2.96	0.41	0.46	9.07	0.41	109.44	0.46	257.64	3.63	43.32	405.84	332.88	1238.04	2.90
10.41	8.39	0.00	0.00	0.00	30.94	8.92	0.33	0.24	6.81	0.20	100.10	0.38	60.06	4.68	34.58	232.96	353.08	957.32	1.87
1.75	0.77	0.00	0.00	0.23	0.00	0.00	0.02	0.03	1.25	0.05	5.13	0.05	2.30	0.16	4.07	48.32	50.98	85.67	0.17
8.76	2.39	0.00	0.00	0.00	46.80	0.78	0.10	0.16	7.02	0.34	29.90	0.30	20.80	1.46	24.70	214.50	318.50	829.40	1.12
8.61	2.22	0.00	0.00	0.00	29.90	0.46	0.09	0.15	6.81	0.31	29.90	0.30	17.25	1.32	19.55	202.40	255.30	537.05	1.08
9.04	2.91	0.00	0.00	0.00	32.50	0.39	0.12	0.16	6.94	0.31	29.90	0.31	24.70	1.48	26.00	218.40	279.50	790.40	1.14
8.65	2.24	0.00	0.00	0.00	72.80	0.78	0.10	0.20	6.86	0.33	29.90	0.36	20.80	1.48	23.40	210.60	276.90	677.30	1.09
3.42	0.53	0.00	0.00	0.00	166.98	1.52	0.13	1.14	2.48	0.33	45.54	1.14	68.31	5.19	45.54	197.34	690.69	1006.94	3.57
8.07	1.13	0.00	0.00	0.00	15.66	4.70	0.49	0.64	5.78	0.28	83.52	1.51	62.64	4.54	62.64	123.54	586.38	910.02	4.96
9.44	0.73	0.00	0.00	0.00	126.27	2.75	0.38	0.86	4.67	0.22	91.50	1.30	237.90	3.84	60.39	186.66	203.13	957.09	3.37
11.44	6.77	0.00	0.00	0.00	36.80	0.00	0.21	0.26	2.86	0.03	42.55	1.10	20.70	3.05	31.05	238.05	265.65	833.75	1.63
5.05	1.03	0.00	0.00	0.37	14.85	0.55	0.09	0.19	1.39	0.03	33.00	0.10	19.80	1.47	16.50	52.25	81.95	188.10	0.34
1.01	0.61	0.00	0.00	0.00	96.36	6.86	0.25	0.10	2.18	0.32	43.80	0.00	4.38	0.88	40.88	108.04	359.16	29.20	0.91
7.69	4.88	0.00	0.00	0.00	3.75	0.75	0.10	0.08	1.75	0.15	20.00	4.48	55.00	1.81	25.00	131.25	162.50	1117.50	1.06
7.54	1.37	0.00	0.00	0.00	255.27	0.13	0.19	0.38	1.51	0.10	46.99	0.77	243.84	2.20	21.59	347.98	173.99	551.18	1.75
14.26	3.01	0.00	0.00	0.00	108.80	0.16	0.99	0.32	4.00	0.11	43.20	0.90	144.00	3.04	24.00	289.60	283.20	1115.20	2.14
9.17	1.75	0.00	0.00	0.00	119.97	2.19	0.35	0.34	2.19	0.12	45.15	0.86	150.93	2.19	23.22	276.06	201.24	888.81	1.90
11.40	2.36	0.00	0.00	0.00	117.04	11.40	0.52	0.30	3.19	0.23	45.60	1.00	144.40	2.13	25.84	335.92	272.08	1080.72	2.17

USDA ID Code	Food Name	Weight in Grams*	Quantity of Units	Unit of Measure	Protein (g)	Fat (g)	Carbohydrate (g)	Kilocalories	Caffeine (g)	Fiber (g)	Cholesterol (mg)	Saturated Fat (g)
	Fast Food-Danish Pastry, Cheese	91.0000	1.000	Each	5.83	24.62	28.69	353.08	0.00	0.00	20.02	5.12
	Fast Food-Danish Pastry, Cinnamo	88.0000	1.000	Each	4.80	16.72	46.85	349.36	0.00	0.00	27.28	3.48
	Fast Food-Danish Pastry, Fruit	94.0000	1.000	Each	4.76	15.93	45.06	334.64	0.00	0.00	18.80	3.32
	Fast Food-Egg and Cheese Sandwic	146.0000	1.000	Each	15.61	19.42	25.93	340.18	0.00	0.00	290.54	6.63
	Fast Food-Egg, Scrambled	94.0000	2.000	Eggs	13.01	15.21	1.96	199.28	0.00	0.00	400.44	5.78
	Fast Food-Enchilada w/ Cheese	163.0000	1.000	Each	9.63	18.84	28.54	319.48	0.00	0.00	44.01	10.60
	Fast Food-Enchilada w/ Cheese an	192.0000	1.000	Each	11.92	17.64	30.47	322.56	0.00	0.00	40.32	9.04
	Fast Food-Enchirito w/ Cheese, B	193.0000	1.000	Each	17.89	16.08	33.79	343.54	0.00	0.00	50.18	7.95
	Fast Food-Fish Fillet, Battered	91.0000	1.000	Each	13.34	11.18	15.44	211.12	0.00	0.46	30.94	2.57
	Fast Food-Fish Sandwich w/ Tarta	158.0000	1.000	Each	16.94	22.77	41.02	431.34	0.00	0.00	55.30	5.23
	Fast Food-Fish Sandwich w/ Tarta	183.0000	1.000	Each	20.61	28.60	47.63	523.38	0.00	0.00	67.71	8.14
	Fast Food-French Toast w/ Butter	135.0000	2.000	Slice	10.34	18.77	36.05	356.40	0.00	0.00	116.10	7.75
	Fast Food-Frijoles w/ Cheese	167.0000	1.000	Cup	11.37	7.78	28.71	225.45	0.00	0.00	36.74	4.07
	Fast Food-Ham and Cheese Sandwich	146.0000	1.000	Each	20.69	15.48	33.35	351.86	0.00	0.00	58.40	6.44
	Fast Food-Ham, Egg, and Cheese S	143.0000	1.000	Each	19.25	16.30	30.95	347.49	0.00	0.00	245.96	7.41
	Fast Food-Hamburger, Double Patt	226.0000	1.000	Each	34.28	26.56	40.27	540.14	0.00	0.00	122.04	10.51
	Fast Food-Hamburger, Double Patt	215.0000	1.000	Each	31.82	32.47	38.74	576.20	0.00	0.00	103.20	12.00
	Fast Food-Hamburger, Double Patt	176.0000	1.000	Each	29.92	27.90	42.93	543.84	0.00	0.00	98.56	10.38
	Fast Food-Hamburger, Large, Sing	218.0000	1.000	Each	25.83	27.36	40.00	512.30	0.00	0.00	87.20	10.42
	Fast Food-Hamburger, Single Patty	106.0000	1.000	Each	12.32	9.77	34.25	272.42	0.00	2.33	29.68	3.56
	Fast Food-Hamburger, Single Patty	90.0000	1.000	Each	12.32	11.82	30.51	274.50	0.00	0.00	35.10	4.14
	Fast Food-Hamburger, Triple Patty	259.0000	1.000	Each	49.99	41.47	28.59	691.53	0.00	0.00	142.45	15.93
	Fast Food-Hot Dog w/ Chili	114.0000	1.000	Each	13.51	13.44	31.29	296.40	0.00	0.00	51.30	4.86
	Fast Food-Hot Dog w/ Corn Flour	175.0000	1.000	Each	16.80	18.90	55.79	460.25	0.00	0.00	78.75	5.16
	Fast Food-Hot Dog, Plain	98.0000	1.000	Each	10.39	14.54	18.03	242.06	0.00	0.00	44.10	5.11
	Fast Food-Ice Milk, Vanilla, Sof	103.0000	1.000	Each	3.89	6.12	24.11	163.77	0.00	0.10	27.81	3.53
	Fast Food-Muffin, English w/ But	63.0000	1.000	Each	4.87	5.76	30.36	189.00	0.00	0.00	12.60	2.43
	Fast Food-Muffin, English w/ Che	115.0000	1.000	Each	15.34	24.27	29.16	393.30	0.00	1.50	58.65	9.86
	Fast Food-Muffin, English w/ Egg	137.0000	1.000	Each	16.69	12.59	26.74	289.07	0.00	1.51	234.27	4.67
	Fast Food-Muffin, English w/ Egg	165.0000	1.000	Each	21.66	30.86	30.97	486.75	0.00	0.00	273.90	12.42
	Fast Food-Nachos w/ Cheese	113.0000	7.000	Each	9.10	18.95	36.33	345.78	0.00	0.00	18.08	7.79
	Fast Food-Nachos w/ Cheese and J	204.0000	7.000	Each	16.81	34.15	60.08	607.92	0.00	0.00	83.64	14.01
	Fast Food-Nachos w/ Cheese, Bean	255.0000	7.000	Each	19.79	30.70	55.82	568.65	0.00	0.00	20.40	12.50
	Fast Food-Nachos w/ Cinnamon and	109.0000	7.000	Each	7.19	35.98	63.39	591.87	0.00	0.00	39.24	18.21
	Fast Food-Onion Rings, Breaded a	83.0000	1.000	Order	3.70	15.51	31.32	275.56	0.00	0.00	14.11	6.96
	Fast Food-Oysters, Battered or B	139.0000	6.000	Each	12.54	17.93	39.88	368.35	0.00	0.00	108.42	4.57
	Fast Food-Pancakes w/ Butter and	232.0000	2.000	Each	8.26	13.99	90.90	519.68	0.00	0.00	58.00	5.85
	Fast Food-Pie, Fried, Fruit (App	85.0000	1.000	Each	2.41	14.37	33.05	266.05	0.00	0.00	12.75	6.51
	Fast Food-Pizza w/ Cheese	63.0000	1.000	Slice	7.68	3.21	20.50	140.49	0.00	0.00	9.45	1.54
	Fast Food-Pizza w/ Cheese, Sausa	79.0000	1.000	Slice	13.01	5.36	21.29	184.07	0.00	0.00	20.54	1.53
	Fast Food-Pizza w/ Pepperoni	71.0000	1.000	Slice	10.12	6.96	19.87	181.05	0.00	0.00	14.20	2.24
	Fast Food-Potato, Baked w/ Chees	296.0000	1.000	Piece	14.62	28.74	46.50	473.60	0.00	0.00	17.76	10.57
	Fast Food-Potato, Baked w/ Chees	299.0000	1.000	Piece	18.42	25.89	44.43	451.49	0.00	0.00	29.90	10.14
	Fast Food-Potato, Baked w/ Chees	339.0000	1.000	Piece	13.66	21.42	46.58	403.41	0.00	0.00	20.34	8.51
	Fast Food-Potato, Baked w/ Chees	395.0000	1.000	Piece	23.23	21.84	55.85	481.90	0.00	0.00	31.60	13.04
	Fast Food-Potato, Baked w/ Sour	302.0000	1.000	Piece	6.67	22.32	50.01	392.60	0.00	0.00	24.16	10.03
	Fast Food-Potato, French Fried I	115.0000	1.000	Large	4.59	18.50	44.36	358.80	0.00	0.00	20.70	8.52
	Fast Food-Potato, French Fried I	115.0000	1.000	Large	4.59	18.50	44.36	357.65	0.00	0.00	16.10	7.63
	Fast Food-Potato, French Fried I	85.0000	1.000	Small	3.66	15.67	33.84	290.70	0.00	2.98	0.00	3.27
	Fast Food-Potato, Mashed	80.0000	0.330	Cup	1.85	0.97	12.90	66.40	0.00	0.00	1.60	0.38
	Fast Food-Potatoes, Hashed Brown	72.0000	0.500	Cup	1.94	9.22	16.15	151.20	0.00	0.00	9.36	4.33
	Fast Food-Salad, w/o Dressing	104.0000	0.750	Cup	1.30	0.07	3.35	16.64	0.00	0.00	0.00	0.01
	Fast Food-Salad, w/o Dressing, w	217.0000	1.500	Cup	8.77	5.79	4.75	101.99	0.00	0.00	97.65	2.97

Page Key: A2 = Baby Food   A2 = Baked Goods   A8 = Beverages   A14 = Breads/Grains and Pasta   A18 = Breakfast Foods/Cereals   A26 = Dairy and Eggs   A40 = Fats and Oils   A42 = Fruits and Vegetables   A52 = Meats and Beans   A60 = Nuts and Seeds   A62 = Frozen Entrees and Packaged Foods   A76 = Restaurant Chains–Fast Foods   A92 = Restaurant Chains–Other   A106 = Seafood and Fish   A110 = Snacks and Sweets   A120 = Soups   A122 = Supplements   A126 = Toppings and Sauces

Monounsaturated Fat (g)	Polyunsaturated Fat (g)	Vitamin D (mg)	Vitamin K (mg)	Vitamin E (mg)	Vitamin A (re)	Vitamin C (mg)	Thiamin (mg)	Riboflavin (mg)	Niacin (mg)	Vitamin B6 (mg)	Folate (mcg)	Vitamin B12 (mg)	Calcium (mg)	Iron (mg)	Magnesium (mg)	Phosphorus (mg)	Potassium (mg)	Sodium (mg)	Zinc (mg)
15.60	2.42	0.00	0.00	0.00	42.77	2.64	0.26	0.21	2.55	0.05	54.60	0.23	70.07	1.85	15.47	80.08	116.48	319.41	0.63
10.60	1.65	0.00	0.00	0.00	5.28	2.55	0.26	0.19	2.20	0.05	54.56	0.22	36.96	1.80	14.08	73.92	95.92	326.48	0.48
10.10	1.57	0.00	0.00	0.00	24.44	1.60	0.29	0.21	1.80	0.06	31.02	0.24	21.62	1.40	14.10	68.62	109.98	332.76	0.48
8.26	2.58	0.00	0.00	0.00	181.04	1.46	0.26	0.57	2.07	0.13	97.82	1.14	224.84	2.98	21.90	302.22	188.34	804.46	1.65
5.54	1.85	1.60	0.00	1.58	251.92	3.10	0.08	0.49	0.20	0.18	52.64	0.95	53.58	2.43	13.16	227.48	138.18	210.56	1.56
6.31	0.81	0.00	0.00	0.00	185.82	0.98	0.08	0.42	1.91	0.39	65.20	0.75	324.37	1.32	50.53	133.66	239.61	784.03	2.51
6.14	1.38	0.00	0.00	0.00	142.08	1.34	0.10	0.40	2.52	0.27	67.20	1.02	228.48	3.07	82.56	167.04	574.08	1319.04	2.69
6.52	0.33	0.00	0.00	0.00	133.17	4.63	0.17	0.69	2.99	0.21	59.83	1.62	218.09	2.39	71.41	223.88	559.70	1250.64	2.76
2.35	5.71	0.00	0.00	0.00	10.92	0.00	0.10	0.10	1.91	0.09	15.47	1.01	16.38	1.92	21.84	155.61	291.20	484.12	0.40
7.69	8.25	0.00	0.00	0.87	30.02	2.84	0.33	0.22	3.40	0.11	85.32	1.07	83.74	2.61	33.18	211.72	339.70	614.62	1.00
8.91	9.42	0.92	0.00	1.83	96.99	2.75	0.46	0.42	4.23	0.11	91.50	1.08	184.83	3.50	36.60	311.10	353.19	938.79	1.17
7.07	2.44	0.00	0.00	0.00	145.80	0.14	0.58	0.50	3.92	0.05	72.90	0.36	72.90	1.89	16.20	145.80	176.85	513.00	0.59
2.62	0.70	0.00	0.00	0.00	70.14	1.50	0.13	0.33	1.49	0.20	111.89	0.68	188.71	2.24	85.17	175.35	604.54	881.76	1.74
6.75	1.37	0.00	0.00	0.29	75.92	2.77	0.31	0.48	2.69	0.20	75.92	0.54	129.94	3.24	16.06	151.84	290.54	770.88	1.37
5.75	1.69	0.00	0.00	0.59	148.72	2.72	0.43	0.56	4.20	0.16	75.79	1.23	211.64	3.10	25.74	346.06	210.21	1005.29	1.99
10.33	2.80	0.00	0.00	0.00	11.30	1.13	0.36	0.38	7.57	0.54	76.84	4.07	101.70	5.85	49.72	314.14	569.52	791.00	5.67
14.13	2.77	0.00	0.00	0.00	4.30	1.08	0.34	0.41	6.73	0.37	83.85	3.33	92.45	5.55	45.15	283.80	526.75	741.75	5.81
12.11	2.34	0.70	0.00	1.32	0.00	0.00	0.33	0.37	8.25	0.32	77.44	2.92	86.24	4.56	36.96	234.08	362.56	554.40	5.72
11.42	2.20	0.00	0.00	0.00	32.70	2.62	0.41	0.37	7.28	0.33	82.84	2.38	95.92	4.93	43.60	233.26	479.60	824.04	4.88
3.40	1.01	0.00	0.00	0.01	9.54	2.23	0.29	0.23	3.91	0.12	51.94	1.09	126.14	2.71	23.32	114.48	251.22	534.24	2.25
5.45	0.92	0.27	0.00	0.50	0.00	0.00	0.33	0.27	3.72	0.06	53.10	0.89	63.00	2.40	18.90	102.60	144.90	387.00	2.00
18.23	2.75	0.00	0.00	0.00	15.54	1.30	0.31	0.54	10.96	0.62	75.11	4.92	64.75	8.31	54.39	393.68	784.77	712.25	10.75
6.60	1.19	0.00	0.00	0.00	5.70	2.74	0.22	0.40	3.74	0.05	72.96	0.30	19.38	3.28	10.26	191.52	166.44	479.94	0.78
9.12	3.50	0.00	0.00	0.00	36.75	0.00	0.28	0.70	4.17	0.09	103.25	0.44	101.50	6.18	17.50	166.25	262.50	973.00	1.31
6.85	1.71	0.00	0.00	0.00	0.00	0.10	0.24	0.27	3.65	0.05	48.02	0.51	23.52	2.31	12.74	97.02	143.08	670.32	1.98
1.81	0.36	0.21	0.00	0.38	51.50	1.13	0.05	0.26	0.31	0.06	12.36	0.21	153.47	0.15	15.45	139.05	168.92	91.67	0.57
1.53	1.35	0.00	0.00	0.13	33.39	0.76	0.25	0.32	2.61	0.04	56.70	0.02	102.69	1.59	13.23	85.05	69.30	386.19	0.42
10.09	2.69	0.00	0.00	0.49	86.25	1.27	0.70	0.25	4.14	0.15	66.70	0.68	167.90	2.25	24.15	186.30	215.05	1036.15	1.68
4.67	1.56	1.10	0.00	0.85	156.18	1.78	0.49	0.45	3.33	0.15	43.84	0.67	150.70	2.44	23.29	269.89	198.65	728.84	1.56
12.75	3.32	0.00	0.00	0.00	171.60	1.49	0.84	0.50	4.46	0.20	54.45	1.37	196.35	3.47	29.70	287.10	293.70	1135.20	2.36
7.99	2.24	0.00	0.00	0.00	91.53	1.24	0.19	0.37	1.54	0.20	10.17	0.82	272.33	1.28	55.37	275.72	171.76	815.86	1.79
14.40	4.02	0.00	0.00	0.00	471.24	1.02	0.12	0.49	2.84	0.37	18.36	1.02	620.16	2.45	108.12	393.72	293.76	1736.04	2.90
10.99	5.69	0.00	0.00	0.00	469.20	4.85	0.23	0.69	3.34	0.41	38.25	1.02	385.05	2.78	96.90	387.60	451.35	1800.30	3.65
11.84	4.13	0.00	0.00	0.00	10.90	7.96	0.19	0.45	3.92	0.17	7.63	1.72	85.02	2.89	19.62	32.70	78.48	439.27	0.59
6.65	0.66	0.00	0.00	0.33	0.83	0.58	0.08	0.10	0.92	0.06	54.78	0.12	73.04	0.85	15.77	86.32	129.48	429.94	0.35
6.92	4.64	0.00	0.00	0.00	108.42	4.17	0.31	0.35	4.42	0.03	30.58	1.01	27.80	4.46	23.63	195.99	182.09	676.93	15.64
5.27	1.95	0.00	0.00	1.39	69.60	3.48	0.39	0.56	3.39	0.12	51.04	0.23	127.60	2.62	48.72	475.60	250.56	1104.32	1.02
5.83	1.16	0.00	0.00	0.37	33.15	1.11	0.10	0.08	0.98	0.03	4.25	0.08	12.75	0.88	7.65	37.40	51.00	324.70	0.17
0.99	0.49	0.00	0.00	0.00	73.71	1.26	0.18	0.16	2.48	0.04	34.65	0.33	116.55	0.58	15.75	112.77	109.62	335.79	0.81
2.54	0.92	0.00	0.00	0.00	101.12	1.58	0.21	0.17	1.96	0.09	32.39	0.36	101.12	1.53	18.17	131.14	178.54	382.36	1.11
3.14	1.16	0.00	0.00	0.00	54.67	1.63	0.13	0.23	3.05	0.06	36.92	0.18	64.61	0.94	8.52	75.26	152.65	266.96	0.52
10.72	6.04	0.00	0.00	0.00	227.92	26.05	0.24	0.21	3.34	0.71	26.64	0.18	310.80	3.02	65.12	319.68	1166.24	381.84	1.89
9.72	4.75	0.00	0.00	0.00	173.42	28.70	0.27	0.24	3.98	0.75	29.90	0.33	307.97	3.14	68.77	346.84	1178.06	971.75	2.15
7.70	4.17	0.00	0.00	0.00	277.98	48.48	0.27	0.27	3.59	0.78	61.02	0.34	335.61	3.32	77.97	345.78	1440.75	484.77	2.03
6.83	0.91	0.00	0.00	0.00	173.80	31.60	0.28	0.36	4.19	0.95	47.40	0.24	110.60	6.12	110.60	497.70	1572.10	699.15	3.79
7.88	3.32	0.00	0.00	0.00	277.84	33.82	0.27	0.18	3.71	0.79	33.22	0.21	105.70	3.11	69.46	184.22	1383.16	181.20	0.91
8.03	0.93	0.00	0.00	0.02	3.45	6.10	0.16	0.05	2.60	0.30	37.95	0.14	18.40	1.55	37.95	152.95	818.80	187.45	0.60
8.23	1.99	0.00	0.00	0.00	3.45	6.10	0.16	0.05	2.60	0.30	37.95	0.14	18.40	1.55	37.95	152.95	818.80	187.45	0.60
9.05	2.66	0.00	0.00	1.04	0.00	9.86	0.07	0.03	2.42	0.31	32.30	0.00	11.90	0.66	33.15	109.65	585.65	168.30	0.40
0.28	0.23	0.00	0.00	0.00	8.00	0.32	0.07	0.04	0.96	0.18	6.40	0.04	16.80	0.38	14.40	44.00	235.20	181.60	0.26
3.86	0.47	0.00	0.00	0.12	2.88	5.47	0.08	0.01	1.07	0.17	7.92	0.01	7.20	0.48	15.84	69.12	267.12	290.16	0.22
0.00	0.03	0.00	0.00	0.00	118.56	24.13	0.03	0.05	0.57	0.08	38.48	0.00	13.52	0.66	11.44	40.56	178.88	27.04	0.22
1.76	0.48	0.00	0.00	0.00	115.01	9.77	0.09	0.17	0.98	0.11	84.63	0.30	99.82	0.67	23.87	132.37	371.07	119.35	1.00

USDA ID Code	Food Name	Weight in Grams*	Quantity of Units	Unit of Measure	Protein (g)	Fat (g)	Carbohydrate (g)	Kilocalories	Caffeine (g)	Fiber (g)	Cholesterol (mg)	Saturated Fat (g)
	Fast Food-Salad, w/o Dressing, w	218.0000	1.500	Cup	17.44	2.18	3.73	104.64	0.00	0.00	71.94	0.59
	Fast Food-Salad, w/o Dressing, w	417.0000	1.500	Cup	16.43	20.85	31.98	379.47	0.00	0.00	50.04	2.59
	Fast Food-Salad, w/o Dressing, w	236.0000	1.500	Cup	14.51	2.48	6.61	106.20	0.00	0.00	179.36	0.66
	Fast Food-Scallops, Breaded and	144.0000	6.000	Each	15.75	19.40	38.49	385.92	0.00	0.00	108.00	4.88
	Fast Food-Shrimp, Breaded and Fr	164.0000	7.000	Each	18.88	24.90	40.00	454.28	0.00	0.00	200.08	5.38
	Fast Food-Steak Sandwich	204.0000	1.000	Each	30.33	14.08	51.96	459.00	0.00	0.00	73.44	3.81
	Fast Food-Submarine Sandwich w/	228.0000	1.000	Each	21.84	18.63	51.05	456.00	0.00	0.00	36.48	6.82
	Fast Food-Submarine Sandwich w/	216.0000	1.000	Each	28.64	12.96	44.30	410.40	0.00	0.00	73.44	7.08
	Fast Food-Submarine Sandwich w/	256.0000	1.000	Each	29.70	27.98	55.37	583.68	0.00	0.00	48.64	5.32
	Fast Food-Sundae, Caramel	155.0000	1.000	Each	7.30	9.27	49.31	303.80	0.00	0.00	24.80	4.51
	Fast Food-Sundae, Hot Fudge	158.0000	1.000	Each	5.64	8.63	47.67	284.40	1.58	0.00	20.54	5.02
	Fast Food-Sundae, Strawberry	153.0000	1.000	Each	6.26	7.85	44.65	267.75	0.00	0.00	21.42	3.73
	Fast Food-Taco	171.0000	1.000	Small	20.66	20.55	26.73	369.36	0.00	0.00	56.43	11.37
	Fast Food-Taco Salad	198.0000	1.500	Cup	13.23	14.77	23.58	279.18	0.00	0.00	43.56	6.83
	Fast Food-Taco Salad w/ Chili Co	261.0000	1.500	Cup	17.41	13.13	26.57	289.71	0.00	0.00	5.22	6.00
	Fast Food-Tostada w/ Guacamole	261.0000	2.000	Each	12.48	23.26	32.02	360.18	0.00	0.00	39.15	9.87
	Fast Food-Tostada, w/ Beans and	144.0000	1.000	Piece	9.60	9.86	26.52	223.20	0.00	0.00	30.24	5.37
	Fast Food-Tostada, w/ Beans, Bee	225.0000	1.000	Piece	16.09	16.94	29.66	333.00	0.00	0.00	74.25	11.48
	Fast Food-Tostada, w/ Beef and C	163.0000	1.000	Piece	18.99	16.35	22.77	314.59	0.00	0.00	40.75	10.40
	Hardee's-Beef, Roast, Big	163.0080	1.000	Each	21.90	13.38	38.93	364.94	0.00	1.09	54.74	6.08
	Hardee's-Beef, Roast, Sandwich	141.7460	1.000	Each	18.65	11.19	38.54	323.28	0.00	0.99	43.52	4.97
	Hardee's-Big Cheese	141.7500	1.000	Each	30.00	30.00	28.00	495.00	0.00	0.00	0.00	0.00
	Hardee's-Big Deluxe	248.1000	1.000	Each	31.00	41.00	46.00	675.00	0.00	0.00	0.00	0.00
	Hardee's-Big Twin	141.7460	1.000	Each	18.84	20.48	27.86	368.70	0.00	1.39	45.06	9.01
	Hardee's-Biscuit	77.9610	1.000	Each	5.00	13.00	35.00	275.00	0.00	0.00	0.00	0.00
	Hardee's-Cheeseburger	100.6310	1.000	Each	17.00	17.00	29.00	335.00	0.00	0.00	0.00	0.00
	Hardee's-Chicken Fillet	191.3580	1.000	Each	27.00	26.00	42.00	510.00	0.00	0.00	0.00	0.00
	Hardee's-Fish Sandwich, Big	191.3580	1.000	Each	20.00	26.00	49.00	514.00	0.00	0.00	0.00	0.00
	Hardee's-Ham & Cheese, Hot	141.7460	1.000	Each	23.00	15.00	37.00	376.00	0.00	0.00	0.00	0.00
	Hardee's-Hamburger	100.0630	1.000	Each	17.00	13.00	29.00	305.00	0.00	0.00	0.00	0.00
	Hardee's-Hot Dog	50.0000	1.000	Each	11.00	22.00	26.00	346.00	0.00	0.00	0.00	0.00
	Jack In The Box-Breakfast Jack	126.0000	1.000	Each	18.74	13.54	29.16	313.44	0.00	0.00	189.52	5.31
	Jack In The Box-Cheeseburger, Ba	242.0000	1.000	Each	35.00	45.00	41.00	705.00	0.00	0.00	113.00	14.90
	Jack In The Box-Cheesecake	99.0000	1.000	Each	8.00	18.00	29.00	309.00	0.00	0.00	63.00	9.40
	Jack In The Box-French Fries, Re	109.0000	1.000	Order	4.00	17.00	45.00	351.00	0.00	0.00	0.00	4.00
	Jack In The Box-French Fries, Sm	68.0000	1.000	Order	3.00	11.00	28.00	219.00	0.00	0.00	0.00	2.50
	Jack In The Box-Jumbo Jack	222.0000	1.000	Each	25.27	26.17	40.61	497.24	0.00	0.00	72.20	10.29
	Jack In The Box-Jumbo Jack w/ Ch	242.0000	1.000	Each	28.47	31.14	40.04	558.74	0.00	0.00	97.87	13.35
	K.F.C.-Breast, Center, Original	103.0000	1.000	Each	25.18	15.26	9.16	260.93	0.00	0.08	86.98	3.81
	K.F.C.-Chicken Sandwich, Colonel	166.0000	1.000	Each	20.80	27.00	39.00	482.00	0.00	1.40	47.00	6.00
	K.F.C.-Drumstick, Original Recipe	57.0000	1.000	Each	11.57	11.57	4.96	168.52	0.00	0.00	58.65	2.48
	K.F.C.-French Fries	77.0000	1.000	Order	3.20	12.00	31.00	244.00	0.00	0.00	2.00	3.00
	K.F.C.-Potatoes, Mashed, and Gra	98.0000	1.000	Each	2.40	2.00	12.00	71.00	0.00	0.00	0.00	1.00
	K.F.C.-Thigh, Original Recipe	95.0000	1.000	Each	15.97	23.95	11.18	324.12	0.00	0.08	102.98	6.39
	K.F.C.-Wing, Original Recipe	53.0000	1.000	Each	11.80	11.00	5.00	172.00	0.00	0.00	59.00	3.00
	McDonald's-Arch Deluxe	239.0000	1.000	Each	28.00	31.00	39.00	550.00	0.00	4.00	90.00	11.00
	McDonald's-Arch Deluxe w/Bacon	247.0000	1.000	Each	32.00	34.00	39.00	590.00	0.00	4.00	100.00	12.00
	McDonald's-Big Mac	215.0000	1.000	Each	25.00	32.00	43.00	560.00	0.00	0.00	103.00	10.10
	McDonald's-Biscuit w/ Spread	75.0000	1.000	Each	5.00	13.00	32.00	260.00	0.00	1.00	1.00	3.00
	McDonald's-Biscuit, Bacon, Egg a	153.0000	1.000	Each	18.00	28.00	36.00	470.00	0.00	1.00	235.00	8.04
	McDonald's-Biscuit, Sausage	118.0000	1.000	Each	11.00	31.00	35.00	470.00	0.00	0.00	44.00	8.00
	McDonald's-Biscuit, Sausage w/ E	175.0000	1.000	Each	19.00	28.00	27.00	440.00	0.00	0.00	260.00	10.00
	McDonald's-Burrito, Breakfast	117.0000	1.000	Each	13.00	19.00	23.00	320.00	0.00	1.00	195.00	7.00

Monounsaturated Fat (g)	Polyunsaturated Fat (g)	Vitamin D (mg)	Vitamin K (mg)	Vitamin E (mg)	Vitamin A (re)	Vitamin C (mg)	Thiamin (mg)	Riboflavin (mg)	Niacin (mg)	Vitamin B$_6$ (mg)	Folate (mcg)	Vitamin B$_{12}$ (mcg)	Calcium (mg)	Iron (mg)	Magnesium (mg)	Phosphorus (mg)	Potassium (mg)	Sodium (mg)	Zinc (mg)
0.68	0.57	0.00	0.00	0.00	95.92	17.44	0.11	0.13	5.89	0.44	67.58	0.20	37.06	1.09	32.70	170.04	446.90	209.28	0.89
4.84	9.09	0.00	0.00	0.00	638.01	38.36	0.29	0.21	3.54	0.33	187.65	1.71	70.89	3.17	50.04	204.33	600.48	1572.09	1.67
0.83	0.50	0.00	0.00	0.00	77.88	9.20	0.12	0.17	1.16	0.14	87.32	3.78	59.00	0.90	37.76	160.48	403.56	488.52	1.27
12.56	0.60	0.00	0.00	0.00	41.76	0.00	0.20	0.85	0.00	0.07	53.28	0.43	18.72	2.04	31.68	292.32	293.76	918.72	1.08
17.38	0.64	0.00	0.00	0.00	36.08	0.00	0.21	0.90	0.00	0.07	36.08	0.15	83.64	2.95	39.36	344.40	183.68	1446.48	1.21
5.34	3.35	0.00	0.00	0.00	44.88	5.51	0.41	0.37	7.30	0.37	89.76	1.57	91.80	5.16	48.96	297.84	524.28	797.64	4.53
8.23	2.28	0.00	0.00	0.00	79.80	12.31	1.00	0.80	5.49	0.14	86.64	1.09	189.24	2.51	68.40	287.28	394.44	1650.72	2.58
1.84	2.61	0.00	0.00	0.00	49.68	5.62	0.41	0.41	5.96	0.32	71.28	1.81	41.04	2.81	66.96	192.24	330.48	844.56	4.38
13.41	7.30	0.00	0.00	0.00	40.96	3.58	0.46	0.33	11.34	0.23	102.40	1.61	74.24	2.64	79.36	220.16	335.36	1292.80	1.87
3.04	1.01	0.31	0.00	0.90	68.20	3.41	0.06	0.29	0.95	0.05	12.40	0.60	189.10	0.22	27.90	217.00	317.75	195.30	0.82
2.34	0.81	0.47	0.00	0.66	56.88	2.37	0.06	0.30	1.07	0.13	9.48	0.65	206.98	0.58	33.18	227.52	395.00	181.70	0.95
2.66	1.03	0.46	0.00	0.78	58.14	1.99	0.06	0.28	0.90	0.08	18.36	0.64	160.65	0.32	24.48	154.53	270.81	91.80	0.66
6.58	0.96	0.00	0.00	0.00	147.06	2.22	0.15	0.44	3.21	0.24	68.40	1.04	220.59	2.41	70.11	203.49	473.67	801.99	3.93
5.17	1.74	0.00	0.00	0.00	77.22	3.56	0.10	0.36	2.46	0.22	83.16	0.63	192.06	2.28	51.48	142.56	415.80	762.30	2.69
4.54	1.54	0.00	0.00	0.00	214.02	3.39	0.16	0.50	2.53	0.52	91.35	0.73	245.34	2.66	52.20	153.99	391.50	884.79	3.29
8.48	3.05	0.00	0.00	0.00	216.63	3.65	0.13	0.57	1.98	0.26	114.84	0.99	422.82	1.62	73.08	232.29	649.89	798.66	4.07
3.05	0.75	0.00	0.00	0.00	84.96	1.30	0.10	0.33	1.32	0.16	43.20	0.69	210.24	1.89	59.04	116.64	403.20	542.88	1.90
3.51	0.61	0.00	0.00	0.00	173.25	4.05	0.09	0.50	2.86	0.25	85.50	1.13	189.00	2.45	67.50	173.25	490.50	870.75	3.17
3.34	0.98	0.00	0.00	0.00	96.17	2.61	0.10	0.55	3.15	0.23	74.98	1.17	216.79	2.87	63.57	179.30	572.13	896.50	3.68
6.08	2.43	0.00	0.00	0.24	0.00	0.00	0.36	0.41	6.57	0.34	29.20	2.98	80.29	4.50	40.14	279.79	389.27	1070.50	7.42
4.97	2.49	0.00	0.00	0.25	0.00	0.00	0.32	0.36	5.72	0.30	24.87	2.60	69.63	3.85	34.81	243.70	323.28	907.67	6.47
0.00	0.00	0.00	0.00	0.00	0.00	0.00	0.00	0.00	0.00	0.00	0.00	0.00	0.00	0.00	0.00	0.00	0.00	1251.00	0.00
0.00	0.00	0.00	0.00	0.00	0.00	0.00	0.00	0.00	0.00	0.00	0.00	0.00	0.00	0.00	0.00	0.00	0.00	1063.00	0.00
7.37	4.10	0.00	0.00	0.74	13.93	2.46	0.23	0.25	5.49	0.22	27.86	1.86	65.55	3.28	28.68	161.41	229.42	475.22	3.77
0.00	0.00	0.00	0.00	0.00	0.00	0.00	0.00	0.00	0.00	0.00	0.00	0.00	0.00	0.00	0.00	0.00	0.00	650.00	0.00
0.00	0.00	0.00	0.00	0.00	0.00	2.00	0.51	0.32	5.50	0.00	0.00	0.00	0.00	0.00	0.00	0.00	0.00	789.00	0.00
0.00	0.00	0.00	0.00	0.00	0.00	0.00	0.00	0.00	0.00	0.00	0.00	0.00	0.00	0.00	0.00	0.00	0.00	360.00	0.00
0.00	0.00	0.00	0.00	0.00	0.00	0.00	0.00	0.00	0.00	0.00	0.00	0.00	0.00	0.00	0.00	0.00	0.00	314.00	0.00
0.00	0.00	0.00	0.00	0.00	0.00	0.00	0.00	0.00	0.00	0.00	0.00	0.00	0.00	0.00	0.00	0.00	0.00	1067.00	0.00
0.00	0.00	0.00	0.00	0.00	0.00	2.00	0.55	0.58	6.40	0.00	0.00	0.00	0.00	0.00	0.00	0.00	0.00	682.00	0.00
0.00	0.00	0.00	0.00	0.00	0.00	0.00	0.00	0.00	0.00	0.00	0.00	0.00	0.00	0.00	0.00	0.00	0.00	744.00	0.00
5.21	2.60	0.00	0.00	0.14	138.50	3.12	0.43	0.49	5.31	0.15	0.00	1.15	184.31	2.60	24.99	322.81	197.85	1079.85	1.87
15.70	8.70	0.00	0.00	0.60	70.00	7.80	0.24	0.48	8.36	0.00	0.00	0.00	200.00	2.80	0.00	0.00	0.00	1240.00	0.00
7.40	1.60	0.00	0.00	0.32	0.00	0.00	0.05	0.24	1.90	0.00	0.00	0.00	88.00	0.30	0.00	0.00	0.00	208.00	0.00
7.00	0.00	0.00	0.00	5.31	0.00	25.80	0.18	0.03	3.61	0.00	0.00	0.00	0.00	0.70	0.00	0.00	0.00	194.00	0.00
7.00	0.00	0.00	0.00	10.36	0.00	16.20	0.11	0.00	2.28	0.00	0.00	0.00	0.00	0.40	0.00	0.00	0.00	121.00	0.00
11.37	2.17	0.00	0.00	0.18	66.78	3.61	0.42	0.31	10.47	0.27	0.00	2.42	120.93	4.06	39.71	235.54	444.00	1023.37	3.79
11.21	1.78	0.00	0.00	0.21	195.74	4.45	0.46	0.34	10.05	0.28	0.00	2.71	242.89	4.09	43.60	365.67	443.96	1482.25	4.27
3.59	1.53	0.00	0.00	0.46	15.26	0.00	0.08	0.13	14.04	0.59	3.81	0.35	16.02	1.22	30.52	238.04	264.75	602.74	1.14
3.90	9.00	0.00	0.00	2.30	14.00	0.00	0.39	0.27	10.64	0.59	29.00	0.31	100.00	3.10	41.00	261.00	297.00	1060.00	1.50
3.06	1.65	0.00	0.00	0.41	14.04	0.00	0.05	0.13	3.39	0.20	4.96	0.18	6.61	0.74	13.22	99.13	129.70	267.65	1.65
7.00	1.00	0.00	0.00	0.00	0.00	15.60	0.15	0.05	1.90	0.00	0.00	0.00	0.00	0.30	0.00	0.00	0.00	139.00	0.00
0.00	0.00	0.00	0.00	0.00	0.00	0.00	0.00	0.03	1.14	0.00	0.00	0.00	16.00	0.20	0.00	0.00	0.00	339.00	0.00
5.59	3.19	0.00	0.00	0.48	27.94	0.00	0.09	0.23	6.55	0.32	7.98	0.29	12.77	1.44	23.15	176.43	223.53	549.24	2.39
6.00	2.00	0.00	0.00	0.00	0.00	0.00	0.03	0.07	2.85	0.00	0.00	0.00	24.00	0.30	0.00	0.00	0.00	383.00	0.00
0.00	0.00	0.00	0.00	0.00	10.00	38.00	0.00	0.00	0.00	0.00	0.00	0.00	6.00	25.00	0.00	0.00	0.00	1010.00	0.00
0.00	0.00	0.00	0.00	0.00	10.00	0.00	0.00	0.00	0.00	0.00	0.00	0.00	6.00	6.00	0.00	0.00	0.00	1150.00	0.00
20.10	1.50	0.00	0.00	0.00	106.00	2.00	0.48	0.41	6.80	0.27	21.00	1.80	256.00	4.00	38.00	314.00	237.00	950.00	4.70
9.00	1.00	0.00	0.00	1.80	0.00	0.00	0.23	0.10	1.52	0.03	6.00	0.10	75.00	1.30	14.00	168.00	100.00	730.00	0.70
15.79	1.96	0.00	0.00	1.47	156.92	0.00	0.35	0.32	2.45	0.17	17.65	0.58	181.44	2.55	30.40	442.33	232.44	1250.00	1.67
17.00	3.00	0.00	0.00	0.00	0.00	0.00	0.45	0.17	3.80	0.00	0.00	0.00	64.00	1.00	0.00	0.00	0.00	1080.00	0.00
20.00	3.00	0.00	0.00	0.00	60.00	0.00	0.45	0.34	3.80	0.00	0.00	0.00	80.00	2.00	0.00	0.00	0.00	1210.00	0.00
0.00	0.00	0.00	0.00	0.00	10.00	15.00	0.00	0.00	0.00	0.00	0.00	0.00	8.00	10.00	0.00	0.00	0.00	600.00	0.00

USDA ID Code	Food Name	Weight in Grams*	Quantity of Units	Unit of Measure	Protein (g)	Fat (g)	Carbohydrate (g)	Kilocalories	Caffeine (g)	Fiber (g)	Cholesterol (mg)	Saturated Fat (g)
	McDonald's-Cheeseburger	116.0000	1.000	Each	15.00	13.00	35.00	320.00	0.00	0.00	50.00	5.00
	McDonald's-Chicken McNuggets	18.5000	1.000	Each	3.33	2.50	2.83	45.00	0.00	0.00	9.17	0.58
	McDonald's-Chicken Sld, Grilled,	257.0000	1.000	Each	21.00	1.50	7.00	120.00	0.00	0.00	45.00	0.00
	McDonald's-Chicken, Crispy, Delu	223.0000	1.000	Each	26.00	25.00	43.00	0.00	0.00	3.00	55.00	4.00
	McDonald's-Chicken, Grilled, Del	223.0000	1.000	Each	27.00	20.00	38.00	300.00	0.00	3.00	50.00	1.00
	McDonald's-Cookies, McDonaldland	56.6990	1.000	Each	3.00	5.00	32.00	180.00	0.00	0.00	0.00	1.00
	McDonald's-Danish, Apple	105.0000	1.000	Each	5.00	16.00	51.00	360.00	0.00	1.60	25.00	4.00
	McDonald's-Danish, Cheese, Iced	110.0000	1.000	Each	7.00	22.00	47.00	410.00	0.00	0.00	47.00	6.00
	McDonald's-Eggs, Scrambled	100.0000	1.000	Each	12.00	10.00	1.00	140.00	0.00	0.00	425.00	3.00
	McDonald's-Fish Filet Deluxe	141.0000	1.000	Each	27.00	28.00	54.00	560.00	0.00	1.09	49.65	5.16
	McDonald's-French Fries, Large	122.0000	1.000	Order	6.00	22.00	57.00	450.00	0.00	0.00	0.00	5.00
	McDonald's-French Fries, Small	68.0000	1.000	Order	3.00	12.00	26.00	220.00	0.00	0.00	0.00	2.50
	McDonald's-French Fries, Super S	176.0000	1.000	Order	8.00	26.00	68.00	540.00	0.00	6.00	0.00	4.50
	McDonald's-Hamburger	102.0000	1.000	Each	13.00	9.00	34.00	260.00	0.00	0.00	30.00	3.50
	McDonald's-Hotcakes w/ Margarine	174.0000	1.000	Each	13.00	19.00	100.00	570.00	0.00	0.00	15.00	3.00
	McDonald's-Ice Crm Cone, Vanilla	90.0000	1.000	Each	4.00	4.50	23.00	150.00	0.00	0.00	20.00	3.00
	McDonald's-McMuffin, Egg	135.0000	1.000	Each	17.61	10.76	27.39	283.70	0.00	1.37	221.09	3.72
	McDonald's-McMuffin, Sausage	135.0000	1.000	Each	15.00	20.00	27.00	345.00	0.00	0.00	57.00	7.00
	McDonald's-McMuffin, Sausage w/	159.0000	1.000	Each	21.00	25.00	27.00	430.00	0.00	0.00	270.00	8.00
	McDonald's-Muffin, Apple Bran, L	114.0000	1.000	Each	6.00	3.00	61.00	300.00	0.00	3.00	0.00	0.50
	McDonald's-Muffin, English w/ Sp	58.0000	1.000	Each	5.00	4.00	26.00	170.00	0.00	1.60	9.00	2.40
	McDonald's-Potatoes, Hash Brown	53.0000	1.000	Each	1.00	7.00	15.00	130.00	0.00	0.00	0.00	1.00
	McDonald's-Quarter Pounder	166.0000	1.000	Each	23.00	21.00	37.00	420.00	0.00	0.00	85.00	8.00
	McDonald's-Quarter Pounder w/ Ch	200.0000	1.000	Each	28.00	30.00	38.00	530.00	0.00	2.00	95.00	13.00
	McDonald's-Salad, Garden	189.0000	1.000	Each	4.00	2.00	6.00	50.00	0.00	0.00	65.00	0.60
	McDonald's-Shake, Chocolate Lowf	294.1240	1.000	Each	11.04	1.71	66.25	321.23	0.00	0.00	10.04	0.70
	McDonald's-Shake, Strawberry Low	294.1240	1.000	Each	11.00	9.00	60.00	360.00	0.00	0.00	10.00	0.60
	McDonald's-Shake, Vanilla Lowfat	294.1240	1.000	Each	11.00	9.00	60.00	360.00	0.00	0.00	10.00	0.60
	McDonald's-Sweet Roll, Cinnamon	95.0000	1.000	Each	7.00	20.00	47.00	400.00	0.00	2.00	75.00	5.00
	Subway-BLT-6″ white	191.0000	1.000	Each	14.00	10.00	38.00	311.00	0.00	3.00	16.00	3.00
	Subway-BMT-6″ Italian	213.0000	1.000	Each	44.00	55.00	83.00	982.00	0.00	5.00	133.00	20.00
	Subway-BMT-6″ Wheat	253.0000	1.000	Each	21.00	22.00	45.00	460.00	0.00	3.00	56.00	7.00
	Subway-BMT-Classic Italian-6″	246.0000	1.000	Each	21.00	21.00	39.00	445.00	0.00	3.00	56.00	8.00
	Subway-Bologna-Deli Sandwich	171.0000	1.000	Each	10.00	12.00	38.00	292.00	0.00	2.00	20.00	4.00
	Subway-Chicken Breast, Roasted	246.0000	1.000	Each	26.00	6.00	41.00	332.00	0.00	3.00	48.00	1.00
	Subway-Chicken Taco Sub-6″ whi	286.0000	1.000	Each	24.00	16.00	43.00	421.00	0.00	3.00	52.00	5.00
	Subway-Club-6″ white	246.0000	1.000	Each	21.00	5.00	40.00	297.00	0.00	3.00	26.00	1.00
	Subway-Club Sandwich-12″ Itali	213.0000	1.000	Each	46.00	22.00	83.00	693.00	0.00	5.00	84.00	7.00
	Subway-Club Sandwich-12″ Wheat	220.0000	1.000	Each	47.00	23.00	89.00	722.00	0.00	6.00	84.00	7.00
	Subway-Cold Cut Combo-12″ Ital	184.0000	1.000	Each	46.00	40.00	83.00	853.00	0.00	5.00	166.00	12.00
	Subway-Cold Cut Combo-12″ Whea	184.0000	1.000	Each	48.00	41.00	88.00	853.00	0.00	6.00	166.00	12.00
	Subway-Cold Cut Trio-6″ white	246.0000	1.000	Each	19.00	13.00	39.00	362.00	0.00	3.00	64.00	4.00
	Subway-Ham-6″ white	232.0000	1.000	Each	18.00	5.00	39.00	287.00	0.00	3.00	28.00	1.00
	Subway-Ham-Deli Sandwich	171.0000	1.000	Each	11.00	4.00	37.00	234.00	0.00	2.00	14.00	1.00
	Subway-Ham and Cheese-12″ Ital	184.0000	1.000	Each	38.00	18.00	81.00	643.00	0.00	5.00	73.00	7.00
	Subway-Ham and Cheese Combo-12	239.0000	1.000	Each	19.00	5.00	45.00	302.00	0.00	3.00	28.00	1.00
	Subway-Italian, Spicy-12″ Ital	213.0000	1.000	Each	42.00	63.00	83.00	1043.00	0.00	5.00	137.00	23.00
	Subway-Italian, Spicy-6″ white	232.0000	1.000	Each	20.00	24.00	38.00	467.00	0.00	3.00	57.00	9.00
	Subway-Meal Ball Sandwich-12″	215.0000	1.000	Each	42.00	44.00	96.00	918.00	0.00	3.00	88.00	17.00
	Subway-Meat Ball Sandwich-12″	224.0000	1.000	Each	44.00	45.00	101.00	947.00	0.00	0.00	88.00	17.00
	Subway-Meatballs-6″ white	260.0000	1.000	Each	18.00	16.00	44.00	404.00	0.00	3.00	33.00	6.00
	Subway-Melt-6″ white	251.0000	1.000	Each	22.00	12.00	40.00	366.00	0.00	3.00	42.00	5.00
	Subway-Pizza Sub-6 white	250.0000	1.000	Each	19.00	22.00	41.00	448.00	0.00	3.00	50.00	9.00

Page Key: A2 = Baby Food   A2 = Baked Goods   A8 = Beverages   A14 = Breads/Grains and Pasta   A18 = Breakfast Foods/Cereals   A26 = Dairy and Eggs   A40 = Fats and Oils   A42 = Fruits and Vegetables   A52 = Meats and Beans   A60 = Nuts and Seeds   A62 = Frozen Entrees and Packaged Foods   A76 = Restaurant Chains–Fast Foods   A92 = Restaurant Chains–Other   A106 = Seafood and Fish   A110 = Snacks and Sweets   A120 = Soups   A122 = Supplements   A126 = Toppings and Sauces

Monounsaturated Fat (g)	Polyunsaturated Fat (g)	Vitamin D (mg)	Vitamin K (mg)	Vitamin E (mg)	Vitamin A (re)	Vitamin C (mg)	Thiamin (mg)	Riboflavin (mg)	Niacin (mg)	Vitamin B6 (mg)	Folate (mcg)	Vitamin B12 (mcg)	Calcium (mg)	Iron (mg)	Magnesium (mg)	Phosphorus (mg)	Potassium (mg)	Sodium (mg)	Zinc (mg)
7.70	1.00	0.00	0.00	0.50	118.00	2.00	0.29	0.21	3.90	0.12	18.00	0.94	199.00	2.30	21.00	177.00	223.00	750.00	2.10
1.67	0.25	0.00	0.00	0.00	0.00	0.00	0.02	0.02	1.27	0.00	0.00	0.00	0.00	0.10	0.00	0.00	0.00	96.67	0.00
0.00	0.00	0.00	0.00	0.00	120.00	40.00	0.00	0.00	0.00	0.00	0.00	0.00	4.00	8.00	0.00	0.00	0.00	240.00	0.00
0.00	0.00	0.00	0.00	0.00	6.00	8.00	0.00	0.00	0.00	0.00	0.00	0.00	6.00	15.00	0.00	0.00	0.00	1060.00	0.00
0.00	0.00	0.00	0.00	0.00	6.00	8.00	0.00	0.00	0.00	0.00	0.00	0.00	6.00	15.00	0.00	0.00	0.00	930.00	0.00
7.00	1.00	0.00	0.00	0.00	0.00	0.00	0.23	0.17	1.90	0.00	0.00	0.00	0.00	1.00	0.00	0.00	0.00	190.00	0.00
11.00	2.00	0.00	0.00	3.80	35.00	15.00	0.30	0.17	2.20	0.03	3.00	0.00	14.00	1.40	8.00	31.00	69.00	290.00	0.20
13.00	2.00	0.00	0.00	0.00	40.00	0.00	0.30	0.26	1.90	0.00	0.00	0.00	32.00	0.80	0.00	0.00	0.00	420.00	0.00
5.00	2.00	0.00	0.00	0.00	100.00	0.00	0.06	0.26	0.00	0.00	0.00	0.00	48.00	1.00	0.00	0.00	0.00	290.00	0.00
10.13	10.72	0.00	0.00	0.00	43.69	0.00	0.30	0.14	2.68	0.10	19.86	0.81	163.84	1.79	26.81	227.39	148.94	1060.00	0.89
15.00	2.00	0.00	0.00	0.00	0.00	15.00	0.23	0.00	2.85	0.00	0.00	0.00	0.00	0.60	0.00	0.00	0.00	290.00	0.00
8.00	1.00	0.00	0.00	0.00	0.00	9.00	0.15	0.00	1.90	0.00	0.00	0.00	0.00	0.20	0.00	0.00	0.00	110.00	0.00
0.00	0.00	0.00	0.00	0.00	0.00	0.00	0.00	0.00	0.00	0.00	0.00	0.00	35.00	8.00	0.00	0.00	0.00	350.00	0.00
5.00	1.00	0.00	0.00	0.00	40.00	4.00	0.30	0.17	3.80	0.00	0.00	0.00	15.00	1.50	0.00	0.00	0.00	580.00	0.00
5.00	5.00	0.00	0.00	0.00	40.00	0.00	0.30	0.34	2.85	0.00	0.00	0.00	80.00	1.00	0.00	0.00	0.00	750.00	0.00
0.00	0.00	0.00	0.00	0.00	6.00	2.00	0.00	0.00	0.00	0.00	0.00	0.00	10.00	2.00	0.00	0.00	0.00	75.00	0.00
5.97	1.27	0.00	0.00	1.76	146.74	0.98	0.46	0.32	3.62	0.16	43.04	0.78	250.43	2.74	32.28	312.07	208.37	723.91	1.76
11.00	2.00	0.00	0.00	0.00	40.00	0.00	0.53	0.26	4.75	0.00	0.00	0.00	160.00	1.50	0.00	0.00	0.00	770.00	0.00
14.00	3.00	0.00	0.00	0.00	100.00	0.00	0.53	0.43	4.75	0.00	0.00	0.00	200.00	2.00	0.00	0.00	0.00	920.00	0.00
0.00	0.00	0.00	0.00	0.00	0.00	0.00	0.00	0.00	0.00	0.00	0.00	0.00	10.00	8.00	0.00	0.00	0.00	380.00	0.00
2.00	1.00	0.00	0.00	0.10	37.00	0.00	0.33	0.14	2.50	0.10	51.00	0.00	151.00	1.60	12.00	60.00	74.00	285.00	0.40
4.00	2.00	0.00	0.00	0.00	0.00	1.20	0.06	0.00	0.76	0.00	0.00	0.00	0.00	0.00	0.00	0.00	0.00	330.00	0.00
11.00	1.00	0.00	0.00	0.00	40.00	3.60	0.38	0.26	6.65	0.00	0.00	0.00	120.00	2.00	0.00	0.00	0.00	645.00	0.00
0.00	0.00	0.00	0.00	0.00	10.00	4.00	0.00	0.00	0.00	0.00	0.00	0.00	15.00	25.00	0.00	0.00	0.00	1290.00	0.00
1.00	0.40	0.00	0.00	0.00	900.00	21.00	0.09	0.10	0.38	0.00	0.00	0.00	32.00	0.80	0.00	0.00	0.00	70.00	0.00
0.90	0.10	0.00	0.00	0.00	92.35	0.00	0.13	0.50	0.40	0.00	0.00	0.00	333.27	0.80	0.00	0.00	0.00	240.92	0.00
0.60	0.10	0.00	0.00	0.00	60.00	0.00	0.12	0.51	0.38	0.00	0.00	0.00	280.00	0.00	0.00	0.00	0.00	170.00	0.00
0.60	0.10	0.00	0.00	0.00	60.00	0.00	0.12	0.51	0.00	0.00	0.00	0.00	280.00	0.00	0.00	0.00	0.00	170.00	0.00
0.00	0.00	0.00	0.00	0.00	10.00	0.00	0.00	0.00	0.00	0.00	0.00	0.00	8.00	8.00	0.00	0.00	0.00	340.00	0.00
0.00	0.00	0.00	0.00	0.00	601.00	15.00	0.00	0.00	0.00	0.00	0.00	0.00	27.00	3.00	0.00	0.00	0.00	945.00	0.00
24.00	7.00	0.00	0.00	5.10	67.00	5.00	0.27	0.34	5.10	0.48	63.00	2.33	64.00	4.30	66.00	308.00	917.00	3139.00	6.10
25.00	7.00	0.00	0.00	0.00	753.00	15.00	0.00	0.00	0.00	0.00	0.00	0.00	44.00	4.00	0.00	0.00	1002.00	3199.00	0.00
0.00	0.00	0.00	0.00	0.00	753.00	15.00	0.00	0.00	0.00	0.00	0.00	0.00	44.00	4.00	0.00	0.00	0.00	1652.00	0.00
0.00	0.00	0.00	0.00	0.00	565.00	14.00	0.00	0.00	0.00	0.00	0.00	0.00	39.00	3.00	0.00	0.00	0.00	744.00	0.00
0.00	0.00	0.00	0.00	0.00	617.00	15.00	0.00	0.00	0.00	0.00	0.00	0.00	35.00	3.00	0.00	0.00	0.00	967.00	0.00
0.00	0.00	0.00	0.00	0.00	1044.00	18.00	0.00	0.00	0.00	0.00	0.00	0.00	118.00	4.00	0.00	0.00	0.00	1264.00	0.00
0.00	0.00	0.00	0.00	0.00	601.00	15.00	0.00	0.00	0.00	0.00	0.00	0.00	29.00	4.00	0.00	0.00	0.00	1341.00	0.00
8.00	4.00	0.00	0.00	1.30	74.00	20.00	0.48	0.33	12.50	0.58	47.00	0.95	58.00	3.10	66.00	384.00	971.00	2717.00	2.50
9.00	4.00	0.00	0.00	4.20	83.00	15.00	0.49	0.35	9.30	0.46	43.00	0.44	96.00	3.20	40.00	247.00	1055.00	2777.00	1.40
15.00	10.00	0.00	0.00	0.90	87.00	17.00	0.36	0.33	3.80	0.20	39.00	1.23	227.00	2.90	28.00	315.00	876.00	2218.00	2.70
15.00	10.00	0.00	0.00	0.90	90.00	18.00	0.37	0.35	3.90	0.21	41.00	1.28	235.00	3.00	29.00	327.00	1010.00	2278.00	2.80
0.00	0.00	0.00	0.00	0.00	649.00	16.00	0.00	0.00	0.00	0.00	0.00	0.00	49.00	4.00	0.00	0.00	0.00	1401.00	0.00
0.00	0.00	0.00	0.00	0.00	601.00	15.00	0.00	0.00	0.00	0.00	0.00	0.00	28.00	3.00	0.00	0.00	0.00	1308.00	0.00
0.00	0.00	0.00	0.00	0.00	565.00	14.00	0.00	0.00	0.00	0.00	0.00	0.00	24.00	3.00	0.00	0.00	0.00	773.00	0.00
8.00	4.00	0.00	0.00	3.80	174.00	17.00	0.53	0.39	3.60	0.34	45.00	0.76	304.00	2.20	50.00	527.00	834.00	1710.00	2.80
8.00	4.00	0.00	0.00	0.00	0.00	0.00	0.00	0.00	0.00	0.00	0.00	0.00	35.00	3.00	0.00	0.00	918.00	1319.00	0.00
28.00	7.00	0.00	0.00	0.00	0.00	0.00	0.00	0.00	0.00	0.00	0.00	0.00	0.00	0.00	0.00	0.00	880.00	2282.00	0.00
0.00	0.00	0.00	0.00	0.00	845.00	15.00	0.00	0.00	0.00	0.00	0.00	0.00	40.00	4.00	0.00	0.00	0.00	1592.00	0.00
17.00	4.00	0.00	0.00	1.00	72.00	19.00	0.33	0.39	9.40	0.40	35.00	3.21	78.00	5.00	47.00	263.00	1210.00	2022.00	6.20
18.00	4.00	0.00	0.00	0.00	0.00	0.00	0.00	0.00	0.00	0.00	0.00	0.00	0.00	0.00	0.00	0.00	1498.00	2082.00	0.00
0.00	0.00	0.00	0.00	0.00	712.00	16.00	0.00	0.00	0.00	0.00	0.00	0.00	32.00	4.00	0.00	0.00	0.00	1035.00	0.00
0.00	0.00	0.00	0.00	0.00	777.00	15.00	0.00	0.00	0.00	0.00	0.00	0.00	93.00	4.00	0.00	0.00	0.00	1735.00	0.00
0.00	0.00	0.00	0.00	0.00	1190.00	16.00	0.00	0.00	0.00	0.00	0.00	0.00	103.00	4.00	0.00	0.00	0.00	1609.00	0.00

USDA ID Code	Food Name	Weight in Grams*	Quantity of Units	Unit of Measure	Protein (g)	Fat (g)	Carbohydrate (g)	Kilocalories	Caffeine (g)	Fiber (g)	Cholesterol (mg)	Saturated Fat (g)
	Subway-Roast Beef-12″ Italian	184.0000	1.000	Each	42.00	23.00	84.00	689.00	0.00	5.00	83.00	8.00
	Subway-Roast Beef-12″ Wheat	189.0000	1.000	Each	41.00	24.00	89.00	717.00	0.00	6.00	75.00	8.00
	Subway-Roast Beef-6″ white	232.0000	1.000	Each	19.00	5.00	39.00	288.00	0.00	3.00	20.00	1.00
	Subway-Roast Beef-Deli Sandwich	180.0000	1.000	Each	13.00	4.00	38.00	245.00	0.00	2.00	13.00	1.00
	Subway-Salad, Club	331.0000	1.000	Each	14.00	3.00	12.00	126.00	0.00	1.00	26.00	1.00
	Subway-Salad, Cold Cut Trio	330.0000	1.000	Each	13.00	11.00	11.00	191.00	0.00	1.00	64.00	3.00
	Subway-Salad, Roast Beef	316.0000	1.000	Each	12.00	3.00	11.00	117.00	0.00	1.00	20.00	1.00
	Subway-Salad, Seafood & Crab	331.0000	1.000	Each	13.00	17.00	10.00	244.00	0.00	2.00	34.00	3.00
	Subway-Salad, Turkey Breast	316.0000	1.000	Each	11.00	2.00	12.00	316.00	0.00	1.00	19.00	1.00
	Subway-Salad, Veggie Delite	260.0000	1.000	Each	2.00	1.00	10.00	51.00	0.00	1.00	0.00	0.00
	Subway-Seafood-12″ Italian	210.0000	1.000	Each	29.00	57.00	94.00	986.00	0.00	5.00	56.00	11.00
	Subway-Seafood-12″ Wheat	219.0000	1.000	Each	31.00	58.00	100.00	1015.00	0.00	2.50	56.00	11.00
	Subway-Seafood & Crab-6″ white	246.0000	1.000	Each	19.00	19.00	38.00	415.00	0.00	3.00	34.00	3.00
	Subway-Steak & Cheese-6″ white	257.0000	1.000	Each	29.00	10.00	41.00	383.00	0.00	3.00	70.00	6.00
	Subway-Steak and Cheese-12″ It	213.0000	1.000	Each	43.00	32.00	83.00	765.00	0.00	6.00	82.00	12.00
	Subway-Tuna-6″ white	246.0000	1.000	Each	18.00	32.00	38.00	527.00	0.00	3.00	36.00	5.00
	Subway-Tuna-Deli Sandwich, lit	178.0000	1.000	Each	11.00	9.00	38.00	279.00	0.00	2.00	16.00	2.00
	Subway-Turkey Breast-12″ Wheat	192.0000	1.000	Each	42.00	20.00	88.00	674.00	0.00	7.00	67.00	6.00
	Subway-Turkey Breast-6″ white	232.0000	1.000	Each	17.00	4.00	40.00	273.00	0.00	3.00	19.00	1.00
	Subway-Turkey Breast-Deli sand	180.0000	1.000	Each	12.00	4.00	38.00	235.00	0.00	2.00	12.00	1.00
	Subway-Turkey Breast & Ham-6″	232.0000	1.000	Each	18.00	5.00	39.00	280.00	0.00	3.00	24.00	1.00
	Subway-Veggie Delight-6″ white	175.0000	1.000	Each	9.00	3.00	38.00	222.00	0.00	3.00	0.00	0.00
	Subway-Veggie Delite-6″ wheat	182.0000	1.000	Each	9.00	4.00	44.00	237.00	0.00	3.00	0.00	0.00
	Taco Bell-Burrito Supreme	198.0000	1.000	Each	20.00	22.00	55.00	440.00	0.00	0.00	33.00	8.00
	Taco Bell-Burrito Supreme, Light	248.0000	1.000	Each	20.00	8.00	50.00	350.00	0.00	0.00	25.00	0.00
	Taco Bell-Burrito, 7-Layer, Light	276.0000	1.000	Each	19.00	9.00	67.00	440.00	0.00	0.00	5.00	0.00
	Taco Bell-Burrito, Bean	206.0000	1.000	Each	15.00	14.00	63.00	387.00	0.00	3.00	9.00	4.00
	Taco Bell-Burrito, Bean, Light	198.0000	1.000	Each	14.00	6.00	55.00	330.00	0.00	0.00	5.00	0.00
	Taco Bell-Burrito, Beef	206.0000	1.000	Each	25.00	21.00	48.00	431.00	0.00	2.00	57.00	8.00
	Taco Bell-Burrito, Chicken, Ligh	170.0000	1.000	Each	12.00	6.00	45.00	290.00	0.00	0.00	30.00	0.00
	Taco Bell-Burrito, Chicken, Supr	248.0000	1.000	Each	18.00	10.00	62.00	410.00	0.00	0.00	65.00	0.00
730	Taco Bell-Cinnamon Twists	28.0000	1.000	Ounce	1.00	6.00	19.00	140.00	0.00	0.00	0.00	0.00
731	Taco Bell-Gordita, Beef, Supreme	154.0000	5.500	Ounce	14.00	13.00	31.00	300.00	0.00	3.00	35.00	6.00
732	Taco Bell-Gordita, Chicken, Gril	154.0000	5.500	Ounce	17.00	14.00	28.00	300.00	0.00	3.00	45.00	5.00
733	Taco Bell-Gordita, Steak, Grille	154.0000	5.500	Ounce	17.00	14.00	27.00	310.00	0.00	3.00	35.00	5.00
734	Taco Bell-MexiMelt, Beef, Big	133.0000	4.750	Ounce	16.00	15.00	23.00	290.00	0.00	4.00	45.00	7.00
	Taco Bell-Nachos	106.0000	1.000	Order	7.00	18.00	37.00	346.00	0.00	1.00	9.00	6.00
	Taco Bell-Nachos Bell Grande	287.0000	1.000	Order	22.00	35.00	61.00	649.00	0.00	4.00	36.00	12.00
735	Taco Bell-Nachos Supreme, Beef,	98.0000	3.500	Ounce	14.00	24.00	45.00	220.00	0.00	9.00	30.00	8.00
	Taco Bell-Pintos 'N Cheese	128.0000	1.000	Each	9.00	9.00	19.00	190.00	0.00	2.00	16.00	4.00
	Taco Bell-Pizza, Mexican	223.0000	1.000	Each	21.00	37.00	40.00	575.00	0.00	3.00	52.00	11.00
	Taco Bell-Salad, Taco	575.0000	1.000	Each	34.00	61.00	55.00	905.00	0.00	4.00	80.00	19.00
	Taco Bell-Salad, Taco w/o Shell	520.0000	1.000	Each	28.00	31.00	22.00	484.00	0.00	3.00	80.00	14.00
	Taco Bell-Salad, Taco, Light	464.0000	1.000	Each	30.00	9.00	35.00	330.00	0.00	0.00	50.00	0.00
	Taco Bell-Salsa	10.0000	1.000	Each	1.00	0.00	4.00	18.00	0.00	0.40	0.00	0.00
	Taco Bell-Taco	78.0000	1.000	Each	10.00	11.00	11.00	183.00	0.00	1.00	32.00	5.00
736	Taco Bell-Taco, Double Decker	140.0000	5.000	Ounce	14.00	15.00	38.00	340.00	0.00	9.00	25.00	6.00
	Taco Bell-Taco, Light	78.0000	1.000	Each	11.00	5.00	11.00	140.00	0.00	1.00	20.00	4.00
	Taco Bell-Taco, Soft	92.0000	1.000	Each	12.00	12.00	18.00	225.00	0.00	2.00	32.00	5.00
	Taco Bell-Taco, Soft, Chicken, L	120.0000	1.000	Each	9.00	5.00	26.00	180.00	0.00	0.00	30.00	0.00
	Taco Bell-Taco, Soft, Light	99.0000	1.000	Each	13.00	5.00	19.00	180.00	0.00	2.00	25.00	4.00
737	Taco Bell-Taco, Soft, Steak, Gri	126.0000	4.500	Ounce	15.00	10.00	20.00	230.00	0.00	2.00	25.00	2.50
738	Taco Bell-Taco, Soft, Steak, Gri	161.0000	5.750	Ounce	16.00	14.00	24.00	290.00	0.00	3.00	35.00	5.00

Page Key: A2 = Baby Food   A2 = Baked Goods   A8 = Beverages   A14 = Breads/Grains and Pasta   A18 = Breakfast Foods/Cereals   A26 = Dairy and Eggs   A40 = Fats and Oils   A42 = Fruits and Vegetables   A52 = Meats and Beans   A60 = Nuts and Seeds   A62 = Frozen Entrees and Packaged Foods   A76 = Restaurant Chains–Fast Foods   A92 = Restaurant Chains–Other   A106 = Seafood and Fish   A110 = Snacks and Sweets   A120 = Soups   A122 = Supplements   A126 = Toppings and Sauces

Monounsaturated Fat (g)	Polyunsaturated Fat (g)	Vitamin D (mg)	Vitamin K (mg)	Vitamin E (mg)	Vitamin A (re)	Vitamin C (mg)	Thiamin (mg)	Riboflavin (mg)	Niacin (mg)	Vitamin B6 (mg)	Folate (mcg)	Vitamin B12 (mcg)	Calcium (mg)	Iron (mg)	Magnesium (mg)	Phosphorus (mg)	Potassium (mg)	Sodium (mg)	Zinc (mg)
9.00	4.00	0.00	0.00	4.40	58.00	5.00	0.23	0.29	4.40	0.42	54.00	2.01	55.00	3.70	57.00	266.00	910.00	2288.00	5.30
9.00	4.00	0.00	0.00	4.50	59.00	5.00	0.24	0.30	4.50	0.43	56.00	2.07	56.00	3.80	59.00	273.00	994.00	2348.00	5.40
0.00	0.00	0.00	0.00	0.00	601.00	15.00	0.00	0.00	0.00	0.00	0.00	0.00	25.00	4.00	0.00	0.00	0.00	928.00	0.00
0.00	0.00	0.00	0.00	0.00	565.00	14.00	0.00	0.00	0.00	0.00	0.00	0.00	23.00	3.00	0.00	0.00	0.00	638.00	0.00
0.00	0.00	0.00	0.00	0.00	1363.00	32.00	0.00	0.00	0.00	0.00	0.00	0.00	26.00	2.00	0.00	0.00	0.00	1067.00	0.00
0.00	0.00	0.00	0.00	0.00	1412.00	33.00	0.00	0.00	0.00	0.00	0.00	0.00	46.00	2.00	0.00	0.00	0.00	1127.00	0.00
0.00	0.00	0.00	0.00	0.00	1363.00	32.00	0.00	0.00	0.00	0.00	0.00	0.00	23.00	2.00	0.00	0.00	0.00	654.00	0.00
0.00	0.00	0.00	0.00	0.00	1366.00	32.00	0.00	0.00	0.00	0.00	0.00	0.00	25.00	2.00	0.00	0.00	0.00	575.00	0.00
0.00	0.00	0.00	0.00	0.00	1363.00	32.00	0.00	0.00	0.00	0.00	0.00	0.00	28.00	2.00	0.00	0.00	0.00	1117.00	0.00
0.00	0.00	0.00	0.00	0.00	1363.00	32.00	0.00	0.00	0.00	0.00	0.00	0.00	23.00	1.00	0.00	0.00	0.00	308.00	0.00
15.00	28.00	0.00	0.00	2.50	107.00	5.00	0.51	0.38	7.00	0.26	91.00	6.54	230.00	4.40	32.00	336.00	641.00	2027.00	5.30
16.00	28.00	0.00	0.00	0.00	0.00	0.00	0.00	0.00	0.00	0.00	0.00	0.00	0.00	0.00	0.00	0.00	557.00	1967.00	0.00
0.00	0.00	0.00	0.00	0.00	604.00	15.00	0.00	0.00	0.00	0.00	0.00	0.00	28.00	3.00	0.00	0.00	0.00	849.00	0.00
0.00	0.00	0.00	0.00	0.00	877.00	18.00	0.00	0.00	0.00	0.00	0.00	0.00	88.00	5.00	0.00	0.00	0.00	1106.00	0.00
12.00	4.00	0.00	0.00	0.80	119.00	6.00	0.33	0.46	5.10	0.38	36.00	2.54	231.00	4.20	43.00	456.00	909.00	1556.00	6.80
0.00	0.00	0.00	0.00	0.00	627.00	15.00	0.00	0.00	0.00	0.00	0.00	0.00	32.00	3.00	0.00	0.00	0.00	875.00	0.00
0.00	0.00	0.00	0.00	0.00	628.00	14.00	0.00	0.00	0.00	0.00	0.00	0.00	26.00	3.00	0.00	0.00	0.00	583.00	0.00
7.00	7.00	0.00	0.00	0.00	0.00	0.00	0.00	0.00	0.00	0.00	0.00	0.00	0.00	0.00	0.00	0.00	605.00	2520.00	0.00
0.00	0.00	0.00	0.00	0.00	601.00	15.00	0.00	0.00	0.00	0.00	0.00	0.00	30.00	4.00	0.00	0.00	0.00	1391.00	0.00
0.00	0.00	0.00	0.00	0.00	565.00	14.00	0.00	0.00	0.00	0.00	0.00	0.00	26.00	3.00	0.00	0.00	0.00	944.00	0.00
0.00	0.00	0.00	0.00	0.00	601.00	15.00	0.00	0.00	0.00	0.00	0.00	0.00	29.00	3.00	0.00	0.00	0.00	1350.00	0.00
0.00	0.00	0.00	0.00	0.00	601.00	15.00	0.00	0.00	0.00	0.00	0.00	0.00	25.00	3.00	0.00	0.00	0.00	3.00	0.00
0.00	0.00	0.00	0.00	0.00	601.00	15.00	0.00	0.00	0.00	0.00	0.00	0.00	32.00	3.00	0.00	0.00	0.00	593.00	0.00
0.00	2.00	0.00	0.00	0.00	26.00	0.40	2.10	3.60	0.00	0.00	0.00	0.00	190.00	4.00	0.00	0.00	501.00	1181.00	0.00
0.00	0.00	0.00	0.00	0.00	600.00	9.00	0.00	0.00	0.00	0.00	0.00	0.00	96.00	1.50	0.00	0.00	0.00	1160.00	0.00
0.00	0.00	0.00	0.00	0.00	350.00	4.80	0.00	0.00	0.00	0.00	0.00	0.00	300.00	2.50	0.00	0.00	0.00	1130.00	0.00
0.00	2.00	0.00	0.00	0.00	0.00	53.00	0.40	2.00	2.80	0.00	0.00	0.00	190.00	4.00	0.00	0.00	495.00	1148.00	0.00
0.00	0.00	0.00	0.00	0.00	300.00	2.40	0.00	0.00	0.00	0.00	0.00	0.00	120.00	2.00	0.00	0.00	0.00	1340.00	0.00
0.00	2.00	0.00	0.00	0.00	0.00	2.00	0.40	0.30	3.20	0.00	0.00	0.00	150.00	3.00	0.00	0.00	380.00	1311.00	0.00
0.00	0.00	0.00	0.00	0.00	200.00	3.60	0.00	0.00	0.00	0.00	0.00	0.00	72.00	1.50	0.00	0.00	0.00	900.00	0.00
0.00	0.00	0.00	0.00	0.00	250.00	4.80	0.00	0.00	0.00	0.00	0.00	0.00	72.00	1.50	0.00	0.00	0.00	1190.00	0.00
0.00	0.00	0.00	0.00	0.00	0.00	0.00	0.00	0.00	0.00	0.00	0.00	0.00	0.00	0.00	0.00	0.00	0.00	190.00	0.00
0.00	0.00	0.00	0.00	0.00	0.00	0.00	0.00	0.00	0.00	0.00	0.00	0.00	0.00	0.00	0.00	0.00	0.00	390.00	0.00
0.00	0.00	0.00	0.00	0.00	0.00	0.00	0.00	0.00	0.00	0.00	0.00	0.00	0.00	0.00	0.00	0.00	0.00	540.00	0.00
0.00	0.00	0.00	0.00	0.00	0.00	0.00	0.00	0.00	0.00	0.00	0.00	0.00	0.00	0.00	0.00	0.00	0.00	550.00	0.00
0.00	0.00	0.00	0.00	0.00	0.00	0.00	0.00	0.00	0.00	0.00	0.00	0.00	0.00	0.00	0.00	0.00	0.00	850.00	0.00
0.00	2.00	0.00	0.00	0.00	0.00	2.00	0.00	0.20	0.60	0.00	0.00	0.00	191.00	1.00	0.00	0.00	159.00	399.00	0.00
0.00	3.00	0.00	0.00	0.00	0.00	58.00	0.10	0.30	2.20	0.00	0.00	0.00	297.00	3.00	0.00	0.00	674.00	997.00	0.00
0.00	0.00	0.00	0.00	0.00	0.00	0.00	0.00	0.00	0.00	0.00	0.00	0.00	0.00	0.00	0.00	0.00	0.00	810.00	0.00
0.00	1.00	0.00	0.00	0.00	0.00	52.00	0.10	0.20	0.40	0.00	0.00	0.00	156.00	1.00	0.00	0.00	384.00	642.00	0.00
0.00	10.00	0.00	0.00	0.00	0.00	31.00	0.30	0.30	3.00	0.00	0.00	0.00	257.00	4.00	0.00	0.00	408.00	1031.00	0.00
0.00	12.00	0.00	0.00	0.00	0.00	75.00	0.50	0.60	4.80	0.00	0.00	0.00	320.00	6.00	0.00	0.00	673.00	910.00	0.00
0.00	2.00	0.00	0.00	0.00	0.00	74.00	0.20	0.40	3.20	0.00	0.00	0.00	290.00	4.00	0.00	0.00	612.00	680.00	0.00
0.00	0.00	0.00	0.00	0.00	1200.00	27.00	0.00	0.00	0.00	0.00	0.00	0.00	120.00	1.50	0.00	0.00	0.00	1610.00	0.00
0.00	0.00	0.00	0.00	0.00	0.00	0.00	0.00	0.10	4.00	0.00	0.00	0.00	36.00	1.00	0.00	0.00	376.00	376.00	0.00
0.00	1.00	0.00	0.00	0.00	0.00	1.00	0.10	0.10	1.20	0.00	0.00	0.00	84.00	1.00	0.00	0.00	159.00	276.00	0.00
0.00	0.00	0.00	0.00	0.00	0.00	15.00	0.00	0.00	0.00	0.00	0.00	0.00	0.00	0.00	0.00	0.00	0.00	750.00	0.00
0.00	1.00	0.00	0.00	0.00	40.00	0.00	0.10	0.10	1.20	0.00	0.00	0.00	0.00	0.00	0.00	0.00	159.00	276.00	0.00
0.00	1.00	0.00	0.00	0.00	0.00	1.00	0.40	0.20	2.80	0.00	0.00	0.00	116.00	2.00	0.00	0.00	196.00	554.00	0.00
0.00	0.00	0.00	0.00	0.00	150.00	4.80	0.00	0.00	0.00	0.00	0.00	0.00	48.00	0.80	0.00	0.00	0.00	570.00	0.00
0.00	1.00	0.00	0.00	0.00	40.00	0.00	0.40	0.20	2.80	0.00	0.00	0.00	48.00	0.60	0.00	0.00	196.00	554.00	0.00
0.00	0.00	0.00	0.00	0.00	0.00	0.00	0.00	0.00	0.00	0.00	0.00	0.00	0.00	0.00	0.00	0.00	0.00	1020.00	0.00
0.00	0.00	0.00	0.00	0.00	0.00	0.00	0.00	0.00	0.00	0.00	0.00	0.00	0.00	0.00	0.00	0.00	0.00	1040.00	0.00

USDA ID Code	Food Name	Weight in Grams*	Quantity of Units	Unit of Measure	Protein (g)	Fat (g)	Carbohydrate (g)	Kilocalories	Caffeine (g)	Fiber (g)	Cholesterol (mg)	Saturated Fat (g)
	Taco Bell-Taco, Soft, Supreme, L	128.0000	1.000	Each	14.00	5.00	23.00	200.00	0.00	0.00	25.00	0.00
	Taco Bell-Taco, Supreme, Light	106.0000	1.000	Each	14.00	5.00	23.00	160.00	0.00	0.00	20.00	0.00
	Taco Bell-Tostada	156.0000	1.000	Each	9.00	11.00	27.00	243.00	0.00	2.00	16.00	4.00
	Wendy's-Cheeseburger Deluxe, Jr.	180.0000	1.000	Each	18.00	17.00	36.00	360.00	0.00	3.00	50.00	6.00
	Wendy's-Cheeseburger, Bacon, Jr.	166.0000	1.000	Each	20.00	19.00	34.00	380.00	0.00	2.00	60.00	7.00
	Wendy's-Cheeseburger, Jr.	130.0000	1.000	Each	17.00	13.00	34.00	320.00	0.00	2.00	45.00	6.00
	Wendy's-Cheeseburger, Kids' Meal	123.0000	1.000	Each	17.00	13.00	33.00	320.00	0.00	2.00	45.00	6.00
	Wendy's-Chicken Club Sandwich	216.0000	1.000	Each	31.00	20.00	44.00	470.00	0.00	2.00	70.00	4.00
	Wendy's-Chicken, Breaded, Sandwi	208.0000	1.000	Each	28.00	18.00	44.00	440.00	0.00	2.00	60.00	3.50
	Wendy's-Chicken, Grilled, Sandwi	189.0000	1.000	Each	27.00	8.00	35.00	310.00	0.00	2.00	65.00	1.50
	Wendy's-Chicken, Spicy, Sandwich	213.0000	1.000	Each	28.00	15.00	43.00	410.00	0.00	2.00	65.00	2.50
	Wendy's-Chili, Large	340.0000	1.000	Each	28.00	9.00	31.00	290.00	0.00	6.00	60.00	4.00
	Wendy's-Chili, Small	227.0000	1.000	Each	19.00	6.00	21.00	190.00	0.00	4.00	40.00	2.00
	Wendy's-French Fries, Biggie	170.0000	1.000	Order	7.00	23.00	61.00	450.00	0.00	0.00	0.00	5.00
	Wendy's-French Fries, Medium	136.0000	1.000	Order	5.00	17.00	50.00	360.00	0.00	0.00	0.00	4.00
	Wendy's-French Fries, Small	91.0000	1.000	Order	3.00	12.00	33.00	240.00	0.00	0.00	0.00	2.00
	Wendy's-Frosty Dairy Dessert, La	402.2200	1.000	Each	15.00	17.00	91.00	570.00	0.00	0.00	70.00	9.00
	Wendy's-Frosty Dairy Dessert, Me	321.7760	1.000	Each	12.00	13.00	76.00	460.00	0.00	0.00	55.00	7.00
	Wendy's-Frosty Dairy Dessert, Sm	241.3320	1.000	Each	9.00	10.00	57.00	340.00	0.00	0.00	40.00	5.00
	Wendy's-Hamburger, Bacon, Big Cl	285.0000	1.000	Each	34.00	30.00	46.00	580.00	0.00	3.00	100.00	12.00
	Wendy's-Hamburger, Big Classic	251.0000	1.000	Each	27.00	23.00	44.00	480.00	0.00	0.00	75.00	7.00
	Wendy's-Hamburger, Jr.	118.0000	1.000	Each	15.00	10.00	34.00	270.00	0.00	2.00	30.00	3.50
	Wendy's-Hamburger, Kids' Meal	111.0000	1.000	Each	15.00	10.00	33.00	270.00	0.00	2.00	30.00	3.50
	Wendy's-Hamburger, Single w/ eve	219.0000	1.000	Each	25.00	20.00	37.00	420.00	0.00	3.00	70.00	6.00
	Wendy's-Hamburger, Single, Plain	133.0000	1.000	Each	24.00	16.00	31.00	360.00	0.00	2.00	65.00	6.00
	Wendy's-Potato, Bkd w/ Bacon and	380.0000	1.000	Each	17.00	17.00	75.00	510.00	0.00	0.00	15.00	4.00
	Wendy's-Potato, Bkd w/ Broccoli	411.0000	1.000	Each	9.00	14.00	77.00	450.00	0.00	0.00	0.00	2.00
	Wendy's-Potato, Bkd w/ Cheese	383.0000	1.000	Each	14.00	24.00	74.00	550.00	0.00	0.00	30.00	8.00
	White Castle-Cheeseburger Sandwi	64.8000	1.000	Each	7.80	11.20	15.53	199.58	0.00	2.70	0.00	0.00
	White Castle-Chicken Sandwich	63.7860	1.000	Each	7.99	7.45	20.49	185.75	0.00	1.73	0.00	0.00
	White Castle-Fish Sandwich, w/o	59.3330	1.000	Each	5.78	4.98	20.87	155.44	0.00	1.41	0.00	0.00
	White Castle-French Fries	96.8300	1.000	Order	2.49	14.70	37.73	301.14	0.00	4.64	0.00	0.00
	White Castle-Hamburger Sandwich	58.5000	1.000	Each	5.88	7.94	15.38	161.27	0.00	2.13	0.00	0.00
	White Castle-Onion Chips	92.1350	1.000	Each	3.72	16.55	38.83	328.66	0.00	3.52	0.00	0.00
	White Castle-Onion Rings	60.1700	1.000	Each	2.91	13.38	26.62	245.49	0.00	2.61	0.00	0.00
	White Castle-Sausage and Egg San	96.2500	1.000	Each	12.55	22.02	16.05	322.37	0.00	3.03	0.00	0.00
	White Castle-Sausage Sandwich	48.6670	1.000	Each	6.67	12.29	13.30	196.10	0.00	1.95	0.00	0.00

Restaurant Chains—Other

USDA ID Code	Food Name	Weight in Grams*	Quantity of Units	Unit of Measure	Protein (g)	Fat (g)	Carbohydrate (g)	Kilocalories	Caffeine (g)	Fiber (g)	Cholesterol (mg)	Saturated Fat (g)
65	Bruegger's Bagels-Bagel, Blueber	101.0000	1.000	Each	10.00	2.00	60.00	300.00	0.00	2.00	0.00	0.00
66	Bruegger's Bagels-Bagel, Cinnamo	101.0000	1.000	Each	10.00	1.50	60.00	290.00	0.00	3.00	0.00	0.00
67	Bruegger's Bagels-Bagel, Egg	101.0000	1.000	Each	10.00	1.00	57.00	280.00	0.00	3.00	25.00	0.50
68	Bruegger's Bagels-Bagel, Everyth	104.0000	1.000	Each	11.00	2.00	58.00	290.00	0.00	2.00	0.00	0.00
69	Bruegger's Bagels-Bagel, Garlic	102.0000	1.000	Each	10.00	1.50	57.00	280.00	0.00	2.00	0.00	0.00
70	Bruegger's Bagels-Bagel, Honey G	103.0000	1.000	Each	11.00	2.50	58.00	300.00	0.00	3.00	0.00	0.50
71	Bruegger's Bagels-Bagel, Onion	102.0000	1.000	Each	10.00	1.50	57.00	280.00	0.00	2.00	0.00	0.00
72	Bruegger's Bagels-Bagel, Plain	101.0000	1.000	Each	10.00	1.50	56.00	280.00	0.00	2.00	0.00	0.00
73	Bruegger's Bagels-Bagel, Poppy S	102.0000	1.000	Each	11.00	1.50	57.00	280.00	0.00	2.00	0.00	0.00
74	Bruegger's Bagels-Bagel, Pumpern	101.0000	1.000	Each	11.00	1.50	56.00	280.00	0.00	4.00	0.00	0.00
75	Bruegger's Bagels-Bagel, Salt	102.0000	1.000	Each	10.00	1.50	55.00	270.00	0.00	2.00	0.00	0.00
76	Bruegger's Bagels-Bagel, Sesame	103.0000	1.000	Each	11.00	2.50	57.00	290.00	0.00	2.00	0.00	0.50
77	Bruegger's Bagels-Bagel, Sun-dri	101.0000	1.000	Each	10.00	1.50	56.00	280.00	0.00	3.00	0.00	0.00
64	Bruegger's Bagels-BLT Sandwich	187.0000	1.000	Each	18.00	18.00	61.00	480.00	0.00	3.00	35.00	7.00
78	Bruegger's Bagels-Chocolate Chunk Brownie	73.0000	1.000	Each	4.00	19.00	39.00	330.00	0.00	2.00	55.00	7.00

Page Key: A2 = Baby Food   A2 = Baked Goods   A8 = Beverages   A14 = Breads/Grains and Pasta   A18 = Breakfast Foods/Cereals   A26 = Dairy and Eggs   A40 = Fats and Oils   A42 = Fruits and Vegetables   A52 = Meats and Beans   A60 = Nuts and Seeds   A62 = Frozen Entrees and Packaged Foods   A76 = Restaurant Chains–Fast Foods   A92 = Restaurant Chains–Other   A106 = Seafood and Fish   A110 = Snacks and Sweets   A120 = Soups   A122 = Supplements   A126 = Toppings and Sauces

Monounsaturated Fat (g)	Polyunsaturated Fat (g)	Vitamin D (mg)	Vitamin K (mg)	Vitamin E (mg)	Vitamin A (re)	Vitamin C (mg)	Thiamin (mg)	Riboflavin (mg)	Niacin (mg)	Vitamin B₆ (mg)	Folate (mcg)	Vitamin B₁₂ (mcg)	Calcium (mg)	Iron (mg)	Magnesium (mg)	Phosphorus (mg)	Potassium (mg)	Sodium (mg)	Zinc (mg)
0.00	0.00	0.00	0.00	0.00	100.00	2.40	0.00	0.00	0.00	0.00	0.00	0.00	48.00	0.60	0.00	0.00	0.00	610.00	0.00
0.00	0.00	0.00	0.00	0.00	100.00	2.40	0.00	0.00	0.00	0.00	0.00	0.00	0.00	0.00	0.00	0.00	0.00	340.00	0.00
0.00	1.00	0.00	0.00	0.00	0.00	45.00	0.10	0.20	0.60	0.00	0.00	0.00	180.00	2.00	0.00	0.00	401.00	596.00	0.00
0.00	0.00	0.00	0.00	0.00	10.00	10.00	0.00	0.00	0.00	0.00	0.00	0.00	18.00	19.00	0.00	0.00	0.00	890.00	0.00
0.00	0.00	0.00	0.00	0.00	8.00	10.00	0.00	0.00	0.00	0.00	0.00	0.00	17.00	19.00	0.00	0.00	0.00	850.00	0.00
0.00	0.00	0.00	0.00	0.00	6.00	2.00	0.00	0.00	0.00	0.00	0.00	0.00	17.00	18.00	0.00	0.00	0.00	830.00	0.00
0.00	0.00	0.00	0.00	0.00	6.00	0.00	0.00	0.00	0.00	0.00	0.00	0.00	17.00	18.00	0.00	0.00	0.00	830.00	0.00
7.00	9.00	0.00	0.00	0.00	20.00	9.00	0.60	0.43	15.20	0.00	0.00	0.00	80.00	8.00	0.00	0.00	470.00	970.00	0.00
0.00	0.00	0.00	0.00	0.00	4.00	10.00	0.00	0.00	0.00	0.00	0.00	0.00	10.00	16.00	0.00	0.00	0.00	840.00	0.00
0.00	0.00	0.00	0.00	0.00	4.00	10.00	0.00	0.00	0.00	0.00	0.00	0.00	10.00	15.00	0.00	0.00	0.00	790.00	0.00
0.00	0.00	0.00	0.00	0.00	0.00	0.00	0.00	0.00	0.00	0.00	0.00	0.00	11.00	15.00	0.00	0.00	0.00	1280.00	0.00
2.00	1.00	0.00	0.00	0.00	150.00	12.00	0.15	0.17	2.85	0.00	0.00	0.00	80.00	4.50	0.00	0.00	660.00	1000.00	0.00
1.00	1.00	0.00	0.00	0.00	100.00	6.00	0.09	0.14	1.90	0.00	0.00	0.00	64.00	3.00	0.00	0.00	440.00	670.00	0.00
15.00	1.00	0.00	0.00	0.00	0.00	12.00	0.30	0.07	3.80	0.00	0.00	0.00	16.00	0.80	0.00	0.00	950.00	280.00	0.00
12.00	1.00	0.00	0.00	0.00	0.00	9.00	0.23	0.03	2.85	0.00	0.00	0.00	16.00	0.60	0.00	0.00	760.00	220.00	0.00
8.00	1.00	0.00	0.00	0.00	0.00	6.00	0.15	0.03	1.90	0.00	0.00	0.00	0.00	0.40	0.00	0.00	510.00	150.00	0.00
4.00	1.00	0.00	0.00	0.00	100.00	0.00	0.23	1.36	0.76	0.00	0.00	0.00	400.00	1.00	0.00	0.00	1040.00	330.00	0.00
3.00	1.00	0.00	0.00	0.00	100.00	0.00	0.15	1.02	0.76	0.00	0.00	0.00	320.00	0.80	0.00	0.00	830.00	260.00	0.00
3.00	0.00	0.00	0.00	0.00	80.00	0.00	0.12	0.77	0.38	0.00	0.00	0.00	240.00	0.60	0.00	0.00	630.00	200.00	0.00
0.00	0.00	0.00	0.00	0.00	15.00	25.00	0.00	0.00	0.00	0.00	0.00	0.00	25.00	30.00	0.00	0.00	0.00	1460.00	0.00
8.00	7.00	0.00	0.00	0.00	60.00	12.00	0.45	0.26	6.65	0.00	0.00	0.00	120.00	3.50	0.00	0.00	500.00	850.00	0.00
0.00	0.00	0.00	0.00	0.00	2.00	2.00	0.00	0.00	0.00	0.00	0.00	0.00	11.00	17.00	0.00	0.00	0.00	610.00	0.00
0.00	0.00	0.00	0.00	0.00	2.00	0.00	0.00	0.00	0.00	0.00	0.00	0.00	11.00	17.00	0.00	0.00	0.00	610.00	0.00
7.00	7.00	0.00	0.00	0.00	60.00	9.00	0.38	0.17	6.65	0.00	0.00	0.00	80.00	3.00	0.00	0.00	430.00	920.00	0.00
7.00	2.00	0.00	0.00	0.00	0.00	0.00	0.38	0.17	5.70	0.00	0.00	0.00	80.00	3.00	0.00	0.00	280.00	580.00	0.00
3.00	8.00	0.00	0.00	0.00	100.00	36.00	0.45	0.17	6.65	0.00	0.00	0.00	80.00	2.50	0.00	0.00	1370.00	1170.00	0.00
3.00	7.00	0.00	0.00	0.00	200.00	60.00	0.30	0.14	4.75	0.00	0.00	0.00	80.00	2.50	0.00	0.00	1310.00	450.00	0.00
6.00	7.00	0.00	0.00	0.00	150.00	36.00	0.30	0.17	3.80	0.00	0.00	0.00	240.00	2.00	0.00	0.00	1210.00	640.00	0.00
0.00	0.00	0.00	0.00	0.00	0.00	0.00	0.00	0.00	0.00	0.00	0.00	0.00	0.00	0.00	0.00	0.00	0.00	361.00	0.00
0.00	0.00	0.00	0.00	0.00	0.00	0.00	0.00	0.00	0.00	0.00	0.00	0.00	0.00	0.00	0.00	0.00	0.00	497.00	0.00
0.00	0.00	0.00	0.00	0.00	0.00	0.00	0.00	0.00	0.00	0.00	0.00	0.00	0.00	0.00	0.00	0.00	0.00	201.00	0.00
0.00	0.00	0.00	0.00	0.00	0.00	0.00	0.00	0.00	0.00	0.00	0.00	0.00	0.00	0.00	0.00	0.00	0.00	193.00	0.00
0.00	0.00	0.00	0.00	0.00	0.00	0.00	0.00	0.00	0.00	0.00	0.00	0.00	0.00	0.00	0.00	0.00	0.00	266.00	0.00
0.00	0.00	0.00	0.00	0.00	0.00	0.00	0.00	0.00	0.00	0.00	0.00	0.00	0.00	0.00	0.00	0.00	0.00	823.00	0.00
0.00	0.00	0.00	0.00	0.00	0.00	0.00	0.00	0.00	0.00	0.00	0.00	0.00	0.00	0.00	0.00	0.00	0.00	566.00	0.00
0.00	0.00	0.00	0.00	0.00	0.00	0.00	0.00	0.00	0.00	0.00	0.00	0.00	0.00	0.00	0.00	0.00	0.00	698.00	0.00
0.00	0.00	0.00	0.00	0.00	0.00	0.00	0.00	0.00	0.00	0.00	0.00	0.00	0.00	0.00	0.00	0.00	0.00	488.00	0.00
0.50	0.50	0.00	0.00	0.00	0.00	0.00	0.00	0.00	0.00	0.00	0.00	0.00	0.00	0.00	0.00	0.00	0.00	480.00	0.00
0.00	0.50	0.00	0.00	0.00	0.00	0.00	0.00	0.00	0.00	0.00	0.00	0.00	0.00	0.00	0.00	0.00	0.00	400.00	0.00
0.50	0.50	0.00	0.00	0.00	0.00	0.00	0.00	0.00	0.00	0.00	0.00	0.00	0.00	0.00	0.00	0.00	0.00	510.00	0.00
0.00	1.00	0.00	0.00	0.00	0.00	0.00	0.00	0.00	0.00	0.00	0.00	0.00	0.00	0.00	0.00	0.00	0.00	700.00	0.00
0.00	0.50	0.00	0.00	0.00	0.00	0.00	0.00	0.00	0.00	0.00	0.00	0.00	0.00	0.00	0.00	0.00	0.00	440.00	0.00
0.50	1.50	0.00	0.00	0.00	0.00	0.00	0.00	0.00	0.00	0.00	0.00	0.00	0.00	0.00	0.00	0.00	0.00	390.00	0.00
0.00	0.50	0.00	0.00	0.00	0.00	0.00	0.00	0.00	0.00	0.00	0.00	0.00	0.00	0.00	0.00	0.00	0.00	430.00	0.00
0.00	1.00	0.00	0.00	0.00	0.00	0.00	0.00	0.00	0.00	0.00	0.00	0.00	0.00	0.00	0.00	0.00	0.00	430.00	0.00
0.00	1.00	0.00	0.00	0.00	0.00	0.00	0.00	0.00	0.00	0.00	0.00	0.00	0.00	0.00	0.00	0.00	0.00	440.00	0.00
0.00	0.50	0.00	0.00	0.00	0.00	0.00	0.00	0.00	0.00	0.00	0.00	0.00	0.00	0.00	0.00	0.00	0.00	390.00	0.00
0.00	0.50	0.00	0.00	0.00	0.00	0.00	0.00	0.00	0.00	0.00	0.00	0.00	0.00	0.00	0.00	0.00	0.00	1670.00	0.00
1.00	1.00	0.00	0.00	0.00	0.00	0.00	0.00	0.00	0.00	0.00	0.00	0.00	0.00	0.00	0.00	0.00	0.00	440.00	0.00
0.00	1.00	0.00	0.00	0.00	0.00	0.00	0.00	0.00	0.00	0.00	0.00	0.00	0.00	0.00	0.00	0.00	0.00	490.00	0.00
0.00	0.00	0.00	0.00	0.00	0.00	0.00	0.00	0.00	0.00	0.00	0.00	0.00	0.00	0.00	0.00	0.00	0.00	820.00	0.00
0.00	0.00	0.00	0.00	0.00	0.00	0.00	0.00	0.00	0.00	0.00	0.00	0.00	0.00	0.00	0.00	0.00	0.00	95.00	0.00

USDA ID Code	Food Name	Weight in Grams*	Quantity of Units	Unit of Measure	Protein (g)	Fat (g)	Carbohydrate (g)	Kilocalories	Caffeine (g)	Fiber (g)	Cholesterol (mg)	Saturated Fat (g)
79	Bruegger's Bagels-Bruegger Bar	94.0000	1.000	Each	5.00	36.00	39.00	490.00	0.00	2.00	5.00	11.00
80	Bruegger's Bagels-Brueggeroons	71.0000	1.000	Each	4.00	18.00	39.00	320.00	0.00	5.00	0.00	16.00
81	Bruegger's Bagels-Cheese, Veggie	244.0000	8.000	Ounce	5.10	13.00	16.00	200.00	0.00	3.20	15.00	4.50
82	Bruegger's Bagels-Chicken Fajita	250.0000	1.000	Each	28.00	10.00	66.00	460.00	0.00	3.00	80.00	4.50
83	Bruegger's Bagels-Chicken Salad,	116.0000	0.500	Cup	24.00	3.00	4.00	140.00	0.00	1.00	95.00	1.00
84	Bruegger's Bagels-Chicken, Aztec	241.0000	8.000	Ounce	8.00	3.50	14.00	120.00	0.00	2.00	15.00	0.50
85	Bruegger's Bagels-Chile Cilantro	246.0000	8.000	Ounce	8.00	7.00	28.00	200.00	0.00	7.00	0.00	1.00
86	Bruegger's Bagels-Chili, The Big	244.0000	8.000	Ounce	13.00	7.00	26.00	220.00	0.00	6.00	20.00	1.50
87	Bruegger's Bagels-Chowder, Bacon	241.0000	8.000	Ounce	4.00	9.00	25.00	190.00	0.00	1.00	10.00	2.50
88	Bruegger's Bagels-Chowder, Clam	241.0000	8.000	Ounce	8.00	7.00	18.00	170.00	0.00	1.00	10.00	2.00
89	Bruegger's Bagels-Cream Cheese,	27.0000	2.000	Tbsp	1.00	8.00	1.00	90.00	0.00	0.00	20.00	5.00
90	Bruegger's Bagels-Cream Cheese,	30.0000	2.000	Tbsp	2.00	10.00	1.00	100.00	0.00	0.00	30.00	6.00
91	Bruegger's Bagels-Cream Cheese,	26.0000	2.000	Tbsp	2.00	4.50	2.00	60.00	0.00	0.00	15.00	3.00
92	Bruegger's Bagels-Crm Chse, Chiv	26.0000	2.000	Tbsp	2.00	9.00	2.00	100.00	0.00	0.00	25.00	4.50
93	Bruegger's Bagels-Crm Chse, Cucu	28.0000	2.000	Tbsp	2.00	9.00	2.00	100.00	0.00	0.00	25.00	4.50
94	Bruegger's Bagels-Crm Chse, Gard	28.0000	2.000	Tbsp	1.00	8.00	1.00	80.00	0.00	0.00	25.00	5.00
95	Bruegger's Bagels-Crm Chse, Gard	27.0000	2.000	Tbsp	2.00	4.50	2.00	60.00	0.00	0.00	15.00	3.00
96	Bruegger's Bagels-Crm Chse, Herb	27.0000	2.000	Tbsp	2.00	4.50	3.00	60.00	0.00	0.00	15.00	3.00
97	Bruegger's Bagels-Crm Chse, Hone	27.0000	2.000	Tbsp	2.00	9.00	3.00	90.00	0.00	0.00	20.00	5.00
98	Bruegger's Bagels-Crm Chse, Jala	30.0000	2.000	Tbsp	1.00	8.00	1.00	80.00	0.00	0.00	20.00	5.00
99	Bruegger's Bagels-Crm Chse, Salm	29.0000	2.000	Tbsp	2.00	9.00	1.00	90.00	0.00	0.00	20.00	5.00
100	Bruegger's Bagels-Crm Chse, Stra	25.0000	2.000	Tbsp	2.00	4.50	5.00	70.00	0.00	0.00	15.00	3.00
101	Bruegger's Bagels-Crm Chse, Sun	27.0000	2.000	Tbsp	2.00	4.50	2.00	60.00	0.00	0.00	15.00	3.00
102	Bruegger's Bagels-Crm Chse, Wild	30.0000	2.000	Tbsp	1.00	8.00	3.00	90.00	0.00	0.00	20.00	5.00
103	Bruegger's Bagels-Cucumber Dill	236.0000	1.000	Each	18.00	15.00	62.00	450.00	0.00	4.00	40.00	8.00
104	Bruegger's Bagels-Garden Veggie,	227.0000	8.000	Ounce	2.00	1.50	11.00	60.00	0.00	2.00	0.00	0.00
105	Bruegger's Bagels-Gumbo, Cajun	241.0000	8.000	Ounce	3.00	4.50	17.00	120.00	0.00	2.00	0.00	1.00
106	Bruegger's Bagels-Hummus	71.0000	1.000	Scoop	5.00	9.00	13.00	150.00	0.00	4.00	0.00	1.50
107	Bruegger's Bagels-Javahhccino	280.0000	12.000	Fl Oz	9.00	3.00	35.00	210.00	0.00	0.00	10.00	3.00
108	Bruegger's Bagels-Kinnow Bruegge	227.0000	8.000	Fl Oz	1.00	0.00	35.00	140.00	0.00	0.00	0.00	0.00
109	Bruegger's Bagels-Leonardo da Ve	220.0000	1.000	Each	19.00	11.00	62.00	420.00	0.00	3.00	30.00	6.00
110	Bruegger's Bagels-Mediterranean	231.0000	1.000	Each	20.00	24.00	74.00	610.00	0.00	8.00	30.00	11.00
111	Bruegger's Bagels-Olivia De Hami	239.0000	1.000	Each	29.00	17.00	62.00	520.00	0.00	3.00	75.00	8.00
112	Bruegger's Bagels-Soup, Chicken	241.0000	8.000	Ounce	10.00	3.50	25.00	170.00	0.00	1.00	40.00	1.00
113	Bruegger's Bagels-Soup, Garden S	247.0000	8.000	Ounce	4.00	6.00	19.00	150.00	0.00	3.00	10.00	3.00
114	Bruegger's Bagels-Soup, Marcello	241.0000	8.000	Ounce	4.00	1.00	18.00	90.00	0.00	2.00	0.00	0.50
115	Bruegger's Bagels-Soup, Turkey L	227.0000	8.000	Ounce	14.00	2.50	17.00	150.00	0.00	7.00	20.00	0.50
116	Bruegger's Bagels-Stew, Ratatoui	244.0000	8.000	Ounce	2.00	9.00	12.00	140.00	0.00	3.00	0.00	1.50
117	Bruegger's Bagels-Strawberry Bru	227.0000	8.000	Fl Oz	0.00	0.00	39.00	150.00	0.00	0.00	0.00	0.00
118	Bruegger's Bagels-Tuna Salad	116.0000	0.500	Cup	12.00	19.00	9.00	260.00	0.00	2.00	30.00	3.00
119	Bruegger's Bagels-Turkey Club Sa	258.0000	1.000	Each	27.00	31.00	58.00	620.00	0.00	3.00	55.00	5.00
120	Bruegger's Bagels-Turkey Orzo, T	241.0000	8.000	Ounce	8.00	3.00	13.00	110.00	0.00	1.00	15.00	0.50
121	Bruegger's Bagels-Turkey, Herby	235.0000	1.000	Each	30.00	13.00	67.00	510.00	0.00	3.00	45.00	5.00
122	Bruegger's Bagels-Turkey, Hot Sh	234.0000	1.000	Each	26.00	8.00	68.00	450.00	0.00	3.00	3.00	3.50
123	Bruegger's Bagels-Turkey, Santa	264.0000	1.000	Each	27.00	9.00	63.00	450.00	0.00	3.00	45.00	4.00
220	Denny's-All American Slam	368.5500	1.000	Serving	38.00	62.00	9.00	712.00	0.00	1.00	686.00	20.00
221	Denny's-Bacon, 4 Strips	28.3500	4.000	Each	12.00	18.00	1.00	162.00	0.00	0.00	36.00	5.00
222	Denny's-Bagel, Dry	85.0000	1.000	Each	9.00	1.00	46.00	235.00	0.00	0.00	0.00	0.00
223	Denny's-Big Texas Chicken Fajita	481.0000	1.000	Serving	49.00	70.00	25.00	1217.00	0.00	8.00	518.00	19.00
224	Denny's-Biscuit & Sausage Gravy	198.4500	1.000	Serving	8.00	21.00	45.00	398.00	0.00	0.00	12.00	6.00
225	Denny's-Biscuit, Buttered	85.0000	1.000	Each	5.00	11.00	39.00	272.00	0.00	0.00	0.00	4.00
226	Denny's-Buttermilk Hotcakes (3)	141.7500	3.000	Each	12.00	7.00	95.00	491.00	0.00	3.00	0.00	1.00
227	Denny's-Chicken Fried Steak & Eg	226.8000	1.000	Serving	22.00	36.00	9.00	430.00	0.00	4.00	440.00	12.00

Monounsaturated Fat (g)	Polyunsaturated Fat (g)	Vitamin D (mg)	Vitamin K (mg)	Vitamin E (mg)	Vitamin A (re)	Vitamin C (mg)	Thiamin (mg)	Riboflavin (mg)	Niacin (mg)	Vitamin B6 (mg)	Folate (mcg)	Vitamin B12 (mcg)	Calcium (mg)	Iron (mg)	Magnesium (mg)	Phosphorus (mg)	Potassium (mg)	Sodium (mg)	Zinc (mg)
0.00	0.00	0.00	0.00	0.00	0.00	0.00	0.00	0.00	0.00	0.00	0.00	0.00	0.00	0.00	0.00	0.00	0.00	440.00	0.00
0.00	0.00	0.00	0.00	0.00	0.00	0.00	0.00	0.00	0.00	0.00	0.00	0.00	0.00	0.00	0.00	0.00	0.00	140.00	0.00
0.00	0.00	0.00	0.00	0.00	0.00	0.00	0.00	0.00	0.00	0.00	0.00	0.00	0.00	0.00	0.00	0.00	0.00	1010.00	0.00
0.00	0.00	0.00	0.00	0.00	0.00	0.00	0.00	0.00	0.00	0.00	0.00	0.00	0.00	0.00	0.00	0.00	0.00	830.00	0.00
0.00	0.00	0.00	0.00	0.00	0.00	0.00	0.00	0.00	0.00	0.00	0.00	0.00	0.00	0.00	0.00	0.00	0.00	440.00	0.00
0.00	0.00	0.00	0.00	0.00	0.00	0.00	0.00	0.00	0.00	0.00	0.00	0.00	0.00	0.00	0.00	0.00	0.00	570.00	0.00
0.00	0.00	0.00	0.00	0.00	0.00	0.00	0.00	0.00	0.00	0.00	0.00	0.00	0.00	0.00	0.00	0.00	0.00	620.00	0.00
0.00	0.00	0.00	0.00	0.00	0.00	0.00	0.00	0.00	0.00	0.00	0.00	0.00	0.00	0.00	0.00	0.00	0.00	810.00	0.00
0.00	0.00	0.00	0.00	0.00	0.00	0.00	0.00	0.00	0.00	0.00	0.00	0.00	0.00	0.00	0.00	0.00	0.00	700.00	0.00
0.00	0.00	0.00	0.00	0.00	0.00	0.00	0.00	0.00	0.00	0.00	0.00	0.00	0.00	0.00	0.00	0.00	0.00	1230.00	0.00
0.00	0.00	0.00	0.00	0.00	0.00	0.00	0.00	0.00	0.00	0.00	0.00	0.00	0.00	0.00	0.00	0.00	0.00	110.00	0.00
0.00	0.00	0.00	0.00	0.00	0.00	0.00	0.00	0.00	0.00	0.00	0.00	0.00	0.00	0.00	0.00	0.00	0.00	120.00	0.00
0.00	0.00	0.00	0.00	0.00	0.00	0.00	0.00	0.00	0.00	0.00	0.00	0.00	0.00	0.00	0.00	0.00	0.00	130.00	0.00
0.00	0.00	0.00	0.00	0.00	0.00	0.00	0.00	0.00	0.00	0.00	0.00	0.00	0.00	0.00	0.00	0.00	0.00	85.00	0.00
0.00	0.00	0.00	0.00	0.00	0.00	0.00	0.00	0.00	0.00	0.00	0.00	0.00	0.00	0.00	0.00	0.00	0.00	85.00	0.00
0.00	0.00	0.00	0.00	0.00	0.00	0.00	0.00	0.00	0.00	0.00	0.00	0.00	0.00	0.00	0.00	0.00	0.00	120.00	0.00
0.00	0.00	0.00	0.00	0.00	0.00	0.00	0.00	0.00	0.00	0.00	0.00	0.00	0.00	0.00	0.00	0.00	0.00	160.00	0.00
0.00	0.00	0.00	0.00	0.00	0.00	0.00	0.00	0.00	0.00	0.00	0.00	0.00	0.00	0.00	0.00	0.00	0.00	150.00	0.00
0.00	0.00	0.00	0.00	0.00	0.00	0.00	0.00	0.00	0.00	0.00	0.00	0.00	0.00	0.00	0.00	0.00	0.00	90.00	0.00
0.00	0.00	0.00	0.00	0.00	0.00	0.00	0.00	0.00	0.00	0.00	0.00	0.00	0.00	0.00	0.00	0.00	0.00	100.00	0.00
0.00	0.00	0.00	0.00	0.00	0.00	0.00	0.00	0.00	0.00	0.00	0.00	0.00	0.00	0.00	0.00	0.00	0.00	120.00	0.00
0.00	0.00	0.00	0.00	0.00	0.00	0.00	0.00	0.00	0.00	0.00	0.00	0.00	0.00	0.00	0.00	0.00	0.00	60.00	0.00
0.00	0.00	0.00	0.00	0.00	0.00	0.00	0.00	0.00	0.00	0.00	0.00	0.00	0.00	0.00	0.00	0.00	0.00	160.00	0.00
0.00	0.00	0.00	0.00	0.00	0.00	0.00	0.00	0.00	0.00	0.00	0.00	0.00	0.00	0.00	0.00	0.00	0.00	100.00	0.00
0.00	0.00	0.00	0.00	0.00	0.00	0.00	0.00	0.00	0.00	0.00	0.00	0.00	0.00	0.00	0.00	0.00	0.00	630.00	0.00
0.00	0.00	0.00	0.00	0.00	0.00	0.00	0.00	0.00	0.00	0.00	0.00	0.00	0.00	0.00	0.00	0.00	0.00	690.00	0.00
0.00	0.00	0.00	0.00	0.00	0.00	0.00	0.00	0.00	0.00	0.00	0.00	0.00	0.00	0.00	0.00	0.00	0.00	930.00	0.00
0.00	0.00	0.00	0.00	0.00	0.00	0.00	0.00	0.00	0.00	0.00	0.00	0.00	0.00	0.00	0.00	0.00	0.00	140.00	0.00
0.00	0.00	0.00	0.00	0.00	0.00	0.00	0.00	0.00	0.00	0.00	0.00	0.00	0.00	0.00	0.00	0.00	0.00	150.00	0.00
0.00	0.00	0.00	0.00	0.00	0.00	0.00	0.00	0.00	0.00	0.00	0.00	0.00	0.00	0.00	0.00	0.00	0.00	0.00	0.00
0.00	0.00	0.00	0.00	0.00	0.00	0.00	0.00	0.00	0.00	0.00	0.00	0.00	0.00	0.00	0.00	0.00	0.00	690.00	0.00
0.00	0.00	0.00	0.00	0.00	0.00	0.00	0.00	0.00	0.00	0.00	0.00	0.00	0.00	0.00	0.00	0.00	0.00	840.00	0.00
0.00	0.00	0.00	0.00	0.00	0.00	0.00	0.00	0.00	0.00	0.00	0.00	0.00	0.00	0.00	0.00	0.00	0.00	1500.00	0.00
0.00	0.00	0.00	0.00	0.00	0.00	0.00	0.00	0.00	0.00	0.00	0.00	0.00	0.00	0.00	0.00	0.00	0.00	1150.00	0.00
0.00	0.00	0.00	0.00	0.00	0.00	0.00	0.00	0.00	0.00	0.00	0.00	0.00	0.00	0.00	0.00	0.00	0.00	1050.00	0.00
0.00	0.00	0.00	0.00	0.00	0.00	0.00	0.00	0.00	0.00	0.00	0.00	0.00	0.00	0.00	0.00	0.00	0.00	890.00	0.00
0.00	0.00	0.00	0.00	0.00	0.00	0.00	0.00	0.00	0.00	0.00	0.00	0.00	0.00	0.00	0.00	0.00	0.00	820.00	0.00
0.00	0.00	0.00	0.00	0.00	0.00	0.00	0.00	0.00	0.00	0.00	0.00	0.00	0.00	0.00	0.00	0.00	0.00	1100.00	0.00
0.00	0.00	0.00	0.00	0.00	0.00	0.00	0.00	0.00	0.00	0.00	0.00	0.00	0.00	0.00	0.00	0.00	0.00	5.00	0.00
0.00	0.00	0.00	0.00	0.00	0.00	0.00	0.00	0.00	0.00	0.00	0.00	0.00	0.00	0.00	0.00	0.00	0.00	580.00	0.00
0.00	0.00	0.00	0.00	0.00	0.00	0.00	0.00	0.00	0.00	0.00	0.00	0.00	0.00	0.00	0.00	0.00	0.00	1420.00	0.00
0.00	0.00	0.00	0.00	0.00	0.00	0.00	0.00	0.00	0.00	0.00	0.00	0.00	0.00	0.00	0.00	0.00	0.00	940.00	0.00
0.00	0.00	0.00	0.00	0.00	0.00	0.00	0.00	0.00	0.00	0.00	0.00	0.00	0.00	0.00	0.00	0.00	0.00	1100.00	0.00
0.00	0.00	0.00	0.00	0.00	0.00	0.00	0.00	0.00	0.00	0.00	0.00	0.00	0.00	0.00	0.00	0.00	0.00	1090.00	0.00
0.00	0.00	0.00	0.00	0.00	0.00	0.00	0.00	0.00	0.00	0.00	0.00	0.00	0.00	0.00	0.00	0.00	0.00	1040.00	0.00
0.00	0.00	0.00	0.00	0.00	390.00	25.80	0.00	0.00	0.00	0.00	0.00	0.00	240.00	3.60	0.00	0.00	0.00	1281.00	0.00
0.00	0.00	0.00	0.00	0.00	0.00	6.00	0.00	0.00	0.00	0.00	0.00	0.00	0.00	0.36	0.00	0.00	0.00	640.00	0.00
0.00	0.00	0.00	0.00	0.00	0.00	0.00	0.00	0.00	0.00	0.00	0.00	0.00	0.00	14.94	0.00	0.00	0.00	495.00	0.00
0.00	0.00	0.00	0.00	0.00	530.00	28.20	0.00	0.00	0.00	0.00	0.00	0.00	220.00	3.06	0.00	0.00	0.00	1817.00	0.00
0.00	0.00	0.00	0.00	0.00	0.00	0.00	0.00	0.00	0.00	0.00	0.00	0.00	0.60	0.18	0.00	0.00	0.00	1267.00	0.00
0.00	0.00	0.00	0.00	0.00	0.00	0.00	0.00	0.00	0.00	0.00	0.00	0.00	0.00	0.00	0.00	0.00	0.00	790.00	0.00
0.00	0.00	0.00	0.00	0.00	0.00	0.00	0.00	0.00	0.00	0.00	0.00	0.00	150.00	1.80	0.00	0.00	0.00	0.00	0.00
0.00	0.00	0.00	0.00	0.00	220.00	0.00	0.00	0.00	0.00	0.00	0.00	0.00	550.00	0.54	0.00	0.00	0.00	861.00	0.00

USDA ID Code	Food Name	Weight in Grams*	Quantity of Units	Unit of Measure	Protein (g)	Fat (g)	Carbohydrate (g)	Kilocalories	Caffeine (g)	Fiber (g)	Cholesterol (mg)	Saturated Fat (g)
228	Denny's-Chicken Fried Steak Skil	737.0000	1.000	Serving	60.00	104.00	119.00	1745.00	0.00	26.00	607.00	28.00
229	Denny's-Cinnamon Swirl French To	340.0000	1.000	Serving	23.00	49.00	124.00	1030.00	0.00	4.00	280.00	21.00
230	Denny's-Cinnamon Swirl Slam	368.5500	1.000	Serving	38.00	78.00	68.00	1105.00	0.00	2.00	635.00	26.00
231	Denny's-Country Fried Potatoes	170.0000	1.000	Serving	3.00	35.00	23.00	515.00	0.00	9.00	8.00	8.00
232	Denny's-Egg Beaters, Egg Substit	56.7000	1.000	Serving	5.00	5.00	1.00	71.00	0.00	0.00	1.00	1.00
233	Denny's-Eggs Benedict	425.2500	1.000	Serving	34.00	46.00	34.00	695.00	0.00	1.00	515.00	11.00
234	Denny's-English Muffin, Dry, 1mu	113.4000	1.000	Each	5.00	1.00	24.00	125.00	0.00	1.00	0.00	0.00
235	Denny's-Flour Tortillas and Sals	156.0000	1.000	Serving	6.00	8.00	50.50	281.00	0.00	4.00	0.00	1.50
236	Denny's-French Slam	397.0000	1.000	Serving	44.00	71.00	58.00	1029.00	0.00	2.00	777.00	20.00
237	Denny's-French Toast (2)	199.0000	2.000	Each	16.00	24.00	54.00	507.00	0.00	3.00	219.00	6.00
238	Denny's-Grand Slam Slugger	340.0000	1.000	Serving	32.00	46.00	58.00	789.00	0.00	2.00	487.00	14.00
239	Denny's-Grits	113.0000	0.500	Cup	2.00	0.00	18.00	80.00	0.00	0.00	0.00	0.00
241	Denny's-Ham, Grilled, sliced	85.0000	3.000	Ounce	15.00	3.00	2.00	94.00	0.00	0.00	23.00	1.00
240	Denny's-Ham'nCheddar Omelette	283.5000	1.000	Each	37.00	45.00	4.00	581.00	0.00	0.00	672.00	8.00
242	Denny's-Hashed Browns	113.4000	1.000	Serving	2.00	14.00	20.00	218.00	0.00	2.00	0.00	2.00
243	Denny's-Kelloggs Dry Cereal	28.3500	1.000	Serving	2.00	0.00	23.00	100.00	0.00	1.00	0.00	0.00
244	Denny's-Lumberjack Slam	538.6500	1.000	Serving	54.00	70.00	118.00	1259.00	0.00	5.00	481.00	18.00
245	Denny's-Meat Lover's Skillet	425.2500	1.000	Serving	41.00	93.00	24.00	1147.00	0.00	7.00	460.00	26.00
246	Denny's-Oatmeal N' Fixins	538.6500	1.000	Serving	13.00	6.00	95.00	460.00	0.00	7.00	11.00	3.00
247	Denny's-One Egg	56.7000	1.000	Each	6.00	10.00	0.50	120.00	0.00	0.00	210.00	3.00
248	Denny's-Original Grand Slam	283.5000	1.000	Serving	34.00	50.00	65.00	795.00	0.00	2.00	460.00	14.00
249	Denny's-Pork Chop & Eggs	354.3800	1.000	Serving	55.00	47.00	6.00	673.00	0.00	0.00	571.00	13.00
250	Denny's-Quaker Oatmeal	113.4000	0.500	Cup	5.00	2.00	18.00	100.00	0.00	3.00	0.00	0.00
251	Denny's-Sausage Gravy	113.4000	1.000	Serving	3.00	10.00	6.00	126.00	0.00	0.00	12.00	2.00
252	Denny's-Sausage, 4 Links	85.0000	4.000	Each	16.00	32.00	0.00	354.00	0.00	0.00	64.00	12.00
253	Denny's-Sirloin Steak & Eggs	255.0000	1.000	Serving	43.00	49.00	1.00	622.00	0.00	1.00	572.00	18.00
254	Denny's-T-bone Steak & Eggs	397.0000	1.000	Serving	73.00	77.00	1.00	991.00	0.00	1.00	657.00	31.00
255	Denny's-Toast, Dry, 1slice	28.3500	1.000	Slice	3.00	1.00	17.00	90.00	0.00	1.00	0.00	0.00
256	Denny's-Two Egg Breakfast	312.0000	1.000	Serving	31.00	67.00	24.00	825.00	0.00	2.00	538.00	17.00
257	Denny's-Ultimate Omelette	368.5500	1.000	Each	30.00	47.00	9.00	594.00	0.00	2.00	639.00	12.00
258	Denny's-Veggie-Cheese Omelette	340.0000	1.000	Each	26.00	39.00	9.00	480.00	0.00	2.00	644.00	13.00
	Dunkin' Donuts-Apple Filled w/ C	79.0000	1.000	Each	5.00	11.00	33.00	250.00	0.00	1.00	0.00	0.00
	Dunkin' Donuts-Bavarian Filled w	79.0000	1.000	Each	5.00	11.00	32.00	240.00	0.00	2.00	0.00	0.00
	Dunkin' Donuts-Blueberry Filled	67.0000	1.000	Each	4.00	8.00	29.00	210.00	0.00	2.00	0.00	0.00
	Dunkin' Donuts-Buttermilk Ring,	74.0000	1.000	Each	4.00	14.00	37.00	290.00	0.00	1.00	10.00	0.00
	Dunkin' Donuts-Cake Ring, Plain	62.0000	1.000	Each	4.00	17.00	25.00	270.00	0.00	1.00	0.00	0.00
	Dunkin' Donuts-Chocolate Rings,	71.0000	1.000	Each	3.50	21.00	34.00	324.00	0.00	1.90	0.00	0.00
	Dunkin' Donuts-Coffee Roll, Glaz	81.0000	1.000	Each	5.00	12.00	37.00	280.00	0.00	2.00	0.00	0.00
	Dunkin' Donuts-Cookie, Chocolate	43.0000	1.000	Each	3.00	10.00	25.00	200.00	0.00	1.00	30.00	0.00
	Dunkin' Donuts-Cookie, Chocolate	43.0000	1.000	Each	3.00	11.00	23.00	210.00	0.00	2.00	30.00	0.00
	Dunkin' Donuts-Cookie, Oatmeal P	46.0000	1.000	Each	3.00	9.00	28.00	200.00	0.00	1.00	25.00	0.00
	Dunkin' Donuts-Croissant, Almond	105.0000	1.000	Each	8.00	27.00	38.00	420.00	0.00	3.00	0.00	0.00
	Dunkin' Donuts-Croissant, Chocol	94.0000	1.000	Each	7.00	29.00	38.00	440.00	0.00	3.00	0.00	0.00
	Dunkin' Donuts-Croissant, Plain	72.0000	1.000	Each	7.00	19.00	27.00	310.00	0.00	2.00	0.00	0.00
	Dunkin' Donuts-Cruller, Glazed F	38.0000	1.000	Each	2.00	8.00	16.00	140.00	0.00	0.00	30.00	0.00
	Dunkin' Donuts-Filled, Jelly	67.0000	1.000	Each	4.00	9.00	31.00	220.00	0.00	1.00	0.00	0.00
	Dunkin' Donuts-Filled, Lemon	79.0000	1.000	Each	4.00	12.00	33.00	260.00	0.00	1.00	0.00	0.00
	Dunkin' Donuts-Muffin, Apple 'n	100.0000	1.000	Each	6.00	8.00	52.00	300.00	0.00	2.00	25.00	0.00
	Dunkin' Donuts-Muffin, Banana Nu	103.0000	1.000	Each	7.00	10.00	49.00	310.00	0.00	3.00	30.00	0.00
	Dunkin' Donuts-Muffin, Blueberry	101.0000	1.000	Each	6.00	8.00	46.00	280.00	0.00	2.00	30.00	0.00
	Dunkin' Donuts-Muffin, Bran w/ R	104.0000	1.000	Each	6.00	9.00	51.00	310.00	0.00	4.00	15.00	0.00
	Dunkin' Donuts-Muffin, Corn	96.0000	1.000	Each	7.00	12.00	51.00	340.00	0.00	1.00	40.00	0.00
	Dunkin' Donuts-Muffin, Cranberry	98.0000	1.000	Each	6.00	9.00	44.00	290.00	0.00	2.00	25.00	0.00

Page Key: A2 = Baby Food   A2 = Baked Goods   A8 = Beverages   A14 = Breads/Grains and Pasta   A18 = Breakfast Foods/Cereals   A26 = Dairy and Eggs   A40 = Fats and Oils
A42 = Fruits and Vegetables   A52 = Meats and Beans   A60 = Nuts and Seeds   A62 = Frozen Entrees and Packaged Foods   A76 = Restaurant Chains–Fast Foods
A92 = Restaurant Chains–Other   A106 = Seafood and Fish   A110 = Snacks and Sweets   A120 = Soups   A122 = Supplements   A126 = Toppings and Sauces

Monounsaturated Fat (g)	Polyunsaturated Fat (g)	Vitamin D (mg)	Vitamin K (mg)	Vitamin E (mg)	Vitamin A (re)	Vitamin C (mg)	Thiamin (mg)	Riboflavin (mg)	Niacin (mg)	Vitamin B6 (mg)	Folate (mcg)	Vitamin B12 (mcg)	Calcium (mg)	Iron (mg)	Magnesium (mg)	Phosphorus (mg)	Potassium (mg)	Sodium (mg)	Zinc (mg)
0.00	0.00	0.00	0.00	0.00	140.00	36.00	0.00	0.00	0.00	0.00	0.00	0.00	130.00	8.10	0.00	0.00	0.00	6184.00	0.00
0.00	0.00	0.00	0.00	0.00	370.00	0.00	0.00	0.00	0.00	0.00	0.00	0.00	180.00	6.48	0.00	0.00	0.00	675.00	0.00
0.00	0.00	0.00	0.00	0.00	540.00	0.00	0.00	0.00	0.00	0.00	0.00	0.00	150.00	5.58	0.00	0.00	0.00	1374.00	0.00
0.00	0.00	0.00	0.00	0.00	0.00	0.00	0.00	0.00	0.00	0.00	0.00	0.00	60.00	1.08	0.00	0.00	0.00	805.00	0.00
0.00	0.00	0.00	0.00	0.00	370.00	0.00	0.00	0.00	0.00	0.00	0.00	0.00	20.00	1.08	0.00	0.00	0.00	138.00	0.00
0.00	0.00	0.00	0.00	0.00	530.00	0.00	0.00	0.00	0.00	0.00	0.00	0.00	190.00	3.96	0.00	0.00	0.00	1718.00	0.00
0.00	0.00	0.00	0.00	0.00	0.00	0.00	0.00	0.00	0.00	0.00	0.00	0.00	80.00	1.80	0.00	0.00	0.00	0.00	0.00
0.00	0.00	0.00	0.00	0.00	150.00	21.00	0.00	0.00	0.00	0.00	0.00	0.00	200.00	2.70	0.00	0.00	0.00	1031.00	0.00
0.00	0.00	0.00	0.00	0.00	530.00	0.00	0.00	0.00	0.00	0.00	0.00	0.00	120.00	5.58	0.00	0.00	0.00	1428.00	0.00
0.00	0.00	0.00	0.00	0.00	130.00	0.00	0.00	0.00	0.00	0.00	0.00	0.00	130.00	3.60	0.00	0.00	0.00	594.00	0.00
0.00	0.00	0.00	0.00	0.00	140.00	0.00	0.00	0.00	0.00	0.00	0.00	0.00	250.00	4.68	0.00	0.00	0.00	1438.00	0.00
0.00	0.00	0.00	0.00	0.00	0.00	0.00	0.00	0.00	0.00	0.00	0.00	0.00	0.00	0.72	0.00	0.00	0.00	520.00	0.00
0.00	0.00	0.00	0.00	0.00	0.00	0.00	0.00	0.00	0.00	0.00	0.00	0.00	0.00	0.72	0.00	0.00	0.00	761.00	0.00
0.00	0.00	0.00	0.00	0.00	390.00	0.00	0.00	0.00	0.00	0.00	0.00	0.00	380.00	2.88	0.00	0.00	0.00	1180.00	0.00
0.00	0.00	0.00	0.00	0.00	30.00	6.60	0.00	0.00	0.00	0.00	0.00	0.00	10.00	0.36	0.00	0.00	0.00	424.00	0.00
0.00	0.00	0.00	0.00	0.00	350.00	9.60	0.00	0.00	0.00	0.00	0.00	0.00	0.00	3.42	0.00	0.00	0.00	276.00	0.00
0.00	0.00	0.00	0.00	0.00	370.00	7.80	0.00	0.00	0.00	0.00	0.00	0.00	230.00	5.22	0.00	0.00	0.00	4028.00	0.00
0.00	0.00	0.00	0.00	0.00	470.00	4.20	0.00	0.00	0.00	0.00	0.00	0.00	220.00	3.42	0.00	0.00	0.00	2507.00	0.00
0.00	0.00	0.00	0.00	0.00	80.00	12.00	0.00	0.00	0.00	0.00	0.00	0.00	250.00	2.70	0.00	0.00	0.00	87.00	0.00
0.00	0.00	0.00	0.00	0.00	20.00	3.60	0.00	0.00	0.00	0.00	0.00	0.00	0.00	0.72	0.00	0.00	0.00	120.00	0.00
0.00	0.00	0.00	0.00	0.00	330.00	0.00	0.00	0.00	0.00	0.00	0.00	0.00	160.00	3.42	0.00	0.00	0.00	2237.00	0.00
0.00	0.00	0.00	0.00	0.00	150.00	0.00	0.00	0.00	0.00	0.00	0.00	0.00	50.00	3.06	0.00	0.00	0.00	1582.00	0.00
0.00	0.00	0.00	0.00	0.00	0.00	0.00	0.00	0.00	0.00	0.00	0.00	0.00	10.00	0.90	0.00	0.00	0.00	175.00	0.00
0.00	0.00	0.00	0.00	0.00	0.00	0.00	0.00	0.00	0.00	0.00	0.00	0.00	10.00	0.18	0.00	0.00	0.00	477.00	0.00
0.00	0.00	0.00	0.00	0.00	4.00	0.00	0.00	0.00	0.00	0.00	0.00	0.00	10.00	1.26	0.00	0.00	0.00	944.00	0.00
0.00	0.00	0.00	0.00	0.00	160.00	1.80	0.00	0.00	0.00	0.00	0.00	0.00	130.00	5.94	0.00	0.00	0.00	632.00	0.00
0.00	0.00	0.00	0.00	0.00	150.00	2.40	0.00	0.00	0.00	0.00	0.00	0.00	200.00	10.80	0.00	0.00	0.00	1003.00	0.00
0.00	0.00	0.00	0.00	0.00	0.00	0.00	0.00	0.00	0.00	0.00	0.00	0.00	30.00	0.72	0.00	0.00	0.00	166.00	0.00
0.00	0.00	0.00	0.00	0.00	170.00	7.80	0.00	0.00	0.00	0.00	0.00	0.00	80.00	3.24	0.00	0.00	0.00	1765.00	0.00
0.00	0.00	0.00	0.00	0.00	320.00	55.20	0.00	0.00	0.00	0.00	0.00	0.00	80.00	3.60	0.00	0.00	0.00	939.00	0.00
0.00	0.00	0.00	0.00	0.00	390.00	16.20	0.00	0.00	0.00	0.00	0.00	0.00	280.00	2.70	0.00	0.00	0.00	535.00	0.00
0.00	0.00	0.00	0.00	0.00	0.00	0.00	0.00	0.00	0.00	0.00	0.00	0.00	0.00	0.00	0.00	0.00	0.00	280.00	0.00
0.00	0.00	0.00	0.00	0.00	0.00	0.00	0.00	0.00	0.00	0.00	0.00	0.00	0.00	0.00	0.00	0.00	0.00	260.00	0.00
0.00	0.00	0.00	0.00	0.00	0.00	0.00	0.00	0.00	0.00	0.00	0.00	0.00	0.00	0.00	0.00	0.00	0.00	240.00	0.00
0.00	0.00	0.00	0.00	0.00	0.00	0.00	0.00	0.00	0.00	0.00	0.00	0.00	0.00	0.00	0.00	0.00	0.00	370.00	0.00
0.00	0.00	0.00	0.00	0.00	0.00	0.00	0.00	0.00	0.00	0.00	0.00	0.00	0.00	0.00	0.00	0.00	0.00	330.00	0.00
0.00	0.00	0.00	0.00	0.00	0.00	0.00	0.00	0.00	0.00	0.00	0.00	0.00	0.00	0.00	0.00	0.00	0.00	383.00	0.00
0.00	0.00	0.00	0.00	0.00	0.00	0.00	0.00	0.00	0.00	0.00	0.00	0.00	0.00	0.00	0.00	0.00	0.00	310.00	0.00
0.00	0.00	0.00	0.00	0.00	0.00	0.00	0.00	0.00	0.00	0.00	0.00	0.00	0.00	0.00	0.00	0.00	0.00	110.00	0.00
0.00	0.00	0.00	0.00	0.00	0.00	0.00	0.00	0.00	0.00	0.00	0.00	0.00	0.00	0.00	0.00	0.00	0.00	100.00	0.00
0.00	0.00	0.00	0.00	0.00	0.00	0.00	0.00	0.00	0.00	0.00	0.00	0.00	0.00	0.00	0.00	0.00	0.00	100.00	0.00
0.00	0.00	0.00	0.00	0.00	0.00	0.00	0.00	0.00	0.00	0.00	0.00	0.00	0.00	0.00	0.00	0.00	0.00	280.00	0.00
0.00	0.00	0.00	0.00	0.00	0.00	0.00	0.00	0.00	0.00	0.00	0.00	0.00	0.00	0.00	0.00	0.00	0.00	220.00	0.00
0.00	0.00	0.00	0.00	0.00	0.00	0.00	0.00	0.00	0.00	0.00	0.00	0.00	0.00	0.00	0.00	0.00	0.00	240.00	0.00
0.00	0.00	0.00	0.00	0.00	0.00	0.00	0.00	0.00	0.00	0.00	0.00	0.00	0.00	0.00	0.00	0.00	0.00	130.00	0.00
0.00	0.00	0.00	0.00	0.00	0.00	0.00	0.00	0.00	0.00	0.00	0.00	0.00	0.00	0.00	0.00	0.00	0.00	230.00	0.00
0.00	0.00	0.00	0.00	0.00	0.00	0.00	0.00	0.00	0.00	0.00	0.00	0.00	0.00	0.00	0.00	0.00	0.00	280.00	0.00
0.00	0.00	0.00	0.00	0.00	0.00	0.00	0.00	0.00	0.00	0.00	0.00	0.00	0.00	0.00	0.00	0.00	0.00	360.00	0.00
0.00	0.00	0.00	0.00	0.00	0.00	0.00	0.00	0.00	0.00	0.00	0.00	0.00	0.00	0.00	0.00	0.00	0.00	410.00	0.00
0.00	0.00	0.00	0.00	0.00	0.00	0.00	0.00	0.00	0.00	0.00	0.00	0.00	0.00	0.00	0.00	0.00	0.00	340.00	0.00
0.00	0.00	0.00	0.00	0.00	0.00	0.00	0.00	0.00	0.00	0.00	0.00	0.00	0.00	0.00	0.00	0.00	0.00	560.00	0.00
0.00	0.00	0.00	0.00	0.00	0.00	0.00	0.00	0.00	0.00	0.00	0.00	0.00	0.00	0.00	0.00	0.00	0.00	560.00	0.00
0.00	0.00	0.00	0.00	0.00	0.00	0.00	0.00	0.00	0.00	0.00	0.00	0.00	0.00	0.00	0.00	0.00	0.00	360.00	0.00

USDA ID Code	Food Name	Weight in Grams*	Quantity of Units	Unit of Measure	Protein (g)	Fat (g)	Carbohydrate (g)	Kilocalories	Caffeine (g)	Fiber (g)	Cholesterol (mg)	Saturated Fat (g)
	Dunkin' Donuts-Muffin, Oat Bran	100.0000	1.000	Each	7.00	11.00	50.00	330.00	0.00	3.00	0.00	0.00
	Dunkin' Donuts-Yeast Ring, Choco	55.0000	1.000	Each	4.00	10.00	25.00	200.00	0.00	1.00	0.00	0.00
	Dunkin' Donuts-Yeast Ring, Glaze	55.0000	1.000	Each	4.00	9.00	26.00	200.00	0.00	1.00	0.00	0.00
265	Einstein Bros.-Almond Delight	360.0000	12.000	Fl Oz	8.00	4.50	29.00	190.00	0.00	0.00	20.00	3.00
266	Einstein Bros.-Almond Delight, I	480.0000	16.000	Fl Oz	7.00	4.00	28.00	180.00	0.00	0.00	15.00	2.50
267	Einstein Bros.-Almond Delight, N	360.0000	12.000	Fl Oz	8.00	0.00	29.00	150.00	0.00	0.00	5.00	0.00
268	Einstein Bros.-Americano	240.0000	8.000	Fl Oz	0.00	0.00	0.00	0.00	0.00	0.00	0.00	0.00
269	Einstein Bros.-Americano, Iced	360.0000	8.000	Fl Oz	0.00	0.00	0.00	0.00	0.00	0.00	0.00	0.00
270	Einstein Bros.-Bagel Chips, Blue	28.0000	1.000	Each	3.00	1.00	19.00	90.00	0.00	1.00	0.00	0.00
271	Einstein Bros.-Bagel Chips, Cinn	28.0000	1.000	Each	3.00	1.00	19.00	90.00	0.00	1.00	0.00	0.00
272	Einstein Bros.-Bagel Chips, Plain	28.0000	1.000	Each	3.00	0.00	18.00	90.00	0.00	1.00	0.00	0.00
273	Einstein Bros.-Bagel Chips, Sour	28.0000	1.000	Each	3.00	1.00	18.00	90.00	0.00	1.00	0.00	0.00
274	Einstein Bros.-Bagel Chips, Sun-	28.0000	1.000	Each	3.00	1.00	17.00	90.00	0.00	1.00	0.00	0.00
275	Einstein Bros.-Bagel Chips, Sunf	28.0000	1.000	Each	3.00	2.00	18.00	100.00	0.00	1.00	0.00	0.00
276	Einstein Bros.-Bagel, Blueberry,	113.0000	1.000	Each	11.00	1.00	77.00	350.00	0.00	3.00	0.00	0.00
277	Einstein Bros.-Bagel, Choc Chip	113.0000	1.000	Each	11.00	3.00	76.00	370.00	0.00	3.00	0.00	2.00
278	Einstein Bros.-Bagel, Cinnamon R	113.0000	1.000	Each	11.00	1.00	78.00	350.00	0.00	2.00	0.00	0.00
279	Einstein Bros.-Bagel, Cinnamon S	106.0000	1.000	Each	10.00	1.00	74.00	330.00	0.00	2.00	0.00	0.00
280	Einstein Bros.-Bagel, Cranberry	113.0000	1.000	Each	10.00	1.00	78.00	350.00	0.00	3.00	0.00	0.00
281	Einstein Bros.-Bagel, Egg	106.0000	1.000	Each	11.00	3.00	69.00	340.00	0.00	2.00	35.00	1.00
282	Einstein Bros.-Bagel, Everything	111.0000	1.000	Each	13.00	2.00	75.00	340.00	0.00	2.00	0.00	0.00
283	Einstein Bros.-Bagel, Garlic, Ch	119.0000	1.000	Each	13.00	3.00	79.00	380.00	0.00	4.00	0.00	1.00
284	Einstein Bros.-Bagel, Honey 8 Gr	106.0000	1.000	Each	11.00	1.00	69.00	320.00	0.00	4.00	0.00	0.00
285	Einstein Bros.-Bagel, Jalapeno	106.0000	1.000	Each	11.00	1.00	71.00	330.00	0.00	2.00	0.00	0.00
286	Einstein Bros.-Bagel, Nutty Bana	113.0000	1.000	Each	11.00	3.00	74.00	360.00	0.00	2.00	0.00	1.00
287	Einstein Bros.-Bagel, Onion, Chp	106.0000	1.000	Each	11.00	1.00	71.00	330.00	0.00	2.00	0.00	0.00
288	Einstein Bros.-Bagel, Plain	106.0000	1.000	Each	11.00	1.00	71.00	320.00	0.00	2.00	0.00	0.00
289	Einstein Bros.-Bagel, Poppy Dip'	111.0000	1.000	Each	12.00	2.00	74.00	350.00	0.00	2.00	0.00	0.00
290	Einstein Bros.-Bagel, Pumpernick	106.0000	1.000	Each	11.00	1.00	68.00	320.00	0.00	3.00	0.00	0.00
291	Einstein Bros.-Bagel, Rye, Marbl	113.0000	1.000	Each	11.00	2.00	73.00	340.00	0.00	3.00	0.00	0.00
292	Einstein Bros.-Bagel, Salt	111.0000	1.000	Each	11.00	1.00	73.00	330.00	0.00	2.00	0.00	0.00
293	Einstein Bros.-Bagel, Sesame Dip	117.0000	1.000	Each	11.00	5.00	75.00	380.00	0.00	3.00	0.00	1.00
294	Einstein Bros.-Bagel, Spinach He	106.0000	1.000	Each	11.00	1.00	68.00	310.00	0.00	3.00	0.00	0.00
295	Einstein Bros.-Bagel, Sun-dried	106.0000	1.000	Each	11.00	1.00	69.00	320.00	0.00	3.00	0.00	0.00
296	Einstein Bros.-Bagel, Sunflower	106.0000	1.000	Each	12.00	5.00	66.00	350.00	0.00	3.00	0.00	1.00
297	Einstein Bros.-Bagel, Veggie Con	106.0000	1.000	Each	11.00	1.00	70.00	320.00	0.00	2.00	0.00	0.00
298	Einstein Bros.-Brownie, Choc Cho	79.5200	2.800	Ounce	3.00	15.00	51.00	346.00	0.00	2.00	18.00	4.00
299	Einstein Bros.-Café Au Lait	360.0000	12.000	Fl Oz	6.00	3.50	9.00	100.00	0.00	0.00	15.00	2.00
300	Einstein Bros.-Café Au Lait, Non	360.0000	12.000	Fl Oz	6.00	0.00	10.00	70.00	0.00	0.00	5.00	0.00
301	Einstein Bros.-Café Latte, Iced	480.0000	16.000	Fl Oz	8.00	4.50	12.00	120.00	0.00	0.00	20.00	3.00
302	Einstein Bros.-Café Latte, Non F	360.0000	12.000	Fl Oz	9.00	0.00	14.00	100.00	0.00	0.00	5.00	0.00
303	Einstein Bros.-Café Latte, Reg	360.0000	12.000	Fl Oz	9.00	5.00	13.00	140.00	0.00	0.00	20.00	3.50
304	Einstein Bros.-Cappuccino	360.0000	12.000	Fl Oz	6.00	3.50	9.00	90.00	0.00	0.00	15.00	2.00
305	Einstein Bros.-Cappuccino, Non F	360.0000	12.000	Fl Oz	6.00	0.00	9.00	60.00	0.00	0.00	5.00	0.00
306	Einstein Bros.-Cheese Melt, Gril	213.0000	1.000	Each	25.00	12.00	74.00	500.00	0.00	3.00	35.00	7.00
307	Einstein Bros.-Chicken Salad, Re	113.6000	4.000	Ounce	16.00	7.00	4.00	150.00	0.00	0.00	45.00	1.50
308	Einstein Bros.-Chili, Turkey, Lo	198.8000	7.000	Ounce	6.00	2.50	9.00	80.00	0.00	3.00	20.00	0.00
309	Einstein Bros.-Chili, Vegetarian	198.8000	7.000	Ounce	3.00	2.00	23.00	120.00	0.00	4.00	0.00	0.00
310	Einstein Bros.-Chix Salad Bagel	324.0000	1.000	Each	28.00	9.00	79.00	510.00	0.00	4.00	45.00	2.00
311	Einstein Bros.-Choc, Hot, Lower	360.0000	12.000	Fl Oz	9.00	7.00	39.00	260.00	0.00	0.00	5.00	6.00
312	Einstein Bros.-Chocolate, Hot, R	360.0000	12.000	Fl Oz	9.00	11.00	39.00	290.00	0.00	0.00	20.00	8.00
313	Einstein Bros.-Chowder, Corn, Am	198.8000	7.000	Ounce	5.00	6.00	25.00	180.00	0.00	2.00	5.00	1.50
314	Einstein Bros.-Chowder, NE Clam	198.8000	7.000	Ounce	9.00	9.00	15.00	170.00	0.00	1.00	25.00	2.50

Page Key: A2 = Baby Food   A2 = Baked Goods   A8 = Beverages   A14 = Breads/Grains and Pasta   A18 = Breakfast Foods/Cereals   A26 = Dairy and Eggs   A40 = Fats and Oils   A42 = Fruits and Vegetables   A52 = Meats and Beans   A60 = Nuts and Seeds   A62 = Frozen Entrees and Packaged Foods   A76 = Restaurant Chains–Fast Foods   A92 = Restaurant Chains–Other   A106 = Seafood and Fish   A110 = Snacks and Sweets   A120 = Soups   A122 = Supplements   A126 = Toppings and Sauces

Monounsaturated Fat (g)	Polyunsaturated Fat (g)	Vitamin D (mg)	Vitamin K (mg)	Vitamin E (mg)	Vitamin A (re)	Vitamin C (mg)	Thiamin (mg)	Riboflavin (mg)	Niacin (mg)	Vitamin B$_6$ (mg)	Folate (mcg)	Vitamin B$_{12}$ (mcg)	Calcium (mg)	Iron (mg)	Magnesium (mg)	Phosphorus (mg)	Potassium (mg)	Sodium (mg)	Zinc (mg)
0.00	0.00	0.00	0.00	0.00	0.00	0.00	0.00	0.00	0.00	0.00	0.00	0.00	0.00	0.00	0.00	0.00	0.00	450.00	0.00
0.00	0.00	0.00	0.00	0.00	0.00	0.00	0.00	0.00	0.00	0.00	0.00	0.00	0.00	0.00	0.00	0.00	0.00	190.00	0.00
0.00	0.00	0.00	0.00	0.00	0.00	0.00	0.00	0.00	0.00	0.00	0.00	0.00	0.00	0.00	0.00	0.00	0.00	230.00	0.00
0.00	0.00	0.00	0.00	0.00	0.00	0.00	0.00	0.00	0.00	0.00	0.00	0.00	0.00	0.00	0.00	0.00	0.00	130.00	0.00
0.00	0.00	0.00	0.00	0.00	0.00	0.00	0.00	0.00	0.00	0.00	0.00	0.00	0.00	0.00	0.00	0.00	0.00	120.00	0.00
0.00	0.00	0.00	0.00	0.00	0.00	0.00	0.00	0.00	0.00	0.00	0.00	0.00	0.00	0.00	0.00	0.00	0.00	135.00	0.00
0.00	0.00	0.00	0.00	0.00	0.00	0.00	0.00	0.00	0.00	0.00	0.00	0.00	0.00	0.00	0.00	0.00	0.00	0.00	0.00
0.00	0.00	0.00	0.00	0.00	0.00	0.00	0.00	0.00	0.00	0.00	0.00	0.00	0.00	0.00	0.00	0.00	0.00	0.00	0.00
0.00	0.00	0.00	0.00	0.00	0.00	0.00	0.00	0.00	0.00	0.00	0.00	0.00	0.00	0.00	0.00	0.00	0.00	105.00	0.00
0.00	0.00	0.00	0.00	0.00	0.00	0.00	0.00	0.00	0.00	0.00	0.00	0.00	0.00	0.00	0.00	0.00	0.00	120.00	0.00
0.00	0.00	0.00	0.00	0.00	0.00	0.00	0.00	0.00	0.00	0.00	0.00	0.00	0.00	0.00	0.00	0.00	0.00	140.00	0.00
0.00	0.00	0.00	0.00	0.00	0.00	0.00	0.00	0.00	0.00	0.00	0.00	0.00	0.00	0.00	0.00	0.00	0.00	120.00	0.00
0.00	0.00	0.00	0.00	0.00	0.00	0.00	0.00	0.00	0.00	0.00	0.00	0.00	0.00	0.00	0.00	0.00	0.00	130.00	0.00
0.00	0.00	0.00	0.00	0.00	0.00	0.00	0.00	0.00	0.00	0.00	0.00	0.00	0.00	0.00	0.00	0.00	0.00	190.00	0.00
0.00	0.00	0.00	0.00	0.00	0.00	0.00	0.00	0.00	0.00	0.00	0.00	0.00	0.00	0.00	0.00	0.00	0.00	510.00	0.00
0.00	0.00	0.00	0.00	0.00	0.00	0.00	0.00	0.00	0.00	0.00	0.00	0.00	0.00	0.00	0.00	0.00	0.00	500.00	0.00
0.00	0.00	0.00	0.00	0.00	0.00	0.00	0.00	0.00	0.00	0.00	0.00	0.00	0.00	0.00	0.00	0.00	0.00	490.00	0.00
0.00	0.00	0.00	0.00	0.00	0.00	0.00	0.00	0.00	0.00	0.00	0.00	0.00	0.00	0.00	0.00	0.00	0.00	490.00	0.00
0.00	0.00	0.00	0.00	0.00	0.00	0.00	0.00	0.00	0.00	0.00	0.00	0.00	0.00	0.00	0.00	0.00	0.00	490.00	0.00
0.00	0.00	0.00	0.00	0.00	0.00	0.00	0.00	0.00	0.00	0.00	0.00	0.00	0.00	0.00	0.00	0.00	0.00	510.00	0.00
0.00	0.00	0.00	0.00	0.00	0.00	0.00	0.00	0.00	0.00	0.00	0.00	0.00	0.00	0.00	0.00	0.00	0.00	820.00	0.00
0.00	0.00	0.00	0.00	0.00	0.00	0.00	0.00	0.00	0.00	0.00	0.00	0.00	0.00	0.00	0.00	0.00	0.00	680.00	0.00
0.00	0.00	0.00	0.00	0.00	0.00	0.00	0.00	0.00	0.00	0.00	0.00	0.00	0.00	0.00	0.00	0.00	0.00	510.00	0.00
0.00	0.00	0.00	0.00	0.00	0.00	0.00	0.00	0.00	0.00	0.00	0.00	0.00	0.00	0.00	0.00	0.00	0.00	510.00	0.00
0.00	0.00	0.00	0.00	0.00	0.00	0.00	0.00	0.00	0.00	0.00	0.00	0.00	0.00	0.00	0.00	0.00	0.00	510.00	0.00
0.00	0.00	0.00	0.00	0.00	0.00	0.00	0.00	0.00	0.00	0.00	0.00	0.00	0.00	0.00	0.00	0.00	0.00	500.00	0.00
0.00	0.00	0.00	0.00	0.00	0.00	0.00	0.00	0.00	0.00	0.00	0.00	0.00	0.00	0.00	0.00	0.00	0.00	520.00	0.00
0.00	0.00	0.00	0.00	0.00	0.00	0.00	0.00	0.00	0.00	0.00	0.00	0.00	0.00	0.00	0.00	0.00	0.00	680.00	0.00
0.00	0.00	0.00	0.00	0.00	0.00	0.00	0.00	0.00	0.00	0.00	0.00	0.00	0.00	0.00	0.00	0.00	0.00	730.00	0.00
0.00	0.00	0.00	0.00	0.00	0.00	0.00	0.00	0.00	0.00	0.00	0.00	0.00	0.00	0.00	0.00	0.00	0.00	690.00	0.00
0.00	0.00	0.00	0.00	0.00	0.00	0.00	0.00	0.00	0.00	0.00	0.00	0.00	0.00	0.00	0.00	0.00	0.00	1790.00	0.00
0.00	0.00	0.00	0.00	0.00	0.00	0.00	0.00	0.00	0.00	0.00	0.00	0.00	0.00	0.00	0.00	0.00	0.00	680.00	0.00
0.00	0.00	0.00	0.00	0.00	0.00	0.00	0.00	0.00	0.00	0.00	0.00	0.00	0.00	0.00	0.00	0.00	0.00	520.00	0.00
0.00	0.00	0.00	0.00	0.00	0.00	0.00	0.00	0.00	0.00	0.00	0.00	0.00	0.00	0.00	0.00	0.00	0.00	520.00	0.00
0.00	0.00	0.00	0.00	0.00	0.00	0.00	0.00	0.00	0.00	0.00	0.00	0.00	0.00	0.00	0.00	0.00	0.00	710.00	0.00
0.00	0.00	0.00	0.00	0.00	0.00	0.00	0.00	0.00	0.00	0.00	0.00	0.00	0.00	0.00	0.00	0.00	0.00	490.00	0.00
0.00	0.00	0.00	0.00	0.00	0.00	0.00	0.00	0.00	0.00	0.00	0.00	0.00	0.00	0.00	0.00	0.00	0.00	193.00	0.00
0.00	0.00	0.00	0.00	0.00	0.00	0.00	0.00	0.00	0.00	0.00	0.00	0.00	0.00	0.00	0.00	0.00	0.00	95.00	0.00
0.00	0.00	0.00	0.00	0.00	0.00	0.00	0.00	0.00	0.00	0.00	0.00	0.00	0.00	0.00	0.00	0.00	0.00	100.00	0.00
0.00	0.00	0.00	0.00	0.00	0.00	0.00	0.00	0.00	0.00	0.00	0.00	0.00	0.00	0.00	0.00	0.00	0.00	125.00	0.00
0.00	0.00	0.00	0.00	0.00	0.00	0.00	0.00	0.00	0.00	0.00	0.00	0.00	0.00	0.00	0.00	0.00	0.00	140.00	0.00
0.00	0.00	0.00	0.00	0.00	0.00	0.00	0.00	0.00	0.00	0.00	0.00	0.00	0.00	0.00	0.00	0.00	0.00	140.00	0.00
0.00	0.00	0.00	0.00	0.00	0.00	0.00	0.00	0.00	0.00	0.00	0.00	0.00	0.00	0.00	0.00	0.00	0.00	95.00	0.00
0.00	0.00	0.00	0.00	0.00	0.00	0.00	0.00	0.00	0.00	0.00	0.00	0.00	0.00	0.00	0.00	0.00	0.00	95.00	0.00
0.00	0.00	0.00	0.00	0.00	0.00	0.00	0.00	0.00	0.00	0.00	0.00	0.00	0.00	0.00	0.00	0.00	0.00	970.00	0.00
0.00	0.00	0.00	0.00	0.00	0.00	0.00	0.00	0.00	0.00	0.00	0.00	0.00	0.00	0.00	0.00	0.00	0.00	540.00	0.00
0.00	0.00	0.00	0.00	0.00	0.00	0.00	0.00	0.00	0.00	0.00	0.00	0.00	0.00	0.00	0.00	0.00	0.00	320.00	0.00
0.00	0.00	0.00	0.00	0.00	0.00	0.00	0.00	0.00	0.00	0.00	0.00	0.00	0.00	0.00	0.00	0.00	0.00	730.00	0.00
0.00	0.00	0.00	0.00	0.00	0.00	0.00	0.00	0.00	0.00	0.00	0.00	0.00	0.00	0.00	0.00	0.00	0.00	1060.00	0.00
0.00	0.00	0.00	0.00	0.00	0.00	0.00	0.00	0.00	0.00	0.00	0.00	0.00	0.00	0.00	0.00	0.00	0.00	160.00	0.00
0.00	0.00	0.00	0.00	0.00	0.00	0.00	0.00	0.00	0.00	0.00	0.00	0.00	0.00	0.00	0.00	0.00	0.00	160.00	0.00
0.00	0.00	0.00	0.00	0.00	0.00	0.00	0.00	0.00	0.00	0.00	0.00	0.00	0.00	0.00	0.00	0.00	0.00	670.00	0.00
0.00	0.00	0.00	0.00	0.00	0.00	0.00	0.00	0.00	0.00	0.00	0.00	0.00	0.00	0.00	0.00	0.00	0.00	820.00	0.00

USDA ID Code	Food Name	Weight in Grams*	Quantity of Units	Unit of Measure	Protein (g)	Fat (g)	Carbohydrate (g)	Kilocalories	Caffeine (g)	Fiber (g)	Cholesterol (mg)	Saturated Fat (g)
315	Einstein Bros.-Cinnamon Bun, Ice	142.0000	5.000	Ounce	11.00	16.00	89.00	545.00	0.00	3.00	20.00	5.00
316	Einstein Bros.-Coffee, Reg	360.0000	12.000	Fl Oz	0.00	0.00	0.00	0.00	0.00	0.00	0.00	0.00
317	Einstein Bros.-Coleslaw, Low Fat	113.6000	4.000	Ounce	2.00	3.50	13.00	90.00	0.00	2.00	5.00	0.50
318	Einstein Bros.-Coleslaw, Low Fat	113.6000	4.000	Ounce	1.00	3.50	13.00	90.00	0.00	2.00	5.00	0.50
319	Einstein Bros.-Cookie, Black & W	113.6000	4.000	Ounce	3.00	12.00	68.00	390.00	0.00	1.00	15.00	3.00
320	Einstein Bros.-Cookie, Chocolate	113.6000	4.000	Ounce	6.00	24.00	68.00	510.00	0.00	2.00	35.00	9.00
321	Einstein Bros.-Cookie, Oatmeal R	113.6000	4.000	Ounce	7.00	18.00	70.00	470.00	0.00	3.00	40.00	4.00
322	Einstein Bros.-Cookie, Peanut Bu	113.6000	4.000	Ounce	10.00	31.00	55.00	540.00	0.00	3.00	40.00	6.00
323	Einstein Bros.-Cookie, Sugar	113.6000	4.000	Ounce	6.00	28.00	28.00	530.00	0.00	1.00	45.00	7.00
324	Einstein Bros.-Cream Cheese, Ch	30.0000	2.000	Tbsp	2.00	9.00	2.00	100.00	0.00	0.00	30.00	6.00
325	Einstein Bros.-Cream Cheese, Pl	30.0000	2.000	Tbsp	2.00	5.00	2.00	60.00	0.00	0.00	15.00	3.00
326	Einstein Bros.-Cream Cheese, Cra	30.0000	2.000	Tbsp	2.00	8.00	5.00	100.00	0.00	0.00	25.00	6.00
327	Einstein Bros.-Cream Cheese, Gar	30.0000	2.000	Tbsp	2.00	9.00	2.00	100.00	0.00	0.00	30.00	6.00
328	Einstein Bros.-Cream Cheese, Jal	30.0000	2.000	Tbsp	2.00	8.00	2.00	90.00	0.00	0.00	25.00	6.00
329	Einstein Bros.-Cream Cheese, Map	30.0000	2.000	Tbsp	2.00	9.00	5.00	100.00	0.00	0.00	25.00	6.00
330	Einstein Bros.-Cream Cheese, Pla	30.0000	2.000	Tbsp	2.00	10.00	2.00	100.00	0.00	0.00	30.00	7.00
331	Einstein Bros.-Cream Cheese, Sal	30.0000	2.000	Tbsp	2.00	8.00	2.00	90.00	0.00	0.00	25.00	6.00
332	Einstein Bros.-Cream Cheese, Str	30.0000	2.000	Tbsp	2.00	8.00	5.00	100.00	0.00	0.00	25.00	6.00
333	Einstein Bros.-Cream Cheese, Sun	30.0000	2.000	Tbsp	2.00	9.00	2.00	100.00	0.00	0.00	30.00	6.00
334	Einstein Bros.-Cream Cheese, Veg	30.0000	2.000	Tbsp	2.00	5.00	2.00	60.00	0.00	0.00	16.00	4.00
335	Einstein Bros.-Cream Cheese, Wil	30.0000	2.000	Tbsp	2.00	5.00	6.00	70.00	0.00	0.00	15.00	4.00
336	Einstein Bros.-Cream Cheese-Hone	30.0000	2.000	Tbsp	2.00	9.00	5.00	100.00	0.00	0.00	25.00	6.00
337	Einstein Bros.-Egg, Scr, & Bacon	225.0000	1.000	Each	30.00	23.00	72.00	620.00	0.00	2.00	395.00	10.00
338	Einstein Bros.-Egg, Scr, & Ham B	248.0000	1.000	Each	34.00	18.00	74.00	590.00	0.00	2.00	405.00	8.00
339	Einstein Bros.-Egg, Scr, & Sausa	250.0000	1.000	Each	31.00	30.00	72.00	690.00	0.00	2.00	415.00	12.00
340	Einstein Bros.-Egg, Scr, & Turk	257.0000	1.000	Each	37.00	19.00	72.00	604.00	0.00	2.00	409.00	8.00
341	Einstein Bros.-Egg, Scr, Bagel S	212.0000	1.000	Each	27.00	16.00	72.00	540.00	0.00	2.00	385.00	7.00
342	Einstein Bros.-Espresso	45.0000	1.500	Fl Oz	0.00	0.00	0.00	1.00	0.00	0.00	0.00	0.00
343	Einstein Bros.-Fruit & Yogurt Cu	227.2000	8.000	Ounce	6.00	1.00	32.00	160.00	0.00	4.00	0.00	0.00
344	Einstein Bros.-Fruit Salad	227.2000	8.000	Ounce	1.00	0.50	25.00	110.00	0.00	2.00	0.00	0.00
345	Einstein Bros.-Fruit Salad, Ruby	113.6000	4.000	Ounce	0.00	0.00	23.00	90.00	0.00	1.00	0.00	0.00
346	Einstein Bros.-Fusilli w/ Olives	170.4000	6.000	Ounce	6.00	23.00	33.00	360.00	0.00	3.00	0.00	3.00
347	Einstein Bros.-Ham/Cheese Bagel	275.0000	1.000	Each	32.00	15.00	79.00	580.00	0.00	3.00	70.00	6.00
348	Einstein Bros.-Ham, Deli, Bagel	305.0000	1.000	Each	37.00	17.00	78.00	620.00	0.00	3.00	85.00	10.00
349	Einstein Bros.-Hummus	30.0000	2.000	Tbsp	2.00	3.50	6.00	60.00	0.00	1.00	0.00	0.50
350	Einstein Bros.-Hummus Bagel Sand	248.0000	1.000	Each	15.00	8.00	86.00	480.00	0.00	5.00	0.00	1.00
351	Einstein Bros.-Hummus, Carrot	57.0000	4.000	Tbsp	3.00	2.00	9.00	60.00	0.00	2.00	0.00	0.00
352	Einstein Bros.-Hummus, Carrot, S	248.0000	1.000	Each	15.00	3.00	83.00	420.00	0.00	5.00	0.00	0.00
353	Einstein Bros.-Intellicino, Iced	480.0000	16.000	Fl Oz	6.00	7.00	13.00	140.00	0.00	0.00	15.00	4.00
354	Einstein Bros.-Intellicino, Low	360.0000	12.000	Fl Oz	7.00	3.50	15.00	120.00	0.00	0.00	5.00	2.50
355	Einstein Bros.-Intellicino, Reg	360.0000	12.000	Fl Oz	7.00	7.00	14.00	150.00	0.00	0.00	15.00	4.50
356	Einstein Bros.-Lox & Bagel	318.0000	1.000	Each	26.00	24.00	77.00	630.00	0.00	3.00	75.00	13.00
357	Einstein Bros.-Mocha, Iced	480.0000	16.000	Fl Oz	7.00	6.00	33.00	210.00	0.00	0.00	15.00	4.00
358	Einstein Bros.-Mocha, Low Fat, R	360.0000	12.000	Fl Oz	8.00	2.50	34.00	190.00	0.00	0.00	5.00	2.00
359	Einstein Bros.-Mocha, Reg	360.0000	12.000	Fl Oz	8.00	6.00	34.00	230.00	0.00	0.00	15.00	4.50
360	Einstein Bros.-Muffin, Apple Dat	56.8000	2.000	Ounce	3.00	2.00	35.00	160.00	0.00	2.00	0.00	0.00
361	Einstein Bros.-Muffin, Banana	56.8000	2.000	Ounce	3.00	12.00	25.00	220.00	0.00	0.00	40.00	2.00
362	Einstein Bros.-Muffin, Blueberry	56.8000	2.000	Ounce	3.00	10.00	25.00	200.00	0.00	0.00	40.00	2.00
363	Einstein Bros.-Muffin, Chocolate	56.8000	2.000	Ounce	3.00	13.00	28.00	240.00	0.00	0.00	40.00	3.00
364	Einstein Bros.-Muffin, Cran Oran	56.8000	2.000	Ounce	4.00	0.50	27.00	130.00	0.00	1.00	0.00	0.00
365	Einstein Bros.-Muffin, Lemon Pop	56.8000	2.000	Ounce	3.00	3.00	28.00	150.00	0.00	0.00	0.00	0.00
366	Einstein Bros.-Muffin, Wildberry	56.8000	2.000	Ounce	3.00	0.50	26.00	120.00	0.00	1.00	0.00	0.00
368	Einstein Bros.-Pastrami, Turkey,	305.0000	1.000	Each	37.00	16.00	78.00	600.00	0.00	3.00	85.00	9.00

Page Key: A2 = Baby Food   A2 = Baked Goods   A8 = Beverages   A14 = Breads/Grains and Pasta   A18 = Breakfast Foods/Cereals   A26 = Dairy and Eggs   A40 = Fats and Oils   A42 = Fruits and Vegetables   A52 = Meats and Beans   A60 = Nuts and Seeds   A62 = Frozen Entrees and Packaged Foods   A76 = Restaurant Chains–Fast Foods   A92 = Restaurant Chains–Other   A106 = Seafood and Fish   A110 = Snacks and Sweets   A120 = Soups   A122 = Supplements   A126 = Toppings and Sauces

Monounsaturated Fat (g)	Polyunsaturated Fat (g)	Vitamin D (mg)	Vitamin K (mg)	Vitamin E (mg)	Vitamin A (re)	Vitamin C (mg)	Thiamin (mg)	Riboflavin (mg)	Niacin (mg)	Vitamin B$_6$ (mg)	Folate (mcg)	Vitamin B$_{12}$ (mcg)	Calcium (mg)	Iron (mg)	Magnesium (mg)	Phosphorus (mg)	Potassium (mg)	Sodium (mg)	Zinc (mg)
0.00	0.00	0.00	0.00	0.00	0.00	0.00	0.00	0.00	0.00	0.00	0.00	0.00	0.00	0.00	0.00	0.00	0.00	656.00	0.00
0.00	0.00	0.00	0.00	0.00	0.00	0.00	0.00	0.00	0.00	0.00	0.00	0.00	0.00	0.00	0.00	0.00	0.00	0.00	0.00
0.00	0.00	0.00	0.00	0.00	0.00	0.00	0.00	0.00	0.00	0.00	0.00	0.00	0.00	0.00	0.00	0.00	0.00	300.00	0.00
0.00	0.00	0.00	0.00	0.00	0.00	0.00	0.00	0.00	0.00	0.00	0.00	0.00	0.00	0.00	0.00	0.00	0.00	300.00	0.00
0.00	0.00	0.00	0.00	0.00	0.00	0.00	0.00	0.00	0.00	0.00	0.00	0.00	0.00	0.00	0.00	0.00	0.00	260.00	0.00
0.00	0.00	0.00	0.00	0.00	0.00	0.00	0.00	0.00	0.00	0.00	0.00	0.00	0.00	0.00	0.00	0.00	0.00	390.00	0.00
0.00	0.00	0.00	0.00	0.00	0.00	0.00	0.00	0.00	0.00	0.00	0.00	0.00	0.00	0.00	0.00	0.00	0.00	360.00	0.00
0.00	0.00	0.00	0.00	0.00	0.00	0.00	0.00	0.00	0.00	0.00	0.00	0.00	0.00	0.00	0.00	0.00	0.00	620.00	0.00
0.00	0.00	0.00	0.00	0.00	0.00	0.00	0.00	0.00	0.00	0.00	0.00	0.00	0.00	0.00	0.00	0.00	0.00	420.00	0.00
0.00	0.00	0.00	0.00	0.00	0.00	0.00	0.00	0.00	0.00	0.00	0.00	0.00	0.00	0.00	0.00	0.00	0.00	130.00	0.00
0.00	0.00	0.00	0.00	0.00	0.00	0.00	0.00	0.00	0.00	0.00	0.00	0.00	0.00	0.00	0.00	0.00	0.00	110.00	0.00
0.00	0.00	0.00	0.00	0.00	0.00	0.00	0.00	0.00	0.00	0.00	0.00	0.00	0.00	0.00	0.00	0.00	0.00	80.00	0.00
0.00	0.00	0.00	0.00	0.00	0.00	0.00	0.00	0.00	0.00	0.00	0.00	0.00	0.00	0.00	0.00	0.00	0.00	135.00	0.00
0.00	0.00	0.00	0.00	0.00	0.00	0.00	0.00	0.00	0.00	0.00	0.00	0.00	0.00	0.00	0.00	0.00	0.00	140.00	0.00
0.00	0.00	0.00	0.00	0.00	0.00	0.00	0.00	0.00	0.00	0.00	0.00	0.00	0.00	0.00	0.00	0.00	0.00	80.00	0.00
0.00	0.00	0.00	0.00	0.00	0.00	0.00	0.00	0.00	0.00	0.00	0.00	0.00	0.00	0.00	0.00	0.00	0.00	100.00	0.00
0.00	0.00	0.00	0.00	0.00	0.00	0.00	0.00	0.00	0.00	0.00	0.00	0.00	0.00	0.00	0.00	0.00	0.00	210.00	0.00
0.00	0.00	0.00	0.00	0.00	0.00	0.00	0.00	0.00	0.00	0.00	0.00	0.00	0.00	0.00	0.00	0.00	0.00	80.00	0.00
0.00	0.00	0.00	0.00	0.00	0.00	0.00	0.00	0.00	0.00	0.00	0.00	0.00	0.00	0.00	0.00	0.00	0.00	100.00	0.00
0.00	0.00	0.00	0.00	0.00	0.00	0.00	0.00	0.00	0.00	0.00	0.00	0.00	0.00	0.00	0.00	0.00	0.00	150.00	0.00
0.00	0.00	0.00	0.00	0.00	0.00	0.00	0.00	0.00	0.00	0.00	0.00	0.00	0.00	0.00	0.00	0.00	0.00	90.00	0.00
0.00	0.00	0.00	0.00	0.00	0.00	0.00	0.00	0.00	0.00	0.00	0.00	0.00	0.00	0.00	0.00	0.00	0.00	80.00	0.00
0.00	0.00	0.00	0.00	0.00	0.00	0.00	0.00	0.00	0.00	0.00	0.00	0.00	0.00	0.00	0.00	0.00	0.00	950.00	0.00
0.00	0.00	0.00	0.00	0.00	0.00	0.00	0.00	0.00	0.00	0.00	0.00	0.00	0.00	0.00	0.00	0.00	0.00	1120.00	0.00
0.00	0.00	0.00	0.00	0.00	0.00	0.00	0.00	0.00	0.00	0.00	0.00	0.00	0.00	0.00	0.00	0.00	0.00	980.00	0.00
0.00	0.00	0.00	0.00	0.00	0.00	0.00	0.00	0.00	0.00	0.00	0.00	0.00	0.00	0.00	0.00	0.00	0.00	1070.00	0.00
0.00	0.00	0.00	0.00	0.00	0.00	0.00	0.00	0.00	0.00	0.00	0.00	0.00	0.00	0.00	0.00	0.00	0.00	750.00	0.00
0.00	0.00	0.00	0.00	0.00	0.00	0.00	0.00	0.00	0.00	0.00	0.00	0.00	0.00	0.00	0.00	0.00	0.00	0.00	0.00
0.00	0.00	0.00	0.00	0.00	0.00	0.00	0.00	0.00	0.00	0.00	0.00	0.00	0.00	0.00	0.00	0.00	0.00	95.00	0.00
0.00	0.00	0.00	0.00	0.00	0.00	0.00	0.00	0.00	0.00	0.00	0.00	0.00	0.00	0.00	0.00	0.00	0.00	10.00	0.00
0.00	0.00	0.00	0.00	0.00	0.00	0.00	0.00	0.00	0.00	0.00	0.00	0.00	0.00	0.00	0.00	0.00	0.00	20.00	0.00
0.00	0.00	0.00	0.00	0.00	0.00	0.00	0.00	0.00	0.00	0.00	0.00	0.00	0.00	0.00	0.00	0.00	0.00	290.00	0.00
0.00	0.00	0.00	0.00	0.00	0.00	0.00	0.00	0.00	0.00	0.00	0.00	0.00	0.00	0.00	0.00	0.00	0.00	1400.00	0.00
0.00	0.00	0.00	0.00	0.00	0.00	0.00	0.00	0.00	0.00	0.00	0.00	0.00	0.00	0.00	0.00	0.00	0.00	1690.00	0.00
0.00	0.00	0.00	0.00	0.00	0.00	0.00	0.00	0.00	0.00	0.00	0.00	0.00	0.00	0.00	0.00	0.00	0.00	65.00	0.00
0.00	0.00	0.00	0.00	0.00	0.00	0.00	0.00	0.00	0.00	0.00	0.00	0.00	0.00	0.00	0.00	0.00	0.00	640.00	0.00
0.00	0.00	0.00	0.00	0.00	0.00	0.00	0.00	0.00	0.00	0.00	0.00	0.00	0.00	0.00	0.00	0.00	0.00	260.00	0.00
0.00	0.00	0.00	0.00	0.00	0.00	0.00	0.00	0.00	0.00	0.00	0.00	0.00	0.00	0.00	0.00	0.00	0.00	780.00	0.00
0.00	0.00	0.00	0.00	0.00	0.00	0.00	0.00	0.00	0.00	0.00	0.00	0.00	0.00	0.00	0.00	0.00	0.00	140.00	0.00
0.00	0.00	0.00	0.00	0.00	0.00	0.00	0.00	0.00	0.00	0.00	0.00	0.00	0.00	0.00	0.00	0.00	0.00	140.00	0.00
0.00	0.00	0.00	0.00	0.00	0.00	0.00	0.00	0.00	0.00	0.00	0.00	0.00	0.00	0.00	0.00	0.00	0.00	135.00	0.00
0.00	0.00	0.00	0.00	0.00	0.00	0.00	0.00	0.00	0.00	0.00	0.00	0.00	0.00	0.00	0.00	0.00	0.00	1240.00	0.00
0.00	0.00	0.00	0.00	0.00	0.00	0.00	0.00	0.00	0.00	0.00	0.00	0.00	0.00	0.00	0.00	0.00	0.00	120.00	0.00
0.00	0.00	0.00	0.00	0.00	0.00	0.00	0.00	0.00	0.00	0.00	0.00	0.00	0.00	0.00	0.00	0.00	0.00	130.00	0.00
0.00	0.00	0.00	0.00	0.00	0.00	0.00	0.00	0.00	0.00	0.00	0.00	0.00	0.00	0.00	0.00	0.00	0.00	135.00	0.00
0.00	0.00	0.00	0.00	0.00	0.00	0.00	0.00	0.00	0.00	0.00	0.00	0.00	0.00	0.00	0.00	0.00	0.00	210.00	0.00
0.00	0.00	0.00	0.00	0.00	0.00	0.00	0.00	0.00	0.00	0.00	0.00	0.00	0.00	0.00	0.00	0.00	0.00	170.00	0.00
0.00	0.00	0.00	0.00	0.00	0.00	0.00	0.00	0.00	0.00	0.00	0.00	0.00	0.00	0.00	0.00	0.00	0.00	180.00	0.00
0.00	0.00	0.00	0.00	0.00	0.00	0.00	0.00	0.00	0.00	0.00	0.00	0.00	0.00	0.00	0.00	0.00	0.00	180.00	0.00
0.00	0.00	0.00	0.00	0.00	0.00	0.00	0.00	0.00	0.00	0.00	0.00	0.00	0.00	0.00	0.00	0.00	0.00	260.00	0.00
0.00	0.00	0.00	0.00	0.00	0.00	0.00	0.00	0.00	0.00	0.00	0.00	0.00	0.00	0.00	0.00	0.00	0.00	220.00	0.00
0.00	0.00	0.00	0.00	0.00	0.00	0.00	0.00	0.00	0.00	0.00	0.00	0.00	0.00	0.00	0.00	0.00	0.00	260.00	0.00
0.00	0.00	0.00	0.00	0.00	0.00	0.00	0.00	0.00	0.00	0.00	0.00	0.00	0.00	0.00	0.00	0.00	0.00	1590.00	0.00

USDA ID Code	Food Name	Weight in Grams*	Quantity of Units	Unit of Measure	Protein (g)	Fat (g)	Carbohydrate (g)	Kilocalories	Caffeine (g)	Fiber (g)	Cholesterol (mg)	Saturated Fat (g)
369	Einstein Bros.-Pastrami, Turkey,	347.0000	1.000	Each	45.00	34.00	77.00	790.00	0.00	3.00	90.00	19.00
367	Einstein Bros.-PB&J Bagel Sandwi	172.0000	1.000	Each	18.00	17.00	99.00	595.00	0.00	4.00	0.00	2.00
370	Einstein Bros.-Peanut Butter, Cr	32.0000	2.000	Tbsp	7.00	16.00	8.00	190.00	0.00	2.00	0.00	2.00
371	Einstein Bros.-Pizza Melt, 3 Che	234.0000	1.000	Each	32.00	18.00	78.00	600.00	0.00	3.00	55.00	10.00
372	Einstein Bros.-Pizza Melt, Peppe	263.0000	1.000	Each	38.00	30.00	79.00	740.00	0.00	3.00	85.00	15.00
373	Einstein Bros.-Pizza Melt, Tomat	277.0000	1.000	Each	32.00	18.00	80.00	610.00	0.00	3.00	55.00	10.00
374	Einstein Bros.-Reuben Bagel Sand	319.0000	1.000	Each	42.00	33.00	82.00	790.00	0.00	5.00	100.00	12.00
375	Einstein Bros.-Salad, Caesar, Ch	269.8000	9.500	Ounce	26.00	37.00	11.00	480.00	0.00	2.00	75.00	8.00
376	Einstein Bros.-Salad, Caesar, La	198.8000	7.000	Ounce	9.00	35.00	10.00	390.00	0.00	2.00	25.00	7.00
377	Einstein Bros.-Salad, Caesar, Re	99.4000	3.500	Ounce	5.00	18.00	7.00	210.00	0.00	1.00	15.00	4.00
378	Einstein Bros.-Salad, Clairemont	113.6000	4.000	Ounce	1.00	4.00	9.00	70.00	0.00	2.00	0.00	0.00
379	Einstein Bros.-Salad, Pasta, Gre	255.6000	9.000	Ounce	12.00	30.00	35.00	270.00	0.00	3.00	45.00	9.00
380	Einstein Bros.-Salad, Pasta, Zit	113.6000	4.000	Ounce	4.00	11.00	20.00	200.00	0.00	2.00	0.00	2.00
381	Einstein Bros.-Salad, Potato & D	113.6000	4.000	Ounce	2.00	0.50	20.00	150.00	0.00	1.00	0.00	0.00
382	Einstein Bros.-Salad, Potato & M	113.6000	4.000	Ounce	2.00	2.50	19.00	110.00	0.00	2.00	0.00	0.00
383	Einstein Bros.-Salad, Potato, Id	113.6000	4.000	Ounce	2.00	7.00	19.00	150.00	0.00	1.00	5.00	1.50
384	Einstein Bros.-Salad, Potato, Ol	113.6000	4.000	Ounce	3.00	8.00	16.00	140.00	0.00	1.00	40.00	1.50
385	Einstein Bros.-Scone, Blueberry	99.4000	3.500	Ounce	8.00	8.50	49.00	295.00	0.00	1.50	20.00	4.50
386	Einstein Bros.-Scone, Cheddar Ch	99.4000	3.500	Ounce	8.00	15.00	37.00	310.00	0.00	2.00	35.00	8.00
387	Einstein Bros.-Scone, Cinnamon	99.4000	3.500	Ounce	8.00	11.00	50.00	325.00	0.00	1.50	20.00	5.50
388	Einstein Bros.-Soup, Bean, Black	198.8000	7.000	Ounce	3.00	1.00	11.00	70.00	0.00	2.00	0.00	0.00
389	Einstein Bros.-Soup, Bean, Monte	198.8000	7.000	Ounce	5.00	2.00	19.00	120.00	0.00	5.00	0.00	0.00
390	Einstein Bros.-Soup, Cheddar & B	198.8000	7.000	Ounce	5.00	10.00	14.00	170.00	0.00	1.00	15.00	3.00
391	Einstein Bros.-Soup, Chicken & R	198.8000	7.000	Ounce	7.00	10.00	15.00	180.00	0.00	1.00	15.00	2.50
392	Einstein Bros.-Soup, Chicken Noo	198.8000	7.000	Ounce	6.00	2.50	13.00	100.00	0.00	1.00	15.00	1.00
393	Einstein Bros.-Soup, Oriental Se	170.4000	6.000	Ounce	7.00	20.00	46.00	390.00	0.00	3.00	0.00	2.50
394	Einstein Bros.-Soup, Pasta Fagio	198.8000	7.000	Ounce	2.00	1.00	11.00	60.00	0.00	1.00	0.00	0.00
395	Einstein Bros.-Soup, Potato, Iri	198.8000	7.000	Ounce	5.00	8.00	19.00	170.00	0.00	1.00	5.00	2.50
396	Einstein Bros.-Soup, Tomato Flor	198.8000	7.000	Ounce	2.00	1.50	14.00	80.00	0.00	2.00	0.00	1.00
397	Einstein Bros.-Soup, Veg, Farmer	198.8000	7.000	Ounce	2.00	0.50	7.00	40.00	0.00	2.00	0.00	0.00
398	Einstein Bros.-Spread, Apricot	28.0000	2.000	Tbsp	0.00	0.00	19.00	75.00	0.00	0.00	0.00	0.00
399	Einstein Bros.-Spread, Butter	14.0000	1.000	Tbsp	0.00	11.00	0.00	100.00	0.00	0.00	30.00	8.00
400	Einstein Bros.-Spread, Butter/Ma	10.0000	1.000	Tbsp	0.00	7.00	0.00	60.00	0.00	0.00	0.00	1.50
401	Einstein Bros.-Spread, Grape Fru	28.0000	2.000	Tbsp	0.00	0.00	19.00	75.00	0.00	0.00	0.00	0.00
402	Einstein Bros.-Spread, Strawberr	28.0000	2.000	Tbsp	0.00	0.00	19.00	75.00	0.00	0.00	0.00	0.00
403	Einstein Bros.-Steamer, Non Fat,	360.0000	12.000	Fl Oz	9.00	0.00	29.00	160.00	0.00	0.00	5.00	0.00
404	Einstein Bros.-Steamer, Reg	360.0000	12.000	Fl Oz	6.00	5.00	30.00	200.00	0.00	0.00	20.00	3.50
405	Einstein Bros.-Syrup, Almond Fla	31.0000	2.000	Tbsp	0.00	0.00	18.00	80.00	0.00	0.00	0.00	0.00
406	Einstein Bros.-Syrup, Caramel Fl	31.0000	2.000	Tbsp	0.00	0.00	18.00	80.00	0.00	0.00	0.00	0.00
407	Einstein Bros.-Syrup, Caramel Fl	31.0000	2.000	Tbsp	0.00	0.00	18.00	80.00	0.00	0.00	0.00	0.00
408	Einstein Bros.-Syrup, Caramel, S	31.0000	2.000	Tbsp	0.00	0.00	0.00	0.00	0.00	0.00	0.00	0.00
409	Einstein Bros.-Syrup, Choc-Hersh	31.0000	2.000	Tbsp	1.00	0.00	24.00	100.00	0.00	0.00	0.00	0.00
410	Einstein Bros.-Syrup, Raspberry	31.0000	2.000	Tbsp	0.00	0.00	18.00	80.00	0.00	0.00	0.00	0.00
411	Einstein Bros.-Syrup, Vanilla, S	31.0000	2.000	Tbsp	0.00	0.00	0.00	0.00	0.00	0.00	0.00	0.00
412	Einstein Bros.-Tabouli, Southwes	284.0000	10.000	Ounce	6.00	1.00	29.00	150.00	0.00	8.00	0.00	0.00
413	Einstein Bros.-Teas, Hot	360.0000	12.000	Fl Oz	0.00	0.00	0.00	1.00	0.00	0.00	0.00	0.00
428	Einstein Bros.-Topping, Chocolat	2.5000	0.500	Tsp	0.00	0.00	2.00	10.00	0.00	0.00	0.00	0.00
429	Einstein Bros.-Topping, Cinnamon	2.5000	0.500	Tsp	0.00	0.00	2.00	10.00	0.00	0.00	0.00	0.00
414	Einstein Bros.-Topping, Nutmeg	2.5000	0.500	Tsp	0.00	0.00	2.00	10.00	0.00	0.00	0.00	0.00
415	Einstein Bros.-Topping, On Top D	31.0000	2.000	Tbsp	0.00	1.50	2.00	20.00	0.00	0.00	0.00	1.00
416	Einstein Bros.-Topping, Vanilla	2.5000	0.500	Tsp	0.00	0.00	2.00	10.00	0.00	0.00	0.00	0.00
417	Einstein Bros.-Tuna Melt	375.0000	1.000	Each	52.00	36.00	78.00	840.00	0.00	3.00	120.00	19.00
418	Einstein Bros.-Tuna Salad	113.6000	4.000	Ounce	21.00	6.00	3.00	150.00	0.00	0.00	30.00	1.00

Page Key: A2 = Baby Food   A2 = Baked Goods   A8 = Beverages   A14 = Breads/Grains and Pasta   A18 = Breakfast Foods/Cereals   A26 = Dairy and Eggs   A40 = Fats and Oils   A42 = Fruits and Vegetables   A52 = Meats and Beans   A60 = Nuts and Seeds   A62 5 Frozen Entrees and Packaged Foods   A76 = Restaurant Chains–Fast Foods   A92 = Restaurant Chains–Other   A106 = Seafood and Fish   A110 = Snacks and Sweets   A120 = Soups   A122 = Supplements   A126 = Toppings and Sauces

Monounsaturated Fat (g)	Polyunsaturated Fat (g)	Vitamin D (mg)	Vitamin K (mg)	Vitamin E (mg)	Vitamin A (re)	Vitamin C (mg)	Thiamin (mg)	Riboflavin (mg)	Niacin (mg)	Vitamin B$_6$ (mg)	Folate (mcg)	Vitamin B$_{12}$ (mcg)	Calcium (mg)	Iron (mg)	Magnesium (mg)	Phosphorus (mg)	Potassium (mg)	Sodium (mg)	Zinc (mg)
0.00	0.00	0.00	0.00	0.00	0.00	0.00	0.00	0.00	0.00	0.00	0.00	0.00	0.00	0.00	0.00	0.00	0.00	1780.00	0.00
0.00	0.00	0.00	0.00	0.00	0.00	0.00	0.00	0.00	0.00	0.00	0.00	0.00	0.00	0.00	0.00	0.00	0.00	663.00	0.00
0.00	0.00	0.00	0.00	0.00	0.00	0.00	0.00	0.00	0.00	0.00	0.00	0.00	0.00	0.00	0.00	0.00	0.00	140.00	0.00
0.00	0.00	0.00	0.00	0.00	0.00	0.00	0.00	0.00	0.00	0.00	0.00	0.00	0.00	0.00	0.00	0.00	0.00	1200.00	0.00
0.00	0.00	0.00	0.00	0.00	0.00	0.00	0.00	0.00	0.00	0.00	0.00	0.00	0.00	0.00	0.00	0.00	0.00	1780.00	0.00
0.00	0.00	0.00	0.00	0.00	0.00	0.00	0.00	0.00	0.00	0.00	0.00	0.00	0.00	0.00	0.00	0.00	0.00	1210.00	0.00
0.00	0.00	0.00	0.00	0.00	0.00	0.00	0.00	0.00	0.00	0.00	0.00	0.00	0.00	0.00	0.00	0.00	0.00	1920.00	0.00
0.00	0.00	0.00	0.00	0.00	0.00	0.00	0.00	0.00	0.00	0.00	0.00	0.00	0.00	0.00	0.00	0.00	0.00	1150.00	0.00
0.00	0.00	0.00	0.00	0.00	0.00	0.00	0.00	0.00	0.00	0.00	0.00	0.00	0.00	0.00	0.00	0.00	0.00	900.00	0.00
0.00	0.00	0.00	0.00	0.00	0.00	0.00	0.00	0.00	0.00	0.00	0.00	0.00	0.00	0.00	0.00	0.00	0.00	500.00	0.00
0.00	0.00	0.00	0.00	0.00	0.00	0.00	0.00	0.00	0.00	0.00	0.00	0.00	0.00	0.00	0.00	0.00	0.00	120.00	0.00
0.00	0.00	0.00	0.00	0.00	0.00	0.00	0.00	0.00	0.00	0.00	0.00	0.00	0.00	0.00	0.00	0.00	0.00	960.00	0.00
0.00	0.00	0.00	0.00	0.00	0.00	0.00	0.00	0.00	0.00	0.00	0.00	0.00	0.00	0.00	0.00	0.00	0.00	350.00	0.00
0.00	0.00	0.00	0.00	0.00	0.00	0.00	0.00	0.00	0.00	0.00	0.00	0.00	0.00	0.00	0.00	0.00	0.00	150.00	0.00
0.00	0.00	0.00	0.00	0.00	0.00	0.00	0.00	0.00	0.00	0.00	0.00	0.00	0.00	0.00	0.00	0.00	0.00	340.00	0.00
0.00	0.00	0.00	0.00	0.00	0.00	0.00	0.00	0.00	0.00	0.00	0.00	0.00	0.00	0.00	0.00	0.00	0.00	210.00	0.00
0.00	0.00	0.00	0.00	0.00	0.00	0.00	0.00	0.00	0.00	0.00	0.00	0.00	0.00	0.00	0.00	0.00	0.00	250.00	0.00
0.00	0.00	0.00	0.00	0.00	0.00	0.00	0.00	0.00	0.00	0.00	0.00	0.00	0.00	0.00	0.00	0.00	0.00	560.00	0.00
0.00	0.00	0.00	0.00	0.00	0.00	0.00	0.00	0.00	0.00	0.00	0.00	0.00	0.00	0.00	0.00	0.00	0.00	670.00	0.00
0.00	0.00	0.00	0.00	0.00	0.00	0.00	0.00	0.00	0.00	0.00	0.00	0.00	0.00	0.00	0.00	0.00	0.00	535.00	0.00
0.00	0.00	0.00	0.00	0.00	0.00	0.00	0.00	0.00	0.00	0.00	0.00	0.00	0.00	0.00	0.00	0.00	0.00	460.00	0.00
0.00	0.00	0.00	0.00	0.00	0.00	0.00	0.00	0.00	0.00	0.00	0.00	0.00	0.00	0.00	0.00	0.00	0.00	680.00	0.00
0.00	0.00	0.00	0.00	0.00	0.00	0.00	0.00	0.00	0.00	0.00	0.00	0.00	0.00	0.00	0.00	0.00	0.00	770.00	0.00
0.00	0.00	0.00	0.00	0.00	0.00	0.00	0.00	0.00	0.00	0.00	0.00	0.00	0.00	0.00	0.00	0.00	0.00	1070.00	0.00
0.00	0.00	0.00	0.00	0.00	0.00	0.00	0.00	0.00	0.00	0.00	0.00	0.00	0.00	0.00	0.00	0.00	0.00	910.00	0.00
0.00	0.00	0.00	0.00	0.00	0.00	0.00	0.00	0.00	0.00	0.00	0.00	0.00	0.00	0.00	0.00	0.00	0.00	320.00	0.00
0.00	0.00	0.00	0.00	0.00	0.00	0.00	0.00	0.00	0.00	0.00	0.00	0.00	0.00	0.00	0.00	0.00	0.00	450.00	0.00
0.00	0.00	0.00	0.00	0.00	0.00	0.00	0.00	0.00	0.00	0.00	0.00	0.00	0.00	0.00	0.00	0.00	0.00	650.00	0.00
0.00	0.00	0.00	0.00	0.00	0.00	0.00	0.00	0.00	0.00	0.00	0.00	0.00	0.00	0.00	0.00	0.00	0.00	870.00	0.00
0.00	0.00	0.00	0.00	0.00	0.00	0.00	0.00	0.00	0.00	0.00	0.00	0.00	0.00	0.00	0.00	0.00	0.00	390.00	0.00
0.00	0.00	0.00	0.00	0.00	0.00	0.00	0.00	0.00	0.00	0.00	0.00	0.00	0.00	0.00	0.00	0.00	0.00	8.00	0.00
0.00	0.00	0.00	0.00	0.00	0.00	0.00	0.00	0.00	0.00	0.00	0.00	0.00	0.00	0.00	0.00	0.00	0.00	100.00	0.00
0.00	0.00	0.00	0.00	0.00	0.00	0.00	0.00	0.00	0.00	0.00	0.00	0.00	0.00	0.00	0.00	0.00	0.00	75.00	0.00
0.00	0.00	0.00	0.00	0.00	0.00	0.00	0.00	0.00	0.00	0.00	0.00	0.00	0.00	0.00	0.00	0.00	0.00	3.00	0.00
0.00	0.00	0.00	0.00	0.00	0.00	0.00	0.00	0.00	0.00	0.00	0.00	0.00	0.00	0.00	0.00	0.00	0.00	17.00	0.00
0.00	0.00	0.00	0.00	0.00	0.00	0.00	0.00	0.00	0.00	0.00	0.00	0.00	0.00	0.00	0.00	0.00	0.00	140.00	0.00
0.00	0.00	0.00	0.00	0.00	0.00	0.00	0.00	0.00	0.00	0.00	0.00	0.00	0.00	0.00	0.00	0.00	0.00	150.00	0.00
0.00	0.00	0.00	0.00	0.00	0.00	0.00	0.00	0.00	0.00	0.00	0.00	0.00	0.00	0.00	0.00	0.00	0.00	10.00	0.00
0.00	0.00	0.00	0.00	0.00	0.00	0.00	0.00	0.00	0.00	0.00	0.00	0.00	0.00	0.00	0.00	0.00	0.00	10.00	0.00
0.00	0.00	0.00	0.00	0.00	0.00	0.00	0.00	0.00	0.00	0.00	0.00	0.00	0.00	0.00	0.00	0.00	0.00	10.00	0.00
0.00	0.00	0.00	0.00	0.00	0.00	0.00	0.00	0.00	0.00	0.00	0.00	0.00	0.00	0.00	0.00	0.00	0.00	20.00	0.00
0.00	0.00	0.00	0.00	0.00	0.00	0.00	0.00	0.00	0.00	0.00	0.00	0.00	0.00	0.00	0.00	0.00	0.00	25.00	0.00
0.00	0.00	0.00	0.00	0.00	0.00	0.00	0.00	0.00	0.00	0.00	0.00	0.00	0.00	0.00	0.00	0.00	0.00	10.00	0.00
0.00	0.00	0.00	0.00	0.00	0.00	0.00	0.00	0.00	0.00	0.00	0.00	0.00	0.00	0.00	0.00	0.00	0.00	20.00	0.00
0.00	0.00	0.00	0.00	0.00	0.00	0.00	0.00	0.00	0.00	0.00	0.00	0.00	0.00	0.00	0.00	0.00	0.00	690.00	0.00
0.00	0.00	0.00	0.00	0.00	0.00	0.00	0.00	0.00	0.00	0.00	0.00	0.00	0.00	0.00	0.00	0.00	0.00	0.00	0.00
0.00	0.00	0.00	0.00	0.00	0.00	0.00	0.00	0.00	0.00	0.00	0.00	0.00	0.00	0.00	0.00	0.00	0.00	0.00	0.00
0.00	0.00	0.00	0.00	0.00	0.00	0.00	0.00	0.00	0.00	0.00	0.00	0.00	0.00	0.00	0.00	0.00	0.00	10.00	0.00
0.00	0.00	0.00	0.00	0.00	0.00	0.00	0.00	0.00	0.00	0.00	0.00	0.00	0.00	0.00	0.00	0.00	0.00	5.00	0.00
0.00	0.00	0.00	0.00	0.00	0.00	0.00	0.00	0.00	0.00	0.00	0.00	0.00	0.00	0.00	0.00	0.00	0.00	0.00	0.00
0.00	0.00	0.00	0.00	0.00	0.00	0.00	0.00	0.00	0.00	0.00	0.00	0.00	0.00	0.00	0.00	0.00	0.00	1610.00	0.00
0.00	0.00	0.00	0.00	0.00	0.00	0.00	0.00	0.00	0.00	0.00	0.00	0.00	0.00	0.00	0.00	0.00	0.00	540.00	0.00

USDA ID Code	Food Name	Weight in Grams*	Quantity of Units	Unit of Measure	Protein (g)	Fat (g)	Carbohydrate (g)	Kilocalories	Caffeine (g)	Fiber (g)	Cholesterol (mg)	Saturated Fat (g)
419	Einstein Bros.-Tuna Salad Bagel	324.0000	1.000	Each	31.00	8.00	78.00	510.00	0.00	4.00	30.00	1.50
420	Einstein Bros.-Turkey, Deli Smok	305.0000	1.000	Each	35.00	16.00	75.00	590.00	0.00	3.00	65.00	9.00
421	Einstein Bros.-Turkey, Smoked, B	275.0000	1.000	Each	30.00	14.00	75.00	550.00	0.00	3.00	45.00	6.00
422	Einstein Bros.-Turkey, Tasty, Ba	279.0000	1.000	Each	26.00	21.00	77.00	600.00	0.00	3.00	90.00	12.00
423	Einstein Bros.-Veg Out Bagel San	248.0000	1.000	Each	14.00	6.00	78.00	420.00	0.00	3.00	20.00	3.00
424	Einstein Bros.-Veggie Cup	170.4000	6.000	Ounce	1.00	20.00	11.00	230.00	0.00	3.00	5.00	3.00
425	Einstein Bros.-Whipped Cream, Li	31.0000	2.000	Tbsp	0.00	2.00	2.00	30.00	0.00	0.00	10.00	1.50
426	Einstein Bros.-Whitefish Bagel S	245.0000	1.000	Each	23.00	22.00	75.00	590.00	0.00	4.00	45.00	4.00
427	Einstein Bros.-Whitefish Salad	56.8000	2.000	Ounce	8.00	14.00	1.00	160.00	0.00	1.00	30.00	2.00
561	Krispy Kreme-Cinnamon Bun	61.0000	1.000	Each	5.00	11.00	26.00	220.00	0.00	4.00	0.00	3.00
562	Krispy Kreme-Cruller, Fudge Iced	48.0000	1.000	Each	2.00	14.00	26.00	240.00	0.00	0.00	0.00	4.00
563	Krispy Kreme-Cruller, Glazed	43.0000	1.000	Each	2.00	14.00	22.00	220.00	0.00	0.00	0.00	3.00
564	Krispy Kreme-Doughnut, Blueberry	59.0000	1.000	Each	4.00	9.00	26.00	200.00	0.00	2.00	0.00	3.00
565	Krispy Kreme-Doughnut, Cake, Blu	67.0000	1.000	Each	2.00	15.00	37.00	300.00	0.00	1.00	0.00	3.00
566	Krispy Kreme-Doughnut, Cake, Dev	54.0000	1.000	Each	2.00	13.00	29.00	240.00	0.00	3.00	0.00	3.00
567	Krispy Kreme-Doughnut, Cake, Fud	56.0000	1.000	Each	3.00	12.00	28.00	230.00	0.00	0.00	0.00	3.00
568	Krispy Kreme-Doughnut, Cake, Sug	52.0000	1.000	Each	3.00	11.00	26.00	220.00	0.00	0.00	0.00	3.00
569	Krispy Kreme-Doughnut, Cake, Tra	48.0000	1.000	Each	3.00	11.00	22.00	200.00	0.00	0.00	0.00	3.00
570	Krispy Kreme-Doughnut, Cinnamon	66.0000	1.000	Each	4.00	9.00	29.00	210.00	0.00	3.00	0.00	3.00
571	Krispy Kreme-Doughnut, Creme Fil	65.0000	1.000	Each	4.00	14.00	32.00	270.00	0.00	2.00	0.00	3.00
572	Krispy Kreme-Doughnut, Crm Fille	65.0000	1.000	Each	4.00	14.00	32.00	270.00	0.00	2.00	0.00	3.00
573	Krispy Kreme-Doughnut, Custard F	76.0000	1.000	Each	4.00	9.00	38.00	250.00	0.00	3.00	0.00	3.00
574	Krispy Kreme-Doughnut, Fdg Iced	54.0000	1.000	Each	3.00	10.00	31.00	220.00	0.00	0.00	0.00	2.50
575	Krispy Kreme-Doughnut, Fudge Ice	57.0000	1.000	Each	3.00	14.00	30.00	260.00	0.00	1.00	0.00	5.00
576	Krispy Kreme-Doughnut, Lemon Fil	64.0000	1.000	Each	4.00	10.00	28.00	210.00	0.00	0.00	0.00	3.00
577	Krispy Kreme-Doughnut, Maple Ice	51.0000	1.000	Each	3.00	9.00	28.00	200.00	0.00	2.00	0.00	2.50
578	Krispy Kreme-Doughnut, Raspberry	57.0000	1.000	Each	4.00	10.00	28.00	210.00	0.00	0.00	0.00	3.00
579	Krispy Kreme-Doughnut, Yeast, Gl	39.0000	1.000	Each	2.00	10.00	17.00	170.00	0.00	0.00	0.00	2.50
	Pizza Hut-Pizza, Cheese, Hand To	70.0000	1.000	Slice	17.00	10.00	27.50	259.00	0.00	0.00	27.50	6.80
	Pizza Hut-Pizza, Cheese, Pan	70.0000	1.000	Slice	15.00	9.00	28.50	246.00	0.00	0.00	17.00	4.50
	Pizza Hut-Pizza, Cheese, Thin'n	70.0000	1.000	Slice	14.00	8.50	18.50	199.00	0.00	0.00	16.50	5.20
	Pizza Hut-Pizza, Pepperoni, Hand	70.0000	1.000	Slice	14.00	11.50	25.00	250.00	0.00	0.00	25.00	6.45
	Pizza Hut-Pizza, Pepperoni, Pan	70.0000	1.000	Slice	14.50	11.00	31.00	270.00	0.00	0.00	21.00	4.50
	Pizza Hut-Pizza, Pepperoni, Pers	250.0000	1.000	Each	37.00	29.00	76.00	675.00	0.00	0.00	53.00	12.50
	Pizza Hut-Pizza, Pepperoni, Thin	70.0000	1.000	Slice	13.00	10.00	18.00	206.50	0.00	0.00	23.00	5.30
	Pizza Hut-Pizza, Super Sprm, Thi	70.0000	1.000	Slice	14.50	10.50	22.00	231.50	0.00	0.00	28.00	5.15
	Pizza Hut-Pizza, Super Supreme,	70.0000	1.000	Slice	16.50	12.50	27.00	278.00	0.00	0.00	27.00	6.50
	Pizza Hut-Pizza, Super Supreme,	70.0000	1.000	Slice	16.50	13.00	26.50	281.50	0.00	0.00	27.50	6.00
	Pizza Hut-Pizza, Supreme, Hand T	70.0000	1.000	Slice	16.00	13.00	25.00	270.00	0.00	0.00	27.50	6.10
	Pizza Hut-Pizza, Supreme, Pan	70.0000	1.000	Slice	16.00	15.00	26.50	294.50	0.00	0.00	24.00	7.00
	Pizza Hut-Pizza, Supreme, Person	250.0000	1.000	Each	33.00	28.00	76.00	647.00	0.00	0.00	49.00	11.20
	Pizza Hut-Pizza, Supreme, Thin'n	70.0000	1.000	Slice	14.00	11.00	20.50	229.50	0.00	0.00	21.00	5.50
	Red Lobster-Calamari, Brded and	141.7460	1.000	Each	13.00	21.00	30.00	360.00	0.00	0.00	140.00	5.60
	Red Lobster-Catfish, Lunch Porti	141.7460	1.000	Each	20.00	10.00	0.00	170.00	0.00	0.00	85.00	2.50
	Red Lobster-Chicken Breast, Skin	113.3970	1.000	Each	26.00	3.00	0.00	140.00	0.00	0.00	70.00	1.00
	Red Lobster-Cod, Atlantic, Lunch	141.7460	1.000	Each	23.00	1.00	0.00	100.00	0.00	0.00	70.00	0.30
	Red Lobster-Crab Legs, King, Lun	453.5900	1.000	Each	32.00	2.00	6.00	170.00	0.00	0.00	100.00	0.50
	Red Lobster-Crab Legs, Snow, Lun	453.5900	1.000	Each	33.00	2.00	1.00	150.00	0.00	0.00	130.00	0.60
	Red Lobster-Flounder, Lunch Port	141.7460	1.000	Each	21.00	1.00	1.00	100.00	0.00	0.00	70.00	0.30
	Red Lobster-Grouper, Lunch Porti	141.7460	1.000	Each	26.00	1.00	0.00	110.00	0.00	0.00	65.00	0.30
	Red Lobster-Haddock, Lunch Porti	141.7460	1.000	Each	24.00	1.00	2.00	110.00	0.00	0.00	85.00	0.30
	Red Lobster-Halibut, Lunch Porti	141.7460	1.000	Each	25.00	1.00	1.00	110.00	0.00	0.00	60.00	0.30
	Red Lobster-Hamburger, Lunch Por	151.1810	1.000	Each	37.00	28.00	0.00	410.00	0.00	0.00	130.00	11.00

Page Key: A2 = Baby Food   A2 = Baked Goods   A8 = Beverages   A14 = Breads/Grains and Pasta   A18 = Breakfast Foods/Cereals   A26 = Dairy and Eggs   A40 = Fats and Oils   A42 = Fruits and Vegetables   A52 = Meats and Beans   A60 = Nuts and Seeds   A62 = Frozen Entrees and Packaged Foods   A76 = Restaurant Chains–Fast Foods   A92 = Restaurant Chains–Other   A106 = Seafood and Fish   A110 = Snacks and Sweets   A120 = Soups   A122 = Supplements   A126 = Toppings and Sauces

Monounsaturated Fat (g)	Polyunsaturated Fat (g)	Vitamin D (mg)	Vitamin K (mg)	Vitamin E (mg)	Vitamin A (re)	Vitamin C (mg)	Thiamin (mg)	Riboflavin (mg)	Niacin (mg)	Vitamin B_6 (mg)	Folate (mcg)	Vitamin B_{12} (mcg)	Calcium (mg)	Iron (mg)	Magnesium (mg)	Phosphorus (mg)	Potassium (mg)	Sodium (mg)	Zinc (mg)
0.00	0.00	0.00	0.00	0.00	0.00	0.00	0.00	0.00	0.00	0.00	0.00	0.00	0.00	0.00	0.00	0.00	0.00	1080.00	0.00
0.00	0.00	0.00	0.00	0.00	0.00	0.00	0.00	0.00	0.00	0.00	0.00	0.00	0.00	0.00	0.00	0.00	0.00	1490.00	0.00
0.00	0.00	0.00	0.00	0.00	0.00	0.00	0.00	0.00	0.00	0.00	0.00	0.00	0.00	0.00	0.00	0.00	0.00	1310.00	0.00
0.00	0.00	0.00	0.00	0.00	0.00	0.00	0.00	0.00	0.00	0.00	0.00	0.00	0.00	0.00	0.00	0.00	0.00	1330.00	0.00
0.00	0.00	0.00	0.00	0.00	0.00	0.00	0.00	0.00	0.00	0.00	0.00	0.00	0.00	0.00	0.00	0.00	0.00	690.00	0.00
0.00	0.00	0.00	0.00	0.00	0.00	0.00	0.00	0.00	0.00	0.00	0.00	0.00	0.00	0.00	0.00	0.00	0.00	340.00	0.00
0.00	0.00	0.00	0.00	0.00	0.00	0.00	0.00	0.00	0.00	0.00	0.00	0.00	0.00	0.00	0.00	0.00	0.00	0.00	0.00
0.00	0.00	0.00	0.00	0.00	0.00	0.00	0.00	0.00	0.00	0.00	0.00	0.00	0.00	0.00	0.00	0.00	0.00	1140.00	0.00
0.00	0.00	0.00	0.00	0.00	0.00	0.00	0.00	0.00	0.00	0.00	0.00	0.00	0.00	0.00	0.00	0.00	0.00	410.00	0.00
0.00	0.00	0.00	0.00	0.00	0.00	0.00	0.00	0.00	0.00	0.00	0.00	0.00	0.00	0.00	0.00	0.00	0.00	160.00	0.00
0.00	0.00	0.00	0.00	0.00	0.00	0.00	0.00	0.00	0.00	0.00	0.00	0.00	0.00	0.00	0.00	0.00	0.00	160.00	0.00
0.00	0.00	0.00	0.00	0.00	0.00	0.00	0.00	0.00	0.00	0.00	0.00	0.00	0.00	0.00	0.00	0.00	0.00	150.00	0.00
0.00	0.00	0.00	0.00	0.00	0.00	0.00	0.00	0.00	0.00	0.00	0.00	0.00	0.00	0.00	0.00	0.00	0.00	160.00	0.00
0.00	0.00	0.00	0.00	0.00	0.00	0.00	0.00	0.00	0.00	0.00	0.00	0.00	0.00	0.00	0.00	0.00	0.00	300.00	0.00
0.00	0.00	0.00	0.00	0.00	0.00	0.00	0.00	0.00	0.00	0.00	0.00	0.00	0.00	0.00	0.00	0.00	0.00	180.00	0.00
0.00	0.00	0.00	0.00	0.00	0.00	0.00	0.00	0.00	0.00	0.00	0.00	0.00	0.00	0.00	0.00	0.00	0.00	280.00	0.00
0.00	0.00	0.00	0.00	0.00	0.00	0.00	0.00	0.00	0.00	0.00	0.00	0.00	0.00	0.00	0.00	0.00	0.00	250.00	0.00
0.00	0.00	0.00	0.00	0.00	0.00	0.00	0.00	0.00	0.00	0.00	0.00	0.00	0.00	0.00	0.00	0.00	0.00	280.00	0.00
0.00	0.00	0.00	0.00	0.00	0.00	0.00	0.00	0.00	0.00	0.00	0.00	0.00	0.00	0.00	0.00	0.00	0.00	150.00	0.00
0.00	0.00	0.00	0.00	0.00	0.00	0.00	0.00	0.00	0.00	0.00	0.00	0.00	0.00	0.00	0.00	0.00	0.00	150.00	0.00
0.00	0.00	0.00	0.00	0.00	0.00	0.00	0.00	0.00	0.00	0.00	0.00	0.00	0.00	0.00	0.00	0.00	0.00	150.00	0.00
0.00	0.00	0.00	0.00	0.00	0.00	0.00	0.00	0.00	0.00	0.00	0.00	0.00	0.00	0.00	0.00	0.00	0.00	150.00	0.00
0.00	0.00	0.00	0.00	0.00	0.00	0.00	0.00	0.00	0.00	0.00	0.00	0.00	0.00	0.00	0.00	0.00	0.00	95.00	0.00
0.00	0.00	0.00	0.00	0.00	0.00	0.00	0.00	0.00	0.00	0.00	0.00	0.00	0.00	0.00	0.00	0.00	0.00	105.00	0.00
0.00	0.00	0.00	0.00	0.00	0.00	0.00	0.00	0.00	0.00	0.00	0.00	0.00	0.00	0.00	0.00	0.00	0.00	150.00	0.00
0.00	0.00	0.00	0.00	0.00	0.00	0.00	0.00	0.00	0.00	0.00	0.00	0.00	0.00	0.00	0.00	0.00	0.00	100.00	0.00
0.00	0.00	0.00	0.00	0.00	0.00	0.00	0.00	0.00	0.00	0.00	0.00	0.00	0.00	0.00	0.00	0.00	0.00	160.00	0.00
0.00	0.00	0.00	0.00	0.00	0.00	0.00	0.00	0.00	0.00	0.00	0.00	0.00	0.00	0.00	0.00	0.00	0.00	95.00	0.00
3.20	0.00	0.00	0.00	0.00	50.00	4.80	0.24	0.25	2.57	0.00	0.00	0.30	300.00	1.50	31.50	220.00	198.00	638.00	2.33
4.50	0.00	0.00	0.00	0.00	45.00	3.60	0.28	0.30	2.47	0.00	0.00	0.30	252.00	1.50	26.25	188.00	160.00	470.00	2.03
3.30	0.00	0.00	0.00	0.00	35.00	2.40	0.20	0.20	2.28	0.00	0.00	0.25	264.00	0.90	21.00	188.00	130.50	433.50	1.80
5.05	0.00	0.00	0.00	0.00	50.00	3.60	0.27	0.26	2.66	0.00	0.00	0.33	176.00	1.40	26.25	156.00	207.50	633.50	1.88
6.50	0.00	0.00	0.00	0.00	50.00	4.20	0.32	0.25	2.57	0.00	0.00	0.30	208.00	1.75	24.50	176.00	202.50	563.50	2.10
16.50	0.00	0.00	0.00	0.00	120.00	10.20	0.56	0.66	7.79	0.00	0.00	0.44	584.00	3.20	52.50	360.00	408.00	1335.00	3.75
4.70	0.00	0.00	0.00	0.00	35.00	3.00	0.21	0.21	2.47	0.00	0.00	0.25	180.00	0.90	19.25	148.00	143.50	493.00	1.73
5.35	0.00	0.00	0.00	0.00	50.00	4.20	0.29	0.22	2.57	0.00	0.00	0.35	184.00	1.35	26.25	168.00	231.50	668.00	2.25
6.00	0.00	0.00	0.00	0.00	55.00	6.00	0.35	0.29	3.52	0.00	0.00	0.41	176.00	1.90	33.25	168.00	258.00	824.00	2.40
7.00	0.00	0.00	0.00	0.00	60.00	5.40	0.38	0.33	3.04	0.00	0.00	0.40	216.00	1.85	31.50	188.00	266.00	723.50	2.70
6.90	0.00	0.00	0.00	0.00	55.00	6.00	0.35	0.26	3.42	0.00	0.00	0.40	192.00	2.25	35.00	184.00	289.00	735.00	2.85
8.00	0.00	0.00	0.00	0.00	60.00	4.80	0.41	0.40	2.85	0.00	0.00	0.38	200.00	1.40	33.25	184.00	290.00	831.50	2.78
16.80	0.00	0.00	0.00	0.00	120.00	10.80	0.59	0.66	7.60	0.00	0.00	0.46	416.00	3.70	52.50	320.00	487.00	1313.00	3.75
5.50	0.00	0.00	0.00	0.00	50.00	4.80	0.30	0.25	2.57	0.00	0.00	0.30	172.00	1.65	29.75	160.00	272.00	664.00	2.33
0.00	1.50	0.00	0.00	0.00	0.00	0.00	0.23	0.14	1.52	0.00	0.00	2.00	0.00	0.60	21.00	360.00	0.00	1150.00	0.90
0.00	1.90	0.00	0.00	0.00	0.00	0.00	0.30	0.14	1.90	0.00	0.00	0.04	0.00	0.00	21.00	160.00	0.00	50.00	0.30
0.00	1.00	0.00	0.00	0.00	0.00	0.00	0.06	0.10	11.40	0.00	0.00	0.08	0.00	0.40	21.00	160.00	0.00	60.00	0.90
0.00	0.60	0.00	0.00	0.00	0.00	0.00	0.03	0.07	0.76	0.00	0.00	0.60	0.00	0.00	28.00	200.00	0.00	200.00	0.30
0.00	1.60	0.00	0.00	0.00	0.00	0.00	0.09	0.17	1.90	0.00	0.00	1.60	48.00	0.00	70.00	320.00	0.00	900.00	6.00
0.00	1.80	0.00	0.00	0.00	0.00	0.00	0.03	0.10	1.90	0.00	0.00	1.60	80.00	0.20	70.00	200.00	0.00	1630.00	6.00
0.00	0.70	0.00	0.00	0.00	0.00	0.00	0.03	0.00	1.52	0.00	0.00	0.30	16.00	0.00	21.00	48.00	0.00	95.00	0.30
0.00	0.50	0.00	0.00	0.00	0.00	0.00	0.06	0.03	1.52	0.00	0.00	0.08	32.00	0.00	28.00	200.00	0.00	70.00	0.30
0.00	1.10	0.00	0.00	0.00	0.00	0.00	0.03	0.07	2.85	0.00	0.00	0.20	0.00	0.00	21.00	160.00	0.00	180.00	0.30
0.00	0.70	0.00	0.00	0.00	0.00	0.00	0.15	0.00	2.85	0.00	0.00	0.30	0.00	0.00	28.00	240.00	0.00	105.00	0.00
0.00	1.00	0.00	0.00	0.00	0.00	0.00	0.06	0.34	7.60	0.00	0.00	1.20	0.00	1.50	28.00	200.00	0.00	115.00	7.50

USDA ID Code	Food Name	Weight in Grams*	Quantity of Units	Unit of Measure	Protein (g)	Fat (g)	Carbohydrate (g)	Kilocalories	Caffeine (g)	Fiber (g)	Cholesterol (mg)	Saturated Fat (g)
	Red Lobster-Langostino, Lunch Po	141.7460	1.000	Each	26.00	1.00	2.00	120.00	0.00	0.00	210.00	0.20
	Red Lobster-Lobster, Live Maine	510.2880	1.000	Each	36.00	8.00	5.00	240.00	0.00	0.00	310.00	1.90
	Red Lobster-Lobster, Rock, Lunch	368.5410	1.000	Each	49.00	3.00	2.00	230.00	0.00	0.00	200.00	0.70
	Red Lobster-Mackerel, Lunch Port	141.7460	1.000	Each	20.00	12.00	1.00	190.00	0.00	0.00	100.00	3.60
	Red Lobster-Monkfish, Lunch Port	141.7460	1.000	Each	24.00	1.00	0.00	110.00	0.00	0.00	80.00	0.20
	Red Lobster-Perch, Atlantic Ocea	141.7460	1.000	Each	24.00	4.00	1.00	130.00	0.00	0.00	75.00	1.10
	Red Lobster-Pollock, Lunch Porti	141.7460	1.000	Each	28.00	1.00	1.00	120.00	0.00	0.00	90.00	0.30
	Red Lobster-Rockfish, Red, Lunch	141.7460	1.000	Each	21.00	1.00	0.00	90.00	0.00	0.00	85.00	0.30
	Red Lobster-Salmon, Norwegian, L	141.7460	1.000	Each	27.00	12.00	3.00	230.00	0.00	0.00	80.00	2.70
	Red Lobster-Salmon, Sockeye, Lun	141.7460	1.000	Each	28.00	4.00	3.00	160.00	0.00	0.00	50.00	1.10
	Red Lobster-Scallops, Deep Sea,	141.7460	1.000	Each	26.00	2.00	2.00	130.00	0.00	0.00	50.00	0.40
	Red Lobster-Shrimp, Lunch Portio	198.4450	1.000	Each	25.00	2.00	2.00	120.00	0.00	0.00	230.00	0.50
	Red Lobster-Snapper, Red, Lunch	141.7460	1.000	Each	25.00	1.00	1.00	110.00	0.00	0.00	70.00	0.40
	Red Lobster-Sole, Lemon, Lunch P	141.7460	1.000	Each	27.00	1.00	1.00	120.00	0.00	0.00	65.00	0.30
	Red Lobster-Steak, Strip, Lunch	255.1440	1.000	Each	47.00	40.00	0.00	560.00	0.00	0.00	150.00	17.00
	Red Lobster-Swordfish, Lunch Por	141.7460	1.000	Each	17.00	4.00	0.00	100.00	0.00	0.00	100.00	1.20
	Red Lobster-Trout, Rainbow, Lunc	141.7460	1.000	Each	23.00	9.00	0.00	170.00	0.00	0.00	90.00	2.50
	Red Lobster-Tuna, Yellow Fin, Lu	141.7460	1.000	Each	32.00	2.00	6.00	180.00	0.00	0.00	70.00	0.50

Seafood and Fish

USDA ID Code	Food Name	Weight in Grams*	Quantity of Units	Unit of Measure	Protein (g)	Fat (g)	Carbohydrate (g)	Kilocalories	Caffeine (g)	Fiber (g)	Cholesterol (mg)	Saturated Fat (g)
	Anchovy, European, Cnd In Oil	28.3500	3.000	Ounce	8.19	2.75	0.00	59.54	0.00	0.00	24.10	0.62
	Bass, Freshwater, Ckd, Dry Heat	62.0000	1.000	Each	14.99	2.93	0.00	90.52	0.00	0.00	53.94	0.62
	Bass, Striped, Ckd, Dry Heat	124.0000	1.000	Each	28.19	3.71	0.00	153.76	0.00	0.00	127.72	0.81
	Bluefish, Ckd, Dry Heat	117.0000	1.000	Each	30.06	6.36	0.00	186.03	0.00	0.00	88.92	1.37
	Catfish, Channel, Farmed, Ckd, D	143.0000	1.000	Each	26.77	11.47	0.00	217.36	0.00	0.00	91.52	2.56
	Catfish, Channel, Wild, Ckd, Dry	143.0000	1.000	Each	26.41	4.08	0.00	150.15	0.00	0.00	102.96	1.06
	Catfish, Fried	87.0000	1.000	Each	15.74	11.60	6.99	199.23	0.00	0.65	70.47	2.86
	Caviar, Black and Red, Granular	16.0000	1.000	Tbsp	3.94	2.86	0.64	40.32	0.00	0.00	94.08	0.65
	Clam, Ckd, Breaded and Fried	85.0000	3.000	Ounce	12.10	9.48	8.78	171.70	0.00	0.00	51.85	2.28
	Clam, Ckd, Moist Heat	85.0000	3.000	Ounce	21.72	1.66	4.36	125.80	0.00	0.00	56.95	0.16
	Clam, Cnd, Drained Solids	160.0000	1.000	Cup	40.88	3.12	8.21	236.80	0.00	0.00	107.20	0.30
	Cod, Atlantic, Ckd, Dry Heat	180.0000	1.000	Each	41.09	1.55	0.00	189.00	0.00	0.00	99.00	0.31
	Cod, Atlantic, Cnd	312.0000	1.000	Can	71.01	2.68	0.00	327.60	0.00	0.00	171.60	0.53
	Crab, Alaska King, Ckd, Moist He	134.0000	1.000	Leg	25.93	2.06	0.00	129.98	0.00	0.00	71.02	0.17
	Crab, Alaska King, Imitation	85.0000	3.000	Ounce	10.22	1.11	8.69	86.70	0.00	0.00	17.00	0.22
	Crab, Blue, Ckd, Moist Heat	118.0000	1.000	Cup	23.84	2.09	0.00	120.36	0.00	0.00	118.00	0.27
	Crab, Blue, Cnd	135.0000	1.000	Cup	27.70	1.66	0.00	133.65	0.00	0.00	120.15	0.34
	Crab, Blue, Crab Cakes	60.0000	1.000	Cake	12.13	4.51	0.29	93.00	0.00	0.00	90.00	0.89
	Crab, Dungeness, Ckd, Moist Heat	85.0000	3.000	Ounce	18.97	1.05	0.81	93.50	0.00	0.00	64.60	0.14
	Crab, Queen, Ckd, Moist Heat	85.0000	3.000	Ounce	20.16	1.28	0.00	97.75	0.00	0.00	60.35	0.15
217	Crawfish, Boiled	85.0000	3.000	Ounce	20.33	1.15	0.00	97.00	0.00	0.00	151.00	0.20
	Crayfish, Farmed, Ckd, Moist Hea	85.0000	3.000	Ounce	14.89	1.11	0.00	73.95	0.00	0.00	116.45	0.19
	Crayfish, Wild, Ckd, Moist Heat	85.0000	3.000	Ounce	14.25	1.02	0.00	69.70	0.00	0.00	113.05	0.15
	Fish Fillets and Sticks, Fried	57.0000	1.000	Piece	8.92	6.97	13.54	155.04	0.00	0.00	63.84	1.80
	Flounder, Ckd, Dry Heat	127.0000	1.000	Each	30.68	1.94	0.00	148.59	0.00	0.00	86.36	0.46
	Grouper, Ckd, Dry Heat	202.0000	1.000	Each	50.18	2.63	0.00	238.36	0.00	0.00	94.94	0.61
	Haddock, Ckd, Dry Heat	150.0000	1.000	Each	36.36	1.40	0.00	168.00	0.00	0.00	111.00	0.26
	Haddock, Smoked	28.3500	1.000	Ounce	7.15	0.27	0.00	32.89	0.00	0.00	21.83	0.05
	Halibut, Ckd, Dry Heat	159.0000	3.000	Ounce	42.44	4.67	0.00	222.60	0.00	0.00	65.19	0.67
	Halibut, Greenland, Ckd, Dry Hea	159.0000	3.000	Ounce	29.29	28.21	0.00	380.01	0.00	0.00	93.81	4.93
	Herring, Ckd, Dry Heat	143.0000	1.000	Each	32.93	16.57	0.00	290.29	0.00	0.00	110.11	3.75
	Herring, Kippered	28.3500	1.000	Ounce	6.97	3.51	0.00	61.52	0.00	0.00	23.25	0.79
	Herring, Pacific, Ckd, Dry Heat	144.0000	1.000	Each	30.25	25.62	0.00	360.00	0.00	0.00	142.56	6.00
	Herring, Pickled	140.0000	1.000	Cup	19.87	25.20	13.50	366.80	0.00	0.00	18.20	3.33

Monounsaturated Fat (g)	Polyunsaturated Fat (g)	Vitamin D (mg)	Vitamin K (mg)	Vitamin E (mg)	Vitamin A (re)	Vitamin C (mg)	Thiamin (mg)	Riboflavin (mg)	Niacin (mg)	Vitamin B6 (mg)	Folate (mcg)	Vitamin B12 (mcg)	Calcium (mg)	Iron (mg)	Magnesium (mg)	Phosphorus (mg)	Potassium (mg)	Sodium (mg)	Zinc (mg)
0.00	0.60	0.00	0.00	0.00	0.00	0.00	0.12	0.00	1.14	0.00	0.00	2.00	16.00	0.80	35.00	160.00	0.00	410.00	1.50
0.00	4.10	0.00	0.00	0.00	0.00	0.00	0.15	0.17	2.85	0.00	0.00	2.00	320.00	0.80	52.50	320.00	0.00	550.00	6.75
0.00	1.40	0.00	0.00	0.00	0.00	0.00	0.00	0.07	3.80	0.00	0.00	0.50	48.00	0.00	87.50	400.00	0.00	1090.00	6.00
0.00	5.40	0.00	0.00	0.00	0.00	0.00	0.15	0.43	5.70	0.00	0.00	0.80	16.00	0.80	21.00	200.00	0.00	250.00	1.20
0.00	0.70	0.00	0.00	0.00	40.00	0.00	0.06	0.14	0.76	0.00	0.00	0.20	0.00	1.00	14.00	64.00	0.00	95.00	0.30
0.00	1.20	0.00	0.00	0.00	0.00	0.00	0.06	0.10	1.52	0.00	0.00	0.30	0.00	0.00	21.00	160.00	0.00	190.00	0.30
0.00	1.00	0.00	0.00	0.00	0.00	0.00	0.06	0.17	0.38	0.00	0.00	1.00	0.00	0.00	28.00	160.00	0.00	90.00	0.30
0.00	0.50	0.00	0.00	0.00	0.00	0.00	0.09	0.10	0.76	0.00	0.00	0.60	0.00	0.00	21.00	120.00	0.00	95.00	0.30
0.00	4.60	0.00	0.00	0.00	0.00	0.00	0.23	0.07	6.65	0.00	0.00	0.20	16.00	0.00	35.00	240.00	0.00	60.00	0.30
0.00	1.80	0.00	0.00	0.00	0.00	0.00	0.38	0.14	7.60	0.00	0.00	2.00	0.00	0.00	35.00	280.00	0.00	60.00	0.30
0.00	1.50	0.00	0.00	0.00	0.00	0.00	0.10	0.10	1.90	0.00	0.00	0.40	0.00	0.00	52.50	240.00	0.00	260.00	1.50
0.00	1.10	0.00	0.00	0.00	0.00	0.00	0.00	0.03	1.90	0.00	0.00	0.50	32.00	0.00	35.00	120.00	0.00	110.00	1.50
0.00	0.60	0.00	0.00	0.00	0.00	0.00	0.06	0.03	4.75	0.00	0.00	0.30	0.00	0.00	21.00	120.00	0.00	140.00	0.30
0.00	0.40	0.00	0.00	0.00	0.00	0.00	0.06	0.10	0.38	0.00	0.00	0.40	0.00	0.00	21.00	64.00	0.00	90.00	0.30
0.00	2.00	0.00	0.00	0.00	0.00	0.00	0.15	0.34	7.60	0.00	0.00	1.20	0.00	2.00	35.00	280.00	0.00	115.00	9.00
0.00	1.00	0.00	0.00	0.00	20.00	0.00	0.06	0.07	3.80	0.00	0.00	0.30	0.00	0.00	28.00	80.00	0.00	140.00	0.60
0.00	4.00	0.00	0.00	0.00	0.00	0.00	0.12	0.17	2.85	0.00	0.00	1.00	80.00	0.00	21.00	200.00	0.00	90.00	0.90
0.00	1.60	0.00	0.00	0.00	0.00	0.00	0.06	0.03	13.30	0.00	0.00	1.60	0.00	0.60	35.00	240.00	0.00	70.00	0.30
1.07	0.73	0.00	0.00	1.42	5.95	0.00	0.02	0.10	5.64	0.06	3.54	0.25	65.77	1.31	19.56	71.44	154.22	1039.88	0.69
1.14	0.84	0.00	0.00	0.00	21.70	1.30	0.06	0.06	0.94	0.09	10.54	1.43	63.86	1.18	23.56	158.72	282.72	55.80	0.51
1.05	1.25	0.00	0.00	0.00	38.44	0.00	0.15	0.05	3.17	0.43	12.40	5.47	23.56	1.34	63.24	314.96	406.72	109.12	0.63
2.69	1.59	0.00	0.00	0.00	161.46	0.00	0.08	0.12	8.48	0.54	2.34	7.28	10.53	0.73	49.14	340.47	558.09	90.09	1.22
5.95	1.99	0.00	0.00	0.00	21.45	1.14	0.60	0.10	3.59	0.23	10.01	4.00	12.87	1.17	37.18	350.35	459.03	114.40	1.50
1.57	0.92	0.00	0.00	0.00	21.45	1.14	0.33	0.10	3.42	0.16	14.30	4.15	15.73	0.50	40.04	434.72	599.17	71.50	0.87
4.88	2.90	0.00	0.00	0.00	6.96	0.00	0.06	0.11	1.98	0.17	26.10	1.65	38.28	1.24	23.49	187.92	295.80	243.60	0.75
0.74	1.19	0.93	0.00	1.12	89.60	0.00	0.03	0.10	0.02	0.05	8.00	3.20	44.00	1.90	48.00	56.96	28.96	240.00	0.15
3.87	2.44	0.00	0.00	0.00	76.50	8.50	0.09	0.20	1.75	0.05	30.60	34.23	53.55	11.82	11.90	159.80	277.10	309.40	1.24
0.14	0.47	0.00	0.00	0.00	145.35	18.79	0.13	0.37	2.85	0.09	24.48	84.06	78.20	23.77	15.30	287.30	533.80	95.20	2.32
0.27	0.88	0.00	0.00	1.60	273.60	35.36	0.24	0.69	5.36	0.18	46.08	158.22	147.20	44.74	28.80	540.80	1004.80	179.20	4.37
0.22	0.52	0.00	0.00	0.54	25.20	1.80	0.16	0.14	4.52	0.50	14.58	1.89	25.20	0.88	75.60	248.40	439.20	140.40	1.04
0.37	0.90	6.55	0.00	0.62	43.68	3.12	0.28	0.25	7.83	0.87	25.27	3.28	65.52	1.53	127.92	811.20	1647.36	680.16	1.81
0.25	0.72	0.00	0.00	0.00	12.06	10.18	0.07	0.08	1.80	0.24	68.34	15.41	79.06	1.02	84.42	375.20	351.08	1436.48	10.21
0.17	0.57	0.00	0.00	0.09	17.00	0.00	0.03	0.03	0.15	0.03	1.36	1.36	11.05	0.33	36.55	239.70	76.50	714.85	0.28
0.33	0.80	0.00	0.00	1.18	2.36	3.89	0.12	0.06	3.89	0.21	59.94	8.61	122.72	1.07	38.94	243.08	382.32	329.22	4.98
0.30	0.59	0.00	0.00	1.35	2.70	3.65	0.11	0.11	1.85	0.20	57.38	0.62	136.35	1.13	52.65	351.00	504.90	449.55	5.43
1.69	1.36	0.00	0.00	0.00	48.60	1.68	0.05	0.05	1.74	0.10	31.80	3.56	63.00	0.65	19.80	127.80	194.40	198.00	2.45
0.18	0.35	0.00	0.00	0.00	26.35	3.06	0.05	0.17	3.08	0.14	35.70	8.82	50.15	0.37	49.30	148.75	346.80	321.30	4.65
0.28	0.46	0.00	0.00	0.00	44.20	6.12	0.09	0.20	2.46	0.14	35.70	8.82	28.05	2.45	53.55	108.80	170.00	587.35	3.05
0.32	0.28	0.00	0.00	0.00	0.00	2.80	0.00	0.07	2.49	0.00	0.00	2.94	26.00	2.67	27.00	280.00	298.00	58.00	1.42
0.21	0.35	0.00	0.00	0.00	12.75	0.43	0.04	0.07	1.42	0.11	9.35	2.64	43.35	0.94	28.05	204.85	202.30	82.45	1.26
0.20	0.31	0.00	0.00	1.28	12.75	0.77	0.04	0.08	1.94	0.07	37.40	1.83	51.00	0.71	28.05	229.50	251.60	79.90	1.50
2.89	1.81	0.00	0.00	0.78	17.67	0.00	0.07	0.10	1.21	0.03	10.37	1.03	11.40	0.42	14.25	103.17	148.77	331.74	0.38
0.30	0.83	0.00	0.00	2.40	13.97	0.00	0.10	0.14	2.77	0.30	11.68	3.19	22.86	0.43	73.66	367.03	436.88	133.35	0.80
0.55	0.81	0.00	0.00	0.00	101.00	0.00	0.16	0.02	0.77	0.71	20.60	1.39	42.42	2.30	74.74	288.86	959.50	107.06	1.03
0.23	0.47	0.00	0.00	0.00	28.50	0.00	0.06	0.08	6.95	0.53	19.95	2.09	63.00	2.03	75.00	361.50	598.50	130.50	0.72
0.05	0.09	0.00	0.00	0.11	6.24	0.00	0.01	0.01	1.44	0.11	4.34	0.45	13.89	0.40	15.31	71.16	117.65	216.31	0.14
1.54	1.49	0.00	0.00	1.73	85.86	0.00	0.11	0.14	11.32	0.64	21.94	2.18	95.40	1.70	170.13	453.15	915.84	109.71	0.84
17.08	2.78	0.00	0.00	0.00	28.62	0.00	0.11	0.16	3.05	0.78	1.59	1.53	6.36	1.35	52.47	333.90	546.96	163.77	0.81
6.85	3.92	0.00	0.00	1.92	44.33	1.00	0.16	0.43	5.89	0.50	16.45	18.79	105.82	2.02	58.63	433.29	599.17	164.45	1.82
1.45	0.83	0.85	0.00	0.28	11.06	0.28	0.04	0.09	1.25	0.12	3.88	5.30	23.81	0.43	13.04	92.14	126.72	260.25	0.39
12.69	4.48	0.00	0.00	0.00	50.40	0.00	0.10	0.37	4.06	0.75	8.64	13.85	152.64	2.07	59.04	420.48	780.48	136.80	0.98
16.73	2.35	23.80	0.00	1.40	361.20	0.00	0.06	0.20	4.62	0.24	3.36	5.98	107.80	1.71	11.20	124.60	96.60	1218.00	0.74

USDA ID Code	Food Name	Weight in Grams*	Quantity of Units	Unit of Measure	Protein (g)	Fat (g)	Carbohydrate (g)	Kilocalories	Caffeine (g)	Fiber (g)	Cholesterol (mg)	Saturated Fat (g)
	Lobster, Northern, Ckd, Moist He	145.0000	1.000	Cup	29.73	0.86	1.86	142.10	0.00	0.00	104.40	0.16
	Lobster, Spiny, Ckd, Moist Heat	163.0000	1.000	Lobster	43.05	3.16	5.09	233.09	0.00	0.00	146.70	0.49
	Mackerel, Ckd, Dry Heat	88.0000	1.000	Each	20.99	15.67	0.00	230.56	0.00	0.00	66.00	3.68
	Mullet, Striped, Ckd, Dry Heat	93.0000	1.000	Each	23.07	4.52	0.00	139.50	0.00	0.00	58.59	1.33
	Mussel, Blue, Ckd, Moist Heat	85.0000	3.000	Ounce	20.23	3.81	6.28	146.20	0.00	0.00	47.60	0.72
	Oyster, Eastern, Breaded and Fri	85.0000	3.000	Ounce	7.45	10.69	9.88	167.45	0.00	0.00	68.85	2.72
	Oyster, Eastern, Cnd	162.0000	1.000	Cup	11.44	4.00	6.33	111.78	0.00	0.00	89.10	1.02
	Oysters, Raw	85.0000	3.000	Ounce	4.44	1.32	4.70	50.15	0.00	0.00	21.25	0.37
	Perch, Atlantic, Ckd, Dry Heat	50.0000	1.000	Each	11.94	1.05	0.00	60.50	0.00	0.00	27.00	0.16
	Perch, Ckd, Dry Heat	46.0000	1.000	Each	11.44	0.54	0.00	53.82	0.00	0.00	52.90	0.11
	Pike, Northern, Ckd, Dry Heat	155.0000	3.000	Ounce	38.27	1.36	0.00	175.15	0.00	0.00	77.50	0.23
	Pike, Walleye, Ckd, Dry Heat	124.0000	1.000	Each	30.43	1.93	0.00	147.56	0.00	0.00	136.40	0.40
	Pollock, Atlantic, Ckd, Dry Heat	151.0000	3.000	Ounce	37.63	1.90	0.00	178.18	0.00	0.00	137.41	0.26
655	Pompano, Cooked	85.0000	3.000	Ounce	20.14	10.32	0.00	179.35	0.00	0.00	54.40	3.82
	Pompano, Florida, Ckd, Dry Heat	88.0000	1.000	Each	20.85	10.68	0.00	185.68	0.00	0.00	56.32	3.96
	Rockfish, Pacific, Ckd, Dry Heat	149.0000	1.000	Each	35.82	2.99	0.00	180.29	0.00	0.00	65.56	0.70
	Roughy, Orange, Ckd, Dry Heat	85.0000	3.000	Ounce	16.02	0.77	0.00	75.65	0.00	0.00	22.10	0.02
	Salmon, Atlantic, Wild, Ckd, Dry	154.0000	3.000	Ounce	39.18	12.52	0.00	280.28	0.00	0.00	109.34	1.94
	Salmon, Chinook, Ckd, Dry Heat	154.0000	3.000	Ounce	39.61	20.61	0.00	355.74	0.00	0.00	130.90	4.94
	Salmon, Chum, Ckd, Dry Heat	154.0000	3.000	Ounce	39.76	7.44	0.00	237.16	0.00	0.00	146.30	1.66
	Salmon, Cnd	369.0000	1.000	Can	75.53	26.97	0.00	564.57	0.00	0.00	162.36	6.05
	Salmon, Coho, Farmed, Ckd, Dry H	143.0000	1.000	Each	34.75	11.77	0.00	254.54	0.00	0.00	90.09	2.77
	Salmon, Coho, Wild, Ckd, Dry Hea	178.0000	3.000	Ounce	41.74	7.65	0.00	247.42	0.00	0.00	97.90	1.87
	Salmon, Coho, Wild, Ckd, Moist H	155.0000	3.000	Ounce	42.41	11.63	0.00	285.20	0.00	0.00	88.35	2.48
	Salmon, Pink, Ckd, Dry Heat	124.0000	3.000	Ounce	31.69	5.48	0.00	184.76	0.00	0.00	83.08	0.89
	Sardine, Atlantic, Cnd In Oil	149.0000	1.000	Cup	36.68	17.06	0.00	309.92	0.00	0.00	211.58	2.28
	Scallop, Breaded and Fried	31.0000	2.000	Large	5.60	3.39	3.14	66.65	0.00	0.00	18.91	0.83
	Scallop, Imitation	85.0000	3.000	Ounce	10.85	0.35	9.03	84.15	0.00	0.00	18.70	0.07
	Scallops, Sauteed	28.3500	3.000	Ounce	9.67	0.33	0.67	50.00	0.00	0.00	20.00	0.00
	Sea Bass, Ckd, Dry Heat	101.0000	1.000	Each	23.87	2.59	0.00	125.24	0.00	0.00	53.53	0.67
	Shark, Ckd, Batter-dipped and Fr	85.0000	3.000	Ounce	15.83	11.75	5.43	193.80	0.00	0.00	50.15	2.73
	Shrimp, Ckd, Breaded and Fried	85.0000	3.000	Ounce	18.18	10.44	9.75	205.70	0.00	0.32	150.45	1.78
	Shrimp, Ckd, Moist Heat	85.0000	3.000	Ounce	17.77	0.92	0.00	84.15	0.00	0.00	165.75	0.25
	Shrimp, Cnd	128.0000	1.000	Cup	29.54	2.51	1.32	153.60	0.00	0.00	221.44	0.47
	Shrimp, Fresh	6.0000	1.000	Slice	1.22	0.10	0.05	6.36	0.00	0.00	9.12	0.02
	Shrimp, Imitation	85.0000	3.000	Ounce	10.53	1.25	7.76	85.85	0.00	0.00	30.60	0.25
	Smelt, Rainbow, Ckd, Dry Heat	85.0000	3.000	Ounce	19.21	2.64	0.00	105.40	0.00	0.00	76.50	0.49
	Snapper, Ckd, Dry Heat	170.0000	1.000	Each	44.71	2.92	0.00	217.60	0.00	0.00	79.90	0.63
	Squid, Fried	85.0000	3.000	Ounce	15.25	6.36	6.62	148.75	0.00	0.00	221.00	1.60
	Sunfish, Ckd, Dry Heat	37.0000	1.000	Each	9.20	0.33	0.00	42.18	0.00	0.00	31.82	0.07
	Swordfish, Ckd, Dry Heat	106.0000	1.000	Piece	26.91	5.45	0.00	164.30	0.00	0.00	53.00	1.49
	Trout, Ckd, Dry Heat	62.0000	1.000	Each	16.51	5.25	0.00	117.80	0.00	0.00	45.88	0.91
	Trout, Rainbow, Farmed, Ckd, Dry	71.0000	1.000	Each	17.23	5.11	0.00	119.99	0.00	0.00	48.28	1.50
	Trout, Rainbow, Wild, Ckd, Dry H	143.0000	1.000	Each	32.78	8.32	0.00	214.50	0.00	0.00	98.67	2.32
	Tuna Salad	205.0000	1.000	Cup	32.88	18.98	19.29	383.35	0.00	0.00	26.65	3.16
	Tuna, Light Meat, Cnd In Oil	171.0000	1.000	Can	49.81	14.04	0.00	338.58	0.00	0.00	30.78	2.62
	Tuna, Light Meat, Cnd In Water	165.0000	1.000	Can	42.09	1.35	0.00	191.40	0.00	0.00	49.50	0.38
	Tuna, Light, Cnd In Water	154.0000	1.000	Cup	39.29	1.26	0.00	178.64	0.00	0.00	46.20	0.35
	Tuna, Skipjack, Ckd, Dry Heat	154.0000	3.000	Ounce	43.44	1.99	0.00	203.28	0.00	0.00	92.40	0.65
	Tuna, White Meat, Cnd In Oil	178.0000	1.000	Can	47.22	14.38	0.00	331.08	0.00	0.00	55.18	2.94
	Tuna, White Meat, Cnd In Water	172.0000	1.000	Can	40.63	5.11	0.00	220.16	0.00	0.00	72.24	1.36
	Tuna, Yellowfin, Ckd, Dry Heat	85.0000	3.000	Ounce	25.47	1.04	0.00	118.15	0.00	0.00	49.30	0.26
	Whitefish, Ckd, Dry Heat	154.0000	1.000	Each	37.68	11.57	0.00	264.88	0.00	0.00	118.58	1.79

Page Key: A2 = Baby Food   A2 = Baked Goods   A8 = Beverages   A14 = Breads/Grains and Pasta   A18 = Breakfast Foods/Cereals   A26 = Dairy and Eggs   A40 = Fats and Oils   A42 = Fruits and Vegetables   A52 = Meats and Beans   A60 = Nuts and Seeds   A62 5 Frozen Entrees and Packaged Foods   A76 = Restaurant Chains–Fast Foods   A92 = Restaurant Chains–Other   A106 = Seafood and Fish   A110 = Snacks and Sweets   A120 = Soups   A122 = Supplements   A126 = Toppings and Sauces

Monounsaturated Fat (g)	Polyunsaturated Fat (g)	Vitamin D (mg)	Vitamin K (mg)	Vitamin E (mg)	Vitamin A (re)	Vitamin C (mg)	Thiamin (mg)	Riboflavin (mg)	Niacin (mg)	Vitamin B₆ (mg)	Folate (mcg)	Vitamin B₁₂ (mcg)	Calcium (mg)	Iron (mg)	Magnesium (mg)	Phosphorus (mg)	Potassium (mg)	Sodium (mg)	Zinc (mg)
0.23	0.13	0.00	0.00	1.45	37.70	0.00	0.01	0.10	1.55	0.12	16.10	4.51	88.45	0.57	50.75	268.25	510.40	551.00	4.23
0.57	1.24	0.00	0.00	0.00	9.78	3.42	0.02	0.10	7.99	0.28	1.63	6.59	102.69	2.30	83.13	373.27	339.04	370.01	11.85
6.17	3.78	0.00	0.00	0.00	47.52	0.35	0.14	0.36	6.03	0.40	1.32	16.72	13.20	1.38	85.36	244.64	352.88	73.04	0.83
1.28	0.86	0.00	0.00	0.00	39.06	1.12	0.09	0.09	5.86	0.46	9.11	0.23	28.83	1.31	30.69	226.92	425.94	66.03	0.82
0.86	1.03	0.00	0.00	0.00	77.35	11.56	0.26	0.36	2.55	0.09	64.26	20.40	28.05	5.71	31.45	242.25	227.80	313.65	2.27
4.00	2.81	0.00	0.00	0.00	76.50	3.23	0.13	0.17	1.40	0.05	26.35	13.29	52.70	5.91	49.30	135.15	207.40	354.45	74.06
0.41	1.20	0.00	0.00	1.38	145.80	8.10	0.24	0.28	2.01	0.16	14.42	30.99	72.90	10.85	87.48	225.18	370.98	181.44	47.34
0.13	0.50	0.00	0.00	0.00	6.80	4.00	0.09	0.06	1.08	0.05	15.30	13.77	37.40	4.91	28.05	79.05	105.40	151.30	32.23
0.40	0.28	0.00	0.00	0.00	7.00	0.40	0.07	0.07	1.22	0.14	5.20	0.58	68.50	0.59	19.50	138.50	175.00	48.00	0.31
0.09	0.22	0.00	0.00	0.00	4.60	0.78	0.04	0.06	0.87	0.06	2.67	1.01	46.92	0.53	17.48	118.22	158.24	36.34	0.66
0.31	0.40	0.00	0.00	0.00	37.20	5.89	0.11	0.12	4.34	0.22	26.82	3.57	113.15	1.10	62.00	437.10	513.05	75.95	1.33
0.47	0.71	0.00	0.00	0.00	29.76	0.00	0.38	0.25	3.47	0.17	21.08	2.86	174.84	2.07	47.12	333.56	618.76	80.60	0.98
0.21	0.94	0.00	0.00	0.00	18.12	0.00	0.08	0.35	6.01	0.50	4.53	5.56	116.27	0.89	129.86	427.33	688.56	166.10	0.91
2.82	1.24	0.00	0.00	0.00	0.00	0.00	0.58	0.13	3.23	0.20	14.71	1.02	36.55	0.57	26.35	289.85	540.60	64.60	0.59
2.92	1.28	0.00	0.00	0.00	31.68	0.00	0.60	0.13	3.34	0.20	15.22	1.06	37.84	0.59	27.28	300.08	559.68	66.88	0.61
0.67	0.88	0.00	0.00	1.86	98.34	0.00	0.06	0.12	5.84	0.40	15.50	1.79	17.88	0.79	50.66	339.72	774.80	114.73	0.79
0.53	0.02	0.00	0.00	0.00	20.40	0.00	0.10	0.15	3.10	0.30	6.80	1.96	32.30	0.20	32.30	217.60	327.25	68.85	0.82
4.16	5.02	0.00	0.00	0.00	20.02	0.00	0.43	0.75	15.52	1.45	44.66	4.70	23.10	1.59	56.98	394.24	967.12	86.24	1.26
8.84	4.10	0.00	0.00	0.00	229.46	6.31	0.06	0.23	15.48	0.71	53.90	4.42	43.12	1.40	187.88	571.34	777.70	92.40	0.86
3.05	1.77	0.00	0.00	0.00	52.36	0.00	0.14	0.34	13.14	0.71	7.70	5.33	21.56	1.09	43.12	559.02	847.00	98.56	0.92
11.66	6.97	0.00	0.00	5.90	195.57	0.00	0.07	0.70	20.22	1.11	36.16	1.11	881.91	3.91	107.01	1202.94	1391.13	1985.22	3.76
5.18	2.80	0.00	0.00	0.00	84.37	2.15	0.14	0.16	10.57	0.82	20.22	4.53	17.16	0.56	48.62	474.76	657.80	74.36	0.67
2.81	2.26	0.00	0.00	1.44	69.42	2.49	0.14	0.25	14.15	1.01	23.14	8.90	80.10	1.09	58.74	573.16	772.52	103.24	1.00
4.19	3.91	0.00	0.00	0.00	49.60	1.55	0.19	0.25	12.06	0.87	13.95	6.94	71.30	1.10	54.25	461.90	705.25	82.15	0.81
1.49	2.15	0.00	0.00	0.00	50.84	0.00	0.25	0.09	10.58	0.29	6.20	4.29	21.08	1.23	40.92	365.80	513.36	106.64	0.88
5.77	7.67	10.13	0.00	0.45	99.83	0.00	0.12	0.34	7.82	0.25	17.58	13.32	569.18	4.35	58.11	730.10	591.53	752.45	1.95
1.40	0.89	0.00	0.00	0.00	6.82	0.71	0.01	0.03	0.47	0.04	11.47	0.41	13.02	0.25	18.29	73.16	103.23	143.84	0.33
0.05	0.18	0.00	0.00	0.00	17.00	0.00	0.01	0.02	0.26	0.03	1.36	1.36	6.80	0.26	36.55	239.70	87.55	675.75	0.28
0.00	0.00	0.00	0.00	0.00	0.00	0.60	0.00	0.00	0.00	0.00	0.00	0.00	8.00	0.00	0.00	0.00	0.00	91.67	0.00
0.55	0.96	0.00	0.00	0.00	64.64	0.00	0.13	0.15	1.92	0.46	5.86	0.30	13.13	0.37	53.53	250.48	331.28	87.87	0.53
5.05	3.15	0.00	0.00	0.00	45.90	0.00	0.06	0.09	2.36	0.26	12.75	1.03	42.50	0.94	36.55	164.90	131.75	103.70	0.41
3.24	4.33	0.00	0.00	0.00	47.60	1.28	0.11	0.12	2.61	0.09	6.89	1.59	56.95	1.07	34.00	185.30	191.25	292.40	1.17
0.17	0.37	0.00	0.00	0.43	56.10	1.87	0.03	0.03	2.20	0.11	2.98	1.27	33.15	2.63	28.90	116.45	154.70	190.40	1.33
0.37	0.97	0.00	0.00	1.19	23.04	2.94	0.04	0.05	3.53	0.14	2.30	1.43	75.52	3.51	52.48	298.24	268.80	216.32	1.61
0.02	0.04	0.23	0.00	0.05	3.24	0.12	0.00	0.00	0.15	0.01	0.18	0.07	3.12	0.14	2.22	12.30	11.10	8.88	0.07
0.19	0.64	0.00	0.00	0.00	17.00	0.00	0.02	0.03	0.14	0.03	1.36	1.36	16.15	0.51	36.55	239.70	75.65	599.25	0.28
0.70	0.97	0.00	0.00	0.00	14.45	0.00	0.01	0.13	1.50	0.14	3.91	3.37	65.45	0.98	32.30	250.75	316.20	65.45	1.80
0.54	1.00	0.00	0.00	0.00	59.50	2.72	0.09	0.00	0.60	0.78	9.86	5.95	68.00	0.41	62.90	341.70	887.40	96.90	0.75
2.34	1.82	0.00	0.00	0.00	9.35	3.57	0.05	0.39	2.21	0.05	11.90	1.05	33.15	0.86	32.30	213.35	237.15	260.10	1.48
0.06	0.12	0.00	0.00	0.00	6.29	0.37	0.03	0.03	0.54	0.05	6.29	0.85	38.11	0.57	14.06	85.47	166.13	38.11	0.74
2.10	1.25	0.00	0.00	0.00	43.46	1.17	0.04	0.13	12.50	0.40	2.44	2.14	6.36	1.10	36.04	357.22	391.14	121.90	1.56
2.59	1.19	0.00	0.00	0.00	11.78	0.31	0.27	0.26	3.58	0.14	9.30	4.64	34.10	1.19	17.36	194.68	287.06	41.54	0.53
1.49	1.65	0.00	0.00	0.00	61.06	2.34	0.17	0.06	6.24	0.28	17.04	3.53	61.06	0.23	22.72	188.86	313.11	29.82	0.35
2.50	2.62	0.00	0.00	0.00	21.45	2.86	0.21	0.14	8.25	0.50	27.17	9.01	122.98	0.54	44.33	384.67	640.64	80.08	0.73
5.92	8.45	0.00	0.00	0.00	55.35	4.51	0.06	0.14	13.74	0.16	16.40	2.46	34.85	2.05	38.95	364.90	364.90	824.10	1.15
5.04	4.94	0.00	0.00	0.00	39.33	0.00	0.07	0.21	21.20	0.19	9.06	3.76	22.23	2.38	53.01	531.81	353.97	85.50	1.54
0.26	0.56	0.00	0.00	0.87	28.05	0.00	0.05	0.12	21.91	0.58	6.60	4.93	18.15	2.52	44.55	268.95	391.05	82.50	1.27
0.25	0.52	0.00	0.00	0.82	26.18	0.00	0.05	0.11	20.45	0.54	6.16	4.60	16.94	2.36	41.58	251.02	364.98	520.52	1.19
0.37	0.62	0.00	0.00	0.00	27.72	1.54	0.06	0.18	28.89	1.51	15.40	3.37	56.98	2.46	67.76	438.90	803.88	72.38	1.62
4.41	6.02	0.00	0.00	0.00	42.72	0.00	0.04	0.14	20.83	0.77	8.19	3.92	7.12	1.16	60.52	475.26	592.74	89.00	0.84
1.34	1.91	0.00	0.00	2.73	10.32	0.00	0.02	0.07	9.98	0.38	3.44	2.01	24.08	1.67	56.76	373.24	407.64	86.00	0.83
0.17	0.31	0.00	0.00	0.00	17.00	0.85	0.43	0.05	10.15	0.88	1.70	0.51	17.85	0.80	54.40	208.25	483.65	39.95	0.57
3.94	4.25	0.00	0.00	0.00	60.06	0.00	0.26	0.23	5.93	0.54	26.18	1.48	50.82	0.72	64.68	532.84	625.24	100.10	1.96

USDA ID Code	Food Name	Weight in Grams*	Quantity of Units	Unit of Measure	Protein (g)	Fat (g)	Carbohydrate (g)	Kilocalories	Caffeine (g)	Fiber (g)	Cholesterol (mg)	Saturated Fat (g)
	Whitefish, Smoked	136.0000	1.000	Cup	31.82	1.26	0.00	146.88	0.00	0.00	44.88	0.31
	Yellowtail, Ckd, Dry Heat	146.0000	3.000	Ounce	43.32	9.81	0.00	273.02	0.00	0.00	103.66	0.00
	Yellowtail, Fresh	187.0000	3.000	Ounce	43.27	9.80	0.00	273.02	0.00	0.00	102.85	2.39

Snacks and Sweets

USDA ID Code	Food Name	Weight in Grams*	Quantity of Units	Unit of Measure	Protein (g)	Fat (g)	Carbohydrate (g)	Kilocalories	Caffeine (g)	Fiber (g)	Cholesterol (mg)	Saturated Fat (g)
	Brownies	28.3500	1.000	Ounce	1.36	4.62	18.12	114.82	0.57	0.60	4.82	1.20
	Candy Bar, Almond Joy	20.0000	1.000	Small Bar	0.84	5.36	11.66	93.40	0.00	0.96	0.80	3.46
	Candy Bar, Alpine White, w/ Almo	35.0000	1.000	Bar	3.50	12.92	17.64	197.40	0.00	1.89	4.20	6.67
	Candy Bar, Butterfinger Bar	174.0000	1.000	Cup	21.66	32.47	114.07	835.20	6.96	4.18	1.74	18.03
	Candy Bar, Chocolate Bar-Krack	41.0000	1.000	Each	2.71	11.77	25.26	217.71	7.38	0.90	7.79	7.42
	Candy Bar, Chocolate, Milk-Sym	42.0000	1.000	Each	3.02	13.78	24.33	232.26	0.00	0.80	9.24	0.00
	Candy Bar, Chocolate, Special Da	41.0000	1.000	Each	2.01	13.28	24.85	226.32	29.93	2.05	0.41	8.32
	Candy Bar, Chocolate-Mr. Goodbar	49.0000	1.000	Each	5.24	17.10	25.33	267.05	9.80	1.72	3.92	7.30
	Candy Bar, Chunky Bar	35.0000	1.000	Each	3.15	10.22	19.99	173.25	10.15	1.68	3.85	8.13
	Candy Bar, Fifth Avenue Bar	57.0000	1.000	Each	5.13	12.14	37.68	280.44	3.99	1.25	3.42	4.50
	Candy Bar, Milky Way	23.0000	1.000	Each	1.04	3.70	16.49	97.29	1.84	0.39	3.22	1.79
	Candy Bar, Mounds	53.0000	1.000	Each	2.01	13.30	31.22	252.81	9.01	3.13	1.06	10.76
	Candy Bar, Nestle Crunch	40.0000	1.000	Each	2.40	10.52	26.08	208.80	9.60	1.04	5.20	6.08
	Candy Bar, Peanut Bar	28.3500	1.000	Ounce	4.39	9.55	13.44	147.99	0.00	1.62	0.00	1.33
	Candy Bar, Peanut Butter Cups-	7.0000	1.000	Miniature	0.72	2.19	3.82	37.87	0.70	0.22	0.35	0.78
	Candy Bar, Snickers	57.0000	1.000	Each	4.56	14.01	33.75	273.03	3.99	1.43	7.41	5.12
	Candy Bar, Three Musketeers	23.0000	1.000	Each	0.74	2.97	17.66	95.68	2.53	0.37	2.53	1.50
	Candy Bar, Twix	57.0000	1.000	Each	2.62	13.90	37.38	284.43	1.71	0.63	2.85	5.07
	Candy Bar, Wafer Bar-Kit Kat	42.0000	1.000	Each	2.98	10.71	26.88	215.88	5.04	0.80	2.52	6.85
	Candy, Butterscotch	28.3500	1.000	Ounce	0.03	0.99	27.02	111.98	0.00	0.00	2.55	0.31
	Candy, Caramels	71.0000	1.000	Package	3.27	5.75	54.67	271.22	0.00	0.85	4.97	4.67
	Candy, Goobers	39.0000	1.000	Package	5.34	13.07	18.99	200.07	8.58	2.38	3.51	4.76
	Candy, Gumdrops	182.0000	1.000	Cup	0.00	0.00	180.00	702.52	0.00	0.00	0.00	0.00
	Candy, Jellybeans	11.0000	10.000	Each	0.00	0.06	10.24	40.37	0.00	0.00	0.00	0.02
	Candy, Lollipop	28.3500	1.000	Ounce	0.00	0.06	27.78	111.70	0.00	0.00	0.00	0.00
	Candy, M&M's Almond	42.0000	1.000	Pkg	4.00	13.00	25.00	230.00	0.00	2.00	5.00	4.00
	Candy, M&M's Peanut	170.0000	1.000	Cup	16.10	44.61	102.78	877.20	18.70	5.78	15.30	17.56
	Candy, M&M's Plain	208.0000	1.000	Cup	9.01	43.95	148.12	1023.36	37.44	5.20	29.12	27.21
	Candy, Peanut Brittle	28.3500	1.000	Ounce	2.13	5.41	19.65	128.43	0.00	0.57	3.69	1.42
	Candy, Praline	39.0000	1.000	Piece	1.09	9.48	24.18	177.06	0.00	0.00	0.00	0.73
	Candy, Raisinets	45.0000	1.000	Package	2.12	7.16	32.04	185.40	11.25	2.30	1.80	3.30
	Candy, Reese's Pieces	47.0000	0.250	Cup	6.49	9.92	28.86	230.77	0.00	1.36	0.94	8.51
	Candy, Skittles Bite Size	205.0000	1.000	Cup	0.39	8.96	185.81	830.25	0.00	0.00	0.00	1.78
	Candy, Taffy	15.0000	1.000	Piece	0.02	0.50	13.71	56.40	0.00	0.00	1.35	0.31
	Candy, Toffee	12.0000	1.000	Piece	0.13	3.94	7.72	65.04	0.00	0.00	12.60	2.45
	Candy, Truffles	12.0000	1.000	Piece	0.68	4.12	5.40	58.56	0.00	0.00	6.24	2.58
	Candy, Twizzlers Strawberry	71.0000	1.000	Package	2.41	1.14	54.95	237.14	0.00	0.99	0.00	0.28
	Candy, York Peppermint Pattie (l	42.0000	1.000	Lg Patty	0.92	2.98	33.64	165.06	0.00	0.84	0.42	1.81
	Candy, York Peppermint Pattie (s	14.0000	1.000	Sm Patty	0.31	0.99	11.21	55.02	0.00	0.28	0.14	0.60
	Chips, Bagel	28.3500	1.000	Ounce	4.00	6.00	20.00	150.00	0.00	1.00	0.00	1.00
	Chips, Banana	28.3500	1.000	Ounce	0.65	9.53	16.56	147.14	0.00	2.18	0.00	8.21
	Chips, Corn	2.2310	1.000	Each	0.15	0.85	1.15	12.31	0.00	0.08	0.00	0.12
	Chips, Doritos-Cheese, Nacho	28.0000	1.000	Ounce	2.00	7.00	17.00	140.00	0.00	1.00	0.00	1.00
	Chips, Doritos-Ranch, Cool	28.0000	1.000	Ounce	2.00	7.00	18.00	140.00	0.00	1.00	0.00	1.00
	Chips, Fritos	28.0000	1.000	Ounce	2.00	10.00	15.00	160.00	0.00	1.00	0.00	1.50
	Chips, Fritos-Barbecue	28.0000	1.000	Ounce	2.00	9.00	16.00	160.00	0.00	1.00	0.00	1.50
	Chips, Pork Skins, Barbecue-flav	28.3500	1.000	Ounce	16.41	9.02	0.45	152.52	0.00	0.00	32.60	3.28
	Chips, Pork Skins, Plain	28.3500	1.000	Ounce	17.38	8.87	0.00	154.51	0.00	0.00	26.93	3.22
	Chips, Potato-Baked Lays	28.0000	1.000	Ounce	2.00	1.50	23.00	110.00	0.00	0.00	0.00	0.00

Monounsaturated Fat (g)	Polyunsaturated Fat (g)	Vitamin D (mg)	Vitamin K (mg)	Vitamin E (mg)	Vitamin A (re)	Vitamin C (mg)	Thiamin (mg)	Riboflavin (mg)	Niacin (mg)	Vitamin B_6 (mg)	Folate (mcg)	Vitamin B_{12} (mcg)	Calcium (mg)	Iron (mg)	Magnesium (mg)	Phosphorus (mg)	Potassium (mg)	Sodium (mg)	Zinc (mg)
0.38	0.39	0.00	0.00	0.27	77.52	0.00	0.04	0.14	3.26	0.53	9.93	4.43	24.48	0.68	31.28	179.52	575.28	1385.84	0.67
0.00	0.00	0.00	0.00	0.00	45.26	4.23	0.26	0.07	12.73	0.28	5.84	1.83	42.34	0.92	55.48	293.46	785.48	73.00	0.98
3.72	2.66	0.00	0.00	0.00	54.23	5.24	0.26	0.07	12.72	0.30	6.92	2.43	43.01	0.92	56.10	293.59	785.40	72.93	0.97
2.54	0.64	0.00	0.00	0.59	1.70	0.00	0.07	0.06	0.49	0.01	5.95	0.02	8.22	0.64	8.79	28.63	42.24	88.45	0.20
1.32	0.30	0.00	0.00	0.00	0.80	0.04	0.01	0.03	0.09	0.01	1.60	0.02	12.20	0.28	13.20	28.00	49.20	29.20	0.16
4.81	0.88	0.00	0.00	0.00	8.75	0.14	0.03	0.15	0.03	0.03	4.55	0.30	80.85	0.20	13.30	81.55	146.30	25.55	0.40
9.67	4.87	0.00	0.00	2.82	0.00	0.00	0.16	0.12	4.35	0.12	46.98	0.02	46.98	1.29	137.46	227.94	662.94	344.52	2.04
3.94	0.37	0.00	0.00	0.00	4.92	0.16	0.02	0.12	0.18	0.01	3.28	0.24	71.75	0.37	22.55	90.61	140.22	56.58	0.50
0.00	0.00	0.00	0.00	0.00	5.46	0.17	0.04	0.16	0.14	0.02	2.94	0.16	90.30	0.50	23.10	105.00	161.70	38.64	0.47
4.59	0.41	0.00	0.00	0.18	1.64	0.00	0.01	0.03	0.16	0.01	0.82	0.00	11.07	0.98	45.51	61.50	122.59	2.87	0.59
5.73	2.35	0.00	0.00	1.34	18.13	0.15	0.08	0.13	1.62	0.04	19.11	0.15	52.92	0.64	42.14	121.52	219.03	73.01	0.89
0.11	1.54	0.00	0.00	0.00	3.85	0.11	0.03	0.14	0.67	0.04	7.70	0.13	50.05	0.44	25.55	72.80	186.90	18.55	0.64
5.70	1.94	0.00	0.00	1.32	8.55	0.11	0.08	0.07	1.97	0.05	21.66	0.07	42.18	0.74	36.48	87.78	169.29	94.05	0.70
1.38	0.14	0.00	0.00	0.15	7.36	0.23	0.01	0.05	0.08	0.01	2.30	0.07	29.90	0.17	7.82	33.12	55.43	55.20	0.16
2.28	0.27	0.00	0.00	0.36	0.53	0.21	0.02	0.03	0.15	0.05	1.59	0.00	7.95	1.11	29.68	48.23	130.91	78.97	0.52
3.44	0.35	0.00	0.00	0.44	8.00	0.12	0.14	0.22	1.58	0.16	31.60	0.15	67.60	0.20	23.20	80.80	137.60	53.20	0.57
4.74	3.02	0.00	0.00	1.30	0.00	0.00	0.03	0.04	2.25	0.05	22.11	0.00	22.11	0.27	32.60	91.29	115.38	44.23	1.17
0.92	0.39	0.00	0.00	0.28	1.33	0.01	0.02	0.01	0.32	0.01	3.85	0.01	5.46	0.08	6.23	14.21	24.64	22.19	0.13
5.96	2.80	0.00	0.00	0.87	22.23	0.34	0.06	0.09	2.39	0.05	22.80	0.09	53.58	0.43	41.04	126.54	184.68	151.62	1.34
0.99	0.10	0.00	0.00	0.15	5.52	0.09	0.01	0.03	0.05	0.00	0.00	0.04	19.32	0.17	6.67	20.93	30.59	44.62	0.13
7.64	0.48	0.00	0.00	0.70	14.25	0.23	0.09	0.13	0.68	0.02	13.68	0.10	51.30	0.46	18.24	68.40	115.14	110.01	0.44
3.11	0.34	0.00	0.00	0.34	20.16	0.29	0.08	0.23	1.07	0.05	59.64	0.07	69.30	0.38	16.38	99.96	122.22	31.50	0.52
0.14	0.02	0.00	0.00	0.02	9.64	0.00	0.00	0.01	0.00	0.00	0.00	0.00	0.85	0.02	0.28	0.85	1.13	104.04	0.01
0.60	0.13	0.00	0.00	0.33	5.68	0.36	0.01	0.13	0.18	0.03	3.55	0.00	97.98	0.10	12.07	80.94	151.94	173.95	0.31
5.75	1.99	0.00	0.00	0.00	0.00	0.00	0.05	0.08	2.03	0.08	3.12	0.11	49.53	0.52	46.41	115.44	195.78	15.99	0.85
0.00	0.00	0.00	0.00	0.00	0.00	0.00	0.00	0.00	0.00	0.00	0.00	0.00	5.46	0.73	1.82	1.82	9.10	80.08	0.00
0.02	0.01	0.00	0.00	0.00	0.00	0.00	0.00	0.00	0.00	0.00	0.00	0.00	0.33	0.12	0.22	0.44	4.07	2.75	0.01
0.00	0.00	0.00	0.00	0.00	0.00	0.00	0.00	0.00	0.00	0.00	0.00	0.00	0.85	0.09	0.85	0.85	1.42	10.77	0.00
0.00	0.00	0.00	0.00	0.00	0.00	0.00	0.00	0.00	0.00	0.00	0.00	0.00	72.00	0.40	0.00	0.00	0.00	20.00	0.00
18.70	7.14	0.00	0.00	4.13	40.80	0.85	0.17	0.29	6.38	0.14	59.50	0.31	171.70	1.96	125.80	387.60	588.20	81.60	3.91
14.31	1.31	0.00	0.00	1.79	110.24	1.04	0.12	0.44	0.46	0.06	12.48	0.56	218.40	2.31	85.28	312.00	553.28	126.88	2.00
2.40	1.33	0.00	0.00	0.46	13.32	0.00	0.05	0.01	0.99	0.03	19.85	0.00	8.51	0.39	14.18	31.47	58.97	128.14	0.27
5.92	2.35	0.00	0.00	0.00	1.95	0.27	0.12	0.02	0.13	0.03	5.46	0.00	12.09	0.46	20.28	42.51	82.29	24.18	0.79
2.67	0.86	0.00	0.00	0.00	4.05	0.09	0.04	0.10	0.18	0.05	2.25	0.09	48.60	0.54	20.25	64.80	231.30	16.20	0.36
0.99	0.47	0.00	0.00	0.98	0.00	0.19	0.05	0.07	1.34	0.03	13.16	0.10	38.54	0.38	20.68	62.04	108.10	69.00	0.36
6.07	0.25	0.00	0.00	0.57	0.00	137.15	0.00	0.04	0.04	0.02	0.00	0.00	0.00	0.02	2.05	4.10	10.25	32.80	0.06
0.14	0.02	0.00	0.00	0.00	4.95	0.00	0.00	0.00	0.00	0.00	0.00	0.00	0.45	0.01	0.15	0.45	0.60	13.35	0.00
1.14	0.15	0.00	0.00	0.00	38.16	0.02	0.00	0.01	0.00	0.00	0.24	0.01	4.08	0.01	0.48	3.96	6.00	22.44	0.02
1.22	0.13	0.00	0.00	0.00	17.16	0.05	0.01	0.03	0.03	0.00	0.12	0.04	18.60	0.12	5.64	21.24	36.60	8.52	0.13
0.00	0.00	0.00	0.00	0.00	0.00	0.00	0.01	0.03	0.07	0.01	0.00	0.00	4.97	0.21	4.26	220.10	45.44	175.37	0.11
1.05	0.08	0.00	0.00	0.00	0.00	0.00	0.00	0.00	0.00	0.00	0.00	0.00	6.30	0.42	0.00	0.00	54.18	10.08	0.00
0.35	0.03	0.00	0.00	0.14	0.00	0.00	0.00	0.01	0.12	0.00	0.56	0.00	2.10	0.14	8.82	13.30	18.06	3.36	0.11
3.00	2.00	0.00	0.00	0.00	0.00	0.00	0.00	0.00	0.00	0.00	0.00	0.00	0.00	0.40	0.00	0.00	0.00	190.00	0.00
0.55	0.18	0.00	0.00	1.53	2.27	1.79	0.03	0.01	0.20	0.07	3.97	4.43	5.10	0.35	21.55	15.88	151.96	1.70	0.21
0.00	0.00	0.00	0.00	0.00	0.00	0.00	0.00	0.00	0.00	0.00	0.00	0.00	5.54	0.02	0.00	0.00	0.00	15.38	0.00
0.00	0.00	0.00	0.00	0.00	0.00	0.00	0.00	0.00	0.00	0.00	0.00	0.00	32.00	0.20	0.00	0.00	0.00	200.00	0.00
0.00	0.00	0.00	0.00	0.00	0.00	0.00	0.00	0.00	0.00	0.00	0.00	0.00	32.00	0.20	0.00	0.00	0.00	170.00	0.00
0.00	0.00	0.00	0.00	0.00	0.00	0.00	0.00	0.00	0.00	0.00	0.00	0.00	0.00	0.00	0.00	0.00	0.00	160.00	0.00
0.00	0.00	0.00	0.00	0.00	0.00	0.00	0.00	0.00	0.00	0.00	0.00	0.00	0.00	0.00	0.00	0.00	0.00	310.00	0.00
4.26	0.98	0.00	0.00	0.00	51.60	0.43	0.02	0.12	0.95	0.05	8.79	0.04	12.19	0.29	0.00	62.37	51.03	756.09	0.20
4.19	1.03	0.00	0.00	0.17	11.06	0.14	0.03	0.08	0.44	0.01	0.00	0.18	8.51	0.25	3.12	24.10	36.00	521.07	0.16
0.00	0.00	0.00	0.00	0.00	0.00	0.00	0.00	0.00	0.00	0.00	0.00	0.00	48.00	0.40	0.00	0.00	0.00	150.00	0.00

USDA ID Code	Food Name	Weight in Grams*	Quantity of Units	Unit of Measure	Protein (g)	Fat (g)	Carbohydrate (g)	Kilocalories	Caffeine (g)	Fiber (g)	Cholesterol (mg)	Saturated Fat (g)
	Chips, Potato-Barbeque	28.0000	1.000	Ounce	2.00	10.00	15.00	160.00	0.00	0.00	0.00	1.50
	Chips, Potato Sticks	28.3500	1.000	Ounce	1.90	9.75	15.11	147.99	0.00	0.96	0.00	2.52
	Chips, Potato, Barbecue-flavor	28.3500	1.000	Ounce	2.18	9.19	14.97	139.20	0.00	1.25	0.00	2.28
	Chips, Potato, Cheese-flavor	28.3500	1.000	Ounce	2.41	7.71	16.36	140.62	0.00	1.47	1.13	2.44
	Chips, Potato, Cheese-flavor-P	28.3500	1.000	Ounce	1.98	10.49	14.35	156.21	0.00	0.95	1.13	2.71
	Chips, Potato, Light	28.3500	1.000	Ounce	2.01	5.90	18.97	133.53	0.00	1.66	0.00	1.18
	Chips, Potato, Light-Pringles	28.3500	1.000	Ounce	1.59	7.29	18.40	142.03	0.00	1.02	0.00	1.45
	Chips, Potato, Plain-Pringles	28.3500	1.000	Ounce	1.67	10.89	14.46	158.19	0.00	1.02	0.00	2.68
	Chips, Potato, Plain, Salted	28.3500	1.000	Ounce	1.98	9.81	15.00	151.96	0.00	1.28	0.00	3.11
	Chips, Potato, Plain, Unsalted	28.3500	1.000	Ounce	1.98	9.81	15.00	151.96	0.00	1.36	0.00	3.11
	Chips, Potato, Reduced Fat-Ruf	28.0000	1.000	Ounce	2.00	6.70	18.00	140.00	0.00	0.00	0.00	1.00
	Chips, Potato, Sour Cream & Onion	28.3500	1.000	Ounce	1.87	10.49	14.54	155.07	0.00	0.34	0.85	2.68
	Chips, Potato, Sour Cream and On	28.3500	1.000	Ounce	2.30	9.61	14.60	150.54	0.00	1.47	1.98	2.52
	Chips, Potato, w/o Salt Added	28.3500	1.000	Ounce	1.82	10.03	14.70	148.27	0.00	1.36	0.00	2.57
	Chips, Sun, original	28.0000	1.000	Ounce	1.00	6.00	20.00	140.00	0.00	0.00	0.00	1.00
	Chips, Taro	28.3500	1.000	Ounce	0.65	7.06	19.31	141.18	0.00	2.04	0.00	1.82
	Chips, Tortilla, Low-Fat, Baked	2.1810	13.000	Chips	0.23	0.08	1.85	8.46	0.00	0.15	0.00	0.00
	Chips, Tortilla, Nacho Flavor	28.3500	1.000	Ounce	2.21	7.26	17.69	141.18	0.00	1.50	0.85	1.39
	Chips, Tortilla, Nacho-flavor, L	28.3500	1.000	Ounce	2.47	4.31	20.30	126.16	0.00	1.36	0.85	0.82
	Chips, Tortilla, Plain	28.3500	1.000	Ounce	1.98	7.43	17.83	142.03	0.00	1.84	0.00	1.42
	Chips, Tortilla, Ranch Flavor	28.3500	1.000	Ounce	2.15	6.75	18.31	138.92	0.00	1.10	0.28	1.29
	Chips, Tortilla, Taco-flavor	28.3500	1.000	Ounce	2.24	6.86	17.89	136.08	0.00	1.50	1.42	1.32
	Chips, Tostitos, Baked	28.0000	1.000	Ounce	2.00	1.00	24.00	110.00	0.00	0.00	0.00	0.00
	Chips, Tostitos, Baked, Salsa &	28.0000	1.000	Ounce	2.00	3.00	21.00	120.00	0.00	0.00	0.00	0.50
	Chocolate, Milk	168.0000	1.000	Cup	11.59	51.58	99.46	861.84	43.68	5.71	36.96	31.05
	Chocolate, Milk, w/ Almonds	41.0000	1.000	Each	3.69	14.10	21.81	215.66	9.02	2.54	7.79	6.96
191	Cliff Bar, Apple Cherry	68.0000	1.000	Each	4.00	2.00	52.00	250.00	0.00	2.00	0.00	0.50
192	Cliff Bar, Apricot	68.0000	1.000	Each	6.00	0.00	55.00	250.00	0.00	2.00	0.00	0.00
193	Cliff Bar, Berry, Real	68.0000	1.000	Each	4.00	2.00	52.00	250.00	0.00	2.00	0.00	0.50
194	Cliff Bar, Chocolate Chip	68.0000	1.000	Each	4.00	3.00	51.00	250.00	0.00	3.00	0.00	0.50
195	Cliff Bar, Chocolate Chip Peanut	68.0000	1.000	Each	12.00	6.00	40.00	250.00	0.00	5.00	0.00	1.00
196	Cliff Bar, Chocolate Espresso	68.0000	1.000	Each	4.00	2.00	52.00	250.00	0.00	2.00	0.00	0.50
197	Cliff Bar, Peanut Butter, Crunch	68.0000	1.000	Each	10.00	4.00	45.00	250.00	0.00	8.00	0.00	1.00
	Cookie Cakes, Devils Food, Fat F	16.0000	1.000	Each	1.00	0.00	13.00	50.00	0.00	0.50	0.00	0.00
	Cookie Cakes, Double Fudge, Fat	16.0000	1.000	Each	1.00	0.00	12.00	50.00	0.00	0.50	0.00	0.00
	Cookies, Butter	28.3500	1.000	Ounce	1.73	5.33	19.53	132.39	0.00	0.21	33.17	3.13
	Cookies, Chocolate Chip, Reduce	0.4480	2.000	Each	1.00	1.25	10.50	50.00	0.00	0.02	0.00	0.02
	Cookies, Chocolate Chip, Dietary	28.3500	1.000	Ounce	1.11	4.76	20.81	127.58	2.27	0.45	0.00	1.19
	Cookies, Chocolate Chip, Lower F	28.3500	1.000	Ounce	1.64	4.37	20.78	128.43	1.98	1.02	0.00	1.08
	Cookies, Chocolate Chip, Soft-ty	28.3500	1.000	Ounce	0.99	6.89	16.75	129.84	1.98	0.91	0.00	2.10
	Cookies, Chocolate Sandwich, Red	12.5000	2.000	Each	0.50	1.25	10.50	50.00	0.00	0.50	0.00	0.25
	Cookies, Creme Sandwich, Reduced	13.0000	2.000	Each	0.50	1.25	10.50	55.00	0.00	0.50	0.00	0.25
	Cookies, Fig Bars	28.3500	1.000	Ounce	1.05	2.07	20.10	98.66	0.00	1.30	0.00	0.32
	Cookies, Fig Newton, Fat Free	29.0000	2.000	Each	1.00	0.00	22.00	100.00	0.00	0.00	0.00	0.00
	Cookies, Gingersnaps	28.3500	1.000	Ounce	1.59	2.78	21.80	117.94	0.00	0.62	0.00	0.69
	Cookies, Molasses	28.3500	1.000	Ounce	1.59	3.63	20.92	121.91	0.00	0.27	0.00	0.91
	Cookies, Oatmeal Raisin, Reduced	13.5000	2.000	Each	1.00	1.25	10.00	55.00	0.00	0.50	0.00	0.00
	Cookies, Oatmeal, Dietary	28.3500	1.000	Ounce	1.36	5.10	19.82	127.29	0.00	0.81	0.00	0.76
	Cookies, Oatmeal, Regular	28.3500	1.000	Ounce	1.76	5.13	19.48	127.58	0.00	0.79	0.00	1.28
	Cookies, Oatmeal, Soft-type	28.3500	1.000	Ounce	1.73	4.17	18.63	115.95	0.00	0.77	1.42	1.03
	Cookies, Oreos, Dietary	28.3500	1.000	Ounce	1.28	6.27	19.19	130.69	0.85	1.17	0.00	1.09
	Cookies, Oreos, Regular	28.3500	1.000	Ounce	1.33	5.84	19.93	133.81	3.69	0.91	0.00	1.04
	Cookies, Oreos, w/ Extra Creme F	28.3500	1.000	Ounce	1.02	7.14	19.31	141.75	1.42	0.57	0.00	1.10

Page Key: A2 = Baby Food   A2 = Baked Goods   A8 = Beverages   A14 = Breads/Grains and Pasta   A18 = Breakfast Foods/Cereals   A26 = Dairy and Eggs   A40 = Fats and Oils   A42 = Fruits and Vegetables   A52 = Meats and Beans   A60 = Nuts and Seeds   A62 5 Frozen Entrees and Packaged Foods   A76 = Restaurant Chains–Fast Foods   A92 = Restaurant Chains–Other   A106 = Seafood and Fish   A110 = Snacks and Sweets   A120 = Soups   A122 = Supplements   A126 = Toppings and Sauces

Monounsaturated Fat (g)	Polyunsaturated Fat (g)	Vitamin D (mg)	Vitamin K (mg)	Vitamin E (mg)	Vitamin A (re)	Vitamin C (mg)	Thiamin (mg)	Riboflavin (mg)	Niacin (mg)	Vitamin B6 (mg)	Folate (mcg)	Vitamin B12 (mcg)	Calcium (mg)	Iron (mg)	Magnesium (mg)	Phosphorus (mg)	Potassium (mg)	Sodium (mg)	Zinc (mg)
0.00	0.00	0.00	0.00	0.00	0.00	6.40	0.00	0.00	0.00	0.00	0.00	0.00	0.00	0.20	0.00	0.00	0.00	300.00	0.00
1.75	5.07	0.00	0.00	1.38	0.00	13.41	0.03	0.03	1.36	0.09	11.34	0.00	5.10	0.64	18.14	48.76	350.69	70.88	0.28
1.85	4.64	0.00	0.00	1.42	6.24	9.61	0.06	0.06	1.33	0.18	23.53	0.00	14.18	0.55	21.26	52.73	357.49	212.63	0.27
2.19	2.71	0.00	0.00	0.00	2.27	15.34	0.05	0.05	1.42	0.10	0.00	0.00	20.41	0.52	21.26	84.77	433.19	224.82	0.26
2.02	5.29	0.00	0.00	0.00	0.00	2.41	0.05	0.03	0.74	0.15	5.10	0.00	31.19	0.45	15.03	46.21	108.01	214.04	0.18
1.36	3.10	0.00	0.00	0.82	0.00	7.29	0.06	0.08	1.98	0.19	7.65	0.00	5.95	0.38	25.23	54.72	494.42	139.48	0.02
1.68	3.82	0.00	0.00	1.42	0.00	3.40	0.05	0.02	1.19	0.22	6.52	0.00	9.64	0.43	17.86	43.66	284.92	121.34	0.17
2.06	5.>6	0.00	0.00	1.38	0.00	2.32	0.06	0.03	0.89	0.04	1.98	0.00	6.80	0.43	16.44	44.51	285.77	185.98	0.17
2.79	3.45	0.00	0.00	1.38	0.00	8.82	0.05	0.06	1.09	0.19	12.76	0.00	6.80	0.46	18.99	46.78	361.46	168.40	0.31
2.79	3.45	0.00	0.00	1.38	0.00	8.82	0.05	0.06	1.09	0.19	12.76	0.00	6.80	0.46	18.99	46.78	361.46	2.27	0.31
0.00	0.00	0.00	0.00	0.00	0.00	0.00	0.00	0.00	0.00	0.00	0.00	0.00	0.00	0.00	0.00	0.00	0.00	130.00	0.00
2.02	5.32	0.00	0.00	0.00	27.78	2.69	0.05	0.03	0.71	0.14	6.52	0.00	18.14	0.40	15.59	47.91	140.62	204.12	0.20
1.74	4.94	0.00	0.00	0.00	5.95	10.57	0.05	0.06	1.14	0.19	17.58	0.28	20.41	0.45	20.98	49.90	377.34	177.19	0.28
1.77	5.15	0.00	0.00	2.23	0.00	11.79	0.04	0.01	1.19	0.14	12.81	0.00	6.80	0.34	16.73	43.38	367.98	2.27	0.30
0.00	0.00	0.00	0.00	0.00	0.00	1.20	0.00	0.00	0.00	0.00	0.00	0.00	0.00	0.00	0.00	0.00	0.00	115.00	0.00
1.26	3.65	0.00	0.00	1.39	0.00	1.42	0.05	0.01	0.15	0.12	5.67	0.00	17.01	0.34	23.81	37.14	214.04	96.96	0.11
0.00	0.00	0.00	0.00	0.00	0.00	0.00	0.00	0.00	0.00	0.00	0.00	0.00	3.69	0.00	0.00	0.00	0.00	10.77	0.00
4.28	1.00	0.00	0.00	0.00	11.62	0.51	0.04	0.05	0.41	0.08	3.97	0.01	41.67	0.41	23.25	69.17	61.24	200.72	0.34
2.54	0.60	0.00	0.00	0.00	11.91	0.06	0.06	0.08	0.12	0.07	7.37	0.00	45.08	0.46	27.50	90.15	77.11	284.35	0.00
4.38	1.03	0.00	0.00	0.39	5.67	0.00	0.02	0.05	0.36	0.08	2.84	0.00	43.66	0.43	24.95	58.12	55.85	149.69	0.43
3.98	0.94	0.00	0.00	0.00	7.65	0.26	0.03	0.07	0.41	0.06	4.82	0.00	39.97	0.41	25.23	67.76	69.17	173.50	0.35
4.05	0.95	0.00	0.00	0.00	25.80	0.26	0.07	0.06	0.57	0.09	5.95	0.00	43.94	0.57	24.95	67.76	61.52	223.11	0.36
0.00	0.00	0.00	0.00	0.00	0.00	0.00	0.00	0.00	0.00	0.00	0.00	0.00	32.00	0.20	0.00	0.00	0.00	200.00	0.00
0.00	0.00	0.00	0.00	0.00	0.00	0.00	0.00	0.00	0.00	0.00	0.00	0.00	32.00	0.20	0.00	0.00	0.00	190.00	0.00
16.75	1.78	0.00	0.00	2.08	92.40	0.67	0.13	0.50	0.54	0.07	13.44	0.66	320.88	2.34	100.80	362.88	646.80	137.76	2.32
5.53	0.93	0.00	0.00	0.77	5.74	0.08	0.02	0.18	0.30	0.02	4.92	0.14	91.84	0.67	36.90	108.24	182.04	30.34	0.55
0.00	0.00	0.00	0.00	0.00	0.00	0.00	0.00	0.00	0.00	0.00	0.00	0.00	0.00	0.00	0.00	0.00	270.00	100.00	0.00
0.00	0.00	0.00	0.00	0.00	0.00	0.00	0.00	0.00	0.00	0.00	0.00	0.00	0.00	0.00	0.00	0.00	250.00	55.00	0.00
0.00	0.00	0.00	0.00	0.00	0.00	0.00	0.00	0.00	0.00	0.00	0.00	0.00	0.00	0.00	0.00	0.00	270.00	100.00	0.00
0.00	0.00	0.00	0.00	0.00	0.00	0.00	0.00	0.00	0.00	0.00	0.00	0.00	0.00	0.00	0.00	0.00	330.00	45.00	0.00
0.00	0.00	0.00	0.00	0.00	0.00	0.00	0.00	0.00	0.00	0.00	0.00	0.00	0.00	0.00	0.00	0.00	220.00	110.00	0.00
0.00	0.00	0.00	0.00	0.00	0.00	0.00	0.00	0.00	0.00	0.00	0.00	0.00	0.00	0.00	0.00	0.00	270.00	100.00	0.00
0.00	0.00	0.00	0.00	0.00	0.00	0.00	0.00	0.00	0.00	0.00	0.00	0.00	0.00	0.00	0.00	0.00	330.00	150.00	0.00
0.00	0.00	0.00	0.00	0.00	0.00	0.00	0.00	0.00	0.00	0.00	0.00	0.00	0.00	0.00	0.00	0.00	0.00	25.00	0.00
0.00	0.00	0.00	0.00	0.00	0.00	0.00	0.00	0.00	0.00	0.00	0.00	0.00	0.00	0.20	0.00	0.00	0.00	70.00	0.00
1.56	0.28	0.00	0.00	0.15	47.63	0.00	0.10	0.10	0.90	0.01	11.06	0.10	8.22	0.63	3.40	28.92	31.47	99.51	0.11
0.02	0.00	0.00	0.00	0.00	0.00	0.00	0.00	0.00	0.00	0.00	0.00	0.00	0.00	0.01	0.00	0.00	0.00	2.63	0.00
1.91	1.43	0.00	0.00	0.70	0.00	0.00	0.10	0.05	0.81	0.01	12.76	0.00	13.04	0.99	5.95	30.90	56.42	3.12	0.13
1.73	1.32	0.00	0.00	0.00	0.00	0.00	0.08	0.08	0.79	0.07	19.85	0.00	5.39	0.87	7.94	23.81	34.87	106.88	0.20
3.69	0.99	0.00	0.00	0.00	0.00	0.00	0.03	0.06	0.46	0.05	11.06	0.00	4.25	0.68	9.92	14.18	26.37	92.42	0.13
0.25	0.00	0.00	0.00	0.00	0.00	0.00	0.00	0.00	0.00	0.00	0.00	0.00	0.00	0.20	0.00	0.00	0.00	95.00	0.00
0.50	0.00	0.00	0.00	0.00	0.00	0.00	0.00	0.00	0.00	0.00	0.00	0.00	12.00	0.10	0.00	0.00	0.00	47.50	0.00
0.85	0.79	0.00	0.00	0.35	1.13	0.09	0.05	0.06	0.53	0.02	7.65	0.03	18.14	0.82	7.65	17.58	58.68	99.22	0.11
0.00	0.00	0.00	0.00	0.00	0.00	0.00	0.00	0.00	0.00	0.00	0.00	0.00	0.00	0.00	0.00	0.00	0.00	115.00	0.00
1.52	0.39	0.00	0.00	0.37	0.00	0.00	0.06	0.08	0.92	0.03	20.41	0.00	21.83	1.81	13.89	23.53	98.09	185.41	0.16
2.02	0.49	0.00	0.00	0.48	0.00	0.00	0.10	0.07	0.86	0.03	20.98	0.00	20.98	1.82	14.74	26.93	98.09	130.13	0.13
0.25	0.25	0.00	0.00	0.00	0.00	0.00	0.00	0.00	0.00	0.00	0.00	0.00	12.00	0.20	0.00	0.00	0.00	67.50	0.00
2.14	1.92	0.00	0.00	0.91	0.28	0.09	0.13	0.06	0.92	0.01	14.74	0.00	15.31	1.15	4.82	34.59	49.61	2.55	0.14
2.84	0.72	0.00	0.00	0.71	0.57	0.14	0.08	0.07	0.63	0.02	12.76	0.00	10.49	0.73	9.36	39.12	40.26	108.58	0.22
2.27	0.62	0.00	0.00	0.00	1.42	0.06	0.05	0.03	0.52	0.03	9.64	0.00	25.52	0.79	8.51	59.25	38.27	98.94	0.12
2.62	2.25	0.00	0.00	1.07	0.00	0.00	0.15	0.08	1.13	0.03	17.58	0.01	27.78	1.34	7.37	56.70	83.63	68.89	0.16
2.43	2.06	0.00	0.00	0.98	0.00	0.00	0.02	0.05	0.59	0.01	12.19	0.01	7.37	1.10	12.76	27.78	49.61	171.23	0.23
3.03	2.66	0.00	0.00	1.27	0.00	0.00	0.02	0.04	0.45	0.01	12.19	0.01	6.80	0.81	9.64	25.80	34.59	139.77	0.18

USDA ID Code	Food Name	Weight in Grams*	Quantity of Units	Unit of Measure	Protein (g)	Fat (g)	Carbohydrate (g)	Kilocalories	Caffeine (g)	Fiber (g)	Cholesterol (mg)	Saturated Fat (g)
	Cookies, Peanut Butter Sandwich,	28.3500	1.000	Ounce	2.84	9.64	14.40	151.67	0.00	0.00	0.00	1.40
	Cookies, Peanut Butter Sandwich,	28.3500	1.000	Ounce	2.49	5.98	18.60	135.51	0.00	0.54	0.00	1.42
	Cookies, Peanut Butter, Regular	28.3500	1.000	Ounce	2.72	6.69	16.70	135.23	0.00	0.51	0.28	1.27
	Cookies, Peanut Butter, Soft-typ	28.3500	1.000	Ounce	1.50	6.92	16.36	129.56	0.00	0.48	0.00	1.74
	Cookies, Raisin, Soft-type	28.3500	1.000	Ounce	1.16	3.86	19.28	113.68	0.00	0.34	0.57	0.98
	Cookies, Shortbread, Pecan	28.3500	1.000	Ounce	1.39	9.21	16.53	153.66	0.00	0.51	9.36	2.32
	Cookies, Shortbread, Plain	28.3500	1.000	Ounce	1.73	6.83	18.29	142.32	0.00	0.51	5.67	1.73
	Cookies, Sugar, Dietary	28.3500	1.000	Ounce	1.16	3.69	21.77	122.19	0.00	0.25	0.00	0.53
	Cookies, Sugar, Regular (include	28.3500	1.000	Ounce	1.45	5.98	19.25	135.51	0.00	0.22	14.46	1.54
	Cookies, Vanilla Sandwich, w/ Cr	28.3500	1.000	Ounce	1.28	5.67	20.44	136.93	0.00	0.43	0.00	0.84
204	Cookies, Wafers, Chocolate	6.0000	1.000	Each	0.40	0.85	4.34	25.98	0.00	0.00	0.12	0.22
	Cookies, Wafers, Vanilla, Higher	28.3500	1.000	Ounce	1.22	5.50	20.16	134.10	0.00	0.57	0.00	1.40
205	Cookies, Wafers, Vanilla, Lower	4.0000	1.000	Each	0.20	0.61	2.94	17.64	0.00	0.00	2.32	0.14
	Cookies, Chocolate Chip, Higher F	28.3500	1.000	Ounce	1.53	6.41	18.94	136.36	3.12	0.71	0.00	2.12
	Cornnuts, Barbecue-flavor	28.3500	1.000	Ounce	2.55	4.05	20.33	123.61	0.00	2.38	0.00	0.73
	Cornnuts, Nacho-flavor	28.3500	1.000	Ounce	2.66	4.03	20.30	124.17	0.00	2.27	0.57	0.73
	Cornnuts, Plain	28.3500	1.000	Ounce	2.41	4.00	20.78	124.46	0.00	1.96	0.00	0.72
	Crackers, Animal	28.3500	1.000	Ounce	1.96	3.91	21.01	126.44	0.00	0.31	0.00	0.98
	Crackers, Classic Golden, Reduce	2.3300	6.000	Each	0.17	0.17	1.83	9.99	0.00	0.00	0.00	0.00
	Crackers, Snack, Cheese, Zesty,	0.9380	32.000	Each	0.09	0.06	0.72	3.75	0.00	0.03	0.16	0.02
	Crackers, Snack, French Onion,	0.9380	32.000	Each	0.06	0.06	0.72	3.75	0.00	0.03	0.72	0.00
	Crackers, Triscuits	4.4290	7.000	Each	0.43	0.71	3.00	20.00	0.00	0.57	0.00	0.14
	Crackers, Triscuits, Low-Fat	4.0000	8.000	Each	0.38	0.38	3.00	16.25	0.00	0.50	0.00	0.06
	Crackers, Wheat Thins	1.8130	16.000	Each	0.13	0.38	1.19	8.75	0.00	0.13	0.00	0.06
	Crackers, Wheat Thins, Low-Fat	1.6110	18.000	Each	0.11	0.22	1.17	6.67	0.00	0.11	0.00	0.03
	Dip, Bean	15.0000	2.000	Tbsp	0.50	0.00	2.00	10.00	0.00	0.50	0.00	0.00
	Dip, Cheese, Nacho	16.5000	2.000	Tbsp	0.00	1.25	2.00	20.00	0.00	0.00	0.00	0.25
	Dip, French Onion	15.0000	2.000	Tbsp	0.50	2.50	1.00	30.00	0.00	0.00	7.50	1.50
259	Doritos, Corn, Toasted	28.0000	1.000	Ounce	2.00	7.00	18.00	140.00	0.00	1.00	0.00	1.50
260	Doritos, Flamin' Hot	28.0000	1.000	Ounce	2.00	7.00	17.00	140.00	0.00	1.00	0.00	1.50
261	Doritos, Nacho, Spicy	28.0000	1.000	Ounce	2.00	4.00	18.00	140.00	0.00	1.00	0.00	1.50
262	Doritos, Pizza Cravers	28.0000	1.000	Ounce	2.00	6.00	18.00	140.00	0.00	1.00	0.00	1.50
263	Doritos, Taco Bell Taco Supreme	28.0000	1.000	Ounce	2.00	7.00	21.00	150.00	0.00	1.00	0.00	1.50
	Doughnut Holes	15.0000	1.000	Each	0.78	3.44	7.62	63.90	0.00	0.00	4.80	0.80
	Egg Custards	282.0000	1.000	Cup	14.38	13.25	30.17	296.10	0.00	0.00	245.34	6.63
	Frostings, Chocolate, Creamy	462.0000	16.000	Ounce	5.08	81.31	291.98	1834.14	9.24	2.77	0.00	25.55
	Frostings, Cream Cheese-flavor	462.0000	16.000	Ounce	0.46	79.93	308.15	1908.06	0.00	0.00	0.00	23.28
	Frostings, Sour Cream-flavor	462.0000	16.000	Ounce	0.46	79.46	312.31	1903.44	0.00	0.46	0.00	23.15
	Frostings, Vanilla, Creamy	462.0000	16.000	Ounce	0.46	77.62	320.63	1935.78	0.00	0.46	0.00	22.59
	Frozen Bar, Fruit and Juice	77.0000	1.000	Each	0.92	0.08	15.55	63.14	0.00	0.00	0.00	0.00
	Frozen Bar, Pops, Ice	52.0000	1.000	Each	0.00	0.00	9.83	37.44	0.00	0.00	0.00	0.00
	Frozen Bar, Popsicles	56.0000	1.000	Each	0.00	0.00	11.00	40.00	0.00	0.00	0.00	0.00
	Frozen Bar, Pudding Pops, Chocol	47.0000	1.000	Each	1.88	2.21	11.94	71.91	0.00	0.19	0.94	0.00
	Frozen Bar, Pudding Pops, Vanill	47.0000	1.000	Each	1.88	2.07	12.60	74.73	0.00	0.00	0.94	0.00
	Frozen Bars, Pops, Gelatin	44.0000	1.000	Each	0.53	0.04	7.35	30.80	0.00	0.00	0.00	0.00
	Frozen Dessert, Brownie, Fudge-H	132.9690	1.000	Cup	6.00	4.00	54.00	280.00	0.00	0.00	10.00	0.00
	Frozen Dessert, Cherry, Bordeaux	132.9690	1.000	Cup	6.00	4.00	46.00	240.00	0.00	0.00	10.00	0.00
	Frozen Dessert, Chocolate Chip-H	132.9690	1.000	Cup	6.00	4.00	48.00	260.00	0.00	0.00	10.00	0.00
	Frozen Dessert, Coffee Toffee-He	132.9690	1.000	Cup	6.00	4.00	50.00	260.00	0.00	0.00	10.00	0.00
	Frozen Dessert, Cookies 'n Cream	132.9690	1.000	Cup	8.00	4.00	48.00	260.00	0.00	0.00	10.00	0.00
	Frozen Dessert, Fudge Swirl, Dou	132.9690	1.000	Cup	6.00	4.00	48.00	260.00	0.00	0.00	10.00	0.00
	Frozen Dessert, Ice Milk, Vanill	65.0000	3.500	Fl Oz	2.47	2.80	14.76	90.35	0.00	0.00	9.10	1.71
	Frozen Dessert, Ice Milk, Vanill	88.0000	0.500	Cup	4.31	2.29	19.18	110.88	0.00	0.00	10.56	1.43

Monounsaturated Fat (g)	Polyunsaturated Fat (g)	Vitamin D (mg)	Vitamin K (mg)	Vitamin E (mg)	Vitamin A (re)	Vitamin C (mg)	Thiamin (mg)	Riboflavin (mg)	Niacin (mg)	Vitamin B₆ (mg)	Folate (mcg)	Vitamin B₁₂ (mcg)	Calcium (mg)	Iron (mg)	Magnesium (mg)	Phosphorus (mg)	Potassium (mg)	Sodium (mg)	Zinc (mg)
4.36	3.41	0.00	0.00	1.63	0.00	0.00	0.10	0.04	1.49	0.02	15.31	0.00	12.19	0.72	14.46	43.66	83.35	116.80	0.29
3.17	1.08	0.00	0.00	0.92	0.28	0.03	0.09	0.07	1.06	0.04	12.47	0.07	15.03	0.74	13.89	53.30	54.43	104.33	0.30
3.51	1.56	0.00	0.00	0.96	0.85	0.00	0.05	0.05	1.21	0.03	17.58	0.01	9.92	0.71	12.76	24.38	47.34	117.65	0.15
3.92	0.90	0.00	0.00	0.00	0.00	0.00	0.07	0.05	0.61	0.01	18.99	0.00	3.40	0.25	9.07	24.66	30.33	95.26	0.16
2.17	0.50	0.00	0.00	0.54	0.28	0.11	0.06	0.06	0.56	0.01	12.47	0.01	13.04	0.65	5.95	23.53	39.69	95.82	0.09
5.28	1.17	0.00	0.00	0.00	0.28	0.00	0.08	0.06	0.70	0.01	17.86	0.00	8.51	0.69	5.10	24.10	20.70	79.66	0.16
3.80	0.92	0.00	0.00	0.91	3.40	0.00	0.09	0.09	0.95	0.02	16.73	0.03	9.92	0.78	4.82	30.62	28.35	128.99	0.15
1.49	1.35	0.00	0.00	0.63	0.00	0.00	0.14	0.07	1.04	0.01	16.44	0.00	7.09	1.14	2.55	20.70	29.48	0.85	0.10
3.36	0.75	0.00	0.00	0.80	7.65	0.03	0.07	0.06	0.76	0.02	12.76	0.05	5.95	0.61	3.40	22.68	17.86	101.21	0.12
2.39	2.14	0.00	0.00	1.02	0.00	0.00	0.07	0.07	0.76	0.01	16.73	0.00	7.65	0.63	3.97	21.26	25.80	98.94	0.11
0.45	0.10	0.00	0.00	0.00	0.12	0.00	0.01	0.02	0.17	0.00	0.66	0.00	1.86	0.24	3.18	7.92	12.60	34.80	0.07
3.14	0.69	0.00	0.00	0.00	0.00	0.00	0.10	0.06	0.84	0.01	12.19	0.01	7.09	0.63	3.40	18.14	30.33	86.75	0.09
0.24	0.15	0.00	0.00	0.00	0.72	0.00	0.01	0.01	0.12	0.01	0.36	0.00	1.92	0.10	0.56	4.16	3.88	12.48	0.01
3.31	0.67	0.00	0.00	0.73	0.00	0.00	0.06	0.08	0.77	0.02	11.91	0.00	7.09	0.80	8.79	30.62	38.27	89.30	0.18
2.09	0.91	0.00	0.00	0.00	9.64	0.11	0.10	0.04	0.43	0.05	0.00	0.00	4.82	0.48	30.90	80.23	81.08	276.70	0.53
2.07	0.91	0.00	0.00	0.00	1.13	4.39	0.10	0.02	0.34	0.06	4.25	0.00	9.92	0.48	30.90	87.60	88.17	179.74	0.51
2.06	0.90	0.00	0.00	0.29	0.00	0.00	0.01	0.04	0.48	0.07	0.00	0.00	2.55	0.47	32.04	77.96	78.81	155.64	0.50
2.17	0.53	0.00	0.00	0.52	0.00	0.00	0.10	0.09	0.98	0.01	24.10	0.01	12.19	0.78	5.10	32.32	28.35	111.42	0.18
0.00	0.00	0.00	0.00	0.00	0.00	0.00	0.00	0.00	0.00	0.00	0.00	0.00	3.99	0.07	0.00	0.00	0.00	23.30	0.00
0.02	0.00	0.00	0.00	0.00	0.00	0.00	0.00	0.00	0.00	0.00	0.00	0.00	1.50	0.02	0.00	0.00	0.00	10.94	0.00
0.02	0.00	0.00	0.00	0.00	0.00	0.00	0.00	0.00	0.00	0.00	0.00	0.00	1.50	0.00	0.00	0.00	0.00	9.06	0.00
0.07	0.21	0.00	0.00	0.00	0.00	0.00	0.00	0.00	0.00	0.00	0.00	0.00	0.00	0.11	0.00	11.43	0.00	24.29	0.00
0.00	0.13	0.00	0.00	0.00	0.00	0.00	0.00	0.00	0.00	0.00	0.00	0.00	0.00	0.13	0.00	15.00	0.00	22.50	0.00
0.03	0.16	0.00	0.00	0.00	0.00	0.00	0.00	0.00	0.00	0.00	0.00	0.00	1.50	0.03	0.00	0.00	0.00	10.63	0.00
0.00	0.08	0.00	0.00	0.00	0.00	0.00	0.00	0.00	0.00	0.00	0.00	0.00	1.33	0.02	0.00	4.44	0.00	12.22	0.00
0.00	0.00	0.00	0.00	0.00	0.00	0.00	0.00	0.00	0.00	0.00	0.00	0.00	0.00	0.10	0.00	0.00	0.00	75.00	0.00
0.00	0.00	0.00	0.00	0.00	0.00	0.00	0.00	0.00	0.00	0.00	0.00	0.00	12.00	0.00	0.00	0.00	0.00	100.00	0.00
0.00	0.00	0.00	0.00	0.00	20.00	0.60	0.00	0.00	0.00	0.00	0.00	0.00	12.00	0.00	0.00	0.00	0.00	52.50	0.00
0.00	5.50	0.00	0.00	0.00	0.00	0.00	0.00	0.00	0.00	0.00	0.00	0.00	0.00	0.00	0.00	0.00	0.00	120.00	0.00
0.00	5.50	0.00	0.00	0.00	0.00	0.00	0.00	0.00	0.00	0.00	0.00	0.00	0.00	0.00	0.00	0.00	0.00	210.00	0.00
0.00	4.50	0.00	0.00	0.00	0.00	0.00	0.00	0.00	0.00	0.00	0.00	0.00	0.00	0.00	0.00	0.00	0.00	210.00	0.00
0.00	5.50	0.00	0.00	0.00	0.00	0.00	0.00	0.00	0.00	0.00	0.00	0.00	0.00	0.00	0.00	0.00	0.00	170.00	0.00
0.00	5.50	0.00	0.00	0.00	0.00	0.00	0.00	0.00	0.00	0.00	0.00	0.00	0.00	0.00	0.00	0.00	0.00	170.00	0.00
1.79	0.39	0.00	0.00	0.00	0.45	0.02	0.03	0.03	0.23	0.00	1.80	0.03	9.00	0.16	2.55	17.55	15.30	60.30	0.07
4.26	0.99	0.00	0.00	0.00	169.20	1.41	0.09	0.64	0.24	0.14	28.20	0.87	315.84	0.85	39.48	318.66	431.46	217.14	1.49
41.67	9.84	0.00	0.00	10.95	914.76	0.00	0.05	0.09	0.55	0.05	0.00	0.00	36.96	6.56	97.02	364.98	905.52	845.46	1.34
41.72	10.86	0.00	0.00	0.00	0.00	0.00	0.05	0.05	0.05	0.00	0.00	0.00	13.86	0.74	9.24	13.86	161.70	180.18	0.00
41.53	10.81	0.00	0.00	0.00	563.64	0.00	0.05	0.09	3.10	0.00	4.62	0.05	9.24	0.32	9.24	18.48	896.28	942.48	0.05
40.52	10.53	0.00	0.00	21.81	1044.12	0.00	0.00	0.05	0.05	0.00	0.00	0.00	13.86	0.51	4.62	180.18	170.94	415.80	0.00
0.00	0.02	0.00	0.00	0.00	2.31	7.32	0.01	0.02	0.12	0.02	4.62	0.00	3.85	0.15	3.08	4.62	40.81	3.08	0.04
0.00	0.00	0.00	0.00	0.00	0.00	0.00	0.00	0.00	0.00	0.00	0.00	0.00	0.00	0.52	0.00	2.08	6.24	0.01
0.00	0.00	0.00	0.00	0.00	0.00	1.20	0.00	0.00	0.00	0.00	0.00	0.00	0.00	0.00	0.00	0.00	0.00	10.00	0.00
0.00	0.00	0.00	0.00	0.01	15.51	0.19	0.02	0.08	0.06	0.01	1.41	0.25	66.27	0.22	9.87	52.64	105.28	77.55	0.17
0.00	0.00	0.00	0.00	0.01	24.44	0.14	0.02	0.09	0.02	0.02	2.35	0.17	60.63	0.03	5.17	47.47	64.86	49.82	0.16
0.00	0.00	0.00	0.00	0.00	0.00	0.00	0.00	0.00	0.00	0.00	0.00	0.00	0.88	0.01	0.44	0.00	0.88	20.24	0.01
0.00	2.00	0.00	0.00	0.00	0.00	0.00	0.06	0.27	0.00	0.00	0.00	0.00	160.00	0.40	0.00	160.00	380.00	140.00	0.00
0.00	2.00	0.00	0.00	0.00	0.00	0.00	0.06	0.34	0.00	0.00	0.00	0.00	160.00	0.00	0.00	200.00	300.00	100.00	0.00
0.00	2.00	0.00	0.00	0.00	0.00	2.40	0.12	0.27	0.00	0.00	0.00	0.00	160.00	0.40	0.00	160.00	320.00	140.00	0.00
0.00	2.00	0.00	0.00	0.00	0.00	2.40	0.12	0.34	0.00	0.00	0.00	0.00	160.00	0.00	0.00	160.00	320.00	160.00	0.00
0.00	2.00	0.00	0.00	0.00	0.00	0.00	0.06	0.34	0.00	0.00	0.00	0.00	240.00	0.00	0.00	200.00	360.00	160.00	0.00
0.00	2.00	0.00	0.00	0.00	0.00	0.00	0.12	0.27	0.00	0.00	0.00	0.00	160.00	0.80	0.00	200.00	420.00	140.00	0.00
0.80	0.10	0.00	0.00	0.00	30.55	0.52	0.04	0.18	0.06	0.05	3.90	0.44	90.35	0.07	9.75	70.85	137.15	55.25	0.29
0.67	0.09	0.00	0.00	0.00	25.52	0.79	0.04	0.18	0.11	0.04	5.28	0.44	138.16	0.05	12.32	106.48	194.48	61.60	0.47

USDA ID Code	Food Name	Weight in Grams*	Quantity of Units	Unit of Measure	Protein (g)	Fat (g)	Carbohydrate (g)	Kilocalories	Caffeine (g)	Fiber (g)	Cholesterol (mg)	Saturated Fat (g)
	Frozen Dessert, Mint Chocolate C	132.9690	1.000	Cup	6.00	4.00	50.00	280.00	0.00	0.00	10.00	0.00
	Frozen Dessert, Neapolitan-Healt	132.9690	1.000	Cup	6.00	4.00	44.00	240.00	0.00	0.00	10.00	0.00
	Frozen Dessert, Pecan, Butter, C	132.9690	1.000	Cup	6.00	4.00	52.00	280.00	0.00	0.00	10.00	0.00
	Frozen Dessert, Praline and Cara	132.9690	1.000	Cup	6.00	4.00	52.00	260.00	0.00	0.00	10.00	0.00
	Frozen Dessert, Rocky Road-Healt	132.9690	1.000	Cup	6.00	4.00	64.00	320.00	0.00	0.00	10.00	0.00
	Frozen Dessert, Sherbet, All Fla	74.0000	0.500	Cup	0.81	1.48	22.50	102.12	0.00	0.00	4.44	0.86
	Frozen Dessert, Sorbet, All Flav	180.0530	0.500	Cup	0.00	0.00	50.01	200.06	0.00	2.00	0.00	0.00
	Frozen Dessert, Sorbet-Ben & Jer	110.0000	0.500	Cup	0.00	0.00	32.00	130.00	0.00	0.00	0.00	0.00
	Frozen Dessert, Vanilla-Healthy	132.9690	1.000	Cup	8.00	4.00	42.00	240.00	0.00	0.00	10.00	0.00
	Frozen Desserts, Pops, Ice, w/ A	52.0000	1.000	Each	0.00	0.00	9.83	37.44	0.00	0.00	0.00	0.00
	Fudge, Brown Sugar w/ Nuts	14.0000	1.000	Piece	0.41	1.41	10.86	55.44	0.00	0.00	0.84	0.25
	Fudge, Chocolate	17.0000	1.000	Piece	0.29	1.45	13.52	64.77	2.38	0.14	2.38	0.88
	Fudge, Chocolate w/ Nuts	19.0000	1.000	Piece	0.65	3.06	13.83	80.94	2.66	0.25	2.66	1.07
	Fudge, Peanut Butter	16.0000	1.000	Piece	0.59	1.04	12.53	59.36	0.00	0.00	0.64	0.24
	Fudge, Vanilla	16.0000	1.000	Piece	0.18	0.86	13.17	59.04	0.00	0.00	2.56	0.54
	Fudge, Vanilla w/ Nuts	15.0000	1.000	Piece	0.44	2.00	11.28	62.25	0.00	0.09	2.10	0.56
	Granola Bars, Hard, Almond	28.3500	1.000	Ounce	2.18	7.23	17.58	140.33	0.00	1.36	0.00	3.55
	Granola Bars, Hard, Chocolate Ch	28.3500	1.000	Each	2.07	4.62	20.44	124.17	0.00	1.25	0.00	3.23
	Granola Bars, Hard, Peanut	28.3500	1.000	Ounce	3.12	6.07	18.06	135.80	0.00	1.22	0.00	0.71
	Granola Bars, Hard, Peanut Butte	28.3500	1.000	Ounce	2.78	6.75	17.66	136.93	0.00	0.82	0.00	0.91
	Granola Bars, Hard, Plain	24.5000	1.000	Each	2.47	4.85	15.78	115.40	0.00	1.30	0.00	0.58
	Granola Bars, Low-Fat	28.0000	1.000	Each	2.00	2.00	21.00	110.00	0.00	1.00	0.00	0.00
	Granola Bars, Soft, Chocolate Ch	42.5000	1.000	Each	3.10	7.06	29.37	178.50	0.00	2.04	0.43	4.33
	Granola Bars, Soft, Nut and Rais	28.3500	1.000	Each	2.27	5.78	18.03	128.71	0.00	1.59	0.28	2.70
	Granola Bars, Soft, Peanut Butte	28.3500	1.000	Each	2.98	4.48	18.26	120.77	0.00	1.22	0.28	1.03
	Granola Bars, Soft, Peanut Butte	28.3500	1.000	Each	2.78	5.67	17.63	122.47	0.00	1.19	0.28	1.58
	Granola Bars, Soft, Plain	28.3500	1.000	Each	2.10	4.88	19.08	125.59	0.00	1.30	0.28	2.05
	Granola Bars, Soft, Raisin	42.5000	1.000	Each	3.23	7.57	28.22	190.40	0.00	1.79	0.43	4.07
	Gum, Bubble-Carefree	3.0000	1.000	Each	0.00	0.00	2.00	10.00	0.00	0.00	0.00	0.00
	Gum, Chewing	3.0000	1.000	Stick	0.00	0.01	2.90	10.23	0.00	0.00	0.00	0.00
	Gum, Chewing, Cinnamon	3.0000	1.000	Each	0.00	0.00	2.00	10.00	0.00	0.00	0.00	0.00
	Gum, Chewing, Mint Flavors	3.0000	1.000	Each	0.00	0.00	2.00	10.00	0.00	0.00	0.00	0.00
	Gum, Chewing, Sugar-Free	1.7000	1.000	Stick	0.00	0.00	1.00	5.00	0.00	0.00	0.00	0.00
	Gum-Carefree	3.0000	1.000	Each	0.00	0.00	2.00	8.00	0.00	0.00	0.00	0.00
	Jello, Gelatin	540.0000	3.000	Ounce	6.48	0.00	75.60	318.60	0.00	0.00	0.00	0.00
	Jerky, Beef, Chopped and Formed	28.3500	1.000	Ounce	9.41	7.26	3.12	116.24	0.00	0.51	13.61	3.08
	Jerky, Slim Jims, Smoked	28.3500	1.000	Ounce	6.10	14.06	1.53	155.93	0.00	0.00	37.71	5.90
	Marshmallows	50.0000	1.000	Cup	0.90	0.10	40.65	159.00	0.00	0.05	0.00	0.03
617	Nutri-Grain Bar, Apple Cinnamon-	37.0000	1.000	Each	2.00	2.80	27.00	136.00	0.00	1.00	0.00	0.60
618	Nutri-Grain Bar, Berry, Mixed-Ke	37.0000	1.000	Each	2.00	3.00	27.00	140.00	0.00	1.00	0.00	0.50
619	Nutri-Grain Bar, Blueberry-Kello	37.0000	1.000	Each	2.00	2.80	27.00	136.00	0.00	1.00	0.00	0.60
620	Nutri-Grain Bar, Cherry-Kellogg'	37.0000	1.000	Each	2.00	2.80	27.00	136.00	0.00	1.00	0.00	6.00
621	Nutri-Grain Bar, Peach-Kellogg's	37.0000	1.000	Each	2.00	2.80	27.00	136.00	0.00	1.00	0.00	0.60
622	Nutri-Grain Bar, Raspberry-Kello	37.0000	1.000	Each	2.00	2.80	27.00	136.00	0.00	1.00	0.00	6.00
623	Nutri-Grain Bar, Strawberry-Kell	37.0000	1.000	Each	2.00	2.80	26.00	140.00	0.00	1.00	0.00	0.60
	Pastries, Toaster, Brown-sugar-c	28.3500	1.000	Ounce	1.45	4.03	19.31	116.80	0.00	0.28	0.00	1.03
	Pastries, Toaster, Fruit	28.3500	1.000	Ounce	1.33	2.89	20.16	111.42	0.00	0.59	0.00	0.43
	Peanuts, Chocolate, Milk, Coated	149.0000	1.000	Cup	19.52	49.92	73.61	773.31	32.78	7.00	13.41	21.75
	Pop Tart, Fruit, Frosted	52.0000	1.000	Each	2.00	5.00	38.00	200.00	0.00	1.00	0.00	1.50
	Popcorn, Air-popped	8.0000	1.000	Cup	0.96	0.34	6.23	30.56	0.00	1.21	0.00	0.05
	Popcorn, Air-popped, White Popco	8.0000	1.000	Cup	0.96	0.34	6.23	30.56	0.00	1.21	0.00	0.05
656	Popcorn, Butter, Golden, Fat, Re	14.0000	3.330	Cup	3.00	4.00	21.00	130.00	0.00	4.00	0.00	0.50
660	Popcorn, Butter-Smartfood	14.0000	3.000	Cup	2.00	9.00	15.00	150.00	0.00	1.00	5.00	2.00

Monounsaturated Fat (g)	Polyunsaturated Fat (g)	Vitamin D (mg)	Vitamin K (mg)	Vitamin E (mg)	Vitamin A (re)	Vitamin C (mg)	Thiamin (mg)	Riboflavin (mg)	Niacin (mg)	Vitamin B₆ (mg)	Folate (mcg)	Vitamin B₁₂ (mcg)	Calcium (mg)	Iron (mg)	Magnesium (mg)	Phosphorus (mg)	Potassium (mg)	Sodium (mg)	Zinc (mg)
0.00	4.00	0.00	0.00	0.00	0.00	0.00	0.12	0.27	0.00	0.00	0.00	0.00	160.00	0.40	0.00	0.00	340.00	160.00	0.00
0.00	2.00	0.00	0.00	0.00	0.00	0.00	0.06	0.34	0.00	0.00	0.00	0.00	160.00	0.00	0.00	200.00	320.00	120.00	0.00
0.00	2.00	0.00	0.00	0.00	0.00	2.40	0.12	0.34	0.00	0.00	0.00	0.00	160.00	0.00	0.00	160.00	300.00	160.00	0.00
0.00	2.00	0.00	0.00	0.00	0.00	0.00	0.06	0.34	0.00	0.00	0.00	0.00	160.00	0.00	0.00	200.00	320.00	140.00	0.00
0.00	2.00	0.00	0.00	0.00	0.00	0.00	0.06	0.34	0.00	0.00	0.00	0.00	160.00	0.00	0.00	200.00	380.00	140.00	0.00
0.39	0.06	0.00	0.00	0.06	10.36	2.29	0.02	0.06	0.04	0.01	3.70	0.14	39.96	0.10	5.92	29.60	71.04	34.04	0.36
0.00	0.00	0.00	0.00	0.00	0.00	24.01	0.00	0.00	0.00	0.00	0.00	0.00	0.00	0.00	0.00	0.00	0.00	20.01	0.00
0.00	0.00	0.00	0.00	0.00	0.00	0.00	0.00	0.00	0.00	0.00	0.00	0.00	80.00	0.00	0.00	0.00	0.00	10.00	0.00
0.00	2.00	0.00	0.00	0.00	0.00	0.00	0.12	0.51	0.00	0.00	0.00	0.00	240.00	0.00	0.00	200.00	360.00	120.00	0.00
0.00	0.00	0.00	0.00	0.00	0.00	5.56	0.00	0.00	0.00	0.00	0.00	0.00	0.00	0.00	0.52	0.00	2.08	6.24	0.01
0.34	0.76	0.00	0.00	0.00	2.38	0.08	0.01	0.01	0.03	0.01	1.54	0.00	15.54	0.25	6.86	12.04	52.36	13.72	0.09
0.44	0.05	0.00	0.00	0.02	7.82	0.03	0.01	0.01	0.02	0.00	0.34	0.01	7.14	0.08	4.25	9.86	17.51	10.54	0.07
0.82	1.03	0.00	0.00	0.08	8.93	0.11	0.01	0.02	0.04	0.02	1.90	0.01	9.50	0.14	8.55	17.67	30.02	11.40	0.14
0.48	0.27	0.00	0.00	0.00	1.60	0.03	0.00	0.01	0.24	0.01	1.76	0.01	6.72	0.04	3.52	10.40	20.96	11.68	0.07
0.25	0.03	0.00	0.00	0.03	8.00	0.03	0.00	0.01	0.00	0.00	0.16	0.01	6.24	0.01	0.80	5.12	8.00	10.72	0.02
0.50	0.83	0.00	0.00	0.07	6.90	0.09	0.01	0.01	0.03	0.01	1.50	0.01	7.05	0.06	4.05	10.65	16.95	9.15	0.08
2.19	1.07	0.00	0.00	0.00	1.13	0.00	0.08	0.02	0.17	0.01	3.40	0.00	9.07	0.71	22.96	64.64	77.40	72.58	0.45
0.75	0.36	0.00	0.00	0.00	1.13	0.03	0.05	0.03	0.16	0.02	3.69	0.00	21.83	0.86	20.41	57.83	71.16	97.52	0.55
1.63	3.37	0.00	0.00	0.32	0.85	0.00	0.05	0.02	0.41	0.02	6.52	0.00	11.06	0.71	31.19	85.05	86.47	78.81	0.59
1.98	3.42	0.00	0.00	0.00	0.57	0.06	0.06	0.03	0.56	0.03	5.10	0.00	11.62	0.68	15.59	39.41	82.50	80.23	0.35
1.07	2.95	0.00	0.00	0.00	3.68	0.22	0.06	0.03	0.39	0.02	5.64	0.00	14.95	0.72	23.77	67.86	82.32	72.03	0.50
0.00	0.00	0.00	0.00	0.00	0.00	0.00	0.00	0.00	0.00	0.00	0.00	0.00	0.00	0.20	0.00	0.00	0.00	70.00	0.00
1.50	0.84	0.00	0.00	0.00	2.13	0.00	0.10	0.06	0.41	0.04	9.35	0.07	39.53	1.08	33.15	97.75	144.50	115.60	0.64
1.20	1.56	0.00	0.00	0.00	1.13	0.00	0.05	0.05	0.74	0.03	8.51	0.07	23.81	0.62	25.80	68.32	111.13	72.01	0.45
1.87	1.21	0.00	0.00	0.00	0.57	0.00	0.07	0.04	0.89	0.03	9.07	0.06	25.80	0.60	24.38	70.88	82.50	115.95	0.53
2.37	1.31	0.00	0.00	0.00	0.57	0.00	0.03	0.03	0.89	0.03	9.36	0.13	22.68	0.55	24.95	74.28	106.88	92.99	0.48
1.08	1.51	0.00	0.00	0.00	0.00	0.00	0.09	0.05	0.15	0.03	6.80	0.11	29.77	0.73	20.98	65.21	92.14	78.81	0.43
1.21	1.36	0.00	0.00	0.00	0.00	0.00	0.10	0.07	0.47	0.04	8.93	0.08	42.93	1.04	30.60	93.50	153.85	119.85	0.55
0.00	0.00	0.00	0.00	0.00	0.00	0.00	0.00	0.00	0.00	0.00	0.00	0.00	0.00	0.00	0.00	0.00	0.00	0.00	0.00
0.00	0.00	0.00	0.00	0.00	0.00	0.00	0.00	0.00	0.00	0.00	0.00	0.00	0.00	0.00	0.00	0.00	0.12	0.18	0.00
0.00	0.00	0.00	0.00	0.00	0.00	0.00	0.00	0.00	0.00	0.00	0.00	0.00	0.00	0.00	0.00	0.00	0.00	0.00	0.00
0.00	0.00	0.00	0.00	0.00	0.00	0.00	0.00	0.00	0.00	0.00	0.00	0.00	0.00	0.00	0.00	0.00	0.00	0.00	0.00
0.00	0.00	0.00	0.00	0.00	0.00	0.00	0.00	0.00	0.00	0.00	0.00	0.00	0.00	0.00	0.00	0.00	0.00	0.00	0.00
0.00	0.00	0.00	0.00	0.00	0.00	0.00	0.00	0.00	0.00	0.00	0.00	0.00	10.80	0.16	5.40	118.80	5.40	226.80	0.16
3.21	0.29	0.00	0.00	0.14	0.00	0.00	0.04	0.04	0.49	0.05	37.99	0.28	5.67	1.54	14.46	115.38	169.25	627.39	2.30
5.80	1.25	0.00	0.00	0.00	47.91	1.93	0.04	0.12	1.29	0.06	0.00	0.28	19.28	0.96	5.95	51.03	72.86	419.58	0.69
0.04	0.03	0.00	0.00	0.00	0.00	0.00	0.00	0.04	0.00	0.00	0.50	0.00	1.50	0.12	1.00	4.00	2.50	23.50	0.02
1.90	0.30	0.00	0.00	0.00	750.00	0.00	0.38	0.43	5.00	0.50	40.00	0.00	14.00	1.80	8.00	40.00	73.00	110.00	1.50
0.00	0.00	0.00	0.00	0.00	750.00	0.00	0.38	0.43	5.00	0.50	40.00	0.00	0.00	1.80	8.00	40.00	0.00	110.00	1.50
1.90	0.30	0.00	0.00	0.00	750.00	0.00	0.38	0.43	5.00	0.00	40.00	0.00	18.00	1.80	8.00	40.00	73.00	110.00	1.50
1.90	0.30	0.00	0.00	0.00	750.00	0.00	0.38	0.43	5.00	0.00	40.00	0.00	18.00	1.80	8.00	40.00	73.00	110.00	1.50
1.90	0.30	0.00	0.00	0.00	750.00	0.00	0.38	0.43	5.00	0.50	40.00	0.00	18.00	1.80	8.00	40.00	73.00	110.00	1.50
1.90	0.30	0.00	0.00	0.00	750.00	0.00	0.38	0.43	5.00	0.00	4.00	0.00	18.00	1.80	8.00	4.00	73.00	110.00	1.50
1.90	0.30	0.00	0.00	0.00	750.00	0.00	0.38	0.43	5.00	0.50	40.00	0.00	17.00	1.80	0.00	40.00	56.00	110.00	1.50
2.28	0.51	0.00	0.00	0.00	63.50	0.03	0.10	0.16	1.30	0.12	8.22	0.06	9.64	1.14	6.80	37.71	32.32	120.20	0.18
1.17	1.10	0.00	0.00	0.65	0.85	0.17	0.08	0.10	1.12	0.11	18.43	0.00	7.37	0.99	5.10	31.47	31.75	118.79	0.19
19.25	6.45	0.00	0.00	3.80	0.00	0.00	0.18	0.25	6.33	0.31	11.92	0.40	154.96	1.95	140.06	315.88	747.98	61.09	2.89
0.00	0.00	0.00	0.00	0.00	100.00	0.00	0.15	0.17	1.90	0.20	20.00	0.00	0.00	1.00	16.00	0.00	170.00	0.00	0.00
0.09	0.15	0.00	0.00	0.01	1.60	0.00	0.02	0.02	0.16	0.02	1.84	0.00	0.80	0.21	10.48	24.00	24.08	0.32	0.28
0.09	0.15	0.00	0.00	0.00	0.24	0.00	0.02	0.02	0.16	0.02	1.84	0.00	0.80	0.21	10.48	24.00	24.08	0.32	0.28
0.00	0.00	0.00	0.00	0.00	0.00	0.00	0.00	0.00	0.00	0.00	0.00	0.00	0.00	0.00	0.00	0.00	0.00	410.00	0.00
0.00	0.00	0.00	0.00	0.00	0.00	0.00	0.00	0.00	0.00	0.00	0.00	0.00	0.00	0.00	0.00	0.00	0.00	240.00	0.00

USDA ID Code	Food Name	Weight in Grams*	Quantity of Units	Unit of Measure	Protein (g)	Fat (g)	Carbohydrate (g)	Kilocalories	Caffeine (g)	Fiber (g)	Cholesterol (mg)	Saturated Fat (g)
	Popcorn, Cakes	10.0000	1.000	Cake	0.97	0.31	8.01	38.40	0.00	0.29	0.00	0.05
	Popcorn, Caramel-coated, w/ Pean	28.3500	0.660	Cup	1.81	2.21	22.88	113.40	0.00	1.08	0.00	0.29
	Popcorn, Caramel-coated, w/o Pea	28.3500	1.000	Ounce	1.08	3.63	22.42	122.19	0.00	1.47	1.42	1.02
657	Popcorn, Cheese, White Cheddar,	14.0000	3.000	Cup	4.00	6.00	19.00	140.00	0.00	4.00	0.00	1.50
658	Popcorn, Cheese, White Cheddar-S	14.0000	2.000	Cup	3.00	12.00	17.00	190.00	0.00	3.00	5.00	2.50
	Popcorn, Cheese-flavor	6.0000	1.000	Cup	1.02	3.65	5.68	57.86	0.00	1.09	1.21	0.71
	Popcorn, Microwave	14.0000	4.000	Cup	0.75	3.00	4.25	42.50	0.00	0.75	0.00	0.75
	Popcorn, Microwave, Low-Fat	14.0000	4.000	Cup	0.67	1.00	3.67	23.33	0.00	0.50	0.00	0.17
659	Popcorn, Microwave, Smart Pop-Re	15.0000	1.000	Cup	3.00	2.00	20.00	105.00	0.00	5.00	0.00	0.00
	Popcorn, Microwave-Pop Secret-94	5.0000	1.000	Serving	1.00	0.00	4.00	20.00	0.00	0.00	0.00	0.00
	Popcorn, Oil-popped	11.0000	1.000	Cup	0.99	3.09	6.29	55.00	0.00	1.10	0.00	0.54
	Popcorn, Oil-popped, White Popco	11.0000	1.000	Cup	0.99	3.09	6.29	55.00	0.00	1.10	0.00	0.54
661	Popcorn, Unpopped, Microwave, Bu	32.0000	2.000	Tbsp	2.70	5.70	19.80	122.00	0.00	4.70	0.00	1.20
662	Popcorn, Unpopped, Microwave, Li	31.0000	2.000	Tbsp	2.60	5.10	18.90	113.00	0.00	4.50	0.00	1.00
663	Popcorn, unpopped, Microwave, No	37.0000	2.000	Tbsp	2.50	12.10	18.70	176.00	0.00	4.50	0.00	2.60
664	Popcorn, Unpopped, Microwave-Sma	30.0000	2.000	Tbsp	2.80	2.10	20.30	92.00	0.00	4.90	0.00	0.40
665	Potato Chips, BBQ, Fat Free-Prin	28.0000	1.000	Ounce	1.00	0.00	15.00	70.00	0.00	1.00	0.00	0.00
666	Potato Chips, Cheezum, Right Cri	51.0000	1.800	Ounce	4.00	24.00	32.00	350.00	0.00	2.00	0.00	6.00
668	Potato Chips, Original, Fat Free	28.0000	1.000	Ounce	1.00	0.00	15.00	70.00	0.00	1.00	0.00	0.00
667	Potato Chips, Original, Right Cr	51.0000	1.800	Ounce	3.00	14.00	36.00	270.00	0.00	2.00	0.00	3.50
	Potato Chips, Pringles, Cheese F	28.3500	1.000	Ounce	1.98	10.49	14.35	156.21	0.00	0.95	1.13	2.71
669	Potato Chips, Ranch, Right Crisp	51.0000	1.800	Ounce	2.00	7.00	18.00	140.00	0.00	1.00	0.00	2.00
670	Potato Chips, S. Cream, Right Cr	51.0000	1.800	Ounce	4.00	23.00	32.00	340.00	0.00	2.00	0.00	6.00
671	Potato Chips, S. Crm/Onion, Fat	28.0000	1.000	Ounce	1.00	0.00	15.00	70.00	0.00	1.00	0.00	0.00
	Power Bar	65.0000	1.000	Each	10.00	2.50	45.00	230.00	0.00	3.00	0.00	0.50
	Pretzels, Cheddar-Combos	28.3500	1.000	Ounce	2.79	4.80	18.85	131.26	0.00	0.00	1.42	0.00
	Pretzels, Hard, Plain, Salted	28.3500	1.000	Ounce	2.58	0.99	22.45	108.01	0.00	0.91	0.00	0.21
	Pretzels, Hard, Plain, Unsalted	28.3500	1.000	Ounce	2.58	0.99	22.45	108.01	0.00	0.79	0.00	0.21
	Pretzels, Hard, Whole-wheat	28.3500	1.000	Ounce	3.15	0.74	23.02	102.63	0.00	2.19	0.00	0.16
	Pudding, Banana	28.3500	1.000	Ounce	0.68	1.02	6.01	36.00	0.00	0.03	0.00	0.16
	Pudding, Bread	252.0000	1.000	Cup	13.10	14.87	61.99	423.36	0.00	0.00	166.32	5.77
	Pudding, Chocolate	28.3500	1.000	Ounce	0.77	1.13	6.46	37.71	1.42	0.28	0.85	0.20
	Pudding, Chocolate, Fat Free	113.0000	0.500	Cup	2.83	0.45	22.71	101.70	0.00	0.90	2.26	0.34
	Pudding, Coconut Cream	140.0000	0.500	Cup	4.34	3.50	24.92	145.60	0.00	0.28	9.80	2.52
	Pudding, Lemon	28.3500	1.000	Ounce	0.03	0.85	7.09	35.44	0.00	0.03	0.00	0.13
	Pudding, Rice	28.3500	1.000	Ounce	0.57	2.13	6.24	46.21	0.00	0.03	0.28	0.33
	Pudding, Tapioca	28.3500	1.000	Ounce	0.57	1.05	5.50	33.74	0.00	0.03	0.28	0.17
	Pudding, Vanilla	28.3500	1.000	Ounce	0.65	1.02	6.21	36.86	0.00	0.03	1.98	0.16
	Pudding, Vanilla, Fat Free	113.0000	0.500	Cup	2.37	0.23	23.17	103.96	0.00	0.11	2.26	0.23
	Raisins, Chocolate, Milk, Coated	180.0000	1.000	Cup	7.38	26.64	122.94	702.00	45.00	7.56	5.40	15.84
	Rice Cakes, Brown Rice, Buckwhea	9.0000	1.000	Cake	0.81	0.32	7.21	34.20	0.00	0.34	0.00	0.06
	Rice Cakes, Brown Rice, Buckwhea	9.0000	1.000	Cake	0.81	0.32	7.21	34.20	0.00	0.00	0.00	0.06
	Rice Cakes, Brown Rice, Corn	9.0000	1.000	Cake	0.76	0.29	7.31	34.65	0.00	0.26	0.00	0.06
	Rice Cakes, Brown Rice, Multigra	9.0000	1.000	Cake	0.77	0.32	7.21	34.83	0.00	0.27	0.00	0.05
	Rice Cakes, Brown Rice, Multigra	9.0000	1.000	Cake	0.77	0.32	7.21	34.83	0.00	0.00	0.00	0.05
	Rice Cakes, Brown Rice, Plain	9.0000	1.000	Cake	0.74	0.25	7.34	34.83	0.00	0.38	0.00	0.05
	Rice Cakes, Brown Rice, Plain, U	9.0000	1.000	Cake	0.74	0.25	7.34	34.83	0.00	0.38	0.00	0.05
	Rice Cakes, Brown Rice, Rye	9.0000	1.000	Cake	0.73	0.34	7.19	34.74	0.00	0.36	0.00	0.05
	Rice Krispie Treats	40.0000	1.000	Cup	1.33	2.00	33.33	160.00	0.00	0.00	0.00	0.00
	Snack Mix, Chex Mix	28.3500	0.660	Cup	3.12	4.90	18.46	120.49	0.00	1.58	0.00	1.57
	Snack Mix, Oriental Mix, Rice-ba	28.3500	1.000	Ounce	4.91	7.25	14.63	155.64	0.00	3.74	0.00	1.07
	Snack Mix, Original Flavor-Doo	56.7000	1.000	Cup	5.84	10.49	36.46	258.55	0.00	3.86	0.57	2.00
	Trail Mix, Regular	150.0000	1.000	Cup	20.70	44.10	67.35	693.00	0.00	0.00	0.00	8.32

Monounsaturated Fat (g)	Polyunsaturated Fat (g)	Vitamin D (mg)	Vitamin K (mg)	Vitamin E (mg)	Vitamin A (re)	Vitamin C (mg)	Thiamin (mg)	Riboflavin (mg)	Niacin (mg)	Vitamin B6 (mg)	Folate (mcg)	Vitamin B12 (mcg)	Calcium (mg)	Iron (mg)	Magnesium (mg)	Phosphorus (mg)	Potassium (mg)	Sodium (mg)	Zinc (mg)
0.09	0.14	0.00	0.00	0.01	0.70	0.00	0.01	0.02	0.60	0.02	1.80	0.00	0.90	0.19	15.90	27.70	32.70	28.80	0.40
0.77	0.93	0.00	0.00	0.43	1.70	0.00	0.01	0.04	0.56	0.05	4.54	0.00	18.71	1.11	22.68	36.00	100.64	83.63	0.35
0.82	1.27	0.00	0.00	0.34	2.84	0.00	0.02	0.02	0.62	0.01	0.57	0.00	12.19	0.49	9.92	23.53	30.90	58.40	0.16
0.00	0.00	0.00	0.00	0.00	0.00	0.00	0.00	0.00	0.00	0.00	0.00	0.00	0.00	0.00	0.00	0.00	0.00	280.00	0.00
0.00	0.00	0.00	0.00	0.00	0.00	0.00	0.00	0.00	0.00	0.00	0.00	0.00	0.00	0.00	0.00	0.00	0.00	310.00	0.00
1.07	1.69	0.00	0.00	0.01	4.84	0.06	0.01	0.03	0.16	0.03	1.21	0.06	12.43	0.25	10.01	39.71	28.71	97.79	0.22
0.00	0.00	0.00	0.00	0.00	0.00	0.00	0.00	0.00	0.00	0.00	0.00	0.00	0.00	0.05	0.00	0.00	0.00	72.50	0.00
0.00	0.00	0.00	0.00	0.00	0.00	0.00	0.00	0.00	0.00	0.00	0.00	0.00	0.00	0.07	0.00	0.00	0.00	55.00	0.00
0.00	0.00	0.00	0.00	0.00	0.00	0.00	0.00	0.00	0.00	0.00	0.00	0.00	0.00	0.00	0.00	0.00	0.00	280.00	0.00
0.00	0.00	0.00	0.00	0.00	0.00	0.00	0.00	0.00	0.00	0.00	0.00	0.00	0.00	0.00	0.00	0.00	0.00	40.00	0.00
0.90	1.48	0.00	0.00	0.01	1.65	0.03	0.01	0.02	0.17	0.02	1.87	0.00	1.10	0.31	11.88	27.50	24.75	97.24	0.29
0.90	1.48	0.00	0.00	0.00	0.22	0.03	0.01	0.02	0.17	0.02	1.87	0.00	1.10	0.31	11.88	27.50	24.75	97.24	0.29
0.00	0.00	0.00	0.00	0.00	0.00	0.00	0.00	0.00	0.00	0.00	0.00	0.00	2.00	0.66	0.00	0.00	0.00	357.00	0.00
0.00	0.00	0.00	0.00	0.00	0.00	0.00	0.00	0.00	0.00	0.00	0.00	0.00	2.00	0.63	0.00	0.00	0.00	321.00	0.00
0.00	0.00	0.00	0.00	0.00	0.00	0.00	0.00	0.00	0.00	0.00	0.00	0.00	2.00	0.62	0.00	0.00	0.00	2.00	0.00
0.00	0.00	0.00	0.00	0.00	0.00	0.00	0.00	0.00	0.00	0.00	0.00	0.00	16.00	0.12	0.00	0.00	0.00	307.00	0.00
0.00	0.00	0.00	0.00	0.00	0.00	0.00	0.00	0.00	0.00	0.00	0.00	0.00	0.00	0.00	0.00	0.00	0.00	160.00	0.00
0.00	0.00	0.00	0.00	0.00	0.00	0.00	0.00	0.00	0.00	0.00	0.00	0.00	0.00	0.00	0.00	0.00	0.00	400.00	0.00
0.00	0.00	0.00	0.00	0.00	0.00	0.00	0.00	0.00	0.00	0.00	0.00	0.00	0.00	0.00	0.00	0.00	0.00	160.00	0.00
0.00	0.00	0.00	0.00	0.00	0.00	0.00	0.00	0.00	0.00	0.00	0.00	0.00	0.00	0.00	0.00	0.00	0.00	260.00	0.00
2.02	5.29	0.00	0.00	0.00	0.00	2.41	0.05	0.03	0.74	0.15	5.10	0.00	31.19	0.45	15.03	46.21	108.01	214.04	0.18
0.00	0.00	0.00	0.00	0.00	0.00	0.00	0.00	0.00	0.00	0.00	0.00	0.00	0.00	0.00	0.00	0.00	0.00	160.00	0.00
0.00	0.00	0.00	0.00	0.00	0.00	0.00	0.00	0.00	0.00	0.00	0.00	0.00	0.00	0.00	0.00	0.00	0.00	290.00	0.00
0.00	0.00	0.00	0.00	0.00	0.00	0.00	0.00	0.00	0.00	0.00	0.00	0.00	0.00	0.00	0.00	0.00	0.00	160.00	0.00
1.50	0.50	0.00	0.00	0.00	0.00	0.00	1.50	1.70	19.00	2.00	200.00	2.00	360.00	3.50	122.50	280.00	0.00	90.00	5.25
0.00	0.00	0.00	0.00	0.00	1.98	0.00	0.09	0.16	0.90	0.01	2.27	0.03	55.85	0.26	6.24	40.54	36.86	316.67	0.21
0.39	0.35	0.00	0.00	0.06	0.00	0.00	0.13	0.18	1.49	0.03	48.48	0.00	10.21	1.22	9.92	32.04	41.39	486.20	0.24
0.39	0.35	0.00	0.00	0.06	0.00	0.00	0.13	0.18	1.49	0.03	23.53	0.00	10.21	1.22	9.92	32.04	41.39	81.93	0.24
0.29	0.24	0.00	0.00	0.00	0.00	0.28	0.12	0.08	1.85	0.08	15.31	0.00	7.94	0.76	8.51	35.44	121.91	57.55	0.18
0.43	0.38	0.00	0.00	0.00	8.51	0.14	0.01	0.04	0.05	0.01	0.57	0.05	24.10	0.04	2.27	19.56	31.19	55.57	0.08
5.42	2.39	0.00	0.00	0.00	163.80	2.02	0.23	0.56	1.58	0.19	32.76	0.00	287.28	2.77	47.88	274.68	564.48	582.12	1.31
0.48	0.41	0.00	0.00	0.04	3.12	0.51	0.01	0.05	0.10	0.01	0.85	0.00	25.52	0.14	5.95	22.68	51.03	36.57	0.12
0.00	0.00	0.00	0.00	0.00	0.00	0.34	0.00	0.00	0.00	0.00	0.00	0.00	89.27	0.60	0.00	85.88	235.04	192.10	0.00
0.73	0.10	0.00	0.00	0.10	70.00	0.98	0.04	0.21	0.13	0.21	5.60	0.36	158.20	0.28	22.40	124.60	222.60	228.20	0.52
0.37	0.32	0.00	0.00	0.00	0.00	0.03	0.00	0.00	0.00	0.00	0.00	0.00	0.57	0.02	0.28	1.42	0.28	39.69	0.01
0.91	0.79	0.00	0.00	0.39	9.92	0.14	0.01	0.02	0.05	0.01	0.85	0.06	14.74	0.09	2.27	19.28	17.01	24.10	0.14
0.45	0.39	0.00	0.00	0.03	0.00	0.20	0.01	0.03	0.09	0.01	0.85	0.06	23.81	0.07	2.27	22.40	27.50	45.08	0.08
0.44	0.38	0.00	0.00	0.04	1.70	0.00	0.01	0.04	0.07	0.00	0.00	0.03	24.95	0.04	2.27	19.28	32.04	38.27	0.07
0.00	0.00	0.00	0.00	0.00	0.00	0.34	0.00	0.00	0.00	0.00	0.00	0.00	85.88	0.05	0.00	115.26	123.17	240.69	0.00
8.53	0.92	0.00	0.00	1.75	12.60	0.36	0.14	0.29	0.72	0.14	9.00	0.32	154.80	3.08	81.00	257.40	925.20	64.80	1.46
0.10	0.10	0.00	0.00	0.00	0.00	0.00	0.01	0.01	0.73	0.01	1.89	0.00	0.99	0.10	13.59	34.20	26.91	10.44	0.23
0.10	0.10	0.00	0.00	0.00	0.00	0.00	0.01	0.01	0.73	0.01	1.89	0.00	0.99	0.10	13.59	34.20	26.91	0.36	0.23
0.10	0.10	0.00	0.00	0.00	0.00	0.00	0.01	0.01	0.58	0.01	1.71	0.00	0.81	0.11	10.26	28.80	24.75	26.19	0.20
0.10	0.13	0.00	0.00	0.00	0.00	0.00	0.01	0.02	0.59	0.01	1.80	0.00	1.89	0.18	12.33	33.30	26.46	22.68	0.23
0.10	0.13	0.00	0.00	0.00	0.00	0.00	0.01	0.02	0.59	0.01	1.80	0.00	1.89	0.18	12.33	33.30	26.46	0.36	0.23
0.09	0.09	0.00	0.00	0.06	0.45	0.00	0.01	0.02	0.70	0.01	1.89	0.00	0.99	0.13	11.79	32.40	26.10	29.34	0.27
0.09	0.09	0.00	0.00	0.01	0.45	0.00	0.01	0.02	0.70	0.01	1.89	0.00	0.99	0.13	11.79	32.40	26.10	2.34	0.27
0.12	0.14	0.00	0.00	0.00	0.00	0.00	0.01	0.01	0.63	0.01	0.45	0.00	1.89	0.16	12.96	34.20	27.99	9.90	0.27
1.33	0.00	0.02	0.00	0.00	200.00	20.00	0.50	0.57	6.33	0.67	0.00	0.67	0.00	1.33	0.00	21.33	26.67	226.67	0.00
0.00	0.00	0.00	0.00	0.00	3.97	13.47	0.44	0.14	4.77	0.44	0.00	3.52	9.92	7.00	17.86	53.01	76.26	288.32	0.59
2.80	3.02	0.00	0.00	2.39	0.00	0.09	0.09	0.04	0.87	0.02	10.77	0.00	15.31	0.69	33.45	74.28	92.99	117.09	0.75
0.00	0.00	0.00	0.00	0.00	24.38	0.06	0.20	0.15	3.04	0.11	22.68	0.01	41.96	1.42	34.02	167.83	157.06	720.66	1.28
18.80	14.48	0.00	0.00	0.00	3.00	2.10	0.69	0.30	7.07	0.45	106.50	0.00	117.00	4.58	237.00	517.50	1027.50	343.50	4.83

USDA ID Code	Food Name	Weight in Grams*	Quantity of Units	Unit of Measure	Protein (g)	Fat (g)	Carbohydrate (g)	Kilocalories	Caffeine (g)	Fiber (g)	Cholesterol (mg)	Saturated Fat (g)
	Trail Mix, Regular, Unsalted	150.0000	1.000	Cup	20.70	44.10	67.35	693.00	0.00	0.00	0.00	8.32
	Trail Mix, Regular, w/ Chocolate	146.0000	1.000	Cup	20.73	46.57	65.55	706.64	0.00	0.00	5.84	8.91
	Trail Mix, Tropical	140.0000	1.000	Cup	8.82	23.94	91.84	569.80	0.00	0.00	0.00	11.87

Soups

USDA ID Code	Food Name	Weight in Grams*	Quantity of Units	Unit of Measure	Protein (g)	Fat (g)	Carbohydrate (g)	Kilocalories	Caffeine (g)	Fiber (g)	Cholesterol (mg)	Saturated Fat (g)
	Soup, Asparagus, Cream Of	248.0000	1.000	Cup	6.32	8.18	16.39	161.20	0.00	0.74	22.32	3.32
	Soup, Bean and Ham-Healthy Choic	212.6200	1.000	Each	12.00	4.00	35.00	220.00	0.00	0.00	5.00	1.00
	Soup, Bean w/ Bacon	264.9000	1.000	Cup	5.48	2.15	16.37	105.96	0.00	9.01	2.65	0.95
	Soup, Bean w/ Ham	243.0000	1.000	Cup	12.61	8.51	27.12	230.85	0.00	11.18	21.87	3.33
	Soup, Bean w/ Hot Dogs	250.0000	1.000	Cup	9.98	6.98	22.00	187.50	0.00	0.00	12.50	2.13
	Soup, Bean w/ Pork	253.0000	1.000	Cup	7.89	5.95	22.80	172.04	0.00	8.60	2.53	1.52
	Soup, Bean, Black	247.0000	1.000	Cup	5.63	1.51	19.81	116.09	0.00	4.45	0.00	0.40
	Soup, Bean, Navy, w/ Ham-Stouffe	283.9200	1.000	Cup	11.02	8.01	31.05	240.36	0.00	0.00	20.03	0.00
	Soup, Beef and Potato-Healthy Ch	212.6200	1.000	Each	9.00	1.00	17.00	110.00	0.00	0.00	20.00	0.00
	Soup, Beef Mushroom	244.0000	1.000	Cup	5.78	3.00	6.34	73.20	0.00	0.24	7.32	1.49
	Soup, Beef Noodle	244.0000	1.000	Cup	4.83	3.07	8.98	82.96	0.00	0.73	4.88	1.15
	Soup, Beef, Chunky	240.0000	1.000	Cup	11.74	5.14	19.56	170.40	0.00	1.44	14.40	2.54
	Soup, Beef, Hearty-Healthy Choic	212.6200	1.000	Each	9.00	1.00	17.00	120.00	0.00	0.00	20.00	0.00
	Soup, Broccoli, Cream Of,-Stouff	283.9200	1.000	Cup	12.02	21.03	16.02	300.45	0.00	0.00	60.09	0.00
	Soup, Broth or Bouillon, Beef	240.0000	1.000	Cup	2.74	0.53	0.10	16.80	0.00	0.00	0.00	0.26
	Soup, Broth or Bouillon, Chicken	244.0000	1.000	Cup	1.34	1.10	1.44	21.96	0.00	0.00	0.00	0.27
	Soup, Cauliflower	253.0000	1.000	Cup	2.89	1.72	10.73	69.15	0.00	0.00	0.00	0.26
	Soup, Celery, Cream Of	248.0000	1.000	Cup	5.68	9.70	14.53	163.68	0.00	0.74	32.24	3.94
	Soup, Cheddar Cheese, Heat'n Ser	307.5800	1.000	Cup	21.70	35.80	21.70	488.23	0.00	0.00	97.65	0.00
	Soup, Cheddar Cheese-Stouffer's	283.9200	1.000	Cup	21.03	31.05	18.03	440.66	0.00	0.00	70.11	0.00
	Soup, Cheese	247.0000	1.000	Cup	5.41	10.47	10.52	155.61	0.00	0.99	29.64	6.67
	Soup, Chicken Gumbo-Stouffer's	283.9200	1.000	Cup	7.01	5.01	9.01	110.17	0.00	0.00	20.03	0.00
	Soup, Chicken Mushroom	244.0000	1.000	Cup	4.39	9.15	9.27	131.76	0.00	0.24	9.76	2.39
	Soup, Chicken Noodle	241.0000	1.000	Cup	4.05	2.46	9.35	74.71	0.00	0.72	7.23	0.65
	Soup, Chicken Noodle, Chunky	240.0000	1.000	Cup	12.72	6.00	17.04	175.20	0.00	3.84	19.20	1.39
	Soup, Chicken Noodle, Heat'n Ser	283.9200	1.000	Cup	13.02	17.03	28.04	320.48	0.00	0.00	60.09	0.00
	Soup, Chicken Noodle, Old Fashio	212.6200	1.000	Each	5.00	2.00	11.00	90.00	0.00	0.00	20.00	0.00
	Soup, Chicken Noodle-Stouffer's	283.9200	1.000	Cup	7.01	7.01	10.02	130.20	0.00	0.00	20.03	0.00
	Soup, Chicken Pasta-Healthy Choi	212.6200	1.000	Each	7.00	2.00	13.00	100.00	0.00	0.00	15.00	0.00
	Soup, Chicken Rice	240.0000	1.000	Cup	2.33	1.37	8.78	57.60	0.00	0.72	2.40	0.31
	Soup, Chicken Rice, Chunky	240.0000	1.000	Cup	12.26	3.19	12.98	127.20	0.00	0.96	12.00	0.96
	Soup, Chicken w/ Dumplings	241.0000	1.000	Cup	5.62	5.52	6.05	96.40	0.00	0.48	33.74	1.30
	Soup, Chicken w/ Rice	241.0000	1.000	Cup	3.54	1.90	7.16	60.25	0.00	0.72	7.23	0.46
	Soup, Chicken w/ Rice-Healthy Ch	212.6200	1.000	Each	5.00	1.00	14.00	90.00	0.00	0.00	10.00	0.00
	Soup, Chicken, Chunky	240.0000	1.000	Cup	12.14	6.34	16.51	170.40	0.00	1.44	28.80	1.90
	Soup, Chicken, Cream Of	248.0000	1.000	Cup	7.46	11.46	14.98	190.96	0.00	0.25	27.28	4.64
	Soup, Chicken, Creamy-Stouffer's	283.9200	1.000	Cup	17.03	8.01	25.04	240.36	0.00	0.00	20.03	0.00
	Soup, Chicken, Hearty-Healthy Ch	212.6200	1.000	Each	7.00	2.00	17.00	110.00	0.00	0.00	25.00	0.00
	Soup, Chili Beef	250.0000	1.000	Cup	6.70	6.60	21.45	170.00	0.00	9.50	12.50	3.35
	Soup, Clam Chowder, Manhattan St	240.0000	1.000	Cup	7.25	3.38	18.82	134.40	0.00	2.88	14.40	2.11
	Soup, Clam Chowder, New England	248.0000	1.000	Cup	9.47	6.60	16.62	163.68	0.00	1.49	22.32	2.95
	Soup, Clam Chowder, New England-	283.9200	1.000	Cup	14.02	23.03	21.03	340.51	0.00	0.00	40.06	0.00
	Soup, Crab	244.0000	1.000	Cup	5.49	1.51	10.30	75.64	0.00	0.73	9.76	0.39
	Soup, Fiesta Mexicali Heat'n Ser	283.9200	1.000	Cup	3.00	1.00	18.03	110.17	0.00	0.00	10.02	0.00
	Soup, Gazpacho	244.0000	1.000	Cup	7.08	0.24	4.39	46.36	0.00	0.49	0.00	0.02
	Soup, Gumbo, Chicken	244.0000	1.000	Cup	2.64	1.44	8.37	56.12	0.00	1.95	4.88	0.32
	Soup, Hot and Sour	244.0000	1.000	Cup	15.00	8.00	5.00	162.00	0.00	0.50	34.00	3.00
	Soup, Instant	240.0000	1.000	Cup	3.00	1.00	7.00	50.00	0.00	0.70	2.00	0.00
	Soup, Lentil w/ ham	248.0000	1.000	Cup	9.28	2.78	20.24	138.88	0.00	0.00	7.44	1.12

Monounsaturated Fat (g)	Polyunsaturated Fat (g)	Vitamin D (mg)	Vitamin K (mg)	Vitamin E (mg)	Vitamin A (re)	Vitamin C (mg)	Thiamin (mg)	Riboflavin (mg)	Niacin (mg)	Vitamin B6 (mg)	Folate (mcg)	Vitamin B12 (mcg)	Calcium (mg)	Iron (mg)	Magnesium (mg)	Phosphorus (mg)	Potassium (mg)	Sodium (mg)	Zinc (mg)
18.80	14.48	0.00	0.00	0.00	3.00	2.10	0.69	0.30	7.07	0.45	106.50	0.00	117.00	4.58	237.00	517.50	1027.50	15.00	4.83
19.77	16.48	0.00	0.00	0.00	7.30	1.90	0.60	0.32	6.44	0.38	94.90	0.00	159.14	4.95	235.06	565.02	946.08	176.66	4.58
3.49	7.22	0.00	0.00	0.00	7.00	10.64	0.63	0.17	2.07	0.46	58.80	0.00	79.80	3.70	134.40	260.40	992.60	14.00	1.64
2.08	2.23	0.00	0.00	0.84	84.32	3.97	0.10	0.27	0.89	0.07	29.76	0.50	173.60	0.87	19.84	153.76	359.60	1041.60	0.92
0.00	1.00	0.00	0.00	0.00	60.00	2.40	0.23	0.17	1.14	0.00	0.00	0.00	48.00	1.00	0.00	220.00	630.00	480.00	0.00
0.93	0.16	0.00	0.00	0.26	5.30	1.06	0.05	0.26	0.40	0.03	7.95	0.03	55.63	1.32	29.14	90.07	325.83	927.15	0.69
3.84	0.95	0.00	0.00	0.00	396.09	4.37	0.15	0.15	1.70	0.12	29.16	0.07	77.76	3.23	46.17	143.37	425.25	972.00	1.07
2.73	1.65	0.00	0.00	0.00	87.50	1.00	0.10	0.08	1.03	0.13	30.00	0.08	87.50	2.35	47.50	165.00	477.50	1092.50	1.18
2.18	1.82	0.00	0.00	0.08	88.55	1.52	0.10	0.03	0.56	0.05	31.88	0.05	80.96	2.05	45.54	131.56	402.27	951.28	1.04
0.54	0.47	0.00	0.00	0.07	49.40	0.74	0.07	0.05	0.54	0.10	24.70	0.02	44.46	2.15	41.99	106.21	274.17	1197.95	1.41
0.00	0.00	0.00	0.00	0.00	0.00	0.00	0.00	0.00	0.19	0.00	0.00	0.00	70.11	3.00	0.00	0.00	570.86	1251.88	0.00
0.00	0.00	0.00	0.00	0.00	0.00	2.40	0.03	0.00	0.38	0.00	0.00	0.00	0.00	0.20	0.00	0.00	100.00	550.00	0.00
1.24	0.12	0.00	0.00	0.00	0.00	4.64	0.05	0.05	0.95	0.05	9.76	0.20	4.88	0.88	9.76	34.16	153.72	941.84	1.46
1.24	0.49	0.00	0.00	0.00	63.44	0.24	0.07	0.05	1.07	0.05	19.52	0.20	14.64	1.10	4.88	46.36	100.04	951.60	1.54
2.14	0.22	0.00	0.00	0.17	261.60	6.96	0.05	0.14	2.71	0.14	13.44	0.62	31.20	2.33	4.80	120.00	336.00	866.40	2.64
0.00	0.00	0.00	0.00	0.00	150.00	9.00	0.06	0.10	1.90	0.00	0.00	0.00	32.00	0.40	0.00	90.00	280.00	540.00	0.00
0.00	0.00	0.00	0.00	0.00	0.00	0.00	0.00	0.01	0.00	0.00	0.00	0.00	2.48	0.00	0.00	0.00	430.64	791.19	0.00
0.22	0.02	0.00	0.00	0.00	0.00	0.00	0.00	0.05	1.87	0.02	4.80	0.17	14.40	0.41	4.80	31.20	129.60	782.40	0.00
0.41	0.37	0.00	0.00	0.02	12.20	0.00	0.00	0.02	0.20	0.02	2.44	0.02	14.64	0.07	4.88	12.20	24.40	1483.52	0.00
0.74	0.64	0.00	0.00	0.00	0.00	2.56	0.08	0.08	0.51	0.03	2.56	0.18	10.24	0.51	2.56	51.22	105.00	842.57	0.26
2.46	2.65	0.00	0.00	0.97	66.96	1.49	0.07	0.25	0.45	0.07	8.43	0.50	186.00	0.69	22.32	151.28	310.00	1009.36	0.20
0.00	0.00	0.00	0.00	0.00	0.00	0.00	0.00	0.02	0.21	0.00	0.00	0.00	4.95	0.11	0.00	0.00	553.33	770.32	0.00
0.00	0.00	0.00	0.00	0.00	0.00	0.00	0.00	0.01	0.19	0.00	0.00	0.00	4.97	0.00	0.00	0.00	510.77	681.02	0.00
2.96	0.30	0.00	0.00	0.00	108.68	0.00	0.02	0.15	0.40	0.02	4.94	0.00	140.79	0.74	4.94	135.85	153.14	958.36	0.64
0.00	0.00	0.00	0.00	0.00	0.00	0.00	0.00	0.00	0.19	0.00	0.00	0.00	160.24	0.10	0.00	0.00	180.27	1422.13	0.00
4.03	2.32	0.00	0.00	0.00	112.24	0.00	0.02	0.12	1.63	0.05	0.24	0.05	29.28	0.88	9.76	26.84	153.72	941.84	0.98
1.11	0.55	0.00	0.00	0.07	72.30	0.24	0.05	0.07	1.40	0.02	21.69	0.14	16.87	0.77	4.82	36.15	55.43	1106.19	0.39
2.66	1.51	0.00	0.00	0.79	122.40	0.00	0.07	0.17	4.32	0.05	38.40	0.31	24.00	1.44	9.60	72.00	108.00	849.60	0.96
0.00	0.00	0.00	0.00	0.00	0.00	6.01	0.00	0.00	0.57	0.00	0.00	0.00	240.36	0.20	0.00	0.00	310.46	1792.69	0.00
0.00	0.00	0.00	0.00	0.00	80.00	12.00	0.03	0.10	1.90	0.00	0.00	0.00	16.00	0.20	0.00	60.00	130.00	540.00	0.00
0.00	0.00	0.00	0.00	0.00	0.00	0.00	0.00	0.00	0.19	0.00	0.00	0.00	80.12	0.10	0.00	0.00	140.21	1281.92	0.00
0.00	0.00	0.00	0.00	0.00	60.00	0.00	0.03	0.00	0.38	0.00	0.00	0.00	0.00	0.00	0.00	0.00	70.00	560.00	0.00
0.60	0.41	0.00	0.00	0.05	0.00	0.00	0.00	0.00	0.34	0.02	0.48	0.07	7.20	0.00	0.00	9.60	9.60	931.20	0.12
1.44	0.67	0.00	0.00	0.10	585.60	3.84	0.02	0.10	4.10	0.05	3.84	0.31	33.60	1.87	9.60	72.00	108.00	888.00	0.96
2.53	1.30	0.00	0.00	0.14	53.02	0.00	0.02	0.07	1.76	0.05	2.41	0.17	14.46	0.63	4.82	60.25	115.68	860.37	0.36
0.92	0.41	0.00	0.00	0.05	65.07	0.24	0.02	0.02	1.13	0.02	0.96	0.14	16.87	0.75	0.00	21.69	101.22	814.58	0.27
0.00	0.00	0.00	0.00	0.00	80.00	6.00	0.03	0.07	1.90	0.00	0.00	0.00	16.00	0.20	0.00	70.00	140.00	510.00	0.00
2.83	1.32	0.00	0.00	0.17	124.80	1.20	0.07	0.17	4.22	0.05	4.32	0.24	24.00	1.66	7.20	108.00	168.00	849.60	0.96
4.46	1.64	0.00	0.00	0.25	94.24	1.24	0.07	0.25	0.92	0.07	7.69	0.55	181.04	0.67	17.36	151.28	272.80	1046.56	0.67
0.00	0.00	0.00	0.00	0.00	0.00	0.00	0.02	0.01	0.19	0.00	0.00	0.00	2.48	0.00	0.00	0.00	510.77	1281.92	0.00
0.00	0.00	0.00	0.00	0.00	200.00	2.40	0.09	0.17	1.90	0.00	0.00	0.00	32.00	0.40	0.00	90.00	190.00	520.00	0.00
2.80	0.28	0.00	0.00	0.18	150.00	4.00	0.05	0.08	1.08	0.15	17.50	0.33	42.50	2.13	30.00	147.50	525.00	1035.00	1.40
0.98	0.12	0.00	0.00	0.10	328.80	12.24	0.05	0.07	1.85	0.26	9.36	7.92	67.20	2.64	19.20	84.00	384.00	1000.80	1.68
2.26	1.09	0.00	0.00	0.15	39.68	3.47	0.07	0.25	1.04	0.12	9.67	10.24	186.00	1.49	22.32	156.24	300.08	992.00	0.79
0.00	0.00	0.00	0.00	0.00	0.00	0.00	0.00	0.01	0.19	0.00	0.00	0.00	2.48	0.10	0.00	0.00	570.86	961.44	0.00
0.68	0.39	0.00	0.00	0.00	51.24	0.00	0.20	0.07	1.34	0.12	14.64	0.20	65.88	1.22	14.64	87.84	326.96	1234.64	1.46
0.00	0.00	0.00	0.00	0.00	0.00	6.01	0.00	0.00	0.19	0.00	0.00	0.00	2.40	1.00	0.00	0.00	430.64	711.07	0.00
0.02	0.07	0.00	0.00	0.46	261.08	7.08	0.05	0.02	0.93	0.15	9.76	0.00	24.40	0.98	7.32	36.60	224.48	739.32	0.24
0.66	0.34	0.00	0.00	0.05	14.64	4.88	0.02	0.05	0.66	0.07	4.88	0.02	24.40	0.90	4.88	24.40	75.64	954.04	0.37
0.30	0.68	0.00	0.00	0.30	0.03	0.60	0.00	0.00	0.00	0.00	0.00	0.00	32.00	1.65	0.00	0.00	0.00	1011.00	0.00
0.00	0.00	0.00	0.00	0.00	0.03	0.03	0.00	0.00	0.00	0.00	0.00	0.00	27.00	0.45	0.00	0.00	0.00	1222.00	0.00
1.29	0.32	0.00	0.00	0.00	34.72	4.22	0.17	0.12	1.36	0.22	49.60	0.30	42.16	2.65	22.32	183.52	357.12	1319.36	0.74

USDA ID Code	Food Name	Weight in Grams*	Quantity of Units	Unit of Measure	Protein (g)	Fat (g)	Carbohydrate (g)	Kilocalories	Caffeine (g)	Fiber (g)	Cholesterol (mg)	Saturated Fat (g)
	Soup, Lentil-Healthy Choice	212.6200	1.000	Each	8.00	1.00	23.00	140.00	0.00	0.00	0.00	0.00
	Soup, Minestrone	241.0000	1.000	Cup	4.27	2.51	11.23	81.94	0.00	0.96	2.41	0.55
	Soup, Minestrone Heat'n Serve-St	283.9200	1.000	Cup	5.01	4.01	18.03	130.20	0.00	0.00	0.00	0.00
	Soup, Minestrone, Chunky	240.0000	1.000	Cup	5.11	2.81	20.74	127.20	0.00	5.76	4.80	1.49
	Soup, Minestrone-Healthy Choice	212.6200	1.000	Each	6.00	1.00	30.00	160.00	0.00	0.00	0.00	0.00
	Soup, Minestrone-Stouffer's	283.9200	1.000	Cup	6.01	3.00	20.03	140.21	0.00	0.00	10.02	0.00
	Soup, Mushroom	253.0000	1.000	Cup	2.23	4.86	11.13	96.14	0.00	0.76	0.00	0.81
	Soup, Mushroom, Cream Of	248.0000	1.000	Cup	6.05	13.59	15.00	203.36	0.00	0.50	19.84	5.13
	Soup, Onion	241.0000	1.000	Cup	3.76	1.74	8.17	57.84	0.00	0.96	0.00	0.27
	Soup, Onion, Cream Of	248.0000	1.000	Cup	6.80	9.37	18.35	186.00	0.00	0.74	32.24	4.04
	Soup, Onion, French-Stouffer's	283.9200	1.000	Cup	4.01	4.01	10.02	100.15	0.00	0.00	0.00	0.00
	Soup, Pea, Green	254.0000	1.000	Cup	12.62	7.04	32.23	238.76	0.00	2.79	17.78	4.01
	Soup, Pea, Split w/ Ham	253.0000	1.000	Cup	10.32	4.40	27.96	189.75	0.00	2.28	7.59	1.77
	Soup, Pea, Split w/ Ham, Chunky	240.0000	1.000	Cup	11.09	3.98	26.81	184.80	0.00	4.08	7.20	1.58
	Soup, Pea, Split, and Ham-Health	212.6200	1.000	Each	10.00	3.00	25.00	170.00	0.00	0.00	10.00	1.00
	Soup, Pea, Split, and Ham-Stouff	283.9200	1.000	Cup	15.02	3.00	35.05	220.33	0.00	0.00	10.02	0.00
	Soup, Potato, Cream Of	248.0000	1.000	Cup	5.78	6.45	17.16	148.80	0.00	0.50	22.32	3.77
	Soup, Potato, Cream Of,-Stouffer	283.9200	1.000	Cup	11.02	13.02	34.05	300.45	0.00	0.00	30.04	0.00
	Soup, Shrimp, Cream Of	248.0000	1.000	Cup	6.82	9.30	13.91	163.68	0.00	0.25	34.72	5.78
	Soup, Sweet & Sour	244.0000	1.000	Cup	3.00	1.00	14.00	72.00	0.00	1.60	5.00	0.00
	Soup, Tomato	248.0000	1.000	Cup	6.10	6.00	22.30	161.20	0.00	2.73	17.36	2.90
	Soup, Tomato Beef w/ noodle	244.0000	1.000	Cup	4.47	4.29	21.15	139.08	0.00	1.46	4.88	1.59
	Soup, Tomato Garden-Healthy Choi	212.6200	1.000	Each	4.00	3.00	22.00	130.00	0.00	0.00	5.00	1.00
	Soup, Tomato Rice	247.0000	1.000	Cup	2.10	2.72	21.93	118.56	0.00	1.48	2.47	0.52
	Soup, Tomato, Garden Heat'n Serv	283.9200	1.000	Cup	4.01	3.00	16.02	110.17	0.00	0.00	10.02	0.00
	Soup, Turkey Noodle	244.0000	1.000	Cup	3.90	2.00	8.64	68.32	0.00	0.73	4.88	0.56
	Soup, Turkey, Chunky	236.0000	1.000	Cup	10.22	4.41	14.07	134.52	0.00	0.00	9.44	1.23
	Soup, Vegetable Beef	253.0000	1.000	Cup	2.93	1.11	8.02	53.13	0.00	0.51	0.00	0.56
	Soup, Vegetable, Beef w/ Barley-	283.9200	1.000	Cup	4.01	13.02	15.02	190.29	0.00	0.00	10.02	0.00
	Soup, Vegetable, Beef-Healthy Ch	212.6200	1.000	Each	8.00	1.00	21.00	130.00	0.00	0.00	15.00	0.00
	Soup, Vegetable, Chicken	241.0000	1.000	Cup	3.62	2.84	8.58	74.71	0.00	0.96	9.64	0.84
	Soup, Vegetable, Chicken, Chunky	240.0000	1.000	Cup	12.31	4.82	18.89	165.60	0.00	0.00	16.80	1.44
	Soup, Vegetable, Chunky	240.0000	1.000	Cup	3.50	3.70	19.01	122.40	0.00	1.20	0.00	0.55
	Soup, Vegetable, Country-Healthy	212.6200	1.000	Each	3.00	1.00	23.00	120.00	0.00	0.00	0.00	0.00
	Soup, Vegetable, Cream Of	260.1000	1.000	Cup	1.90	5.70	12.30	106.64	0.00	0.52	0.00	1.43
	Soup, Vegetable, Garden-Healthy	212.6200	1.000	Each	3.00	1.00	18.00	100.00	0.00	0.00	0.00	0.00
	Soup, Vegetable, Tomato	241.0000	1.000	Cup	1.90	0.82	9.74	53.02	0.00	0.48	0.00	0.36
	Soup, Vegetable, Turkey	241.0000	1.000	Cup	3.08	3.04	8.63	72.30	0.00	0.48	2.41	0.89
	Soup, Vegetable, Turkey-Healthy	212.6200	1.000	Each	4.00	3.00	17.00	110.00	0.00	0.00	15.00	1.00
	Soup, Vegetable, Vegetarian	241.0000	1.000	Cup	2.10	1.93	11.98	72.30	0.00	0.48	0.00	0.29
	Soup, Vegetable, Vegetarian-Stou	283.9200	1.000	Cup	6.01	2.00	20.03	120.18	0.00	0.00	0.00	0.00
	Soup, Won-Ton	241.0000	1.000	Cup	14.00	7.00	14.00	182.00	0.00	0.90	53.00	2.00

Supplements

USDA ID Code	Food Name	Weight in Grams*	Quantity of Units	Unit of Measure	Protein (g)	Fat (g)	Carbohydrate (g)	Kilocalories	Caffeine (g)	Fiber (g)	Cholesterol (mg)	Saturated Fat (g)
3	Boost Plus, Chocolate	240.0000	8.000	Fl Oz	14.00	14.00	45.00	360.00	0.00	0.00	0.00	2.00
4	Boost Plus, Strawberry	240.0000	8.000	Fl Oz	14.00	14.00	45.00	360.00	0.00	0.00	0.00	2.00
5	Boost Plus, Vanilla	240.0000	8.000	Fl Oz	14.00	14.00	45.00	360.00	0.00	0.00	0.00	2.00
6	Boost, Chocolate	240.0000	8.000	Fl Oz	10.00	4.00	40.00	240.00	0.00	0.00	5.00	0.50
7	Boost, Chocolate Mocha	240.0000	8.000	Fl Oz	10.00	4.00	40.00	240.00	0.00	0.00	5.00	0.50
8	Boost, Strawberry	240.0000	8.000	Fl Oz	10.00	4.00	40.00	240.00	0.00	0.00	5.00	0.50
9	Boost, Vanilla	240.0000	8.000	Fl Oz	10.00	4.00	40.00	240.00	0.00	0.00	5.00	0.50
430	Enlive-Ross Labs	243.0000	8.000	Fl Oz	10.00	0.00	65.00	300.00	0.00	0.00	3.00	0.00
431	Ensure Fiber with FOS-Ross Labs	240.0000	8.000	Fl Oz	8.80	6.10	42.00	250.00	0.00	2.80	0.00	0.00
432	Ensure Glucerna OS-Ross Labs	240.0000	8.000	Fl Oz	10.00	11.00	22.00	220.00	0.00	2.00	0.00	1.00

Page Key: A2 = Baby Food   A2 = Baked Goods   A8 = Beverages   A14 = Breads/Grains and Pasta   A18 = Breakfast Foods/Cereals   A26 = Dairy and Eggs   A40 = Fats and Oils   A42 = Fruits and Vegetables   A52 = Meats and Beans   A60 = Nuts and Seeds   A62 5 Frozen Entrees and Packaged Foods   A76 = Restaurant Chains–Fast Foods   A92 = Restaurant Chains–Other   A106 = Seafood and Fish   A110 = Snacks and Sweets   A120 = Soups   A122 = Supplements   A126 = Toppings and Sauces

Monounsaturated Fat (g)	Polyunsaturated Fat (g)	Vitamin D (mg)	Vitamin K (mg)	Vitamin E (mg)	Vitamin A (re)	Vitamin C (mg)	Thiamin (mg)	Riboflavin (mg)	Niacin (mg)	Vitamin B6 (mg)	Folate (mcg)	Vitamin B12 (mcg)	Calcium (mg)	Iron (mg)	Magnesium (mg)	Phosphorus (mg)	Potassium (mg)	Sodium (mg)	Zinc (mg)
0.00	0.00	0.00	0.00	0.00	60.00	2.40	0.06	0.03	0.38	0.00	0.00	0.00	0.00	0.60	0.00	0.00	160.00	480.00	0.00
0.70	1.11	0.00	0.00	0.07	233.77	1.21	0.05	0.05	0.94	0.10	36.15	0.00	33.74	0.92	7.23	55.43	313.30	910.98	0.75
0.00	0.00	0.00	0.00	0.00	0.00	0.00	0.00	0.00	0.00	0.00	0.00	0.00	0.00	0.20	0.00	0.00	310.46	1191.79	0.00
0.91	0.26	0.00	0.00	0.72	434.40	4.80	0.05	0.12	1.18	0.24	52.80	0.00	60.00	1.78	14.40	110.40	612.00	864.00	1.44
0.00	0.00	0.00	0.00	0.00	60.00	15.00	0.12	0.14	1.52	0.00	0.00	0.00	32.00	0.60	0.00	130.00	440.00	520.00	0.00
0.00	0.00	0.00	0.00	0.00	0.00	0.00	0.00	0.00	0.19	0.00	0.00	0.00	0.00	0.20	0.00	0.00	370.56	1281.92	0.00
2.25	1.54	0.00	0.00	0.63	0.00	1.01	0.28	0.10	0.51	0.03	5.06	0.25	65.78	0.51	5.06	75.90	199.87	1019.59	0.08
2.98	4.61	0.00	0.00	1.34	37.20	2.23	0.07	0.27	0.92	0.07	9.92	0.50	178.56	0.60	19.84	156.24	270.32	917.60	0.64
0.75	0.65	0.00	0.00	0.29	0.00	1.21	0.02	0.02	0.60	0.05	15.18	0.00	26.51	0.67	2.41	12.05	67.48	1053.17	0.60
3.27	1.59	0.00	0.00	0.07	69.44	2.48	0.10	0.27	0.60	0.07	22.32	0.50	178.56	0.69	22.32	153.76	310.00	1004.40	0.62
0.00	0.00	0.00	0.00	0.00	0.00	0.00	0.02	0.02	0.00	0.00	0.00	0.00	240.36	0.00	0.00	0.00	170.26	2073.11	0.00
2.18	0.53	0.00	0.00	0.18	58.42	2.79	0.15	0.28	1.35	0.10	7.87	0.43	172.72	2.01	55.88	238.76	375.92	970.28	1.75
1.80	0.63	0.00	0.00	0.00	45.54	1.52	0.15	0.08	1.47	0.08	2.53	0.25	22.77	2.28	48.07	212.52	399.74	1006.94	1.32
1.63	0.58	0.00	0.00	0.14	487.20	6.96	0.12	0.10	2.52	0.22	4.56	0.24	33.60	2.14	38.40	177.60	304.80	964.80	3.12
0.00	0.00	0.00	0.00	0.00	100.00	6.00	0.15	0.14	1.90	0.00	0.00	0.00	16.00	0.60	0.00	190.00	450.00	460.00	0.00
0.00	0.00	0.00	0.00	0.00	0.00	0.00	0.01	0.00	0.38	0.00	0.00	0.00	240.36	0.20	0.00	0.00	570.86	1191.79	0.00
1.74	0.57	0.00	0.00	0.10	66.96	1.24	0.07	0.25	0.64	0.10	9.18	0.50	166.16	0.55	17.36	161.20	322.40	1061.44	0.67
0.00	0.00	0.00	0.00	0.00	0.00	0.00	0.00	0.01	0.19	0.00	0.00	0.00	2.08	0.10	0.00	0.00	791.19	1422.13	0.00
2.68	0.35	0.00	0.00	0.87	54.56	1.24	0.07	0.22	0.52	0.45	9.92	1.04	163.68	0.60	22.32	146.32	248.00	1036.64	0.79
0.00	0.00	0.00	0.00	0.00	30.00	16.80	0.00	0.00	0.00	0.00	0.00	0.00	27.00	0.45	0.00	0.00	0.00	1292.00	0.00
1.61	1.12	0.00	0.00	2.60	109.12	67.70	0.12	0.25	1.51	0.17	20.83	0.45	158.72	1.81	22.32	148.80	448.88	744.00	0.30
1.73	0.68	0.00	0.00	0.78	53.68	0.00	0.07	0.10	1.88	0.10	19.52	0.20	17.08	1.12	7.32	56.12	219.60	917.44	0.76
0.00	0.00	0.00	0.00	0.00	100.00	6.00	0.06	0.10	1.14	0.00	0.00	0.00	32.00	0.40	0.00	70.00	440.00	510.00	0.00
0.59	1.36	0.00	0.00	0.79	76.57	14.82	0.07	0.05	1.06	0.07	13.59	0.00	22.23	0.79	4.94	34.58	330.98	815.10	0.52
0.00	0.00	0.00	0.00	0.00	0.00	0.00	0.00	0.00	0.19	0.00	0.00	0.00	240.36	0.30	0.00	0.00	430.64	1051.58	0.00
0.81	0.49	0.00	0.00	0.05	29.28	0.24	0.07	0.07	1.39	0.05	19.52	0.15	12.20	0.95	4.88	48.80	75.64	814.96	0.59
1.77	1.09	0.00	0.00	0.00	715.08	6.37	0.05	0.12	3.59	0.31	11.09	2.12	49.56	1.91	23.60	103.84	361.08	922.76	2.12
0.46	0.05	0.00	0.00	0.03	22.77	1.27	0.03	0.03	0.46	0.05	7.59	0.25	12.65	0.86	22.77	35.42	75.90	1001.88	0.28
0.00	0.00	0.00	0.00	0.00	0.00	0.00	0.00	0.00	0.19	0.00	0.00	0.00	240.36	0.10	0.00	0.00	340.51	1251.88	0.00
0.00	0.00	0.00	0.00	0.00	150.00	15.00	0.09	0.10	1.90	0.00	0.00	0.00	32.00	0.40	0.00	120.00	360.00	530.00	0.00
1.28	0.60	0.00	0.00	0.07	265.10	0.96	0.05	0.05	1.23	0.05	4.82	0.12	16.87	0.87	7.23	40.97	154.24	944.72	0.36
2.16	1.01	0.00	0.00	0.00	600.00	5.52	0.05	0.17	3.29	0.10	12.00	0.24	26.40	1.46	9.60	105.60	367.20	1068.00	2.16
1.58	1.39	0.00	0.00	0.60	588.00	6.00	0.07	0.07	1.20	0.19	16.56	0.00	55.20	1.63	7.20	72.00	396.00	1010.40	3.12
0.00	0.00	0.00	0.00	0.00	200.00	6.00	0.06	0.07	1.52	0.00	0.00	0.00	32.00	0.40	0.00	100.00	380.00	540.00	0.00
2.55	1.48	0.00	0.00	1.25	2.60	3.90	1.22	0.10	0.52	0.03	7.80	0.13	31.21	0.52	10.40	54.62	96.24	1170.45	0.26
0.00	0.00	0.00	0.00	0.00	350.00	9.00	0.09	0.07	0.76	0.00	0.00	0.00	16.00	0.40	0.00	0.00	230.00	560.00	0.00
0.29	0.07	0.00	0.00	0.77	19.28	5.78	0.05	0.05	0.75	0.05	9.64	0.00	7.23	0.60	19.28	28.92	98.81	1091.73	0.17
1.33	0.67	0.00	0.00	0.14	243.41	0.00	0.02	0.05	1.01	0.05	4.82	0.17	16.87	0.77	4.82	40.97	175.93	906.16	0.60
0.00	1.00	0.00	0.00	0.00	150.00	4.80	0.03	0.03	0.38	0.00	0.00	0.00	16.00	0.20	0.00	140.00	540.00	0.00
0.82	0.72	0.00	0.00	0.80	301.25	1.45	0.05	0.05	0.92	0.05	10.60	0.00	21.69	1.08	7.23	33.74	209.67	821.81	0.46
0.00	0.00	0.00	0.00	0.00	0.00	0.00	0.00	0.00	0.19	0.00	0.00	0.00	0.00	0.10	0.00	0.00	400.60	911.37	0.00
0.00	0.00	0.00	0.00	0.00	100.00	3.60	0.00	0.00	0.00	0.00	0.00	0.00	29.00	1.50	0.00	0.00	0.00	543.00	0.00
0.00	0.00	0.00	0.00	0.00	0.00	0.00	0.00	0.00	0.00	0.00	0.00	0.00	0.00	0.00	0.00	0.00	350.00	200.00	0.00
0.00	0.00	0.00	0.00	0.00	0.00	0.00	0.00	0.00	0.00	0.00	0.00	0.00	0.00	0.00	0.00	0.00	350.00	200.00	0.00
0.00	0.00	0.00	0.00	0.00	0.00	0.00	0.00	0.00	0.00	0.00	0.00	0.00	0.00	0.00	0.00	0.00	350.00	200.00	0.00
0.00	0.00	0.00	0.00	0.00	0.00	0.00	0.00	0.00	0.00	0.00	0.00	0.00	0.00	0.00	0.00	0.00	400.00	130.00	0.00
0.00	0.00	0.00	0.00	0.00	0.00	0.00	0.00	0.00	0.00	0.00	0.00	0.00	0.00	0.00	0.00	0.00	400.00	130.00	0.00
0.00	0.00	0.00	0.00	0.00	0.00	0.00	0.00	0.00	0.00	0.00	0.00	0.00	0.00	0.00	0.00	0.00	400.00	130.00	0.00
0.00	0.00	0.00	0.00	0.00	0.00	0.00	0.00	0.00	0.00	0.00	0.00	0.00	0.00	0.00	0.00	0.00	400.00	130.00	0.00
0.00	0.00	1.50	20.00	3.00	118.12	24.00	0.38	0.34	2.00	0.40	80.00	1.20	60.00	2.70	8.00	20.00	40.00	65.00	3.80
0.00	0.00	2.50	20.00	2.50	118.12	30.00	0.38	0.43	5.00	0.50	100.00	1.50	350.00	4.50	100.00	300.00	370.00	200.00	3.80
0.00	0.00	2.50	20.00	10.00	118.12	60.00	0.38	0.43	5.00	0.50	100.00	1.50	250.00	4.50	100.00	250.00	370.00	210.00	3.80

USDA ID Code	Food Name	Weight in Grams*	Quantity of Units	Unit of Measure	Protein (g)	Fat (g)	Carbohydrate (g)	Kilocalories	Caffeine (g)	Fiber (g)	Cholesterol (mg)	Saturated Fat (g)
433	Ensure Glucerna Snack Bars-Ross	38.0000	1.000	Bar	6.00	4.00	24.00	140.00	0.00	4.00	3.00	1.00
434	Ensure High Calcium-Ross Labs	240.0000	8.000	Fl Oz	12.00	6.00	31.00	225.00	0.00	0.00	0.00	0.50
435	Ensure High Protein-Ross Labs	240.0000	8.000	Fl Oz	12.00	6.00	30.80	225.00	0.00	0.00	0.00	0.64
436	Ensure Light-Ross Labs	240.0000	8.000	Fl Oz	10.00	3.00	33.30	200.00	0.00	0.00	3.00	0.31
437	Ensure Nutrition Bars-Ross Labs	35.0000	1.000	Bar	6.00	3.00	21.00	130.00	0.00	0.00	3.00	1.00
438	Ensure Plus-Ross Labs	240.0000	8.000	Fl Oz	13.00	11.40	50.10	355.00	0.00	0.00	3.00	0.00
439	Ensure Powder-Ross Labs	240.0000	8.000	Fl Oz	9.00	9.00	34.00	250.00	0.00	0.00	0.00	0.00
440	Ensure Pudding-Ross Labs	120.0000	4.000	Ounce	4.00	5.00	27.00	170.00	0.00	0.00	0.00	0.00
441	Ensure-Ross Labs	240.0000	8.000	Fl Oz	8.80	6.10	40.00	250.00	0.00	0.00	3.00	0.00
677	Power Bar, Apple Cinnamon	65.0000	1.000	Each	10.00	2.50	45.00	230.00	0.00	3.00	0.00	0.50
678	Power Bar, Banana	65.0000	1.000	Each	9.00	2.00	45.00	230.00	0.00	3.00	0.00	0.50
679	Power Bar, Berry, Wild	65.0000	1.000	Each	10.00	2.50	45.00	230.00	0.00	3.00	0.00	0.50
680	Power Bar, Chocolate	65.0000	1.000	Each	10.00	2.00	45.00	230.00	0.00	3.00	0.00	0.50
681	Power Bar, Harvest, Apple Crisp	65.0000	1.000	Each	7.00	4.00	45.00	240.00	0.00	4.00	0.00	0.50
682	Power Bar, Harvest, Cherry Crunc	65.0000	1.000	Each	7.00	4.00	45.00	240.00	0.00	4.00	0.00	0.50
683	Power Bar, Harvest, Chocolate	65.0000	1.000	Each	7.00	4.00	45.00	240.00	0.00	4.00	0.00	1.00
684	Power Bar, Harvest, Strawberry	65.0000	1.000	Each	7.00	4.00	45.00	240.00	0.00	4.00	0.00	0.50
685	Power Bar, Malt Nut	65.0000	1.000	Each	10.00	2.50	45.00	230.00	0.00	3.00	0.00	0.50
686	Power Bar, Mocha	65.0000	1.000	Each	10.00	2.50	45.00	230.00	0.00	3.00	0.00	1.00
687	Power Bar, Oatmeal Raisin	65.0000	1.000	Each	10.00	2.50	45.00	230.00	0.00	3.00	0.00	0.50
688	Power Bar, Peanut Butter	65.0000	1.000	Each	10.00	2.50	45.00	230.00	0.00	3.00	0.00	0.50
673	Power Bar, Power Gel, Fruit, Tro	41.0000	1.400	Ounce	0.00	0.00	28.00	110.00	0.00	0.00	0.00	0.00
674	Power Bar, Power Gel, Lemon Lime	41.0000	1.400	Ounce	0.00	0.00	28.00	110.00	0.00	0.00	0.00	0.00
675	Power Bar, Power Gel, Straw-Bana	41.0000	1.400	Ounce	0.00	0.00	28.00	110.00	0.00	0.00	0.00	0.00
676	Power Bar, Power Gel, Vanilla	41.0000	1.400	Ounce	0.00	0.00	28.00	110.00	0.00	0.00	0.00	0.00
698	Slim-Fast Bar, Chocolate, Dutch	34.0000	1.200	Ounce	5.00	5.00	20.00	140.00	0.00	2.00	1250.00	2.00
699	Slim-Fast Bar, Peanut Butter	34.0000	1.200	Ounce	6.00	5.00	19.00	150.00	0.00	2.00	1250.00	3.00
700	Slim-Fast Powder, Chocolate	28.0000	1.000	Ounce	5.00	1.00	20.00	100.00	0.00	2.00	750.00	0.50
701	Slim-Fast Powder, Chocolate Malt	28.0000	1.000	Ounce	5.00	1.00	20.00	100.00	0.00	2.00	750.00	0.50
702	Slim-Fast Powder, Strawberry	28.0000	1.000	Ounce	5.00	0.50	20.00	100.00	0.00	2.00	750.00	0.00
703	Slim-Fast Powder, Vanilla	28.0000	1.000	Ounce	5.00	0.50	20.00	100.00	0.00	2.00	750.00	0.00
740	Tiger Bar, Café Mocha	65.0000	1.000	Each	10.00	2.00	43.00	200.00	0.00	3.00	0.00	0.50
741	Tiger Bar, Chocolate	65.0000	1.000	Each	10.00	2.00	43.00	200.00	0.00	3.00	0.00	0.50
742	Tiger Bar, Vanilla	65.0000	1.000	Each	10.00	2.00	43.00	200.00	0.00	3.00	0.00	0.50
751	Ultra Slim-Fast Bar, Choc Chip C	28.0000	1.000	Ounce	1.00	4.00	16.00	120.00	0.00	2.00	0.00	2.00
752	Ultra Slim-Fast Bar, Peanut Butt	28.0000	1.000	Ounce	2.00	4.00	19.00	120.00	0.00	2.00	0.00	2.00
753	Ultra Slim-Fast Bar, Peanut Cara	28.0000	1.000	Ounce	1.00	4.00	22.00	120.00	0.00	2.00	500.00	2.00
754	Ultra Slim-Fast Powder, Café Moc	33.0000	1.200	Ounce	5.00	1.00	24.00	120.00	0.00	5.00	5.00	0.50
755	Ultra Slim-Fast Powder, Chocolat	33.0000	1.200	Ounce	5.00	2.00	24.00	120.00	0.00	5.00	5.00	1.00
756	Ultra Slim-Fast Powder, Chocolat	33.0000	1.200	Ounce	5.00	1.00	24.00	120.00	0.00	5.00	5.00	0.50
757	Ultra Slim-Fast Powder, Chocolat	33.0000	1.200	Ounce	5.00	1.00	24.00	110.00	0.00	5.00	5.00	0.50
758	Ultra Slim-Fast Powder, Chocolat	33.0000	1.200	Ounce	5.00	1.00	24.00	120.00	0.00	6.00	750.00	0.00
759	Ultra Slim-Fast Powder, Fruit Ju	31.0000	1.100	Ounce	5.00	1.00	24.00	120.00	0.00	5.00	4.00	0.00
760	Ultra Slim-Fast Powder, Strawber	33.0000	1.200	Ounce	5.00	0.50	25.00	120.00	0.00	4.00	5.00	0.00
761	Ultra Slim-Fast Powder, Vanilla	33.0000	1.200	Ounce	5.00	0.50	22.00	110.00	0.00	6.00	5.00	0.00
762	Ultra Slim-Fast, Juice Base, Rtd	350.0000	11.500	Fl Oz	7.00	1.50	46.00	220.00	0.00	5.00	10.00	0.50
763	Ultra Slim-Fast, Juice Base, Rtd	350.0000	11.500	Fl Oz	7.00	1.50	48.00	220.00	0.00	5.00	10.00	0.50
764	Ultra Slim-Fast, Juice Base, Rtd	350.0000	11.500	Fl Oz	7.00	1.50	47.00	220.00	0.00	5.00	10.00	0.50
765	Ultra Slim-Fast, Rtd, Choc Fudge	350.0000	11.000	Fl Oz	10.00	3.00	42.00	220.00	0.00	5.00	5.00	1.00
766	Ultra Slim-Fast, Rtd, Choc Royal	350.0000	11.000	Fl Oz	10.00	3.00	38.00	220.00	0.00	5.00	5.00	1.00
770	Ultra Slim-Fast, Rtd, Chocolate,	350.0000	11.000	Fl Oz	10.00	3.00	42.00	220.00	0.00	5.00	5.00	1.00
767	Ultra Slim-Fast, Rtd, Coffee	350.0000	11.000	Fl Oz	10.00	3.00	38.00	220.00	0.00	5.00	5.00	0.50
768	Ultra Slim-Fast, Rtd, Strawberry	350.0000	11.000	Fl Oz	10.00	3.00	42.00	220.00	0.00	5.00	5.00	1.00

Page Key: A2 = Baby Food   A2 = Baked Goods   A8 = Beverages   A14 = Breads/Grains and Pasta   A18 = Breakfast Foods/Cereals   A26 = Dairy and Eggs   A40 = Fats and Oils   A42 = Fruits and Vegetables   A52 = Meats and Beans   A60 = Nuts and Seeds   A62 5 Frozen Entrees and Packaged Foods   A76 = Restaurant Chains–Fast Foods   A92 = Restaurant Chains–Other   A106 = Seafood and Fish   A110 = Snacks and Sweets   A120 = Soups   A122 = Supplements   A126 = Toppings and Sauces

Monounsaturated Fat (g)	Polyunsaturated Fat (g)	Vitamin D (mg)	Vitamin K (mg)	Vitamin E (mg)	Vitamin A (re)	Vitamin C (mg)	Thiamin (mg)	Riboflavin (mg)	Niacin (mg)	Vitamin B6 (mg)	Folate (mcg)	Vitamin B12 (mcg)	Calcium (mg)	Iron (mg)	Magnesium (mg)	Phosphorus (mg)	Potassium (mg)	Sodium (mg)	Zinc (mg)
0.00	0.00	1.50	12.00	10.00	118.12	60.00	0.23	0.26	3.00	0.30	60.00	0.90	250.00	2.70	60.00	150.00	60.00	75.00	2.25
0.00	0.00	3.50	28.00	5.00	118.12	42.00	0.38	0.43	5.00	0.50	120.00	1.80	400.00	4.50	100.00	250.00	500.00	290.00	6.00
0.00	0.00	2.50	20.00	4.00	118.12	30.00	0.38	0.43	5.00	0.50	100.00	1.50	300.00	4.50	100.00	250.00	500.00	290.00	5.70
0.00	0.00	2.50	20.00	2.50	118.12	30.00	0.38	0.43	5.00	0.50	100.00	1.50	250.00	4.50	100.00	250.00	370.00	200.00	3.80
0.00	0.00	1.50	10.00	2.00	67.64	21.00	0.23	0.26	3.00	0.30	60.00	0.90	250.00	2.70	60.00	150.00	200.00	115.00	2.30
0.00	0.00	2.50	20.00	2.50	118.12	30.00	0.38	0.43	5.00	0.50	100.00	1.50	200.00	4.50	100.00	200.00	440.00	240.00	3.80
0.00	0.00	1.25	10.00	1.88	58.62	37.50	0.38	0.43	5.00	0.50	100.00	1.50	125.00	2.25	50.00	125.00	370.00	200.00	2.82
0.00	0.00	1.00	12.00	2.00	45.09	9.00	0.23	0.26	3.00	0.30	60.00	1.20	100.00	2.70	40.00	100.00	180.00	135.00	3.00
0.00	0.00	2.50	20.00	2.50	118.12	30.00	0.38	0.43	5.00	0.50	100.00	1.50	300.00	4.50	100.00	300.00	370.00	200.00	3.80
1.50	0.50	0.00	0.00	0.00	0.00	0.00	0.00	0.00	0.00	0.00	0.00	0.00	0.00	0.00	0.00	0.00	110.00	90.00	0.00
1.00	0.50	0.00	0.00	0.00	0.00	0.00	0.00	0.00	0.00	0.00	0.00	0.00	0.00	0.00	0.00	0.00	200.00	90.00	0.00
1.50	0.50	0.00	0.00	0.00	0.00	0.00	0.00	0.00	0.00	0.00	0.00	0.00	0.00	0.00	0.00	0.00	110.00	90.00	0.00
0.50	1.00	0.00	0.00	0.00	0.00	0.00	0.00	0.00	0.00	0.00	0.00	0.00	0.00	0.00	0.00	0.00	145.00	90.00	0.00
0.00	0.00	0.00	0.00	0.00	0.00	0.00	0.00	0.00	0.00	0.00	0.00	0.00	0.00	0.00	0.00	0.00	0.00	80.00	0.00
0.00	0.00	0.00	0.00	0.00	0.00	0.00	0.00	0.00	0.00	0.00	0.00	0.00	0.00	0.00	0.00	0.00	0.00	80.00	0.00
0.00	0.00	0.00	0.00	0.00	0.00	0.00	0.00	0.00	0.00	0.00	0.00	0.00	0.00	0.00	0.00	0.00	0.00	80.00	0.00
0.00	0.00	0.00	0.00	0.00	0.00	0.00	0.00	0.00	0.00	0.00	0.00	0.00	0.00	0.00	0.00	0.00	0.00	80.00	0.00
1.00	1.00	0.00	0.00	0.00	0.00	0.00	0.00	0.00	0.00	0.00	0.00	0.00	0.00	0.00	0.00	0.00	110.00	90.00	0.00
1.50	0.50	0.00	0.00	0.00	0.00	0.00	0.00	0.00	0.00	0.00	0.00	0.00	0.00	0.00	0.00	0.00	145.00	90.00	0.00
1.00	1.00	0.00	0.00	0.00	0.00	0.00	0.00	0.00	0.00	0.00	0.00	0.00	0.00	0.00	0.00	0.00	180.00	120.00	0.00
1.00	1.00	0.00	0.00	0.00	0.00	0.00	0.00	0.00	0.00	0.00	0.00	0.00	0.00	0.00	0.00	0.00	150.00	110.00	0.00
0.00	0.00	0.00	0.00	0.00	0.00	0.00	0.00	0.00	0.00	0.00	0.00	0.00	0.00	0.00	0.00	0.00	40.00	50.00	0.00
0.00	0.00	0.00	0.00	0.00	0.00	0.00	0.00	0.00	0.00	0.00	0.00	0.00	0.00	0.00	0.00	0.00	40.00	50.00	0.00
0.00	0.00	0.00	0.00	0.00	0.00	0.00	0.00	0.00	0.00	0.00	0.00	0.00	0.00	0.00	0.00	0.00	40.00	50.00	0.00
0.00	0.00	0.00	0.00	0.00	0.00	0.00	0.00	0.00	0.00	0.00	0.00	0.00	0.00	0.00	0.00	0.00	40.00	50.00	0.00
0.00	0.00	0.00	0.00	0.00	0.38	15.00	5.00	0.43	1.50	0.40	40.00	2.50	40.00	0.50	16.00	4.50	40.00	80.00	3.75
0.00	0.00	0.00	0.00	0.00	0.38	15.00	1.50	0.40	1.50	0.40	40.00	2.50	40.00	0.50	16.00	4.50	40.00	80.00	3.75
0.00	0.00	0.00	0.00	0.00	0.45	18.00	7.00	0.26	1.20	0.60	100.00	2.50	150.00	0.40	100.00	6.30	100.00	110.00	4.50
0.00	0.00	0.00	0.00	0.00	0.45	18.00	7.00	0.26	1.20	0.60	100.00	2.50	150.00	0.40	100.00	6.30	100.00	120.00	4.50
0.00	0.00	0.00	0.00	0.00	0.45	18.00	7.00	0.26	1.20	0.60	100.00	2.50	150.00	0.40	100.00	6.30	100.00	130.00	4.50
0.00	0.00	0.00	0.00	0.00	0.45	18.00	7.00	0.26	1.20	0.60	100.00	2.50	150.00	0.40	100.00	6.30	100.00	130.00	4.50
0.00	0.00	0.00	0.00	0.00	0.00	0.00	0.00	0.00	0.00	0.00	0.00	0.00	0.00	0.00	0.00	0.00	0.00	90.00	0.00
0.00	0.00	0.00	0.00	0.00	0.00	0.00	0.00	0.00	0.00	0.00	0.00	0.00	0.00	0.00	0.00	0.00	0.00	90.00	0.00
0.00	0.00	0.00	0.00	0.00	0.00	0.00	0.00	0.00	0.00	0.00	0.00	0.00	0.00	0.00	0.00	0.00	0.00	90.00	0.00
0.00	0.00	0.00	0.00	0.00	750.00	9.00	0.15	0.26	3.00	0.30	60.00	0.90	150.00	2.70	0.00	150.00	110.00	40.00	0.60
0.00	0.00	0.00	0.00	0.00	750.00	9.00	0.23	0.26	3.00	0.30	60.00	0.90	150.00	2.70	16.00	150.00	100.00	45.00	0.60
0.00	0.00	0.00	0.00	0.00	0.23	6.00	3.00	0.26	0.90	0.30	60.00	1.00	150.00	0.00	0.00	2.70	150.00	35.00	0.60
0.00	0.00	0.00	0.00	0.00	750.00	27.00	0.45	0.17	10.00	0.60	100.00	2.10	150.00	6.30	100.00	100.00	210.00	110.00	4.50
0.00	0.00	0.00	0.00	0.00	750.00	27.00	0.45	0.17	10.00	0.60	100.00	2.10	150.00	6.30	100.00	100.00	340.00	100.00	4.50
0.00	0.00	0.00	0.00	0.00	750.00	27.00	0.45	0.17	10.00	0.60	100.00	2.10	150.00	6.30	100.00	100.00	220.00	100.00	4.50
0.00	0.00	0.00	0.00	0.00	750.00	27.00	0.45	0.17	10.00	0.60	100.00	2.10	150.00	6.30	100.00	100.00	280.00	130.00	4.50
0.00	0.00	0.00	0.00	0.00	0.45	27.00	10.00	0.17	2.10	0.60	100.00	4.00	150.00	0.50	100.00	100.00	100.00	120.00	4.50
0.00	0.00	0.00	0.00	0.00	750.00	27.00	0.45	0.17	10.00	0.60	100.00	2.10	150.00	6.30	100.00	200.00	210.00	110.00	4.50
0.00	0.00	0.00	0.00	0.00	750.00	27.00	0.45	0.17	10.00	0.60	100.00	2.10	150.00	6.30	100.00	100.00	170.00	130.00	4.50
0.00	0.00	0.00	0.00	0.00	750.00	27.00	0.45	0.17	10.00	0.60	100.00	2.10	150.00	6.30	100.00	100.00	140.00	130.00	4.50
0.00	0.00	0.00	0.00	0.00	2500.00	60.00	0.38	0.43	5.00	0.50	100.00	1.50	250.00	4.50	100.00	250.00	200.00	240.00	3.75
0.00	0.00	0.00	0.00	0.00	2500.00	60.00	0.38	0.43	5.00	0.50	100.00	1.50	250.00	4.50	100.00	250.00	190.00	260.00	3.75
0.00	0.00	0.00	0.00	0.00	2500.00	60.00	0.38	0.43	5.00	0.50	100.00	1.50	250.00	4.50	100.00	250.00	200.00	240.00	3.75
0.00	0.00	0.00	0.00	0.00	1750.00	21.00	0.53	0.60	7.00	0.70	120.00	2.10	400.00	2.70	140.00	350.00	530.00	300.00	2.25
0.00	0.00	0.00	0.00	0.00	1750.00	21.00	0.53	0.60	7.00	0.70	120.00	2.10	400.00	2.70	140.00	350.00	530.00	220.00	2.25
0.00	0.00	0.00	0.00	0.00	1750.00	21.00	0.53	0.60	7.00	0.70	120.00	2.10	400.00	2.70	140.00	350.00	530.00	220.00	2.25
0.00	0.00	0.00	0.00	0.00	1750.00	21.00	0.53	0.60	7.00	0.70	120.00	2.10	400.00	2.70	140.00	350.00	500.00	300.00	2.25
0.00	0.00	0.00	0.00	0.00	1750.00	21.00	0.53	0.60	7.00	0.70	120.00	2.10	400.00	2.70	140.00	350.00	450.00	460.00	2.25

USDA ID Code	Food Name	Weight in Grams*	Quantity of Units	Unit of Measure	Protein (g)	Fat (g)	Carbohydrate (g)	Kilocalories	Caffeine (g)	Fiber (g)	Cholesterol (mg)	Saturated Fat (g)
769	Ultra Slim-Fast, Rtd, Vanilla	350.0000	11.000	Fl Oz	10.00	3.00	38.00	220.00	0.00	5.00	5.00	1.00
771	Viactiv-Calcium Chew, Caramel	2.0000	1.000	Each	0.00	0.50	4.00	20.00	0.00	0.00	0.00	0.00
772	Viactiv-Calcium Chew, Chocolate	2.0000	1.000	Each	0.00	0.50	4.00	20.00	0.00	0.00	0.00	0.00
773	Viactiv-Calcium Chew, Mochaccino	2.0000	1.000	Each	0.00	0.50	4.00	20.00	0.00	0.00	0.00	0.00
774	Viactiv-Energy Bar, Fruit Crispy	30.0000	1.000	Each	4.00	2.00	22.00	120.00	0.00	0.00	0.00	0.00
775	Viactiv-Energy Bar, Fruit Crispy	30.0000	1.000	Each	4.00	2.00	20.00	120.00	0.00	0.00	0.00	0.00
776	Viactiv-Energy Bar, Hearty, Appl	45.0000	1.000	Each	6.00	4.50	29.00	180.00	0.00	0.00	0.00	3.50
777	Viactiv-Energy Bar, Hearty, Choc	45.0000	1.000	Each	6.00	4.50	29.00	180.00	0.00	0.00	0.00	3.50
778	Viactiv-Energy Fruit Smoothie, F	240.0000	8.000	Fl Oz	0.00	0.00	37.00	150.00	0.00	0.00	0.00	0.00
779	Viactiv-Energy Fruit Smoothie, S	240.0000	8.000	Fl Oz	0.00	0.00	28.00	110.00	0.00	0.00	0.00	0.00
780	Viactiv-Energy Fruit Spritzer, C	240.0000	8.000	Fl Oz	0.00	0.00	22.00	90.00	0.00	0.00	0.00	0.00
781	Viactiv-Energy Fruit Spritzer, C	240.0000	8.000	Fl Oz	0.00	0.00	22.00	90.00	0.00	0.00	0.00	0.00
	Vitamin Supplement, Centrum	1.0000	1.000	Each	0.00	0.00	0.00	0.00	0.00	0.00	0.00	0.00
782	Vitamin Supplement, Maximum One-	2.0000	1.000	Each	0.00	0.00	0.00	0.00	0.00	0.00	0.00	0.00
	Vitamin Supplement, One-A-Day	1.0000	1.000	Each	0.00	0.00	0.00	0.00	0.00	0.00	0.00	0.00
	Vitamin Supplement, StressTab	1.0000	1.000	Each	0.00	0.00	0.00	0.00	0.00	0.00	0.00	0.00
783	Vitamin Supplement, Theragram	2.0000	1.000	Each	0.00	0.00	0.00	0.00	0.00	0.00	0.00	0.00
784	Vitamite	240.0000	1.000	Cup	3.00	5.00	14.00	110.00	0.00	0.00	0.00	1.50

Toppings and Sauces

USDA ID Code	Food Name	Weight in Grams*	Quantity of Units	Unit of Measure	Protein (g)	Fat (g)	Carbohydrate (g)	Kilocalories	Caffeine (g)	Fiber (g)	Cholesterol (mg)	Saturated Fat (g)
	Apple Butter	282.0000	1.000	Cup	1.10	0.00	120.61	487.86	0.00	4.23	0.00	0.00
	Catsup	240.0000	1.000	Cup	3.65	0.86	65.50	249.60	0.00	3.12	0.00	0.12
	Catsup, Low Sodium	240.0000	1.000	Cup	3.65	0.86	65.50	249.60	0.00	3.12	0.00	0.12
	Gravy, Au Jus, Cnd	149.0000	0.250	Cup	2.86	0.48	5.96	38.14	0.00	0.00	0.00	0.24
	Gravy, Beef, Cnd	233.0000	1.000	Cup	8.74	5.50	11.21	123.49	0.00	0.93	6.99	2.68
	Gravy, Chicken, Cnd	238.0000	1.000	Cup	4.59	13.59	12.90	188.02	0.00	0.95	4.76	3.36
	Gravy, Mushroom, Cnd	238.4000	1.000	Cup	3.00	6.46	13.04	119.20	0.00	0.95	0.00	0.95
	Gravy, Turkey, Cnd	298.0000	0.250	Cup	6.20	5.01	12.16	121.58	0.00	0.95	4.77	1.48
	Gravy, Unspecified Type	298.0000	0.250	Cup	3.22	1.99	14.38	86.26	0.00	0.00	0.00	0.71
	Honey	339.0000	1.000	Cup	1.02	0.00	279.34	1030.56	0.00	0.68	0.00	0.00
	Jams and Preserves	20.0000	1.000	Tbsp	0.07	0.01	13.77	55.60	0.00	0.22	0.00	0.00
	Jellies	300.0000	1.000	Cup	0.60	0.09	211.41	849.00	0.00	3.00	0.00	0.06
	Marmalade, Orange	320.0000	1.000	Cup	0.96	0.00	212.16	787.20	0.00	0.64	0.00	0.00
	Mustard	5.0000	1.000	Tbsp	0.00	0.00	0.00	0.00	0.00	0.00	0.00	0.00
	Relish, Pickle, Hamburger	15.0000	1.000	Tbsp	0.09	0.08	5.17	19.35	0.00	0.48	0.00	0.01
	Relish, Pickle, Hot Dog	15.0000	1.000	Tbsp	0.23	0.07	3.50	13.65	0.00	0.23	0.00	0.01
	Relish, Pickle, Sweet	245.0000	1.000	Cup	0.91	1.15	85.87	318.50	0.00	2.70	0.00	0.15
	Salsa	16.5170	2.000	Tbsp	0.00	0.00	2.50	10.01	0.00	0.00	0.00	0.00
	Salt Substitute	4.8000	0.250	Tsp	0.00	0.00	0.00	0.00	0.00	0.00	0.00	0.00
	Salt, Table	292.0000	1.000	Cup	0.00	0.00	0.00	0.00	0.00	0.00	0.00	0.00
	Sauce, A-1 Steak	31.3000	2.000	Tbsp	0.00	0.01	5.00	19.00	0.00	0.50	0.00	0.00
	Sauce, Barbecue	250.0000	1.000	Cup	4.50	4.50	32.00	187.50	0.00	3.00	0.00	0.68
	Sauce, Marinara	250.0000	0.500	Cup	4.00	8.37	25.45	170.00	0.00	0.00	0.00	1.20
	Sauce, Mustard, Chinese	15.0000	1.000	Tbsp	1.00	1.00	1.00	11.00	0.00	0.40	0.00	0.00
	Sauce, Soy (Tamari)	18.0000	1.000	Tbsp	0.93	0.01	1.53	9.54	0.00	0.00	0.00	0.00
	Sauce, Spaghetti	249.0000	0.500	Cup	4.53	11.88	39.67	271.41	0.00	8.47	0.00	1.70
	Sauce, Spaghetti, w/ Garlic & He	113.0000	1.000	Cup	2.00	0.59	9.00	40.00	0.00	0.00	0.00	0.00
	Sauce, Spaghetti-Prego	146.0000	1.000	Cup	3.56	4.15	26.11	154.31	0.00	3.56	0.00	1.19
	Sauce, Spaghetti-Ragu	146.0000	1.000	Cup	3.56	4.75	20.18	130.57	0.00	3.56	0.00	1.78
	Sauce, Teriyaki	288.0000	1.000	Cup	17.08	0.00	45.94	241.92	0.00	0.29	0.00	0.00
	Sauce, White	263.8000	0.500	Cup	10.21	13.45	21.39	240.06	0.00	0.00	34.29	6.41
	Sauce, Worcestershire	34.0000	2.000	Tbsp	0.00	0.00	6.00	23.00	0.00	0.00	0.00	0.00
	Sugar, Brown	220.0000	1.000	Cup	0.00	0.00	214.06	827.20	0.00	0.00	0.00	0.00
	Sugar, Granulated	200.0000	1.000	Cup	0.00	0.00	199.80	774.00	0.00	0.00	0.00	0.00

Monounsaturated Fat (g)	Polyunsaturated Fat (g)	Vitamin D (mg)	Vitamin K (mg)	Vitamin E (mg)	Vitamin A (re)	Vitamin C (mg)	Thiamin (mg)	Riboflavin (mg)	Niacin (mg)	Vitamin B6 (mg)	Folate (mcg)	Vitamin B12 (mcg)	Calcium (mg)	Iron (mg)	Magnesium (mg)	Phosphorus (mg)	Potassium (mg)	Sodium (mg)	Zinc (mg)
0.00	0.00	0.00	0.00	0.00	1750.00	21.00	0.53	0.60	7.00	0.70	120.00	2.10	400.00	2.70	140.00	350.00	450.00	460.00	2.25
0.00	0.00	2.50	40.00	0.00	0.00	0.00	0.00	0.00	0.00	0.00	0.00	0.00	500.00	0.00	0.00	0.00	0.00	10.00	0.00
0.00	0.00	2.50	40.00	0.00	0.00	0.00	0.00	0.00	0.00	0.00	0.00	0.00	500.00	0.00	0.00	0.00	0.00	10.00	0.00
0.00	0.00	2.50	40.00	0.00	0.00	0.00	0.00	0.00	0.00	0.00	0.00	0.00	500.00	0.00	0.00	0.00	0.00	10.00	0.00
0.00	0.00	0.00	0.00	33.00	0.00	120.00	0.00	0.00	0.00	2.00	400.00	6.00	0.00	0.00	0.00	0.00	0.00	65.00	0.00
0.00	0.00	0.00	0.00	33.00	0.00	120.00	0.00	0.00	0.00	2.00	400.00	6.00	0.00	0.00	0.00	0.00	0.00	80.00	0.00
0.00	0.00	2.50	40.00	0.00	0.00	0.00	0.00	0.00	0.00	2.00	400.00	6.00	330.00	1.80	0.00	66.66	0.00	90.00	15.00
0.00	0.00	2.50	40.00	0.00	0.00	0.00	0.00	0.00	0.00	2.00	400.00	6.00	330.00	1.80	0.00	66.66	0.00	90.00	15.00
0.00	0.00	0.00	0.00	0.00	0.00	60.00	0.00	0.00	0.00	2.00	400.00	6.00	300.00	0.00	0.00	0.00	0.00	15.00	0.00
0.00	0.00	0.00	0.00	0.00	0.00	60.00	0.00	0.00	0.00	2.00	400.00	6.00	300.00	0.00	0.00	0.00	0.00	5.00	0.00
0.00	0.00	0.00	0.00	0.00	0.00	60.00	0.00	0.00	0.00	2.00	400.00	6.00	0.00	0.00	0.00	0.00	0.00	70.00	0.00
0.00	0.00	0.00	0.00	0.00	0.00	60.00	0.00	0.00	0.00	2.00	400.00	6.00	0.00	0.00	0.00	0.00	0.00	70.00	0.00
0.00	0.00	5.00	0.00	10.00	1000.00	60.00	1.50	1.70	20.00	2.00	400.00	6.00	162.00	18.00	100.00	109.00	40.00	0.00	15.00
0.00	0.00	0.25	0.00	20.00	1000.00	60.00	1.50	1.70	20.00	2.00	400.00	6.00	130.00	18.00	100.00	0.00	37.50	0.00	15.00
0.00	0.00	5.00	0.00	10.00	1000.00	60.00	1.50	1.70	20.00	2.00	400.00	6.00	0.00	0.00	0.00	0.00	0.00	0.00	0.00
0.00	0.00	0.00	0.00	10.00	0.00	500.00	10.00	0.00	100.00	5.00	400.00	12.00	0.00	18.00	0.00	0.00	0.00	0.00	0.00
0.00	0.00	0.25	0.00	20.00	1100.00	120.00	3.00	3.40	30.00	3.00	400.00	9.00	40.00	27.00	100.00	0.00	7.50	0.00	15.00
0.00	0.00	0.00	0.00	0.00	0.00	0.00	0.00	0.00	0.00	0.00	0.00	0.00	0.00	0.00	0.00	0.00	110.00	120.00	0.00
0.00	0.00	0.00	0.00	0.03	33.84	1.97	0.06	0.06	0.31	0.14	2.82	0.00	39.48	0.87	14.10	28.20	256.62	11.28	0.17
0.14	0.36	0.00	0.00	3.53	244.80	36.24	0.22	0.17	3.29	0.43	36.00	0.00	45.60	1.68	52.80	93.60	1154.40	2846.40	0.55
0.14	0.36	0.00	0.00	3.53	244.80	36.24	0.22	0.17	3.29	0.43	36.00	0.00	45.60	1.68	52.80	93.60	1154.40	48.00	0.55
0.19	0.02	0.00	0.00	0.00	0.00	2.38	0.05	0.14	2.15	0.02	4.77	0.24	9.54	1.43	4.77	71.52	193.10	119.20	2.38
2.24	0.19	0.00	0.00	0.14	0.00	0.00	0.07	0.09	1.54	0.02	4.66	0.23	13.98	1.63	4.66	69.90	188.73	1304.80	2.33
6.07	3.57	0.00	0.00	0.38	264.18	0.00	0.05	0.10	1.05	0.02	4.76	0.24	47.60	1.12	4.76	69.02	259.42	1373.26	1.90
2.79	2.43	0.00	0.00	0.00	0.00	0.00	0.07	0.14	1.60	0.05	28.61	0.00	16.69	1.57	4.77	35.76	252.70	1358.88	1.67
2.15	1.17	0.00	0.14	0.00	0.00	0.00	0.05	0.19	3.10	0.02	4.77	0.24	9.54	1.67	4.77	69.14	259.86	1375.57	1.91
0.78	0.39	0.00	0.00	0.00	0.00	1.83	0.05	0.11	0.78	0.03	3.40	0.18	36.60	0.26	10.46	49.67	65.35	1422.02	0.26
0.00	0.00	0.00	0.00	0.00	0.00	1.70	0.00	0.14	0.41	0.07	6.78	0.00	20.34	1.42	6.78	13.56	176.28	13.56	0.75
0.01	0.00	0.00	0.00	0.00	0.20	1.76	0.00	0.00	0.01	0.00	6.60	0.00	4.00	0.10	0.80	2.20	15.40	6.40	0.01
0.03	0.06	0.00	0.00	0.00	6.00	2.70	0.00	0.09	0.12	0.06	3.00	0.00	24.00	0.60	18.00	15.00	192.00	84.00	0.12
0.00	0.00	0.00	0.00	0.00	16.00	15.36	0.03	0.03	0.16	0.03	115.20	0.00	121.60	0.48	6.40	19.20	118.40	179.20	0.13
0.00	0.00	0.00	0.00	0.00	0.00	0.00	0.00	0.00	0.00	0.00	0.00	0.00	0.00	0.00	0.00	0.00	0.00	75.00	0.00
0.04	0.02	0.00	0.00	0.00	4.05	0.35	0.00	0.01	0.09	0.00	0.15	0.00	0.60	0.17	1.05	2.55	11.40	164.40	0.02
0.03	0.02	0.00	0.00	0.00	2.55	0.15	0.01	0.01	0.08	0.00	0.15	0.00	0.75	0.19	2.85	6.00	11.70	163.65	0.03
0.51	0.29	0.00	0.00	0.10	39.20	2.45	0.00	0.07	0.56	0.05	2.45	0.00	7.35	2.13	12.25	34.30	61.25	1986.95	0.34
0.00	0.00	0.00	0.00	0.00	40.04	1.80	0.00	0.00	0.00	0.00	0.00	0.00	0.00	0.00	0.00	0.00	0.00	120.12	0.00
0.00	0.00	0.00	0.00	0.00	0.00	0.00	0.00	0.00	0.00	0.00	0.00	0.00	0.00	0.00	0.00	0.00	2440.00	0.00	0.00
0.00	0.00	0.00	0.00	0.00	0.00	0.00	0.00	0.00	0.00	0.00	0.00	0.00	70.08	0.96	2.92	0.00	23.36	113173.36	0.29
0.00	0.00	0.00	0.00	0.00	32.00	4.80	0.00	0.00	0.00	0.00	0.00	0.00	12.00	0.30	0.00	0.00	0.00	454.00	0.00
1.93	1.70	0.00	0.00	2.78	217.50	17.50	0.08	0.05	2.25	0.20	10.00	0.00	47.50	2.25	45.00	50.00	435.00	2037.50	0.50
4.28	2.29	0.00	0.00	0.00	240.00	32.00	0.11	0.15	3.97	0.62	33.75	0.00	45.00	2.00	60.00	87.50	1060.00	1572.50	0.67
0.00	0.00	0.00	0.00	0.00	0.00	0.00	0.00	0.00	0.00	0.00	0.00	0.00	12.00	0.30	0.00	0.00	0.00	188.00	0.00
0.00	0.01	0.00	0.00	0.00	0.00	0.00	0.01	0.02	0.60	0.03	2.79	0.00	3.06	0.36	6.12	19.80	32.40	1028.70	0.07
6.07	3.25	0.00	0.00	6.22	306.27	27.89	0.14	0.15	3.75	0.88	53.78	0.00	69.72	1.62	59.76	89.64	956.16	1235.04	0.52
0.00	0.00	0.00	0.00	0.00	56.00	18.00	0.00	0.00	0.00	0.00	0.00	0.00	24.00	0.80	0.00	0.00	0.00	390.00	0.00
0.00	0.00	0.00	0.00	0.00	356.10	21.37	0.00	0.00	0.00	0.00	0.00	0.00	85.46	0.71	0.00	0.00	0.00	724.07	0.00
0.00	0.00	0.00	0.00	0.00	178.05	1.42	0.00	0.00	0.00	0.00	0.00	0.00	56.98	0.71	0.00	0.00	0.00	652.85	0.00
0.00	0.00	0.00	0.00	0.00	0.00	0.00	0.09	0.20	3.66	0.29	57.60	0.00	72.00	4.90	175.68	443.52	648.00	11039.04	0.29
4.70	1.69	0.00	0.00	0.00	92.33	2.64	0.08	0.45	0.53	0.07	15.83	1.06	424.72	0.26	263.80	255.89	443.18	796.68	0.55
0.00	0.00	0.00	0.00	0.00	0.00	4.20	0.00	0.00	0.00	0.00	0.00	0.00	43.00	1.50	0.00	0.00	0.00	333.00	0.00
0.00	0.00	0.00	0.00	0.00	0.00	0.00	0.02	0.02	0.18	0.07	2.20	0.00	187.00	4.20	63.80	48.40	761.20	85.80	0.40
0.00	0.00	0.00	0.00	0.00	0.00	0.00	0.00	0.04	0.00	0.00	0.00	0.00	2.00	0.12	0.00	4.00	4.00	2.00	0.06

USDA ID Code	Food Name	Weight in Grams*	Quantity of Units	Unit of Measure	Protein (g)	Fat (g)	Carbohydrate (g)	Kilocalories	Caffeine (g)	Fiber (g)	Cholesterol (mg)	Saturated Fat (g)
	Sugar, Powdered	120.0000	1.000	Cup	0.00	0.12	119.40	466.80	0.00	0.00	0.00	0.02
	Syrup, Corn, Dark	328.0000	1.000	Cup	0.00	0.00	251.25	924.96	0.00	0.00	0.00	0.00
	Syrup, Corn, High-fructose	310.0000	1.000	Cup	0.00	0.00	235.60	871.10	0.00	0.00	0.00	0.00
	Syrup, Corn, Light	328.0000	1.000	Cup	0.00	0.00	251.25	924.96	0.00	0.00	0.00	0.00
	Syrup, Malt	384.0000	1.000	Cup	23.81	0.00	273.79	1221.12	0.00	0.00	0.00	0.00
	Syrup, Maple	315.0000	1.000	Cup	0.00	0.63	211.68	825.30	0.00	0.00	0.00	0.13
	Syrup, Pancake, Lo Cal	240.0000	1.000	Cup	0.00	0.00	106.32	393.60	0.00	0.00	0.00	0.00
	Syrup, Pancake, w/ 2% Maple	315.0000	1.000	Cup	0.00	0.32	219.24	834.75	0.00	0.00	0.00	0.06
	Syrup, Pancake, w/ Butter	315.0000	1.000	Cup	0.00	5.04	233.42	932.40	0.00	0.00	12.60	3.18
	Toppings, Butterscotch or Caramel	41.0000	2.000	Tbsp	0.62	0.04	27.02	103.32	0.00	0.37	0.41	0.05
	Toppings, Caramel	16.6800	1.000	Tbsp	0.27	0.00	13.01	51.71	0.00	0.00	0.00	0.00
	Toppings, Chocolate	304.0000	1.000	Cup	13.98	27.06	191.22	1064.00	18.24	8.51	6.08	12.10
	Toppings, Fudge, Hot	19.0180	1.000	Tbsp	1.00	2.00	11.01	70.07	0.00	0.00	0.00	0.50
	Toppings, Marshmallow Cream	28.3500	1.000	Ounce	0.23	0.09	22.40	91.29	0.00	0.03	0.00	0.02
	Toppings, Nuts in Syrup	328.0000	1.000	Cup	14.76	72.16	175.15	1338.24	0.00	5.25	0.00	6.43
	Toppings, Pineapple	340.0000	1.000	Cup	0.34	0.34	225.76	860.20	0.00	3.40	0.00	0.07
	Toppings, Strawberry	340.0000	1.000	Cup	0.68	0.34	225.42	863.60	0.00	3.40	0.00	0.03

Page Key: A2 = Baby Food   A2 = Baked Goods   A8 = Beverages   A14 = Breads/Grains and Pasta   A18 = Breakfast Foods/Cereals   A26 = Dairy and Eggs   A40 = Fats and Oils
A42 = Fruits and Vegetables   A52 = Meats and Beans   A60 = Nuts and Seeds   A62 = Frozen Entrees and Packaged Foods   A76 = Restaurant Chains–Fast Foods
A92 = Restaurant Chains–Other   A106 = Seafood and Fish   A110 = Snacks and Sweets   A120 = Soups   A122 = Supplements   A126 = Toppings and Sauces

Monounsaturated Fat (g)	Polyunsaturated Fat (g)	Vitamin D (mg)	Vitamin K (mg)	Vitamin E (mg)	Vitamin A (re)	Vitamin C (mg)	Thiamin (mg)	Riboflavin (mg)	Niacin (mg)	Vitamin B6 (mg)	Folate (mcg)	Vitamin B12 (mcg)	Calcium (mg)	Iron (mg)	Magnesium (mg)	Phosphorus (mg)	Potassium (mg)	Sodium (mg)	Zinc (mg)
0.04	0.06	0.00	0.00	0.00	0.00	0.00	0.00	0.00	0.00	0.00	0.00	0.00	1.20	0.07	0.00	2.40	2.40	1.20	0.04
0.00	0.00	0.00	0.00	0.00	0.00	0.00	0.03	0.03	0.07	0.03	0.00	0.00	59.04	1.21	26.24	36.08	144.32	508.40	0.13
0.00	0.00	0.00	0.00	0.00	0.00	0.00	0.00	0.06	0.00	0.00	0.00	0.00	0.00	0.09	0.00	0.00	0.00	6.20	0.06
0.00	0.00	0.00	0.00	0.00	0.00	0.00	0.03	0.03	0.07	0.03	0.00	0.00	9.84	0.16	6.56	6.56	13.12	396.88	0.07
0.00	0.00	0.00	0.00	0.00	0.00	0.00	0.04	1.50	31.18	1.92	46.08	0.00	234.24	3.69	276.48	906.24	1228.80	134.40	0.54
0.19	0.32	0.00	0.00	0.00	0.00	0.00	0.03	0.03	0.09	0.00	0.00	0.00	211.05	3.78	44.10	6.30	642.60	28.35	13.10
0.00	0.00	0.00	0.00	0.00	0.00	0.00	0.02	0.02	0.05	0.00	0.00	0.00	2.40	0.05	0.00	103.20	7.20	480.00	0.05
0.09	0.16	0.00	0.00	0.00	0.00	0.00	0.03	0.06	0.06	0.00	0.00	0.00	15.75	0.22	6.30	31.50	18.90	192.15	0.72
1.48	0.19	0.00	0.00	0.09	47.25	0.00	0.03	0.03	0.06	0.00	0.00	0.00	6.30	0.28	6.30	31.50	9.45	308.70	0.13
0.01	0.00	0.00	0.00	0.00	11.07	0.12	0.00	0.04	0.02	0.00	0.82	0.04	21.73	0.08	2.87	19.27	34.44	143.09	0.08
0.00	0.00	0.00	0.00	0.00	0.00	0.00	0.00	0.00	0.00	0.00	0.00	0.00	2.34	0.00	0.00	4.67	5.67	11.01	0.03
11.73	0.85	0.00	0.00	8.88	12.16	0.61	0.18	0.67	0.91	0.18	12.16	0.64	246.24	3.95	155.04	410.40	1100.48	1051.84	2.07
0.00	0.00	0.00	0.00	0.00	0.00	0.00	0.00	0.00	0.00	0.00	0.00	0.00	36.03	0.20	0.00	0.00	0.00	35.03	0.00
0.02	0.01	0.00	0.00	0.00	0.00	0.00	0.00	0.00	0.02	0.00	0.28	0.00	0.85	0.06	0.57	2.27	1.42	13.89	0.01
16.30	45.03	0.00	0.00	2.85	13.12	3.61	0.59	0.39	1.34	0.62	68.88	0.00	131.20	3.44	206.64	364.08	685.52	137.76	3.41
0.10	0.17	0.00	0.00	0.00	6.80	199.24	0.10	0.03	0.31	0.07	10.20	0.00	74.80	1.63	6.80	27.20	1077.80	214.20	1.63
0.03	0.17	0.00	0.00	0.48	6.80	84.66	0.03	0.07	0.85	0.07	6.80	0.00	81.60	3.30	13.60	44.20	248.20	71.40	1.67

Cholesterol Content of Food

Item	Serving size	Cholesterol (mg/serving)	Item	Serving size	Cholesterol (mg/serving)
Beef			Ice cream		
Ground, medium-fat, pan-fried	3 oz	75	Premium	½ cup	70
			Low-fat	½ cup	20
Steak	3 oz	75	Lamb, leg, meat only	3 oz	76
Thin sliced	5 slices (21 g)	9	Liver		
Butter	1 pat (5 g)	11	Chicken, simmered	3 oz	38
Cheese			Beef, pan-fried	3 oz	409
Cheddar	½ cup (66 g)	69	Lobster	1 cup	104
Cottage, 2% fat	½ cup (113 g)	10	Margarine	1 Tbsp	0
Cream	1 Tbsp	16	Milk, fluid		
Hard (asiago, Parmesan)	1 oz	20	Buttermilk	1 cup	9
			Condensed	½ cup	52
Chicken			Reduced-fat, 2%	1 cup	18
Breast, no skin	3 oz	47	Non-fat	1 cup	4
Breast, with skin	3 oz	50	Whole	1 cup	33
Dark meat, no skin	3 oz	87	Oysters, raw	3 oz	21
Dark meat, with skin	3 oz	90	Pork		
Clam	3 oz	57	Bacon	3 slices (19 g)	16
Crab meat	3 oz	62	Chopped	3 oz	14
Cream, whipping, heavy	½ cup	82	Ham slices	1 oz	16
Egg			Tenderloin	3 oz	69
Whole	1 large	213	Sausage	1 oz	20
White only	¼ cup	0	Shrimp	3 oz	165
Fish			Sour cream	½ cup	51
Halibut	3 oz	65	Turkey		
Salmon	3 oz	88	Breast, with skin	3 oz	83
Tuna, yellowfin	3 oz	50	Dark meat, roasted	3 oz	77
Yellowtail	3 oz	102	Light meat, roasted	3 oz	81
Frozen yogurt	½ cup	5	Veal	3 oz	100

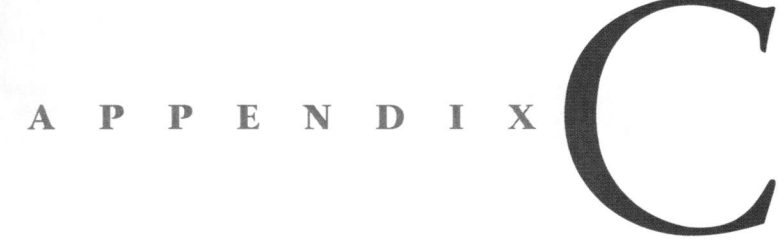

APPENDIX C

Dietary Fiber in Selected Plant Foods

Food	Amount	Weight (g)	Total dietary fiber (g)	Noncellulose polysaccharides (g)	Cellulose (g)	Lignin
Apple	1 medium					
Flesh		138	1.96	1.29	0.66	0.01
Skin		100	3.71	2.21	1.01	0.49
Banana	1 small	119	2.08	1.33	0.44	0.31
Beans						
Baked	1 cup	255	18.53	14.45	3.59	0.48
Green, cooked	1 cup	125	4.19	2.31	1.61	0.26
Bread						
White	1 slice	25	0.68	0.50	0.18	Trace
Whole grain	1 slice	25	2.13	1.49	0.33	0.31
Broccoli, cooked	1 cup	155	6.36	4.53	1.78	0.05
Brussels sprouts, cooked	1 cup	155	4.43	3.08	1.24	0.11
Cabbage, cooked	1 cup	145	4.10	2.55	1	0.55
Carrots, cooked	1 cup	155	5.74	3.44	2.29	Trace
Cauliflower, cooked	1 cup	125	2.25	0.84	1.41	Trace
Cereals						
All-Bran	1 oz	30	8.01	5.35	1.80	0.86
Corn Flakes	1 cup	25	2.75	1.82	0.61	0.33
Grapenuts	¼ cup	30	2.10	1.54	0.38	0.17
Puffed Wheat	1 cup	15	2.31	1.55	0.39	0.37
Rice Krispies	1 cup	30	1.34	1.04	0.23	0.07
Shredded Wheat	1 biscuit	25	3.07	2.20	0.66	0.21
Special K	1 cup	30	1.64	1.10	0.22	0.32
Cherries	10 cherries	68	0.84	0.63	0.17	0.05
Cookies						
Ginger	4 snaps	28	0.56	0.41	0.08	0.07
Oatmeal	4 cookies	52	2.08	1.64	0.21	0.22
Plain	4 cookies	48	0.80	0.68	0.05	0.06
Corn	1 cup	165	7.82	7.11	0.51	0.20
Canned	1 cup	165	9.39	8.20	1.06	0.13

Continued.

Food	Amount	Weight (g)	Total dietary fiber (g)	Noncellulose polysaccharides (g)	Cellulose (g)	Lignin
Flour						
Bran	1 cup	100	44	32.70	8.05	3.23
White	1 cup	115	3.62	2.90	0.69	0.03
Whole grain	1 cup	120	11.41	7.50	2.95	0.96
Grapefruit	½ cup	100	0.44	0.34	0.04	0.06
Jam, strawberry	1 Tbsp	20	0.22	0.17	0.02	0.03
Lettuce	⅛ head	100	1.53	0.47	1.06	Trace
Marmalade, orange	1 Tbsp	20	0.14	0.13	0.01	Trace
Onions, raw, sliced	1 cup	100	2.10	1.55	0.55	Trace
Orange	1 cup	200	0.58	0.44	0.08	0.06
Parsnips, raw, diced	1 cup	100	4.90	3.77	1.13	Trace
Peach, flesh and skin	1 medium	100	2.28	1.46	0.20	0.62
Peanuts	1 oz	30	2.79	1.92	0.51	0.36
Peanut butter	1 Tbsp	16	1.21	0.90	0.31	Trace
Pear	1 medium					
Flesh		164	4	2.16	1.10	0.74
Skin		100	8.59	3.72	2.18	2.67
Peas, canned	1 cup	170	13.35	8.85	3.91	0.60
Peas, raw or frozen	1 cup	100	7.75	5.48	2.09	0.18
Plums	1 medium	66	1	0.65	0.15	0.20
Potato, raw	1 medium	135	4.73	3.36	1.38	Trace
Raisins	1 oz	30	1.32	0.72	0.25	0.35
Strawberries	1 cup	149	2.65	1.39	1.04	0.22
Tomato						
Raw	1 medium	135	1.89	0.88	0.61	0.41
Canned, drained	1 cup	240	2.04	1.08	0.89	0.07
Turnips, raw	1 medium	100	2.20	1.50	0.70	Trace

Data from Southgate DAT and others: A guide to calculating intakes of dietary fiber, *J Hum Nutr* 30:303, 1976.

D

Sodium and Potassium Content of Foods, 100 g, Edible Portion

Food and description	Sodium (mg)	Potassium (mg)
Almonds		
Dried	4	773
Roasted and salted	198	773
Apple brown betty	153	100
Apple butter	2	252
Apple juice, canned or bottled	1	101
Apples		
Raw, pared	1	110
Frozen, sliced, sweetened	14	68
Applesauce, canned, sweetened	2	65
Apricot nectar, canned (approx. 40% fruit)	Trace	151
Apricots		
Raw	1	281
Canned, syrup pack, light	1	239
Dried, sulfured, cooked, fruit and liquid	8	318
Asparagus		
Cooked spears, boiled, drained	1	183
Canned spears, green		
Regular pack, solids and liquid	236[a]	166
Special dietary pack (low-sodium), solids and liquid	3	166
Frozen		
Cuts and tips, cooked, boiled, drained	1	220
Spears, cooked, boiled, drained	1	238
Avocados, raw, all commercial varieties	4	604
Bacon, cured, cooked, broiled or fried, drained	1021	236
Bacon, Canadian, cooked, broiled or fried, drained	2555	432
Baking powders		
Home use		
Straight phosphate	8220	170

For table notes, see p. D147.

Continued.

Food and description	Sodium (mg)	Potassium (mg)
Special low-sodium preparations	6	10,948
Bananas, raw, common	1	370
Barbecue sauce	815	174
Bass, black sea, raw	68	256
Beans, common, mature seeds, dry		
White		
Cooked	7	416
Canned, solids and liquid, with pork and tomato sauce	463	210
Red, cooked	3	340
Beans, lima		
Immature seeds		
Cooked, boiled, drained	1	422
Canned		
Regular pack, solids and liquid	236[a]	222
Special dietary pack (low-sodium), solids and liquid	4	222
Frozen, thin-seeded types, commonly called *baby limas,* cooked, boiled, drained	129	394
Mature seeds, dry, cooked	2	612
Beans, mung, sprouted seeds, cooked, boiled, drained	4	156
Beans, snap		
Green		
Cooked, boiled, drained	4	151
Canned		
Regular pack, solids and liquid	236[a]	95
Special dietary pack (low-sodium), solids and liquid	2	95
Frozen, cut, cooked, boiled, drained	1	152
Yellow or wax		
Cooked, boiled, drained	3	151
Canned		
Regular pack, solids and liquid	236[a]	95
Special dietary pack (low-sodium), solids and liquid	2	95
Frozen, cut, cooked, boiled, drained	1	164
Beans and frankfurters, canned	539	262
Beef		
Retail cuts, trimmed to retail level		
Round	60	370
Rump	60	370
Hamburger, regular ground, cooked	47	450
Beef and vegetable stew, canned	411	174
Beef, corned, boneless		
Cooked, medium-fat	1740	150
Canned corned-beef hash (with potato)	540	200
Beef, dried, cooked, creamed	716	153
Beef potpie, commercial, frozen, unheated	366	93
Beet greens, common, cooked, boiled, drained	76	332
Canned		
Regular pack, solids and liquid	236[a]	167
Special dietary pack (low-sodium), solids and liquid	46	167
Beverages, alcoholic		
Beer, alcohol 4.5% by volume (3.6% by weight)	7	25

Food and description	Sodium (mg)	Potassium (mg)
Gin, rum, vodka, whisky		
80 proof (33.4% alcohol by weight)	1	2
86 proof (36.0% alcohol by weight)	1	2
90 proof (37.9% alcohol by weight)	1	2
94 proof (39.7% alcohol by weight)	1	2
100 proof (42.5% alcohol by weight)	1	2
Wines		
Dessert, alcohol 18.8% by volume (15.3% by weight)	4	75
Table, alcohol 12.2% by volume (9.9% by weight)	5	92
Biscuit dough, commercial, frozen	910	86
Biscuit mix, with enriched flour, and biscuits baked from mix		
Dry form	1300	80
Made with milk	973	116
Biscuits, baking powder, made with enriched flour	626	117
Blackberries, including dewberries, boysenberries, and youngberries, raw	1	170
Blackberries, canned, solids and liquid		
Water pack, with or without artificial sweetener	1	115
Syrup pack, heavy	1	109
Blueberries		
Raw	1	81
Frozen, not thawed, sweetened	1	66
Bluefish, cooked		
Baked or broiled	104	—
Fried	146	—
Boston brown bread	251	292
Bouillon cubes or powder	24,000	100
Boysenberries, frozen, not thawed, sweetened	1	105
Bran, added sugar and malt extract	1060	1070
Bran flakes (40% bran), added thiamine	925	—
Bran flakes with raisins, added thiamine	800	—
Brazil nuts	1	715
Bread crumbs, dry, grated	736	152
Bread stuffing mix and stuffings prepared from mix, dry form	1331	172
Breads		
Cracked wheat	529	134
French or Vienna, enriched	580	90
Italian, enriched	585	74
Raisin	365	233
Rye, American (⅓ rye, ⅔ clear flour)	557	145
White enriched, made with 3% to 4% nonfat dry milk	507	105
Whole wheat, made with 2% nonfat dry milk	527	273
Broccoli		
Cooked spears, boiled, drained	10	267
Frozen, spears, cooked, boiled, drained	12	220
Brussels sprouts, frozen, cooked, boiled, drained	14	295
Buffalo fish, raw	52	293
Bulgur (parboiled wheat), canned, made from hard red winter wheat		
Unseasoned[b]	599	87
Seasoned[c]	460	112

Continued.

Food and description	Sodium (mg)	Potassium (mg)
Butter[d]	987	23
Buttermilk, fluid, cultured (made from skim milk)	130	140
Cabbage		
Common varieties (Danish, domestic, and pointed types)		
Raw	20	233
Cooked, boiled until tender, drained, shredded, cooked in small amount of water	14	163
Red, raw	26	268
Cabbage, Chinese (also called *celery cabbage* or *petsai*)	23	253
Cakes		
Baked from home recipes		
Angel food	283	88
Fruit cake, made with enriched flour, dark	158	496
Gingerbread, made with enriched flour	237	454
Plain cake or cupcake, without icing	300	79
Pound, modified	178	78
Frozen, commercial, devil's food, with chocolate icing	420	119
Candy		
Caramels, plain or chocolate	226	192
Chocolate, sweet	33	269
Chocolate-coated, chocolate fudge	228	193
Gum drops, starch jelly pieces	35	5
Hard	32	4
Marshmallows	39	6
Peanut bars	10	448
Carp, raw	50	286
Carrots		
Raw	47	341
Canned		
Regular pack, solids and liquid	236[a]	120
Special dietary pack (low-sodium), solids and liquid	39	120
Cashew nuts	15[e]	464
Catfish, freshwater, raw	60	330
Cauliflower		
Cooked, boiled, drained	9	206
Frozen, cooked, boiled, drained	10	207
Caviar, sturgeon, granular	2200	180
Celery, all, including green and yellow varieties		
Raw	126	341
Cooked, boiled, drained	88	239
Chard, Swiss, cooked, boiled, drained	86	321
Cheese straws	721	63
Cheeses		
Natural cheeses		
Cheddar (domestic type)	700	82
Cottage (large or small curd)		
Creamed	229	85
Uncreamed	290	72
Cream	250	74
Parmesan	734	149

Food and description	Sodium (mg)	Potassium (mg)
Swiss (domestic)	710	104
Pasteurized process cheese, American	1136[f]	80
Pasteurized process cheese spread, American	1625[f]	240
Cherries		
Raw, sweet	2	191
Canned		
Sour, red, solids and liquid, water pack	2	130
Sweet, solids and liquid, syrup pack, light	1	128
Frozen, not thawed, sweetened	2	130
Chicken, all classes		
Light meat without skin, cooked, roasted	64	411
Dark meat without skin, cooked, roasted	86	321
Chicken potpie, commercial, frozen, unheated	411	153
Chicory, Witloof (also called *French* or *Belgian endive*), bleached head (forced), raw	7	182
Chili con carne, canned, with beans	531	233
Chocolate, bitter or baking	4	830
Chocolate syrup, fudge-type	89	284
Chop suey, with meat, canned	551	138
Chow mein, chicken (without noodles), canned	290	167
Citron, candied	290	120
Clams, raw		
Soft meat only	36	235
Hard or round, meat only	205	311
Clams, canned, including hard, soft, razor, and unspecified solids and liquid	—	140
Cocoa and chocolate-flavored beverage powders		
Cocoa powder with nonfat dry milk	525	800
Mix for hot chocolate	382	605
Cocoa, dry powder, high-fat or breakfast		
Plain	6	1522
Processed with alkali	717	651
Coconut cream (liquid expressed from grated coconut meat)	4	324
Coconut meat, fresh	23	256
Cod		
Cooked, broiled	110	407
Dehydrated, lightly salted	8100	160
Coffee, instant, water-soluble solids		
Dry powder	72	3256
Beverage	1	36
Coleslaw, made with French dressing (commercial)	268	205
Collards, cooked, boiled, drained, leaves (including stems) cooked in small amount of water	25	234
Cookie dough, plain, chilled in roll, baked	548	48
Cookies		
Assorted, packaged, commercial	365	67
Butter, thin, rich	418	60
Gingersnaps	571	462
Molasses	386	138
Oatmeal with raisins	162	370
Sandwich-type	483	38
Vanilla wafer	252	72

Continued.

Food and description	Sodium (mg)	Potassium (mg)
Corn, sweet		
Cooked, boiled, drained, white and yellow, kernels, cut off cob before cooking	Trace	165
Canned		
Regular pack, cream style, white and yellow, solids and liquid	236[a]	(97)
Special dietary pack (low-sodium), cream style, white and yellow, solids and liquid	2	(97)
Frozen, kernels cut off cob, cooked, boiled, drained	1	184
Corn fritters	477	133
Corn grits, degermed, enriched, dry form	1	80
Corn products used mainly as ready-to-eat breakfast cereals		
Corn flakes, added nutrients	1005	120
Corn, puffed, added nutrients	1060	—
Corn, rice and wheat flakes, mixed, added nutrients	950	—
Cornbread mix and cornbread baked from mix, made with egg, milk	744	127
Cornmeal, white or yellow, degermed, enriched, dry form	1	120
Cornstarch	Trace	Trace
Cowpeas, including black-eyed peas		
Immature seeds, canned, solids and liquid	236[a]	352
Young pods, with seeds, cooked, boiled, drained	3	196
Crab, canned	1000	110
Crackers		
Butter	1092	113
Graham, plain	670	384
Saltines	(1100)	(120)
Sandwich-type, peanut-cheese	992	226
Soda	1100	120
Cranberries, raw	2	82
Cranberry juice cocktail, bottled (approx. 33% cranberry juice)	1	10
Cranberry sauce, sweetened, canned, strained	1	30
Cream, fluid, light, coffee or table, 20% fat	43	122
Cream substitutes, dried, containing cream, skim milk (calcium-reduced), and lactose	575	—
Cream puffs with custard filling	83	121
Cress, garden, raw	14	606
Croaker, Atlantic, cooked, baked	120	323
Cucumbers, raw, pared	6	160
Custard, baked	79	146
Dates, domestic, natural and dry	1	648
Doughnuts, cake-type	501	90
Duck, domesticated, raw, flesh only	74	285
Eggplant, cooked, boiled, drained	1	150
Eggs, chicken		
Raw		
Whole, fresh, and frozen	122	129
Whites, fresh and frozen	146	139
Yolks, fresh	52	98
Endive (curly endive and escarole), raw	14	294
Farina		
Enriched		
Regular		
Dry form	2	83

Food and description	Sodium (mg)	Potassium (mg)
Cooked	144	9
Quick-cooking, cooked	165	10
Instant-cooking, cooked	188	13
Nonenriched, regular, dry form	2	83
Figs, canned, solids and liquid, syrup pack, light	2	152
Flatfishes (flounders, soles, sand dabs), raw	78	342
Fruit, cocktail, canned, solids and liquid, water pack, with or without artificial sweetener	5	168
Garlic, cloves, raw	19	529
Ginger root, fresh	6	264
Gizzard, chicken, all classes, cooked, simmered	57	211
Goose, domesticated, flesh only, cooked, roasted	124	605
Gooseberries, canned, solids and liquid, syrup pack, heavy	1	98
Grapefruit		
Raw, pulp, pink, red, white, all varieties	1	135
Canned, juice, sweetened	1	162
Grapefruit juice and orange juice, blended, canned, sweetened	1	184
Grapes, raw, American-type (slip skin), such as Concord, Delaware, Niagara, Catawba, and Scuppernong	3	158
Grape juice, canned or bottled	2	116
Guavas, whole, raw, common	4	289
Haddock, cooked, fried	177	348
Hake, including Pacific hake, squirrel hake, and silver hake or whiting, raw	74	363
Halibut, Atlantic, and Pacific, cooked, broiled	134	525
Ham croquette	342	83
Heart, beef, lean, cooked, braised	104	232
Herring		
Raw, Pacific	74	420
Smoked, hard	6231	157
Honey, strained or extracted	5	51
Horseradish, prepared	96	290
Ice cream and frozen custard, regular (approx. 17% fat)	63[g]	181
Ice cream cones	232	244
Ice milk	68[g]	195
Jams and preserves	12	88
Kale, cooked, boiled, drained, leaves including stems	43	221
Kingfish; southern, gulf, and northern (whiting); raw	83	250
Lake herring (cisco), raw	47	319
Lamb, retail cuts	70	290
Lemon juice, canned or bottled, unsweetened	1	141
Lettuce, raw crisphead varieties such as iceberg, New York, and Great Lakes strains	9	175
Lime juice, canned or bottled, unsweetened	1	104
Liver, beef, cooked, fried	184	380
Lobster, northern, canned or cooked	210	180
Loganberries, canned, solids and liquid, syrup pack, light	1	111
Macadamia nuts	—	164
Macaroni, unenriched, dry form	2	197
Macaroni and cheese, canned	304	58
Margarine[h]	987	23
Marmalade, citrus	14	33

Continued.

Food and description	Sodium (mg)	Potassium (mg)
Milk, cow		
Fluid (pasteurized and raw)		
Whole, 3.5% fat	50	144
Skim	52	145
Canned, evaporated (unsweetened)	118	303
Dry, skim (nonfat solids), regular	532	1745
Malted		
Dry powder	440	720
Beverage	91	200
Chocolate drink, fluid, commercial		
Made with skim milk	46	142
Made with whole (3.5% fat) milk	47	146
Molasses, cane		
First extraction or light	15	917
Third extraction or blackstrap	96	2927
Muffin mixes, corn, and muffins baked from mixes		
Made with egg, milk	479	110
Made with egg, water	346	104
Mushrooms		
Raw	15	414
Canned, solids and liquid	400	197
Muskmelons, raw, cantaloupes, other netted varieties	12	251
Mussels, Atlantic and Pacific, raw, meat only	289	315
Mustard greens, cooked, boiled, drained	18	220
Mustard, prepared		
Brown	1307	130
Yellow	1252	130
Nectarines, raw	6	294
New Zealand spinach, cooked, boiled, drained	92	463
Noodles, egg noodles, enriched, cooked	2	44
Oat products used mainly as hot breakfast cereals, oatmeal or rolled oats		
Dry form	2	352
Cooked	218	61
Oat products used mainly as ready-to-eat breakfast cereals, with or without corn, puffed added nutrients	1267	—
Ocean perch, Atlantic (redfish)		
Raw	79	269
Cooked, fried	153	284
Ocean perch, Pacific, raw	63	390
Oils, salad or cooking	0	0
Okra		
Raw	3	249
Cooked, boiled, drained	2	174
Olives, pickled, canned or bottled		
Green	2400	55
Ripe, Ascolano (extra large, mammoth, giant jumbo)	813	34
Ripe, salt-cured, oil-coated, Greek style	3288	—
Onions, mature (dry), raw	10	157
Onions, young green (bunching varieties), raw, bulb and entire top	5	231

Food and description	Sodium (mg)	Potassium (mg)
Oranges, raw, peeled fruit, all commercial varieties	1	200
Orange juice		
Raw, all commercial varieties	1	200
Canned, unsweetened	1	199
Frozen concentrate, unsweetened, diluted with 3 parts water, by volume	1	186
Oysters		
Raw, meat only, Eastern	73	121
Cooked, fried	206	203
Frozen, solids and liquid	380	210
Oyster stew, commercial frozen, prepared with equal volume of milk	366	176
Pancake and waffle mixes and pancakes baked from mixes, plain and buttermilk, made with egg, milk	564	154
Parsnips, cooked, boiled, drained	8	379
Peaches		
Raw	1	202
Canned, solids and liquid, water pack, with or without artificial sweetener	2	137
Frozen, sliced, sweetened, not thawed	2	124
Peanut butters made with small amounts of added fat, salt	607	670
Peanuts		
Roasted with skins	5	701
Roasted and salted	418	674
Pears		
Raw, including skin	2	130
Canned, solids and liquid, syrup pack, light	1	85
Peas, green, immature		
Cooked, boiled, drained	1	196
Canned, Alaska (early or June peas)		
Regular pack, solids and liquid	236[a]	96
Special dietary pack (low-sodium), solids and liquid	3	96
Frozen, cooked, boiled, drained	115	135
Peas, mature seeds, dry, whole, raw	35	1005
Peas and carrots, frozen, cooked, boiled, drained	84	157
Pecans	Trace	603
Peppers, hot, chili, mature, red, raw, pods excluding seeds	25	564
Peppers, sweet, garden varieties, immature, green, raw	13	213
Perch, yellow, raw	68	230
Pickles, cucumber, dill	1428	200
Pie crust or plain pastry, made with enriched flour, baked	611	50
Pies, baked, pie crust made with unenriched flour		
Apple	301	80
Cherry	304	105
Mincemeat	448	178
Pumpkin	214	160
Pike, walleye, raw	51	319
Pineapple		
Raw	1	146
Frozen chunks, sweetened, not thawed	2	100
Pizza, with cheese, from home recipe, baked		
With cheese topping	702	130

Continued.

Food and description	Sodium (mg)	Potassium (mg)
With sausage topping	729	168
Plate dinners, frozen, commercial, unheated		
Beef pot roast, whole oven-browned potatoes, peas, corn	259	244
Chicken, fried; mashed potatoes; mixed vegetables (carrots, peas, corn, beans)	344	112
Meat loaf with tomato sauce, mashed potatoes, peas	393	115
Turkey, sliced; mashed potatoes, peas	400	176
Plums		
Raw, Damson	2	299
Canned, solids and liquid, purple (Italian prunes), syrup pack, light	1	145
Popcorn, popped		
Plain	(3)	—
Oil and salt added	1940	—
Pork, fresh, retail cuts, trimmed to retail level, loin	65	390
Pork, lightly cured, commercial, ham, medium-fat class, separable, lean, cooked, roasted	930	326
Pork, cured, canned ham, contents of can	(1100)	(340)
Potatoes		
Cooked, boiled in skin	3[i]	407
Dehydrated mashed, flakes without milk		
Dry form	89	1600
Prepared, water, milk, table fat added	231	286
Pretzels	1680[j]	130
Prunes, dehydrated (low moisture), stewed	2	353
Pudding mixes and puddings made from mixes, with starch base		
With milk, cooked	129	136
With milk, without cooking	124	129
Pumpkin, canned	2	240
Radishes, raw, common	18	322
Raisins, natural (unbleached), cooked, fruit and liquid, added sugar	13	355
Raspberries		
Canned, solids and liquid, water pack, with or without artificial sweetener, red	1	114
Frozen, red, sweetened, not thawed	1	100
Rennin products		
Tablet (salts, starch, rennin enzyme)	22,300	—
Rhubarb, cooked, added sugar	2	203
Rice		
Brown		
Raw	9	214
Cooked	282	70
White (fully milled or polished), enriched, common commercial varieties, all types		
Raw	5	92
Cooked	374	28
Rice products used mainly as ready-to-eat breakfast cereals		
Rice flakes, added nutrients	987	180
Rice, puffed; added nutrients, without salt	2	100
Rice, puffed or open-popped, presweetened, honey and added nutrients	706	—
Rockfish, including black, canary, yellowtail, rasphead, and bocaccio, cooked, oven-steamed	68	446
Roe, cooked, baked or broiled, cod and shad[k]	73	132
Rolls and buns, commercial, ready-to-serve		
Danish pastry	366	112

Food and description	Sodium (mg)	Potassium (mg)
Hard rolls, enriched	625	97
Plain (pan rolls), enriched	506	95
Sweet rolls	389	124
Rusk	246	161
Rutabagas, cooked, boiled, drained	4	167
Rye, flour, medium	(1)	203
Rye wafers, whole grain	882	600
Salad dressings, commercial[l]		
Blue and Roquefort cheese		
Regular	1094	37
Special dietary (low-calorie), low-fat (approx. 5 kcal/tsp)	1108	34
French		
Regular	1370	79
Special dietary (low-calorie), low-fat (approx. 5 kcal/tsp)	787	79
Mayonnaise	597	34
Thousand Island		
Regular	700	113
Special dietary (low-calorie, approx. 10 kcal/tsp)	700	113
Salmon, coho (sliver)		
Raw	48[m]	421
Canned, solids and liquid	351[n]	339
Salt port, raw	1212	42
Salt sticks, regular-type	1674	92
Sandwich spread (with chopped pickle)		
Regular	626	92
Special dietary (low-calorie, approx. 5 kcal/tsp)	626	92
Sardines, Atlantic, canned in oil, drained solids	823	590
Sardines, Pacific, in tomato sauce, solids and liquid	400	320
Sauerkraut, canned, solids and liquid	747[o]	140
Sausage, cold cuts, and luncheon meats		
Bologna, all samples	1300	230
Frankfurters, raw, all samples	1100	220
Luncheon meat, pork, cured ham or shoulder, chopped, spiced or unspiced, canned	1234	222
Pork sausage, links or bulk, cooked	958	269
Scallops, bay and sea, cooked, steamed	265	476
Soups, commercial, canned		
Beef broth, bouillon, and consommé, prepared with equal volume of water	326	54
Chicken noodle, prepared with equal volume of water	408	23
Tomato		
Prepared with equal volume of water	396	94
Prepared with equal volume of milk	422	167
Vegetable beef, prepared with equal volume of water	427	66
Soy sauce	7325	366
Spaghetti, enriched, cooked, tender stage	1	61
Spaghetti, in tomato sauce with cheese, canned	382	121
Spinach		
Cooked, boiled, drained	50	324
Canned		
Regular pack, drained solids	236[a]	250

Continued.

Food and description	Sodium (mg)	Potassium (mg)
Special dietary pack (low-sodium), solids and liquid	34	250
Frozen, chopped, cooked, boiled, drained	52	333
Squash, summer, all varieties, cooked, boiled, drained	1	141
Squash, frozen		
Summer, yellow crookneck, cooked, boiled, drained	3	167
Winter, heated	1	207
Strawberries		
Raw	1	164
Frozen, sweetened, not thawed, sliced	1	112
Sturgeon, cooked, steamed	108	235
Succotash (corn and lima beans), frozen, cooked, boiled, drained	38	246
Sugars, beet or cane, brown	30	344
Sweet potatoes		
Cooked, all, baked in skin	12	300
Canned, liquid pack, solids and liquid, regular pack in syrup	48	(120)
Dehydrated flakes, prepared with water	45	140
Tangerines, raw (Dancy variety)	2	126
Tapioca, dry	3	18
Tapioca desserts, tapioca cream pudding	156	135
Tartar sauce, regular	707	78
Tea, instant (water-soluble solids), carbohydrate added		
Dry powder	—	4530
Beverage	—	25
Tomato catsup, bottled	1042[p]	363
Tomato juice, canned or bottled		
Regular pack	200	227
Special dietary pack (low-sodium)	3	227
Tomato juice cocktail, canned or bottled	200	221
Tomato puree, canned		
Regular pack	399	426
Special dietary pack (low-sodium)	6	426
Tomatoes, ripe		
Raw	3	244
Canned, solids and liquid, regular pack	130	217
Tongue, beef, medium-fat, cooked, braised	61	164
Tuna, canned		
In oil, solids and liquid	800	301
In water, solids and liquid	41[q]	279[q]
Turkey, all classes		
Light meat, cooked, roasted	82	411
Dark meat, cooked, roasted	99	398
Turkey potpie, commercial, frozen, unheated	369	114
Turnips, cooked, boiled, drained	34	188
Turnip greens, leaves, including stems		
Canned, solids and liquid	236[a]	243
Frozen, cooked, boiled, drained	17	149
Veal, retail cuts, untrimmed	80	500
Vinegar, cider	1	100
Waffles, frozen, made with enriched flour	644	158

Food and description	Sodium (mg)	Potassium (mg)
Walnuts		
Black	3	460
Persian or English	2	450
Watercress leaves including stems, raw	52	282
Watermelon, raw	1	100
Wheat flours		
Whole (from hard wheats)	3	370
Patent		
All-purpose or family flour, enriched	2	95
Self-rising flour, enriched (anhydrous monocalcium phosphate used as a baking acid)[r]	1079	—[s]
Wild rice, raw	7	220
Yeast		
Baker's, compressed	16	610
Brewer's, debittered	121	1894
Yogurt, made from whole milk	47	132
Zweiback	250	150

Numbers in parentheses denote values input, usually from another form of the food or from a similar food. Dashes denote lack of reliable data for a constituent believed to be present in measurable amount. Values are selected from Watt BK, Merril AL: *Composition of foods—raw, processed, prepared,* Agriculture Handbook No. 8, Washington, DC, December 1963, U.S. Department of Agriculture.

[a]Estimated average based on addition of salt in the amount of 0.6% of the finished product.

[b]Processed, partially debranned, whole-kernel wheat with salt added.

[c]Processed, partially debranned, whole-kernel wheat with chicken fat, chicken stock base, dehydrated onion flakes, salt, monosodium glutamate, and herbs.

[d]Values apply to unsalted butter. Unsalted butter contains less than 10 mg of either sodium or potassium per 100 g. Value for vitamin A is the year-round average.

[e]Applies to unsalted nuts. For salted nuts, value is approximately 200 mg/100 g.

[f]Values for phosphorus and sodium are based on use of 1.5% anhydrous disodium phosphate as the emulsifying agent. If emulsifying agent does not contain either phosphorus (P) or sodium (Na), the content of these two nutrients in milligrams per 100 g is as follows:

Food	Na	P
American process cheese	650	444
Swiss process cheese	681	540
American cheese food	—	427
American cheese spread	1139	548

[g]Value for product without added salt.

[h]Values apply to salted margarine. Unsalted margarine contains less than 10 mg/100 g of either sodium or potassium. Vitamin A value based on the minimum required to meet federal specifications for margarine with vitamin A added, 15,000 IU/lb.

[i]Applies to product without added salt. If salt is added, an estimated average value for sodium is 236 mg/100 g.

[j]Sodium content is variable. For example, very thick pretzel sticks contain about twice the average amount listed.

[k]Prepared with butter or margarine, lemon juice, or vinegar.

[l]Values apply to products containing salt. For those without salt, sodium content is low, ranging from less than 10 to 50 mg/100 g; the amount usually is indicated on the label.

[m]Sample dipped in brine contained 215 mg sodium/100 g.

[n]For product canned without added salt, value is approximately the same as for raw salmon.

[o]Values for sauerkraut and sauerkraut juice are based on salt content of 1.9% and 2.0%, respectively, in the finished products. The amounts in some samples may vary significantly from the estimate.

[p]Applies to regular pack. For special dietary pack (low-sodium), values range from 5 to 35 mg/100 g.

[q]One sample with salt added contained 875 mg of sodium/100 g and 275 mg of potassium.

[r]The acid ingredient most commonly used in self-rising flour. When sodium and pyrophosphate in combination with either anhydrous monocalcium phosphate or calcium carbonate is used, the value for calcium is approximately 120 mg/100 g; for phosphorus, 540 mg; for sodium, 1360 mg.

[s]90 mg of potassium/100 g contributed by flour. Small quantities of additional potassium may be provided by other ingredients.

Salt-Free Seasoning Guide

FISH

Breaded, Battered Fillets

Dry mustard, onion, oregano, basil, garlic, thyme

Broiled Steaks or Fillets

Chili, curry powder, tarragon

Fillets in Butter Sauce

Thyme, chervil, dill, fennel

Fish Soup

Italian seasoning, bay leaf, thyme, tarragon

Fish Cakes

Tarragon, savory, dry mustard, white pepper, red pepper, oregano

BEEF

Swiss Steak

Rosemary, black pepper, bay leaf, thyme, clove

Roast Beef

Basil, oregano, bay leaf, nutmeg, tarragon, marjoram

Beef Stew

Chili powder, bay leaf, tarragon, caraway, marjoram

Meatballs

Garlic, thyme, basil, oregano, onion, black pepper, dry mustard

Beef Stroganoff

Red pepper, onion, garlic, nutmeg, curry powder

POULTRY AND VEAL

Fried Chicken

Basil, oregano, garlic, onion, dill, sesame seed, nutmeg

Roast Chicken or Turkey

Ginger, garlic, onion, thyme, tarragon

Chicken Croquettes

Dill, curry, chili, cumin, tarragon, oregano

Veal Patties

Italian seasoning, tarragon, dill, onion, sesame seed

Barbecue Chicken

Garlic, clove, allspice, dry mustard, basil, oregano

GRAVIES AND SAUCES

Barbecue

Bay leaf, thyme, red pepper, cinnamon, ginger, allspice, dry mustard, chili powder

Brown

Chervil, onion, bay leaf, thyme, nutmeg, tarragon

Chicken

Dry mustard, ginger, garlic, marjoram, thyme, bay leaf

Cream

White pepper, dry mustard, curry powder, dill, onion, paprika, tarragon, thyme

SOUPS

Chicken

Thyme, savory, ginger, clove, white pepper, allspice

Clam Chowder

Basil, oregano, nutmeg, white pepper, thyme, garlic powder

Mushroom

Ginger, oregano, thyme, tarragon, bay leaf, black pepper, chili powder

Onion

Curry, caraway, marjoram, garlic, cloves

Tomato

Bay leaf, thyme, Italian seasoning, oregano, onion, nutmeg

Vegetable

Italian seasoning, paprika, caraway, rosemary, thyme, fennel

SALADS

Chicken

Curry, chili powder, Italian seasoning, thyme, tarragon

Coleslaw

Dill, caraway, poppy, dry mustard, ginger

Fish or Seafood

Dill, tarragon, ginger, dry mustard, red pepper, onion, garlic

Macaroni

Dill, basil, thyme, oregano, dry mustard, garlic

Potato

Chili powder, curry, dry mustard, onion

PASTA, BEANS, AND RICE

Baked Beans

Dry mustard, chili powder, clove, onion, ginger

Rice and Vegetables

Curry, thyme, onion, paprika, rosemary, ginger, garlic

Spanish Rice

Cumin, oregano, basil, Italian seasoning

Spaghetti

Italian seasoning, nutmeg, oregano, basil, red pepper, tarragon

Rice Pilaf

Dill, thyme, savory, black pepper

VEGETABLES

Asparagus

Ginger, sesame seed, basil, onion

Broccoli

Italian seasoning, marjoram, basil, nutmeg, onion, sesame seed

Cabbage

Caraway, onion, nutmeg, allspice, clove

Carrots

Ginger, nutmeg, onion, dill

Cauliflower

Dry mustard, basil, paprika, onion

Tomatoes

Oregano, chili powder, dill, onion

Spinach

Savory, thyme, nutmeg, garlic, onion

Exchange Lists
for Meal Planning

Foods are listed with their serving sizes, which are usually measured after cooking. When you begin, measuring the size of each serving will help you learn to "eyeball" correct serving sizes.

The following chart shows the amount of nutrients in one serving from each list:

Groups/lists	Carbohydrate (g)	Protein (g)	Fat (g)	Calories
CARBOHYDRATE GROUP				
Starch	15	3	0-1	80
Fruit	15	—	—	60
Milk				
Fat-free, low-fat	12	8	0-3	90
Reduced-fat	12	8	5	120
Whole	12	8	8	150
Other carbohydrates	15	Varies	Varies	Varies
Nonstarchy vegetables	5	2	—	25
MEAT AND MEAT SUBSTITUTES GROUP				
Very lean	—	7	0-1	35
Lean	—	7	3	55
Medium-fat	—	7	5	75
High-fat	—	7	8	100
FAT GROUP	—	—	5	45

Common Measurements

3 tsp = 1 Tbsp
4 Tbsp = ¼ cup
5⅓ Tbsp = ⅓ cup

4 oz = ½ cup
8 oz = 1 cup
1 cup = ½ pint

STARCH LIST

Cereals, grains, pasta, breads, crackers, snacks, starchy vegetables, and cooked beans, peas, and lentils are starches. In general, one starch is as follows:

- ½ cup of cooked cereal, grain, or starchy vegetable
- ⅓ cup of cooked rice or pasta

- 1 oz of a bread product, such as 1 slice of bread
- ¾ to 1 oz of most snack foods (Some snack foods may also have added fat).

Nutrition Tips

1. Most starch choices are good sources of B vitamins.
2. Foods made from whole grains are good sources of fiber.
   - A serving from the Bread list, on average, has 1 g of fiber.

■ A serving from the Cereals and Grains list or the Crackers and Snacks list, on average, has 2 g of fiber.

■ A serving from the Starchy Vegetables list, on average, has 3 g of fiber.

3. Beans, peas, and lentils are good sources of protein and fiber.

■ A serving from this group, on average, has 6 g of fiber.

Selection Tips

1. Choose starches made with little fat as often as you can.
2. Starchy vegetables prepared with fat count as one starch and one fat.
3. For many starchy foods (e.g., bagels, muffins, dinner rolls, buns), a general rule of thumb is 1 oz equals one carbohydrate serving. However, bagels or muffins range widely in size. Check the size you eat. Also, use the Nutrition Facts on food labels when available.
4. Beans, peas, and lentils are also found on the Meat and Meat Substitutes list.
5. A waffle or pancake is about the size of a compact disc (CD) and about ¼ inch thick.
6. Because starches often swell in cooking, a small amount of uncooked starch becomes a much larger amount of cooked food.
7. Most of the serving sizes are measured or weighed after cooking.
8. For specific information, check Nutrition Facts on the food label.

One starch exchange equals 15 g of carbohydrate, 3 g of protein, 0 to 1 g of fat, and 80 calories.

Bread

Bagel, 4 oz	¼ (1 oz)
Bread, reduced-calorie	2 slices (1½ oz)
Bread, white, whole wheat, pumpernickel, rye	1 slice (1 oz)
Bread sticks, crisp, 4 inches × ½ inch	4 (⅔ oz)
English muffin	½
Hot dog or hamburger bun	½ (1 oz)
Naan, 8 × 2 inch	¼
Pancake, 4 inches across, ¼ inch thick	1
Pita, 6 inches across	½
Roll, plain, small	1 (1 oz)
Raisin bread, unfrosted	1 slice (1 oz)
Tortilla, corn, 6 inches across	1
Tortilla, flour, 6 inches across	1
Tortilla, flour, 10 inches across	⅓
Waffle, 4½ inches square or across, reduced-fat	1

Cereals and Grains

Bran cereals	½ cup
Bulgur	½ cup
Cereals, cooked	½ cup
Cereals, unsweetened, ready-to-eat	¾ cup
Cornmeal (dry)	3 Tbsp
Couscous	⅓ cup
Flour (dry)	3 Tbsp
Granola, low-fat	¼ cup
Grape-Nuts	¼ cup
Grits	½ cup
Kasha	½ cup
Millet	⅓ cup
Muesli	¼ cup
Oats	½ cup
Pasta	⅓ cup
Puffed cereal	1½ cups
Rice, white or brown	⅓ cup
Shredded Wheat	½ cup
Sugar-frosted cereal	½ cup
Wheat germ	3 Tbsp

Starchy Vegetables

Baked beans	⅓ cup
Corn	½ cup
Corn on the cob, large	½ cob (5 oz)
Mixed vegetables with corn, peas, or pasta	1 cup
Peas, green	½ cup
Plantain	½ cup
Potato, baked with skin	¼ large (3 oz)
Potato, boiled	½ cup or ½ medium (3 oz)
Potato, mashed	½ cup
Squash, winter (acorn, butternut, pumpkin)	1 cup
Yam, sweet potato, plain	½ cup

Crackers and Snacks

Animal crackers	8
Graham crackers, 2½-inch square	3
Matzoh	¾ oz
Melba toast	4 slices
Oyster crackers	24
Popcorn (popped, no fat added, or low-fat microwave)	3 cups
Pretzels	¾ oz

Rice cakes, 4 inches across	2
Saltine-type crackers	6
Snack chips, fat-free or baked (tortilla, potato)	15-20 (¾ oz)
Whole wheat crackers, no fat added	2-5 (¾ oz)

Beans, Peas, and Lentils

(count as 1 starch exchange, plus 1 very lean meat exchange)

Beans and peas (garbanzo, pinto, kidney, white, split, black-eyed)	½ cup
Lima beans	⅔ cup
Lentils	½ cup
Miso ✎	3 Tbsp

Starchy Foods Prepared with Fat

(count as 1 starch exchange, plus 1 fat exchange)

Biscuit, 2½ inches across	1
Chow mein noodles	½ cup
Corn bread, 2-inch cube	1 (2 oz)
Crackers, round butter-type	6
Croutons	1 cup
French-fried potatoes, oven-baked (see also the Fast Foods list)	1 cup (2 oz)
Granola	¼ cup
Hummus	⅓ cup
Muffin, 5 oz	⅕ (1 oz)
Popcorn, microwaved	3 cups
Sandwich crackers, cheese or peanut butter filling	3
Snack chips (potato, tortilla)	9-13 (¾ oz)
Stuffing, bread (prepared)	⅓ cup
Taco shell, 6 inches across	2
Waffle, 4 inches square or across	1
Whole wheat crackers, fat added	4-6 (1 oz)

✎ = 400 mg or more sodium per exchange.

FRUIT LIST

Fresh, frozen, canned, and dried fruits and fruit juices are on this list. In general, one fruit exchange is as follows:

- 1 small fresh fruit (4 oz)
- ½ cup of canned or fresh fruit or unsweetened fruit juice
- ¼ cup of dried fruit

Nutrition Tips

1. Fresh, frozen, and dried fruits have about 2 g of fiber per choice. Fruit juices contain very little fiber.

2. Citrus fruits, berries, and melons are good sources of vitamin C.

Selection Tips

1. Count ½ cup cranberries or rhubarb sweetened with sugar substitutes as free foods.
2. Read the Nutrition Facts on the food label. If one serving has more than 15 g of carbohydrate, you will need to adjust the size of the serving you eat or drink.
3. Portion sizes for canned fruits are for the fruit and a small amount of juice.
4. Whole fruit is more filling than fruit juice and may be a better choice.
5. Food labels for fruits may contain the words *no sugar added* or *unsweetened*. This means that no sucrose (table sugar) has been added.
6. Generally, fruit canned in extra light syrup has the same amount of carbohydrate per serving as the *no sugar added* or the juice pack. All canned fruits on the fruit list are based on one of these three types of packaging.

One fruit exchange equals 15 g of carbohydrate and 60 calories. The weight includes skin, core, seeds, and rind.

Fruit

Apple, unpeeled, small	1 (4 oz)
Applesauce, unsweetened	½ cup
Apples, dried	4 rings
Apricots, fresh	4 whole (5½ oz)
Apricots, dried	8 halves
Apricots, canned	½ cup
Banana, small	1 (4 oz)
Blackberries	¾ cup
Blueberries	¾ cup
Cantaloupe, small	⅓ melon (11 oz) or 1 cup cubes
Cherries, sweet, fresh	12 (3 oz)
Cherries, sweet, canned	½ cup
Dates	3
Figs, fresh	1½ large or 2 medium (3½ oz)
Figs, dried	1½
Fruit cocktail	½ cup
Grapefruit, large	½ (11 oz)
Grapefruit sections, canned	¾ cup
Grapes, small	17 (3 oz)
Honeydew melon	1 slice (10 oz) or 1 cup cubes
Kiwi	1 (3½ oz)

Mandarin oranges, canned	¾ cup
Mango, small	½ fruit (5½ oz) or
	½ cup
Nectarine, small	1 (5 oz)
Orange, small	1 (6½ oz)
Papaya	½ fruit (8 oz) or
	1 cup cubes
Peach, medium, fresh	1 (4 oz)
Peaches, canned	½ cup
Pear, large, fresh	½ (4 oz)
Pears, canned	½ cup
Pineapple, fresh	¾ cup
Pineapple, canned	½ cup
Plums, small	2 (5 oz)
Plums, canned	½ cup
Plums, dried (prunes)	3
Raisins	2 Tbsp
Raspberries	1 cup
Strawberries	1¼ cup whole berries
Tangerines, small	2 (8 oz)
Watermelon	1 slice (13½ oz) or
	1¼ cup cubes

Fruit Juice, Unsweetened

Apple juice/cider	½ cup
Cranberry juice cocktail	⅓ cup
Cranberry juice cocktail, reduced-calorie	1 cup
Fruit juice blends, 100% juice	⅓ cup
Grape juice	⅓ cup
Grapefruit juice	½ cup
Orange juice	½ cup
Pineapple juice	½ cup
Prune juice	⅓ cup

MILK LIST

Different types of milk and milk products are on this list. Cheeses are on the Meat and Meat Substitutes list, and cream and other dairy fats are on the Fat list. Based on the amount of fat they contain, milks are divided into fat-free/low-fat milk, reduced-fat milk, and whole milk. One choice of these includes the following:

Type of Milk	Carbohydrate (g)	Protein (g)	Fat (g)	Calories
Fat-free/low-fat (½% or 1%)	12	8	0-3	90
Reduced-fat (2%)	12	8	5	120
Whole	12	8	8	150

Nutrition Tips

1. Milk and yogurt are good sources of calcium and protein. Check the Nutrition Facts on the food label.
2. The higher the fat content of milk and yogurt, the greater the amount of saturated fat and cholesterol. Choose lower-fat varieties.
3. For those who are lactose intolerant, look for lactose-reduced or lactose-free varieties of milk. Check the food label for total amount of carbohydrate per serving.

Selection Tips

1. 1 cup equals 8 fluid oz or ½ pint.
2. Look for chocolate milk, rice milk, frozen yogurt, and ice cream on the Sweets, Desserts, and Other Carbohydrates list.
3. Nondairy creamers are on the Free Foods list.

One milk exchange equals 12 g of carbohydrate and 8 g of protein.

Fat-Free and Low-Fat Milk

(0-3 g fat/serving)

Fat-free milk	1 cup
½% milk	1 cup
1% milk	1 cup
Buttermilk, low-fat or fat-free	1 cup
Evaporated fat-free milk	½ cup
Fat-free dry milk	⅓ cup dry
Soy milk, low-fat or fat-free	1 cup
Yogurt, fat-free, flavored, sweetened with nonnutritive sweetener and fructose	⅔ cup (6 oz)
Yogurt, plain, fat-free	⅔ cup (6 oz)

Reduced-Fat

(5 g fat/serving)

2% milk	1 cup
Soy milk	1 cup
Sweet acidophilus milk	1 cup
Yogurt, plain, low-fat	¾ cup

Whole Milk

(8 g fat/serving)

Whole milk	1 cup
Evaporated whole milk	½ cup
Goat's milk	1 cup
Kefir	1 cup
Yogurt, plain (made from whole milk)	¾ cup

SWEETS, DESSERTS, AND OTHER CARBOHYDRATES LIST

You can substitute food choices from this list for a starch, fruit, or milk choice on your meal plan. Some choices will also count as one or more fat choices.

Nutrition Tips

1. These foods can be substituted for other carbohydrate-containing foods in your meal plan, even though they contain added sugars or fat. However, they do not contain as many important vitamins and minerals as the choices on the Starch, Fruit, and Milk lists.
2. When choosing these foods, include foods from the other lists to eat balanced meals.

Selection Tips

1. Because many of these foods are concentrated sources of carbohydrate and fat, saturated fat, and *trans* fat, the portion sizes are often very small.
2. Look for the words *hydrogenated* or *partially hydrogenated* on the ingredient label. The lower down on the list these words appear, the fewer *trans* fats there are.
3. Be sure to check the Nutrition Facts on the food label. It is your most accurate source of information.
4. Many fat-free or reduced-fat products made with fat replacers contain carbohydrate. When eaten in large amounts, they may need to be counted. Talk with your dietitian to determine how to count these in your meal plan.
5. Look for fat-free salad dressings in smaller amounts on the Free Foods list.

One carbohydrate exchange equals 15 g of carbohydrate, or 1 starch, or 1 fruit, or 1 milk.

Food	Serving Size	Exchanges per Serving
Angel food cake, unfrosted	1/12th cake (about 2 oz)	2 carbohydrates
Brownie, small, unfrosted	2-inch square (about 1 oz)	1 carbohydrate, 1 fat
Cake, unfrosted	2-inch square (about 1 oz)	1 carbohydrate, 1 fat
Cake, frosted	2-inch square (about 2 oz)	2 carbohydrates, 1 fat
Cookie or sandwich cookie with crème filling	2 small (about 2/3 oz)	1 carbohydrate, 1 fat
Cookies, sugar-free	3 small or 1 large (3/4-1 oz)	1 carbohydrate, 1-2 fats
Cranberry sauce, jellied	1/4 cup	1 1/2 carbohydrates
Cupcake, frosted	1 small (about 2 oz)	2 carbohydrates, 1 fat
Doughnut, plain cake	1 medium (1 1/2 oz)	1 1/2 carbohydrates, 2 fats
Doughnut, glazed	3 3/4 inches across (2 oz)	2 carbohydrates, 2 fats
Energy, sport, or breakfast bar	1 bar (1 1/3 oz)	1 1/2 carbohydrates, 0-1 fat
Energy, sport, or breakfast bar	1 bar (2 oz)	2 carbohydrates, 1 fat
Fruit cobbler	1/2 cup (3 1/2 oz)	3 carbohydrates, 1 fat
Fruit juice bars, frozen, 100% juice	1 bar (3 oz)	1 carbohydrate
Fruit snacks, chewy (puréed fruit concentrate)	1 roll (3/4 oz)	1 carbohydrate
Fruit spreads, 100% fruit	1 1/2 Tbsp	1 carbohydrate
Gelatin, regular	1/2 cup	1 carbohydrate
Gingersnaps	3	1 carbohydrate
Granola or snack bar, regular or low-fat	1 bar (1 oz)	1 1/2 carbohydrates
Honey	1 Tbsp	1 carbohydrate
Ice cream	1/2 cup	1 carbohydrate, 2 fats
Ice cream, light	1/2 cup	1 carbohydrate, 1 fat
Ice cream, low-fat	1/2 cup	1 1/2 carbohydrates
Ice cream, fat-free, no sugar added	1/2 cup	1 carbohydrate
Jam or jelly, regular	1 Tbsp	1 carbohydrate
Milk, chocolate, whole	1 cup	2 carbohydrates, 1 fat
Pie, fruit, 2 crusts	1/6 of 8-inch commercially prepared pie	3 carbohydrates, 2 fats

Food	Serving Size	Exchanges per Serving
Pie, pumpkin or custard	⅛ of 8-inch commercially prepared pie	2 carbohydrates, 2 fats
Pudding, regular (made with reduced-fat milk)	½ cup	2 carbohydrates
Pudding, sugar-free or sugar-free and fat-free (made with fat-free milk)	½ cup	1 carbohydrate
Reduced-calorie meal replacement (shake)	1 can (10-11 oz)	1½ carbohydrates, 0-1 fat
Rice milk, low-fat or fat-free, plain	1 cup	1 carbohydrate
Rice milk, low-fat, flavored	1 cup	1½ carbohydrates
Salad dressing, fat-free ✎	¼ cup	1 carbohydrate
Sherbet, sorbet	½ cup	2 carbohydrates
Spaghetti sauce or pasta sauce, canned ✎	½ cup	1 carbohydrate, 1 fat
Sports drinks	8 oz (1 cup)	1 carbohydrate
Sugar	1 Tbsp	1 carbohydrate
Sweet roll or Danish	1 (2½ oz)	2½ carbohydrates, 2 fats
Syrup, light	2 Tbsp	1 carbohydrate
Syrup, regular	1 Tbsp	1 carbohydrate
Syrup, regular	¼ cup	4 carbohydrates
Vanilla wafers	5	1 carbohydrate, 1 fat
Yogurt, frozen	½ cup	1 carbohydrate, 0-1 fat
Yogurt, frozen, fat-free	⅓ cup	1 carbohydrate
Yogurt, low-fat with fruit	1 cup	3 carbohydrates, 0-1 fat

✎ = 400 mg or more of sodium per exchange.

NONSTARCHY VEGETABLE LIST

Vegetables that contain small amounts of carbohydrate and calories are on this list. Vegetables contain important nutrients. Try to eat at least 2 or 3 vegetable choices each day. In general, one vegetable exchange is as follows:

- ½ cup of cooked vegetables or vegetable juice
- 1 cup of raw vegetables

If you eat 3 cups or more of raw vegetables or 1½ cups of cooked vegetables at one meal, count them as 1 carbohydrate choice.

Nutrition Tips

1. Fresh and frozen vegetables have less added salt than canned vegetables. Drain and rinse canned vegetables if you want to remove some salt.
2. Choose more dark-green and dark-yellow vegetables, such as spinach, broccoli, romaine, carrots, chilies, and peppers.
3. Broccoli, Brussels sprouts, cauliflower, greens, peppers, spinach, and tomatoes are good sources of vitamin C.
4. Vegetables contain 1 to 4 g of fiber per serving.

Selection Tips

1. A 1-cup portion of broccoli is about the size of a light bulb.
2. Tomato sauce is different from spaghetti sauce, which is on the Sweets, Desserts, and Other Carbohydrates list.
3. Canned vegetables and juices are available without added salt.
4. Starchy vegetables such as corn, peas, winter squash, and potatoes that contain larger amounts of calories and carbohydrates are on the Starch list.

One vegetable exchange (½ cup cooked or 1 cup raw) equals 5 g of carbohydrate, 2 g of protein, 0 g of fat, and 25 calories.

Foods

Artichoke
Artichoke hearts
Asparagus
Bean sprouts
Beans (green, wax, Italian)
Beets
Broccoli
Brussels sprouts
Cabbage
Carrots
Cauliflower
Celery
Cucumber

Eggplant
Green onions or scallions
Greens (collard, kale, mustard, turnip)
Kohlrabi
Leeks
Mixed vegetables (without corn, peas, or pasta)
Mushrooms
Okra
Onions
Pea pods
Peppers (all varieties)
Radishes

Salad greens (endive, escarole, lettuce, romaine, spinach)
Sauerkraut ✐
Spinach
Summer squash
Tomato
Tomato sauce ✐
Tomato/vegetable juice ✐
Tomatoes, canned
Turnips
Water chestnuts
Watercress
Zucchini

✐ = 400 mg or more sodium per exchange.

MEAT AND MEAT SUBSTITUTES LIST

Meat and meat substitutes that contain both protein and fat are on this list. In general, one meat exchange is as follows:

- 1 oz of meat, fish, poultry, or cheese
- ½ cup of beans, peas, or lentils

Based on the amount of fat they contain, meats are divided into very lean, lean, medium-fat, and high-fat lists. This is done so that you can see which ones contain the least amount of fat. One ounce (one exchange) of each of these includes the following:

Type of Meat	Carbohydrate (g)	Protein (g)	Fat (g)	Calories
Very lean	0	7	0-1	35
Lean	0	7	3	55
Medium-fat	0	7	5	75
High-fat	0	7	8	100

Nutrition Tips

1. Choose very lean and lean meat choices whenever possible. Items from the high-fat group are high in saturated fat, cholesterol, and calories and can raise blood cholesterol levels.
2. Beans, peas, and lentils are good sources of fiber, about 3 g per serving.
3. Some processed meats, seafood, and soy products may contain carbohydrate when consumed in large amounts. Check the Nutrition Facts on the label to see if the amount is close to 15 g. If so, count it as a carbohydrate choice as well as a meat choice.

Selection Tips

1. Weigh meat after cooking and removing bones and fat; 4 oz of raw meat is equal to 3 oz of cooked meat. Some examples of meat portions are as follows:
   - 1 oz cheese = 1 meat choice and is about the size of a 1-inch cube or 4 cubes the size of dice
   - 2 oz meat = 2 meat choices, such as the following:
     1 small chicken leg or thigh
     ½ cup cottage cheese or tuna

- 3 oz meat = 3 meat choices and is about the size of a deck of cards, such as the following:
  1 medium pork chop
  1 small hamburger
  ½ of a whole chicken breast
  1 unbreaded fish fillet
2. Limit your choices from the high-fat group to three times per week or less.
3. Most grocery stores stock Select and Choice grades of meat. The Select grades of meat are the leanest. The Choice grades contain a moderate amount of fat, and Prime cuts of meat have the highest amount of fat.
4. *Hamburger* may contain added seasoning and fat, but ground beef does not.
5. Read labels to find products that are low in fat and cholesterol (5 g of fat or less per serving).
6. Dried beans, peas, and lentils are also found on the Starch list.
7. Peanut butter, in smaller amounts, is also found on the Fat list.
8. Bacon, in smaller amounts, is also found on the Fat list.
9. Don't be fooled by ground beef packages that say X% lean (e.g., 90% lean). This is the percentage of fat by weight, NOT the percentage of calories from fat. A 3.5-oz patty of this raw ground beef has about half its calories from fat.
10. Meatless burgers are in the Combination Foods list (3 oz of soy-based burger = ½ carbohydrate + 2 very lean meats; 3 oz of vegetable- and starch-based burger = 1 carbohydrate + 1 lean meat).

One exchange equals 0 g of carbohydrate, 7 g of protein, 0-1 g of fat, and 35 calories.

Meal Planning Tips

1. Bake, roast, broil, grill, poach, steam, or boil meat and fish rather than frying.
2. Place meat on a rack so that the fat will drain off during cooking.
3. Use a nonstick spray and a nonstick pan to brown or fry foods.
4. Trim off visible fat or skin before or after cooking.
5. If you add flour, bread crumbs, coating mixes, fat, or marinades when cooking, ask your dietitian how to count it in your meal plan.

One exchange equals 0 g of carbohydrate, 7 g of protein, 3 g of fat, and 55 calories.

Very Lean Meat and Substitutes List

- One very lean meat exchange is equal to any one of the following items:

Poultry: Chicken or turkey (white meat, no skin), Cornish hen (no skin)	1 oz
Fish: Fresh or frozen cod, flounder, haddock, halibut, trout, lox (smoked salmon); ✐ tuna, fresh or canned in water	1 oz
Shellfish: Clams, crab, lobster, scallops, shrimp, imitation shellfish	1 oz
Game: Duck or pheasant (no skin), venison, buffalo, ostrich	1 oz
Cheese with 1 g of fat or less per ounce:	
Fat-free or low-fat cottage cheese	¼ cup
Fat-free cheese	1 oz
Other	
Processed sandwich meats with 1 g of fat or less per ounce, such as deli thin, shaved meats, chipped beef, ✐ turkey ham	1 oz
Egg whites	2
Egg substitutes, plain	¼ cup
Hot dogs with 1 g of fat or less per ounce ✐	1 oz
Kidney (high in cholesterol)	1 oz
Sausage with 1 g of fat or less per ounce	1 oz

- Count the following items as one very lean meat and one starch exchange:

Beans, peas, lentils (cooked)	½ cup

✐ = 400 mg or more sodium per exchange.

Lean Meat and Substitutes List

■ One lean meat exchange is equal to any one of the following items:

Beef: USDA Select or Choice grades of lean beef trimmed of fat, such as round, sirloin, and flank steak; tenderloin; roast (rib, chuck, rump); steak (T-bone, porterhouse, cubed); ground round   1 oz

Pork: Lean pork, such as fresh ham; canned, cured, or boiled ham; Canadian bacon; ✏ tenderloin, center loin chop   1 oz

Lamb: Roast, chop, or leg   1 oz

Veal: Lean chop, roast   1 oz

Poultry: Chicken, turkey (dark meat, no skin), chicken (white meat, with skin), domestic duck or goose (well-drained of fat, no skin)   1 oz

Fish

Herring (uncreamed or smoked)   1 oz

Oysters   6 medium

Salmon (fresh or canned), catfish   1 oz

Sardines (canned)   2 medium

Tuna (canned in oil, drained)   1 oz

Game: Goose (no skin), rabbit   1 oz

Cheese:

4.5%-fat cottage cheese   ¼ cup

Grated Parmesan   2 Tbsp

Cheeses with 3 g of fat or less per ounce   1 oz

Other

Hot dogs with 3 g of fat or less per ounce ✏   1½ oz

Processed sandwich meat with 3 g of fat or less per ounce, such as turkey pastrami or kielbasa   1 oz

Liver, heart (high in cholesterol)   1 oz

✏ = 400 mg or more sodium per exchange.

One exchange equals 0 g of carbohydrate, 7 g of protein, 5 g of fat, and 75 calories.

Medium-Fat Meat and Substitutes List

■ One medium-fat meat exchange is equal to any one of the following items:

Beef: Most beef products fall into this category (ground beef, meat loaf, corned beef, short ribs, Prime grades of meat trimmed of fat, such as prime rib)   1 oz

Pork: Top loin, chop, Boston butt, cutlet   1 oz

Lamb: Rib roast, ground   1 oz

Veal: Cutlet (ground or cubed, unbreaded)   1 oz

Poultry: Chicken (dark meat, with skin), ground turkey or ground chicken, fried chicken (with skin)   1 oz

Fish: Any fried fish product   1 oz

Cheese with 5 g of fat or less per ounce

Feta   1 oz

Mozzarella   1 oz

Ricotta   ¼ cup (2 oz)

Other

Egg (high in cholesterol, limit to 3 per week)   1

Sausage with 5 g of fat or less per ounce   1 oz

Tempeh   ¼ cup

Tofu   4 oz or ½ cup

One exchange equals 0 g of carbohydrate, 7 g of protein, 8 g of fat, and 100 calories.

High-Fat Meat and Substitutes List

Remember that these items are high in saturated fat, cholesterol, and calories and may raise blood cholesterol levels if eaten on a regular basis.

■ One high-fat meat exchange is equal to any one of the following items:

Pork: Spareribs, ground pork, pork sausage	1 oz
Cheese: All regular cheeses, such as American, 🔪 cheddar, Monterey Jack, Swiss	1 oz
Other	
Processed sandwich meats with 8 g of fat or less per ounce, such as bologna, pimento loaf, salami	1 oz
Sausage, such as bratwurst, Italian, knockwurst, Polish, smoked	1 oz
Hot dog (turkey or chicken) 🔪	1 (10/lb)
Bacon	3 slices (20 slices/lb)
Peanut butter (contains unsaturated fat)	1 Tbsp

■ Count the following items as 1 high-fat plus 1 fat exchange:

Hot dog (beef, pork, or combination) 🔪	1 (10/lb)

🔪 = 400 mg or more sodium per exchange.

FAT LIST

Fats are divided into three groups, based on the main type of fat they contain: monounsaturated, polyunsaturated, and saturated. Monounsaturated and polyunsaturated fats in the foods we eat are linked with good health benefits. Saturated fats and fats called *trans* fatty acids (or *trans* unsaturated fatty acids) are linked with heart disease. In general, one fat exchange is as follows:

■ 1 tsp of regular margarine or vegetable oil
■ 1 Tbsp of regular salad dressing

Nutrition Tips

1. All fats are high in calories. Limit serving sizes for good nutrition and health.
2. Nuts and seeds contain small amounts of fiber, protein, and magnesium.
3. If blood pressure is a concern, choose fats in the unsalted form to help lower sodium intake, such as unsalted peanuts.

Selection Tips

1. Check the Nutrition Facts on food labels for serving sizes. One fat exchange is based on a serving size containing 5 g of fat.
2. The Nutrition Facts on food labels usually list total fat grams and saturated fat grams per serving. When most of the calories come from saturated fat, the food fits into the Saturated Fats list.
3. Occasionally the Nutrition Facts on food labels list monounsaturated and/or polyunsaturated fats in addition to total and saturated fats. If more than half the total fat is monounsaturated, the food fits into the Monounsaturated Fats list; if more than half is polyunsaturated, the food fits into the Polyunsaturated Fats list.
4. When selecting fats to use with your meal plan, consider replacing saturated fats with monounsaturated fats.
5. When selecting regular margarine, choose those with liquid vegetable oil as the first ingredient. Soft margarines are not as saturated as stick margarines and are healthier choices.
6. Avoid foods on the Fat list (such as margarines) listing hydrogenated or partially hydrogenated fat as the first ingredient because these foods contain higher amounts of *trans* fatty acids.
7. When selecting reduced- or lower-fat margarines, look for liquid vegetable oil as the second ingredient. Water is usually the first ingredient.
8. When used in smaller amounts, bacon and peanut butter are counted as fat choices. When used in larger amounts, they are counted as high-fat meat choices.

9. Fat-free salad dressings are on the Sweets, Desserts, and Other Carbohydrates list and the Free Foods list.
10. See the Free Foods list for nondairy coffee creamers, whipped topping, and fat-free products, such as margarines, salad dressings, mayonnaise, sour cream, cream cheese, and nonstick cooking spray.

One fat exchange equals 5 g of fat and 45 calories.

Monounsaturated Fats List

Avocado, medium	2 Tbsp (1 oz)
Oil (canola, olive, peanut)	1 tsp
Olives	
Ripe (black)	8 large
Green, stuffed ✐	10 large
Nuts	
Almonds, cashews	6 nuts
Mixed (50% peanuts)	6 nuts
Peanuts	10 nuts
Pecans	4 halves
Peanut butter, smooth or crunchy	½ Tbsp
Sesame seeds	1 Tbsp
Tahini or sesame paste	2 tsp

✐ = 400 mg or more sodium per exchange.

Polyunsaturated Fats List

Margarine	
Stick, tub, or squeeze	1 tsp
Lower-fat spread (30%-50% vegetable oil)	1 Tbsp
Mayonnaise	
Regular	1 tsp
Reduced-fat	1 Tbsp
Nuts: walnuts, English	4 halves
Oil (corn, safflower, soybean)	1 tsp
Salad dressing	
Regular ✐	1 Tbsp
Reduced-fat	2 Tbsp
Miracle Whip salad dressing	
Regular	2 tsp
Reduced-fat	1 Tbsp
Seeds: pumpkin, sunflower	1 Tbsp

✐ = 400 mg or more sodium per exchange.

Saturated Fats List

Bacon, cooked	1 slice (20 slices/lb)
Bacon, grease	1 tsp
Butter	
Stick	1 tsp
Whipped	2 tsp
Reduced-fat	1 Tbsp
Chitterlings, boiled	2 Tbsp (½ oz)
Coconut, sweetened, shredded	2 Tbsp
Coconut milk	1 Tbsp
Cream, half and half	2 Tbsp
Cream cheese	
Regular	1 Tbsp (½ oz)
Reduced-fat	1½ Tbsp (¾ oz)
Fatback or salt pork ✐	See below*
Shortening or lard	1 tsp
Sour cream	
Regular	2 Tbsp
Reduced-fat	3 Tbsp

*Use a piece 1 inch × 1 inch × ¼ inch if you plan to eat the fatback cooked with vegetables. Use a piece 2 inch × 1 inch × ½ inch when eating only the vegetables with the fatback removed.

✐ = 400 mg or more sodium per exchange.

FREE FOODS LIST

A *free food* is any food or drink that contains less than 20 calories or less than or equal to 5 g of carbohydrate per serving. Foods with a serving size listed should be limited to 3 servings per day. Be sure to spread them out throughout the day. If you eat all 3 servings at one time, it could raise your blood glucose level. Foods listed without a serving size can be eaten whenever you like.

Fat-Free or Reduced-Fat Foods

Cream cheese, fat-free	1 Tbsp (½ oz)
Creamers, nondairy, liquid	1 Tbsp
Creamers, nondairy, powdered	2 tsp
Mayonnaise, fat-free	1 Tbsp
Mayonnaise, reduced-fat	1 tsp
Margarine spread, fat-free	4 Tbsp
Margarine spread, reduced-fat	1 tsp
Miracle Whip, fat-free	1 Tbsp
Miracle Whip, reduced-fat	1 tsp
Nonstick cooking spray	
Salad dressing, fat-free or low-fat	1 Tbsp
Salad dressing, fat-free, Italian	2 Tbsp
Sour cream, fat-free, reduced-fat	1 Tbsp
Whipped topping, regular	1 Tbsp
Whipped topping, light or fat-free	2 Tbsp

Sugar-Free Foods

Candy, hard, sugar-free	1 candy
Gelatin dessert, sugar-free	
Gelatin, unflavored	
Gum, sugar-free	
Jam or jelly, light	2 tsp
Sugar substitutes*	
Syrup, sugar-free	2 Tbsp

*Sugar substitutes, alternatives, or replacements that are approved by the Food and Drug Administration (FDA) are safe to use. Common brand names include the following:

Equal (aspartame)	Sweet One (acesulfame K)
Splenda (sucralose)	Sweet-10 (saccharin)
Sprinkle Sweet (saccharin)	Sugar Twin (saccharin)
	Sweet 'N Low (saccharin)

Drinks

Bouillon, broth, consommé 🖋	
Bouillon or broth, low-sodium	
Carbonated or mineral water	
Club soda	
Cocoa powder, unsweetened	1 Tbsp
Coffee	
Diet soft drinks, sugar-free	
Drink mixes, sugar-free	
Tea	
Tonic water, sugar-free	

🖋 = 400 mg or more sodium per exchange.

Condiments

Catsup	1 Tbsp
Horseradish	
Lemon juice	
Lime juice	
Mustard	
Pickle relish	1 Tbsp
Pickles, dill 🖋	1½ medium
Pickles, sweet (bread and butter)	2 slices
Pickles, sweet (gherkin)	¾ oz
Salsa	¼ cup
Soy sauce, regular or light 🖋	1 Tbsp
Taco sauce	1 Tbsp
Vinegar	
Yogurt	2 Tbsp

🖋 = 400 mg or more sodium per exchange.

Seasonings

Flavoring extracts
Garlic
Herbs, fresh or dried
Pimento
Spices
Tabasco or hot pepper sauce
Wine, used in cooking
Worcestershire sauce

Be careful with seasonings that contain sodium or are salts, such as garlic or celery salt, and lemon pepper.

COMBINATION FOODS LIST

Many of the foods we eat are mixed together in various combinations. These combination foods do not fit into any one exchange list. Often it is hard to tell what is in a casserole dish or prepared food item. This is a list of exchanges for some typical combination foods. This list helps you fit these foods into your meal plan. Ask your dietitian for information about any other combination foods you would like to eat.

Food	Serving Size	Exchanges per Serving
Entrees		
Tuna noodle casserole, lasagna, spaghetti with meatballs, chili with beans, macaroni and cheese 🖋	1 cup (8 oz)	2 carbohydrates 2 medium-fat meats
Chow mein (without noodles or rice) 🖋	2 cups (16 oz)	1 carbohydrate 2 lean meats
Tuna or chicken salad	½ cup (3½ oz)	½ carbohydrate 2 lean meats 1 fat

Food	Serving Size	Exchanges per Serving
Frozen entrees and meals		
Dinner-type meal 🖋	Generally 14-17 oz	3 carbohydrates 3 medium-fat meats 3 fats
Meatless burger, soy-based	3 oz	½ carbohydrate 2 lean meats
Meatless burger, vegetable- and starch-based	3 oz	1 carbohydrate 1 lean meat
Pizza, cheese, thin crust 🖋	¼ of 12-inch (6 oz)	2 carbohydrates 2 medium-fat meats 1 fat
Pizza, meat topping, thin crust 🖋	¼ of 12-inch (6 oz)	2 carbohydrates 2 medium-fat meats 2 fats
Pot pie 🖋	1 (7 oz)	2½ carbohydrates 1 medium-fat meat 3 fats
Entrée or meal with less than 340 calories 🖋	About 8-11 oz	2-3 carbohydrates 1-2 lean meats
Soups		
Bean 🖋	1 cup	1 carbohydrate 1 very lean meat
Cream (made with water) 🖋	1 cup (8 oz)	1 carbohydrate 1 fat
Instant 🖋	6 oz prepared	1 carbohydrate
Instant with beans/lentils 🖋	8 oz prepared	2½ carbohydrates 1 very lean meat
Split pea (made with water) 🖋	½ cup (4 oz)	1 carbohydrate
Tomato (made with water) 🖋	1 cup (8 oz)	1 carbohydrate
Vegetable beef, chicken noodle, or other broth type 🖋	1 cup (8 oz)	1 carbohydrate

🖋 = 400 mg or more sodium per exchange.

FAST FOODS* LIST

Food	Serving Size	Exchanges per Serving
Burrito with beef 🖋	1 (5-7 oz)	3 carbohydrates 1 medium-fat meat 1 fat
Chicken nuggets 🖋	6	1 carbohydrate 2 medium-fat meats 1 fat
Chicken breast and wing, breaded and fried 🖋	1 each	1 carbohydrate 4 medium-fat meats 2 fats

*Ask at your fast-food restaurant for nutrition information about your favorite fast foods or check web sites.

Food	Serving Size	Exchanges per Serving
Chicken sandwich, grilled 🖊	1	2 carbohydrates 3 very lean meats
Chicken wings, hot 🖊	6 (5 oz)	1 carbohydrate 3 medium-fat meats 4 fats
Fish sandwich/tartar sauce 🖊	1	3 carbohydrates 1 medium-fat meat 3 fats
French fries 🖊	1 medium serving (5 oz)	4 carbohydrates 4 fats
Hamburger, regular	1	2 carbohydrates 2 medium-fat meats
Hamburger, large 🖊	1	2 carbohydrates 3 medium-fat meats 1 fat
Hot dog with bun 🖊	1	1 carbohydrate 1 high-fat meat 1 fat
Individual pan pizza 🖊	1	5 carbohydrates 3 medium-fat meats 3 fats
Pizza, cheese, thin crust 🖊	¼ 12-inch (about 6 oz)	2½ carbohydrates 2 medium-fat meats
Pizza, meat, thin crust 🖊	¼ 12-inch (about 6 oz)	2½ carbohydrates 2 medium-fat meats 1 fat
Soft-serve cone	1 small (5 oz)	2½ carbohydrates 1 fat
Submarine sandwich 🖊	1 sub (6-inch)	3 carbohydrates 1 vegetable 2 medium-fat meats 1 fat
Submarine sandwich (less than 6 g fat) 🖊	1 sub (6-inch)	2½ carbohydrates 2 lean meats
Taco, hard or soft shell 🖊	1 (3-3½ oz)	1 carbohydrate 1 medium-fat meat 1 fat

🖊 = 400 mg or more sodium per exchange.

The Exchange Lists are the basis of a meal-planning system designed by a committee of the American Diabetes Association and The American Dietetic Association. Although designed primarily for people with diabetes and others who must follow special diets, the Exchange Lists are based on principles of good nutrition that apply to everyone. Copyright 2003 American Diabetes Association, Inc., The American Dietetic Association. Used with permission.

Meal Plan

Meal Plan for: _____

Dietitian: _____

Date: _____

Phone: _____

Carbohydrate   Grams _____   Percent _____
Protein   _____   _____
Fat   _____   _____
Calories   _____

Time	Number of Exchanges/Choices	Menu Ideas	Menu Ideas
	Carbohydrate group _____ Starch _____ Fruit _____ Milk _____ Meat group _____ Fat group		
	Carbohydrate group _____ Starch _____ Fruit _____ Milk ✓ Vegetables _____ Meat group _____ Fat group		
	Carbohydrate group _____ Starch _____ Fruit _____ Milk ✓ Vegetables _____ Meat group _____ Fat group		

PLANNING INDIVIDUALIZED DIETS USING EXCHANGE LISTS

Step 1: Conduct Nutrition History

A 4-hour or 3-day recall (see Chapter 17) can be used to determine usual food intake. Categorize intake into exchanges (or servings) from each list at each meal and snack. Translate into kcalories and grams of carbohydrate, protein, and fat from exchanges. Round off kcalorie level to the nearest 50 or 100 kcalories. Calculations of food intake are not precise enough to allow more accuracy, and patients may consume an extra 50 to 60 kcalories/day from free foods (see Exchange Lists). When in doubt, round up instead of down. Determine percentages of carbohydrate, protein, and fat in current intake.

To determine total kcalories, add up the number of exchanges actually consumed from each Exchange Group. Multiply the number of exchanges by the number of kcalories in each Exchange Group.

Number of exchanges from starch list	=	____	×	80 kcal	= ____
Number of exchanges from fruit list	=	____	×	60 kcal	= ____
Number of exchanges from milk list	=	____	×	80 kcal (skim)	= ____
	=	____	×	120 kcal (low-fat)	= ____
	=	____	×	150 kcal (whole)	= ____
Number of exchanges from vegetable list	=	____	×	25 kcal	= ____
Number of exchanges from meat groups	=	____	×	35 kcal (very lean)	= ____
	=	____	×	55 kcal (lean)	= ____
	=	____	×	75 kcal (medium-fat)	= ____
	=	____	×	100 kcal (high-fat)	= ____
Number of exchanges from fat list	=	____	×	45 kcal	= ____
				TOTAL KCAL	____

Using the total number of each Exchange Group, calculate the grams of carbohydrate (CHO), protein (PRO) and fat (FAT).

	Number of Exchanges CHO			Number of Exchanges PRO			Number of Exchange FAT		
Bread list	____ × 15 g	=	____ g	____ × 2 g	=	____ g	____ × 0-3 g	=	____ g
Fruit list	____ × 15 g	=	____ g	____ × 0 g	=	____ g	____ × 0 g	=	____ g
Milk list									
Skim	____ × 12 g	=	____ g	____ × 8 g	=	____ g	____ × 0 g	=	____ g
Low-fat	____ × 12 g	=	____ g	____ × 8 g	=	____ g	____ × 5 g	=	____ g
Whole	____ × 12 g	=	____ g	____ × 8 g	=	____ g	____ × 8 g	=	____ g
Vegetable list	____ × 5 g	=	____ g	____ × 2 g	=	____ g	____ × 0 g	=	____ g
Meat list									
Very lean	____ × 0 g	=	____ g	____ × 7 g	=	____ g	____ × 0-1 g	=	____ g
Lean	____ × 0 g	=	____ g	____ × 7 g	=	____ g	____ × 3 g	=	____ g
Medium-fat	____ × 0 g	=	____ g	____ × 7 g	=	____ g	____ × 5 g	=	____ g
High-fat	____ × 0 g	=	____ g	____ × 7 g	=	____ g	____ × 8 g	=	____ g
Fat group	____ × 0 g	=	____ g	____ × 0 g	=	____ g	____ × 5 g	=	____ g
	TOTAL	____		TOTAL	____		TOTAL	____	

Take total kcalories from above and determine the percentage of the diet that is carbohydrate, protein, and fat:

A.

Multiply total grams CHO	× 4 kcal	=	____ kcal
Multiply total grams PRO	× 4 kcal	=	____ kcal
Multiply total grams FAT	× 9 kcal	=	____ kcal
	TOTAL		____ kcal

B. Divide each nutrient's total kcalories by the total kcalories for the day, and multiply by 100 to get the percentage of kcalories.

Kcal from CHO	× 100 = % kcal from CHO	_____	×	100	=	_____ Total kcal
Kcal from PRO	× 100 = % kcal from PRO	_____	×	100	=	_____ Total kcal
Kcal from FAT	× 100 = % kcal from FAT	_____	×	100	=	_____ Total kcal

Step 2: Calculate Daily Kilocalorie Requirements

Kcalorie needs are based on age, weight, and activity level. Use the Harris-Benedict equation to calculate energy needs. Round figure to nearest 100 kcalories. Subtract kcalories if weight loss is desired. Reducing kcaloric intake by 500 kcal/day will theoretically produce a 1 lb weight loss per week. Never reduce kcaloric level to below that required for basal energy needs.

Example: CG is a 62-year-old female with type 2 diabetes. She is 5′5″ tall (medium frame), and weighs 140 lb. CG walks 10 to 12 miles per week at the mall.

$$655.1 + [9.6 \times wt\ (kg)] + [1.8 \times ht\ (cm)] - [4.7 \times age\ (yrs)]$$
$$655.1 + [9.6 \times 63.6\ kg] + [1.8 \times 165.1\ cm] - [4.7 \times 62]$$
$$655.1 + 610.6 + 297.2 - 291.4 = 1271.5\ kcal$$
$$1271.5\ kcal \times 1.3\ (activity\ factor) = 1652.95\ kcal$$
$$Round\ off\ to\ 1700\ kcal$$

If weight loss is desired, subtract 500 kcal: $1700 - 500 = 1200$ kcalories, which is below her basal energy needs of 1271.5 kcal. Adjust to 1300 kcalories if weight loss is determined to be a treatment goal.

Step 3: Determine Distribution of Carbohydrate, Protein, and Fat Kilocalories

This should be based on the patient's usual intake, blood glucose levels, blood lipid levels, and treatment goals.

Example: CG's 24-hr recall indicates an intake of approximately 1500 kcal distributed into 17% protein, 30% fat, and 53% carbohydrate. Her pertinent lab values: glycosylated hemoglobin is 6%, cholesterol 210 mg/dl, LDL cholesterol 179 mg/dl, HDL cholesterol 55 mg/dl. Although her lipid levels are at the high end of normal or just slightly above normal, her exercise and eating habits appear to be sufficient to control her blood glucose levels. In this case, you would distribute her kcalories in the same pattern as found in her diet recall:

$$Carbohydrate:\ 1500\ kcal \times 0.53 = 795\ kcal \div 4\ kcal/gm = 199\ gm$$
$$Protein:\ 1500\ kcal \times 0.17 = 255\ kcal \div 4\ kcal/gm = 64\ gm$$
$$Fat:\ 1500\ kcal \times 0.30 = 450\ kcal \div 9\ kcal/gm = 50\ gm$$

Step 4: Determine Servings from Each Exchange List

These calculations are based on the amount of carbohydrate, protein, and fat in each exchange list and the patient's preferences for foods within each list or group. The type of milk the patient uses should be calculated into the meal plan. Skim milk and low-fat milks are recommended, but whole milk can be used if the patient will not drink the others. Although lean meats should be encouraged, when calculating fat grams per meat serving, use the fat value that best represents actual intake. People do not need to add or subtract fat exchanges when using different meat categories.

Example: CG's usual eating pattern indicates she uses the following amounts from the milk, vegetable, and fruit exchange groups:

	Servings	Carbohydrate (g)	Protein (g)	Fat (g)	Kcal
Milk, skim	1	12	8	1	90
Vegetables	4	20	8	0	100
Fruits	4	60	0	0	240
CARBOHYDRATE SUBTOTAL		92	16	1	430

The starch exchange list is the only group remaining that provides carbohydrates. To determine the number of servings to be used from this group, subtract the total grams of carbohydrate (92 g) from the milk, vegetable, and fruit lists from the total grams of carbohydrate (199 g) in the meal plan. This amount is divided by 15 g carbohydrate/serving in the starch list.

	Servings	Carbohydrate (g)	Protein (g)	Fat (g)	Kcal
Carbohydrate Subtotal		92	24	1	460
Starches	7	105	21	7	560
PROTEIN SUBTOTAL		197	45	8	1020

The meat exchange list is the only group remaining that provides protein. To determine the number of servings to be used from this group, subtract the total grams of protein (48 g) from the milk, vegetable, and starch lists from the total grams of protein (56 g) in the meal plan. This amount is divided by 7 g protein/serving in the meat list.

	Servings	Carbohydrate (g)	Protein (g)	Fat (g)	Kcal
Protein Subtotal		197	45	8	1020
Meat/lean	4	0	28	12	220
FAT SUBTOTAL		197	73	20	1240

The fat exchange list is the only group remaining that provides fat. To determine the number of servings to be used from this group, subtract the total grams of fat (20 g) from the milk, starch, and meat lists from the total grams of fat (50 g) in the meal plan. This amount is divided by 5 gm fat/serving in the fat list.

	Servings	Carbohydrate (g)	Protein (g)	Fat (g)	Kcal
Fat Subtotal		197	73	20	1240
Fats	6	0	0	30	270
TOTAL		197	73	50	1510

Note: When calculating the number of servings from each exchange list, round to the nearest whole number. It is usually impractical to calculate and plan half servings from the lists.

The daily distribution of servings from the exchange list is as follows. These servings can now be divided into the appropriate number of meals and snacks per day.

Exchange list group	Servings	Carbohydrate (g)	Protein (g)	Fat (g)	Kcal
Carbohydrates	12				
Starches	7	105	21	7	560
Fruit	4	60	0	0	240
Milk (skim)	1	0	0	30	270
Vegetables	4	20	8	1	90
Meats/lean	4	0	28	12	220
Fats	6	0	0	30	270

Modified from American Dietetic Association: *Exchange lists for meal planning,* Alexandria, VA, 2003, American Diabetes Association; American Dietetic Association: *Handbook of clinical dietetics,* ed 2, New Haven, 1992, Yale University Press; Davis JR, Sherer K: *Applied nutrition and diet therapy for nurses,* ed 2, Philadelphia, 1994, Saunders; American Dietetic Association: Nutrition recommendations and principles for people with diabetes mellitus, *J Am Diet Assoc* 94:504, 1994; and Tinker LF, Heins JM, Holler HJ: Commentary and translation: 1994 nutrition recommendations for diabetes, *J Am Diet Assoc* 94:507, 1994.

Canada's Food Guide to Healthy Eating

These guidelines were developed as the key messages to be communicated to healthy Canadians, older than 4 years of age:

1. Enjoy a VARIETY of foods.
2. Emphasize cereals, breads, other grain products, vegetables, and fruit.
3. Choose lower-fat dairy products, leaner meats, and food prepared with little or no fat.
4. Achieve and maintain a healthy body weight by enjoying regular physical activity and healthy eating.
5. Limit salt, alcohol, and caffeine intake.

Health   Santé
Canada   Canada

CANADA'S
Food Guide

TO HEALTHY EATING
FOR PEOPLE FOUR YEARS
AND OVER

Enjoy a variety
of foods from each
group every day.

Choose lower-
fat foods
more often.

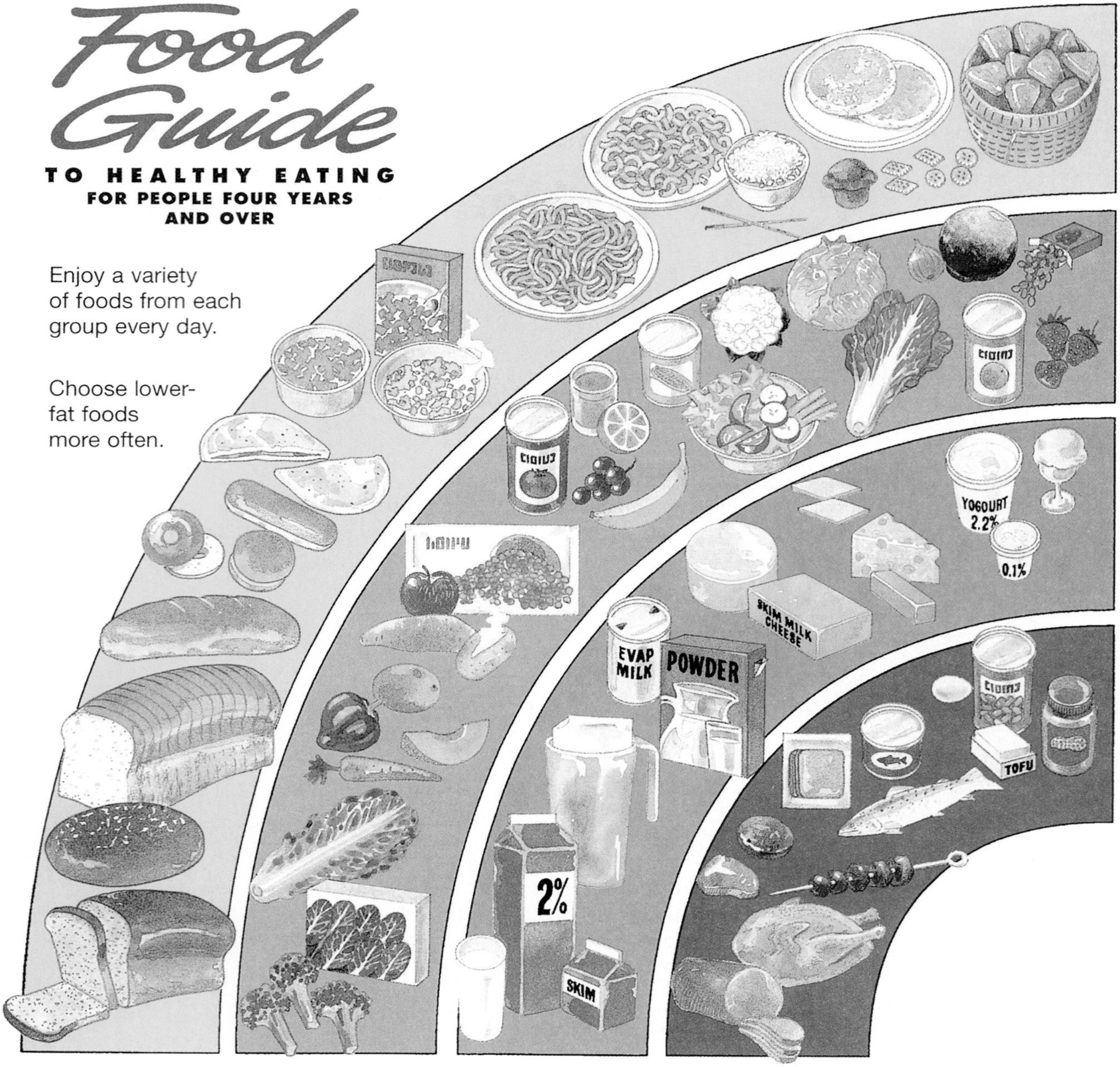

Grain Products
Choose whole grain
and enriched
products more often.

Vegetables and Fruit
Choose dark green and
orange vegetables and
orange fruit more often.

Milk Products
Choose lower-fat milk
products more often.

Meat and Alternatives
Choose leaner meats,
poultry and fish, as well
as dried peas, beans
and lentils more often.

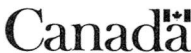

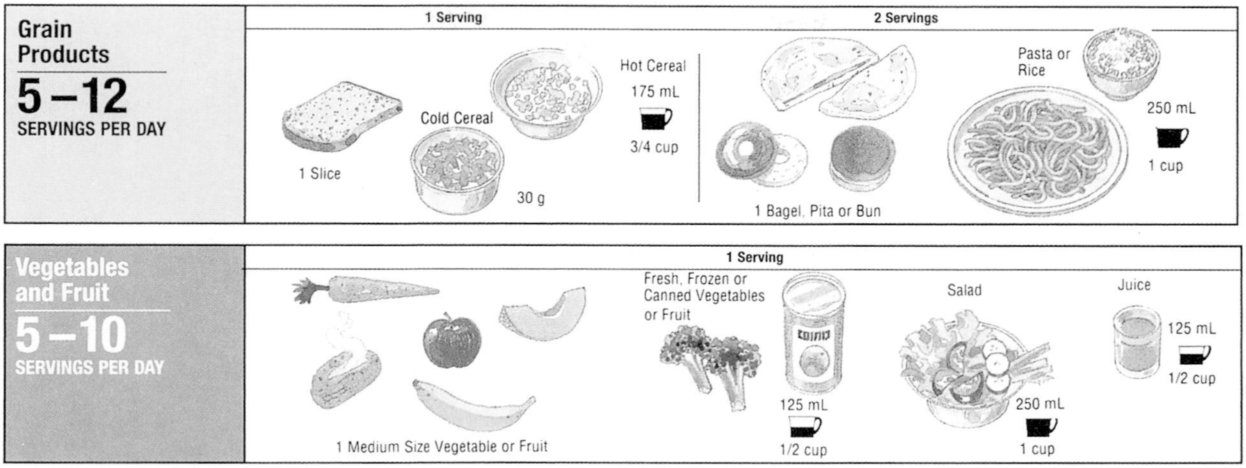

Grain Products

5–12

SERVINGS PER DAY

1 Serving

1 Slice

Cold Cereal

30 g

Hot Cereal
175 mL
3/4 cup

2 Servings

1 Bagel, Pita or Bun

Pasta or Rice

250 mL
1 cup

Vegetables and Fruit

5–10

SERVINGS PER DAY

1 Serving

1 Medium Size Vegetable or Fruit

Fresh, Frozen or Canned Vegetables or Fruit

125 mL
1/2 cup

Salad

250 mL
1 cup

Juice

125 mL
1/2 cup

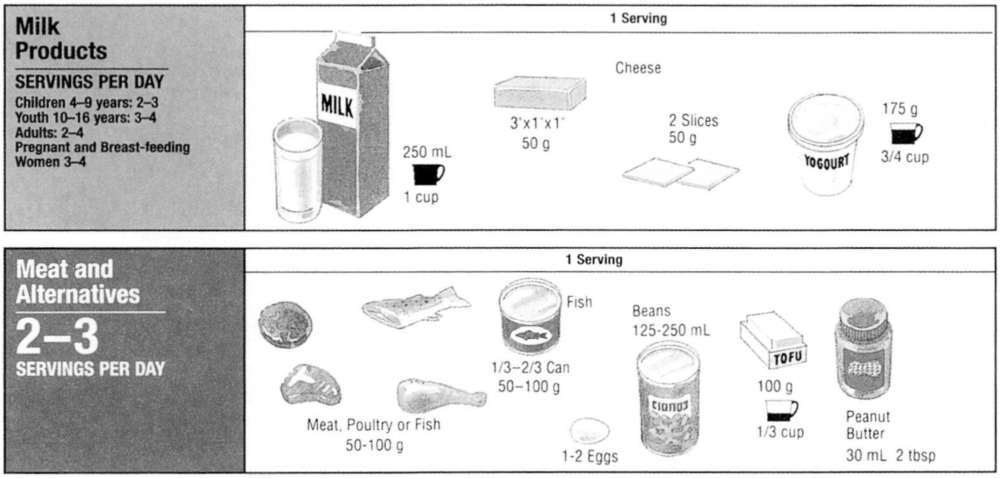

Milk Products

SERVINGS PER DAY

Children 4–9 years: 2–3
Youth 10–16 years: 3–4
Adults: 2–4
Pregnant and Breast-feeding Women 3–4

1 Serving

MILK

250 mL
1 cup

Cheese

3"x1"x1"
50 g

2 Slices
50 g

YOGOURT

175 g
3/4 cup

Other Foods

Taste and enjoyment can also come from other foods and beverages that are not part of the 4 food groups. Some of these foods are higher in fat or calories, so use these foods in moderation.

Meat and Alternatives

2–3

SERVINGS PER DAY

1 Serving

Meat, Poultry or Fish
50-100 g

1-2 Eggs

Fish
1/3–2/3 Can
50–100 g

Beans
125-250 mL

125 mL
1/3 cup

TOFU
100 g

Peanut Butter
30 mL 2 tbsp

Different People Need Different Amounts of Food

The amount of food you need every day from the 4 food groups and other foods depends on your age, body size, activity level, whether you are male or female and if you are pregnant or breast-feeding. That's why the Food Guide gives a lower and higher number of servings for each food group. For example, young children can choose the lower number of servings, while male teenagers can go to the higher number. Most other people can choose servings somewhere in between.

Consult *Canada's Physical Activity Guide to Healthy Active Living* to help you build physical activity into your daily life.

Enjoy eating well, being active and feeling good about yourself. That's VITALITÉ

© Minister of Public Works and Government Services Canada, 1997
Cat. No. H39-252/1992E   ISBN 0-662-19648-1
No changes permitted. Reprint permission not required.

Calculation Aids and Conversion Tables

More than 185 years ago a group of French scientists set up the metric system of weights and measures. Today, with refinements over years of use, it is called the *Système International* (SI). Here are a few conversion factors to help you make transitions in your necessary calculations.

METRIC SYSTEM OF MEASUREMENT

Like our money system, this is a simple decimal system based on units of 10. It is uniform and used internationally.

Weight Units
  1 kilogram (kg) = 1000 grams (gm or g)
  1 g = 1000 milligrams (mg)
  1 mg = 1000 micrograms (mcg or μg)

Length Units
  1 meter (m) = 100 centimeters (cm)
  1000 m = 1 kilometer (km)

Volume Units
  1 liter (L) = 1000 milliliters (ml)
  1 ml = 1 cubic centimeter (cc)

Temperature Units
  Celsius (C) scale, based on 100 equal units between 0° C (freezing point of water) and 100° C (boiling point of water); this scale is used entirely in all scientific work.

Energy Units
  Kilocalorie (kcal) = Amount of energy required to raise 1 kg water 1° C
  Kilojoule (kJ) = Amount of energy required to move 1 kg mass 1 m by a force of 1 newton
  1 kcal = 4.184 kJ

BRITISH/AMERICAN SYSTEM OF MEASUREMENT

Our customary system is a confusion of units with no uniform relationships. It is not a decimal system, but rather a collection of different units collected in usage and language over time. It is predominantly used in America.

Weight Units
  1 pound (lb) = 16 ounces (oz)

Length Units
  1 foot (ft) = 12 inches (in)
  1 yard (yd) = 3 feet (ft)

Volume Units
  3 teaspoons (tsp) = 1 tablespoon (Tbsp)
  16 Tbsp = 1 cup
  1 cup = 8 fluid ounces (fl oz)
  4 cups = 1 quart (qt)
  5 cups = 1 imperial quart (qt) (Canada)

Temperature Units
  Fahrenheit (F) scale, based on 180 equals units between 32° F (freezing point of water) and 212° F (boiling point of water) at standard atmospheric pressure

CONVERSIONS BETWEEN MEASUREMENT SYSTEMS

Weight
  1 oz = 28.35 g
  2.2 lb = 1 kg

Length
  1 in = 2.54 cm
  1 ft = 30.48 cm
  39.37 in = 1 m

Volume

1.06 qt = 1 L

0.85 imperial qt = 1 L (Canada)

Temperature

Boiling point of water: 100° C; 212° F

Body temperature: 37° C; 98.6° F

Freezing point of water: 0° C; 32° F

Interconversion Formulas

Fahrenheit temperature (°F) = $\frac{9}{5}$ (°C + 32)

Celsius temperature (°C) = $\frac{5}{9}$ (°F − 32)

RETINOL EQUIVALENTS

The following definitions and equivalences that are internationally agreed on provide a basis for calculating retinol equivalent conversions.

Definitions

International units (IU) and retinol equivalents (RE) are defined as follows:

1 IU = 0.3 mg retinol (0.0003 mg)

1 IU = 0.6 mg beta-carotene (0.0006 mg)

1 RE = 6 mg retinol

1 RE = 6 mg beta-carotene

1 RE = 12 mg other provitamin A carotenoids

1 RE = 3.33 IU retinol

1 RE = 10 IU beta-carotene

Conversion Formulas

On the basis of weight, beta-carotene is one half as active as retinol; on the basis of structure, the other provitamin carotenoids are one fourth as active as retinol. In addition, retinol is more completely absorbed in the intestine, whereas the provitamin carotenoids are much less well utilized, with an average absorption of about one third. Therefore in overall activity, beta-carotene is one sixth as active as retinol, and the other carotenoids are one twelfth as active. These differences in utilization provide the basis for the 1:6:12 relationship shown in the equivalences given and in the following formulas for calculating retinol equivalents from values of vitamin A, beta-carotene, and other active carotenoids, expressed either as international units or micrograms.

If retinol and beta-carotene are given in micrograms, the following equation results:

Micrograms of retinol +

(Micrograms of beta-carotene ÷ 6) = RE

If both are given as IU, the following equation is used:

(International units of retinol ÷ 3.33) +

(International units of beta-carotene ÷ 10) = RE

If beta-carotene and other carotenoids are given in micrograms, the following equation is used:

(Micrograms of beta-carotene ÷ 6) +

(Micrograms of other carotenoids ÷ 12) = RE

Approximate Metric Conversions		
When you know. . .	**. . . Multiply by . . .**	**. . . to find . . .**
WEIGHT		
Ounces	28	Grams
Pounds	0.45	Kilograms
LENGTH		
Inches	2.5	Centimeters
Feet	30	Centimeters
Yards	0.9	Meters
Miles	1.6	Kilometers
VOLUME		
Teaspoons	5	Millimeters
Tablespoons	15	Millimeters
Fluid ounces	30	Millimeters
Cups	0.24	Liters
Pints	0.47	Liters
Quarts	0.95	Liters
TEMPERATURE		
Fahrenheit temperature	$\frac{5}{9}$ (after subtracting 32)	Celsius temperature

I

Infant and Child Growth Charts

**UNITED STATES
CENTERS FOR DISEASE CONTROL
AND PREVENTION (CDC)**

CDC Growth Charts: United States

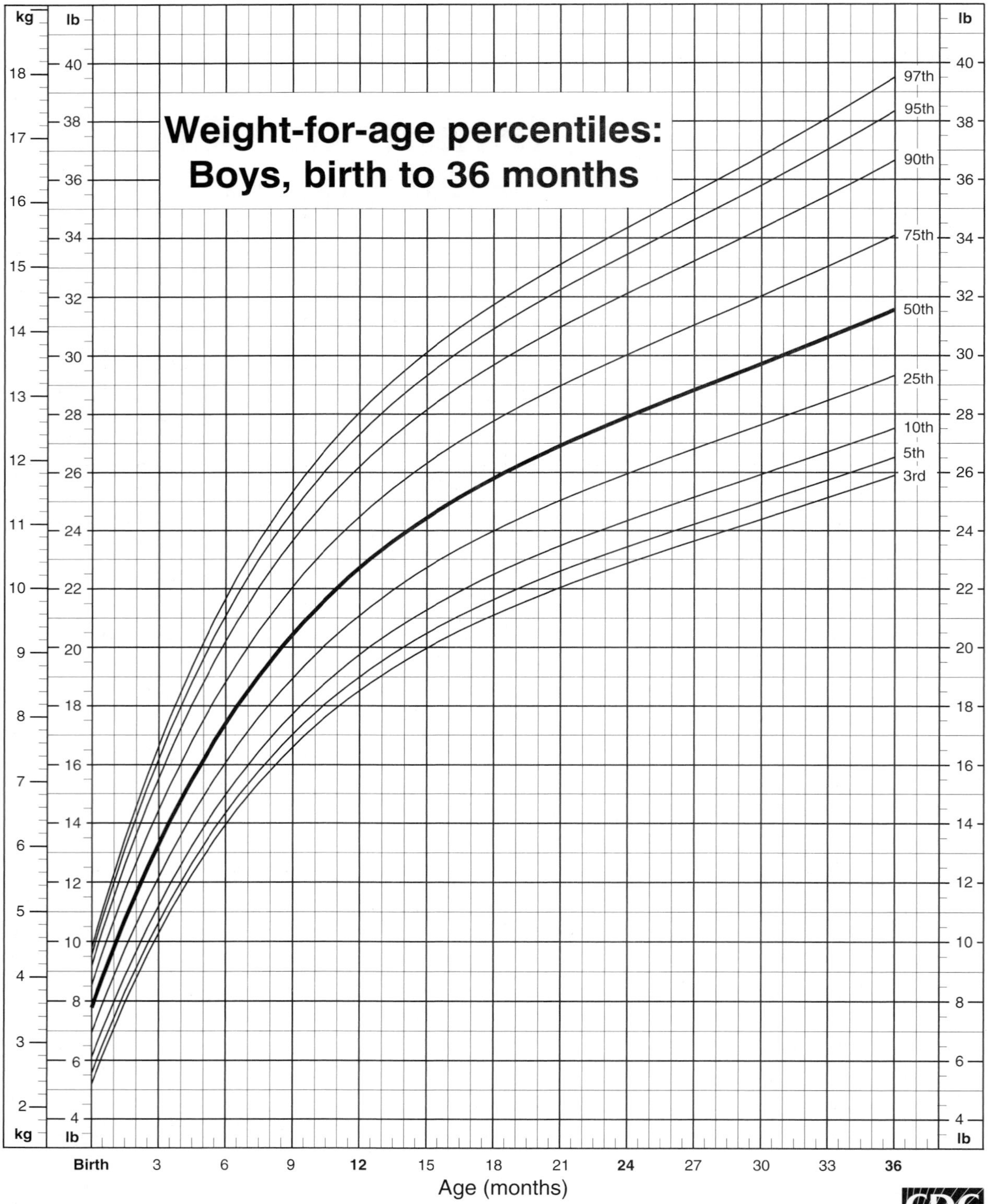

Weight-for-age percentiles: Boys, birth to 36 months

Age (months)

Published May 30, 2000.
SOURCE: Developed by the National Center for Health Statistics in collaboration with
the National Center for Chronic Disease Prevention and Health Promotion (2000).

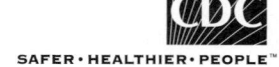

SAFER · HEALTHIER · PEOPLE™

CDC Growth Charts: United States

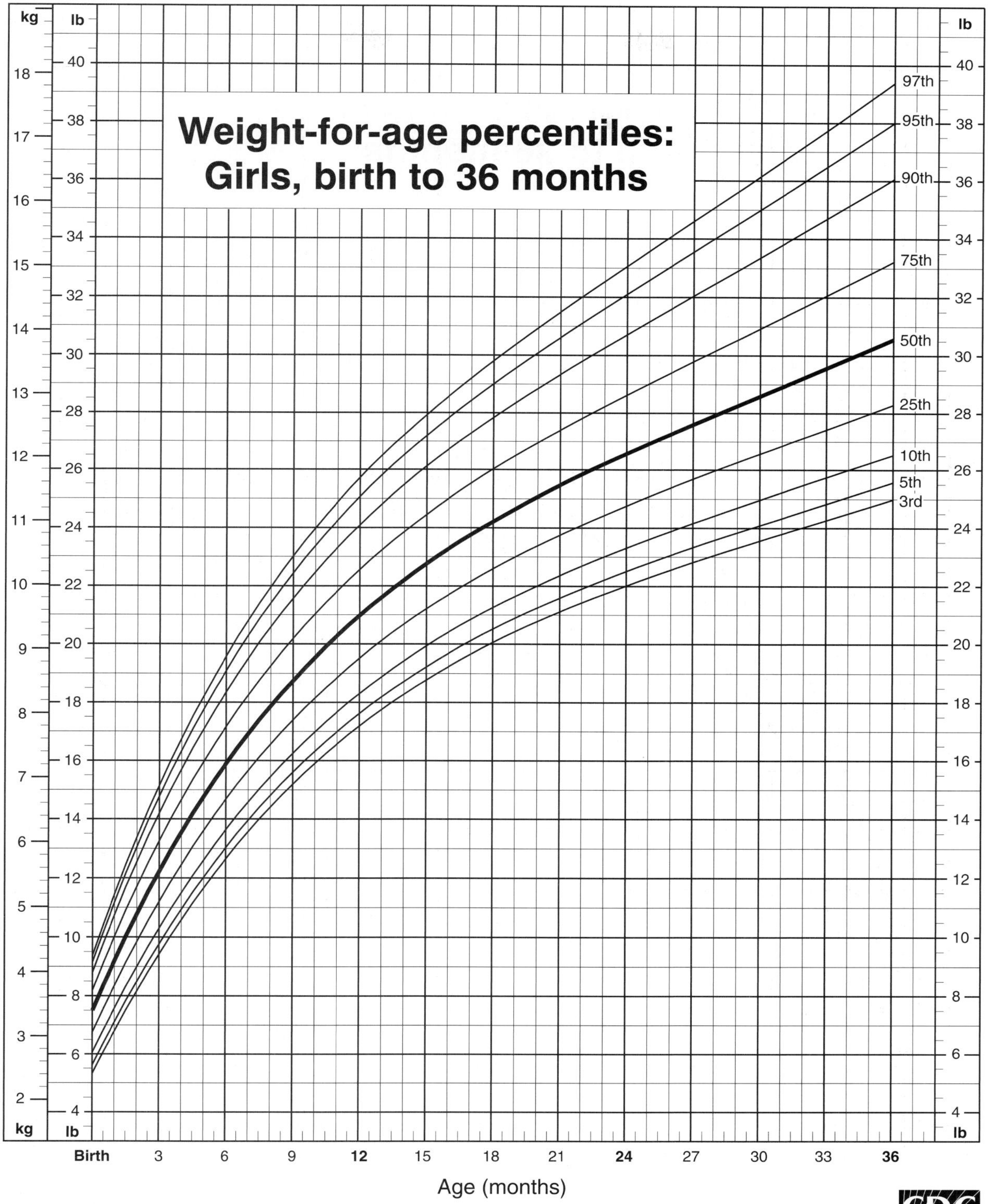

Weight-for-age percentiles: Girls, birth to 36 months

Age (months)

Published May 30, 2000.
SOURCE: Developed by the National Center for Health Statistics in collaboration with
the National Center for Chronic Disease Prevention and Health Promotion (2000).

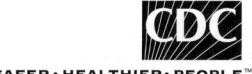

SAFER · HEALTHIER · PEOPLE™

CDC Growth Charts: United States

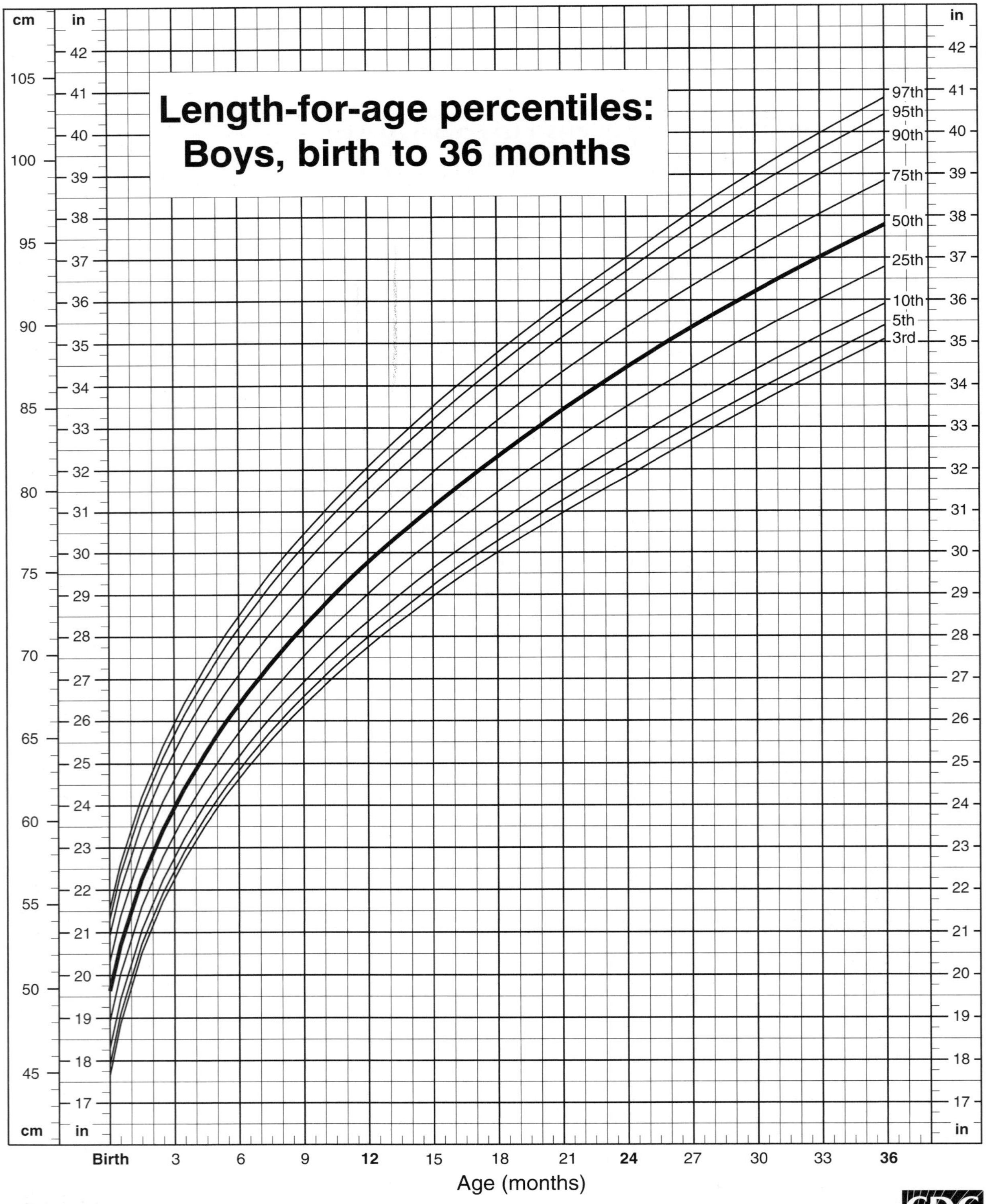

Length-for-age percentiles: Boys, birth to 36 months

97th
95th
90th
75th
50th
25th
10th
5th
3rd

Age (months)

Birth 3 6 9 12 15 18 21 24 27 30 33 36

Published May 30, 2000.
SOURCE: Developed by the National Center for Health Statistics in collaboration with
the National Center for Chronic Disease Prevention and Health Promotion (2000).

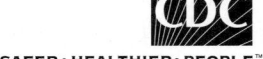

SAFER · HEALTHIER · PEOPLE™

CDC Growth Charts: United States

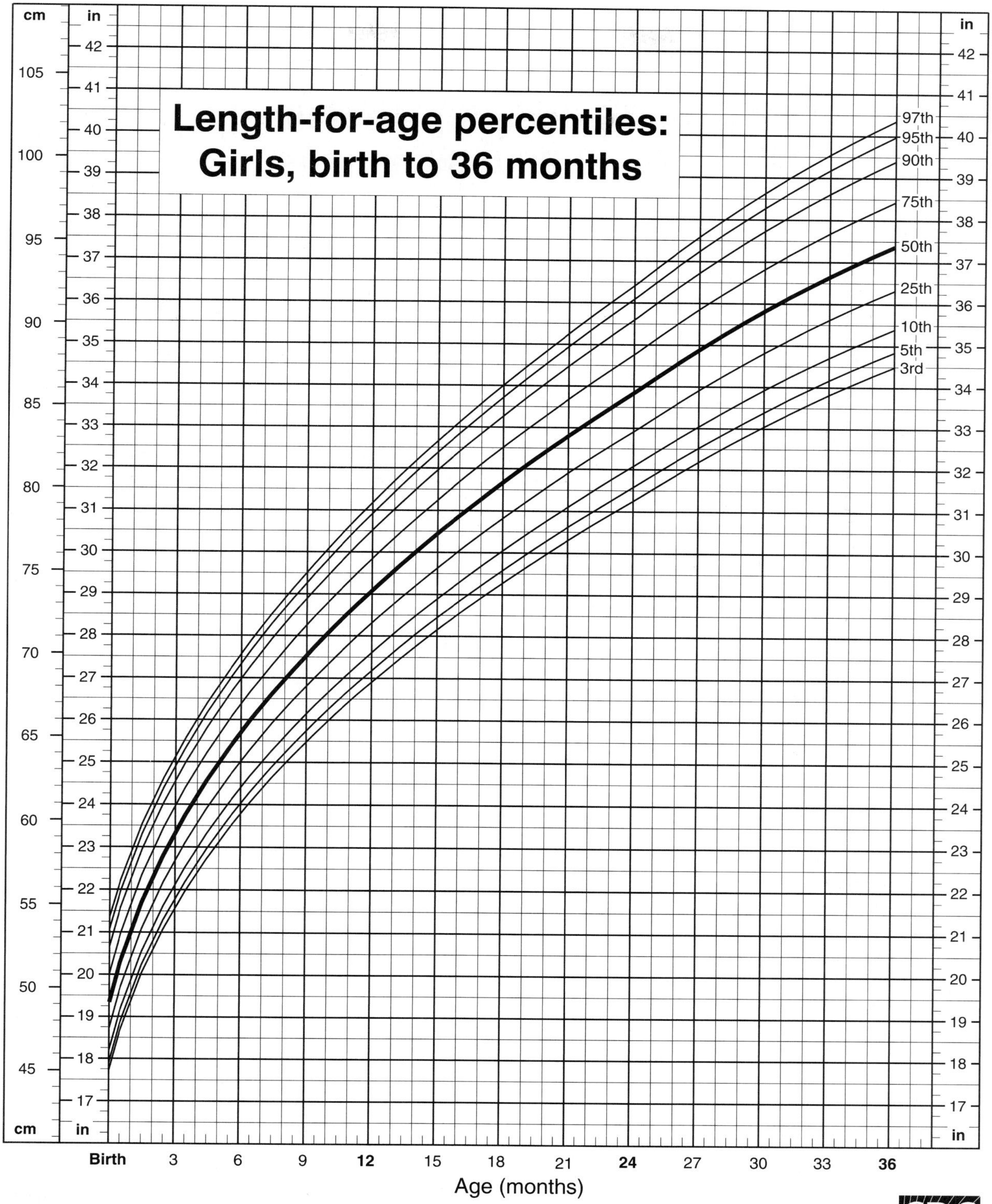

Length-for-age percentiles:
Girls, birth to 36 months

97th
95th
90th
75th
50th
25th
10th
5th
3rd

Age (months)

Birth   3   6   9   12   15   18   21   24   27   30   33   36

Published May 30, 2000.
SOURCE: Developed by the National Center for Health Statistics in collaboration with
the National Center for Chronic Disease Prevention and Health Promotion (2000).

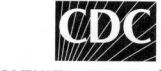

SAFER ∙ HEALTHIER ∙ PEOPLE™

CDC Growth Charts: United States

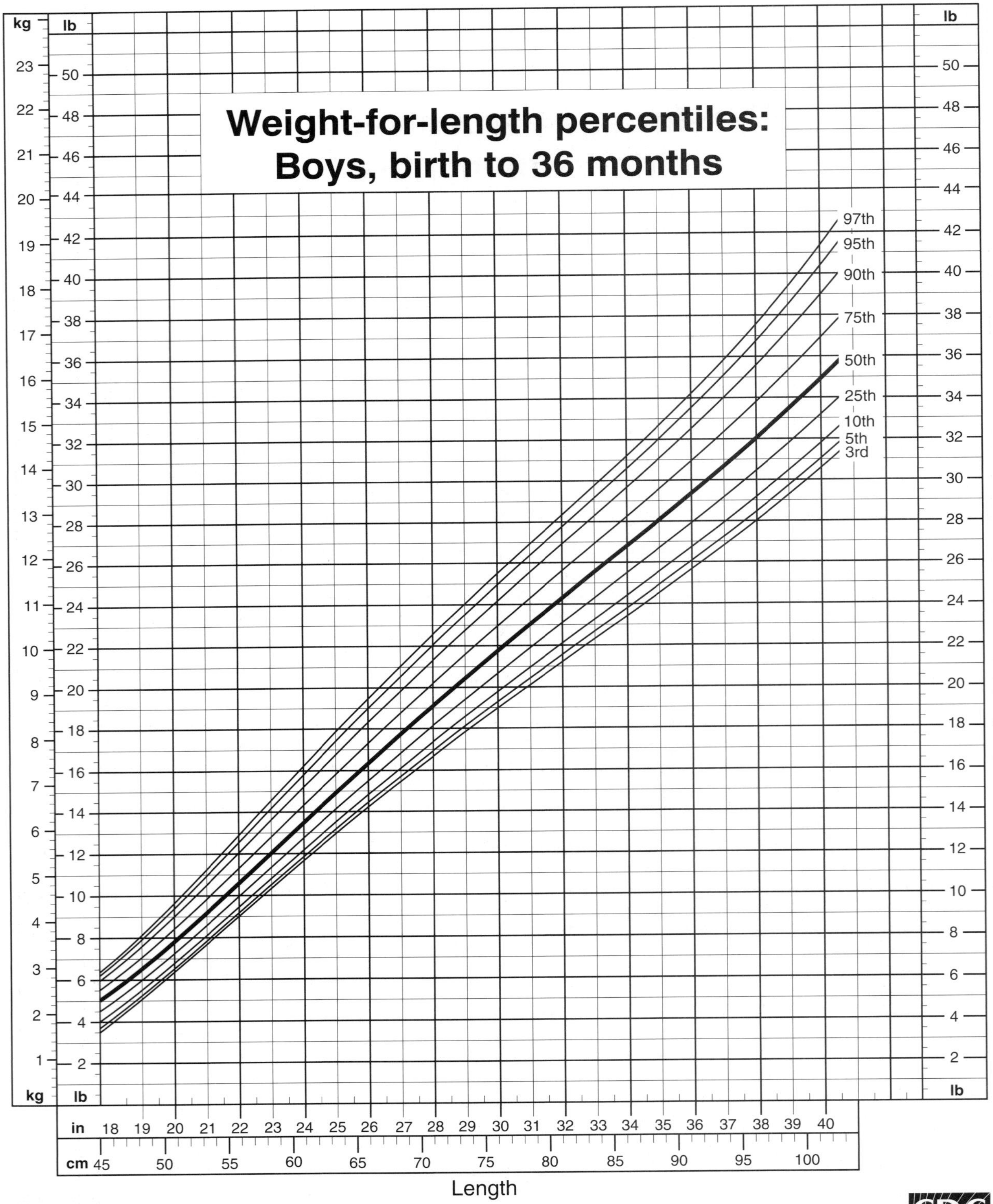
Weight-for-length percentiles:
Boys, birth to 36 months
kg
lb
97th
95th
90th
75th
50th
25th
10th
5th
3rd
in
cm
Length

Published May 30, 2000. (modified 6/8/00).
SOURCE: Developed by the National Center for Health Statistics in collaboration with the National Center for Chronic Disease Prevention and Health Promotion (2000).

CDC
SAFER • HEALTHIER • PEOPLE™

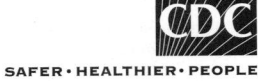

CDC Growth Charts: United States

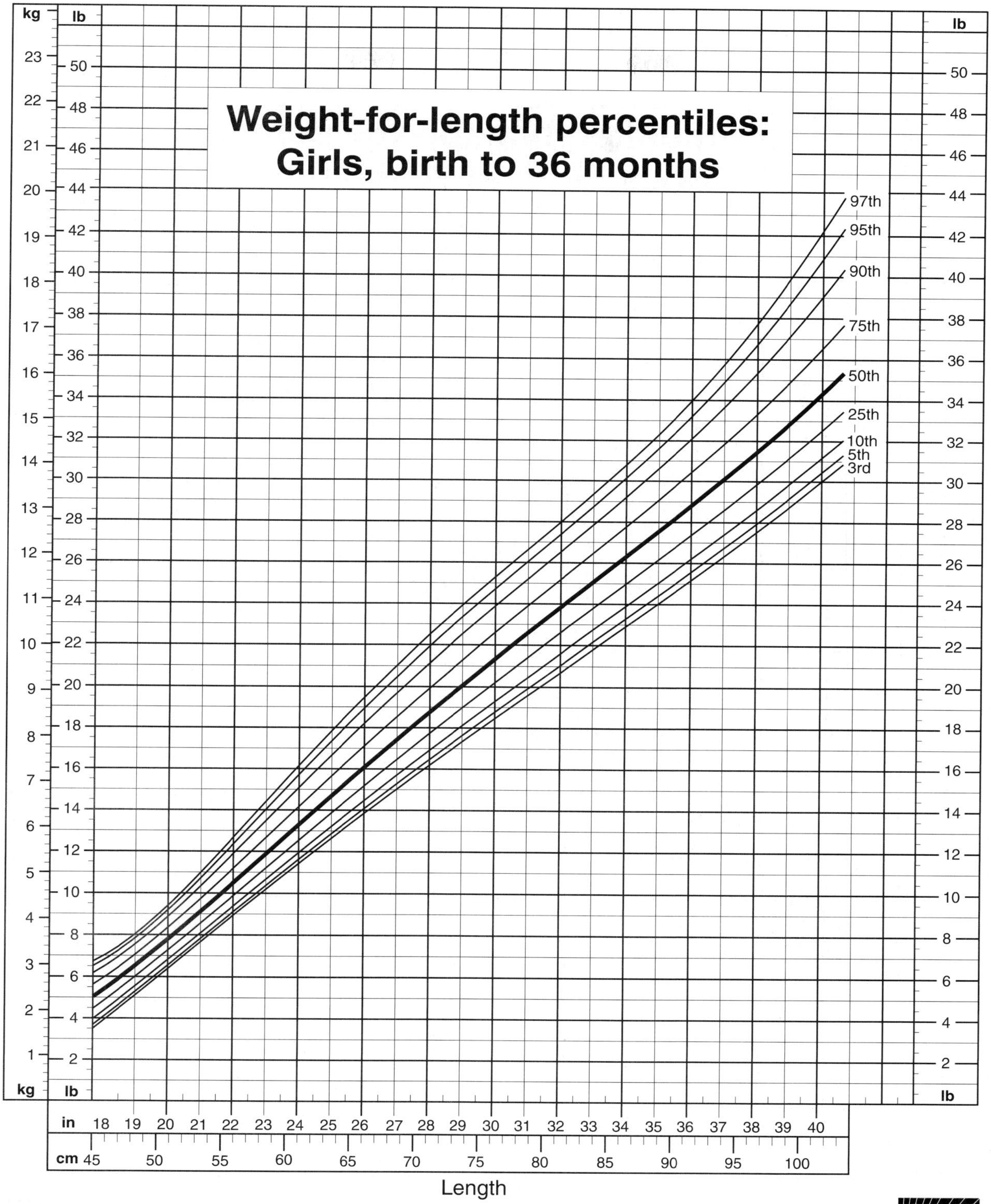

Weight-for-length percentiles: Girls, birth to 36 months

97th
95th
90th
75th
50th
25th
10th
5th
3rd

Length

Published May 30, 2000. (modified 6/8/00).
SOURCE: Developed by the National Center for Health Statistics in collaboration with
    the National Center for Chronic Disease Prevention and Health Promotion (2000).

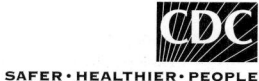

SAFER·HEALTHIER·PEOPLE™

CDC Growth Charts: United States

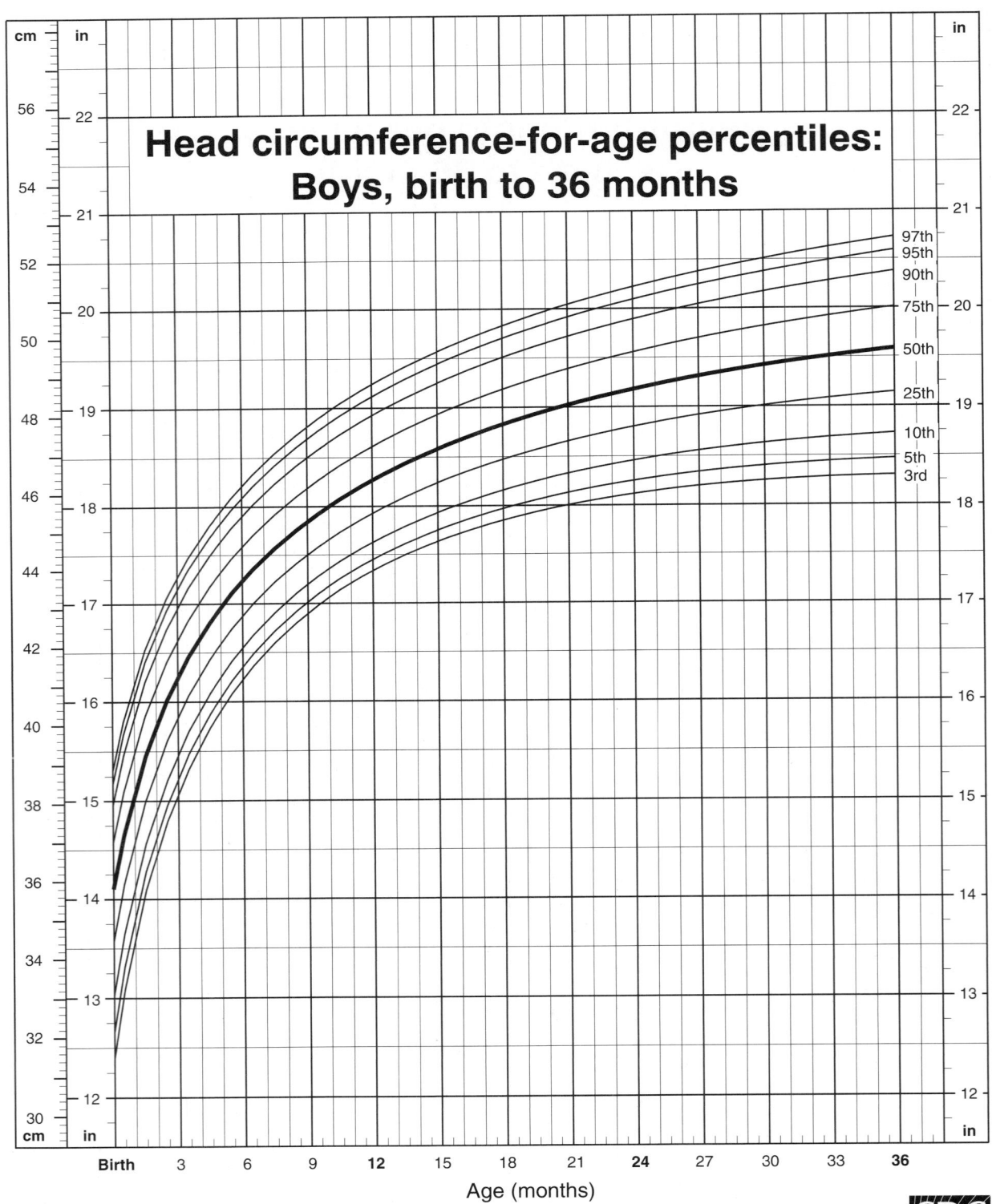

Head circumference-for-age percentiles:
Boys, birth to 36 months

Age (months)

Published May 30, 2000.
SOURCE: Developed by the National Center for Health Statistics in collaboration with
   the National Center for Chronic Disease Prevention and Health Promotion (2000).

SAFER · HEALTHIER · PEOPLE™

CDC Growth Charts: United States

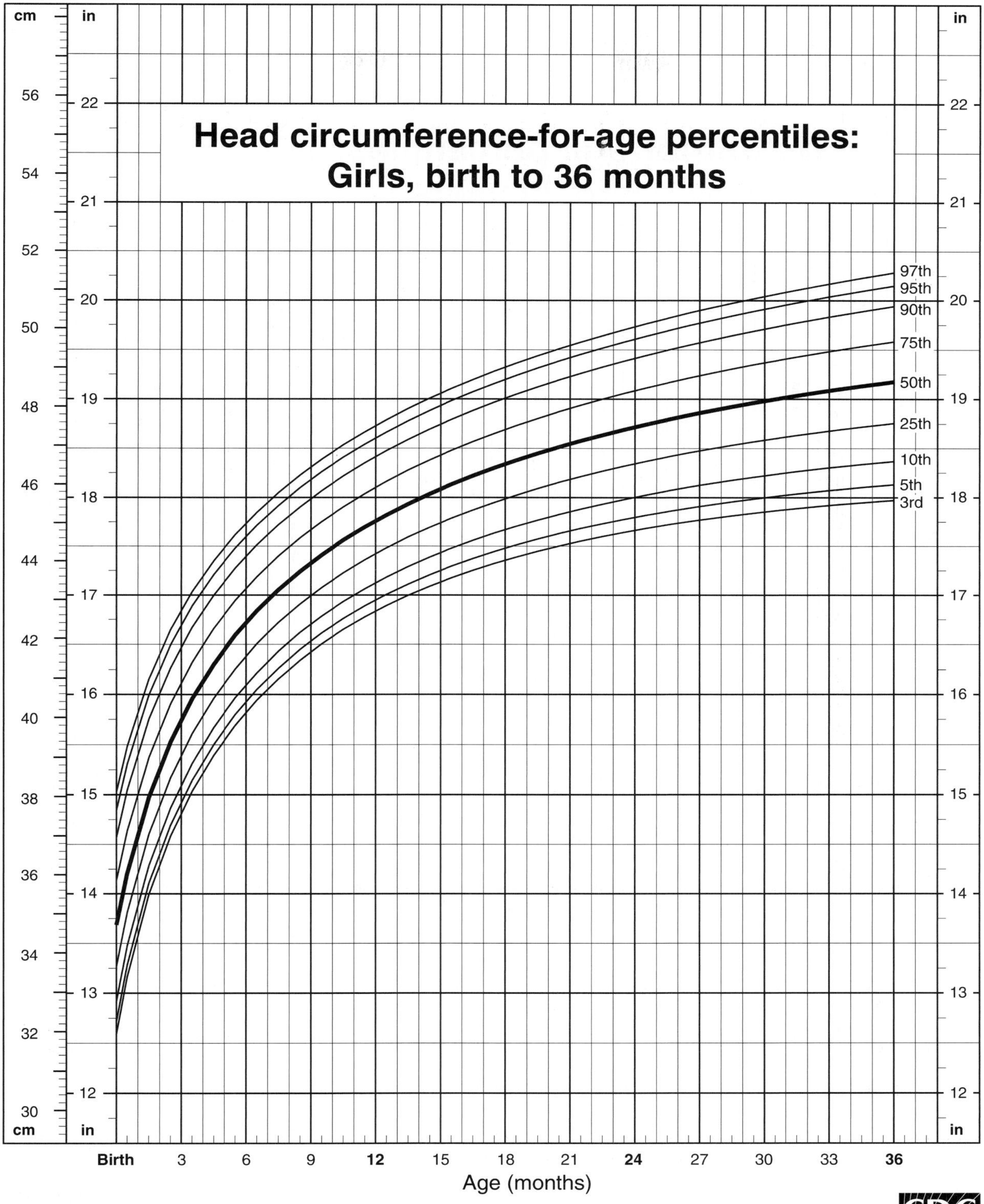

Head circumference-for-age percentiles: Girls, birth to 36 months

Axis labels — left: cm / in, with cm values 30, 32, 34, 36, 38, 40, 42, 44, 46, 48, 50, 52, 54, 56 and in values 12, 13, 14, 15, 16, 17, 18, 19, 20, 21, 22

Right axis: in — 12, 13, 14, 15, 16, 17, 18, 19, 20, 21, 22

Percentile curves (top to bottom): 97th, 95th, 90th, 75th, 50th, 25th, 10th, 5th, 3rd

Bottom axis: Birth, 3, 6, 9, 12, 15, 18, 21, 24, 27, 30, 33, 36

Age (months)

Published May 30, 2000.
SOURCE: Developed by the National Center for Health Statistics in collaboration with
the National Center for Chronic Disease Prevention and Health Promotion (2000).

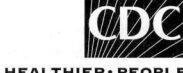
SAFER · HEALTHIER · PEOPLE™

CDC Growth Charts: United States

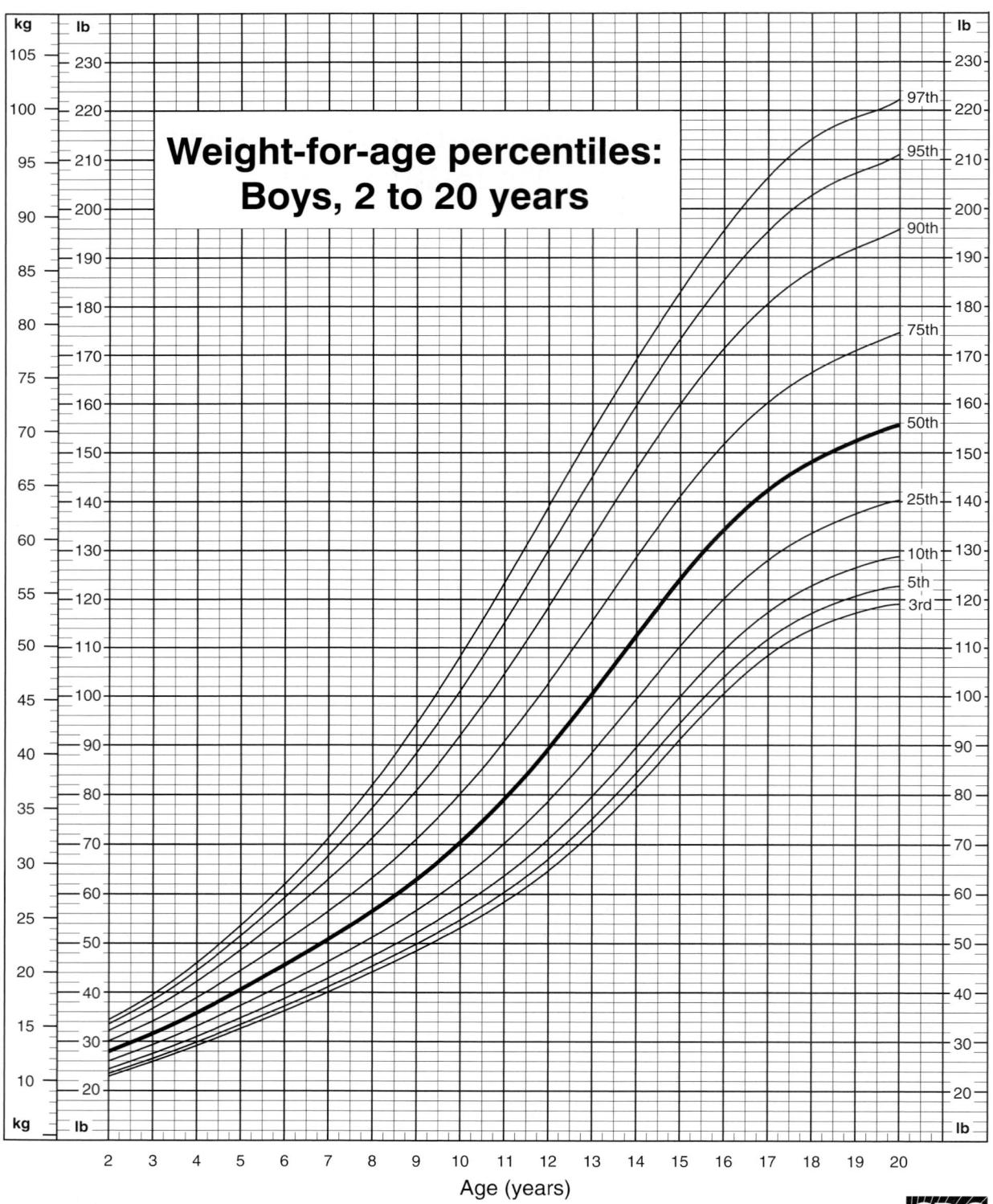

Weight-for-age percentiles: Boys, 2 to 20 years

Age (years)

Published May 30, 2000.
SOURCE: Developed by the National Center for Health Statistics in collaboration with
the National Center for Chronic Disease Prevention and Health Promotion (2000).

SAFER · HEALTHIER · PEOPLE™

CDC Growth Charts: United States

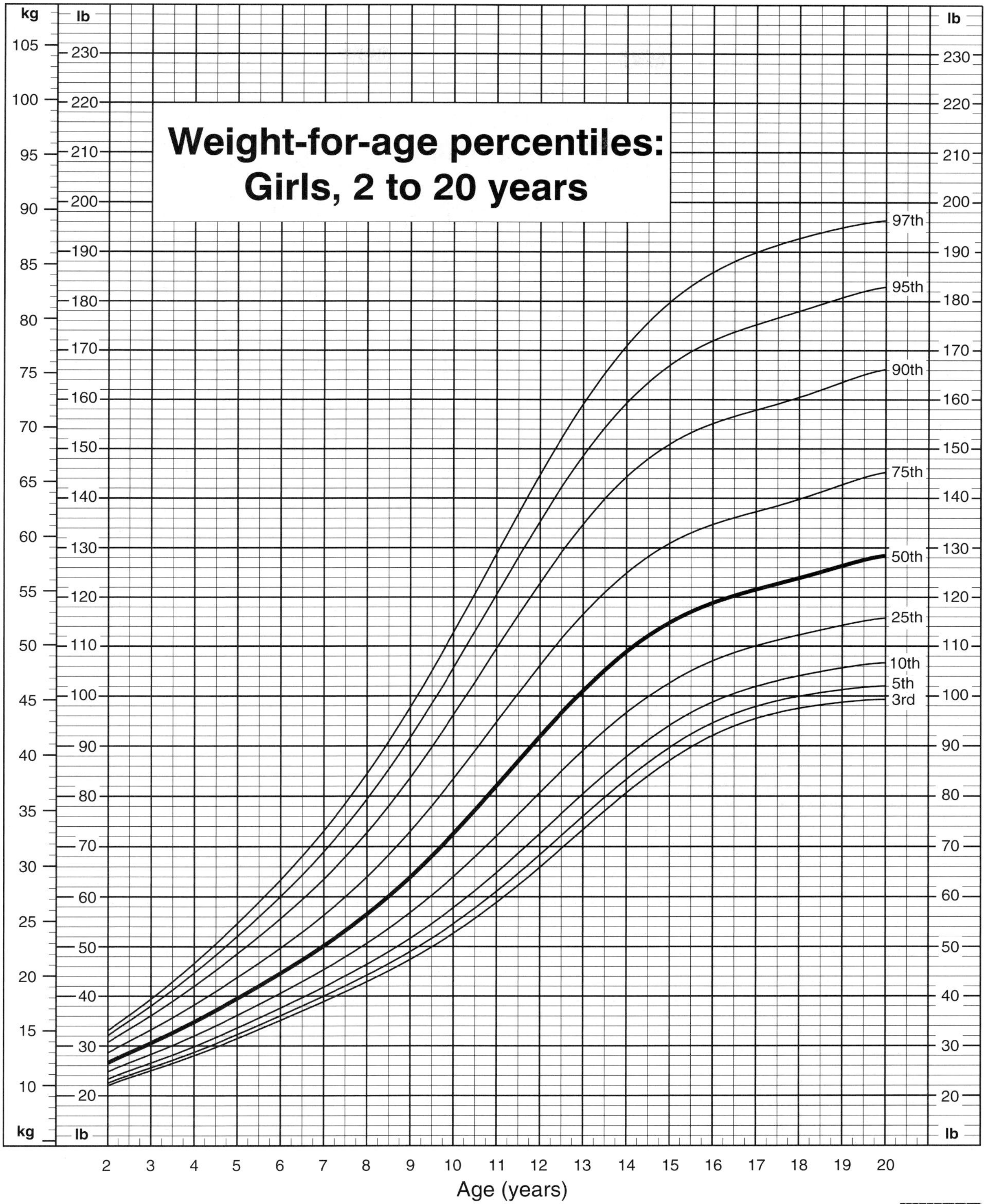

Weight-for-age percentiles: Girls, 2 to 20 years

97th
95th
90th
75th
50th
25th
10th
5th
3rd

Age (years)

Published May 30, 2000.
SOURCE: Developed by the National Center for Health Statistics in collaboration with
the National Center for Chronic Disease Prevention and Health Promotion (2000).

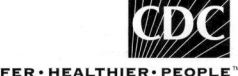

SAFER · HEALTHIER · PEOPLE™

CDC Growth Charts: United States

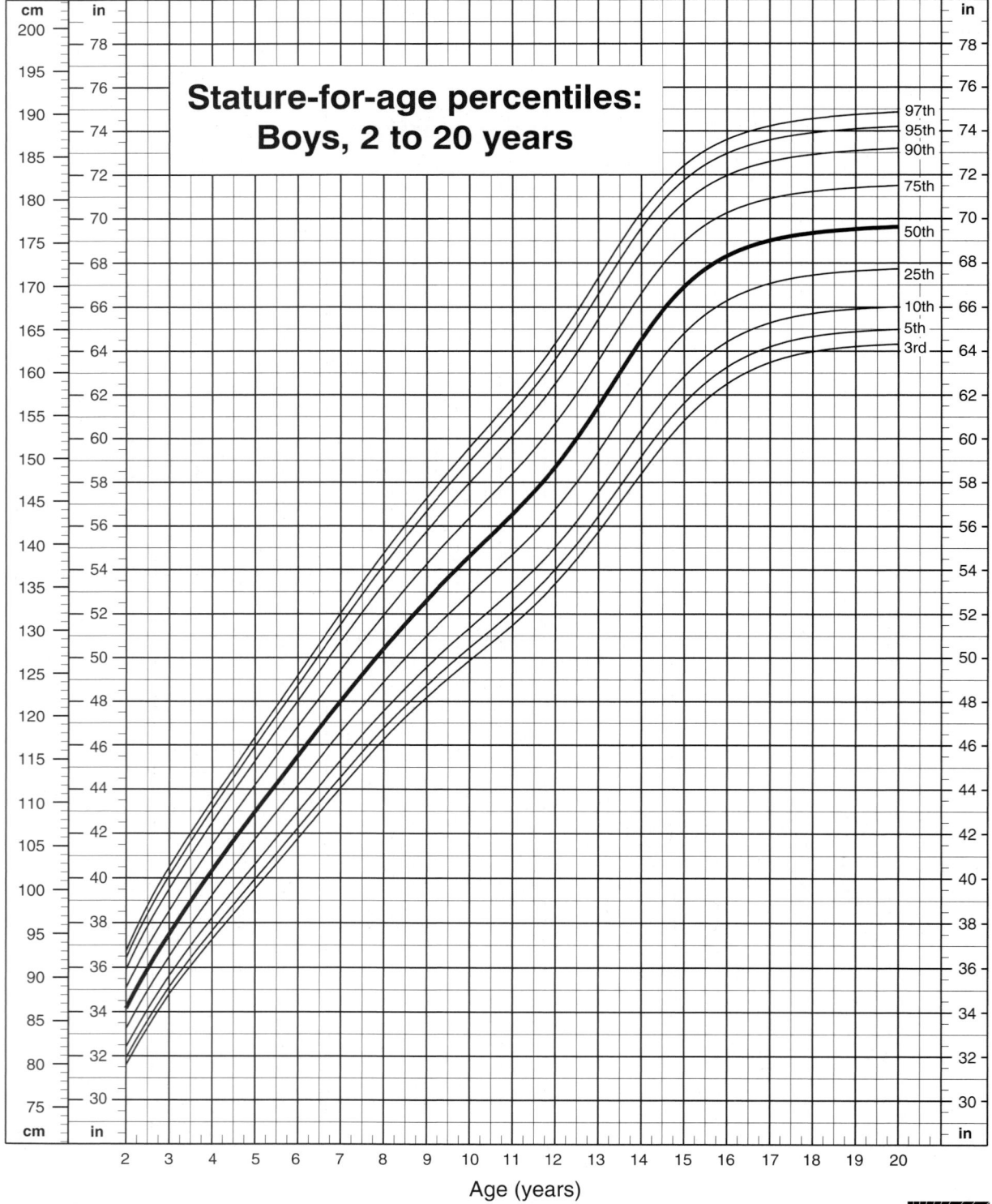

**Stature-for-age percentiles:
Boys, 2 to 20 years**

Age (years)

Published May 30, 2000.
SOURCE: Developed by the National Center for Health Statistics in collaboration with
the National Center for Chronic Disease Prevention and Health Promotion (2000).

CDC

SAFER · HEALTHIER · PEOPLE™

CDC Growth Charts: United States

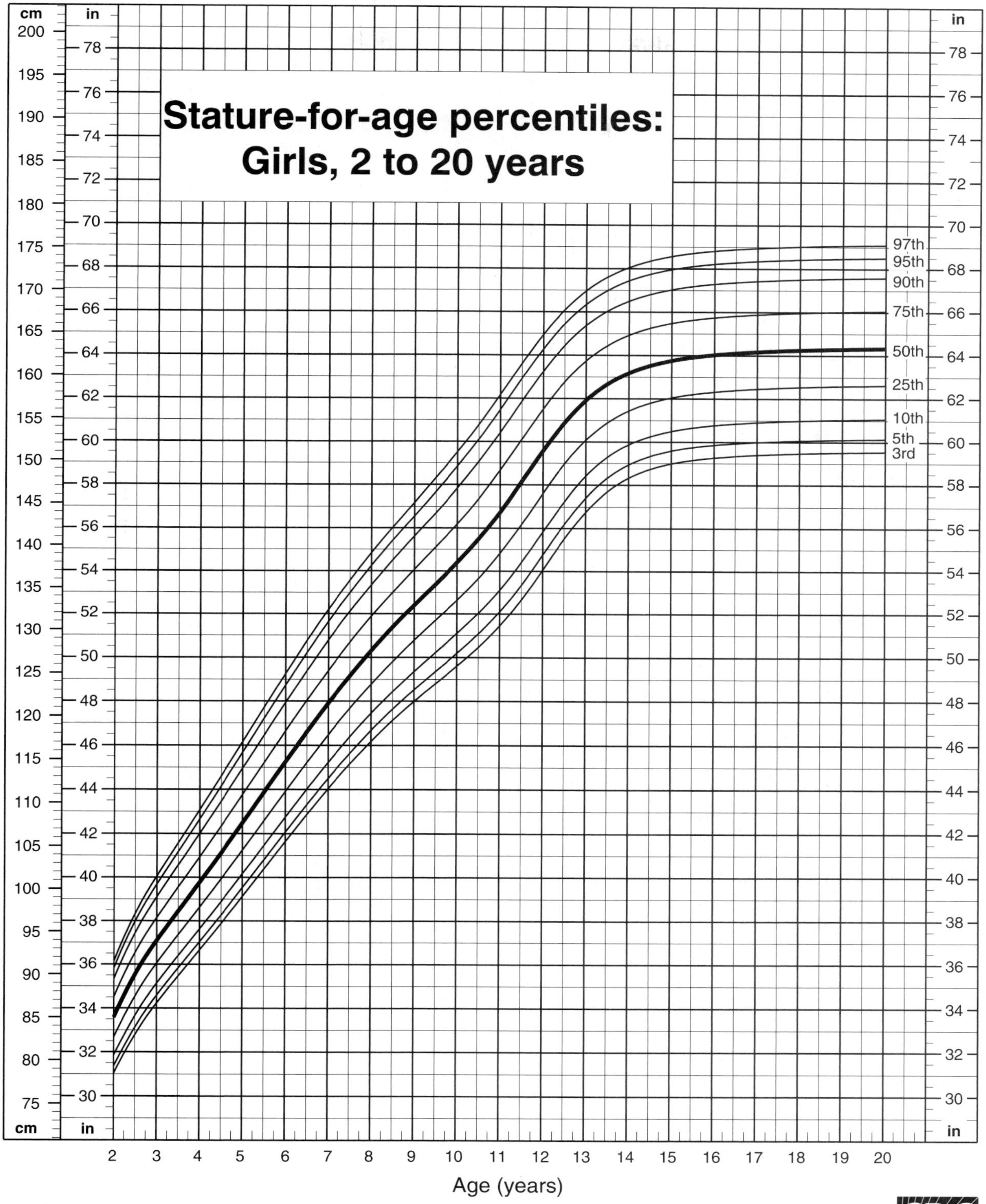

Stature-for-age percentiles: Girls, 2 to 20 years

Age (years)

97th
95th
90th
75th
50th
25th
10th
5th
3rd

Published May 30, 2000.
SOURCE: Developed by the National Center for Health Statistics in collaboration with
the National Center for Chronic Disease Prevention and Health Promotion (2000).

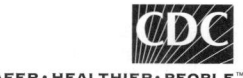

SAFER · HEALTHIER · PEOPLE™

CDC Growth Charts: United States

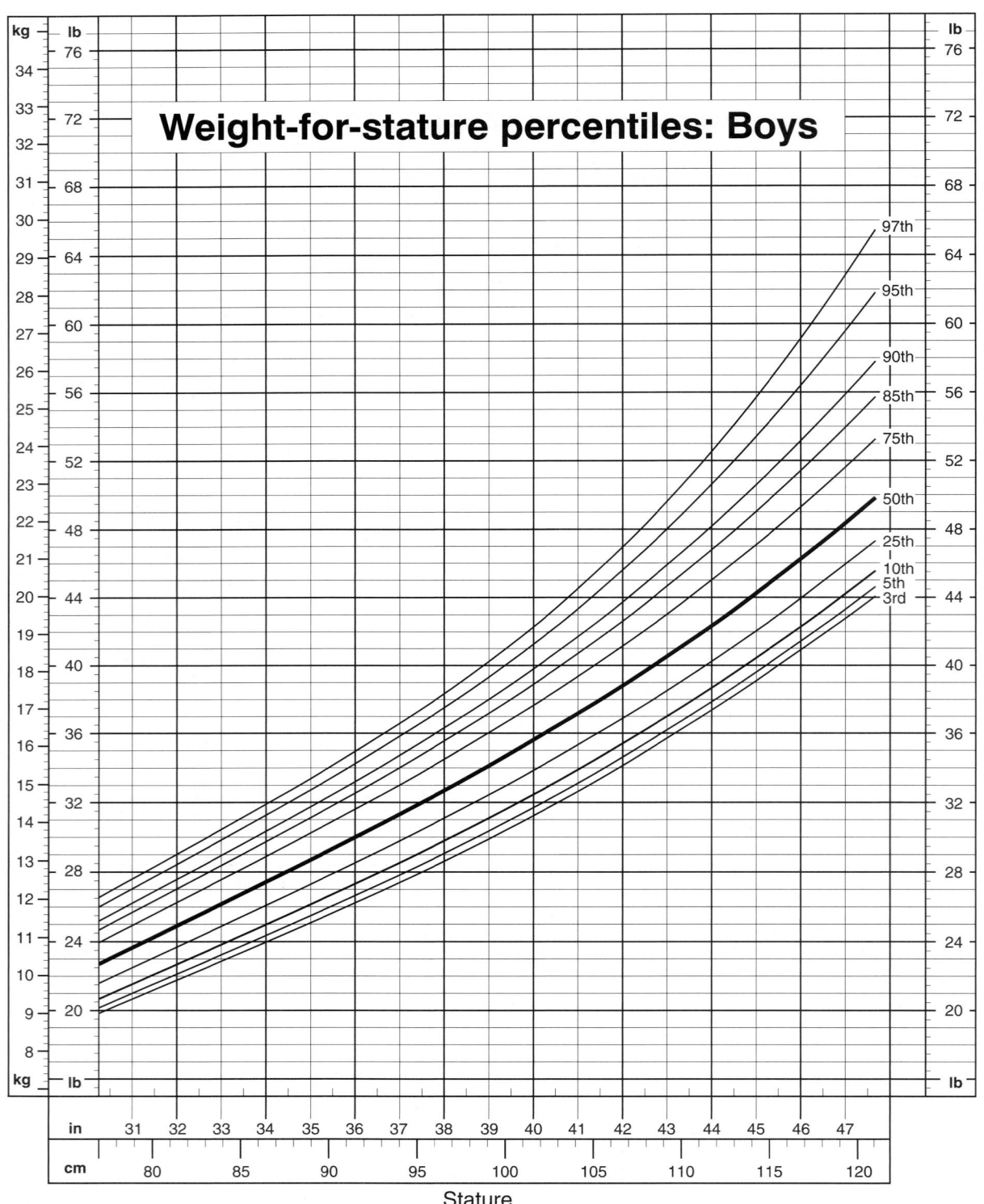

Weight-for-stature percentiles: Boys

Stature

Published May 30, 2000. (modified 11/21/00).
SOURCE: Developed by the National Center for Health Statistics in collaboration with
       the National Center for Chronic Disease Prevention and Health Promotion (2000).

SAFER · HEALTHIER · PEOPLE™

CDC Growth Charts: United States

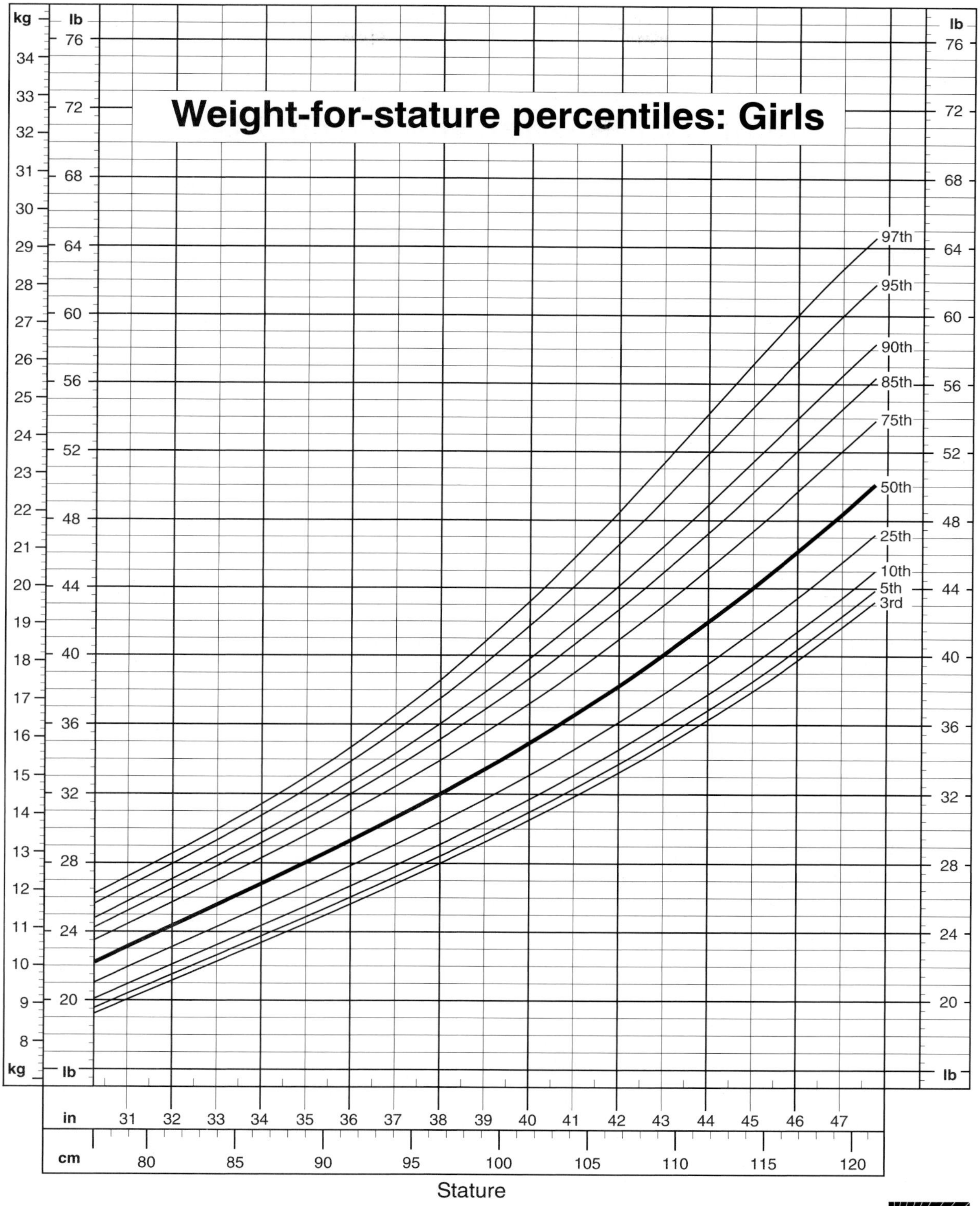
Weight-for-stature percentiles: Girls
kg
lb
34
33
32
31
30
29
28
27
26
25
24
23
22
21
20
19
18
17
16
15
14
13
12
11
10
9
8
76
72
68
64
60
56
52
48
44
40
36
32
28
24
20
97th
95th
90th
85th
75th
50th
25th
10th
5th
3rd
in
31
32
33
34
35
36
37
38
39
40
41
42
43
44
45
46
47
cm
80
85
90
95
100
105
110
115
120
Stature

Published May 30, 2000. (modified 11/21/00).

SOURCE: Developed by the National Center for Health Statistics in collaboration with the National Center for Chronic Disease Prevention and Health Promotion (2000).

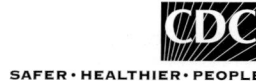

CDC SAFER • HEALTHIER • PEOPLE™

CDC Growth Charts: United States

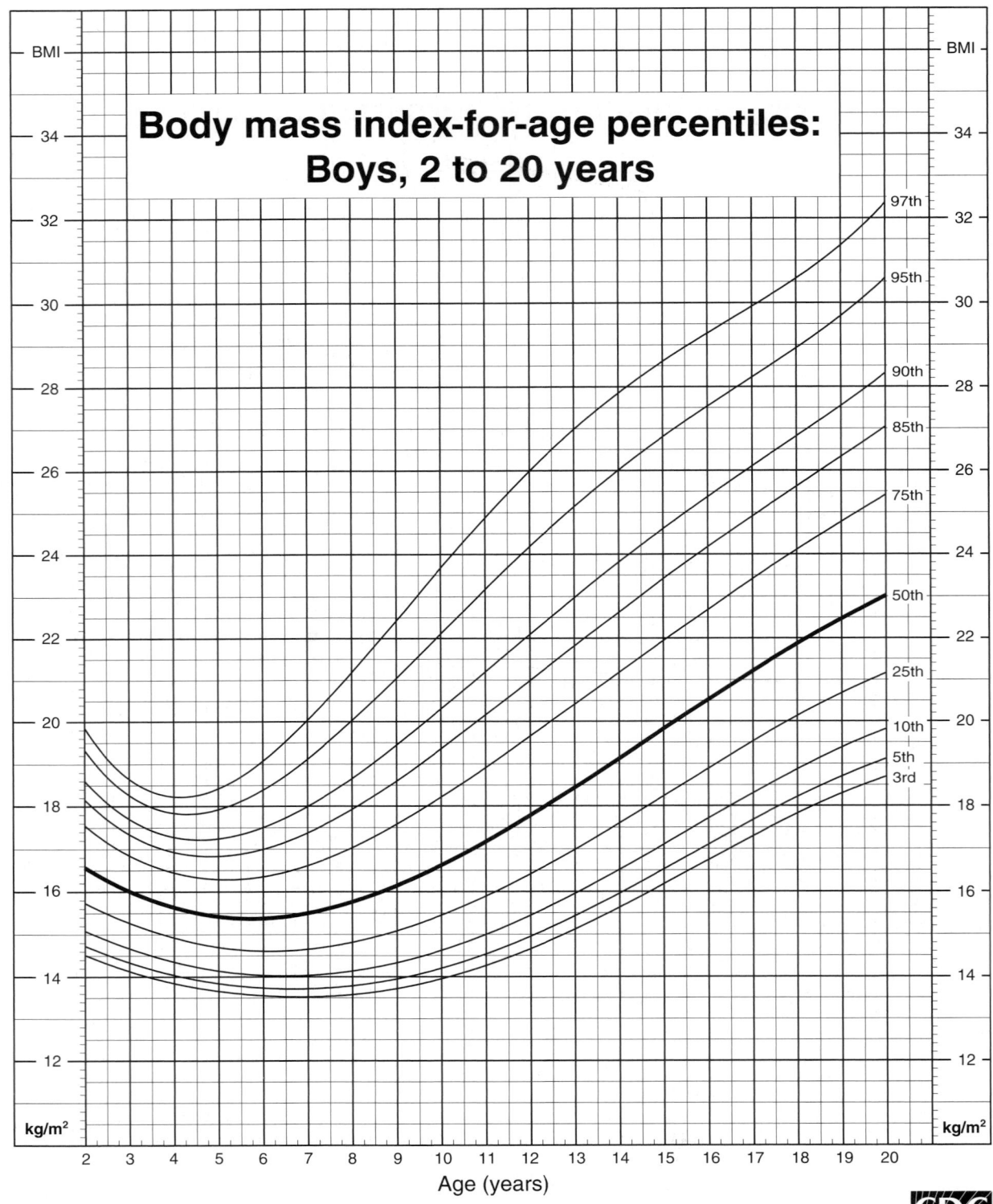

**Body mass index-for-age percentiles:
Boys, 2 to 20 years**

Published May 30, 2000.
SOURCE: Developed by the National Center for Health Statistics in collaboration with
the National Center for Chronic Disease Prevention and Health Promotion (2000).

SAFER · HEALTHIER · PEOPLE™

CDC Growth Charts: United States

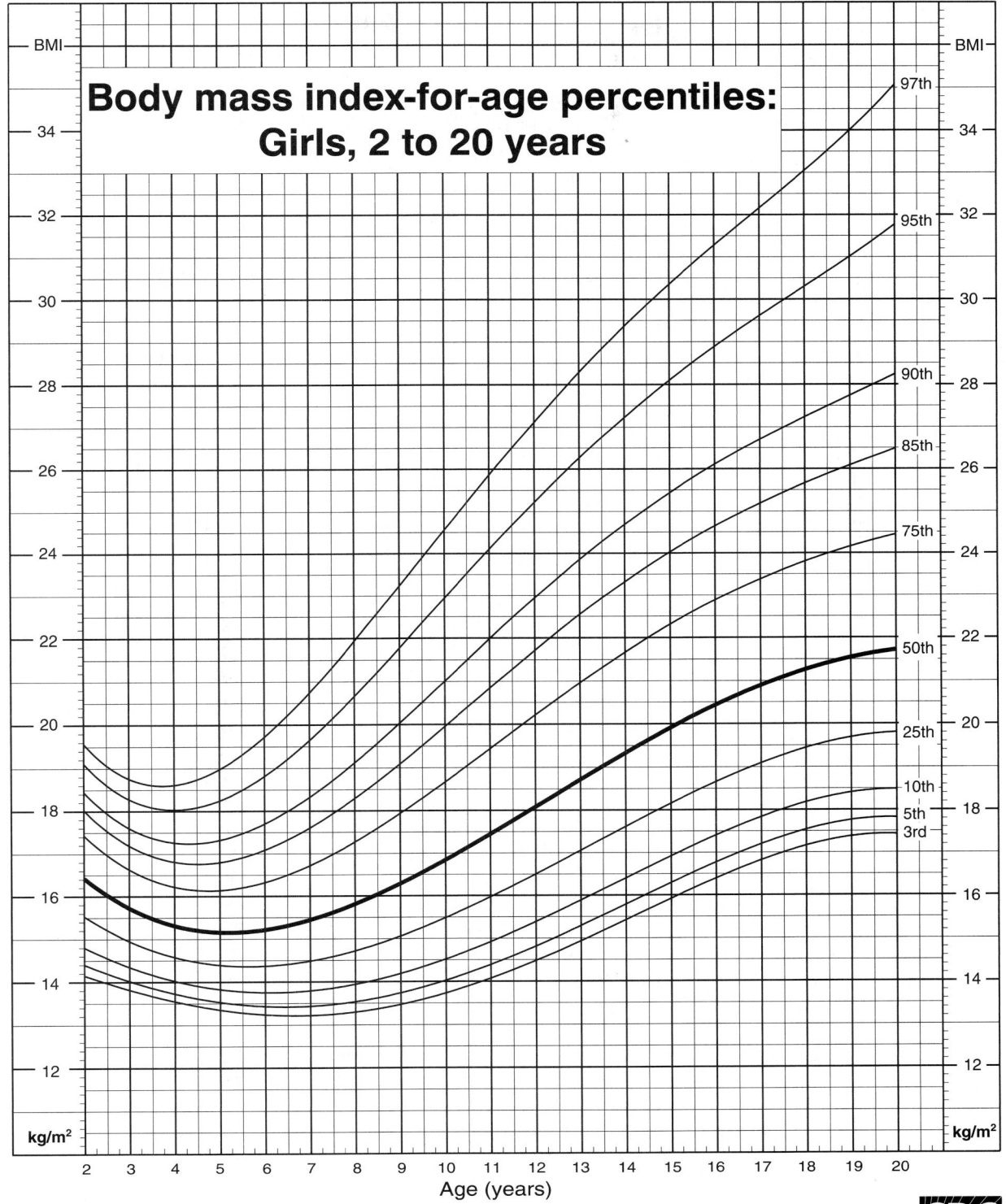

**Body mass index-for-age percentiles:
Girls, 2 to 20 years**

Published May 30, 2000.
SOURCE: Developed by the National Center for Health Statistics in collaboration with
the National Center for Chronic Disease Prevention and Health Promotion (2000).

SAFER · HEALTHIER · PEOPLE™

Cultural Dietary Patterns and Religious Dietary Practices

Only foods that are specifically associated with these cultural groups are noted. Individuals may also consume typical American foods, as dietary adaptations are common. Assumptions of dietary patterns cannot be made, but knowledge of these unique foods provides a common understanding of the range of possible food choices.

Cultural Dietary Patterns

Culture	Bread, cereal, rice, and pasta group	Vegetable group
Native American	Blue corn flour (ground dried blue corn kernels) used to make cornbread, mush dumplings; fruit dumplings (walakshi); fry bread (biscuit dough deep fried); ground sweet acorn; hominy; tortillas; wheat and rye products; wild rice	Artichokes, cacti, chili, mushrooms, nettles, onions, potatoes, pumpkin, squash, sweet potatoes, tomatoes, wild greens, turnips, and yucca
Northern European	Barley, hops, oat, rice, rye, and wheat products	Artichokes, asparagus, beets, Brussels sprouts, cabbage, carrots, cauliflower, celery, cucumbers, eggplant, fennel, green peppers, kale, leeks, mushrooms, olives, onions, peas, potatoes, radishes, spinach, turnips, and watercress
Southern European	Cornmeal, rice, and wheat products	Arugula, artichokes, asparagus, broccoli, cabbage, cardoon, cauliflower, celery, chicory, cucumber, eggplant, endive, escarole, fennel, kale, kohlrabi, mushrooms, mustard greens, olives, pimentos, potatoes, radicchio, Swiss chard, turnips, and zucchini
Central European and Russian	Barley, buckwheat, corn, millet, oats, potato starch, rice, rye, and wheat products	Asparagus, beets, Brussels sprouts, cabbage, carrots, cauliflower, celery, chard, cucumbers, eggplant, endive, kohlrabi, leeks, mushrooms, olives, onions, parsnips, peppers, potatoes, radishes, sorrel, spinach, and turnips
African American (Southern United States)	Biscuits; cornbread as spoon bread, corn pone, hush puppies, or grits; and rice	Broccoli, cabbage, corn; leafy greens including dandelion greens, kale, mustard greens, collard greens, and turnips, okra, pumpkin, potatoes, spinach, squash, sweet potatoes, tomatoes, and yams
Mexican	Corn (tortillas, masa harina), wheat, and rice products; sweet bread	Cactus (nopales), calabaza criolla, chili peppers, corn, jicama, onions, peas, plantains, squashes (chayote, pumpkin, etc.), tomatillos, tomatoes, yams, and yucca root (cassava or manioc)
Central American	Corn (tamales, tortillas), rice, and wheat products	Asparagus, beets, cabbage, calabaza, chayote, chili peppers, corn, cucumbers, eggplant, hearts of palm, leeks, loroco flowers, onions, pacaya buds, plantains, pumpkin, spinach, sweet peppers, tomatillos, watercress, yams, yucca, and yucca flowers

Fruit group	Milk, yogurt, cheese group	Meat, poultry, fish, dry beans, eggs, and nuts groups	Fats, oils, and sweets
Dried wild berries, cherries and grapes, berries, elderberries, persimmons, plums, and rhubarb	None in traditional diet	Bear, buffalo, deer, elk, moose, rabbit, and squirrel. Duck, goose, quail, and wild turkey. A variety of fish, legumes, nuts, and seeds	Tallow and lard Maple sugar and pine sugar
Apples, apricots, cherries, currants, gooseberries, grapes, lemons, melons, oranges, peaches, pears, plums, prunes, raspberries, rhubarb, and strawberries	Cheese (made from cow, sheep, and goat milk), cream, milk, sour cream, and yogurt	Beef, lamb, oxtail, pork, rabbit, veal, and venison. Chicken, duck, goose, pheasant, pigeon, quail, and turkey. A wide variety of fish, legumes, and nuts	Butter, lard, margarine, olive oil, vegetable oil, and salt pork Honey and sugar
Apples, apricots, bananas, cherries, citron, dates, figs, grapefruit, grapes, lemons, medlars, peaches, pears, pineapples, prunes, pomegranates, quinces, oranges, raisins, and tangerines	Cheese (made from cow, sheep, buffalo, and goat milk), and milk	Beef, goat, lamb, pork, and veal. Chicken, duck, goose, pigeon, turkey, and woodcock. A variety of fish, shellfish, legumes, and nuts	Butter, lard, olive oil, and vegetable oil Honey and sugar
Apples, apricots, a variety of berries, currants, dates, grapes, grapefruit, lemons, melons, oranges, peaches, pears, plums, prunes, quinces, raisins, rhubarb, and strawberries	Buttermilk, cheese, cream, milk, sour cream, and yogurt	Beef, boar, hare, lamb, pork, sausage, veal, and venison. Chicken, Cornish hen, duck, goose, grouse, partridge, pheasant, quail, squab, and turkey. A variety of fish, shellfish, legumes, and nuts	Butter, bacon, chicken fat, flaxseed oil, lard, olive oil, salt pork, and vegetable oil Honey, sugar, and molasses
Apples, bananas, berries, fruit juices, peaches, and watermelon	Buttermilk and some cheese	Beef, pork and pork products including scrapple (cornmeal and pork), chitterlings (pork intestines), bacon, pig feet and ears. Fried meats and poultry, organ meats (kidney, liver, tongue, tripe); fish (catfish, crawfish, salmon, shrimp, tuna); frogs, rabbit, squirrel, and a variety of legumes and nuts	Butter and lard Honey, molasses, and sugar
Avocadoes, bananas, cactus fruit, carambola, casimiroa, cherimoya, coconut, granadilla, guanabana, guava, lemons, limes, mamey, mangoes, melon, oranges, papaya, pineapple, strawberries, sugar cane, and zapote	Cheese, flan, sour cream, and milk	Beef, goat, pork, chicken, turkey, firm-fleshed fish, shrimp, and a variety of legumes	Bacon fat, lard (manteca), salt pork, dairy cream Sugar and panocha (raw brown cane sugar)
Apples, avocadoes, bananas, breadfruit, cherimoya, coconut, grapes, guava, mameys, mangoes, nances, oranges, papaya, passion fruit, pejibaye, pineapples, prunes, raisins, tamarind, tangerines, and zapote	Cheese, cream, and milk	Beef, iguana, lizards, pork, and venison. Chicken, duck, turkey and a variety of fish, shellfish, and legumes	Butter, lard, vegetable oils, and shortening Honey, sugar, and sugar syrup

Continued.

Cultural Dietary Patterns—*cont'd*

Culture	Bread, cereal, rice, and pasta group	Vegetable group
Caribbean Islands	Cassava bread; cornmeal (surrulitos); oatmeal; rice, and wheat products	Arracacha, arrowroot, black-eyed peas, cabbage, calabaza, callaloo, cassava, chilis, corn, cucumbers, eggplant, malangas, okra, onions, palm hearts, peppers, radishes, spinach, squashes, sweet potatoes, taro, and yams
Cuban and Puerto Rican	Rice; starchy green bananas, usually fried (plantains)	Beets, breadfruit, chayote, chili peppers, eggplant, onion, tubers (yucca), white yams (boniato)
South American	Amaranth (corn, rice, quinoa) and wheat products	Ahipa, arracacha, calabaza, cassava, green peppers, hearts of palm, kale, okra, oca, onions, rosella, squash, sweet potatoes, yacon, and yams
Chinese	Rice and related products (flour, cakes, and noodles); noodles made from barley, corn, and millet; wheat and related products (breads, noodles, spaghetti, stuffed noodles [won ton], and filled buns [bow])	Bamboo shoots, cabbage (napa), celery, Chinese turnips (lo bok), dried day lilies, dry fungus (Black Juda's ear); leafy green vegetables including kale, cress, mustard greens (gai choy), chard (bok choy), amaranth greens (yin choy), wolfberry leaves (gou gay), and Chinese broccoli (gai lan); eggplant, lotus tubers, okra, snow peas, stir-fried vegetables (chow yuk), taro roots, white radish (daikon), yams, and yam beans
Japanese	Rice and rice products, rice flour (mochiko), noodles (comen/soba), buckwheat, and millet	Artichoke, asparagus, bamboo shoots (takenoko), burdock (gobo), cabbage (nappa), eggplant, horseradish (wasabi), mizuna, mushrooms (shiitake, matsutake, nameko), Japanese parsley (seri), lotus root (renkon), pickled cabbage (kimchee), pickled vegetables, seaweed (laver, nori, wakame, kombu), snow peas, spinach, sweet potato, vegetable soup (mizutaki), watercress, white radish (daikon)

Fruit group	Milk, yogurt, cheese group	Meat, poultry, fish, dry beans, eggs, and nuts groups	Fats, oils, and sweets
Acerola cherries, akee, avocadoes, bananas, breadfruit, caimito, cherimoya, citron, coconuts, cocoplum, gooseberries, granadilla, grapefruit, guava, guanabana, jackfruit, kumquats, lemons, limes, mamey, mangoes, oranges, papayas, pineapple, plantains, pomegranates, raisins, sapodilla, sugar cane, and tamarind	Cheese and milk	Beef, goat, pork, chicken, turkey, and a variety of fish, shellfish, and legumes	Butter, coconut oil, lard, and olive oil Sugar cane products
Coconuts, guava, mango, oranges (sweet and sour), prune and mango paste	Flan, hard cheese (queso de mano)	Chicken, fish, (all kinds and preparations including smoked, salted, canned, and fresh), shellfish, legumes (all kinds especially black beans), pork (fried), sausage (chorizo), calf brain, beef tongue	Olive and peanut oil, lard Coconut
Avocado, abiu, acerola, apples, banana, caimito, casimiroa, cherimoya, feijoa, guava, grapes, jackfruit, jabitocaba, lemons, limes, lulo, mammea, mango, melon, olives, oranges, palm fruits, papaya, passion fruit, peaches, pineapple, pitanga, quince, sapote, and strawberries	Cheese and milk	Beef, frog, goat, guinea pig, llama, mutton, pork, and rabbit. Chicken, duck, turkey and a variety of fish, shellfish, and nuts	Palm oil, olive oil, and butter Sugar cane, brown sugar, and honey
Apples, bananas, custard apples, coconuts, dates, longan, figs, grapes, kumquats, lime, litchi, mango, muskmelon, oranges, papaya, passion fruit, peaches, persimmons, pineapple, plums, pomegranates, pomelos, tangerines, and watermelon	Milk (cow, buffalo, and soymilk)	Beef, lamb, and pork. Chicken, duck, quail, squab, a large variety of fish and shellfish, in addition to legumes and nuts	Lard; peanut, soy, sesame, and rice oil Honey, rice or barley malt, palm sugar, sorghum sugar, and dehydrated cane juice
Pearlike apple (nasi), apricots, bananas, cherries, figs, grapefruit (yuzu), kumquats, lemons, limes, persimmons, plums, pineapple, strawberries, and tangerine (mikan)	Milk, butter, and ice cream	Beef, deer, lamb, pork, rabbit, veal. Fish and shellfish including dried fish with bones, raw fish (sashimi), and fish cake (kamaboko). A variety of poultry (chicken, duck, goose, turkey) and legumes (black beans, red beans, soybeans—as tofu, fermented soybean, and sprouts)	Lard; soy, sesame, rapeseed, and rice oil Honey and sugar

Continued.

Cultural Dietary Patterns—*cont'd*

Culture	Bread, cereal, rice, and pasta group	Vegetable group
Korean	Barley, buckwheat, millet, rice, and wheat products	Bamboo shoots, bean sprouts, beets, cabbage, chives, chrysanthemum leaves, cucumber, eggplant, fern, green onion, green pepper, leeks, lotus root, mushrooms, onion, perilla, seaweed, spinach, sweet potato, turnips, water chestnuts, watercress, and white radishes
Filipino	Noodles, rice, rice flour (mochiko), stuffed noodles (won ton), white bread (pan de sal)	Amaranth, bamboo shoots, beets, burdock root, cassava, Chinese celery, dark green leafy vegetables (malunggay and salvyot), eggplant, garlic, green pepper, hearts of palm, hyacinth bean, kamis, leek, mushrooms, okra, onion, sweet potatoes (camotes), turnips, and root crop (gabi)
Pacific Islanders	Rice and wheat products	Arrowroot, bitter melon, burdock root, cabbage, carrot, cassava, daikon, eggplant, ferns, green pepper, horseradish, jute, kohlrabi, leeks, lotus root, mustard greens, green onion, seaweed, spinach, squashes, sweet potato, taro, water chestnuts, and yams
South Asian	Rice, wheat, buckwheat, corn, millet, and sorghum products	Agathi flowers, amaranth, artichokes, bamboo shoots, beets, bitter melon, Brussels sprouts, cabbage, collard greens, cucumbers, drumstick plant, eggplant, lotus root, manioc, mushrooms, okra, pandanus, plantain flowers, sago palm, spinach, squash, turnips, yams, water chestnuts, water convolus, and water lilies
Jewish (both cultural and religious customs)	Bagel, buckwheat groats (kasha), dumplings made with matzoh meal (matzoh balls or knaidelach), egg bread (challah), noodle or potato pudding (kugel), crepe filled with farmer cheese and/or fruit (blintz), unleavened bread or large cracker made with wheat flour and water (matzoh)	Potato pancakes (latkes); vegetable stew made with sweet potatoes, carrots, prunes, and sometimes brisket (tzimmes); beet soup (borscht)

Data from Kittler PG, Sucher KP: *Food and culture*, ed 4, Belmont, CA, 2004, Brooks/Cole, a division of Thomson Learning; and Grodner M, Long S, DeYoung S: *Foundations and clinical applications of nutrition: a nursing approach*, ed 3, St Louis, 2004, Mosby.

Fruit group	Milk, yogurt, cheese group	Meat, poultry, fish, dry beans, eggs, and nuts groups	Fats, oils, and sweets
Apples, Asian pears, cherries, dates, grapes, melons, oranges, pears, persimmons, plums, and tangerines	Very little, if any, consumption	Beef, oxtail, pork, chicken, pheasant, and a variety of fish, shellfish, legumes, and nuts	Sesame seed oil and vegetable oil Honey and sugar
Apples, avocado, bananas, bitter melon (ampalaya), breadfruit, coconut, guavas, jackfruit, limes, mangoes, papaya, pod fruit (tamarind), pomelos, rambutan, rhubarb, star fruit, tamarind, tangelo (naranghita), and watermelon	White cheese, evaporated cow or goat milk, and soymilk	Beef, carabao, goat, pork, monkey, organ meats, and rabbit. Fish, dried fish (dilis), egg roll (lumpia), fish sauce (alamang and bagoong); legumes such as mung beans, bean sprouts, chickpeas; and soybean curd (tofu)	Coconut oil, lard, and vegetable oil Brown and white sugar, coconut, and honey
Acerola cherries, apples, apricot, avocado, bananas, breadfruit, coconut, guava, jackfruit, kumquat, litchis, loquat, mango, melons, papaya, passion fruit, peaches, pear, pineapple, plum, prune, strawberries, and tamarind	Very little, if any, consumption	Beef, pork, chicken, duck, squab, turkey, and a variety of fish, shellfish, and legumes	Butter, coconut oil, lard, sesame oil, and vegetable oil Sugar
Apples, apricots, avocados, bananas, coconut, dates, figs, grapes, guava, jackfruit, limes, litchis, loquats, mangoes, melon, nongus, oranges, papaya, peaches, pears, persimmons, pineapple, plums, pomegranate, pomelos, starfruit, sugar cane, tangerines, and watermelon	Milk (evaporated and fermented products); cheese, and milk-based desserts	Beef, goat, mutton, pork, chicken, duck, and a variety of fish, seafood, legumes, and nuts	Coconut oil, ghee, mustard oil, peanut oil, sesame seed oil, and sunflower oil Sugar cane, jaggery, and molasses
		A mixture of fish formed into balls and poached (gefilte fish); smoked salmon (lox)	Chicken fat

Religious Dietary Practices

	Seventh-Day Adventist	Buddhist	Eastern Orthodox
Beef		Avoided by most devout	
Pork	Prohibited or strongly discouraged	Avoided by most devout	
All meat	Avoided by most devout	Avoided by most devout	Permitted but some restrictions apply
Eggs/dairy	Permitted but avoided at some observances	Permitted but avoided at some observances	Permitted but some restrictions apply
Fish	Avoided by most devout	Avoided by most devout	Permitted but some restrictions apply
Shellfish	Prohibited or strongly discouraged	Avoided by most devout	Permitted but avoided at some observances
Meat and dairy at same meal			
Leavened foods			
Ritual slaughter of animals			
Alcohol	Prohibited or strongly discouraged		
Caffeine	Prohibited or strongly discouraged		

From Kittler PG, Sucher KP: *Food and culture*, ed 4, Belmont, CA, 2004, Brooks/Cole, a division of Thomson Learning.

Hindu	Jewish	Mormon	Moslem	Roman Catholic
Prohibited or strongly discouraged				
Avoided by most devout	Prohibited or strongly discouraged		Prohibited or strongly discouraged	
Avoided by most devout	Permitted but some restrictions apply		Permitted but some restrictions apply	Permitted but some restrictions apply
Permitted but avoided at some observances	Permitted but some restrictions apply			
Permitted but some restrictions apply	Permitted but some restrictions apply			
Permitted but some restrictions apply	Prohibited or strongly discouraged			
	Prohibited or strongly discouraged			
	Permitted but some restrictions apply			
	Practiced		Practiced	
Avoided by most devout		Prohibited or strongly discouraged	Prohibited or strongly discouraged	
		Prohibited or strongly discouraged	Avoided by most devout	

Answers to Chapter Challenge Questions

CHAPTER 1
True-False
1. T
2. F
3. F
Multiple Choice
1. a
2. d
3. a

CHAPTER 2
True-False
1. F
2. T
3. F
4. T
5. F
6. T
Multiple Choice
1. d
2. b
3. d

CHAPTER 3
True-False
1. F
2. T
3. F
4. F
5. T
Multiple Choice
1. a
2. d
3. b

CHAPTER 4
True-False
1. F
2. T
3. F
4. F
5. F
6. F
7. T
8. T
9. T
10. T
Multiple Choice
1. a
2. d
3. c

CHAPTER 5
True-False
1. F
2. T
3. F
4. T
5. F
6. F
7. T
Multiple Choice
1. d
2. a, c, d
3. c
4. b
5. d
6. a

CHAPTER 6
True-False
1. F
2. F
3. T
4. F
5. F
6. F
Multiple Choice
1. b
2. c
3. c
4. c
5. d
6. c

CHAPTER 7
True-False
1. F
2. F
3. T
4. F
5. T
6. T
Multiple Choice
1. c
2. c
3. d

CHAPTER 8
True-False
1. T
2. T
3. F
4. T
5. F
6. F
7. F
Multiple Choice
1. c
2. a
3. b

CHAPTER 9
Matching
1. k
2. g
3. n
4. a
5. l
6. b
7. f
8. h
9. i
10. p
11. d
12. o
13. j
14. c
15. e
16. m

CHAPTER 10
True-False
1. T
2. F
3. F
4. T
5. F
6. F
7. T
8. T
9. T
10. T
Multiple Choice
1. a
2. d
3. b
4. d
5. c

CHAPTER 11
True-False
1. F
2. F
3. F
4. F
5. F
Multiple Choice
1. d
2. c
3. b

CHAPTER 12
True-False
1. F
2. F
3. F
4. F
5. T
6. F
7. F
Multiple Choice
1. d
2. c
3. b, d
4. a, b, c, d

CHAPTER 13
True-False
1. F
2. F
3. F
4. T
5. F
6. F
7. F
8. T
Multiple Choice
1. a, b, c, d
2. c

CHAPTER 14
True-False
1. F
2. T
3. T
4. T
5. F
6. F

Multiple Choice
1. d
2. a, c, d
3. a, b
4. b
5. c

CHAPTER 15
True-False
1. F
2. F
3. T
4. T
5. F
Multiple Choice
1. a, b, c, d
2. a
3. b

CHAPTER 16
True-False
1. F
2. F
3. T
4. F
5. F
6. T
7. T
8. F
9. T
Multiple Choice
1. b
2. d
3. a, b, c
4. a, c
5. c

CHAPTER 17
True-False
1. T
2. F
3. T
4. F
5. F
6. F
7. F

Multiple Choice
1. a, b, c, d
2. a, b, c, d
3. a, b, c, d
4. a, d

CHAPTER 18
True-False
1. F
2. F
3. F
4. F
5. F
6. T
7. T
8. T
9. T
Multiple Choice
1. d
2. b
3. c
4. b

CHAPTER 19
True-False
1. T
2. F
3. F
4. F
5. T
6. T
7. T
8. F
9. F
10. F
Multiple Choice
1. b, c
2. a, c
3. a

CHAPTER 20
True-False
1. F
2. F
3. F
4. T
5. T
6. T
7. T
8. F
9. F
10. F
Multiple Choice
1. c
2. a, b, c, d

CHAPTER 21
True-False
1. T
2. F
3. F
4. T
5. T
6. F
7. T
8. F
9. T
10. T
Multiple Choice
1. b, d
2. b, c, d
3. a, b, c

CHAPTER 22
True-False
1. T
2. T
3. F
4. T
5. T
6. F
7. F
8. F
9. F
10. T
Multiple Choice
1. a
2. b
3. a
4. a, b, c, d
5. a, b, c, d

CHAPTER 23
True-False
1. F
2. T
3. T
4. F
5. T
6. F
7. F
8. F
9. T
10. T
Multiple Choice
1. b
2. c
3. b
4. a
5. d
6. b
7. d
8. d
9. a

Glossary

acetone A major ketone compound that results from fat breakdown for energy in uncontrolled diabetes; persons with diabetes periodically do urinary acetone tests to monitor status of their diabetes control.

adipose (L. *adeps*, fat; *adiposus*, fatty) Fat present in cells of adipose (fatty) tissue.

adipose tissue Storage site for excess fat.

aerobic capacity (Gr. *aer*, air or gas) Requiring oxygen to proceed. Milliliters of oxygen consumed per kilogram of body weight per minute, as influenced by body composition.

albumin (L. *albus*, white) A major protein in many animal and plant tissues; specialized plasma protein maintaining normal blood pressure.

aldosterone A potent hormone of the outside layer of the adrenal glands that acts on the distal nephron tubule to cause reabsorption of sodium in an ion exchange with potassium. The aldosterone mechanism is essentially a sodium-conserving mechanism but also indirectly conserves water because water absorption follows the sodium resorption.

aldosteronoma Excess secretion of aldosterone from the adrenal cortex. Symptoms and complications include sodium retention, potassium wasting (loss in the urine), alkalosis, weakness, paralysis, polyuria, polydipsia, hypertension, and cardiac arrhythmias.

allergens Food proteins eliciting an immune system response, or "allergic reaction." Symptoms may include itching, swelling, hives, diarrhea, difficulty breathing, or anaphylaxis in the worst cases.

allergy (Gr. *allos*, other; *ergon*, work) A state of hypersensitivity to particular substances in the environment that work on the body tissues to produce problems in functions of affected tissues; the agent involved (allergen) may be a certain food eaten or a substance such as pollen inhaled.

amino acids Nitrogen-bearing compounds that form the structural units of protein. The various food proteins, when digested, yield their specific constituent amino acids, which are then available for use by the cells to synthesize specific tissue proteins.

aminopeptidase Specific protein-splitting enzyme secreted by small glands in the walls of the small intestine that breaks off the nitrogen-containing amino (—NH₂) end of the peptide chain, producing smaller chained peptides and free amino acids.

anabolism (an-A-bol-iz-um) Metabolic process of building large substances from smaller parts.

anaerobic (Gr. *an-*, without; *aer*, air; *bios*, life) A microorganism that can live and grow in an oxygen-free environment.

anemia (Gr. *an-*, negative prefix; *haima*, blood) Blood condition characterized by a decreased number of circulating red blood cells, hemoglobin, or number of volume-packed red blood cells.

anencephaly (Gr. *an*, not; *enkephalos*, the brain) Congenital absence of the brain resulting from the incomplete closure of the upper end of the neural tube.

angina pectoris (L. *angina*, severe pain; *pectus*, breast) Spasmodic, choking chest pain resulting from lack of oxygen to the heart muscle, symptom of a heart attack; also may be caused by severe effort or excitement.

anorexia nervosa (Gr. *an-*, negative prefix; *orexis*, appetite) Extreme psychophysiologic aversion to food resulting in life-threatening weight loss. A psychiatric eating disorder resulting from a morbid fear of fatness in which the person's distorted body image is reflected as fat when the body is actually malnourished and extremely thin from self-starvation.

anthropometric measurements Physical measurements of the human body used for health assessment including height, weight, skinfold thickness, and circumference (head, hip, waist, wrist, mid-arm muscle).

antibody Any of numerous protein molecules produced by B cells as a primary immune defense for attaching to specific related antigens.

antidiuretic hormone (ADH) A hormone of the pituitary gland that acts on the distal nephron tubule to conserve water by causing its reabsorption; also called *vasopressin*.

antigen (antibody + Gr. *gennan*, to produce) Any foreign or "nonself" substances, such as toxins, viruses, bacteria, and foreign proteins, that stimulate the production of antibodies specifically designed to counteract their activity.

anuria (Gr. *an-*, negative prefix; *ouron*, urine) An absence of urine, indicating kidney shutdown or failure.

ascites (Gr. *askites*, from; *askos*, bag) Outflow and accumulation of serous (blood and lymph serum) fluid in the abdominal cavity; also known as *abdominal* or *peritoneal dropsy*.

ascorbic acid Chemical name for vitamin C from its ability to cure scurvy.

atherosclerosis (Gr. *athere*, gruel; *skleros*, hard) The underlying pathology of coronary heart disease; characterized by the formation of yellow cheeselike fatty streaks containing cholesterol that develop into hardened plaques in the inner lining of major blood vessels such as the coronary arteries.

atrophy (Gr. *a-*, negative prefix; *trophē*, nourishment) A wasting away.

azotemia (Gr. *a-*, negative prefix; *zoe*, life; *azote*, nitrogen; *haima*, blood) An excess of urea and other nitrogenous substances in the blood.

basal energy expenditure (Gr. *basis*, base) The amount of energy needed by the body for maintenance of life when a person is at digestive, physical, and emotional rest. This basal metabolic rate (BMR) is reported as the percent of variation in the person above or below the normal number of kilocalories required for a person of like height, weight, sex, and age.

beriberi (Singhalese for "I can't, I can't") A disease of the peripheral nerves caused by a deficiency of thiamin (vitamin B$_1$) characterized by pain (neuritis) and paralysis of legs and arms, cardiovascular changes, and edema.

bile (L. *bilis*, bile) A fluid secreted by the liver and transported to the gallbladder for concentration and storage; released into the duodenum with the entry of fat to facilitate enzymatic fat digestion by acting as an emulsifying agent.

blood urea nitrogen (BUN) A basic test of nephron function by measuring its ability to normally filter urea nitrogen, a product of protein metabolism, from the blood.

body composition The relative sizes of the four basic body compartments that make up the total body: lean body mass (muscle mass), fat, water, and bone.

body mass index (BMI) Body weight in kilograms divided by the square of height in meters (kg/m^2). Correlates with body fatness and health risk associated with obesity.

brush border Cells that are located on the microvilli within the lining of the intestinal tract. The microvilli are tiny hairlike projections that protrude from the mucosal cells that help increase surface area for the digestion and absorption of nutrients.

bulimia nervosa (L. *bous*, ox; *limos*, hunger) A psychiatric eating disorder related to a person's fear of fatness, in which cycles of gorging on large quantities of food are followed by self-induced vomiting and use of diuretics and laxatives to maintain a "normal" body weight.

cachexia (Gr. *kakos*, bad; *hexis*, habit) A specific profound effect caused by malnutrition and a disturbance in glucose and fat metabolism usually seen in patients with terminal cancer or AIDS; general poor health indicated by an emaciated appearance.

Cajun (Derivative, *Acadian*) Group of people with an enduring tradition whose French-Catholic ancestors established permanent communities in the southern Louisiana coastal waterways after being expelled from Acadia (now Nova Scotia, Canada) by the reigning English in the late eighteenth century; developed unique food pattern from blend of native French influence and mix of Creole cooking found in the new land.

calcitriol The activated hormone form of vitamin D.

calorie (L. *calor*, heat) A measure of heat. The *energy* required to do the work of the body is measured as the amount of *heat* produced by the body's work. The energy value of food is expressed as the number of kilocalories a specified portion of the food will yield when oxidized in the body.

callus (L. *callositis*, callus, bone) Unorganized meshwork of newly grown, woven bone developed on a pattern of original clot of fibrin, formed after fracture or surgery, and normally replaced in the healing process by hard adult bone.

carboxypeptidase (L. *carbo-*, carbon; *oxy*, oxygen) A specific protein-splitting enzyme secreted in inactive form in the pancreas that is activated by trypsin in the small intestine to break off the acid (*carboxyl*, COOH) end of the peptide chain, producing smaller chained peptides and free amino acids.

carotene A group name of three red and yellow pigments (alpha-, beta-, and gamma-carotene) found in dark green and yellow vegetables and fruits. The one most important to human nutrition is beta-carotene because the body can convert it to vitamin A, thus making it a primary source of the vitamin.

catabolism (Gr. *katabole*, a throwing down) The process by which body tissues are broken down, the opposite of *anabolism*. Catabolism includes all the processes in which complex substances are progressively broken down into simpler ones, usually with the release of energy. Together, anabolism and catabolism constitute metabolism, which is the coordinated operation of anabolic (building up) and catabolic (breaking down) processes into a dynamic balance of energy and substance.

cellulitis   Diffuse inflammation of soft or connective tissues (e.g., in the foot) from injury, bruises, or pressure sores that lead to infection; poor care may result in ulceration and abscess or gangrene.

cerebrovascular accident   (L. *cerebrum*, brain; *vas*, vessel) A stroke, caused by arteriosclerosis in a blood vessel in the brain that cuts off oxygen supply to the affected portion of brain tissue, thus paralyzing body muscle actions controlled by the affected brain area.

cholecalciferol   The chemical name for vitamin D in its inactive dietary form; often shortened to *calciferol*.

cholesterol   (Gr. *chole*, bile; *steros*, solid) A fat-related compound, a sterol, synthesized only in animal tissues; a normal constituent of bile and a principal constituent of gallstones. In the body, cholesterol is synthesized mainly in the liver. In the diet, it is found only in animal food sources. In human body metabolism, cholesterol is important as a precursor of various steroid hormones, such as sex hormones and adrenal corticoids. In disordered lipid metabolism, however, it is a major factor in atherosclerosis, the underlying disease process in coronary arteries that leads to heart attacks.

chronic dieting syndrome   The cyclic pattern of weight loss by dieting to achieve an unnatural but culturally ideal body thinness, then regaining weight by compulsive food binges in response to stress, anxiety, and hunger. This abnormal psychophysiologic food pattern becomes chronic, changing the person's natural body metabolism and relative body composition to the abnormal state of a "metabolically obese" person of normal weight.

chylomicron   (kye-lo-MY-cron) Lipoprotein formed in the intestinal cell composed of triglycerides, cholesterol, phospholipids, and protein. Allows for absorption of fat into the lymphatic circulatory system before entering blood circulation.

chyme   (Gr. *chymos*, juice) Semifluid food mass in the gastrointestinal tract following gastric digestion.

chymotrypsin   (Gr. *chymos*, semifluid food mass from digestion; *trypein*, enzyme trypsin) One of the protein-splitting and milk-curdling pancreatic enzymes activated in the small intestine from the precursor chymotrypsinogen; breaks specific amino acid peptide linkages of protein.

cobalamin   The chemical name for the B-complex vitamin B_{12}; found mainly in animal protein food sources so deficiencies seen mostly among strict vegetarians (vegans). It is closely related to amino acid me-

tabolism and formation of the heme portion of hemoglobin. Absence of its necessary absorbing agent in the gastric secretions, intrinsic factor, leads to pernicious anemia and degenerative effects on the nervous system, which require monthly cobalamin injections, bypassing the intestinal absorption defect.

collagen disease   (Gr. *kolla*, glue; *gennan*, to produce) A disease attacking collagen tissues, the protein substance of the white fibers (collagenous fibers) of skin, tendon, bone, cartilage, and other connective tissues; any of a group of diseases that cause widespread changes in the connective tissue, such as rheumatoid arthritis, lupus erythematosus, scleroderma, and rheumatic fever.

colloidal osmotic pressure (COP)   Fluid pressure produced by the protein molecules in the plasma and in the cell. Because proteins are large molecules, they do not pass through the separating membranes of the capillary cells. Thus they remain in their respective compartments exerting a constant osmotic pull that protects vital plasma and cell fluid volumes in these areas.

colostrum   (L. *colostrum*, premilk) A thin, yellow fluid first secreted by the mammary gland a few days before and after childbirth, preceding the mature breast milk. It contains up to 20% protein including a large amount of lactalbumin, more minerals, and less lactose and fat than mature milk, and immunoglobulins that represent the antibodies found in maternal blood.

complex carbohydrates   Large, complex molecules of carbohydrates composed of many sugar units (polysaccharides). Complex forms of dietary carbohydrates are starch, which is digestible and provides a major energy source, and dietary fiber, which is indigestible (humans lack the necessary enzymes) and thus provides important bulk in the diet.

conditionally indispensable amino acids   These are normally considered dispensable amino acids because the body can make them. However, under certain circumstances, such as illness, the body cannot make them in high enough quantities and they become indispensable in the diet.

congestive heart failure   Chronic condition of gradually weakening heart muscle unable to pump normal blood flow through the heart-lung circulation, resulting in congestion of fluids in the lungs.

coronary heart disease   Term designating the overall medical problem resulting from the underlying disease of atherosclerosis in the coronary arteries serving the heart muscle tissue with blood oxygen and nutrients.

creatinine   Nitrogen-carrying product of tissue protein breakdown, excreted in the urine.

Cushing's syndrome Excess secretion of glucocorticoids from the adrenal cortex. Symptoms and complications include protein loss, obesity, fatigue, osteoporosis, edema, excess hair growth, diabetes, and skin discoloration.

dehiscence (L. *dehiscere,* to gape) A splitting open; the separation of layers of a surgical wound—partial, superficial, or complete—with total disruption requiring resuturing.

dialysis (Gr. *dia,* through; *lysis,* dissolution) The process of separating crystalloids (crystal-forming substances) and colloids (gluelike substances) in solution by the difference in their rates of diffusion through a semipermeable membrane; crystalloids (e.g., blood sugar and other simple metabolites), pass through readily and colloids (e.g., plasma proteins) pass through slowly or not at all.

Dietary Reference Intakes (DRIs) A system of reference values that can be used for assessing and planning diets for healthy populations and many other purposes. These values encompass the Recommended Dietary Allowances (RDAs), which have been published by the National Academy of Sciences since 1941.

dietetics Management of diet and the use of food; the science concerned with the nutritional planning and preparation of foods.

dipeptidase Specific final enzyme in the protein-splitting system that produces the last two free amino acids.

diverticulitis (L. *divertere,* to turn aside) Inflammation of pockets of tissue (diverticuli) in the lining of the mucous membrane of the colon.

dysphagia (Gr. *dys-,* painful; *phagein,* to eat) Difficulty in swallowing.

edema (Gr. *oidema,* swelling) An unusual accumulation of fluid in the interstitial (small structural spaces between tissue parts) spaces of the body.

elemental formula A nutrition-support formula composed of simple elemental nutrient components that require no further digestive breakdown and thus are readily absorbed; formulas with the protein as free amino acids and the carbohydrate as the simple sugar glucose.

emulsifier An agent that breaks down large fat globules into smaller, uniformly distributed particles; action accomplished in the intestine chiefly by bile acids, which lower the surface tension of the fat particles, breaking the fat into many smaller droplets, thus greatly increasing the surface area of fat and facilitating contact with the fat-digesting enzymes.

enteral (Gr. *enteron,* intestine) A mode of feeding that uses the gastrointestinal tract through oral or tube feeding.

enzyme (Gr. *en,* in; *zyme,* leaven) Specific proteins produced in cells that digest or change specific nutrients in specific chemical reactions without being changed themselves in the process. Their action is therefore that of a *catalyst.* Digestive enzymes in the gastrointestinal secretions act on food substances to break them down into simpler compounds. An enzyme usually is named according to the substance (substrate) on which it acts, with common word ending of *-ase;* for example, sucrase is the specific enzyme for sucrose, which it breaks down into glucose and fructose.

ergogenic (Gr. *ergon,* work; *gennan,* to produce) Tendency to increase work output; various substances that increase work or exercise capacity and output.

essential hypertension An inherent form of high blood pressure with no specific discoverable cause, considered to be familial; also called *primary hypertension.*

exudate (L. *exsudare,* to sweat out) Various materials (e.g., cells, cellular debris, and fluids), usually resulting from inflammation, that have escaped from the blood vessels and are deposited in or on the surface tissues; protein content is high.

fatty acid The major structural component of lipids.

fetal alcohol syndrome Combination of physical and mental birth defects in infants born to mothers who abused alcohol during pregnancy.

filé powder Substance made from ground sassafras leaves and serves both to season and thicken the dish being made.

Food Guide Pyramid A visual pattern of the current basic five food groups (bread/cereal, 6 to 11 servings; vegetable, 3 to 5 servings; fruit, 2 to 4 servings; milk-cheese, 2 to 3 servings; meat/dry beans/egg, 2 to 3 servings), arranged in a pyramid shape to indicate proportionate amounts of daily food choices. The largest food group, bread/cereal, forms the entire foundation. The next two narrowing tiers indicate relatively fewer daily portions of vegetables and fruits, and then of the milk/cheese and meat/dry beans/egg groups. The small tip at the pyramid top indicates sparing use of fats, oils, and sweets.

gastroscopy (*gastro,* stomach; *scopy,* to view or see) examination of upper intestinal tract using a flexible tube with a small camera on the end. The tube is about 9 mm in diameter and takes color pictures as well as biopsy samples, if necessary.

glomerulus (L. *glomus,* ball, cluster) First section of the nephron, a cluster of capillary loops cupped in the nephron head that serves as an initial filter.

glucagon (Gr. *glykys,* sweet; *gonē,* seed) A hormone secreted by the α cells of the pancreatic islets of Langerhans in response to hypoglycemia; it has an opposite, balancing effect to that of insulin, raising the blood sugar; thus it is used as a quick-acting antidote for a low blood sugar reaction of insulin. It also counteracts the overnight fast during sleep hours by breaking down liver glycogen to keep blood sugar levels normal and maintain an adequate energy supply for normal nerve and brain function.

gluconeogenesis (Gr. *gluco*, glucose; *neos*, new; *genesis*, generation, birth, gloo-ko-nee-oh-JEN-uh-sis) Formation of glucose from noncarbohydrate substances such as amino acids.

glycerides Chemical group name for fats, from their base substance glycerol; formed from the glycerol base with one, two, or three fatty acids attached to make monoglycerides, diglycerides, and triglycerides. Glycerides are the principal constituents of adipose tissue and are found in animal and vegetable fats and oils.

glycogen (Gr. *glykys*, sweet; *gennan*, to produce) A polysaccharide, the main storage form of carbohydrate, largely stored in the liver and to a lesser extent in muscle tissue.

glycogenesis (Gr. *glykys*, sweet; *genesis*, generation, birth) Formation of stored glycogen from glucose.

goiter (L. *gutter*, throat) An enlarged thyroid gland caused by lack of sufficient available iodine to produce the thyroid hormone thyroxine.

health A state of optimal physical, mental, and social well-being; relative freedom from disease or disability.

health promotion (A.S. *hal*, hale, sound; L. *promovere*, to move forward) Active involvement in behaviors or programs that advance positive well-being.

Heimlich maneuver A first-aid maneuver to relieve a person who is choking from blockage of the breathing passageway by a swallowed foreign object or food particle. Standing behind the person, clasp the victim around the waist, placing one fist just under the sternum (breastbone) and grasping the fist with the other hand. Then make a quick, hard, thrusting movement inward and upward to dislodge the object.

hematuria (Gr. *haima*, blood; *ouron*, urine) The abnormal presence of blood in the urine.

hemoglobin (Gr. *haima*, blood; L. *globus*, globe) A conjugated protein in red blood cells; composed of a compact rounded mass of polypeptide chains forming *globin*, the protein portion, attached to an iron-containing red pigment called *heme*. Carries oxygen in the blood to cells.

homeostasis (Gr. *homoios*, like, unchanging; *stasis*, standing, stable) The state of relative dynamic equilibrium within the body's internal environment; a balance achieved through the operation of various interrelated physiologic mechanisms.

hyperglycemia (Gr. *hyper*, above; *glykys*, sweet) Elevated blood sugar above normal limits.

hypertension High blood pressure.

hypoglycemia (Gr. *hypo-*, below; *glykys*, sweet; *haima*, blood) An abnormally low blood sugar level that may lead to muscle tremors, cold sweat, headache, and confusion; a serious condition in diabetes management that requires immediate sugar intake to counteract, followed by a snack of complex carbohydrate food (e.g., bread or crackers) and a protein (e.g., lean meat, peanut butter, or cheese) to maintain the normal blood sugar.

immunocompetence (L. *immunis*, free, exempt) The ability or capacity to develop an immune response (i.e., antibody production or cell-mediated immunity) following exposure to an antigen.

jambalaya A dish of Creole origin, combining rice, chicken, ham, pork, sausage, broth, vegetables, and seasonings.

ketoacidosis Excess production of ketones, a form of metabolic acidosis that occurs in uncontrolled diabetes or starvation from burning body fat for energy fuel; a continuing uncontrolled state can result in coma and death.

ketones Chemical name for a class of organic compounds, including three ketoacid bases (e.g., acetone), that occur as intermediate products of fat metabolism.

ketosis The accumulation of ketones, intermediate products of fat metabolism, in the blood.

kilocalorie (Fr. *chilioi*, thousand; L. *calor*, heat) The general term *calorie* refers to a unit of heat measure and is used alone to designate the *small calorie*. The calorie used in nutritional science and the study of metabolism is the *large calorie* (which equals 1000 calories) or kilocalorie, to be more accurate and avoid the use of very large numbers in calculations.

lactated Ringer's solution Sterile solution of calcium chloride, potassium chloride, sodium chloride, and sodium lactate in water given to replenish fluid and electrolytes; developed by English physiologist Sidney Ringer (1835-1910).

life expectancy The number of years a person of a given age may expect to live. Life expectancy is affected by environment, gender, and race.

linoleic acid Essential fatty acid with 18 carbon atoms and two double bonds. Found in vegetable oils.

linolenic acid Essential fatty acid with 18 carbon atoms and three double bonds. Found in soybean, canola, and flaxseed oil.

lipectomy (Gr. *lipos*, fat; *ektomē*, excision) Surgical removal of subcutaneous fat by suction through a tube inserted into a surface incision, or by removing larger amounts of subcutaneous fat by major surgical incision.

lipids   (Gr. *lipos*, fat) The chemical group name for organic substances of a fatty nature. The lipids include fats, oils, waxes, and other fat-related compounds such as cholesterol and lipoproteins.

lipogenesis   (Gr. *lipos*, fat; *genesis*, generation, birth) Formation of fat.

lipoproteins   Chemical complexes of fat and protein that serve as the major carriers of lipids in the plasma. They vary in density according to the size of the fat load being carried; the lower the density, the higher the fat load. The combination package with water-soluble protein makes possible the transport of non–water-soluble fatty substances in the water-based blood circulation.

macrosomia   (Gr. *macro*, large; *sōma*, body) Excessive fetal growth resulting in an abnormally large infant carrying high risk of perinatal mortality.

major minerals   The group of minerals that are required by the body in amounts of more than 100 mg/day. The seven major minerals in the body are calcium, phosphorus, sodium, potassium, magnesium, chlorine, and sulfur.

menopause   (Gr. *men*, month; *pauses*, cessation) The end of menstrual activity and capacity to bear children.

metabolism   (Gr. *metabole*, to turn about, change, or alter) The sum of all chemical changes that take place in the body by which it maintains itself and produces energy for its functioning. Products of the various reactions are called *metabolites*.

micelles   Packages of free fatty acids, monoglycerides, and bile salts. The non–water-soluble fat particles are found in the middle of the package, whereas the water-soluble part faces outward and allows for the absorption of fat into the intestinal mucosal cell.

microvilli   (Gr. *mikros*, small; L. *villus*, tuft of hair) Exceedingly small hairlike projections covering all villi on the surface of the small intestine and greatly extending the total absorbing surface area; visible through electron microscope.

mucosal folds   (L. *mucus*, mucosa) Large visible folds of the mucous lining of the small intestine that increase the absorbing surface area.

mutation   (L. *mutare*, to change) A permanent transmissible change in a gene.

myocardial infarction   (Gr. *mys*, muscle; *kardia*, heart; L. *infarcire*, to stuff in) A heart attack; caused by failure of the heart muscle to maintain normal blood circulation because of blockage of coronary arteries with fatty cholesterol plaques that cut off

delivery of oxygen to the affected part of the heart muscle.

neoplasm   (Gr. *neos*, new; *plasma*, formation) Any new or abnormal cellular growth, specifically one that is uncontrolled and aggressive.

nephron   (Gr. *nephros*, kidney) Microscopic anatomic and functional unit of the kidney that selectively filters and reabsorbs essential blood factors, secretes hydrogen ions as needed for maintaining acid-base balance, then reabsorbs water to protect body fluids and forms and excretes a concentrated urine for elimination of wastes. There are approximately 1 million nephrons in each kidney.

nephrosis   (Gr. *nephros*, kidney) A nephrotic syndrome caused by degenerative lesions of the renal tubules of the nephrons, especially the thin basement membrane of the glomerulus that helps support the capillary loops; marked by edema, albuminuria, and decreased serum albumin.

niacin   Chemical name for a B vitamin discovered in relation to the deficiency disease pellagra, largely a skin disorder; important as a coenzyme factor in many cell reactions related to energy and protein metabolism.

nutrition   (L. *nutritic*, nourishment) The sum of the processes involved in taking in nutrients and assimilating and using them to maintain body tissue and provide energy; a foundation for life and health.

nutritional science   The body of science, developed through controlled research, that relates to the processes involved in nutrition: international, community, and clinical.

oliguria   (Gr. *oligos*, little; *ouron*, urine) The secretion of small amounts of urine in relation to fluid intake.

organic farming   Farming methods that use natural means of pest control by choosing hardy plant varieties that resist diseases and introduce beneficial insects to thrive and help control entrenched populations of destructive ones, thus avoiding dependence on stronger and stronger pesticides as resistant insects multiply; also uses time-tested natural means of enriching soil (e.g., crop rotation and cycling plant mulch and manure for a healthier soil and pesticide-free foods).

osmosis   (Gr. *osmos*, a thrusting) Passage of a solvent such as water through a membrane that separates solutions of different concentrations, tending to equalize the concentration pressures of the solutions on both sides of the membrane.

osteodystrophy   (Gr. *osteon*, bone; *dys*, painful, disordered, abnormal; *trephein*, to nourish) Bone disease resulting from defective bone formation. The general term *dystrophy* applies to any disorder arising from faulty nutrition.

osteoporosis (Gr. *osteon*, bone; *poros*, passage, pore) Abnormal thinning of the bone, producing a porous, fragile, latticelike bone tissue of enlarged spaces that is prone to fracture or deformity.

pancreatic amylase Major starch-splitting enzyme secreted by the pancreas and acting in the small intestine.

pancreatic lipase (Gr. *lipos*, fat) A major fat-splitting enzyme produced by the pancreas and secreted into the small intestine to digest fat.

pandemic (Gr. *pan*, all; *dēmos*, people) A widespread epidemic that is distributed through a region, a continent, or the world.

pantothenic acid (Gr. *pantothen*, from all sides, in every corner) A B-complex vitamin widely distributed in nature and occurring throughout the body tissues. Its one role, a major one, is as an essential constituent of the body's main activating agent, coenzyme A. This special compound has extensive metabolic responsibility in activating a number of compounds in many tissues; it is a key energy metabolism substance in every cell.

parasite (Gr. *para*, along side; *sitos*, food, grain; *parasitos*, one who eats at another's table; in ancient Greece, a term for a person who received free meals in return for amusing or flattering conversation). An organism that lives in or on an organism of another species known as the host, from whom all life-cycle nourishment is obtained.

parenteral (Gr. *para*, alongside, accessory, beyond; *enteron*, intestine) A mode of feeding that does not use the gastrointestinal tract but instead provides nutritional support by intravenous delivery of nutrient solutions.

parotid glands (Gr. *para*, beyond, beside; *ous*, ear) The largest of three pairs of salivary glands situated near the ear. The parotid glands lie, one on each side, above the angle of the jaw, below and in front of the ear. They continually secrete saliva, which passes along the duct of the gland and into the mouth through an opening in the inner cheek, level with the second upper molar tooth. Normal saliva flow facilitates the chewing and swallowing of food and prevents dry mouth problems.

pellagra (L. *pelle*, skin; Gr. *agra*, seizure) Deficiency disease caused by a lack of dietary niacin and an inadequate amount of protein containing the amino acid tryptophan, a precursor of niacin. Pellagra is characterized by skin lesions that are aggravated by sunlight, and by gastrointestinal, mucosal, neurologic, and mental symptoms. The four Ds often associated with pellagra are dermatitis, diarrhea, dementia, and death.

pepsin (Gr. *pepsis*, digestion) The main gastric enzyme specific for proteins. Pepsin begins breaking large protein molecules into shorter chain polypeptides; gastric hydrochloric acid is necessary to activate.

peritoneal cavity (Gr. *per*, around; *teinein*, to stretch) A strong, smooth, serous membrane lining the abdominal and pelvic walls and undersurface of the diaphragm, forming a sac enclosing the body's vital visceral organs. *Peritoneal dialysis* is a form of dialysis through the peritoneum into and out of the peritoneal cavity.

pharynx (Gr. *pharynx*, throat) The muscular membranous passage between the mouth and posterior nasal passages and the larynx and esophagus.

photosynthesis (Gr. *photos*, light; *synthesis*, putting together) Process by which plants containing chlorophyll are able to manufacture carbohydrate by combining CO_2 from air and water from soil. Sunlight is used as energy; chlorophyll is a catalyst. $6\ CO_2 + 6\ H_2O + \text{Energy} \rightarrow \text{Chlorophyll} \rightarrow C_6H_{12}O_6 + 6\ O_2$.

phylloquinone A fat-soluble vitamin of the K group found in green plants or prepared synthetically.

plasma protein Any of a number of protein substances carried in the circulating blood. A major one is *albumin*, which maintains the fluid volume of the blood through its colloidal osmotic pressure.

portal (L. *porta*, a portal or doorway) An entrance or gateway; for example, the portal blood circulation designates the entry of blood vessels from the intestines into the liver, carrying nutrients for major liver metabolism, then draining into the body's main systemic circulation to deliver metabolic products to body cells.

proenzyme An inactive precursor (forerunner substance from which another substance is made) that is converted to the active enzyme by the action of an acid, another enzyme, or other means. Also called *zymogen*.

prohormone A precursor substance that the body converts to a hormone; for example, a cholesterol compound in the skin is first irradiated by sunlight and then converted through successive enzyme actions in the liver and kidney into the vitamin D hormone, which then regulates calcium absorption and bone development. Only a few food sources of vitamin D are found in food fats (e.g., cream, butter, egg yolks), but it occurs in other processed foods (e.g., breakfast cereals and milk) through enrichment.

proteinuria (Gr. *protos*, first, protein; *ouron*, urine) An abnormal excess of serum proteins such as albumin in the urine.

pulmonary edema (L. *pulmonis*, lung; Gr. *oidēma*, swelling) Accumulation of fluid in lung tissues.

purines (L. *purum*, pure; Gr. *ouron*, urine) Nitrogen-containing compounds that yield uric acid as a metabolic end product eliminated in the urine.

pyridoxine The chemical name of vitamin B_6. In its activated phosphate form, B_2-PO_4, pyridoxine functions as an important coenzyme factor in many reactions in cell metabolism related to amino acids, glucose, and fatty acids. Clinically, pyridoxine deficiency produces a specific anemia and disturbances of the central nervous system.

Ramadan (Ar. *ramadān*, the hot month) The ninth month of the Muslim year, a period of daily fasting from sunrise to sunset.

Recommended Dietary Allowances (RDAs) Recommended daily allowances of nutrients and energy intake for population groups according to age and sex, with defined weight and height. They are established and reviewed periodically by a representative group of nutritional scientists, in relation to current research. These standards vary little among the developed countries.

registered dietitian (RD) A professional dietitian, accredited with an academic degree of undergraduate or graduate study who has passed required registration examinations administered by the American Dietetic Association.

rennin Milk-curdling enzyme of the gastric juice of human infants and young animals such as calves. Do not confuse with *renin*, an important enzyme produced by the kidney that plays a vital role in producing angiotensin, a potent vasoconstrictor and stimulant for release of the hormone aldosterone from the adjacent adrenal glands.

resting energy expenditure The amount of energy needed by the body for maintenance of life at rest over a 24-hour period. Often used interchangeably with basal energy expenditure, but is actually slightly higher.

retinol (L. *retina*, from *rēte*, net, eye vision; suffix *-ol*, an alcohol) The chemical name of vitamin A; derived from its vision function relating to the retina of the eye, the back inner lining of the eyeball that "catches" the lens light refractions to form images interpreted by the optic nerve and brain and makes the necessary light-dark adaptations.

riboflavin Chemical name of one of the early B vitamins, discovered in relation to an early vitamin-deficiency syndrome called *ariboflavinosis* and evidenced mainly in breakdown of skin tissues and resulting infections; role as a coenzyme factor in many cell reactions related to energy and protein metabolism.

rickets (Gr. *rhachitis*, a spinal complaint) A disease of childhood characterized by softening of the bones from an inadequate intake of vitamin D and insufficient exposure to sunlight; also associated with impaired calcium and phosphorus metabolism.

saccharide (L. *saccharum*, sugar) Chemical name for sugar molecules. May occur as single molecules in monosaccharides (glucose, fructose, maltose), as two molecules in disaccharides (sucrose, lactose, maltose), or as multiple molecules in polysaccharides (starch, dietary fiber, glycogen).

salivary amylase (Gr. *amylon*, starch) A starch-splitting enzyme in the mouth, commonly called *ptyalin* (Gr. *ptyalon*, spittle) that is secreted by the salivary glands.

saturated (L. *saturare*, to fill) State of being filled; state of fatty acid components of fats being filled in all their available carbon bonds with hydrogen, making the fat harder and more solid. Such solid food fats are generally from animal sources.

scurvy A vitamin-deficiency disease caused by a lack of vitamin C. It is a hemorrhagic disease with diffuse tissue bleeding, painful limbs and joints, thickened bones, skin discoloration from tissue bleeding; bones fracture easily, wounds do not heal, gums are swollen and bleed, and teeth loosen.

senescence (L. *senescere*, to grow old) The process or condition of growing old.

simple carbohydrates Sugars with a simple structure of one or two single-sugar (saccharide) units. A monosaccharide is composed of one sugar unit; a disaccharide is composed of two sugar units.

sorbitol A sugar alcohol formed in mammals from glucose and converted to fructose. Named for its initial discovery in nature, it is found in ripe berries of the tree *Sorbus acuparia* and also occurs in small quantities in various other berries, cherries, plums, and pears. Produced in food industry laboratories for use as a sweetener in candies, chewing gum, beverages, and other foodstuffs; side effect of diarrhea limits use.

spina bifida (L. *spina*, spine; *bifidus*, cleft into two parts or branches) Congenital defect in the embryonic-fetal closing of the neural tube to form a portion of the lower spine, leaving the spine unclosed and the spinal cord open in various degrees of exposure and damage.

steatorrhea (Gr. *steatos*, fat; *rhoia*, flow) Fatty diarrhea; excessive amounts of fat in the feces often caused by malabsorption diseases.

steroids (Gr. *stereos*, solid; L. *-ol*, *oleum*, oil) Group name for lipid-based sterols, including hormones, bile acids, and cholesterol.

stoma (Gr. *stoma*, mouth, opening) The opening established in the abdominal wall, connecting with the ileum or colon, for elimination of intestinal wastes after surgical removal of diseased portions of the intestines.

sugar alcohols Nutritive sweeteners that provide 4 kcal per gram; sorbitol, mannitol, and xylitol. Produced in food industry laboratories for use as sweeteners in candies, chewing gum, beverages, and other foodstuffs; side effect of diarrhea limits use.

sustainable agriculture A system of agriculture that combines traditional conservation-minded farming techniques with modern technologies. Sustainable systems use modern equipment, certified seed, and soil and water conservation practices, with emphasis on rotating crops, building up the soil, diversifying crops and livestock, and controlling pests naturally. Major goals are safe soil preservation and avoiding heavy dependence on pesticides and chemical fertilizers.

teratogen (Gr. *teratos*, monster; *gennan*, to produce) Drug or substance causing birth defect.

thiamin Chemical name of a major B-complex vitamin; also called *vitamin B$_1$*, discovered in relation to the classic deficiency disease beriberi; important in body metabolism as a coenzyme factor in many cell reactions related to energy metabolism.

tocopherol (Gr. *tokos*, childbirth; *pherein*, to carry) The chemical name for vitamin E, so named by early investigators because their initial work with rats indicated a reproductive function, not true with humans. In humans Vitamin E functions as a strong antioxidant that preserves structural membranes such as cell walls.

trace elements The group of elements, also called *micronutrients*, that are required by the body in smaller amounts of less than 100 mg/day. The 10 trace elements in the body are iron, iodine, zinc, copper, manganese, chromium, cobalt, selenium, molybdenum, and fluoride.

triglycerides Chemical name for fats in the body or in food; compound of three fatty acids attached to a glycerol base.

trypsin (Gr. *trypein*, to rub; *pepsis*, digestion) A protein-splitting enzyme, secreted as the inactive proenzyme *trypsinogen* in the pancreas, activated and acting in the small intestine to reduce proteins to shorter chain polypeptides and dipeptides.

urea Chief nitrogen-carrying product of dietary protein metabolism; appears in blood, lymph, and urine.

varices Dilated blood vessels within the wall of the esophagus used to redirect blood flow from the liver. During cirrhosis, blood flow is significantly reduced in the liver. As a result, alternative pathways form, expand, and crowd the esophagus. These vessels can continue to expand to the point of rupturing and can lead to death.

villi (L. *villus*, tuft of hair) Small protrusions from the surface of a membrane; fingerlike projections covering mucosal surfaces of the small intestine that further increase the absorbing surface area; visible through a regular microscope.

virus (L. *virus*, poison; *virion*, individual virus particle) A minute microscopic infectious organism characterized by lack of independent metabolism and by the ability to reproduce with genetic continuity only within a living host. Each particle (virion) consists basically of nucleic acids (genetic material) and a protein shell that protects and contains the genetic material and any enzymes present.

wean (Middle English, 1000 AD, *wenen*, to accustom) To gradually accustom a young child to food other than the mother's milk or a bottle-fed substitute formula as the child's natural need to suckle wanes.

xerostomia (Gr. *xeros*, dry; *stoma*; mouth) Dryness of the mouth from lack of normal secretions.

Index

L

M

NOTES

NOTES

MOSBY'S NutriTrac, VERSION III

Welcome to *Mosby's NutriTrac, Version III*—the most innovative nutrient analysis program for students. The following walks the user through the program, screen by screen, and highlights its features and capabilities.

The Main Start-Up Screen

This is a new screen in the *NutriTrac* program, serving as a navigational tool for the user to access the main features of the program. These features include the Main Menu, Intake Record, Energy Expenditure, and Explore Foods.

Main Menu

The following options and activities are available from the Main Menu screen.

Personal Profiles

This is where the user enters all of his or her vital statistics, including name; height; weight; age; gender; whether pregnant, lactating, or not pregnant; ID#; instructor name; and class time. Within this Personal Profiles section, the user will choose one of the following options.

- *New*—Enables user to create a new profile.
- *Edit*—Enables user to modify an existing profile.
- *Delete*—Enables user to delete an existing profile.

This screen also features a new body mass index (BMI) calculator. The user simply enters his or her vital statistics, then clicks this button. The program will automatically calculate the user's BMI and display it onscreen.

Analysis Tools

This section includes the following activities in the *NutriTrac* program.

- *Intake Record*—Here the user enters all of the food he or she has consumed for up to 31 days.
- *Detailed Energy Expenditure*—Here the user enters all of the activities he or she has performed for up to 31 days. A new "Search" function has been added in this section of *NutriTrac* to help the user sift through the wide variety of activities that have also been added in this new version.
- *Weight Management Planner*—This tool helps the user analyze the balance of food intake and energy expenditure required to reach his or her goal weight. It also shows the time required to safely reach this goal.

Exploring Foods/Nutrients

This feature allows the user to look up dietary information within the database (this new version incorporates the latest Dietary Reference Intake [DRI] values!) by choosing one of the following options.

- *Explore Foods*—Read the nutritional details of any food in the database.
- *NutriTrac Top 20*—Provides the top 20 foods that have the highest nutrient density for any nutrient selected by the user.

Intake Record

Foods

This is the main feature for entering food intake. Under this heading, the user will find the following options.

- *Category*—Allows the user to select a category of food from which to search. Scroll down the list to see all of the categories available. The automatic default is to "None"; the program will search the entire database for the selected food.
- *Search For*—The user can search the database for a particular food in one of three ways: Contains, Starts w/, and Code. First, the user types in the food name in the "Search for" box, then chooses Contains, Starts w/, or Code. Then the user clicks the "Search for" button and the program searches the entire database according to the search criteria.
  - *Contains*—The name of the food contains the word or partial word that the user typed into the "Search for" box. For example,

if the user types "butter" or "but" in the box, the program will bring up such foods as peanut butter, apple butter, and buttermilk.
  - *Starts w/*—This search option will list foods the user is searching for that start with the word the user types into the "Search for" box. For example, if the user types "ice" in the box, the program will bring up such foods as ice cream, iced tea, and ice milk.
  - *Code*—Each food has been assigned a code. The user can enter this code in the "Search for" box and the program will bring up that food. (A listing of these codes is available in appendix form in some of the texts that *NutriTrac* is packaged with.)
- *Add Selected Food to Intake*—The user clicks this button when he or she wishes to add a particular food to the meal profile (in the "Your Intake" section of the screen).

Your Intake

This feature contains the various foods the user has entered into his or her meal profile. It is also here that the user selects which day (up to 31) and which meal (Breakfast, Lunch, Dinner, or Snacks) he or she is entering food for. Other features in this section include the following.

- *Copy Meal*—Allows the user to copy a meal and move it to the intake record for 1 or more other days.
- *Standard Foods*—By clicking the *Standard Foods* box, the user can create groups of foods that are eaten regularly as part of a particular meal. For example, someone who always consumes orange juice and toast for breakfast could designate these foods as a standard "group" and then add cereal, eggs, or any other food on a day-to-day basis. The *Add Standard Foods* button is clicked by the user to add a created Standard Foods list to the current meal.
- *Remove Food*—Deletes a food from the meal profile.

Analysis Boxes

These boxes are found beneath the "Your Intake" box, in the bottom right corner of the "Intake Analysis" screen. This is the food analysis portion of the program, based on the latest DRI values and some Recommended Dietary Allowance (RDA) values (if DRI values had not been published by the time of printing of *NutriTrac Version III*). The user can choose to analyze a particular food, a complete meal, a complete day, or an average of his or her entire food intake record. The food analysis options include the following.

- *Nutrients*—Provides values for 33 nutrients.
- *Calorie Pie*—Breaks down calorie sources from fat, carbohydrate, and protein.
- *DRIs/Other*—Analyzes the percentage of DRIs/RDAs in the food intake. (NOTE: By press time for *NutriTrac Version III*, the National Academy of Sciences had not published DRIs for kilocalories (kcals), protein, carbohydrates, fats, fatty acids, and fiber; therefore RDA values are provided for these in this version of *NutriTrac*.)
- *USDA Food Guide Pyramid*—Illustrates the number of servings the user consumed from each group in the pyramid versus the number of servings the USDA recommends is consumed from each group in the pyramid.
- *Fat Pie*—Analyzes the fat content of the user's food intake by breaking it down into three categories: saturated, monounsaturated, and polyunsaturated.
- *RNIs/Other*—Compares the user's food intake against the Canadian Recommended Nutrient Intake (RNI) and provides the results of this analysis in bar graph form.
- *Spreadsheet*—Provides a spreadsheet of all of the nutrient values for a particular meal. The user can also sort the foods in that meal from highest to lowest based on a particular nutrient selected by the user.

Detailed Energy Expenditure

This feature allows the user to analyze energy expenditure based on activities performed.

Activities

Under this heading, the user has two types of activities to choose from.
1. *Common*—These are common, everyday activities for most people.

Continued on inside back cover.